Clinics in Developmental Medicine
DISEASES OF THE NERVOUS SYSTEM IN CHILDHOOD
3rd Edition

Clinics in Developmental Medicine

Diseases of the Nervous System in Childhood

3rd Edition

edited by

JEAN AICARDI

with
MARTIN BAX
and
CHRISTOPHER GILLBERG

2009
Mac Keith Press
Distributed by Wiley-Blackwell

© 2009 Mac Keith Press
6 Market Road, London N7 9PW

Editor: Hilary Hart
Managing Director, Mac Keith Press*:* Caroline Black
Sub Editor/Design: Pat Chappelle

Indexer: Jill Halliday
Cover/Title Design: John Morgan Studio

First edition 1992
Second edition 1998
Third edition 2009

British Library Cataloguing-in-Publication data:
A catalogue record for this book is available from the British Library

ISBN: 978 1 898683 59 9

Printed by The Lavenham Press Ltd, Water Street, Lavenham, Suffolk

Mac Keith Press is supported by **Scope**

CONTENTS

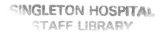

AUTHORS' APPOINTMENTS

EDITOR

Jean Aicardi
Formerly Department of Neurologic and Metabolic Diseases, Hôpital Robert-Debré, Paris, France; *and* Honorary Professor of Child Neurology, Institute of Child Health, London, England

CO-EDITORS

Martin Bax
Emeritus Reader in Child Health, Imperial College London (Chelsea and Westminster Campus), London, England

Christopher Gillberg
Professor of Child and Adolescent Psychiatry, University of Göteborg, Göteborg, Sweden

CONTRIBUTORS

Alexis Arzimanoglou
Head of the Epilepsy Program, Department of Child Neurology and Metabolic Diseases, University Hospital Robert Debré, Paris, France

J Keith Brown
Paediatric Neurologist, Edinburgh, Scotland

Linda S de Vries
Professor in Neonatal Neurology, Wilhelmina Children's Hospital, Utrecht, The Netherlands

Folker Hanefeld
Formerly Professor of Paediatrics, Georg August University, Goettingen, Germany

Cheryl Hemingway
Consultant Paediatric Neurologist, Great Ormond Street Hospital for Children, London, England

Ingeborg Krägeloh-Mann
Professor of Paediatrics, Director, Department of Paediatric Neurology and Developmental Medicine, University Children's Hospital, Tübingen, Germany

Hermione Lyall
Consultant Paediatrician, Infectious Diseases, *and* Chief of Service, Paediatrics, Imperial College Healthcare NHS Trust, London, England

Carey Matsuba
Clinical Assistant Professor, Department of Paediatrics, Division of Developmental Paediatrics, University of British Columbia, Vancouver, BC, Canada

Robert A Minns
Professor of Paediatric Neurology and Academic Head, Child Life and Health, College of Medicine and Veterinary Medicine, The University of Edinburgh, Edinburgh, Scotland

Kathryn North
Douglas Burrows Professor, Discipline of Paediatrics and Child Health, Faculty of Medicine, University of Sydney; Head, Neurogenetics Research Unit, *and* Deputy Head, Institute for Neuromuscular Research, The Children's Hospital at Westmead, Sydney, NSW, Australia

Hélène Ogier (de Baulny)
Centre de références des maladies métaboliques, Assistance Publique des Hôpitaux de Paris, Hôpital Robert Debré, Paris, France

Anne O'Hare
Section of Child Life and Health, University of Edinburgh, Edinburgh, Scotland

Robert Ouvrier
Petre Foundation Professor of Paediatric Neurology, The University of Sydney, *and* Head, The Institute for Neuromuscular Research, The Children's Hospital at Westmead, Sydney, NSW, Australia

Lloyd Shield
Formerly Senior Neurologist, Children's Neuroscience Centre, Royal Children's Hospital, Parkville, Victoria, Australia

PREFACE TO THIRD EDITION

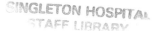

Diseases of the nervous system in infancy and childhood have a profound impact on the life of patients and their families and are probably the most disruptive of all paediatric ailments. Around 20–30% of hospitalized paediatric patients have a neurological problem, either as a sole or as an associated complaint. However, many well-educated paediatricians not infrequently feel uncomfortable and hesitant about how to treat children and what to tell to parents of patients with neurological disorders.

Diseases of the Nervous System in Childhood is meant for physicians with an interest in paediatric neurological diseases, whether paediatricians, neurologists, child neurologists or physicians dedicated to developmental medicine, and deals only with diseases of the nervous system (as indicated by its title). It is resolutely clinically oriented but, when necessary, some notions concerning pathogenesis and mechanisms are provided.

This third edition has been extensively updated to cover the tremendous volume of new information collected over the past 10 years, while trying to maintain the size of the book within reasonable limits. In spite of considerable efforts the speed of acquisition of new information is such that no textbook can pretend to be really up to date with respect to the very latest data. Electronic databases fulfil the need for 'last minute' results, but in a fragmentary and often uncritical manner. Books, on the other hand, aim to give a different, more global and balanced overview of a subject, taking into account the relative importance of the various parts, and assessing and selecting the material in the light of the experience of authors. I believe this synthetic and critical process is more essential than ever in view of the abundance of the material available.

The rapid increase of new data necessitated some rearrangements of this book. Unlike in the earlier editions where I had principally edited all the chapters, I felt this was no longer possible and invited Dr Martin Bax and Professor Christopher Gillberg to be co-editors with me, and they viewed all the material. In addition, whereas previously I had taken responsibility for the majority of chapters, we decided it was necessary to invite more collaborators to author certain chapters. We are very grateful to those who have given their time and knowledge for the completion of the book.

As before we have not included a chapter on the neurological examination of infants and children. Excellent books and monographs on these topics are available (e.g. Cioni and Mercuri 2008). We have also omitted the chapter on fetal neurology as this highly specialized area of paediatric neurology is also well covered by a number of texts (e.g. Hill and Volpe 1989, Levene et al. 2001).

I wish to introduce this book with a few remarks, based on a 40-year experience, on what could be termed the 'philosophy' of paediatric neurological examination. In this age of ubiquitous technology, I strongly believe that collection of clinical data and their correct interpretation remain as essential as ever.

In the first place, the eminent importance of history taking needs to be re-emphasized, as the history of the disease – as well as that of the child from conception and that of his/her family – forms the initial and most important step of the diagnostic approach. For most conditions, the diagnosis is established by thorough clinical history even before, and much more frequently than by, examination (Dooley et al. 2003). History taking is a difficult art requiring careful listening, patience, clinical acumen and understanding. It also necessitates a thorough knowledge of which information is worth looking for, and constant attention to possibly revealing words that may occasionally emerge out of a casual or even apparently irrelevant conversation.

This emphasis on history taking does not in any way minimize the essentiality of neurological examination, which should be as thorough as possible and largely guided by historical data. However, in children, and especially in infants or neonates, it cannot be conducted systematically as in adults. Attempts at 'adult-type' examination will lead to crying and fussing. Much of the examination should not require that the child be lying, as the lying position will often frighten the child by reminding him/her of previous unpleasant experiences and prevent the gathering of more important information on central nervous system functioning. After all, the vertical posture has been a major evolutionary acquisition and, since the emergence of Homo erectus, most human activities take place in the standing position.

Indeed, a major part of examination, and one too often neglected, consists of watching the spontaneous activity of the child. While an early example of observation is of neonatal and early infantile general movements, which have been shown to have predictive value (Ferrari et al. 1990, Einspieler and Prechtl 2005), later observation should be watching children's spontaneous activity with special emphasis on how they relate to their surroundings and to other children or adults, the duration of their capacity of attention, and their verbal or preverbal communication. Playing or interacting with the child is the best manner of assessing CNS function and provides information not only on purely neurological function but also on behavioural problems, which is clearly essential for the diagnosis of the behavioural syndromes that are currently taking a major place in child pathology. Advantage can be taken as often as possible of video-recording for prolonged observation of children's behaviour and is also particularly useful for the precise study of transient events such as seizures as it allows leisurely and repeated analysis of the ictal phenomena.

It cannot be overemphasized that the basic role of the nervous system is to produce not just reflexes but above all complex and adaptive behaviours that are much more informative on the status of the central nervous system than elementary responses to imposed stimuli. This is best achieved by prolonged observation of the qualitative aspects of the spontaneous activities of the children or infants. All too often, the child is examined but not looked at.

Spectacular advances in medical technologies made over the past decades have revolutionized and enormously increased our diagnostic possibilities, both pre- and postnatally (and recently even in pre-implantation diagnosis), and also improved follow-up surveillance far beyond what could be imagined 20 years ago. Neuroimaging, especially MRI, has become an almost routine investigation, and with continuing improvements and new developments such as diffusion-weighted MRI, tensor tractography, functional MRI and MR spectrography can now provide information not only on the anatomy but also on the function of some of the central nervous system structures. Biochemical progress in the molecular structure of proteins and the advent of molecular genetics allow a precise diagnosis of many genetic disorders even in the absence of clinical manifestations, representing an entirely new field opening new perspectives in diagnosis and prevention. However, at the same time, the availability of these multiple techniques has made the task of choosing among the possibilities offered much more difficult. Investigations should not be performed indiscriminately or systematically but only after formulation of one (or a limited number) of diagnostic hypotheses, arising mainly from history and clinical findings, with a view to validate or reject them on the basis of their confrontation by clinical and laboratory data. Clinical medicine is and must remain an intellectual process whereby all sources of information, whether clinical stricto sensu or arising from technical aids, are used to formulate a diagnosis that will lead to the best possible care of the patient. One's last task is to communicate and discuss our, sometimes complex, findings with the patient and their family. I hope this new edition of *Diseases of the Nervous System in Childhood* will help the clinician to carry out his/her tasks effectively.

JEAN AICARDI
Paris, September 2008

REFERENCES

Cioni G, Mercuri E (2008) *Neurological Assessment in the First Two Years of Life. Clinics in Developmental Medicine No. 176.* London: Mac Keith Press.

Dooley JM, Gordon KE, Wood EP, et al. (2003) The utility of the physical examination and investigations in the pediatric neurology consultation. *Pediatr Neurol* 28: 96–9.

Einspieler C, Prechtl HF (2005) Prechtl's assessment of general movements: a diagnostic tool for the functional assessment of the young nervous system. *Ment Retard Dev Disabil Res Rev* 11: 61–7.

Ferrari F, Cioni G, Prechtl HF (1990) Qualitative changes of general movements in preterm infants with brain lesions. *Early Hum Dev* 23: 193–231.

Hill A, Volpe JJ (1989) *Fetal Neurology: International Review of Child Neurology.* Philadelphia : Lippincott, Williams & Wilkins.

Levene MI, Chervenak FA, Whittle M, eds. (2001) *Fetal and Neonatal Neurology and Neurosurgery, 3rd edn.* London: Churchill Livingstone.

PART I

NEONATAL NEUROLOGY

1
NEUROLOGICAL DISEASES IN THE PERINATAL PERIOD

Linda S de Vries

This chapter deals with the period that extends from the onset of labour – covering abnormal intrapartum events – to the end of the neonatal period, conventionally limited to the first 28 days after birth. The majority of the neurological problems of that period arise during the first 10 days after birth. Intracranial haemorrhages and hypoxia–ischaemia dominate the neurology of the perinatal period, though it must be emphasized that they do not account for all the neurological problems of this period and that their predominance should not lead one to miss other important diagnoses such as metabolic or neuromuscular diseases.

The pre- and perinatal periods are nowadays more often considered as a continuum rather than two separate periods. Indeed, prenatal factors such as intrauterine growth restriction, prenatal hypoxia of whatever origin, prenatal inflammation and preterm birth all play a considerable role in the determination of many perinatal disorders. The response of the central nervous system (CNS) to the stress of the birth process and adaptation to extrauterine challenges are also of importance.

The two major pathological conditions encountered in the perinatal period – haemorrhage and hypoxia–ischaemia – are not totally separate entities. They often coexist, and they share some common causes and precipitating factors. However, other mechanisms such as mechanical trauma or coagulopathies can provoke haemorrhage without hypoxia, and the pathology and mechanisms are sufficiently different to warrant separate description.

INTRACRANIAL HAEMORRHAGE IN THE PERINATAL PERIOD

The epidemiology of intracranial haemorrhage has changed considerably over the past three decades. The incidence of traumatic haemorrhage, mainly subdural in location, has markedly decreased as a result of progress in obstetric practices. At the same time the relative frequency of intraventricular haemorrhage (IVH) has increased, as it is mainly a disorder of preterm infants and many more of these sometimes very immature babies survive than used to be the case. Over the last decade a marked decrease has been noted in the incidence of IVH in preterm infants, which can be mainly attributed to improved obstetric care, with increased use of antenatal steroids, as well as improvement in neonatal care with availability of artificial surfactant and better strategies to support respiratory function.

Modern imaging techniques, such as ultrasonography and especially magnetic resonance imaging (MRI), have made it possible to make an in vivo diagnosis of IVH and subarachnoid haemorrhage with much greater precision than was previously possible. Indeed many such haemorrhages would have remained undetected without the use of these imaging techniques.

There are two main groups of neonatal intracranial haemorrhage. Subdural haemorrhage is mainly of traumatic origin and occurs in term babies often of high birthweight (Welch and Strand 1986). Towner et al. (1999) looked at the effect of mode of delivery in nulliparous women on neonatal intracranial injury. They found that the rate of intracranial haemorrhage was higher among infants delivered by ventouse extraction, forceps, or caesarean section during labour than among infants delivered spontaneously, but the rate among infants delivered by caesarean section before labour was not higher, suggesting that the common risk factor for haemorrhage is abnormal labour. Intraparenchymal haemorrhage is also occasionally traumatic in origin and occurs in the same category of infants (Pierre-Kahn et al. 1986). This type of lesion has also been detected on antenatal imaging, related in some cases to alloimmune thrombocytopenia. Spontaneous intraparenchymal haemorrhage of unknown cause has been reported by Sandberg et al. (2001) in 11 infants. Eight required surgical decompression, and 4 of the 11 developed a motor deficit. IVH predominates in the preterm population (Volpe 2008). Other types of haemorrhage, e.g. subarachnoid, are often associated with IVH, but will often remain undetected when imaging is restricted to ultrasonography. Intraparenchymal haemorrhage, especially thalamic haemorrhage, may be due to sino-venous thrombosis in association with IVH (Wu et al. 2003).

INTRACRANIAL HAEMORRHAGE OTHER THAN IVH

SUBDURAL HAEMORRHAGE
Subdural haemorrhage may result from tentorial tear with rupture of the straight sinus or the vein of Galen, or smaller afferent veins; from occipital osteodiastasis with damage to the occipital sinus or cerebellar veins; from tear of the falx with involvement of the inferior sagittal sinus; or from injury to the bridging veins between the convexity of the hemispheres and the superior sagittal sinus, or between the transverse or sigmoid sinus and the base of the brain (Govaert 1993, Volpe 2001). In the first two situations,

the haemorrhage occurs in the posterior fossa, whereas in the other cases it is supratentorial, located adjacent to the convexity in the case of injury to the bridging veins, to the hemispheral fissure in falx laceration, and at the base of the brain with rupture of the veins draining into the lateral sinus.

Rupture is caused by excessive head moulding in vertex presentation or to excessive traction on the aftercoming head in breech presentation (Pape and Wigglesworth 1979). Localized trauma with skull fracture by forceps application is rare (Pierre-Kahn et al. 1986). Tentorial haemorrhage can also occur as a consequence of ventouse extraction (Hanigan et al. 1990, Govaert 1993). A subdural haemorrhage associated with a frontal lobar haemorrhage without apparent trauma has also been reported.

The *clinical features* are variable depending on the location and acuteness of the haemorrhage. In acute cases of *posterior fossa haemorrhage*, there can be massive bleeding with compression of vital brainstem structures, manifested by stupor or coma, nuchal rigidity, opisthotonus, eye deviation, bradycardia and apnoeic spells. Seizures occur in 36% of cases (Govaert 1993). A tense fontanelle, generalized hypotonia or hypertonia, skew eye deviation, facial palsy and unequal pupils may be observed. Of the 90 infants reviewed by Govaert (1993), a fatal outcome occurred in 15 unoperated and 3 operated cases. Sequelae include hydrocephalus, but outflow obstruction can be temporary and can be treated by insertion of a subcutaneous reservoir into the lateral ventricle. In subacute cases, the onset of neurological symptoms is delayed for 12 hours or more. Irritability, stupor, a bulging fontanelle and respiratory irregularities may suggest the diagnosis (Menezes et al. 1983, Fenichel et al. 1984). Diagnosis by ultrasound is possible, provided that the collection is large enough. CT and especially MRI better define the size and exact localization of the haematoma (Menezes et al. 1983, Govaert 1993, Sandberg et al. 2001). Surgical treatment is effective but adhesions may evolve leading to the development of hydrocephalus, requiring shunt insertion. Vinchon et al. (2005) relieved the subdural haemorrhage by percutaneous needle aspiration in 5 out of 7 infants who required surgical decompression of the clot.

Supratentorial haematoma of the convexity does not usually produce an immediate dramatic clinical picture. In typical cases, focal seizures or asymmetry in tone or both occur on the second or third day of life (Deonna and Oberson 1974, Sandberg et al. 2001). The occurrence of a IIIrd nerve palsy manifested by a dilated, nonreactive pupil on the side of the haematoma is characteristic. Minor subdural haematomas over the convexity may only give minimal clinical signs (Whitby et al. 2004).

In cases of subdural haemorrhage, the cerebrospinal fluid (CSF) is usually bloody. Lumbar punctures should no longer be used for the diagnosis of intracerebral haemorrhage, in view of the different imaging techniques available nowadays.

Basal subdural haemorrhage due to lateral tentorial injury results in collection of blood underneath the temporal lobe and/or occipital lobes. Govaert (1993) reviewed 21 cases confirmed by CT that presented in a similar way to convexity haematomas. Such cases are sometimes associated with arterial stroke due to compression of the middle cerebral artery (Govaert et al. 1992b).

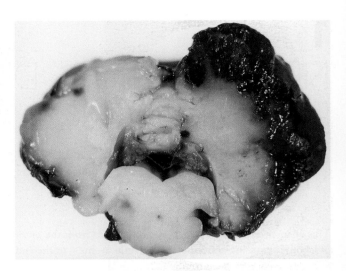

Fig. 1.1. Cerebellar haemorrage in infant born at 29 weeks gestational age, weighing 1500 g. Death at age 5 days. (Courtesy Dr J-C. Larroche, Maternité Port Royal, Paris.)

Similar cases have been seen involving the posterior cerebral artery (Deonna and Prod'hom 1980).

INTRACEREBELLAR HAEMORRHAGE
Intracerebellar haemorrhage has many features in common with posterior fossa subdural haematoma. Its mechanism is different as it seems to be related to hypoxia and ischaemia rather than to mechanical trauma, although it may be caused by occipital osteodiastasis or traumatic cerebellar injury (Welch and Strand 1986, De Campo 1989). It is often associated with IVH. It is frequent in series of low birthweight preterm infants (Fig. 1.1) and it is now increasingly recognized with routine MRI of all very low birthweight infants in some neonatal intensive care units (Merrill et al. 1998, Limperopoulos et al. 2005). Twenty-five of the 35 infants reported by Limperopoulos had a unilateral hemispheric haemorrhage. It may originate as dissection from IVH into the fourth ventricle or from the subarachnoid space into the cerebellar parenchyma, or represent primary intracerebellar haematoma or haemorrhagic infarction (Takashima and Becker 1989). The possible role of bands used for fixation of face masks has been suggested in the past, but this appears unlikely as the incidence was found to be similar when masks were not applied (Paneth et al. 1994). This type of haemorrhage appears to occur more often in the very immature preterm infant with a gestational age below 27 weeks (Limperopoulos et al. 2005). Neurological manifestations are generally overshadowed by symptoms and signs of hypoxia–ischaemia or respiratory distress. Apnoea, bradycardia and a falling haematocrit are frequent features. Ultrasonography can be diagnostic when the lesion is large or when care is taken to use the posterolateral fontanelle as the acoustic window (Merrill et al. 1998). CT and MRI will give better definition of the extent of the lesion. Obstructive hydrocephalus is common even following surgical evacuation of the collection and may be associated with the development of a cerebellar cyst communicating

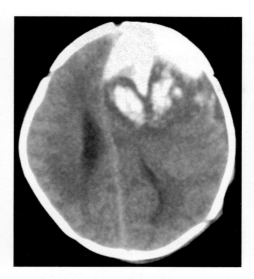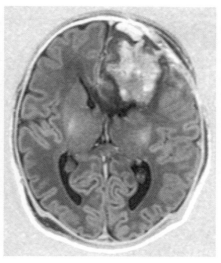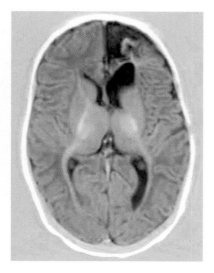

Fig. 1.2. Term infant, uncomplicated ventouse delivery. *(Left)* CT, day 1, showing intraparenchymal haemorrhage and subdural haematoma with shift of the midline. *(Middle)* MRI (inversion recovery), end of the first week following neurosurgical intervention, still showing a large parenchymal haemorrhage and slight asymmetry of the signal in the posterior limb of the internal capsule. *(Right)* Repeat MRI at 3 months shows ex-vacuo dilatation and resolution of the haemorrhage. There is a slight delay in myelination of the anterior limb of the anterior capsule. Outcome at 36 months was good.

with the fourth ventricle (Huang and Shen 1991). Clinically, cerebellar deficit may be seen as a sequela (Williamson et al. 1985). Cerebellar haemorrhage has also been seen as a complication of extracorporeal membrane oxygenation (Bulas et al. 1991) and in some infants with organic acidurias (Fischer et al. 1981, Dave et al. 1984). Cerebellar atrophy has also recently been reported as a common sequela of severe immaturity, and this atrophy is probably preceded by a cerebellar haemorrhage in the neonatal period or supratentorial white matter damage (Bodensteiner and Johnsen 2005, Johnsen et al. 2005, Messerschmidt et al. 2005, Srinivasan et al. 2006).

INTRAPARENCHYMAL HAEMORRHAGE

Intraparenchymal haemorrhage is virtually always associated with subarachnoid haemorrhage. In most cases it involves a single lobe and may result from trauma or haemorrhagic infarction (Pierre-Kahn et al. 1986, Hayashi et al. 1987, Huang and Robertson 2004). In five term-born infants studied by Pierre-Kahn et al. (1986) the haematoma communicated with the subdural space and the clot was surrounded by marked to massive cerebral oedema (Fig. 1.2). Breech delivery, and mechanically difficult delivery in general, was a major causal factor, although intraparenchymal haemorrhage has also been reported in uncomplicated vaginal deliveries (Sandberg et al. 2001). Clotting defects, and especially neonatal allo- and isoimmune thrombocytopenia may play an auxiliary role (Hanigan et al. 1995, Berkowitz et al. 2006). The symptomatology resembles that of subdural haematoma (Fenichel et al. 1984, Govaert 1993), with a symptom-free period of sometimes more than 24 hours, followed by focal signs and symptoms of raised intracranial pressure. Variable focal signs depend on the lobe involved and may include convulsions, asymmetry in tone and ocular signs.

Surgical evacuation is indicated when symptoms of increased intracranial pressure are present, associated with a midline shift on neuroimaging. A residual cavity in the brain may not cause any symptoms or may be associated with a focal deficit (Pasternak et al. 1980). A similar picture may be seen with haemorrhagic brain infarction.

THALAMIC HAEMORRHAGE

Thalamic haemorrhage (Fig. 1.3) is a rare form of neonatal intraparenchymal haemorrhage (Fenichel et al. 1984, Primhak and Smith 1985, Trounce et al. 1985, Adams et al. 1988b, de Vries et al. 1992b). The haemorrhage can be associated with an IVH (Roland et al. 1990, Govaert et al. 1992a, Govaert 1993, Monteiro et al. 2001, Wu et al. 2003) or limited to the thalamus and neighbouring structures. It was recently shown by Wu et al. (2003) that a sinovenous thrombosis should be suspected when the thalamic haemorrhage is associated with an IVH. Some venous congestion in the periventricular white matter or even venous infarction can be present on the side of the thalamic haemorrhage. With power Doppler through the anterior and posterior fontanelle, or better with CT or magnetic resonance venography, one is nowadays able to confirm the sinovenous thrombosis, and some will consider the use of anticoagulants. Infants with thalamic haemorrhage tend to present with seizures between days 2 and 14, following a normal delivery. Eye signs could include vertical upward gaze palsy, eye deviation toward the lesion, ipsilateral saccadic paresis and a flat visual evoked response, and they have all been attributed to the fronto-mesencephalic optic pathway (Trounce et al. 1985). Although the course may appear favourable in early infancy, Monteiro et al. (2001) reported that epilepsy with continuous spike-waves during sleep was related to primary neonatal thalamic haemorrhage. In a review of the literature they reported occurrence of epilepsy in 13 of 28 infants. A less favourable outcome was also reported by Campistol et al.

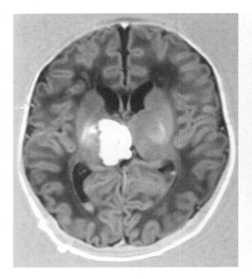
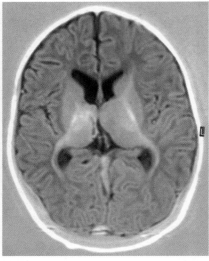

Fig. 1.3. Thalamic haemorrhage associated with sinovenous thrombosis. Coronal inversion recovery image *(far left)* shows a small amount of intraventricular blood, and a large haemorrhage in the right thalamus, which has almost completely resolved on the repeat MRI, performed at 3 months *(left)*.

(1994). Unilateral thalamic haemorrhage should not be confused with the more severe condition of *bilateral thalamic and basal ganglia involvement* in term infants with 'near-total acute asphyxia' (Barkovich 1992, Rutherford et al. 1995), which can also be haemorrhagic (Kreusser et al. 1984, Voit et al. 1987).

Brainstem haemorrhage is rarely of traumatic origin. At least one case of spontaneous brainstem haemorrhage, with diaphragmatic paralysis and lower cranial nerve involvement, is on record (Blazer et al. 1989).

PRIMARY SUBARACHNOID HAEMORRHAGE
Haemorrhage within the subarachnoid space, not being the result of extension from an intraventricular, subdural or intraparenchymal haemorrhage is common, based on the fact that bloody or xanthochromic CSF is frequently found when performing a lumbar puncture during the first few days after birth. A significant subarachnoid haemorrhage, also visible on CT, is much less common. Escobedo et al. (1975) found that only 29% of infants <2000 g at birth who had a bloody CSF at lumbar puncture had a subarachnoid haemorrhage detectable by CT. Subarachnoid haemorrhage can be of either traumatic or asphyxic cause. These were found respectively in 16 and 17 of 48 cases reported by Govaert (1993), while 10 cases remained of undetermined origin.

Clinical manifestations are often lacking. In some, irritability and seizures, sometimes presenting as apnoeic spells, are noted, typically on the second day after birth in otherwise well infants (Volpe 2008). Outcome is favourable, although development of posthaemorrhagic ventricular dilatation can occur. Diagnosis is difficult using ultrasound unless the posterolateral window is used, but is better made with CT or MRI, showing blood in the posterior interhemispheric fissure and in the region of the vein of Galen and on the tentorium (Govaert et al. 1990, Paneth et al. 1994).

Haemorrhagic disease of the newborn should no longer be seen with prophylactic administration of vitamin K, but is still reported in the literature in countries where prophylaxis is not yet common practice or in infants with specific problems like alpha-1 antitrypsin deficiency, Alagille syndrome and other problems leading to malabsorption of orally administered vitamin K (Vorstman et al. 2003, Danielsson et al. 2004, Ijland et al. 2008).

Other coagulation disorders may be responsible for severe intracranial haemorrhage in the neonatal period. Haemophilia can produce subdural intraparenchymal haemorrhage, subgaleal haemorrhage or IVH (Kletzel et al. 1989, Chalmers 2004). Thrombocytopenia is reviewed in Chapter 22.

EPIDURAL HAEMATOMA AND RARE TYPES OF NEONATAL
INTRACRANIAL HAEMORRHAGE
Epidural haematoma is a rare condition in newborn infants and is usually caused by mechanical trauma during or sometimes after delivery by a fall at home or out of an incubator (Choux et al. 1975, Gama and Fenichel 1985, Negishi et al. 1989).

Cephalhaematoma is commonly associated and communicates with the extradural blood collection through a skull fracture. Signs of progressive CNS dysfunction are usually delayed and may be absent altogether. Ultrasonography is not very helpful, and the diagnosis will usually be made by CT or MRI (see Fig. 1.2). Surgical evacuation is usually indicated. The collection tends to liquefy rapidly leading to a differential density within it (Aoki 1990). Conservative treatment is possible in asymptomatic infants and in those with only mild symptoms (Pozzati and Tognetti 1986).

Other rare types of haemorrhage in the newborn infant include subgaleal haemorrhage with extensive blood loss (Kilani and Wetmore 2006), and haemorrhages related to vascular malformations such as Osler–Weber–Rendu (Morgan et al. 2002) and the vein of Galen (Chapter 14) and congenital tumours.

GERMINAL MATRIX–INTRAVENTRICULAR HAEMORRHAGE (GMH-IVH)

This type of haemorrhage is especially common in the very low birthweight infant. The haemorrhage may subsequently rupture into the lateral ventricule. IVH is less common in the term infant

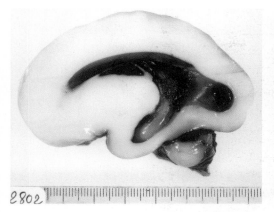

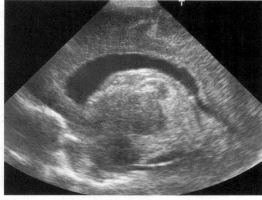

2802

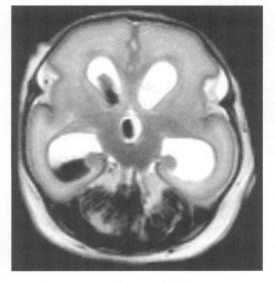

Fig. 1.4. *(Above left)* Intraventricular haemorrhage in an infant born at 27 weeks gestational age (birthweight 940 g; death at 36 hours after birth). Sagittal cut of brain demonstrates large clot occupying entire ventricular cavity. (Courtesy Dr J-C. Larroche, Maternité Port Royal, Paris.)
(Above right) Ultrasound scan of another infant shows a clot (hyperintense) in the lateral ventricle.
(Left) T$_2$-weighted MRI in a third infant, performed during the first week, shows a large intraventricular haemorrhage with ventricular dilatation and blood in both cerebellar hemispheres.

and is then more likely to start off in the choroid plexus, rather than the germinal matrix, which has shown almost complete involution at term equivalent age. With routine use of cranial ultrasound, the incidence could be assessed and was approximately 40% in the early 1980s, but had decreased to about 20% in the '90s (Papile et al. 1978, Batton et al. 1994, Heuchan et al. 2002, Horbar et al. 2002). Less mature infants are more at risk to develop a haemorrhage, and it was shown by Perlman and Volpe (1986) that 60% of infants weighing <1000 g at birth developed GMH-IVH, compared to only 20% of larger infants (Fig. 1.4).

The majority of cases of GMH-IVH in preterm infants originate in the subependymal germinal matrix, the highly cellular area that gives rise to neurons and glia during gestation and involutes before term. In infants of less than 28 weeks gestational age, haemorrhage is often located to that part of the matrix overlying the body of the caudate nucleus, while in those over 28 weeks it more commonly overlies the head of the caudate. Haemorrhages arise in the region of the germinal matrix. IVH results when the ependyma ruptures. Parenchymal haemorrhage, often referred to as grade IV haemorrhage, was initially considered to be an extension of the haemorrhage with rupture of the ependyma. It is nowadays considered more likely to be due to im-

paired function of the medullary veins draining the white matter (Takashima et al. 1986, Gould et al. 1987), and the terms 'venous infarction' or 'haemorrhagic parenchymal infarction' appear to be more appropriate. Various staging systems have been devised (Papile et al. 1987, Volpe 2008). The staging system according to Volpe is shown in Table 1.1. Like Volpe, I prefer to use a separate notation for associated (haemorrhagic) lesions in the white matter, than to use the term 'grade IV haemorrhage'. A parenchymal haemorrhagic lesion is often noted to develop following on from an IVH, which may lead to impaired venous drainage into the terminal vein. The lesion is mostly unilateral and at the side of the IVH. It is important to note both the site and extent of the lesion (Rademaker et al. 1994, de Vries et al. 2001, Bassan et al. 2006). Most of the parenchymal lesions will develop in the parietal white matter, but some occur in the anterior white matter or in the germinal matrix in the temporal white matter (Fig. 1.5). Associated lesions that have mainly been diagnosed at post-mortem examination include *pontine neuronal necrosis*, encountered in 46% of cases, and this was associated with *pontosubicular necrosis* in 20% (Armstrong et al. 1987).

Sequelae of GMH-IVH include posthaemorrhagic ventricular dilatation (PHVD) and infantile hydrocephalus. PHVD is considered to be due to adhesive arachnoiditis. It is more common

TABLE 1.1
Staging system for germinal matrix-intraventricular haemorrhage (GMH-IVH)*

Description	Generic term
Grade I: Germinal matrix haemorrhage	GMH-IVH
Grade II: Intraventricular haemorrhage without ventricular dilatation	GMH-IVH
Grade III: Intraventricular haemorrhage with acute ventricular dilatation (clot fills >50% of ventricle)	GMH-IVH and ventriculomegaly
Intraparenchymal lesion (IPL) – describe size, location	IPL

*Volpe (2008)

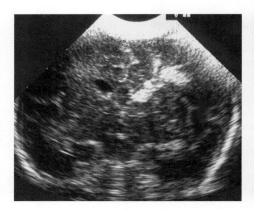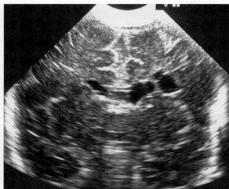

Fig. 1.5. Preterm infant, gestational age 29 weeks. Cranial ultrasound, coronal views during first week *(left)* and at term age equivalent *(right)* show intraventricular haemorrhage with associated parenchymal haemorrhage (venous infarction), which resolved and led to cystic formation that remained separate from the lateral ventricle. The child did not develop hemiplegia.

in infants who had a large haemorrhage, where blood has passed through the aqueduct and through the foramina of Luschka and Magendie into the basal cisterns. Acute outflow obstruction is less common but does occur and is usually due to a clot obstructing the aqueduct.

When the haemorrhage is restricted to the germinal matrix (grade I) one can see subsequent development of a germinal matrix cyst. These tend to resolve over the next 3–6 months and appear to be of little clinical consequence. However, destruction of neuron and glial cell precursors may have deleterious consequences on subsequent brain development.

The precise nature and origin of GMH-IVH remains uncertain. While some groups have suggested that the capillaries in the germinal matrix do not rupture easily, others have claimed that they can due to the fact that the vessels are immature in structure with little evidence of basement membrane protein, and are of relatively large diameter (Grunnet 1989). Pape and Wigglesworth (1979) suggested from their injection studies that capillary bleeding was more prominent than terminal vein rupture. A recent anatomical analysis of the developing cerebral vasculature was unable to show precapillary arteriole-to-venous shunts (Anstrom et al. 2002).

Risk factors can be prenatal, intrapartum and neonatal in origin. Histological signs of amniotic infection have been shown to increase the risk of GMH-IVH. Increased serum levels of

interleukin 1β, IL-6 and IL-8 have been found to be associated with severe IVH in extremely preterm infants (Yanowitz et al. 2002, Heep et al. 2003, Tauscher et al. 2003). There is still no agreement about the effect of the mode of delivery on the occurrence of GMH-IVH. Some suggest a protective effect of an elective caesarean section, but others were unable to support this. In a recent cohort study, a protective effect of a caesarean section was seen for only the most immature infants <27 weeks gestation (Thorp et al. 2001). Neonatal transport to a tertiary referral unit was also shown to be a risk factor in the same cohort study.

Haemodynamic factors play an important role. The immature brain is considered vulnerable to fluctuations in blood pressure due to limitations in autoregulation of cerebral blood flow (CBF) (Lou 1988). Impaired autoregulation renders the cerebral circulation 'pressure-passive' and hence unprotected from any wide swings or changes in blood pressure. An increase in systemic pressure can probably produce rupture of capillaries (Perlman et al. 1983, van Bel et al. 1987, Miall-Allen et al. 1989). This is especially likely to occur if a period of hypotension and ischaemia with injury of the germinal matrix vessels precedes the peaks of hypertension. The fluctuating pattern may be exaggerated in hypovolaemia (Pryds 1991). Several groups have shown that arterial hypotension precedes the development of GMH-IVH (Miall-Allen et al. 1989, Watkins et al. 1989), with the haemorrhage occurring during a period of reperfusion. Osborn et al. (2003) showed a low flow in the superior vena cava, detected during the first few hours of life, preceding an IVH. Perlman et al. (1983) and Miall-Allen et al. (1989) have emphasized the importance of fluctuating cerebral blood flow, as estimated from the blood flow velocity in the pericallosal branch of the anterior cerebral artery. Muscle paralysis was noted to stabilize the fluctuating blood flow pattern and was followed by a reduction in GMH-IVH (Perlman et al. 1985). Pneumothorax, a complication of artificial ventilation, is associated with both a dramatic increase in blood flow velocity – which returns to normal with resolution of the pneumothorax – and GMH-IVH (Hill et al. 1982b, Kuban and Volpe 1993). Better respiratory control, avoiding the situation where the infant is 'fighting the ventilator', and the more common successful use of nasal continuous positive airway pressure help to avoid sudden changes in blood pressure.

Asphyxia, i.e. hypoxia with hypercapnia, is another important aetiological factor. It aggravates the circulatory disorders by increasing blood flow and disturbs autoregulation. Low Apgar scores at 1 and 5 minutes and low umbical arterial pH have been associated with subsequent development of GMH-IVH (Perlman et al. 1996).

GMH-IVH mainly occurs within the first 3 days after delivery and is rarely noted to develop beyond the first week after birth, in contrast with periventricular leukomalacia (McDonald et al. 1984, Funato et al. 1992) (see below). Rare cases may occur prenatally (de Vries et al. 1998).

CLINICAL MANIFESTATIONS

The onset of GMH-IVH has been noted to occur earlier in preterm infants weighing <1000 g than in larger ones. Perlman and Volpe (1986) found that the onset in such infants was 10 ± 8 hours, as opposed to the second or third day in larger infants. Clinical symptoms are not too common and the diagnosis is most often made using routine cranial ultrasound. Ultrasound diagnosis is accurate in 92% of cases with an IVH and in 85% of cases with a haemorrhage restricted to the germinal matrix (Szymonowicz et al. 1984). CT and lumbar puncture are no longer recommended in making the diagnosis. Electroencephalography is not particularly helpful in making the diagnosis, although a change in the background pattern may precede the development of the haemorrhage (Connell et al. 1988). The presence of positive rolandic sharp waves has a good correlation with presence of GMH-IVH (Clancy and Tharp 1984) but correlates even better with white matter lesions such as periventricular leukomalacia and is thus nonspecific (Marret et al. 1986, 1992). The number of bursts per hour counted on the continuous amplitude integrated EEG is also helpful with regard to prognosis (Hellström-Westas et al. 2001).

Three clinical syndromes can be recognized in preterm infants not paralysed or heavily sedated on the ventilatator (Volpe 2001). The first one is known as *catastrophic deterioration*, noted by a sudden deterioration in the baby's clinical state, for example an increase in oxygen or ventilatory requirement, a fall in blood pressure and/or acidosis. The fontanelle may be tense or even bulging, and clinical seizures may be noted. More often, however, a drop in haematocrit is seen without a clear change in the infant's condition. The *saltatory syndrome* is more common and gradual in onset, presenting with a change in spontaneous general movements. The third and most frequent presentation is *asymptomatic*: 25–50% of infants with GMH-IVH have no obvious clinical signs. On careful neurological assessment impaired clinical signs, like visual tracking, a tight popliteal angle and later development of roving eye movements, decrease in tone and poor motility have been shown to correlate with GMH-IVH (Dubowitz et al. 1981).

COURSE AND SEQUELAE

Onset of GMH-IVH is within five hours after birth in 40% of the infants (Paneth et al. 1993), and 90% of cases can be detected by the fourth day after birth (Volpe 2008). However, the haemorrhage may only reach its maximal extent within three to five days of diagnosis.

The course may be rapidly lethal, especially when the haemorrhage is large and associated with a parenchymal haemorrhagic infarction. These very severe haemorrhages are no longer common; the mortality rate among 214 preterm infants with a large intraventricular and/or parenchymal haemorrhagic infarction seen at our centre was 33% (Brouwer et al. 2008).

Posthaemorrhagic ventricular dilatation (PHVD) may occur shortly after a large IVH, due to a large obstructing clot, but it is more common to see the development over the next 10–20 days. Having a large IVH is an indication for sequential ultrasound examinations, as it is well known that the larger the haemorrhage the higher the risk of developing PHVD. Without sequential ultrasound examinations, severe ventricular dilatation may develop without any clinical symptoms or a rapid increase in head circumference, as the extracerebral space is large in the very preterm infant. Once it has been recognized that the ventricles are starting to enlarge, the baseline size should be measured using ultrasound. The most widely adopted measurement system is that of Levene and Starte (1981). This 'ventricular index' is the distance between the midline and the lateral border of the ventricle measured in a coronal view in the plane of the third ventricle. Another useful measurement is the depth of the frontal horn taken just in front of the thalamic notch, a height >3 mm being used to define ventriculomegaly and one >6 mm to suggest PHVD (Davies et al. 2000).

The incidence of PHVD is less than 10% following a small haemorrhage and 15–25% after a moderate haemorrhage, but 65–100% following a severe haemorrhage (Hill and Volpe 1981b). Of 87 infants with GMH-IVH followed up by Hill and Volpe (1981a), 20 had rapidly progressive ventricular dilatation with signs of increased intracranial pressure, 47 had no ventricular dilatation, and 20 had progressive hydrocephalus without evidence of increased intracranial pressure. In 9 of these infants, hydrocephalus stabilized with or without resolution of ventriculomegaly. The remaining 11 had progressive dilatation following a stable period of 2 weeks to 3 months and eventually required insertion of a ventriculo-peritoneal shunt. In a more recent study by Murphy et al. (2002), a total of 248 very low birthweight infants had a GMH-IVH and a quarter of these developed PHVD. Spontaneous arrest was seen in 38%. Of the remaining 62%, 48% required non-surgical therapy while 34% required surgical intervention and 18% died.

Raised CSF pressure can cause symptoms. These include visual disturbance, seizures, feed intolerance and apnoea. In the long term, pressure-induced destruction of neuronal tissue can lead to motor impairment and learning disability (mental retardation). Short-term adverse effects on the nervous system have been confirmed using somatosensory and visual evoked potentials, Doppler estimates of cerebral blood flow velocity and near-infrared spectroscopy (Soul et al. 2004). They showed a pronounced effect of CSF removal on cerebral perfusion, irrespective of the opening pressure and the amount of fluid removed. The impact of removal of CSF on cerebral tissue was also assessed using advanced volumetric 3D-MRI, showing an increase in both cortical grey and myelinated white matter volume (Hunt et al. 2003). CSF hypoxanthine levels and soluble Fas were noted to be raised in infants with PHVD and especially so in those with associated periventricular leukomalacia (Felderhoff-Mueser et al. 2003).

In spite of all these data, there is no direct evidence that early drainage of CSF alters the natural history or outcome of PHVD. In a large retrospective multicentre study from the Netherlands, 95 infants with a large IVH (grade III) were compared for early [treatment started before exceeding the 97th centile by more than 4 mm (usually referred to as reaching the P 97 + 4 mm line)] versus late intervention (treatment started after crossing the 97 + 4 mm line) (de Vries et al. 2002). There was a significant reduction in requirement for shunt insertion in the early intervention group. There was also a trend for a better neurodevelopmental outcome but this did not reach statistical significance. A prospective randomized controlled trial allocating the infants to early versus late insertion of a reservoir has been done. The initial data of the drainage intervention fibrinolytic therapy (DRIFT) study showed a reduced need for shunt insertion, 22% vs around 60% in the ventriculomegaly and acetazolamide multicentre studies (Whitelaw et al. 2003), but this reduction was not confirmed in the subsequent randomized controlled trial, which was discontinued due to the large number of secondary IVHs in the group allocated to DRIFT (Whitelaw et al. 2007). No significant differences were seen between the 34 infants allocated to DRIFT and the 36 treated by tapping of cerebrospinal fluid by reservoir. We have now started a prospective randomized study, randomizing for early or later placement of a subcutaneous reservoir.

Development of neurodevelopmental sequelae depends mainly on the size of the initial haemorrhage and of involvement of the periventricular white matter. Older studies reported that 50–75% of those with a large haemorrhage (Papile et al. 1983) compared to only 16% of those with a small haemorrhage (Catto-Smith et al. 1985) have an adverse outcome. However, several studies (Weisglas-Kuperus et al. 1987, Fazzi et al. 1992, Vohr et al. 1992, van de Bor et al. 2004) have also shown that even infants with a small GMH-IVH have a higher incidence of dis-

ability than those without. Vasileiadis et al. (2004) showed a 16% reduction in cortical volume at near term age in 23 preterm infants with an uncomplicated IVH. Krishnamoorthy et al. (1990) confirmed in a large prospective study the association of GMH-IVH with neurodevelopmental sequelae. They stressed the importance of early ventriculomegaly as a predictor of motor sequelae. Ventriculomegaly may also, however, be due to associated white matter lesions, which probably play a more important role in determining outcome than a haemorrhage that is restricted to the lateral ventricle (Kuban et al. 1999). The outcome of infantile hydrocephalus in preterm infants with a gestational age below 33 weeks was recently reported by Persson et al. (2005, 2006), showing that the prevalence came down to 6 per 1000 livebirths but 88% of the infants went on to develop cerebral palsy. The outcome of infants with parenchymal haemorrhage depends very much on the size and especially the site of the lesion. The mortality in series reporting the outcome of large parenchymal haemorrhages is high, 59% in one study (Guzzetta et al. 1986), with 86% of the survivors suffering hemiplegia or spastic quadriplegia. Single large porencephalic cysts are now less common, in our experience. Smaller parenchymal haemorrhages that are only partly communicating with the lateral ventricle are more often seen nowadays, and the outcome appears to be better. Of 45 babies found to have a unilateral intraparenchymal lesion more than 1 cm in diameter, 17 did not have any motor sequelae at all at follow-up (de Vries et al. 2001). Early prediction of hemiplegia is now possible, using MRI at 40–42 weeks postmenstrual age (Cowan and de Vries 2005). At term, myelination should be present in the posterior limb of the internal capsule; babies who have asymmetry or lack of myelination in the posterior limb of the internal capsule at term went on to develop hemiplegia (de Vries et al. 1999). Diffusion tensor MRI can be used to visualize the tracts at an even earlier stage (Counsell et al. 2007).

PREVENTION
The decreasing frequency of GMH-IVH in most centres is difficult to attribute to one single factor. Administration of antenatal corticosteroids is according to several studies the most important protective factor for development of GMH-IVH (Shankaran et al. 1996, Crowley 2000). The effect may be due to a direct maturational effect on the brain, but other factors may also be involved, like the reduction of the severity of lung disease and the decreased need for inotropes after birth. It is not recommended to repeat the courses of antenatal corticosteroids, as a negative effect on brain growth has been shown in animal models as well as in newborn infants (Modi et al. 2001, Kanagawa et al. 2006). Betamethasone instead of dexamethasone is recommended as the latter was associated with an increased incidence of periventricular leukomalacia (Baud et al. 1999). Many more infants are no longer ventilated for hyaline membrane disease but manage on the newer nasal chronic positive airway pressure (CPAP) systems. Surfactant is sometimes given following the so-called InSurE procedure, where the infant is intubated, given endotracheal surfactant and then extubated. Not having to be ventilated has led to less handling and the elimination of procedures during

which fluctuations of cerebral blood flow will occur, like endotracheal suctioning. When ventilation is required more care is taken to avoid the infant fighting the ventilator (Shaw et al. 1993). An increased risk of developing GMH-IVH using high frequency ventilation has been suggested but was not found to be significant in a recent systematic review (Henderson-Smart et al. 2003).

Pharmacological intervention may be promising, especially the prophylactic use of indomethacin, immediately after birth. The results of a meta-analysis, involving 19 trials and a total of 2872 infants showed a significant reduction in the incidence of grade III and IV haemorrhages, with a pooled risk ratio (RR) of 0.66 and a 95% confidence interval (CI) of 0.53–0.82 (Fowlie and Davis 2002). The children of the original cohort studied by Ment et al. (1994a,b) were re-assessed at 8 years of age and no effect of indomethacin was seen on long-term outcome (Vohr et al. 2003). It was of interest though that male preterm subjects randomly assigned to saline tended to have lower Peabody Picture Vocabulary Test–Revised scores than did all of the other preterm groups. Using functional MRI to assess long-term influences of early indomethacin exposure on language processing, a significant treatment-by-gender effect was demonstrated in three brain regions: the left inferior parietal lobule, the left inferior frontal gyrus (Broca's area), and the right dorsolateral prefrontal cortex (Ment et al. 2006). Another large trial (Schmidt et al. 2001) was also unable to show an improvement in survival without sensory impairment at 18 months, despite a reduction in incidence of severe GMH-IVH.

Phenobarbitone was the first drug used postnatally in the prevention of GMH-IVH. The first studies were promising, but a meta-analysis of nine trials was unable to show a reduction in the incidence or severity of GMH-IVH (RR 1.04; 95% CI 0.66–1.24) (Whitelaw and Odd 2007).

Other drugs like ethamsylate and vitamin E are considered to have a stabilizing effect on the fragile vessels in the germinal matrix. Ethamsylate looked promising at first, but a multicentre study was unable to show a protective effect (Fish et al. 1990, EC Ethamsylate Trial Group 1994). The data for vitamin E are controversial.

The use of magnesium sulphate given prenatally has been studied extensively and the data obtained give different results (Weintraub et al. 2001, Mittendorf et al. 2002). No reduction in the incidence of either a small or a large GMH-IVH was found in two recent large randomized multicentre studies (Crowther et al. 2003, Rouse et al. 2008), although long-term follow-up did show an improvement in gross motor function, but no significant reduction in development of cerebral palsy.

GMH-IVH IN TERM NEWBORN INFANTS
GMH-IVH in term babies is uncommon. There is some dispute about the site of origin (Pagano et al. 1990). Some consider that these haemorrhages originate in the choroid plexus (Lacey and Terplan 1982). Recently attention has been drawn to sinovenous thrombosis as an underlying problem, with some of these children having associated unilateral thalamic haemorrhage and venous

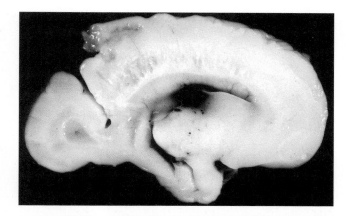

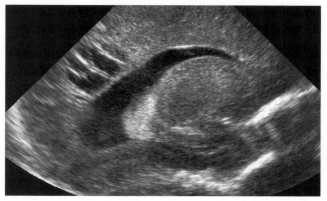

Fig. 1.6. Periventricular leukomalacia. *(Top)* Infant born at 28 weeks gestational age (birthweight 945 g), who died age 2 weeks: pathological specimen with multiple small cavities in periventricular location. (Courtesy Dr J-C Larroche, Maternité Port Royal, Paris.)
(Bottom) Ultrasound scan of a different infant, sagittal cut: multiple cavities visible alongside ventricular cavity.

congestion of true infarction (Roland et al. 1990, Wu et al. 2003).

Wu et al. studied 29 term infants with an IVH. Twenty-six of these had a sinovenous thrombosis. Four of the 5 who also had a thalamic haemorrhage compared to 5 of the 21 who did not have an associated thalamic haemorrhage had a sinovenous thrombosis (p=0.03). Sepsis, cyanotic heart defect and coagulopathy may all be predisposing factors.

Performing power Doppler through the posterior fontanelle and especially obtaining MR venography during the MR examination will help to clarify the origin of the IVH. There is not yet agreement about the role of fibrinolytic therapy in newborn infants with a sinovenous thrombosis, and a multicentre study is warranted and will start shortly (Kuhle et al. 2006).

The features and course of an IVH in a term infant – as well as hydrocephalus and other complications – are similar to those in the preterm infant.

PERIVENTRICULAR LEUKOMALACIA

The most common hypoxic–ischaemic lesion in the preterm infant is periventricular leukomalacia (PVL) (Fig. 1.6). This

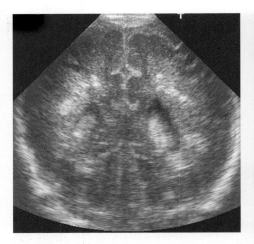 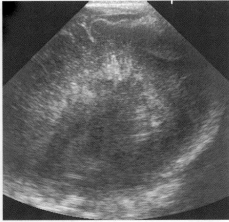

Fig. 1.7. Preterm infant, gestational age 30 weeks. Cranial ultrasound performed on day 1: *(left)* coronal view through the anterior fontanelle, and *(right)* parasagittal view through the posterior fontanelle. Severe 'patchy' echogenicity is seen in both views.

TABLE 1.2
Staging system for periventricular leukomalacia (PVL)

Description	Generic term

Grade I: transient periventricular echodensities persisting for >7 days
    a) homogeneous PVE
    b) inhomogeneous PVE
	PVE

Grade II: PVE evolving into small localized fronto-parietal cystic lesions	Localized c-PVL
Grade III: PVE evolving into extensive periventricular cystic lesions	Extensive c-PVL
Grade IV: densities extending into the deep white matter, evolving into extensive subcortical cysts	SCL

PVE = periventricular echogenicity; c-PVL = cystic PVL; SCL = subcortical leukomalacia.

condition was also reported by Miller et al. (2000) in term infants. The term was coined by Banker and Larroche in 1962, with softening (malacia) of the white (leukos) matter. Most of the infants in this study were born at more than 28 weeks gestation and were several weeks old at the time of death. Anoxic events were recorded in all. Pathological examination was able to show bilateral, although not necessarily symmetrical, coagulation necrosis adjacent to the external angle of the lateral ventricles. In more recent years the classical pattern is less often recognized and in a study by Paneth et al. (1990) only 3 out of 15 infants with white matter necrosis showed the classical changes of PVL. A distinction is nowadays made (Volpe 2008) between the more *focal* type of white matter damage – with cystic lesions limited to the regions of the trigone and occipital horns, involving the optic radiations, sometimes extending more anteriorly in the fronto-parietal white matter – and the more *diffuse* type, which is now more commonly referred to as leukoencephalopathy or periventricular white matter injury (PWMI) rather than PVL (Leviton and Gilles 1984, Back 2006). While evolution into cystic lesions, well visualized with cranial ultrasound, is the hallmark of the focal type, more diffuse changes in signal intensity on MRI represent a more appropriate technique to diagnose the more diffuse white matter disease (Counsell et al. 2003).

Cystic periventricular leukomalacia (c-PVL) was first diagnosed using cranial ultrasound in 1982 (Hill et al. 1982a). The lesions were haemorrhagic in older pathology studies in about 25% of the cases (Levene et al. 1983). The incidence of c-PVL has been noted to have decreased over the last decade (Hamrick et al. 2004) from 5–10% to below 1% in some centres.

NEUROIMAGING CORRELATES
The initial changes seen with ultrasound are areas of increased periventricular echogenicity (PVE), which is a very subjective finding (Fig. 1.7). Some suggest assessing PVE by comparing it to the echogenicity of the choroid plexus. The duration of the PVE should be taken into account, and the longer they exist the more likely they represent a mild degree of PVL. It may also help to look at the homogeneity of the PVE. In the case of inhomogeneity ('patchy' PVE), it is more likely that one is dealing with white matter damage, and the patchy areas often correlate with small petechial haemorrhages on MRI (Sie et al. 2000b, Childs et al. 2001). PVL can be graded into four subgroups (de Vries et al. 1992a) (Table 1.2). Grade I can be further divided into two subgroups, (a) homogeneous, and (b) inhomogeneous (patchy) PVE.

Several MRI studies have shown that there is poor correlation between PVE and signal intensity changes in the white matter

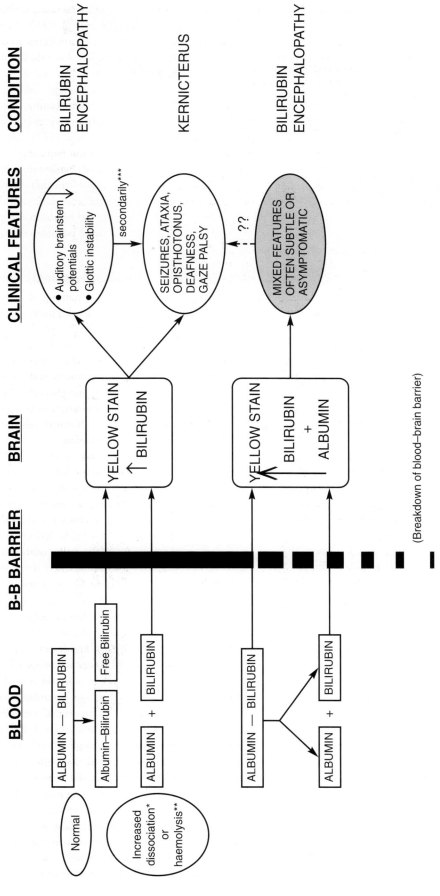

Fig. 1.13. Schematic representation of the relationship between albumin, free and bound bilirubin, and kernicterus or bilirubin encephalopathy. [Modified from Hansen and Bratild (1986).]

(*) May be due to drugs (*e.g.* sulfonamides), low albumin levels, and perhaps other factors such as acidosis: also observed in Crigler–Najjar syndrome (glucuronyl transferase deficiency). Except in the latter case is almost exclusively observed in preterm infants.

(**) Generally due to Rh haemolytic disease or ABO incompatibility.

(***) Intervention might be possible at this point to prevent neurological involvement.

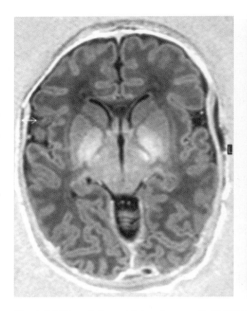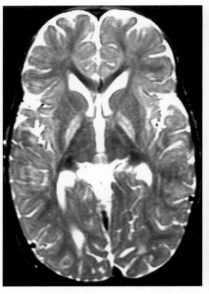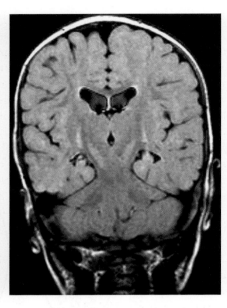

Fig. 1.14. Term infant with kernicterus. *(Left)* MRI (inversion recovery) during the first week shows increased signal intensity in the globus pallidus. *(Middle)* T₂-weighted spin-echo sequence at 18 months shows increased signal intensity in the same region as well as severe atrophy. *(Right)* Coronal FLAIR sequence shows increased signal of the globus pallidus as well as of the subthalamic nuclei.

remains impossible to predict which infant will exhibit bilirubin toxicity (Watchko and Oski 1992). In the study by Govaert et al. (2003), 5 preterm infants of 25–29 weeks gestational age presented with total serum bilirubin (TSB) levels below commonly advised exchange transfusion thresholds. Mixed acidosis was present in 3 infants around the TSB peak. The bilirubin/albumin molar ratio was >0.5 in all, in the absence of displacing drugs. All failed to pass bedside hearing screen tests and had severe hearing loss on auditory brain response testing. Four of the 5 infants presented with severe developmental delay as a result of dyskinetic cerebral palsy and hearing loss.

Some evidence (Perlman and Frank 1988) suggests that bilirubin might enter the brain in a reversible manner and might be responsible for 'subclinical neurotoxicity' that may either be transient or evolve into definitive neuronal damage. This hypothesis is based mainly on alterations of auditory and visual evoked potentials with hyperbilirubinaemia (Nakamura et al. 1985). Evoked potentials may return to normal following exchange transfusion (Chin et al. 1985, Hung 1989, Deliac et al. 1990). If this hypothesis were to be confirmed, it would be possible to contemplate exchange transfusion on the basis of clinical and electrophysiological signs rather than solely on bilirubin levels (Perlman and Frank 1988), but the evidence is far from complete and the method difficult to use in practice. A similar attempt using MRI (Palmer and Smith 1990) remained inconclusive.

CLINICAL MANIFESTATIONS
The classical picture of the term infant with typical kernicterus is not common in developed countries, although there appeared to be a slight increase following the changes of guidelines in the 1990s allowing higher bilirubin levels before initiating treatment (Ebbesen 2000). The increase in the number of cases of kernic-terus was considered by Ebbesen to have been caused by, inter alia, (i) a decreased awareness of the pathological signs, (ii) a change in the assessment of the risk of bilirubin encephalopathy, and (iii) difficulty in estimating the degree of jaundice in certain groups of immigrants. Furthermore, immigration and intermarriage allowed the spread of glucose-6-phosphate dehydrogenase (G-6-PD) deficiency mutants to geographic areas distant from its place of origin and thus transformed severe neonatal jaundice associated with G-6-PD deficiency into a global problem (Kaplan and Hammerman 1998). The first neurological signs develop between 48 hours and 4 days of age with feeding difficulties and a high-pitched cry, followed by hypertonus, extensor spasms and, in rare cases, clonic seizures. Hyperthermia is frequent (Connolly and Volpe 1990). A similar, though less acute picture can occur in preterm infants between 4 and 7 days of age. Following the acute stage, hypotonia sets in. Later on, the classic tetrad of Perlstein (1960) – choreoathetosis, supranuclear ophthalmoplegia frequently affecting vertical more than horizontal eye movements, sensorineural hearing loss and enamel hypoplasia – may evolve progressively, although in many cases one or several features are absent and hearing loss may be isolated (de Vries et al. 1985). Deafness and choreoathetosis may appear later, even in the absence of neurological signs in the neonatal period. Abnormal MRI signal from the pallidum (Fig. 1.14) has been observed in the neonatal period in several such cases (Martich-Kross et al. 1995, Yokochi 1995, Worley et al. 1996, Groenendaal et al. 2004). Residual cognitive deficits are possible. Severe mental retardation is uncommon.

Several authors have entertained the possibility that bilirubin toxicity in preterm infants may remain inapparent in the neonatal period but be responsible for delayed development, hearing problems and motor or learning difficulties in childhood (Ritter et al. 1982, Nakamura et al. 1985). Van de Bor et al. (1989) found a relationship between the occurrence of cerebral palsy (of undescribed type), as well as of minor developmental anomalies, and hyperbilirubinaemia in the first few days of life. In this large study, each increase in bilirubin level by 50 µmol/L (2.9 mg/dL) was associated with a small increase in the frequency of neurological sequelae. Similar conclusions were drawn from a large cohort of 2575 infants, born in 12 centres in the USA between January 1, 1994, and December 31, 1997 (Oh et al. 2003). A significant association was found between peak total serum bilirubin (mg/dL) and death or neurodevelopmental impairment [odds ratio (OR) 1.068; 95% CI 1.03–1.11], Psychomotor Developmental Index <70 (OR 1.057; 95% CI 1.00–1.12), and hearing impairment requiring hearing aids (OR 1.138; 95% CI 1.00–1.30). Other large studies (Scheidt et al. 1991, Seidman et al. 1991, Graziani et al. 1992a, O'Shea et al. 1992) did not confirm a relationship between neonatal bilirubin concentrations and developmental problems or intelligence. A relationship with hearing loss seeems better established (de Vries et al. 1985, Govaert et al. 2003).

The *diagnosis* of classical kernicterus is easy but the significance of a history of neonatal hyperbilirubinaemia, even moderate, in the neonatal period in a child with cerebral palsy, hearing loss or cognitive difficulties is impossible to interpret. Modern imaging is increasingly being used in kernicterus (Martich-Kriss et al. 1995, Yokochi et al. 1995, Groenendaal et al. 2004). Increased signal in the pallidum is best seen in neonates using T_1-weighted sequences, while in infancy MRI, usually but not in all cases, shows signal changes on T_2-weighted images from the hippocampus, thalamus and pallidum but not from the putamen, in agreement with pathological data (Yilmaz et al. 2001).

THERAPY
The treatment of kernicterus in term infants with haemolysis rests on the prevention of excessive hyperbilirubinaemia. Exchange transfusion is indicated for infants with erythroblastosis at a level of 340 µmol/L (20 mg/dL) (Watchko 2005). Prevention and prenatal treatment of blood group incompatibility (Whittle 1992) has resulted in almost complete disappearance of this problem. In a study by Watchko and Claassen (1994) only 3 of 81 infants had demonstrated kernicterus at relatively low bilirubin levels. Half of the remaining 78 infants had bilirubin levels in excess of those recommended by the National Institute of Child Health and Human Development, so the indications for exchange remain uncertain (American Academy of Pediatrics Subcommittee on Hyperbilirubinemia 2004, Wennberg et al. 2006). In preterm infants, exchange transfusion is of uncertain value and there is no agreement as to the levels at which it should be performed (Newman and Maisels 1992, Watchko and Maisels 2003). Although relatively safe, the procedure carries certain risks (Keenan et al. 1985).

Phototherapy effectively limits the neonatal increase in bilirubin in preterm infants. The technique is safe (Brown et al. 1985, Lipsitz et al. 1985), and breakdown products do not seem to produce bilirubin encephalopathy (Scheidt et al. 1991) while lower-ing peak levels of bilirubin by an average of 70 µmol/L (4 mg/dL). The value of mesoporphyrin inhibitors of bilirubin production is being tested and encouraging results have been reported (Valaes et al. 1994, Kappas et al. 1995), for instance in infants with G-6-PD deficiency (Kappas et al. 2001).

High levels of bilirubin may induce some behavioural changes in the absence of encephalopathy (Telzrow et al. 1980, Escher-Graub and Fricker 1986) but these are probably of limited significance.

METABOLIC INSULTS: NEONATAL ASPECTS

Metabolic disorders are considered in Chapter 8. Only the specific aspects of metabolic problems in the newborn infant are discussed here.

NEONATAL HYPOGLYCAEMIA
There is a lot of discussion about the definition of hypoglycaemia and the cut-off value of safe glucose levels in the newborn infant (Cornblath et al. 2000). The conventional definition of significant hypoglycaemia in the neonate is a blood sugar level of less than 1.1 mmol/L (20 mg/dL). Related to a paper by Koh et al. (1988), values below 2.6 mmol/L are now also considered to be potentially deleterious to the developing brain. Both figures are rather arbitrary as some infants may be symptomatic with levels of 1.6–2.2 mmol/L (30–40 mg/dL) while many others do not have symptoms even at levels well below 1.1 mmol/dL). Other factors such as the rate of fall of glucose and the duration of low glucose levels and associated hypoxia–ischaemia are thus important. Asymptomatic, transient hypoglycaemia can be detected in 11% of all newborn babies during the first hours post partum before oral feeding is initiated (Fenichel 1983), especially in those with intrauterine growth restriction or birth asphyxia or in those born to diabetic or toxaemic mothers (Cornblath and Schwartz 1991). The incidence of symptomatic hypoglycaemia is certainly much lower.

MECHANISMS AND PATHOLOGY
The mechanisms of neonatal hypoglycaemia are diverse. Rare infants suffer from grave conditions like nesidioblastosis. In the majority, especially in small for gestational age neonates, an imbalance between a relatively large brain that consumes glucose as its primary fuel and a small liver depleted of glycogen reserves seems to compromise supply to the CNS. The absence of symptoms in many infants with hypoglycaemia may be related to the fact that the newborn brain can oxidize other fuels than glucose, such as ketone bodies, lactic acid and fatty acids. Brain dysfunction with seizures and coma is not associated with a significant fall in high-energy phosphate compounds, a situation that also occurs with hypoxia (Petroff et al. 1988).

The pathology of hypoglycaemia is reminiscent of that of hypoxia, with which it is often associated (Collins and Leonard 1984). Neuronal loss involves not only the brain but also anterior horn cells of the spinal cord, but it usually predominates in the posterior part of the cerebrum (Anderson et al. 1967). Recent imaging studies have confirmed this observation (Spar et al. 1994, Barkovich et al. 1998, Traill et al. 1998, Filan et al. 2006).

CLINICAL FEATURES

Neurological manifestations of neonatal hypoglycaemia include apnoea, jitteriness, high-pitched cry, cyanosis, vomiting, seizures and coma, isolated or in any combination. The occurrence of symptoms seems to depend more on the duration of hypoglycaemia than on its degree (Koivisto et al. 1972). Several types can be observed. In the first few hours of life, an 'adaptive' hypoglycaemia frequently occurs in infants of diabetic mothers, those with erythroblastosis fetalis, and many preterm asphyxiated infants. Most cases with onset in the first 12 hours of life remain asymptomatic. Secondary hypoglycaemia usually occurs in the later part of the first day of life and is seen in severely asphyxiated infants born at or before term (Collins and Leonard 1984). The part played by hypoglycaemia in such cases is difficult to disentangle from that of the primary disorder. The classical type is seen primarily in small for gestational age infants. Symptoms are present in about 20% of such cases. They appear in the latter part of the first day or in the second day.

The outlook depends on severity and duration of hypoglycaemia and on therapy. Recurrent hypoglycaemia, on the other hand, is usually associated with hyperinsulinism, glycogenoses, fructose intolerance, or other disorders of carbohydrate metabolism or regulation. Congenital hypopituitarism, although infrequent, is an important cause because recognition is essential to avoid recurrences and mental retardation. Symptomatic hypoglycaemia in otherwise healthy breastfed term newborn infants has also been reported and is seen in children where the breast-milk intake is insufficient and additional intake is not given (Moore and Perlman 1999). Breastfed children are known to have lower blood glucose concentrations and higher ketone body concentrations on days 2 and 3 of life than formula-fed infants (Hawdon et al. 1994).

The outcome of neonatal hypoglycaemia is serious, with one study (Koivisto et al. 1972) showing cognitive or motor sequelae in about half of symptomatic patients, while only 6% of asymptomatic children had neurodevelopmental abnormalities at follow-up. Pildes et al. (1974) found that the average IQ of patients with symptomatic hypoglycaemia was lower than that of controls. Focal epilepsy may be an isolated sequela (Boulloche et al. 1987). Duvanel et al. (1999) also noted an adverse effect following repeated episodes of hypoglycaemia in small for gestational age preterm infants. Recent studies suggest that lasting effects may follow relatively mild hypoglycaemia. Koh et al. (1988) reported delayed nerve conduction velocities in children with marginal hypoglycaemia that persisted after correction of the metabolic defect. Lucas et al. (1988) found that children who had prolonged biochemical hypoglycaemia had a 3–14 point disadvantage on the Bayley scale as compared with normoglycaemic children, although this was a retrospective study with consequent limitations.

TREATMENT

Treatment of neonatal hypoglycaemia consists of the intravenous administration of 0.5–1.0 g/kg of glucose as a 25% solution at a rate of 1 mL/min, followed by continuous infusion of 8–10 mg/kg/min. The bolus injection should be used only in case of emergency and should always be associated with an increase in the glucose intake following the bolus. The underlying cause must be determined. Asymptomatic infants should probably have their glycaemia corrected by continuous infusion when blood glucose is below 2.2 mmol/L (40 mg/L) (Hawdon et al. 1994, Mehta 1994, Deshpande and Ward Platt 2005).

HYPOGLYCORRHACHIA WITHOUT HYPOGLYCAEMIA

Hypoglycorrhachia without hypoglycaemia (De Vivo et al. 1991) is a rare condition whose importance lies in the possibility of active treatment and in its diagnostic difficulties. The disorder is caused by deficiency of the carrier protein GLUT-1 that transports glucose from blood to CSF (Seidner et al. 1998). It is transmitted as an autosomal recessive trait and usually manifests clinically from the end of the first month onwards. GLUT-1 deficiency syndrome is caused by haploinsufficiency of the blood–brain barrier hexose carrier. Truly neonatal cases are known (Brockmann et al. 2001). The major clinical features are seizures, but ataxia, paroxysmal disturbances of consciousness and even periodic weakness have been observed. A low CSF lactate level may be a clue. Treatment by ketogenic diet prevents neurological deficit and has been successfully maintained for several years.

HYPERGLYCAEMIA

Marked hyperglycaemia occurs occasionally in neonates with CNS disturbances (Cornblath and Schwartz 1991) and has a grave prognostic significance. Idiopathic neonatal hyperglycaemia is exceptional (Lewis and Mortimer 1964).

DISTURBANCES OF ELECTROLYTE METABOLISM IN THE NEONATAL PERIOD

HYPOCALCAEMIA AND HYPOMAGNESAEMIA

Hypocalcaemia is defined as a blood calcium level <1.75 mmol/L (7 mg/dL) and is often associated with hypomagnesaemia, a magnesium level <0.6 mmol/L (1.5 mg/dL). Two distinct forms of neonatal hypocalcaemia form the bulk of the cases seen in the neonatal period, but both have become very rare with improved neonatal care, total parenteral nutrition in the preterm infant and improved cow milk formulae.

Early hypocalcaemia occurs before 48 hours of age mainly in preterm infants, infants of diabetic mothers, and those who are small for gestational age or have suffered asphyxia. Between 21% and 60% of such infants have calcium levels <1.75 mmol/L (7 mg/dL) or ionized calcium levels <0.75–0.85 mmol/L (3–3.5 mg/dL). This form has no symptoms of its own, and any clinical manifestation observed is likely to be due to the primary condition of the infant.

Late hypocalcaemia presents at between 5 and 10 days of life, typically in infants fed cow milk formulae with a high phosphorus content. The excess phosphate load cannot be completely excreted by the immature kidney and the resulting hyperphosphataemia

resonance signal in the internal capsule predicts poor neurodevelopmental outcome in infants with hypoxic–ischemic encephalopathy. *Pediatrics* 102: 323–8.

Rutherford M, Counsell S, Allsop J, et al. (2004) Diffusion-weighted magnetic resonance imaging in term perinatal brain injury: a comparison with site of lesion and time from birth. *Pediatrics* 114: 1004–14.

Sandberg DI, Lamberti-Pasculli M, Drake JM, et al. (2001 Spontaneous intraparenchymal hemorrhage in full-term neonates. *Neurosurgery* 48: 1042–8; discussion 1048–9.

Scheidt PC, Graubard BI, Nelson KB, et al. (1991) Intelligence at six years in relation to neonatal bilirubin level. Follow-up of the National Institute of Child Health and Human Development Clinical Trial on Phototherapy. *Pediatrics* 87: 797–805.

Schmidt B, Davis P, Moddemann D, et al. (2001) Long-term effects of indomethacin prophylaxis in extremely-low-birth-weight infants. *N Engl J Med* 344: 1966–72.

Schneider H, Ballowitz L, Schachinger H, et al. (1975) Anoxic encephalopathy with predominant involvement of basal ganglia, brain stem and spinal cord in the perinatal period. Report on seven newborns. *Acta Neuropathol* 32: 287–98.

Schumacher RE, Weinfeld IJ, Bartlett RH (1989) Neonatal vocal cord paralysis following extracorporeal membrane oxygenation. *Pediatrics* 84: 793–6.

Seidman DS, Paz I, Stevenson DK, et al. (1991) Neonatal hyperbilirubinemia and physical and cognitive performance at 17 years of age. *Pediatrics* 88: 828–33.

Seidner G, Alvarez MG, Yeh JI, et al. (1998) GLUT-1 deficiency syndrome caused by haploinsufficiency of the blood–brain barrier hexose carrier. *Nat Genet* 18: 188–91.

Shadid M, Moison R, Steendijk P, et al. (1998) The effect of antioxidative combination therapy on post hypoxic–ischemic perfusion, metabolism, and electrical activity of the newborn brain. *Pediatr Res* 44: 119–24.

Shankaran S, Bauer CR, Bain R, et al. (1996) Prenatal and perinatal risk and protective factors for neonatal intracranial hemorrhage. National Institute of Child Health and Human Development Neonatal Research Network. *Arch Pediatr Adolesc Med* 150: 491–7.

Shankaran S, Laptook AR, Ehrenkranz RA, et al. (2005) Whole-body hypothermia for neonates with hypoxic–ischemic encephalopathy. *N Engl J Med* 353: 1574–84.

Shankaran S, Langer JC, Kazzi SN, et al. (2006) Cumulative index of exposure to hypocarbia and hyperoxia as risk factors for periventricular leukomalacia in low birth weight infants. *Pediatrics* 118: 1654–9.

Shaw NJ, Cooke RW, Gill AB, et al. (1993) Randomised trial of routine versus selective paralysis during ventilation for neonatal respiratory distress syndrome. *Arch Dis Child* 69: 479–82.

Shen EY, Huang CC, Chyou SC, et al. (1986) Sonographic finding of the bright thalamus. *Arch Dis Child* 61: 1096–9.

Shortland D, Trounce JQ, Levene MI (1987) Hyperkalaemia, cardiac arrhythmias and cerebral lesions in high risk neonates. *Arch Dis Child* 62: 1139–43.

Sie LT, van der Knaap MS, Oosting J, et al. (2000a) Patterns of hypoxic–ischaemic brain damage after prenatal, perinatal or postnatal asphyxia. *Neuropediatrics* 31: 128–36.

Sie LT, van der Knaap MS, van Wezel-Meijler G, et al. (2000b) Early MR features of hypoxic–ischemic brain injury in neonates with periventricular densities on sonograms. *AJNR* 21: 852–61.

Soul JS, Eichenwald E, Walter G, et al. (2004) CSF removal in infantile posthemorrhagic hydrocephalus results in significant improvement in cerebral hemodynamics. *Pediatr Res* 55: 872–6.

Spar JA, Lewine JD, Orrison WW (1994) Neonatal hypoglycemia: CT and MR findings. *AJNR* 15: 1477–8.

Sreenan C, Bhargava R, Robertson CM (2000) Cerebral infarction in the term newborn: clinical presentation and long-term outcome. *J Pediatr* 137: 351–5.

Srinivasan L, Allsop J, Counsell SJ, et al. (2006) Smaller cerebellar volumes in very preterm infants at term-equivalent age are associated with the presence of supratentorial lesions. *AJNR* 27: 573–9.

Stern L, Cashore WJ (1989) Cellular mechanisms of bilirubin encephalopathy in the newborn. In: French JH, Harel S, Casaer P, eds. *Child Neurology and Developmental Disabilities*. Baltimore: Paul Brookes, pp. 103–6.

Stromme JH, Nesbakken R, Normann T, et al. (1969) Familial hypomagnesemia. Biochemical, histological and hereditary aspects studied in two brothers. *Acta Paediatr Scand* 58: 433–44.

Szymonowicz G, Schaffler K, Kussen LJ, Yu VYH (1984) Ultrasound and necropsy study of periventricular hemorrhage in preterm infants. *Arch Dis Child* 59: 637–42.

Takashima S, Becker LE (1989) Relationship between abnormal respiratory control and perinatal brainstem and cerebellar infarctions. *Pediatr Neurol* 5: 211–5.

Takashima S, Takashi M, Ando Y (1986) Pathogenesis of periventricular white matter haemorrhage in preterm infants. *Brain Dev* 8: 25–30.

Tauscher MK, Berg D, Brockmann M et al. (2003) Association of histologic chorioamnionitis, increased levels of cord blood cytokines, and intracerebral hemorrhage in preterm neonates. *Biol Neonate* 83: 166–70.

Telzrow RW, Snyder DM, Tronick E, et al. (1980) The behavior of jaundiced infants undergoing phototherapy. *Dev Med Child Neurol* 22: 317–26.

Thoresen M, Wyatt J (1997) Keeping a cool head, post-hypoxic hypothermia—an old idea revisited. *Acta Paediatr* 86: 1029–33.

Thoresen M, Penrice J, Lorek A, et al. (1995) Mild hypothermia after severe transient hypoxia–ischemia ameliorates delayed cerebral energy failure in the newborn piglet. *Pediatr Res* 37: 667–70.

Thorp JA, Jones PG, Clark RH, et al. (2001) Perinatal factors associated with severe intracranial hemorrhage. *Am J Obstet Gynecol* 185: 859–62.

Towbin A (1969) Latent spinal cord and brain stem injury in newborn infants. *Dev Med Child Neurol* 11: 54–68.

Towner D, Castro MA, Eby-Wilkens E, Gilbert WM (1999) Effect of mode of delivery in nulliparous women on neonatal intracranial injury. *N Engl J Med* 341: 1709–14.

Traill Z, Squier M, Anslow P (1998) Brain imaging in neonatal hypoglycaemia. *Arch Dis Child Fetal Neonatal Ed* 79: F145–7.

Trauner DA, Chase C, Walker P, Wulfeck B (1993) Neurologic profiles of infants and children after perinatal stroke. *Pediatr Neurol* 9: 383–6.

Trounce JQ, Dodd KL, Fawer CL, et al. (1985) Primary thalamic haemorrhage in the newborn: a new clinical entity. *Lancet* 1: 190–2.

Trounce JQ, Shaw DE, Levene MI, Rutter N (1988) Clinical risk factors and periventricular leukomalacia. *Arch Dis Child* 63: 17–22.

Truwit CL, Barkovich AJ, Koch TK, Ferriero DM (1992) Cerebral palsy: MR findings in 40 patients. *AJNR* 13: 67–78.

Tsang RC (1972) Neonatal magnesium disturbances—a review. *Am J Dis Child* 124: 282–93.

Tsuji M, Saul P, du Plessis A, et al. (2000) Cerebral intravascular oxygenation correlates with mean arterial pressure in critically ill premature infants. *Pediatrics* 108: 625–32.

Valaes T, Petmezaki S, Henschke C, et al. (1994) Control of jaundice in preterm newborns by an inhibitor of bilirubin production: studies with tin-mesoporphyrin. *Pediatrics* 93: 1–11.

Van Bel F, van de Bor M, Stijnen T, et al. (1987) Aetiological role of cerebral blood-flow alterations in development and extension of peri-intraventricular haemorrhage. *Dev Med Child Neurol* 29: 601–14.

Van Bel F, Shadid M, Moison RM, et al. (1998) Effect of allopurinol on postasphyxial free radical formation, cerebral hemodynamics, and electrical brain activity. *Pediatrics* 101: 185–93.

van de Bor M, den Ouden L (2004) School performance in adolescents with and without periventricular–intraventricular hemorrhage in the neonatal period. *Semin Perinatol* 28: 295–303.

van de Bor M, Van Zeben-Van der Aa TM, Verloove-Vanhorick SP, et al. (1989) 'Hyperbilirubinemia in preterm infants and neurodevelopmental outcome at 2 years of age: results of a national collaborative survey. *Pediatrics* 83: 915–20.

Van den Hout BM, Eken P, van der Linden D, et al. (1998) Visual, cognitive and neurodevelopmental outcome at 5⅓ years of age in neonatal haemorrhagic/ischaemic brain lesions. *Dev Med Child Neurol* 40: 820–8.

van Haastert IC, de Vries LS, Helders PJM, et al. (2008) Gross motor functional abilities in preterm children with cerebral palsy due to periventricular leukomalacia. *Dev Med Child Neurol* 50: 684–9.

Vannucci RC, Yager JY (1992) Glucose, lactic acid, and perinatal hypoxic–ischemic brain damage. *Pediatr Neurol* 8: 3–12.

Vasileiadis GT, Gelman N, Han VK, et al. (2004) Uncomplicated intraventricular hemorrhage is followed by reduced cortical volume at near-term age. *Pediatrics* 114: e367–72.

Vasta I, Kinali M, Messina S, et al. (2005) Can clinical signs identify newborns with neuromuscular disorders? *J Pediatr* 146: 73–9.

Verma U, Tejani N, Klein S, et al. (1997) Obstetric antecedents of intraventricular hemorrhage and periventricular leukomalacia in the low-birth-weight neonate. *Am J Obstet Gynecol* 176: 275–81.

Vinchon M, Pierrat V, Tchofo PJ, et al. (2005) Traumatic intracranial hemorrhage in newborns. *Childs Nerv Syst* 21: 1042–148.

Visudhiphan P, Visudtibhan A, Chiemchanya S, Khongkhatithum C (2005) Neonatal seizures and familial hypomagnesemia with secondary hypocalcemia. *Pediatr Neurol* 33: 202–5.

Vohr BR, Garcia-Coll C, Flanagan P, Oh W (1992) Effects of intraventricular hemorrhage and socioeconomic status on perceptual, cognitive, and neurologic status of low birth weight infants at 5 years of age. *J Pediatr* 121: 280–85.

Vohr BR, Allan WC, Westerveld M, et al. (2003) School-age outcomes of very low birth weight infants in the indomethacin intraventricular hemorrhage prevention trial. *Pediatrics* 111: e340–6.

Voit T, Lemburg P, Neuen E, et al. (1987) Damage of thalamus and basal ganglia in asphyxiated full-term neonates. *Neuropediatrics* 18: 176–81.

Volpe JJ (2008) *Neurology of the Newborn, 5th edn.* Philadelphia: WB Saunders.

Volpe JJ, Pasternak JF (1977) Parasagittal cerebral injury in neonatal hypoxic–ischemic encephalopathy. Clinical and neuroradiologic features. *J Pediatr* 91: 472–6.

Vorstman EB, Anslow P, Keeling DM, et al. (2003) Brain haemorrhage in five infants with coagulopathy. *Arch Dis Child* 88: 1119–21.

Waller S, Kurzawinski T, Spitz L, et al. (2004) Neonatal severe hyperparathyroidism: genotype/phenotype correlation and the use of pamidronate as rescue therapy. *Eur J Pediatr* 163: 589–94.

Watchko JF (2005) Vigintiphobia revisited. *Pediatrics* 115: 1747–53.

Watchko JF, Claassen D (1994) Kernicterus in premature infants: current prevalence and relationship to NICHD Phototherapy Study exchange criteria. *Pediatrics* 93: 996–9.

Watchko JF, Maisels MJ (2003) Jaundice in low birthweight infants: pathobiology and outcome. *Arch Dis Child Fetal Neonatal Ed* 88: F455–8.

Watchko JF, Oski FA (1992) Kernicterus in preterm newborns: past, present, and future. *Pediatrics* 90: 707–15.

Watkins AMC, West CR, Cooke RWI (1989) Blood pressure and cerebral haemorrhage and ischaemia in very low birthweight infants. *Early Hum Dev* 19: 103–10.

Weinstein D, Margalioth EJ, Navot D, et al. (1983) Neonatal fetal death following cesarian section secondary to hyperextended head in breech presentation. *Acta Obstet Gynecol Scand* 62: 629–31.

Weintraub Z, Solovechick M, Reichman B, et al. (2001) Effect of maternal tocolysis on the incidence of severe periventricular/intraventricular haemorrhage in very low birthweight infants. *Arch Dis Child Fetal Neonatal Ed* 85: F13–7.

Weisglas-Kuperus N, Uleman-Vleeschdrager M, Baerts W (1987) Ventricular haemorrhages and hypoxic–ischaemic lesions in preterm infants: neurodevelopmental outcome at 3½ years. *Dev Med Child Neurol* 29: 623–9.

Welch K, Strand R (1986) Traumatic parturitional intracranial haemorrhage. *Dev Med Child Neurol* 28: 156–64.

Wennberg RP, Ahlfors CE, Bhutani VK, et al. (2006) Toward understanding kernicterus: a challenge to improve the management of jaundiced newborns. *Pediatrics* 117: 474–85.

Whitby EH, Griffiths PD, Rutter S, et al. (2004) Frequency and natural history of subdural haemorrhages in babies and relation to obstetric factors. *Lancet* 363: 846–51.

Whitelaw A, Odd D (2007) Postnatal phenobarbital for the prevention of intraventricular hemorrhage in preterm infants. *Cochrane Database Syst Rev* 2007 (4): CD000691.

Whitelaw A, Pople I, Cherian S, et al. (2003) Phase 1 trial of prevention of hydrocephalus after intraventricular hemorrhage in newborn infants by drainage, irrigation, and fibrinolytic therapy. *Pediatrics* 111: 759–65.

Whitelaw A, Evans D, Carter M, et al. (2007) Randomized clinical trial of prevention of hydrocephalus after intraventricular hemorrhage in preterm infants: brain-washing versus tapping fluid. *Pediatrics* 119: 1071–8.

Whittle MJ (1992) Rhesus haemolytic disease. *Arch Dis Child* 67: 65–8.

Williamson WD, Percy AK, Fishman MA, et al. (1985) Cerebellar hemorrhage in the term neonate: developmental and neurologic outcome. *Pediatr Neurol* 1: 356–60.

Wiswell TE, Graziani LJ, Kornhauser MS, et al. (1996) Effects of hypocarbia on the development of cystic periventricular leukomalacia in premature infants treated with high frequency jet ventilation. *Pediatrics* 98: 918–24.

Worley G, Erwin CW, Goldstein RF, et al. (1996) Delayed development of sensorineural hearing loss after neonatal hyperbilirubinemia: a case report with brain magnetic resonance imaging. *Dev Med Child Neurol* 38: 271–7.

Wu YW, Colford JM (2000) Chorioamnionitis as a risk factor for cerebral palsy. *JAMA* 284: 1417–24.

Wu YW, Miller SP, Chin K, et al. (2002) Multiple risk factors in neonatal sinovenous thrombosis. *Neurology* 59: 438–40.

Wu YW, Hamrick SE, Miller SP, et al. (2003) Intraventricular hemorrhage in term neonates caused by sinovenous thrombosis. *Ann Neurol* 54: 123–6.

Yamano T, Fujiwara S, Matsukawa S, et al. (1992) Cervical cord birth injury and subsequent development of syringomyelia: a case report. *Neuropediatrics* 23: 327–8.

Yanowitz TD, Jordan JA, Gilmour CH, et al. (2002) Hemodynamic disturbances in premature infants born after chorioamnionitis: association with cord blood cytokine concentrations. *Pediatr Res* 51: 310–6.

Yilmaz Y, Alper G, Kilicoglu G, et al. (2001) Magnetic resonance imaging findings in patients with severe neonatal indirect hyperbilirubinemia. *J Child Neurol* 16: 452–5.

Yokochi K (1995) Magnetic resonance imaging in children with kernicterus. *Acta Paediatr* 84: 937–9.

Yoon BY, Jun JK, Romero R, et al. (1997) Amniotic fluid inflammatory cytokines (interleukin-6, interleukin-1beta, and tumor necrosis factor-alpha), neonatal brain white matter lesions, and cerebral palsy. *Am J Obstet Gynecol* 177: 19–26.

Young RSK, Towfighi J, Marks KH (1983) Focal necrosis of the spinal cord in utero. *Arch Neurol* 40: 654–5.

Younkin D, Medoff-Cooper B, Guillet R, et al. (1988) In vivo 31P nuclear magnetic resonance measurement of chronic changes in cerebral metabolites following neonatal intraventricular hemorrhage. *Pediatrics* 82: 331–6.

Zifko U, Hartmann M, Girsch W, et al. (1995) Diaphragmatic paresis in newborns due to phrenic nerve injury. *Neuropediatrics* 26: 281–4.

PART II

CNS MALFORMATIONS, CHROMOSOMAL ABNORMALITIES, NEUROCUTANEOUS SYNDROMES AND SKULL MALFORMATIONS

2

MALFORMATIONS OF THE CENTRAL NERVOUS SYSTEM

Malformations of the CNS have tended to be of interest only to neuropathologists and not to clinicians. The emergence of new concepts on teratogenesis drawn from experimental embryology, the study of animal models and other new techniques of investigation over the past two decades have excited the interest of other neurology specialists. With the advent of CT, then MRI, the diagnosis of many malformations has become feasible in the living patient and clinicians have become interested in their study (Peter and Fieggen 1999). An early diagnosis has practical implications because it allows a precise prognosis to be made, and, in the case of genetically determined malformations, it is essential for genetic counselling. The development of techniques for prenatal diagnosis of fetal abnormalities has coincided with liberalization in attitudes toward abortion, allowing termination of pregnancies in which the fetus is proved to be affected. This has raised considerable ethical and practical problems but the whole perspective of congenital brain defects has been transformed. Novel methods of prefertilization/preimplantation diagnosis have also become available. Further advances in developmental neurobiology will enable us not only to answer fundamental questions about mammalian and, especially, human brain development but also hopefully to develop methods for the prevention, and perhaps the treatment, of at least some developmental brain defects (for reviews, see Caviness et al. 2003, Rakic and Zecevik 2003). For a detailed account of the range of CNS malformations, their causes and pathology, the reader is referred to Harding and Copp (1997).

DEFINITIONS, FREQUENCY, AETIOLOGICAL FACTORS

The formation of the brain is such a fantastically complex process that it is not difficult to understand that it can be disturbed at any stage by a number of factors.

The term 'malformation', in this chapter, will designate any gross morphological abnormality of the CNS that dates to the embryonic or fetal period, regardless of its established or supposed mechanism (Evrard et al. 1984, Friede 1989). Some malformations are due to a deviation in the normal morphogenetic processes that may result from faulty genetic information or from interference with the harmonious development of correct genetic information. Another mechanism that can lead to malformation, in the broad sense used in this text, is damage to normally formed structures followed by faulty repair (Marin-Padilla 1999, 2000). Malformations of this type generally occur late in pregnancy. However, purely destructive processes such as cystic softening or so-called 'clastic' porencephaly that do not modify the general structure of the nervous system do not belong in the group of malformations. Because repair mechanisms in the fetus are morphologically quite different from what they are later, in particular due to lack of glial proliferation, lesions incurred before the 20th week of pregnancy were once often regarded as resulting from 'arrest of development' or abnormal development. Such applies with at least some of the cases of schizencephaly (formerly termed malformative porencephaly) (see below), which was formerly thought to be due to arrest in development of the cerebral mantle but can result from an early destructive process, perhaps of vascular origin. Secondary repair without cicatrization results in the formation of a cleft whose lips may be fused in a pial–ependymal 'seam'. The cleft interferes with neuronal migration, if it is not yet completed, producing secondary abnormalities of migration (Menezes et al. 1988), thus illustrating the intricate relationship between external insults and errors of development, as well as the possible late consequences of temporally remote injuries.

Malformations are one of the commonest problems of child neurology. Statistical data suggest that 25% of conceptuses are affected by a developmental CNS disturbance and such disturbances account for a high percentage of fetal deaths (Williams and Caviness 1984). In postnatal life, it has been estimated that 40% of deaths in the first year are related in some way to CNS malformations (Evrard et al. 1984). Skjaerven et al. (1999) found a mortality rate of 20% for patients with CNS malformation in Norway; deaths were predominantly in infants under 2 years, but an excess rate was still noticeable between 12 and 14 years of age. In addition, recent studies indicate that many major neurological problems, such as cerebral palsy, are more frequently of prenatal than of postnatal origin (Volpe 2001) and that a substantial proportion of the prenatal cases are due to malformations. Likewise, prenatal abnormalities are often the origin of perinatal problems (Freeman and Nelson 1988) traditionally attributed to birth trauma or asphyxia.

The *aetiology* of CNS malformations remains obscure in most cases. It is generally held that the timing of an insult to the fetus is more important than the nature of the insult itself in determining the type of resulting malformations, and that the same noxious agent operating at different periods can produce distinct malformation patterns. However, some teratogenic agents tend preferentially to produce certain patterns of anomalies, as shown by the effects of alcohol or of some antiepileptic drugs on the CNS. Thus sodium valproate tends to produce abnormal closure of the neural tube (Lindhout and Schmidt 1986), which is not the case with other anticonvulsant agents, although carbamazepine has also been incriminated (Rosa 1991).

Congenital malformations may be the result of *environmental causes* of infectious, toxic (Bingol et al. 1987), or physical (e.g. X-rays) nature; such account for about 5% of malformations. Retinoic acid (Lammer et al. 1985), other drugs including antiepileptic agents (Dodson 1989), toluene encephalopathy (Hersh et al. 1985) and the fetal alcohol syndrome (Hoyme et al. 2005, Autti-Rämö et al. 2006) are well-studied examples.

The role attributed to *genetic factors* in the development of malformations has been increasing as a result of progress in genetics. Common malformations are less commonly monogenic, although new diagnostic techniques tend to increase the proportion of cases seen to be due to minor chromosomal anomalies such as microdeletions, especially subtelomeric rearrangements (Shapira et al. 1997). Chromosomal aberrations and an increasing number of gene mutations can be causes. In recent years, however, a number of CNS malformations related to single-gene mutations have been recognized. In addition some malformations such as harelip, cleft palate and limb defects are much more frequent in offspring of women with the same malformations, but do not follow a mendelian pattern (Skjaerven et al. 1999). Polygenic inheritance, allowing for a multifactorial aetiology with interacting environmental and genetic factors, may be the cause in 20% of cases, whereas well-defined environmental teratogens have only a minor role (3.5%), even though new teratogenic agents continue to be discovered.

About 60% of all CNS malformations are of unknown cause (Cordero 1994).

The *mechanisms* of malformations are still poorly understood despite important progress in the field (Evrard et al. 1989, Walshe 1995, Sarnat and Flores-Sarnat 2001a, Barth 2003b). As already mentioned there are three major possibilities: (1) the scheme ('blueprint') of CNS development is incorrect from the start because of inheritance, chromosomal anomaly, point mutations, larger DNA rearrangements or other factors resulting in modified and improper instructions; (2) the basic design is normal but the instructions are incorrectly carried out because of traductional or post-traductional abnormalities, external interference with the processes of development, or haphazard accidents in the complex chain of events leading to a normal CNS; (3) the basic design is normal and it is normally carried out, only to be damaged secondarily with subsequent repair leading to major morphological changes in the CNS. Such changes may be difficult to distinguish morphologically from primary malformations.

From a didactic point of view, the likely date of occurrence of malformations allows one to separate them into two broad groups: (1) malformations that arise during the first five months of pregnancy – when major morphogenetic events, such as division of telencephalon into cerebral vesicles or neural tube closure, are taking place – and affect organogenesis and histogenesis, i.e. proliferation and migration of neurons leading to defective corticogenesis; (2) malformations that arise during the latter months of gestation, when all major cerebral components are in place and maturing. Most of these malformations are the secondary result of destructive processes such as ischaemia or infections (Larroche 1986). However, minor primary malformations can still arise because late migration, lamination and synaptogenesis can be interfered with (Sarnat 1987).

Peripheral malformations commonly accompany CNS abnormalities. For example, associated heart malformations are frequent and 7% of children with congenital heart disease also have CNS malformations. Even outside well-defined malformation complexes, certain peripheral and visceral congenital anomalies tend to co-exist, whereas other associations are rare (Natowicz et al. 1988). Thus, neural tube defects are not associated with conotruncal abnormalities and are more frequent with spina bifida than with anencephaly or cephalocele. There exists also an association between CNS malformations and more general disturbances in development, abnormalities being 2.5 times more frequent in patients with intrauterine growth retardation than in the general population (Khoury et al. 1988).

NORMAL DEVELOPMENT OF THE CENTRAL NERVOUS SYSTEM

Only a brief outline of the embryological development of the CNS will be given. The reader is referred for more complete information to classical studies (Sarnat 1987, Barkovich et al. 1992, McConnell 1992). Table 2.1 presents a schematic overview of the main stages of CNS embryogenesis. The regulation of CNS development, a fantastically complex process, is controlled by many factors, especially genetic ones. A major role is played by a large number of proteins coded for or regulated by genes (homeobox genes and transcription factors) that determine gradients of differentiation (antero-posterior and dorsoventral) and govern the definition of major organizational territories. These mechanisms are still largely obscure and their study is beyond the scope of this book.

During the second week of embryogenesis, the three layers of ectoderm, mesoderm and entoderm are formed (Fig. 2.1). By 2 weeks the midline ectoderm, under the inductive influence of the underlying mesoderm, becomes the neural plate that further develops into the neural groove, then the *neural tube*. During the fourth week, the neural tube closes. The process of closure begins in the middle part of the tube and proceeds towards the extremities. Neural cell adhesion molecules play a central role in the process of closure (Sarnat and Flores-Sarnat 2002, 2004). Closure of the neural tube is determined by dorsal induction from the mesoderm. Before closure of the tube, on day 9, the anlagen of

TABLE 2.1
Major stages of CNS development

Stage	Peak time of occurrence	Major morphological events in cerebrum	Major morphological events in cerebellum	Main corresponding disorders*
Uterine implantation	1 wk			
Separation of 3 layers	2 wks	Neural plate		Enterogenous cysts and fistulae
Dorsal induction 　Neurulation	3–4 wks	Neural tube, neural crest and derivatives. Closure of anterior (d 24) and posterior (d 29) neuropores	Paired alar plates	Anencephaly, encephalocele, craniorachischisis, spina bifida, meningoceles
Caudal neural tube formation	4–7 wks	Canalization and regressive differentiation of cord	Rhombic lips (d 35), cerebellar plates	Diastematomyelia, Dandy–Walker syndrome, Cerebellar hypoplasia
Ventral induction	5–6 wks	Forebrain and face (cranial neural crest). Cleavage of prosencephalon into cerebral vesicles (d 33). Optic placodes (d 26), olfactory placodes. Diencephalon	Fusion of cerebellar plates	Holoprosencephaly, median cleft face syndrome
Neuronal and glial proliferation	8–16 wks	Cellular proliferation in ventricular and subventricular zone (interkinetic migration). Early differentiation of neuroblasts and glioblasts.	Migration of Purkinje cells (9–10 w). Migration of external granule layer (10–11 w)	Microcephaly, megalencephaly
Migration	12–20 wks	Radial migration and accessory pathways (e.g. corpus gangliothalamicum). Formation of corpus callosum	Dendritic tree of Purkinje cells (16–25 w)	Lissencephaly–pachygyria (types I and II), Zellweger syndrome, glial heterotopia, microgyria (some forms), agenesis of corpus callosum
Organization**	24 wks to postnatal	Late migration (to 5 months). Alignment, orientation and layering of cortical neurons. Synaptogenesis. Glial proliferation/differentation well into postnatal life	Monolayer of Purkinje cells (16–28 w). Migration of granules to form internal granular layer (to postnatal life)	Minor cortical dysplasias, dendritic/synaptic abnormalities, microgyria (some forms)
Myelination	24 wks to 2 yrs postnatally			Dysmyelination, clastic insults

*Disorders do not necessarily correspond to abnormal development. They may also result from secondary destruction/disorganization.
**Programmed cellular death takes place throughout the second half of pregnancy and the first year of extrauterine life.

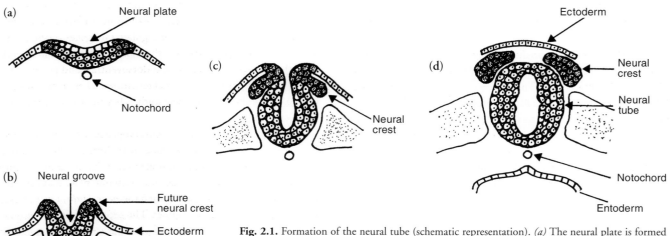

Fig. 2.1. Formation of the neural tube (schematic representation). *(a)* The neural plate is formed by thickening of the ectoderm under induction from the notochord. *(b)* The neural groove appears. The anlagen of the neural crest are visible. *(c)* The neural crest is well formed and its cells will migrate laterally to their targets. *(d)* Closure of the neural tube begins in the central region; the extremities (anterior and posterior neuropores) will close later. Closure allows the tube to be covered by ectoderm and mesenchymal tissue.

the future rhombencephalon, mesencephalon, prosencephalon and otic placodes become apparent at its anterior part. Simultaneously, clusters of cells along the lateral margins of the neural tube separate to form the paired *neural crests* that will give rise to major structures of the peripheral nervous system, meninges, melanocytes and face.

The posterior part of the neural plate and notocord has a different fate: it forms a mass of cells that will canalize and undergo the process of regressive differentation to form the lower spinal cord.

By 32–33 days, the prosencephalon has formed the telencephalic vesicles and the diencephalon has differentiated, so that four identifiable cellular masses are present by 8 weeks, in the region of the basal ganglia. The process of vesicle formation probably results from *ventral induction* by the notocord, but intimate mechanisms of induction are not fully understood.

From about 30 days, the major inductive processes are completed and cellular differentiation begins. Multiplication of primitive cells that are going to form both neurons and glia occurs, mostly in the vicinity of the lumen of the neural tube in the ventricular and, to a lesser extent, the subventricular zone. Mitoses take place in the deeper cellular layers (Caviness et al. 2003). Division of the cells is asymmetrical: one daughter cell migrates toward the outside during telophase, then comes back to the deep region to initiate another cycle; the so-called *intrakinetic migration* remains in the ventricular zone. The other cell leaves the ventricular zone to initiate its journey towards the cortical plate. Proliferation of neuroblasts reaches its greater rate at 15 weeks gestation and then decreases to essentially stop by 20 weeks. Proliferation exceeds the ultimate requirements so that it is intimately related to the poorly understood process of *programmed cell death by apoptosis*. The activity of the apoptotic process increases at the same time as proliferation diminishes. The actual proportion of dying cells in humans is not precisely known. It seems to be variable depending on location and might in some regions affect as many as 30–50% of the cells formed.

Corticogenesis has been particularly studied over the past two decades. In the late embryonic period (45–50 days gestation), primitive corticopetal fibres arrive via the diencephalic sulcus and expand under the telencephalic pia; neurons appear within these fibres to form the primordial plexiform layer (PPL) (Bentivoglio et al. 2003) or preplate. The PPL precedes the *migration of neurons that form the cortical plate* and serves as scaffolding for subsequently migrating cells. The migrating neurons split the cortical zone into a superficial part that will constitute the molecular layer or layer I formed mostly of Cajal–Retzius cells and their processes (Sarnat and Flores-Sarnat 2002, Rakic and Zecevic 2003) and a deep layer termed the *subplate* (or layer VII) that disappears before the end of intrauterine life. Cajal–Retzius cells play an important role in the ultimate fate of pyramidal cells, probably by secreting reelin (Crino 2001, Assadi et al. 2003). The majority of them disappear by apoptosis before 1 year of age. Subplate neurons act as a relay for corticopetal thalamic axons before cells of the cortical fourth layer are functional. Later migrating cells, that will form layers II to VI of the definitive cortex, migrate in

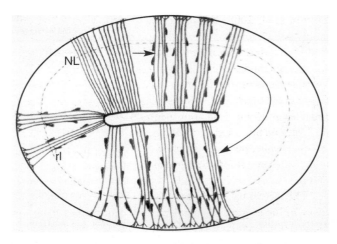

Fig. 2.2. Schematic representation of neuronal migration along radial glial guides. Transverse section of neural tube. (Courtesy Prof. P Evrard, Cliniques Saint-Luc, Brussels.)

NL: Embryonic stage—regularly aligned glial guides. *First arrow:* migration of neurons destined to deep cortical layers along glial guides now grouped in fascicles. *Curved arrow:* late stages of neuronal migration (layers II and III). Progressive defasciculation of glial guides.

rl: Situation in the reeler mutant mouse in which no defasciculation takes place.

an 'inside out' manner, that is to say the most recently generated late-migrating cells form the most superficial layer (layer II) of the cortical plate, whereas large pyramidal cells of layers V and VI migrate early.

Most neurons destined for the cerebral cortex migrate between the 10th and 18th gestational weeks, and the full complement of cortical neurons is essentially completed by 20 weeks. However, cellular migration continues at a slower pace throughout pregnancy, and some cells, e.g. cerebellar and hippocampal granules, migrate postnatally (Sarnat 1987). Some cortical neurogenesis persists througout life especially in the mesial temporal lobe and the cerebellum (Gage 2002).

Neuronal migration is a complex process that differs depending on neuron types. *Radial migration* involves a majority (probably 75%) of precursor cells destined to become pyramidal neurons. These migrate radially along glial guides that extend from the ventricular (proliferative) zone to the pial surface of the neural tube and derived structures (Rakic 1981, Williams and Caviness 1984) (Fig. 2.2). Glial guides are later converted into astrocytes, thus marking the end of radial migration. Several cells use the same glial fibre in their migration, which may be responsible for the columnar organization of the cortex universally found in mammals (Rockel et al. 1980), the column representing the functional units of the cortex. These functional units in different species differ by their numbers rather than by their basic organization. Not all neurons follow faithfully a particular glial guide. Other precursor cells destined to become interneurons leave their guide to migrate in a perpendicular direction (Walsh 1995, Caviness et al. 2003) and a few may move to a neighbouring guide. Some cells originate in the ganglionic eminences in the basal forebrain and migrate tangentially (Jimenez et al. 2002,

Bystron et al. 2005, Kanatani et al. 2005). They follow still poorly known routes, possibly along axonal fasciculi, to the cortical plate. Most appear to be interneurons, mostly gabaergic, whereas pyramidal (glutamatergic) cells migrate radially. These multiple routes may explain how multiple postmigratory neurons from a single clonal origin disperse over wide cortical areas (Walsh and Cepko 1993). Migrating neuroblasts are guided to their final location by a series of signalling systems, especially biochemical ones, which are under the control of multiple genes, currently under intensive study (Sarnat and Flores-Sarnat 2002, Crino 2004).

The second half of gestation is characterized by a rapid increase in the length and complexity of dendrites and axons, by the establishment of synapses, and by maturation and fine organization of the cortex. The result is a rapid increase in weight of the brain and the process of sulcation necessary to accomodate the massively increasing surface area of the cortex. Secondary and tertiary sulci appear between the 7th and 9th months of gestation, and most gyri are present by 28 weeks. The full laminar structure of the cortex is complete by birth. Reduction of the number and density of synapses resulting from development of neuronal processes and from programmed cell death by apoptosis also plays a major role in giving its final shape to the central nervous system. Dendrites, axons and synapses develop at a tremendous rate, and many of the synapses then formed will eventually disappear. Development of dendrites, axonal arborizations and dendritic spines continues until the fourth year of life. *Glial development* is a complex process, various precursors having different fates. Some develop into radiating glial fibres used by migrating neurons. Many astrocytes are produced by the persisting periventricular proliferative zone after the end of neuronal migration (Gressens et al. 1992). Myelin begins to be deposited at about 30 weeks but most of the process of myelin formation is postnatal (Yakovlev and Lecours 1967, Brody et al. 1987).

DISTURBANCES OF NORMAL DEVELOPMENT

As expected from the complexity of the processes involved, there is an almost infinite variety of abnormalities of CNS development. I will consider successively disorders of neurulation and caudal tube formation (blastopathies), disorders of ventral induction, and those of cortical development (corticogenesis).

DISORDERS OF NEURULATION AND CAUDAL NEURAL TUBE FORMATION (BLASTOPATHIES)

Disorders of neurulation and caudal neural tube formation include all forms of failure of the neural tube to close completely, with secondary abnormal development of the mesenchymal structures enclosing the CNS, from anencephaly to sacral myelomeningocele and sacral agenesis. In the absence of tube closure, the posterior mesenchyme does not develop so that there is no bony structure covering the neuroectoderm. The basic anomaly may be nondisjunction of the neural gutter from overlying epithelium, resulting in myelomeningocele or dermal sinus.

Premature disjunction could be responsible for lipomyelocele or juxtamedullary or subpial lipoma. This in turn could result from a defect in the cell adhesion molecules. Other mechanisms include abnormal canalization or regression of the caudal end of the cord resulting in abnormalities of the filum and abnormal splitting of the notochord responsible for spinal–enteric cysts and diastematomyelia.

The term *dysraphism* indicates, in its complete form, persistent continuity between posterior neuroectoderm and cutaneous ectoderm. Dysraphism comprises several varieties. Cranial dysraphism includes *anencephaly* and *cephaloceles*. Spinal dysraphism designates *spina bifida cystica* and *occulta*, with several subtypes. The basic mechanism appears to be a lack of closure of the neural tube, perhaps related to a defect in the cell adhesion molecules, rather than secondary reopening or rupture of the neural tube.

The causes of dysraphism remain obscure. They seem to be sufficiently similar to allow all types to be considered together even though there may be some differences (for example the recurrence risks may not be equal for spina aperta, anencephaly or cephaloceles). Genetic factors are important. Usually they fit in with a polygenic or multifactorial model, but a small minority (<10%) may follow a mendelian type of inheritance with recessive and even X-linked transmission (Baraitser and Burn 1984). Environmental factors have been repeatedly stressed although the search for specific agents has been disappointing. Young maternal age and low socioeconomic level seem to play a part. The role of vitamin deficiency – especially *folic acid*, initially proposed by Smithells et al. (1981) – has been demonstrated (Green 2002, Yerbi 2003), and a reduction of up to 70% of the incidence of spina bifida can be obtained (Mitchell et al. 2004) with the administration of multivitamin and/or folic acid preparations starting from the very onset of pregnancy. This may also be beneficial for other, non-neural tube, malformations (Botto et al. 2004). A common polymorphism of the gene that codes for methylene tetrahydrofolate reductase may significantly increase the risk of neural tube defect (Volcik et al. 2003). It has been confirmed that administration of multiple vitamin supplements containing folic acid sharply reduces – by up to 72% (Berry et al. 1999) – the incidence of neural tube defects if commenced at least 28 days before conception and continued for the first two months of pregnancy (MRC Study Research Group 1991, Czeizel and Dudás 1992). Systematic administration of folic acid (4 mg/day) is strongly recommended (Yerby 2003). Unfortunately, more than half of pregnancies are unplanned so the actual efficacy in population studies is much lower (Ray et al. 2002, Ward et al. 2004). This has led in several countries to fortification of cereal foods with folic acid (Olney and Mulinare 2002, Mitchell et al. 2004).

Maternal fever (Finnell et al. 1993), drugs (Lindhout and Schmidt 1986), other chemicals and X-irradiation have also been incriminated. Valproic acid has been implicated. Valproate and valproic acid are associated with spina bifida in up to 1–2% of pregnancies in women on the drug. Thus it is preferable to use another agent if treatment cannot be discontinued.

The empirical risks of recurrence for untreated mothers who have given birth to a child with neural tube defects vary between

1.5% and 5%. The risk is about 6% for women with two children with spina bifida. For anencephaly the risk may be higher, up to 10% of siblings of anencephalics having neural tube defects of various types. The transmission of anencephaly appears to be matrilineal, and the recurrence rate for maternal half-siblings is the same as for full siblings.

The *incidence* of neural tube defects is widely variable in different parts of the world, being low in Japan and reaching 3% in the British Isles (Luciano 1987). The incidence is 10 times higher in early abortuses (Botto et al. 2005) and 24 times higher in stillborn infants (Wiswell et al. 1990). Secular changes in occurrence have long been known (Stone 1987, Botto et al. 2005). Anencephaly is 3–7 times more frequent in girls than in boys, but the sex ratio is about equal in low spina bifida (Seller 1987). Currently, there is a sharp decrease in the frequency of neural tube defects in Western countries, which is due in part to, but may not be entirely explained by, the practice of prenatal diagnosis followed by termination.

The respective frequencies of the various types are variable and with the practice of termination are difficult to assess. Stoll et al. (1988) in eastern France found an incidence of of 0.62 per 1000 for spina bifida, 0.33 per 1000 for anencephaly, and 0.14 per 1000 for cephaloceles.

Prenatal diagnosis of the open forms of neural tube defect is possible by ultrasonography and by determination of alpha-fetoprotein (AFP) in the amniotic fluid obtained by amniocentesis (Botto et al. 1999, 2005). AFP represents 90% of total serum globulins in the fetus. With open tube defects, it leaks into the amniotic fluid and hence into maternal blood. Determination of AFP levels in amniotic fluid obtained by amniocentesis at 16–18 weeks gestational age permits detection of over 99% of fetuses with neural tube defects. False positives are often, but not always, associated with other severe fetal abnormalities. They can be avoided by simultaneous determination of acetylcholinesterase.

AFP levels in maternal serum at 13–16 weeks gestation are used as a screening test for neural tube defects, and the routine determination of AFP is recommended, the more so as it is also used in the 'triple or quadruple test' for the detection of Down syndrome. Normal adult levels are below 10 ng/mL and increase during pregnancy up to 500 ng/mL. Levels greater than 1000 ng/mL at 15–20 weeks gestational age are highly suggestive of neural tube defect. However, there is a high incidence of false positives, and even the finding of two abnormal levels of AFP without a 'benign' explanation (e.g. multiple pregnancy, wrong dates) is associated with a benign outcome of pregnancy in 40% of instances, and only 10% of such fetuses have a neural tube defect. On the other hand, false negatives are also known to occur so the value is not absolute.

Ultrasonography is used as a routine procedure for the detection of fetal malformations. It permits detection of over 98% of cases of anencephaly from the age of about 12–14 weeks. For spina bifida (Fig. 2.3), similar figures are reached in the best hands at 16–20 weeks but qualified personnel and adequate material are not available everywhere (Govaert and de Vries 1997). Careful search for a deformity of the frontal bone ('lemon sign')

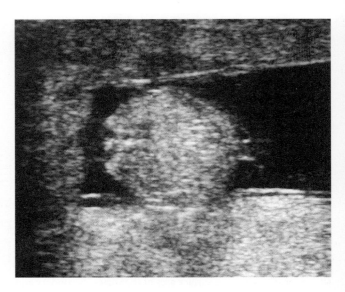

Fig. 2.3. Spina bifida aperta (antenatal diagnosis at 18 weeks of amenorrhoea). Axial cut showing absence of neurulation of neural plate *(left side of photograph)*, which is denser than rest of fetal body and limited on both sides by a well-defined ridge. (Courtesy Dr M-C Aubry, Maternité Port-Royal, Paris.)

and of cerebellar compression due to the associated Chiari malformation ('banana sign') helps considerably to make a correct diagnosis (Van den Hof et al. 1990). False positive results occur uncommonly (Chard and Macintosh 1992). Antenatal diagnosis of cephaloceles and meningoceles is relatively easy. Currently, ultrasonography is the best tool for antenatal diagnosis of neural tube defects if performed by a well-trained operator as it is reliable and non-invasive. If no certainty is gained, amniocentesis with AFP and acetylcholinesterase determination should be performed. In addition, any examination of amniotic fluid taken for another indication should include AFP determination. Many investigators think that amniocentesis can be avoided if a good ultrasonogram can be obtained but others are reluctant to abandon it completely.

CRANIAL DYSRAPHISM
This heading includes anencephaly and cephaloceles/encephaloceles.

Anencephaly
Anencephaly is a lethal condition that is progressively disappearing from most developed countries because its early antenatal diagnosis is easy. Anencephaly results from failure of the cephalic folds to fuse into a neural tube with resulting degeneration of the neural cells and absence of mesodermal tissue dorsal to the neural elements so that the bony skull does not develop. Partial forms with preservation of some telencephalic structures may be due to the fact that there are multiple sites of anterior neuropore closure (Golden and Chernoff 1995). Marin-Padilla (1991) proposed that the primary defect is in the segmental division of the anterior part of the embryo, with resultant hypoplasia of the sphenoid bone. This could produce secondary skull bone abnormalities variably resulting in absence of formation of the skull vault or,

in less severe cases, in a hypoplastic posterior fossa. In this view, CNS abnormalities are secondary: the defective skull results in failure of tube formation because of the wide gap between the lips of the neural gutter. Exposure then leads to secondary destruction of the brain.

The spinal cord, brainstem and cerebellum are present, and part of the diencephalon may also be preserved. Failure of fusion of vertebrae (rachischisis) and herniation of cerebral tissue (exencephaly) are frequently associated. There may be evidence of secondary degeneration of some previously formed structures.

Automatisms of suction and Moro reflexes are usually present, and some infants exhibit seizures that may be similar to infantile spasms. Anencephalic infants usually die in a few hours to weeks. The anterior hypophysis of anencephalic infants is ectopic or absent. The syndrome of panhypopituitarism with microphthalmia is probably related to anencephaly (Kaplowitz and Bodurtha 1993).

Atelencephaly differs from anencephaly by the presence of a normally formed skull. There is no organized neural structure above the diencephalic level, the telencephalon being reduced to a small mass of anarchically disposed neurons and glial cells. Surprisingly, such atelencephalic brains can occasionally produce typical epileptic EEG discharges, recordable from the scalp (Danner et al. 1985), a phenomenon also observed in cases of hydranencephaly. Accessory brains are a rare anomaly that may present with prenatal mass lesions (Harris et al. 1994a). *Aprosencephaly* is a more severe variant in which diencephalic structures are not preserved (Harris et al. 1994b).

Encephaloceles or cephaloceles and cranium bifidum

These abnormalities satisfy the criteria for dysraphism, i.e. a mesenchymal defect with herniation of dura, cerebral or cerebellar tissue or ventricles is apparent. Although anterior cephaloceles may be more closely related to disorders of ventral rather than dorsal induction (see below), they are considered here for convenience. Cephaloceles are frequently associated with other malformations such as agenesis of the corpus callosum or abnormal gyration (Martinez-Lage et al. 1996). *Cephaloceles* are 3–16 times less common than spina bifida cystica (Olney and Mulinare 2002, Siffel et al. 2003). In Western countries, 85% of cephaloceles are posteriorly located (Fig. 2.4), whereas in Asia anterior cephaloceles are more common. Isolated *cranium bifidum*, which is a simple skull defect without prolapse of meninges or brain, is rare and clinically insignificant. Atretic cephaloceles are regarded as formes frustes of meningoencephaloceles. They commonly occur in the parietal and occipital regions (Yokota et al. 1988) and may present as a large posterior fontanelle. They may occur in the Walker–Warburg, Meckel–Gruber and Joubert syndromes. Most cephaloceles contain some brain tissue (encephaloceles). Cranial meningoceles contain only meninges and CSF without neural tissue.

Cranial meningoceles are less common than cephaloceles. Small posterior meningoencephaloceles are usually covered by a normal scalp. Larger ones may be covered by abnormal skin with angiomas or by a thin membrane. The presence of a hair collar

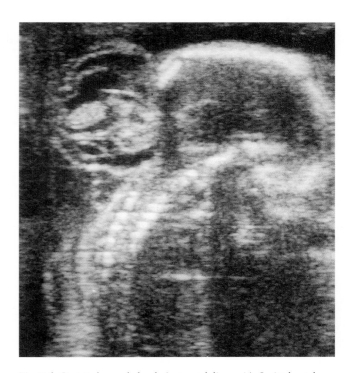

Fig. 2.4. Occipital encephalocele (antenatal diagnosis). Sagittal cut showing normal cranial vault anteriorly *(right side of photograph)* and large encephalocele protruding posteriorly with content of mixed echodensity *(left side)*. (Courtesy Dr M-C Aubry, Maternité Port-Royal, Paris.)

may be a marker of cranial dysraphism. They are genetically related to other neural tube defects. Some forms are part of mendelian syndromes (Table 2.2).

Posterior cephaloceles may contain infratentorial or supratentorial brain structures or both (Siffel et al. 2003, Tubbs et al. 2003b). The bony defect may be of any size and is located above or below the tentorium. Cerebellar ectopia may be associated – the *Chiari III malformation* (see Table 2.3). Of 147 occipital cephaloceles studied by Lorber and Schofield (1979), only 25% were pure meningoceles; hydrocephalus was present in half the cases, and 16% had other anomalies, in particular agenesis of the corpus callosum. Parietal cephaloceles are much rarer and even more frequently associated with other malformations. Posterior cephaloceles seem to result from dysraphism in most cases. However, postinductional occurrence is possible.

Subtorcular occipital cephaloceles are usually associated with severe cerebellar developmental defects (Chapman et al. 1989).

The prognosis of posterior cephaloceles is poor (Brown and Sheridan-Pereira 1992). In the series of Lorber and Schofield (1979), 90% of infants died and 50% of survivors were retarded. Fifty per cent of operated infants survived but two thirds of them remained disabled. Hydrocephalus was present in over half the cases.

Anterior cephaloceles include several types: sphenoidal, protruding through the body of the sphenoid; and fronto-ethmoidal, subdivided into nasoethmoidal, nasofrontal, nasoorbital, interfrontal and posterior orbital types (Mahapatra and Agrawal 2006). They are sometimes associated with supratentorial defects

TABLE 2.2
Main syndromes with encephalocele

Syndrome	Main features	Inheritance*	References
Meckel–Gruber syndrome	See text	AR (at least 3 different loci)	Gazioglu et al. (1998), Morgan et al. (2002), Chao et al. (2005)
Dandy–Walker syndrome	See text	Sporadic (rare familial cases)	Hirsch et al. (1984), Pascual-Castroviejo et al. (1991), Klein et al. (2003)
Walker–Warburg syndrome	See text	?	Yamaguchi et al. (1993), Parisi and Dobyns (2003)
Joubert syndrome	See text	AR (at least 3 different loci)	Edwards et al. (1988), Valente et al. (2005)
Goldenhar–Gorlin syndrome	Orofacial abnormalities, preauricular tags, epibulbar dermoids	Sporadic	Aleksic et al. (1983)
Tectocerebellar dysraphia with occipital cephalocele	Inverted cerebellum, hypoplastic vermis, mental retardation	Sporadic	Hori (1994), Dehdashti et al. (2004)
Occipital cephalocele, myopia and retinal dysplasia (Knobloch syndrome)		AR (at least 2 different loci)	Menzel et al. (2004)
Chromosomal syndromes, in particular trisomy 13	Chapter 4	?	See Chapter 4
Median cleft face syndrome	Anterior cephalocele	?	Naidich et al. (1990)
Roberts syndrome	Anterior cephalocele in some cases	AR	Freeman et al. (1974)
Syndrome of cranial and limb defects secondary to aberrant tissue bands; amniotic bands syndrome		Sporadic	Urich and Herrick (1985), Moerman et al. (1992)

*AR = autosomal recessive.

such as callosal agenesis. Their overall prognosis is considerably better than that of the posterior anomalies. There is no increased risk of recurrence in siblings. They are usually revealed easily at birth by the presence of a visible deformity, especially in the naso-frontal and interfrontal types. Sphenoidal cephaloceles produce pharyngeal obstruction in association with hypertelorism and/or labial fissure and with optic nerve abnormalities (coloboma or optic atrophy). An endocrinological syndrome of deficit in somato-trophin, gonadotrophin or antidiuretic hormone secretion is noted in half the cases. Recurrent meningitis has been observed (Izquierdo and Gil-Carcedo 1988). Diagnosis is suggested by ex-amination of the pharynx and is confirmed by skull X-rays and CT showing herniation of the third ventricle. Surgery is indicated. Basal cephaloceles (Morioka et al. 1995) may be associated with optic disc anomalies and hormonal disturbances.

Nasofrontal cephaloceles produce nasal obstruction and, rarely, CSF leakage. They may be detected only after 2 years of age. Their prognosis depends on the nature of the content. The so-called nasal glioma (Younus and Coode 1986) is a small nasal cephalo-cele that has become separated from the base of the brain.

Lipomas of the corpus callosum may have an anterosuperior extension that represents a mild form of cephalocele protruding in the region of the bregma. They should be distinguished from angiomas and dermoid cysts of the anterior fontanelle, melan-

otic progonoma and ectopic brain tissue. Dermoid cysts of the anterior fontanelle can be adherent to the sagittal sinus, and great care should be exercised in their exeresis (Chapter 13).

Anterobasal temporal cephaloceles extending into the pterygo-palatine fossa through a bony defect at the base of the greater wing of the sphenoid may be responsible for resistant epilepsy (Leblanc et al. 1991). They are often associated with ocular abnormalities (Morioka et al. 1995) and may produce CSF otorrhoea and re-current meningitis.

Cephaloceles are uncommonly part of a *defined syndrome* (Friede 1989), although they are frequently associated with other birth defects: cleft palate, microphthalmia, holoprosencephaly, agenesis of the corpus callosum and cerebellar defects. The most common of the many syndromes that include cephalocele as a necessary or prominent feature are listed in Table 2.2. *Meckel–Gruber syndrome* is the most frequent of these (Gazioglu et al. 1998). It consists of polydactyly, polycystic kidneys, retinal dys-plasia and hydrocephalus, in addition to the CNS features: prosen-cephalic dysgenesis, occipital cephalocele and rhombic roof dysgenesis (Ahdab-Barmada and Claassen 1990). The clinical ex-pression of this autosomal recessive syndrome is variable even within the same sibship, and cases may be wrongly diagnosed as Dandy–Walker syndrome or congenital hydrocephalus when the expression is incomplete. There is a good ceorrelation between imaging and pathological data (Chao et al. 2005). At least three genes (*MKS1–3*) can be responsible (Morgan et al. 2002), and prenatal diagnosis by sonography is possible from 12–13 weeks (Mittermayer et al. 2004).

The *treatment* of cephaloceles is surgical. Surgery is sometimes indicated on an emergency basis when there is leakage of CSF. In other cases it is elective. The results depend on the volume of brain tissue contained in the cephalocele and on associated malformations (Brown and Sheridan-Pereira 1992).

SPINAL DYSRAPHISM

The term 'spinal dysraphism' applies to a heterogeneous group of spinal abnormalities with the common feature of imperfect formation of the midline mesenchymal, bony and neural structures. Despite its decreasing incidence, it remains a frequent problem thought to affect 300,000 persons worldwide. In almost all cases spinal dysraphism manifests as spina bifida in which there is dysraphism of the osseous structures resulting in incomplete closure of the spinal canal. Some investigators have argued that secondary rupture, rather than absence of closure, is the cause in some cases.

Spina bifida cystica

Spina bifida cystica (Fig. 2.5) is the commonest type of spinal dysraphism and includes *myeloschisis*, *myelomeningocele* and *meningocele*. Except in the last of these, nervous structures are exposed without skin covering. In spina bifida occulta the neural elements are covered by skin and do not protrude above the level of the back.

Myelomeningocele and myeloschisis, which constitute 95% of the cases of overt spinal dysraphism, are basically identical, but differ by the fact that myeloschisis is flat while myelomeningocele is bulging. In both cases, there is no mesenchyme behind the spinal cord, which has remained flat with a median groove corresponding to the open ependymal canal. The skin is in direct continuity with the meninges that attach to the lateral limits of the plate (Botto et al. 1999). Variable abnormalities are associated. Diastematomyelia is present in 31–46% of instances, the slit being cephalic to the cele in 31%, at the level of the cele in 22% and caudal to it in 25% of cases. In rare patients, the cele is located to one hemicord or involves the two hemicords at different levels, producing very asymmetrical clinical findings.

Hydrosyringomyelia is present in 33–75% of cases and is often associated with severe scoliosis. Hydrocephalus occurs in 90% of cases and frequently has a prenatal onset (Girard et al. 2003, Biggio et al. 2004, Wyldes and Watkinson 2004).

Hydromyelia typically distends the entire length of the spinal canal from the obex down the central canal to the upper pole of the neural plate. CSF may remain within the central canal or penetrate into the spinal cord, so the distinction between syringomyelia and hydromyelia is somewhat artificial (Breningstall et al. 1992). In all cases, the cord is stuck in a low position. The meninges are extremely thin and rupture easily with a resulting high risk of infection. In cases left untreated, epithelialization takes place over the meningeal membrane and neural plate. The

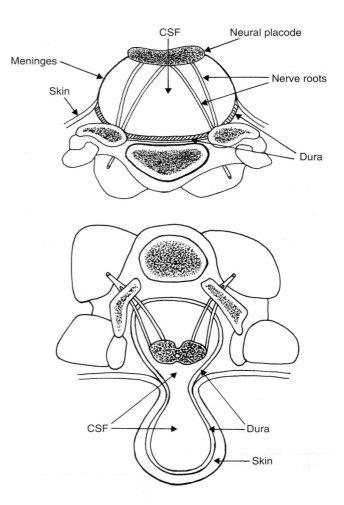

Fig. 2.5. *(Top)* Myelomeningocele. The neural placode has not undergone neurulation and is in direct continuity with the rest of the dorsal ectoderm. A thin membrane, representing the leptomeninx and easily torn open, connects the placode to the skin. Note the absence of the posterior arch of vertebra and of any form of mesenchymal derivate behind the neural tissue.

(Bottom) Meningocele. The spinal cord is completely formed. The meninges are covered with skin. In some cases, the neural roots may have an abnormal course and enter the meningocele before exiting from the spinal canal which remains uncovered with mesenchyma behind the neural tissue.

process may leave scarring, with a fibrous band kinking and compressing the cord. In some cases, epidermoid or dermoid cysts result from skin cell inclusion in the scar, often associated with small lipomas detectable by MRI better than by CT. Segmental infarction of the cord may occur. Myeloceles are lumbar or thoracolumbar in more than half the cases, and lumbosacral in over 25%. Cervical and thoracic locations together account for around 11% of cases (Matson 1969).

Cranial anomalies are often associated with myelomeningoceles, especially Chiari II malformation, which is present in 70% of cases (Table 2.3).

Chiari I malformation (Fig. 2.6a), on the other hand, is not associated with spina bifida and is uncommonly symptomatic during childhood (Tubbs et al. 2003a). It may be associated with

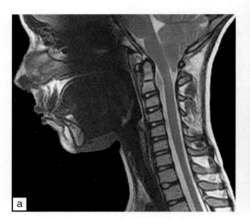
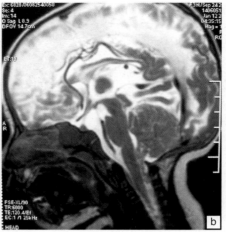

Fig. 2.6. (a) Chiari I malformation. Dorsal extension of cerebellar tonsils below the level of the foramen magnum. The lowermost part of the cerebellar tonsils enters the spinal canal below the level of the occipital bone.

(b) Chiari II malformation. Cerebellar tissue going down in the spinal canal as far as the second cervical vertebra. Note elongation of brainstem and enlarged interthalamic commissure.

TABLE 2.3
Chiari (Cleland–Chiari, Arnold–Chiari) malformations

Type	Main features	Associated anomalies	Neurological features	References
Type I[1]	Downward displacement of lower cerebellum, especially tonsils, elongated 4th ventricle and lower brainstem, in the absence of intracranial space-occupying lesion	Platybasia, basilar impression, syringomyelia (20% of cases), hydrocephalus (40% of cases), no spina bifida or myelomeningocele	Mainly adolescents and adults. Features related to hydrocephalus or syringomyelia. Cervical compression with quadriplegia, apnoea, headaches possible even in young children (Itoh *et al.* 1988); rarely familial (Stovner *et al.* 1992)	Itoh *et al.* (1988), Tan *et al.* (1995), Tubbs et al. (2003a,b)
Type II	Downward displacement of cerebellar vermis or tonsils along the dorsal aspect of cervical spinal cord. Kinking of posterior aspect of spinal cord at level of C2–C3 vertebrae	Myelomeningocele in over 95% of cases. Posterior fossa and midbrain abnormalities, aqueductal stenosis, meningeal anomalies (see text). Abnormal cortical gyration[2]	Manifest from newborn period by signs related to hydrocephalus and myelomeningocele. Dysfunction of lower cranial nerves, respiration and swallowing. Paralysis of upper limbs due to cervical compression	Friede (1989), McLone and Dias (2003), Stevenson (2004)
Type III	Downward displacement of cerebellum into a posterior cephalocele with elongation and herniation of 4th ventricle	Cervical spina bifida or posterior cranium bifidum or both	Manifest from newborn period. Analogous to type II	Friede (1989)
Type IV	Cerebellar hypoplasia[3]	See text	See text	Friede (1989)

[1]Chronic tonsillar herniation (Friede 1989, Cama *et al.* 1995) secondary to hydrocephalus is difficult to separate completely from Chiari 1 deformity. Friede requires that cerebellar herniation is associated with one other component, *e.g.* elongated medulla. With or without brainstem elongation, quadriplegia or even sudden death following minor trauma may occur.
[2]Crowding of convolutions without architectonic abnormality.
[3]Although included in Chiari's original description, not a part of the Chiari deformity as understood now.

malformations of the base of the skull and upper cervical spine (Chapter 5), and with syringomyelia in about half the cases. The diagnosis can be made by ultrasonography (Govaert and de Vries 1997), but is determined more precisely by MRI, which shows the low position and elongation of the lower brainstem (Mikulis et al. 1992). Symptoms may result from medullary compression and be precipitated by trauma. They variably include headache, dysfunction of the lower cranial nerves, cerebellar signs, and pain in the neck and occipital region. Somnolence and episodes of apnoea are sometimes observed (Keefover et al. 1995, Yglesias et al. 1996). Treatment for symptomatic cases is by surgical de-

compression of the posterior fossa and gives satisfactory results (Navarro et al. 2004, Schijman and Steinbok 2004).

Chiari II malformation (Fig. 2.6b) is the most common variant of the Cleland–Chiari malformation (Cama et al. 1995, Stevenson 2004). It consists of partial dislocation of medulla and cerebellum, especially the vermis, into the cervical canal, overriding the upper spinal cord. The dorsal aspect of the medulla forms a kink at the bulbospinal junction. Cerebellar tissue may descend as far down as C3 level. The fourth ventricle is elongated and partially herniated into the cervical canal. There is often a defect in the posterior arch of the atlas, and a fibrous band is often

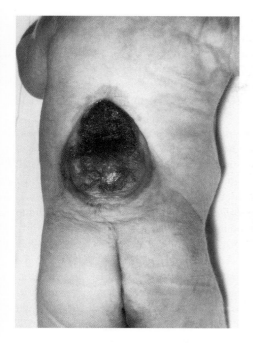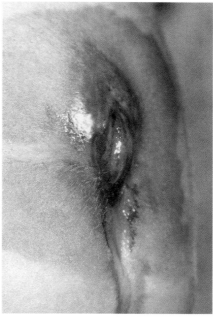

Fig. 2.7. Myelomeningoceles. *(Far left)* Dorso-lumbar lesion, associated with paraplegia and hydrocephalus. *(Left)* Lumbosacral lesion, clearly showing the non-neurulated cord. (Courtesy Dr F Renault, Hôpital Trousseau, Paris.)

present at the level of the foramen magnum and may compress the medulla. The posterior fossa is small, with scalloping and erosion of the posteromedial part of the petrous pyramids. The so-called lacunar skull (Luckenschädel) is present in up to 85% of cases with Chiari II malformation. It does not necessarily predict a low intelligence. The brainstem is elongated and the colliculi are fused and beaked. The cerebellar hemispheres may develop anteriorly, surrounding the brainstem. There is a large massa intermedia and, not infrequently, heterotopias of hemispheral grey matter. A microgyric appearance of the cortex is often reported, but microscopic examination indicates a normal cortical architecture, so the appearance is due to mechanical factors rather than a true malformation. The falx cerebri and tentorium are hypoplastic. Extradural malformations of the duodenum, heart and oesophagus may accompany the neural deformity. The Chiari II malformation is associated with hydrocephalus in over 90% of cases. In reported series, hydrocephalus was due to aqueductal stenosis in 30–73% of cases. Its cause was unclear in the remaining cases, although occlusion of the foramen of Magendie may be responsible. An imbalance between CSF production and resorption is another possible mechanism. The choroid plexuses may be hypertrophic. Exceptionally, massive plexus hypertrophy can cause isolation of a lateral ventricle with consequent localized hydrocephalus (Chadduck and Glasier 1989). Ventricular dilatation is present from birth in 50–75% of infants, suggesting that the apparent development of hydrocephalus following repair of myelomeningocele is probably not causally related to operation.

The mechanism of Chiari II malformation is unknown. Downward traction by the tethered spinal cord is no longer an accepted theory. The main factor is thought to be leakage of CSF during pregnancy (Boltshauser 2004), the resulting hydrostatic dysequilibrium leading to descent of the posterior fossa structures into the upper spinal canal. Descent of posterior fossa structures occurs only in late pregnancy, suggesting that intrauterine surgery might prevent it. Marin-Padilla (1991) believes that the primary defect is in the development of the mesenchyma of cephalic somites with hypoplasia of the basisphenoid resulting in a small posterior fossa.

The various abnormalities that accompany Chiari II deformity can be well demonstrated by CT and even better by MRI. A complete imaging study of the spinal lesion (Altman and Altman 1987, Davis et al. 1988) is not necessary before primary repair, except when markedly asymmetrical signs are found. It is mandatory when reoperation on a previously treated patient is contemplated or when secondary deterioration occurs. MRI precisely indicates the relationship between the skin and the neural plate, root position, and intrinsic cord pathology such as diastematomyelia or hydromyelia.

• *Clinical features and complications of spina bifida cystica.* At birth the appearance of the defect is that of a sac-like structure covered by a thin membrane that is often ruptured, with CSF leak. The surrounding skin is often angiomatous (Fig. 2.7). Older unrepaired lesions are partially epithelialized. The neurological manifestations of myelomeningocele include: (1) the direct consequences of the spinal malformation; (2) those of hydrocephalus and hindbrain anomalies; and (3) those of associated neural and extraneural abnormalities.

The *consequences* of the spinal lesion depend on the level of the myelocele, which in over 80% of cases is located to the lumbosacral area. Children exhibit varying degrees of flaccid, areflexic paralysis and sensory deficits that may be asymmetrical, especially in high lesions. The pattern is usually a mixture of upper and lower motor neuron dysfunction. Motor deficit is often patchy. A sensory level is more constant and permits accurate determination of the upper limit of the lesion. After months and years, wasting, poor cutaneous circulation and trophic changes become prominent. Retractions lead to stiffness and deformities, and poor ossification is associated with fractures that may heal in awkward positions. The sphincter and detrusor functions are compromised in all cases. With lesions above L3 level, there is complete paraplegia. The lower limbs are completely flaccid but straight. Sensory deficits are present distal to the L3 or L4 dermatomes. Ambulation is impossible. In lower lumbar lesions, hip flexors, hip adductors and knee extensors are preserved. Hip dislocation is frequently present from birth, and flexion contracture of the hip results in flexion of the limbs at the hips with extension of the knee. With appropriate treatment, ambulation with aids is often possible. Lesions of the upper sacral roots are compatible with ambulation with minimal or no aids. However, there is variable involvement of the feet, so that most patients have at least some degree of deformity. With sacral lesions lower than S3, the function of the lower extremities is normal but there is saddle anaesthesia and sphincter dysfunction.

Sensory abnormalities may result in trophic changes of the skin, fractures with exuberant callus formation, or arthropathy.

Motor and sensory abnormalities are fixed following the early weeks of life. During the first 48 hours, a rapid deterioration of motor function is often noted, which is probably explained by mechanical trauma to the neural plate during the birth process and/or by exposure. Conversely, rapid improvement may occur following closure. Late postoperative deterioration is not part of the natural history of myelomeningoceles but is suggestive of complications (Hunt 1990). These include constriction of the reconstituted arachnoid tube, tethering of the spinal cord by scarring, hydrosyringomyelia, segmental cord infarction, and cord compression by a cyst or lipoma. In such cases, CT or MRI exploration may shed light on the cause of disturbances and lead to effective treatment.

Sphincter disturbances are of two major types, often coexisting (Fernandes et al. 1994). When the lesion is below S3 level, bladder and anal sphincters are paralysed and there is anaesthaesia of the rectum and lower urinary tract. Dribbling is present in one third of patients: the bladder is distended, with absent detrusor activity on cystometry (Borzyskowsky 1990), and manual expression of urine is easy. In the larger group of higher lesions, detrusor contractions are weak and there is outlet obstruction at the external sphincter as a result of impaired coordination between its activity and that of the detrusor. Bladder sensation is variable. This results in high resting vesical pressure with bladder trabeculation and, eventually, dilatation of the upper urinary tract. Bacteriuria is observed in 50% of 2-year-old children; urinary tract infection leads to chronic pyelonephritis and is the most frequent cause of mortality and morbidity in these patients (Hunt and Whitaker 1987, Borzyskowski 1990).

Hydrocephalus is a major complication of myelomeningocele. Simple nonprogressive ventricular dilatation does not raise great difficulties. Progressive hydrocephalus is often present despite a normal head-growth curve. Normal pressure hydrocephalus may occur in some patients with myelomeningocele and these infants may benefit from shunting procedures. Hydrocephalus is present at birth in 85–95% of cases as shown by ultrasonography. It is not observed with sacral defects. Clinical manifestations of progressive hydrocephalus in myelocele patients usually have no special feature (Chapter 6). Peculiar manifestations, however, may result from involvement of lower cranial nerves, which appears to be due to a combination of brainstem abnormalities and hydrocephalus.

Upper respiratory tract obstruction due to vocal cord paralysis, and *central apnoea* have long been recognized complications of the Chiari II malformation and represent a major cause of death in such patients (Papasozomenos and Roessmann 1981). Other respiratory difficulties can occur and are collectively known as *central ventilatory dysfunction* (CVD). CVD includes, in addition to obstruction of respiratory pathways, increased periodic breathing during sleep (Ward et al. 1986a) and central apnoea (Oren et al. 1986). Some children have a decreased or absent response to hypoxia and hypercapnia (Ward et al. 1986b, Petersen et al. 1995). The incidence of CVD in hydrocephalus patients varies from 5.7% (Hays et al. 1989) to 20% (Kirk et al. 2000). Onset of symptoms is within 1 month of birth in two thirds of cases. In all cases of CVD, hydrocephalus is present. Symptoms may include stridor alone, or stridor associated with cyanotic spells and/or apnoeic episodes. The prognosis is poor: 19 of the 35 patients of Hays et al. died before 30 months of age. CVD may fluctuate and disappear. In several cases correction of shunt dysfunction has alleviated the symptoms of CVD, suggesting that high intracranial pressure with brainstem compression may be a cause (Hays et al. 1989). In some cases, there appears to be a wider pattern of dysfunction of lower cranial nerves, which includes dysphagia, bradycardia, poor head control and weakness of the upper extremities that may be resolved by lowering intracranial pressure.

Such cases of infantile brainstem syndrome require urgent investigation. Sleep-related apnoeas are common. Deray et al. (1995) found abnormal polysomnographic studies in 14 of 16 symptomatic patients. Abnormal polysomnographic studies are frequent. Systematic polygraphic sleep studies should therefore be obtained. Severe abnormalities are associated with additional pathology such as myelomalacia and severe spinal stenosis. Most asymptomatic patients have normal studies and do well without surgery. However, Petersen et al. (1995) concluded that pneumogram and 10% CO_2 challenge did not reliably predict which infants will present symptoms. Taylor et al. (1996) emphasized the value of brainstem evoked potentials, whose abnormalities are well correlated to respiratory problems and neurological sequelae.

Treatment of CVD may require tonsillectomy or tracheostomy, alone or with surgical decompression of the posterior fossa (Navarro et al. 2004). However, current practice is based on clinical anecdotal experience and no first class evidence is so far available (Tubbs and Oakes 2004). Dysphagia alone does not require surgical treatment and is of favourable prognosis.

Another peculiar complication of hydrocephalus due to myelomeningocele is the late appearance of a marked and *evolutive scoliosis with progressive paresis*. Such neurological manifestations should be recognized early because revision of a malfunctioning shunt can improve dramatically the deficits (Hoffman et al. 1987).

Mental retardation is generally a consequence of hydrocephalus, although associated malformations may play a role. The date of shunting, number of shunt revisions and, especially, the occurrence of CNS infections have a major bearing on ultimate intelligence level. Shunted infected patients, especially those with ventriculitis, do significantly less well. Seizures often occur in patients with hydrocephalus due to myelomeningocele (Talwar et al. 1995).

• *Management of spina bifida cystica.* The management of spina bifida cystica raises difficult problems, and no completely satisfactory solution is at hand. Prevention is certainly the best form of therapy. Primary prevention with vitamins and folic acid is efficacious and without danger. Multivitamin preparations containing folic acid are mandatory for pregnant women who have had an affected child, and are probably indicated for all pregnancies (MRC Study Research Group 1991). Prenatal diagnosis is currently the most effective means of preventing the birth of affected infants; screening of maternal serum for AFP, although recommended, is not cost-effective in areas where the incidence of spina bifida is relatively low. For the delivery of affected fetuses, preventive caesarian section is not universally recommended and vaginal delivery remains acceptable.

The *indications for repair* of myelomeningocele have changed over the years. In the 1960s, emergency repair was advocated for all cases. In the '70s, several investigators reported that cases with a very poor prognosis – i.e. high lumbar lesion with marked kyphosis, total flaccid paraplegia and bladder paralysis, major associated defects, and a head circumference at least 2 cm above the 90th centile – fared poorly despite modern techniques (Lorber 1975). Unoperated infants have a 2-year survival rate of 0–4%. Many clinicians are now reluctant to 'select' patients for operation, unless perhaps in extreme cases such as small preterm, feeble infants. Indeed, long-term catastrophes can occur in unoperated infants, and a number of children with several adverse criteria have been able to live productive lives. In fact, operation aims essentially at preserving function rather than life and is currently performed in most cases. Surgery may be performed in the neonatal period or be delayed for up to 3 months. The defect should then be dressed in a sterile way. A prospective study to assess the value of early versus late operation has been launched in the USA (*Lancet* 2004).

Prenatal closure of open defects has been performed in a number of cases in an attempt to improve the functional motor and urological outcome and to reduce the frequency and severity of Chiari II malformation (Walsh and Adzyck 2003, Kaufman 2004, Tulipan 2004, Zambelli et al. 2007). Its efficacy has not been proved and the risks need to be fully assessed. Hydrocephalus requiring shunting is frequent (Bruner et al. 2004). According to one study, the risk of complications of preterm birth in 100 cases was not significantly higher than in control preterm births (Hamdan et al. 2004).

The method of surgical closure is also variable. Current techniques permit better mobility of the cord vis-à-vis the bony and cutaneous coverings. Closure of the defect makes the baby easier to handle, reduces the risk of ascending infection, and may improve motor and sensory function. Secondary tethering of the cord occurs in 10% of patients who develop delayed symptoms, and will require further operation. Delayed closure may be used for large defects (Ersahin and Yurtseven 2004) or for small, feeble infants.

Operation is but the first step in the management of spina bifida (Kaufman 2004). The variety of problems that confront myelomeningocele patients is such that their successful management requires a team of specialists, including paediatric surgeon, paediatrician, urologist, physiotherapist and psychologist (Kaufman 2004). Neurosurgical management following repair includes, in about 90% of cases, *shunting of progressive hydrocephalus* and, occasionally, posterior fossa decompression in case of cervical spinal compression with respiratory difficulties and lower cranial nerve paralyses (see above).

Contracture deformities of the lower limbs demand physiotherapy, bracing, or orthopaedic operations such as muscle transplants or joint arthrodeses. The hips should be carefully monitored as dislocation is a common occurrence.

Urological problems are of paramount importance in the surveillance and treatment of spina bifida patients. The reader is referred to the works of Borzyskowski (1990) and Snodgrass and Adams (2004). Prevention of urinary infections and protection of the kidneys are essential aims. The latter is especially important in the cases of a spastic, irritable bladder with vesicoureteral reflux and may require surgical attention. Urinary continence remains a problem. Appropriate education and monitoring may be effective in a number of cases. The rest will have to use different methods. Bladder expression, if the bladder capacity is sufficient and there is no vesicoureteric reflux, may be effective in a small number of children (Borzyskowski 1990, Kothari et al. 1995). Drug treatment with propantheline bromide or phenyloxybenzamine is of little value, and continuous catheter drainage is variably evaluated. Transurethral resection may have a small place in treatment. Penile appliances in boys and, especially, clean intermittent bladder catheterization are the main techniques for dealing with incontinence. Surgical urinary diversion by various techniques can achieve a high rate of success (Chulamorkodt et al. 2004, Snodgrass and Adams 2004). Infection and dilatation of the upper urinary tract are a major cause of morbidity and mortality in spina bifida patients. Therefore, early and regular monitoring of the urinary tract with urine cultures, intravenous pyelograms and cystograms are an essential part of management. Anal incontinence is less of a problem and can usually be managed successfully with enemas and training. Urodynamic assessment of children with neuropathic bladder (Rickwood 1990) is useful to determine the type of bladder dysfunction and, consequently, the management. Conservative and surgical management has been reviewed in great detail by Borzyskowski (1990) and Stephenson and Mundy (1990).

The prognosis of myelomeningocele remains serious even though many individuals are able to live useful lives.

• *Meningoceles.* Meningoceles share the essential pathological features of myelomeningoceles but the mesenchymal defect is covered with skin and the spinal cord is normal. Herniation through the posterior bone and muscle defect is limited to the meninges. In some cases, roots may run in the wall of the meningocele or cross its cavity. At operation, the surgeon must carefully check any 'fibrous' tract, and the operating microscope and electrical stimulation are essential tools.

Meningoceles are never associated with hydrocephalus. The anatomical distribution is the same as that of myelomeningoceles. Meningoceles are sessile or pedunculated. In the latter cases, the dura and arachnoid tend to fuse at the neck of the sac, and the development of adhesions may partially obliterate the communication that normally exists between the sac and the subarachnoid space (Friede 1989). In pedunculated lesions, the bony defect tends to be limited to one or two posterior arches.

Clinically, meningoceles are marked by protrusion of the skin over a fluctuating mass. Often the skin cover is abnormal and flat angiomas are present. Neurological examination is negative. Meningoceles do not require immediate repair, and elective closure later in childhood is generally preferable.

Ventral meningoceles are much rarer. The main localization is sacral, and the lesions may be of large size and are associated with partial sacral aplasia. Anterior sacral meningoceles may be dominantly inherited (Gardner and Albright 2006). They usually go unnoticed during childhood, although they may provoke rectal compression and chronic constipation (Ashley and Wright 2006). *Currarino syndrome* (Emans et al. 2005) includes a triad of sacral agenesis, anorectal malformations and presacral meningocele and/or other presacral masses such as teratoma. Communication with the CSF is frequent with neurological complications (Cretolle et al. 2006). It is due to dominant mutation in the homeogene *HLXB9* (Merello et al. 2006). Currarino syndrome is one form of the *caudal regression syndrome* (Singh et al. 2005), which is variably expressed by various abnormalities of the distal segments of the spinal cord and lower vertebrae with neurological and sphincter abnormalities. About 1% of the cases are associated with maternal diabetes (Zaw and Stone 2002). The most severe form is *sirenomyelia*. Partial or total sacral agenesis is a more common expression. Wilmshurst et al. (1999) reviewed the clinical and radiological features of 22 cases and detailed the problems of management.

Lateral meningoceles are herniations of an abnormally thin dura through the enlarged lateral foramina. They are seen with neurofibromatosis in association with scalloping of the vertebral bodies (Chapter 3).

Spina bifida occulta (occult spinal dysraphism)
The term 'spina bifida occulta' applies to cases of spinal dysraphism in which there is no herniation of the neural structures or envelopes through the mesenchymal defect (Fig. 2.8). This definition includes the split notochord syndrome, dorsal dermal sinuses, fibrolipomas of the filum terminale and diastematomyelia. Lipomas and lipomyelomeningoceles do not exactly fulfil the criteria for occult dysraphism as they produce definite protrusion of the skin, and the cord lesion is very similar to that of classical

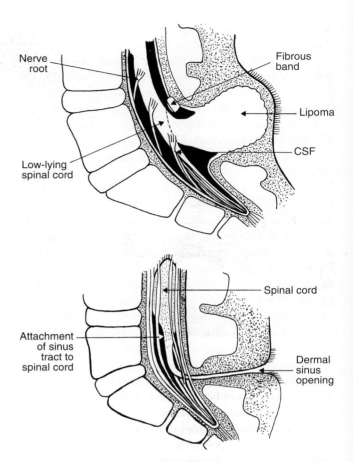

Fig. 2.8. Occult dysraphism. *(Top)* Lipomyelomeningocele. The lipoma is implanted on a low-lying spinal cord which is often incompletely neurulated. The intradural lipoma is in direct continuity with the subcutaneous lipoma. There is a variable degree of meningeal herniation through the bony defect. In most cases the lesion is asymmetrical. *(Bottom)* Congenital dermal sinus. The sinus tract ascends two or more vertebral bodies. It may end on the low-lying spinal cord, as shown here, or in a dermoid cyst.

myelomeningocele. However, they will be described in this section because their clinical symptomatology is not very different from that of other forms of occult dysraphism.

The clinical presentation of spina bifida occulta is variable. Lipomas, lipomeningoceles, diastematomyelia and the tethered cord syndrome share many common features, and their clinical manifestations will be described together. Cutaneous abnormalities such as angiomas, dimples, tags, sinuses or abnormal hairy areas are extremely frequent and suggestive diagnostic cues (Henriques et al. 2005). In all cases, detailed neuroradiological examination is necessary to assess the extent and nature of lesions. Plain X-rays, CT with and without metrizamide and MRI are all used. MRI is the best technique as it permits study in several planes. Sonography of the spine and cord may also be useful although it is less precise (Robinson et al. 2005). Hydrocephalus is not a feature of occult spinal dysraphism. Only rarely is Chiari type II malformation associated with dysraphism (Tubbs and Oakes 2004).

• *The split notochord syndrome.* This syndrome results from splitting of the notochord during embryogenesis with persistent

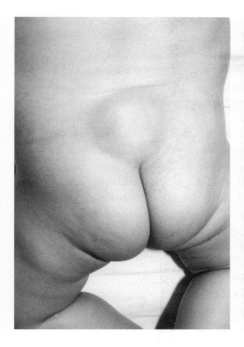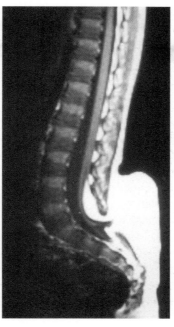

Fig. 2.9. Lipomyelomeningocele. *(Far left)* Skin-covered low-lying lipomatous mass. *(Left)* MRI: the intraspinal mass is in continuity with subcutaneous lipoma. Note low termination of spinal cord on upper pole of lipoma. (Courtesy Dr Kling Chong, Great Ormond Street Hospital, London.)

communication between gut and the dorsal skin. Communication is usually only partial between gut and vertebrae or the spinal cord. The total form (dorsal enteric fistula) is rare. Intraspinal enteric cysts are found mainly in the upper thoracic region. They are lined by digestive epithelium, can produce spinal compression and should be surgically treated (Rebhandl et al. 1998).

• *Dorsal dermal sinuses* are epithelium-lined dermal tubes that course from the skin surface toward the CNS. Many of them terminate on the dura. Others pierce the dura and terminate in an intradural dermoid cyst located two or more vertebrae above the cutaneous orifice (Martinez-Lage et al. 1995, Soto-Ares et al. 2001). Twenty to 30 per cent of intradural dermoids are associated with a dermal sinus. Dermal sinuses are mainly located at both extremities of the spinal canal. Of 127 sinuses reported by Wright (1971), 72 were in the lumbosacral region, 30 in the occipital area, and only 14 at the thoracic or cervical levels. Dermal sinuses are easily mistaken for pilonidal sinuses. If not clearly superficial, such tracts should be explored radiologically but never by a probe or by injection of contrast material. CT or MRI can visualize the tract as a line of increased density with an ascending orientation, and dermoid cysts are best shown by MRI. The tract may pass between two spinous processes without producing any bony defect. Dermal sinuses are frequently revealed by a complication, usually purulent meningitis that is often relapsing or recurrent. Intraspinal suppuration occasionally occurs. In any case of recurrent meningitis or meningitis due to unusual pathogens, careful examination of the spine and occipital region is mandatory. Shaving of the nuchal area may show a tiny, punctiform defect that may discharge fluid material. In some cases, chemical meningitis, with polymorphs in the CSF but no infecting organisms, results from fissuration of an intradural dermoid. I have seen chronic hydrocephalus as a result of basilar block, due

to chemical meningitis, in two children. After antibiotic treatment of meningitis, resection of the tract should be performed after careful radiological assessment.

• *Lumbosacral lipomas* are collections of partially encapsulated fat and connective tissue, and, in many cases, are associated with failure of fusion of the posterior bony structures. They may be of three types: intradural lipomas, lipomyelomeningoceles, and fibrolipomas of the filum terminale. Bulsara et al. (2001) reported 114 cases: 22 involved the filum terminale, 64% were lipomyelomeningoceles and 16% were intraspinal lipomas. Arai et al. (2001) reported on 120 lumbar lipomas, 47 of which were asymptomatic.

Intradural lipomas are rare tumours, representing less than 1% of all spinal tumours, and may be cervical, thoracic or lumbar. They are of soft consistency and almost half of them have an extramedullary, extradural component. The spinal canal may be normal or expanded locally and there may be a narrow spina bifida. They can produce cord compression but there is no visible anomaly on the back.

Lipomyelomeningoceles consist of a lipoma or lipofibroma attached to the dorsal surface of the open, non-neurulated spinal cord, under an intact skin cover. The lipoma bulges in the lumbosacral region and merges peripherally with the normal subcutaneous fat. It is generally asymmetrical and, in its most common location, deviates the buttock sulcus to one side. The lipoma may extend cephalad into the spinal canal, overriding the dorsal aspect of the neurulated cord, and is sometimes accompanied by a dermoid or epidermoid cyst. A meningocele is frequently associated with the lipoma (Fig. 2.9). The meningocele protrudes opposite an asymmetrical lipoma and produces a rotation of the neural plate. The spinal canal is open posteriorly so that the subcutaneous lipoma continues directly with the intraspinal part.

There is usually a fibrous band or arch between the last lamina cephalad to the defect. The cord is often kinked on this band, which has to be divided to free the neural structures. In all cases, the caudal end of the cord is tethered in a low position below the L2 level (Hirsch and Pierre-Kahn 1988, Kanev et al. 1990, Pierre-Kahn et al. 1997). Bony abnormalities with errors of segmentation, osseous bars or partial sacral agenesis are present in over 40% of cases. Cutaneous abnormalities in the form of tags, angiomas or blind sinuses are often present. CT and MRI are essential for determining, before surgical treatment, the exact anatomical details of the lesion. Cutaneous abnormalities are present in almost 90% of patients and a preopoerative neurological deficit in one or both lower limbs in 57% (congenital in 22%). Sphincter disturbances, motor deficits and urinary problems are common before operation but may also appear following surgery. Many lesions remain asymptomatic, and whether these should be surgically treated remains a disputed issue (Naidich et al. 1983, Hirsch and Pierre-Kahn 1988, Harrison et al. 1990, Pierre-Kahn et al. 1997). However, progressive neurological deterioration is frequent (Cochrane et al. 2000). Among 93 patients followed up for 5 years or more (Pierre-Kahn et al. 1997), progression of neurological abnormalities was observed in 59% and was rapid in 43%. Following surgery, performed in 50% of the patients, there was significant improvement that, however eroded with time. Fifty-three per cent of their patients were symptom-free after 5 years.

The *tight filum terminale syndrome* is marked by a low position (below L2 level) of the conus medullaris (James and Lassman 1981, Cornette et al. 1998) and is characterized by neurological and orthopaedic abnormalities. Traction on the spinal cord and repeated microtrauma may be responsible for the late appearance of neurological signs. Although the condition is often asymptomatic, it can produce neurological and especially urinary symptoms. Tethering can result from multiple causes in addition to lipomyelomeningoceles, including sequelae of operation for open spina bifida, diastematomyelia or short filum terminale. The tight filum terminale is often associated with a lipoma and results from abnormal canalization of the terminal cord. It may be associated with a small cyst. However, fibrolipomas of the filum are most often incidental findings. The diagnosis of tight filum is difficult as the bony defect is of limited extent or absent altogether. CT and especially MRI (Bale et al. 1986, Bulsara et al. 2004) are most effective for diagnosis of a tight filum because it may be so closely applied to the posterior wall of the meningeal sac as to be invisible on myelography. Hendrick et al. (1977) found a lipoma in 23% of their patients with tight filum, a cyst in 3%, and scoliosis or kyphoscoliosis in 25%. Surgical treatment may prevent progression of symptoms (Komagata et al. 2004).

• *Diastematomyelia* consists of a sagittal cleft dividing the spinal cord into two 'half-cords' each surrounded by its own pia mater (Fig. 2.10). The cleft may extend through the full thickness of the cord or only partially through the dorsal half of the cord (partial syringomyelia) (Hilal et al. 1974, Schijman 2003). The cleft is usually located between T9 and S1 but cervical location has

been reported (Simpson and Rose 1987). A bony spur is present in about half the cases (James and Lassman 1981). The spur may be partial, purely cartilaginous or fibrous. It impales the cord or cauda equina so that the conus is fixed in a low position as a result of the differential growth between vertebral column and spinal cord. The two cords reunite below the cleft in 90% of cases (Hilal et al. 1974).

In about 40% of cases, both the arachnoid and dura form separate tubes around each half-cord for a limited number of segments. There are thus two dural layers between the half-cords. It is in this form that there is a fibrous or bony spur that lies at the lowermost end of the cleft. In the remaining cases, the two half-cords lined by pia mater lie side-by-side in a single arachnoid tube surrounded by undivided dura. Such cases do not have a septum and usually remain asymptomatic (James and Lassman 1981). A *tight filum* is present in about half the patients, and 5% have multiple spurs.

The vertebral column is grossly abnormal in over 90% of patients with diastematomyelia. The spinal canal is widened, errors of segmentation of the vertebral bodies are present in 85% of cases, spina bifida is frequent, and *scoliosis* is marked in over half the cases. In the experience of Hilal et al. (1974), 4.9% of 392 cases of scoliosis resulted from diastematomyelia. Prenatal diagnosis is possible (Pierre-Kahn et al. 2003).

Cutaneous abnormalities are present in 75% of patients. Typically, a tuft of hair or a dimple overlies the defect, but a lipoma, angioma or dermal sinus may also occur.

Diastematomyelia, the tethered cord syndrome and lipomyelomeningocele have many common neurological features. Two clinical neurological presentations are encountered. The first is a picture of congenital atrophy, weakness, and deformity of one lower limb, or of both limbs with a marked unilateral preponderance. Reflexes are depressed or abolished in the affected territory, and sphincter disturbances of the type seen in low spina bifida are present, especially with lipomyelomeningocele. The asymmetry is highly suggestive of spinal dysraphism, especially if associated with cutaneous anomalies, a palpable bony defect or kyphoscoliosis. Such a picture demands plain X-ray and myelography, CT or MRI of the spinal canal.

A *second presentation* is with progressive neurological deficit that may appear at any age and can be superimposed on a previously fixed picture. A mixture of peripheral and central signs and cutaneous abnormalities is characteristic. This syndrome may occur following trauma, or spontaneously following a growth spurt or a rapid increase in weight. Occasionally, a severe neurological syndrome develops suddenly with marked or massive paraplegia or quadriplegia. Following such an event, recuperation is poor, even with operation (Albright et al. 1989).

The *treatment of the tethered cord syndrome* is of variable difficulty. Its aim is to free the spinal cord from its low and posterior attachment without injury to the neural placode or roots. This aim is attained rather easily in uncomplicated diastematomyelia, for which liberation of the spur is usually sufficient. It is more difficult to divide a tight filum, as roots may be difficult to distinguish from fibrous tracts, and electrical stimulation is

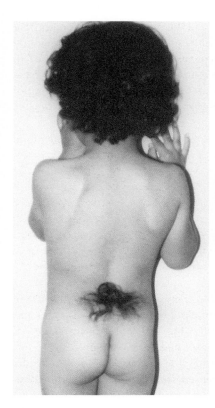
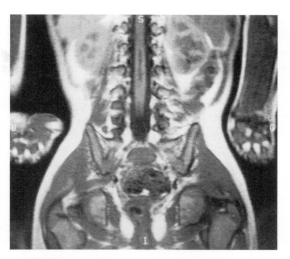
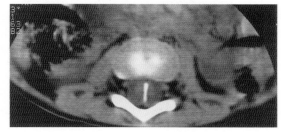

Fig. 2.10. Diastematomyelia in a 20-month-old boy. Note hair tuft on midline in the lumbar region. *(Top right)* MRI (T$_1$-weighted sequence, frontal cut). Cord is divided into two halves that reunite below midline septum. There is low attachment of the cord at L4–L5 level. *(Bottom right)* Axial cut demonstrates sagitally oriented bony septum. (Courtesy Dr D Renier, Prof. J-F Hirsh, Hôpital des Enfants Malades, Paris.)

invaluable. Untethering of the cord is indicated when recent motor, sensory or sphincter dysfunction is present. and can be effective when no neural damage has set in (Haberl et al. 2004, Wehby et al. 2004, Royo-Salvador et al. 2005). Urological complications are a major problem in many cases of spina bifida occulta. They should be systematically monitored, as early treatment is essential for prevention of upper urinary tract problems.

OTHER DEVELOPMENTAL ABNORMALITIES RELATED TO
SPINAL DYSRAPHISM
Abnormalities that have a more or less distant relationship to spinal dysraphism include syringomyelia, sacral agenesis and other manifestations of the caudal regression syndrome (Nievelstein et al. 1994), and congenital defects of the skull with or without defect of the scalp. These anomalies probably arise through different mechanisms and only superficially resemble dysraphic states.

Syringomyelia
Syringomyelia is defined as a tubular cavitation within the spinal cord. In theory it differs from hydromyelia, which is a dilatation of the cord central canal lined with ependyma, whereas the syringomyelic cavity is lined by glial cells. However, the distinction is difficult in practice, and it may be simpler to refer to all intraspinal cavities of non tumoural nature as hydrosyringomyelia (Gower et al. 1994), especially as the diagnosis is now frequently made by MRI demonstrating cavitation in vivo (van Hall et al. 1992, Gower et al. 1994). Hydrosyringomyelic cavities are of variable length. Tashiro et al. (1987) found a cervical cavity in 69% of their cases, total length cavitation in 6%, and cavitation limited to the lumbar cord in 3%. The cavities may or may not be in communication with the fourth ventricle. Some may extend into the medulla and pons, with resulting involvement of lower cranial nerves and nuclei (syringomyelobulbia). Cavitation may be of variable location and diameter within the cord, which is frequently distended by cyst fluid. Experience with CT has shown that most syringomyelic cavities are opacified by intrathecally injected contrast, even if only after a few hours, indicating communication with the subarachnoid space. Syringomyelia is very often associated with Chiari I malformation and hydrocephalus, which may play an important role in its mechanism. The thrust of the CSF wave has been thought to be responsible for the slow progressive downward extension of the cavity within the spinal cord (Gower et al. 1994). However, the exact mechanism that produces syringomyelia is uncertain (Levine 2004). Syringomyelia can be a consequence of spinal trauma. It has also been reported in association with postmeningitic spinal arachnoiditis (Caplan et al. 1990).

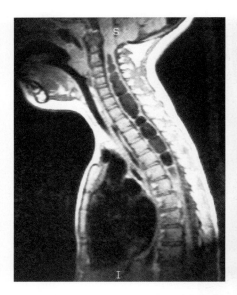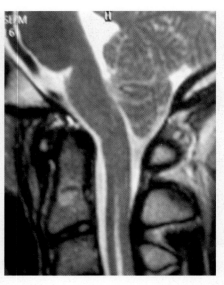

Fig. 2.11. Syringomyelia. *(Left)* Massive cavitation of the spinal cord in a 5½-year-old girl with only minimal symptoms and signs. (Courtesy Dr D Renier, Prof. J-F Hirsch, Hôpital des Enfants Malades, Paris.) *(Right)* Asymptomatic syrinx visible in the spinal cord, associated with Chiari I malformation.

Because most of the lesions involve the cervical cord, involvement of the upper limbs tends to be prominent. The central location of the cavity explains why temperature and pain sensation are electively disturbed, as the fibres that convey these sensations cross through the central white matter. Interference with fibres concerned with pain perception is responsible for the frequently observed trophic disturbances.

The condition is sporadic, although occasional familial forms have been reported (Busis and Hochberg 1985). The disease is rarely symptomatic in children, although symptoms have been observed as early as 2 years of age (Tashiro et al. 1987). Adolescent onset is common with up to 40% of patients first seen in their second decade (Mariani et al. 1991).

The *clinical manifestations* may include painless whitlows and occasionally Charcot's joints as a manifestation of the classical sensory disturbances in a suspended topography. Later, paralysis and more complete sensory disturbances develop in the upper limbs, where abolition of deep tendon reflexes is an early sign. Pyramidal tract signs are frequently found in the lower limbs. With bulbar involvement, rotary nystagmus and other signs of hemibulbar syndrome may be present (Gower et al. 1994). Stridor and laryngospasm have been reported. Scoliosis is a major and early manifestation. Tashiro et al. (1987) found scoliosis to be present before 10 years of age in 19% of their cases.

The introduction of modern neuroimaging has considerably increased the frequency of the diagnosis and indicated more variability of clinical features (Schijman 2003). Many cases are discovered on the occasion of imaging studies and remain asymptomatic for long periods. Classical suspended dissociated hypoaesthesia appears to be uncommon, deep tendon reflexes may be preserved in the upper limbs, and nystagmus may be downbeating rather than rotatory (Tashiro et al. 1987, Pou Serradell and Mares Segura 1988). Chiari I malformation was present in over

half the cases in the latter series and basilar impression in 27%. Symptoms tend to be uncharacteristic for a very long time. Scoliosis is often the reason for imaging studies. Syringomyelia associated with myelomeningocele is usually asymptomatic (Breningstall et al. 1992). Acute presentation with sudden paraplegia is rare (Zager et al. 1990). Syringobulbia is often associated with spinal cord cavities but occasionally occurs alone. Onset is often many years before diagnosis. Symptoms and signs may include occipital headache, vertigo, auditory failure, nystagmus and lower nerve involvement.

The diagnosis of syringobulbomyelia is based on imaging techniques. Myelography has been supplanted by CT and, especially, by MRI (Lee et al. 1985) (Fig. 2.11). These methods allow full visualization of the cavity and separation of true syringomyelia from intraspinal tumours. They also allow assessment of the efficacy of surgical treatment by measuring the size of the syrinx before and after operation, and spontaneous resolution has been reported (Sudo et al. 1990).

Regular monitoring of the patients is essential. In many cases, there is no or only very slow progression and operation is not indicated. Surgical treatment is indicated even in the absence of clinical manifestations if Chiari I malformation is present (Mariani et al. 1991, Gower et al. 1994), or in the presence of clinical symptoms and signs. Posterior fossa decompression with dural opening is the generally preferred method (Attal et al. 2004, Arruda et al. 2004). A success rate of 72% was obtained in a large series of 96 patients (Navarro et al. 2004). Recurrence is not infrequent (Mariani et al. 1991). For resistant cases, shunting of the cystic cavity may be considered (Goel and Desai 2000). Indications of shunting treatment need further assessment.

Cysts of the arachnoid mater may develop dorsal to the spinal cord and may produce signs of compression (Chang et al. 2004, Sharma et al. 2004). The cysts often extend over several vertebral

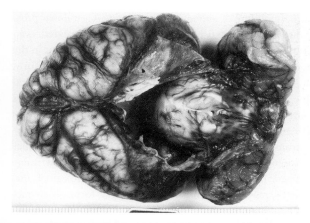

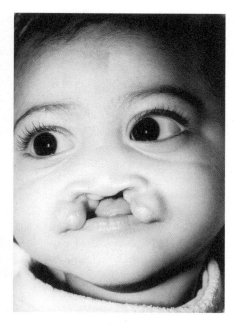

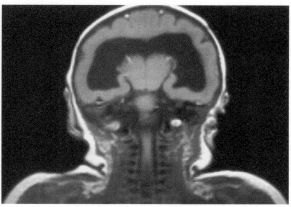

Fig. 2.12. Holoprosencephly. *(Top left)* Brain of an infant who died at 6 hours of life. Note small size of brain with no division of hemispheres and presence of a dorsal cyst (opened). (Courtesy Dr J-C Larroche, Maternité Port Royal, Paris.) *(Top right)* Infant with holoprosencephaly with median cleft lip. *(Left)* T₁-weighted MRI showing single telencephalic ventricle and fused thalami.

segments and communicate with the subarachnoid space by a small opening. Because of their posterior location they may go undetected by conventional myelography if the patient is not placed in the prone position. Such cysts are found in adolescents with kyphosis. They are best demonstrated by MRI. A syndrome of spinal arachnoid cyst, lymphoedema of the feet and a double row of eyelashes has been described (Schwartz et al. 1980). Richaud (1988) has reviewed in detail malformations of the spinal meninges in children.

Congenital defects of the skull and scalp
Aplasia of the scalp can occur alone or in combination with bone defects. Scalp defects are mainly located to the vertex. They are common in the trisomy 13 syndrome (Chapter 4). Isolated skull defects may be located to the vertex in association with scalp aplasia. A large posterior fontanelle is present in several conditions including the Walker–Warburg syndrome (see below) and represents a minor form of cephalocele. Symmetrical parietal foramina, sometimes referred to as the 'Catlin mark', may be large and palpable or visible only on skull X-rays. They are transmitted as a dominant mendelian trait. Aplasia of the sphenoidal greater wing occurs in neurofibromatosis and can produce pulsatile exophthalmos.

Small scalp defects can be closed but large ones require grafting. Bony defects of small size may be left alone. Large defects require surgical closure.

DISORDERS OF VENTRAL INDUCTION
This term designates those malformations that result from induction failure involving the cephalic mesoderm, the adjacent neuroectoderm and associated neural crest derivatives, and the entodermal anlagen for facial structures. Induction failure is probably time-specific as ventral induction is completed prior to the 33rd post fecundation day. The major defect is failure of the primary cerebral vesicle (telencephalon) to cleave and expand laterally. Midline facial defects that are frequently associated are a simultaneous consequence of the same defect involving the facial structures.

Holoprosencephaly (or Pprosencephaly)
These terms are used synonymously to designate the most common form of ventral induction defect. The term *arhinencephaly* is improper as abnormal development of the rhinencephalic structures and, in particular, absence of the olfactory bulbs and stems can exist in brains with complete separation of the hemispheres (Kobori et al. 1987), although they are virtually always lacking with incomplete forebrain division. Holoprosencephaly means an undivided anterior brain (Fig. 2.12). The severity of the abnormality is variable (Probst 1979, DeMyer 1987, Oba and Barkovich 1995). Three major types are classically described: *alobar*, *semilobar* and *lobar holoprosencephaly*. In fact intermediate forms exist between these types and holoprosencephaly encompasses a spectrum of malformations.

The birth incidence is variable with the populations. It is low, of the order of 1 per 18,000, in Western countries but reaches 6 per 10,000 livebirths in Japan (Matsunaga and Shiota 1987). The total frequency, including abortuses, is much higher as only 3% of fetuses with holoprosencephaly survive to delivery (Cohen et al. 1989).

The defect may have multiple causes. Genetic factors are known to be operative in some cases. They include mainly chromosomal abnormalities, which accounted for about 40% of liveborn infants with holoprosencephaly in a large Californian population study; half of these had trisomy 13 (Croen et al. 1996, Hahn and Plawner 2004). However, Stashinko et al. (2004) found that only 9% of their 104 patients had chromosomal anomalies, suggesting that the populations studied differed. Several other abnormalities have been reported. Other associated syndromes of multiple malformations include Pallister–Hall, Smith–Lemli–Opitz and cardiovelofacial syndromes. Familial *cases with normal chromosomes* also occur. At least 12 loci have been implicated (Roessler et al. 1998), and mutations in 8 genes have been identified (Ming and Muenke 2002); at least two of the mutated genes encode proteins of the sonic hedgehog pathway. Mutations have been identified in only 15–20% of patients with normal chromosomes and in <5% of sporadic cases of holoprosencephaly (Nanni et al. 1999). Dominant inheritance, especially due to mutation of the *SHH* gene, appears more common than recessive transmission. Environmental influences are important, in particular maternal diabetes mellitus. About 1% of diabetic mothers may bear children with holoprosencephaly, and the incidence of the condition among offspring of diabetic mothers is at least 100 times that in the general population (Barr et al. 1983). Prenatal exposure to various toxins has been reported, e.g. alcohol and antiepileptic agents (Ronen and Andrews 1991, Cohen and Shiota 2002).

Alobar holoprosencephaly refers to a completely undivided, very small forebrain that assumes the shape of a horseshoe in the concavity of which lies a dorsal sac. This structure contains little neocortex, the concavity of the horseshoe being made of entorhinal cortex (Probst 1979, Friede 1989). The thalami are fused on the midline (Simon et al. 2000b). The brainstem and cerebellum are well developed. Hydrocephalus is often associated. Such brain anomalies may be associated with extremely severe facial defects and ocular abnormalities. In cyclopia, a rapidly lethal condition, there is a single orbit with fused ocular globes. In cases of ethmocephaly, the nose is absent, replaced by a proboscis that is located above the level of the closely placed orbits. Cebocephaly patients present with an abnormal nose with single nostril. The most frequent type is holoprosencephaly with median cleft lip in which the premaxillary bone anlage is missing (Fig. 2.12). There is marked osseous hypotelorism. Such patients may live for several months or years, in contrast to those affected by the previously mentioned types.

In *semilobar holoprosencephaly*, there is no dorsal sac and the brain is divided into two hemispheres in its posterior part, while anteriorly abnormal transverse convolutions bridge the median fissure (Fig. 2.12). The thalami are fused in the midline. In the most evoluted forms, sometimes termed type A semilobar prosencephaly, the two hemispheres seem to be fully separated, even anteriorly. However, interhemispheric bridging is present in the anterior frontal region and there is no corpus callosum anteriorly, while the splenium may be present. Anteriorly, the cerebral mantle invaginates deeply with both grey and white matter layers crossing the midline after having lined a more or less sinuous 'interhemispheric' fissure (Oba and Barkovich 1995). The sinuous fissure may be a cue for the diagnosis by CT of semilobar holoprosencephaly. MRI permits differentiation of the interhemispheric bridging from a true corpus callosum on sagittal cuts.

Lobar prosencephaly, in its fully developed forms, is characterized by almost complete separation of the hemispheres. Probst (1979) prefers not to classify it as holoprosencephaly, but it is included in the latter group by most investigators (Oba and Barkovich 1995). In this form, the hemispheres are fairly well separated; only the most anterior and ventral part is undivided. The genu of the corpus callosum is thin and the frontal horns are often rudimentary. The central grey nuclei are also partially or completely fused. The cases of telencephalic pseudo-monoventricle with a large cavum septum pellucidum in association with atresia of the frontal horns and various other abnormalities (Poll-Thé and Aicardi 1985) probably belong to this type.

In addition to these classic types, a less common type is now recognized (Lewis et al. 2002, Simon et al. 2002, Takahashi et al. 2003) in which there is failure of separation of the posterior frontal and parietal lobes whereas the frontal and occipital poles are well separated. The term *syntelencephaly* is used to designate such cases.

The frequency of the individual types was recently studied in a review of 83 children. Half had semilobar type and each of the other forms accounted for 15% of cases (Hahn and Plawner 2004).

Associated malformations are common and include congenital heart disease, scalp defects, and polydactyly, in which case a chromosomal defect is likely. Holoprosencephaly may be a part of several malformation syndromes, including Meckel–Gruber syndrome (Paetau et al. 1985) and Aicardi syndrome (Sato et al. 1987). Isolated forms are not, as a rule, part of a chromosomal syndrome.

The *diagnosis* of holoprosencephaly is easy when facial abnormalities are present (Burck et al. 1981, De Myer 1987). In addition to those described above, there may be bilateral cleft lip and palate with hypoplasia of the median tubercle or trigonocephaly with orbital hypotelorism. However, the face may be normal in the less severe forms. Microcephaly is a feature common to most forms unless aqueductal stenosis, with resulting hydrocephalus, is present (Nyberg et al. 1987). Endocrine dysfunction, especially diabetes insipidus (Hasegawa et al. 1990), and adrenal and growth hormone deficiency, can contribute to the mortality and morbidity of holoprosencephaly.

Imaging studies, especially MRI, confirm the diagnosis and permit detailed analysis of the abnormalities including those of the basal ganglia (Simon et al. 2000b). Diagnosis can also be made by ultrasonography when the fontanelle is open (Govaert and de Vries 1997).

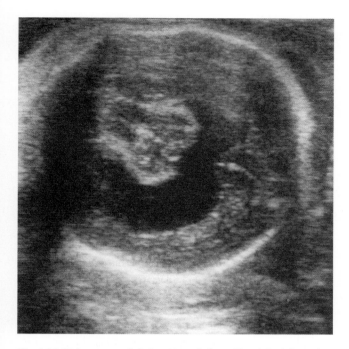

Fig. 2.13. Holoprosencephaly in a 29-week fetus: dilated single horseshoe ventricle (fetal forehead facing bottom of photograph). (Courtesy Dr M-C Aubry, Maternité Port Royal, Paris.)

Infants with the most severe types rarely survive the neonatal period. Most surviving infants are severely retarded, and develop seizures that are often infantile spasms with hypsarrhythmia. Neurological manifestations are highly variable, and some patients may survive into adulthood. A child presenting with spastic diplegia has been reported (Shanks and Wilson 1988). However, mental retardation, usually of a severe degree, is constant, particularly in cases that are symptomatic early. The occurrence of endocrinological abnormalities such as diabetes insipidus and growth hormone deficiency is possible. Hydrocephalus is present in 40% of patients with holoprosencephaly, especially when no facial abnormalities are associated.

Prenatal diagnosis of holoprosencephaly can be made from the 16th week of pregnancy by ultrasonography (Fig. 2.13). In the series of Nyberg et al. (1987) holoprosencephaly accounted for 19% of all cases of hydrocephalus diagnosed prenatally. Twenty-nine per cent of the diagnosed cases had normal facial features, emphasizing the importance of not relying excessively on facial appearance. Orbital hypotelorism is the most reliable diagnostic feature for antenatal diagnosis. However, the sensitivity of sonography for the detection of the less severe forms is relatively low (Stashinko et al. 2004). In addition, for a single dominant mutation there is considerable variation in the phenotype (Hehr et al. 2004). Prenatal MRI (Sonigo et al. 1998) can permit detection of the minor forms. Minor features such as single central incisor or anosmia seen in members of a proband's family suggests the probability of a genetic form.

The empirical recurrence risk for a couple who have had an affected offspring is said to be 6%. However, this figure is probably biased and results from the averaging of data from genetic

cases with different patterns of transmission and nongenetic cases.

Treatment includes that of seizures and endocrinopathies, together with appropriate education and family support.

CONDITIONS RELATED TO HOLOPROSENCEPHALY
Arhinencephaly without holoprosencephaly is occasionally encountered at autopsy in the brains of individuals with mentally retardation. Other malformations, especially microgyrias or heterotopias, are associated (Kobori et al. 1987). Holoprosencephaly may be unilateral.

Familial isolated agenesis of the olfactory stems, also known as Kallmann syndrome, is discussed with migration disorders (see below).

MEDIAN CLEFT FACE SYNDROMES
The median cleft face syndromes are a group of conditions whose visible common denominator is hypertelorism. Several cases are associated with other ventral induction abnormalities, the commonest of which is anterior cranium bifidum. Hypertelorism is a frequent feature in cases of corpus callosum agenesis, sometimes with cleft lip, bifid nose or similar anomalies (Aicardi et al. 1987). Anterior cephaloceles of various locations may be found, and these are frequently accompanied by extensive cortical and other malformations (Leech and Shuman 1986). A similar picture can obtain with lipomas of the corpus callosum.

DISORDERS OF CORTICAL DEVELOPMENT
Abnormal development of the cortex (Table 2.4; see also Chapter 15) is an extremely common cause of neurodevelopmental disorders. The high frequency of such abnormalities has become evident with the development of modern neuroimaging, especially MRI, and their role as a cause of epilepsy, cerebral palsy and mental retardation now appears greater than that of perinatally acquired damage. The terms commonly used for the description of these abnormalities are multiple and confusing. Pathological terms are often used to designate conditions diagnosed by imaging techniques. Such terms as 'cortical dysplasia' are used either in a general sense to refer to any type of abnormally developed cortex, or in the more restricted meaning of disorder of cortical organization. The term 'migration disorders' is often wrongly applied to abnormalities limited to final cortical organization.

To avoid such confusion in this section I will use the term *developmental cortical abnormalities* for all types. The term 'malformations of cortical development' has been widely accepted with the same meaning (Barkovich et al. 1996, 2001a) but malformations are *the result of* an error of development and it seems difficult to apply it to the process of development itself. The terms 'migration disorders' and 'organization disorders' will be used only for abnormalities of the corresponding stages of corticogenesis.

Several systems of classification of cortical malformations have been proposed. The most commonly used is that of Barkovich et al. (1996, 2001a) that divides these malformations into three groups according to the supposed timing of determination and mechanisms of formation of the various types: disorders of

TABLE 2.4
Main disorders of cortical development*

Malformations due to abnormal neuronal and glial proliferation, differentiation or apoptosis
- Decreased proliferation/increased apoptosis
  - Microcephaly
  - Microlissencephaly
- Increased proliferation
  - Megalencephaly
  - Hemimegalencephaly

Malformations due to abnormal migration
- Heterotopia
  - Subependymal
  - Subcortical
  - Marginal glioneuronal
- Lissencephaly/subcortical band heterotopia spectrum
  - LIS1 lissencephaly
  - Other lissencephalies
  - Subcortical band heterotopia
  - Others
- Cobblestone complex
  - With muscular dystrophy syndromes
    - Walker–Warburg syndrome
    - Muscle–eye–brain disease
    - Fukuyama congenital dystrophy
  - Without muscular dystrophy

Malformations due to abnormal organization
- Polymicrogyria1
  - With schizencephaly
  - Without schizencephaly
- Cortical dysplasias
  - Architectural and cytoarchitectural
  - Taylor type (with balloon cells)

Unclassified malformations
- With metabolic disorders
  - Mitochondrial
  - Peroxisomal
- Others

*Modified from Barkovich et al. (2001a).
Several mechanisms may be operative in a single case.
1May be a postmigrational abnormality in some cases.

---

neuroglial proliferation/differentiation and apoptosis; malformations due to abnormal *migration*; and malformations due to abnormal cortical *organization* (including late neuronal migration). Table 2.4 shows a simplified form of this classification. Other systems based on pathology, clinical presentation or genetic and molecular processes (Sarnat and Flores-Sarnat 2001b, 2002, 2004; Clark 2004) have been proposed. From a clinical point of view, a simple scheme separating *diffuse* and *localized* cortical malformations is useful. Diffuse abnormalities (e g. lisssencephaly) are responsible for generalized seizures, especially infantile spasms, severe neurological signs and mental retardation; localized abnormalities (e.g. focal cortical dysplasias) are mostly responsible for focal epilepsy usually of early onset (Fauser et al. 2006), which may not be accompanied by cognitive or neurological deficits, and have a much better outlook. Only symptomatic therapy is possible for diffuse cortical abnormalities, whereas effective surgical treatment may be available for many cases of focal dysplasia. Some diffuse abnormalities may result from metabolic defects (e.g. Zellweger syndrome) (Raoul et al. 2003). Multifocal

dysplasias can also produce a picture similar to that of diffuse malformations.

The classification of Barkovich et al. schematically indicates the most likely mechanisms for each type of cortical malformation. The different stages of corticogenesis described above are, in fact, interdependent and overlapping. The fate of precursor cells is determined before they migrate (McConnell and Kaznowski 1991), and this determination has a bearing on the subsequent processes of migration and organization. Thus, abnormal cells, e.g. in tuberous sclerosis or in some types of 'cortical dysplasia', often do not migrate to their normal position and/or fail to establish normal connectivity. Likewise, disorders of cell proliferation are frequently associated with abnormal migration, e.g. in pachygyria or agyria. As a result, it may be difficult to determine which step of cortical development is mainly interfered with in individual cases, and classifications may be to some extent arbitrary. Thus, hemimegalencephaly and microcephaly are often associated with abnormal migration, and subcortical heterotopias frequently coexist with overlying cortical abnormalities. Several anomalies are often simultaneously present in the same brain, and microdysgenesis (Meencke and Veith 1992) may be present together with subcortical and cortical developmental abnormalities. Some disorders do not fit easily in the proposed scheme; for example, a high proportion of cases of microcephaly or macrocephaly may not be disorders of cortical development and may be be due to destructive or other mechanisms rather than developmental diseases. Moreover, even in some developmental errors the mechanisms supposed to be responsible are mostly speculative and it is likely that many cortical developmental abnormalities are due to associations or interactions of several known or unknown mechanisms. I will describe successively the various anomalies attributed to the different mechanisms.

DISORDERS OF PROLIFERATION/DIFFERENTIATION
This section focuses on those cases in which disorders of proliferation and differentiation are the dominant abnormality, although they rarely occur in isolation. The phenomenon of programmed cell death, which is thought to affect between 30% and 50% of formed neurons, may play an important role, while destructive processes may be responsible for loss of cerebral volume and may be difficult to distinguish from maldevelopment because of the peculiar features of the repair processes in fetal life (Marin-Padilla 2000). *Tuberous sclerosis*, which belongs to the category of proliferation/differentiation diseases, is described in Chapter 3, because of the prominence of the cutaneous manifestations.

Microcephaly/micrencephaly
Microcephaly is variably defined as head circumference more than two standard deviations below the mean (Barkovich et al. 2001a) or below the 3rd centile (Haslam 2000), although the latter is termed extreme microcephaly by Barkovich et al. (2001a). Both definitions obviously include normal individuals. *Micrencephaly*, on the other hand, theoretically refers to a small brain (Friede 1989) but in practice the two definitions are equivalent. All authors admit that children with moderately small heads (between

2 and 3 SD below the mean) are frequently normal, but there is statistically an increased prevalence of mild microcephaly among children with learning disabilities. Mental retardation may be more common when a small head is associated with growth retardation. However, even patients with head circumference between 3 and 4 SD below the mean may have a normal intelligence.

The aetiology of microcephaly is diverse (Opitz and Holt 1990). Many cases, termed *secondary microcephaly*, are the result of acquired clastic lesions or other pathological processes incurred during pregnancy or even later, during the period of rapid head and brain growth that takes place in the first years of life (Hughes and Miskin 1986). A significant proportion of cases are apparently *primary* and are mostly of genetic origin. The mechanisms of such cases are imperfectly known. Insufficient cell proliferation is only one of these mechanisms, which conceivably can include excessive embryofetal cell death. Genetic microcephaly may belong to several entities. Sugimoto et al. (1993) found that 44 of 55 cases were of genetic origin, the rest being due to a variety of nongenetic developmental errors.

Primary microcephaly (also called 'true' microcephaly or 'microcephalia vera') is inherited in a recessive manner (Suri 2003). Its incidence varies with populations depending in part on the frequency of consanguineous marriages. The degree of microcephaly is usually marked (at 3 SD and often 5–6 SD below the mean), with a narrow, receding forehead and a pointed vertex, giving a peculiar clinical and radiological appearance. Paradoxically, individuals with microcephalia vera do not exhibit gross neurological signs, but hyperkinetic behaviour and disturbances of fine motor coordination are frequently present (Accardo and Whitman 1988). Seizures do not occur in typical cases. Some degree of mental retardation is present but it is usually mild and most children can acquire at least a simplified language. This is all the more remarkable as the brain weight may be as little as 500 g in the adult.

From a pathological point of view, the brain convolutions look normal and the cortex is thin. There is severe depletion of neurons in layers II and III (Evrard et al. 1989).

Mirocephalia vera is genetically heterogeneous. Recessive inheritance is the rule. Six loci (*MCPH1–5*) have been mapped and two genes identified (Suri 2003). In one third of families in Suri's study no linkage was demonstrated, indicating further heterogeneity. A third gene has been recently identified in a similar condition common in the Amish community. The gene at the *MCPH1* locus codes for a protein, microcephalin, involved in brain growth. In heterozygotes, the gene might be responsible for mild mental retardation, sometimes with a relatively small head.

In other cases of microcephaly, the cortex is abormally thick and shows only a small number of abnormal convolutions. These cases have been termed *microlissencephaly* (Barkovich et al. 1998) or *oligogyric microcephaly* (Dobyns and Barkovich 1999). Several subtypes probably exist (Ross et al. 2001). They differ clinically from primary microcephaly by the presence of profound mental retardation, seizures and neurological signs and sometimes ocular or other abnormalities (Silengo et al. 1992, Kroon et al. 1996). MRI of the brain shows variable abnormalities of the cortical gyri

in addition to the small size of the brain and poor development of the frontal lobes (Steinlin et al. 1991, Sugimoto et al. 1993, Sztriha et al. 2004). Other rare types are microcephly with cerebellar hypoplasia (Kato et al. 1999, Ross et al. 2001, Barth 2003a) and the Neu–Laxova syndrome (Manning et al. 2004).

These cases are part of a heterogeneous group of 'microcephaly plus'. Tolmie et al. (1987) found that only 1 of 29 cases they studied had 'microcephalia vera', whereas the other patients had more complex clinical features, including seizures and/or spasticity. Most cases were apparently recessive (Harbord et al. 1989). Others types may be dominantly inherited (Burton 1981). In still other cases, an array of associated anomalies was found, including congenital nephrotic syndrome (Nishikawa et al. 1997), a short jejuno-ileum (Nézelof et al. 1976), callosal agenesis and severe disturbances of migration (King et al. 1995). Familial cases with intracranial calcification masquerading as intrauterine infection (Aicardi–Goutières syndrome) are of especial interest because they mimic prenatal infections and the diagnosis of a familial condition is easily missed in such instances (Baraitser et al. 1983).

At the other end of the spectrum are rare cases of clinically silent, dominantly transmitted microcephaly (Haslam and Smith 1979, Accardo and Whitman 1988).

Cases with or without neurodevelopmental disturbances with chromosomal instability (Seemanova et al. 1985) or primary combined immunodeficiency (Berthet et al. 1994) are rare. An exhaustive list of syndromes with microcephaly is given by Friede (1989).

An extreme variant of microcephaly is that of *radial microbrain*. According to Evrard et al. (1989) the weight of brain in such cases can be as low as 16–50 g. The radial brain columns are almost normal but their number is markedly decreased. Such cases are distinct from atelencephaly in which there is no cortical structure.

Microcephaly is also a feature of a vast number of *chromosomal abnormalities*, of dysmorphic syndromes with mental retardation, and of syndromes with dwarfism such as Seckel syndrome. The pathology of such cases is usually poorly known. Some of these syndromes are genetically determined.

The *diagnosis* of microcephaly is easy in extreme cases but may be difficult in mild ones. The size of the head is normally variable on an individual and familial basis. Measurement of head size is imprecise, and the commonly used occipitofrontal circumference is only imperfectly correlated to brain volume, so that better indices have been sought using radiological measurements (Gooskens et al. 1989). However, head circumference remains the common simple method for evaluating brain size. In children, head circumference increases rapidly with the growth of the brain, so appropriate growth curves should be used for infants and children of average birthweight and for healthy and sick preterm infants (Gross et al. 1983). In normal infants, the weight of the brain trebles within the first year of life, and repeated measurements of head circumference are an essential part of examination.

The differential diagnosis with total craniosynostosis does not raise real problems, and the shape of skull, exophthalmia, normal

TABLE 2.5
Causes of macrocephaly other than internal hydrocephalus

Of extracerebral origin or due to the presence of alien tissue
- Pericerebral effusions, post-traumatic or of unknown origin (benign subdural effusions, external hydrocephalus) (Chapter 6)
- Congenital anomalies of intra- or extracerebral veins (aneurysm of the vein of Galen; other abnormalities of venous drainage) (Chapter 14)
- Achondroplasia and other skeletal dysplasias: osteopetrosis, Pyle disease, thanatophoric dwarfism (macrocephaly probably results in part from abnormal venous damage and resulting hydrocephalus) (Chapter 5)
- Osteogenesis imperfecta (especially type III) (Tsipouras et al. 1986)
- Tumours, congenital or acquired (Chapter 13)
- Intracranial cysts, especially giant arachnoid cysts in infants (Chapter 13)
- Agenesis of corpus callosum[1]

Due to increased volume of brain or envelopes
Megalencephaly of anatomical origin
- Tumours (diffuse astrocytomas or gliomatosis)
- Neurocutaneous syndromes (Chapters 3, 14)
    - Neurofibromatosis type 1
    - Tuberous sclerosis[2]
    - Proteus syndrome
    - Haemangiomatosis (Klippel–Trenaunay, Sturge–Weber, Bannayan–Riley–Ruvalcaba syndromes)
    - Cowden syndrome
    - Macrocephaly–cutis marmorata syndrome (Giuliano et al. 2004)
- Dysmorphic syndromes
    - Cerebral gigantism (Sotos syndrome) (Chapter 4)
    - Beckwith–Wiedemann syndrome
    - Macrocephaly and dilated Virchow–Robin spaces (Groeschel et al. 2006)
    - Macrocephaly–mental retardation–short stature
- Primary megalencephaly (usually nonfamilial, associated with abnormalities of brain architecture, including hemimegalencephaly[3]
- Variants of normal (often familial and unassociated with brain abnormalities)

Metabolic megalencephaly (Chapter 8)
- Leukodystrophies (Canavan–van Bogaert and Alexander disease, megalencephalic leukodystrophy with cysts)
- GM2 gangliosidosis (Tay–Sachs, Sandhoff diseases)
- Mucopolysaccharidoses
- Organic acidurias, especially glutaric aciduria types I and II, 2-oxyglutaric aciduria (Hoffmann et al. 1991, Brismar and Ozand 1995)
Macrocephalies of unknown origin
- Autism and developmental language disorder (Herbert et al. 2004)[4]

[1]Usually classified as hydrocephalus, often nonprogressive.
[2]Macrocephaly is unusual, in contrast to neurofibromatosis type 1.
[3]Hemimegalencephaly more commonly results in neurodevelopmental abnormalities than in macrocephaly.
[4]Macrocephaly develops postnatally.

development, signs of increased intracranial pressure and plain X-rays of the skull make the diagnosis obvious. The most important issue in diagnosis is to differentiate acquired (clastic) micrencephaly from genetic types. Marked neurological involvement, severe mental retardation, and a history of abnormal prenatal or perinatal events in the face of moderate microcephaly support a clastic origin, while the reverse features favour a genetic microcephaly. However, clinical features leave considerable room for uncertainty. The demonstration of destructive changes by neuroimaging is of great value. A normal CT, on the contrary, does not exclude an acquired origin.

Antenatal diagnosis may be difficult, especially in the absence of associated malformations, and errors by excess or by default have been frequent. Simple measurement of the biparietal diameter is not sufficient as it may be low in fetuses with sagittal craniosynostosis or marked intrauterine molding. Repeated examinations with full attention to skull shape are essential.

The prognosis of microcephaly is variable. Because certain children have relatively good intellectual potential, a sustained effort to educate them is worthwhile. Special schooling is unavoidable although an exceptional child will do well even with head circumference as low as 6 SD below the mean (personal case).

Macrocephaly

Macrocephaly, like microcephaly, is defined by reference to head circumference, the arbitrary limit of two standard deviations above the age norm being often accepted. With this statistical criterion, the definition includes normal individuals as well as a collection of diverse and totally unrelated entities (Table 2.5). A majority of the cases of macrocephaly are not due to abnormal brain development but will be considered here as the large head is a common and striking feature. Lorber and Priestley (1981) studied 510 children with head circumference above the 98th centile. Seventy-five per cent of these had hydrocephalus and increased intracranial pressure, 3% had specific syndromes, and 20% had primary megalencephaly with normal pressure. Only 13% of the this last group had mental retardation or neurological abnormalities. The major diagnostic consideration is hydro-

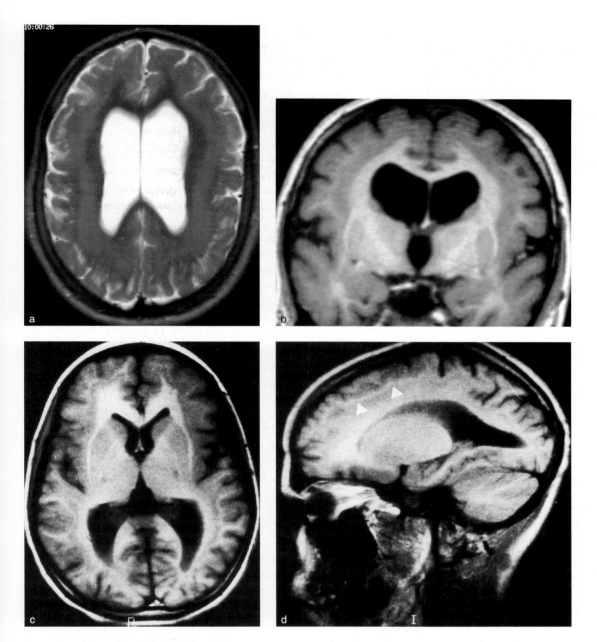

Fig. 2.20. Subcortical band heterotopia ('double cortex'). *(a)* MRI axial cut shows thick, continuous band with same signal as the cortex. *(b)* Coronal cut: in this patient there is also ventricular dilatation predominating anteriorly. *(c,d)* MRI, T$_1$-weighted sequence – *(c)* axial cut, *(d)* sagittal cut – demonstrates a thin band of white matter lying between the true cortex and the thin laminar heterotopia of grey matter *(arrows)*.

The differential diagnosis is with other conditions in which a thick and poorly sulcated cortex is present. Pachygyria due to *LIS1* mutation is only a mild grade of lissencephaly, not a differential diagnosis. Certain fetal disorders, in particular cytomegalovirus infection, can produce an apparently pachygyric cortex associated histologically with polymicrogyria. Periventricular calcification may be associated with abnormal gyration. In such cases, the microconvolutions may be apposed and give a pachygyric appearance.

Prenatal diagnosis is not possible by sonography in late pregnancy, as only tertiary sulci appear at that time (Toi et al. 2004). DNA studies may show a mutated or missing *LIS1* gene. Chromosome studies and MRI of the parents (especially the mother) should be performed in search of laminar heterotopias in order to help determine the risk of recurrence.

• *Subcortical band heteropia and lissencephaly due to DCX mutation.* Band heterotopias (Barkovich et al. 1994, Franzoni et al. 1995) or 'double cortex' (Livingston and Aicardi 1990, Palmini et al. 1991) are a disorder of migration in which a superficial cortex, which may be grossly normal or show an aberrant gyration, is separated by a thin layer of white matter from a band of grey matter whose separation from the underlying white matter is straight as in agyria–pachygyria (Fig. 2.20). Patients with this anomaly often have seizures that may be focal or generalized, sometimes in the form of the Lennox–Gastaut syndrome, and EEG anomalies (Hashimoto et al. 1993, Parmeggiani et al. 1994). The degree of mental involvement is quite variable and some patients develop normally (Livingston and Aicardi 1990, Ianetti et al. 1993). Barkovich et al. (1994) in a detailed study of 27 cases found a significant inverse correlation between the intellectual level and the thickness of the heterotopic band; an apparently normal cortex was associated with a better development but this seems to be variable. The band has been found to be able to generate paroxysmal EEG activity, and increased blood flow as demonstrated by SPECT studies indicates activation of the cortex.

The condition is due in a vast majority of cases to mutations in the sex-linked *DCX* gene that codes for doublecortin (des Portes et al. 1998, Gleeson et al. 1999). However, the same mutation in boys may give rise to classical lissencephaly (Pilz et al. 1998). The mutation is very variably expressed in women and even in some males (Cardoso et al. 2000, Gleeson 2000) and may thus be difficult to recognize. Therefore, when genetic counselling is requested by families with a lissencephalic boy, a careful search for band heterotopia by MRI and, if necessary for a *DCX* mutation, must be done in the mother and sisters. Families are known in which an affected mother has given birth to boys with lissencephaly and girls with band heterotopias (Pinard et al. 1994). Rare cases of band heterotopia are associated with *LIS1* missense mutations and with a milder phenotype (Leventer et al. 2001).

From the imaging point of view also, the severity of expression in girls varies from thick subcortical bands, sometimes covered by an abnormal cortex, to hardly detectable thin bands that may be visible only under localized cortical areas. Unilateral and partial band heterotopias may be difficult to recognize and may require special cuts and reformatting on MRI for detection (Gallucci et al. 1991). In boys, the picture is of classical lissencephaly similar to that of *LIS1* cases. However, the anterior part of the cortex is smoother than the posterior part, as opposed to what obtains in patients wiith *LIS1* mutations.

The epilepsy associated with band heterotopias may be amenable to drug therapy. It may also be refractory. Surgical resection has been attempted to no avail.

The *Baraitser–Winter syndrome* includes dysmorphic features and brain abnormalities that consist of classical lissencephaly or of subcortical band heterotopias (Rossi et al. 2003).

• *Pachygyria*. This type represents a less severe end of the lissencephaly spectrum and probably results from similar mechanisms. However, it is heterogeneous and may belong to several syndromes. Clinically pachygyria presents with similar symptoms of variable but lesser severity. MRI shows thickening of the cortex and linear separartion between the cortex and the white matter.

• *Other forms and syndromes of lissencephaly.* Several less common variants of lissencephaly are important to recognize because of different genetic and prognostic consequences (Hennekam and Barth 2003, Raoul et al. 2003) (Table 2.7).

Microlissencephaly consists of extreme congenital microcephaly and agyria or pachygyria with a thick cortex. At least five or six types that may be recessively transmitted have been described with variable thickness of the cortex, localization of any existing sulci, and presence of associated abnormalities such as cerebellar hypoplasia, brainstem atrophy and enlarged ventricles (Ross et al. 2002, Dobyns and Leventer 2003, Sztriha et al. 2004). Some authors (Dobyns and Barkovich 1999) separate these cases from 'oligogyric microcephaly' (Hanefeld 1999), which they consider a form of primary microcephaly rather than a disorder of migration. One of these syndromes may be associated with a mutation of the *reelin* gene (Hong et al. 2000, Crino 2001).

Lissencephaly with cerebellar hypoplasia is another extreme microcephaly with a rudimentary two-layer cerebral cortex and severe hypoplasia of the cerebellum (Ross et al. 2001, Sztriah et al. 2005). It seems to be recessively inherited.

Lissencephaly with corpus callosum agenesis is genetically heterogeneous. Some cases may belong to the *LIS1* group or to that of the microlissencephalies.

X-linked lissencephaly with ambiguous genitalia (XLAG) is a congenital disorder with microcephaly, severe developmental delay, tendency to hypothermia, absence of the corpus callosum and multiple brain anomalies (Berry-Kravis and Israel 1994, Dobyns et al. 1999). Hypoplasia of the genitalia rather than agenesis may be present. XLAG is due to mutations of the aristaless homeobox gene *ARX* on chromosome X33.2 (Uyanik et al. 2003), whose other mutations can also produce several neurological syndromes (Kato et al. 2004, Suri 2005), including X-linked mental retardation (*MRX54*), agenesis of the corpus callosum with abnormal genitalia (see below), and Partington syndrome of mental retardation, ataxia and dystonia, depending on the type of mutation.

Interestingly, lissencephaly with neonatal seizures and severe neurodevelopmental abnormalities has been found to be associated with absence of glutamine (Chapter 8).

The cobblestone complex (Table 2.7)
This term has replaced the previously used denomination of 'type 2 lissencephaly'. In this group of malformations the cortex has a granular surface, and a polymicrogyric appearance is frequently visible together with areas devoid of gyri. The mechanism of formation is primarily that of excess migration of neurons beyond a defective glial limiting membrane (Williams et al. 1984, Dobyns et al. 1996) into the subpial space (Haltia et al. 1997). It is thus completely different from that of classical lissencephaly. In addition, *involvement of muscle* is present in almost all diseases of this group, which include the Walker–Warburg syndrome, muscle–eye–brain disease and Fukuyama congenital muscular dystrophy (Barkovich et al. 1998).

• *Walker–Warburg syndrome* (Cormand et al. 2001) is a complex syndrome that consists of cobblestone cortex (often with areas of polymicrogyria), ocular abnormalities, cerebellar malformations and severe muscular dystrophy. The cortex has the appearance of

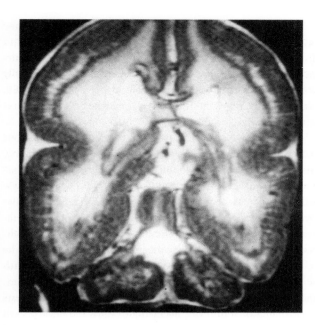

Fig. 2.21. Cobblestone complex (type II lissencephaly). T₂-weighted MRI showing thick, smooth cortex. The underlying thin white band may represent multiple small cysts. Note massive hydrocephalus and absence of the cerebellar vermis.

a double cortical layer due to the presence of the subcortical heterotopic islands, which may be striking (Fig. 2.21). The meninges are thick and have a milky appearance due to massive mesenchymal proliferation, especially around the brainstem. The cerebellum is small and lacks a vermis. The pyramidal tracts are usually absent, and in 75% of cases hydrocephalus is present. It is usually due to fibrosis of the abnormal meninges, but aqueductal stenosis has been reported (Bordarier et al. 1984). There is often fusion of the frontal poles and of the molecular surfaces of cerebellar lamellae. Microscopically, there is complete disruption of cortical architecture, the cortical plate consisting of a variable thickness of poorly oriented cells separated by trabeculae of gliomesenchymal tissue in continuity with that of the meninges. Multiple islands of heterotopic grey matter are aligned parallel to the cortical surface, separated from the overlying cortex by a thin layer of white matter in which thin blood vessels are tangentially aligned. Fibroglial tissue isolates glomerular or trabecular formations of neural cells (Takashima et al. 1987). The cerebellum is totally disorganized. The vermis is usually missing, and multiple cortical round cysts are seen that can be visualized by MRI (D'Amico et al. 2006). Walker–Warburg syndrome is a genetic disorder transmitted as an autosomal recessive character (Dobyns et al. 1985, 1989); it has been shown to be associated with mutations of the *POMT1* gene on chromosome 1p32–34 (Cormand et al. 1999, Beltran-Valero de Bernabe et al. 2002, Balci et al. 2005). Beltran-Valero de Bernabe et al. (2004) have described cases due to mutation in the *fukutin* gene with the same clinical presentation, and more heterogeneity is likely (Chapter 21). However, no mutation is found in the majority of cases (Currier et al. 2005).

The clinical features (Dobyns et al. 1985, Dobyns and Leventer 2003) include severe neurological dysfunction from birth; eye abnormalities with retinal dysplasia in all cases, and microphthalmia and anomalies of the anterior segment (Peters' anomaly, cataracts, persistence of primitive vitreous body) in most; and the presence in some cases of a posterior cephalocele or large posterior fontanelle. Infants with severe neurological abnormalities and hydrocephalus in association with eye anomalies are highly suspect of having type II lissencephaly, which is a relatively common cause of genetic hydrocephalus.

On MRI (Fig. 2.21) the cobblestone cortex appears as moderately thickened, with an irregular or pebbled surface and grey–white interface (van der Knaap et al. 1997). The brainstem is atrophic, and the vermis is small or aplastic. Small, rounded cerebellar cortical cysts are often present (Aida et al. 1994). Walker–Warburg syndrome has been rarely associated with adducted thumbs and aqueductal stenosis (Bordarier et al. 1984) and should be distinguished from the X-linked Becker syndrome (Chapter 6) as the genetic implications are different. Prenatal diagnosis is possible on the basis of hydrocephalus, cephalocele and eye abnormalities (microphthalmia and/or retinal detachment) (Rhodes et al. 1992) and may be confirmed by gene study (Gasser et al. 1998). Muscle involvement is an integral part of cases of type II lissencephaly (Barkovich 1998), although an occasional case with normal eyes and muscle is on record (Dobyns et al. 1996). Widespread necrosis of fibres is present in all muscles, the appearance being reminiscent of that in severe muscular dystrophies. It appears likely that the cerebro-oculo-muscular syndrome (COMS) is closely related to or identical with the Walker–Warburg syndrome.

• *Muscle–eye–brain disease.* In this disease, described by Santavuori et al. (1989, 1998), brain dysfunction is usually less severe. Eye abnormalities mainly consist of severe myopia but may also include such complications as glaucoma and visual failure (Pihko et al. 1995, Haltia et al. 1997). The ventricles are widely dilated and the septum is usually absent. The disease is present at birth but is apparently progressive as shown by the flattening of the ERG after infancy. Flash-evoked potentials are of high amplitude in three quarters of the patients. Mutation of the *POMGnT1* gene mapping to chromosome 1p34–p32 has been demonstrated (Cormand et al. 1999), but heterogeneity has also been shown (Chapter 21).

• *Fukuyama congenital muscular dystrophy* is from the neurological point of view a less severe presentation of the cobblestone cortex group, although severe mental retardation is marked and eye abnormalities are frequent. The clinical presentation is dominated by muscular impairment (Chapter 21). The disorder is recessively inherited and caused by mutation in the gene *FTCD* that codes for the protein fukutin mapping to chromosome 9q31.

• *Glioneural heterotopias* seem to be minor forms of similar abnormalities in the subpial space. These are common in malformed brains but may also occur in brains of normal individuals (Dambska et al. 1986, Hirano et al. 1992). These lesions consist of irregularly shaped nodules of variable size, sometimes of sheets of astrocytes and neurons overlying the molecular layer. *Nodular cortical dysplasia*, also called *status verrucosus*, consists of circumscribed cortical deformities presenting as hemispherical protrusions, 1–2 mm in diameter, on the cortical surface (Friede 1989, Iida et al. 1994); they comprise a core of radial myelinated fibres that projects into the superficial layers and splits as a fountain-head producing a bulge of the upper layers. These nodules, when limited in number, are probably asymptomatic. Similar deformities in large number are present in the brains of patients with glutaric aciduria type 2 (Goodman and Frerman 1984). Together with other abnormalities, they are a common pathological feature of the fetal alcohol syndrome.

The *prognosis of the cobblestone syndromes* is poor, especially that of the Walker–Warburg type. Most affected infants die in a few weeks or months, an occasional patient living to a few years. Patients with severe hydrocephalus should receive a shunt to avoid monstrous growth of the head, but the ultimate prognosis remains dismal. However, the outcome of muscle–eye–brain disease and of Fukuyama dystrophy is less severe, and a spectrum of severity from lethal cases to cases of congenital muscular dystrophy or even limb–girdle dystrophy with normal brain and cognition may be observed (D'Amico et al. 2006).

Kallmann syndrome

A peculiar migration abnormality is the cause of the Kallmann syndrome, comprising anosmia due to absence of olfactory bulb stalks and gyri, hypogonadism, and often mild mental retardation (Christian 1982). This syndrome is genetically heterogeneous but usually transmitted as an X-linked recessive trait. Two genes [*KALIG1*, localized to Xp22.3 (White et al. 1983); and *KALIG2*, a fibroblast growth factor receptor (FGFR1) gene], confirm the genetic heterogneity (Sato et al. 2004, Albuisson et al. 2005). The migration defects involve the olfactory axons and gonadotrophin releasing hormone-secreting neurons that originate from the olfactory placode and normally migrate through the ethmoid to the olfactory bulbs, which do not develop if not reached by axons. The migration of these cells in Kallmann syndrome is blocked in the nasal area because of lack of adhesion molecules, which play a major role in olfactory axon development. Absence of the olfactory bulbs can be visualized by MRI (Truwit et al. 1993).

Disorders of Cortical Organization

According to the classification of Barkovich, this category also includes some disorders of late migration. Like in the other categories, some of the conditions included depend on mechanisms other than disturbed organization. Many cases of focal cortical dysplasia, for example, show abnormal cells of both neuronal and glial origin, indicating abnormal cell differentiation.

The terms *microgyria* and *polymicrogyria* (PMG) refer to an abnormal appearance of cortical gyri that seem to be crowded, too narrow, and form an abnormal convolutional pattern (Fig.

2.22). The macroscopic aspect, however, is variable. In some cases, broad convolutions are apparent that may be difficult to distinguish from areas of pachygyria by looking only at the surface of the brain, but the cortical ribbon is characteristically polymicrogyric with fusion of the molecular layers (Friede 1989, Harding and Copp 1997). Microgyria may be generalized, unilateral, multifocal or focal.

Two major histological types of PMG are observed, but transitional or mixed types are frequent. The most commonly encountered, clearly a developmental disorder, is *unlayered microgyria* (Ferrer 1984, Harding and Copp 1997), in which a single cell layer undulates between the white matter and the molecular layer. In *classical four-layer microgyria*, a first layer of small pyramidal cells underneath the molecular layer is separated by a cell-poor layer from the deep layer containing the large pyramids. The cell-poor layer corresponds to normal layers IV and V, with which it merges at the limits of the microgyric cortex (Williams and Caviness 1984, Evrard et al. 1989). This appearance suggests a postmigrational disorder, occurring towards the fifth or sixth month of pregnancy, with secondary laminar necrosis that could be due to perfusion failure and resulting hypoxia. The occurrence of classical PMG following abnormal events occurring after midgestation such as severe trauma, carbon monoxide intoxication or maternal asphyxia (Larroche 1986, Barth 2003b), and its occurrence in only one member of a monozygous twin pair (Sugama and Kusano 1994), supports this interpretation. Evrard et al. (1989) found two peak periods for perfusion failure: between 20 and 24 weeks, and during the last 10 weeks of gestation.

Perfusion failure may also be responsible for the microgyria that is seen with fetal infections (Marques-Dias et al. 1984), which can produce vascular damage (Barkovich and Lindan 1994) or circulatory insufficiency, and for that located at the margin of porencephalic defects. However, some PMGs may form slightly before the end of the migrational process and may result from an insult to superficial layers, damaging the glial guides before later migrating cells have completed their migration (Dvorak et al. 1978). In these cases, neurons, arrested in their migration, are visible under the area of microgyric cortex (Lyon and Beaugerie 1988, Evrard et al. 1989). Several cases of familial, probably genetically determined cases are on record. Several cases associated with large deletions of the DiGeorge critical region of chromosome 22q11.2 have been described (Bingham et al. 1998, Worthington et al. 2000), suggesting that this might be a factor favouring the occurrence of PMG. Other rare types of PMG are seen in the Zellweger syndrome (Raoul et al. 2003) (Chapter 8) and in some other unusual syndromes such as Delleman syndrome (Moog et al. 2005, Pascual-Castroviejo et al. 2005).

Generalized polymicrogyria

Generalized PMGs may occur in isolation or as part of multiple malformation syndromes. They manifest by epileptic seizures, by mental retardation, often of a severe degree, and by bilateral neurological deficits. MRI can permit recognition of PMG when there is rippling of the brain surface, and fine interdigitations can be made out at the interface of grey and white matter (Raybaud

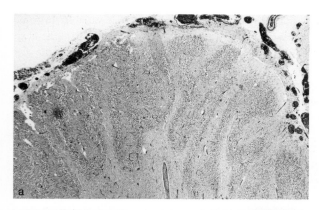

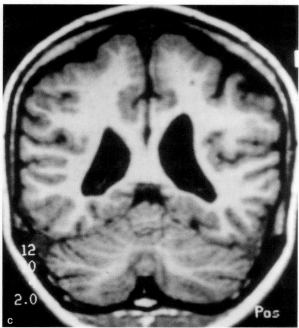

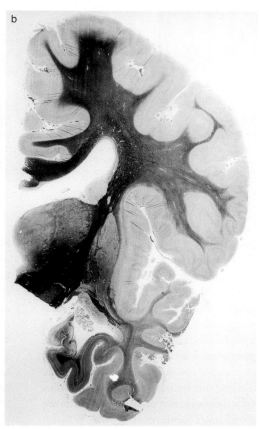

Fig. 2.22. Polymicrogyria. *(a)* Polymicrogyric cortex. Note undulating band of neurons without intervening sulci, indicating that the external appearance of the brain may be that of broad convolutions reminiscent of pachygyria. (Courtesy Dr J-C Larroche, Maternité Port Royal, Paris.) *(b)* Low-power view of coronal section of one hemisphere at midthalamic level, showing the excessively folded and fused miniconvolutions of polymicrogyric cortex. (Courtesy Dr B Harding, Institute of Neurology, London.) *(c)* MRI showing extensive areas of apparent polymicrogyria in upper part of both hemispheres predominating with striated appearance suggesting the existence of miniconvolutions. (Courtesy Dr Kling Chong, Great Ormond Street Hospital, London.)

et al. 1996), but these signs may not be present except on high-resolution MRI and the appearance may then wrongly suggest lissencephaly. PMG should be distinguished from ulegyria, the sclerotic, atrophic convolutions occurring as a late result of hypoxic–ischaemic damage. These present in transverse sections as mushrooms because hypoxic damage is more prominent deep in sulci than on the crown of convolutions. They can occasionally be identified on MRI, but clinical history is essential for diagnosis.

Unilateral polymicrogyria
Cases of *microgyria involving a whole hemisphere* are uncommon. The affected hemisphere is usually small, and the gyral pattern is abnormal throughout. Most patients have congenital hemiparesis but cognitive development is variably affected or may be

normal. In some of these children a distinctive syndrome of seizures especially drop attacks, associated with episodes of continuous spike and wave complexes on EEG in slow sleep (CSWS) has been described (Guerrini et al. 1996a, Caraballo et al. 2004). However, this syndrome does not necessarily herald intractability of seizures, which often stop in a few months or before adolescence, or a poor cognitive outcome (Guerrini et al. 1996b, Caraballo et al. 2004), that may depend in part on the duration of the paroxysmal EEG activity. Consequently, radical surgery or callosotomy should be considered only following an unsuccessful full trial of medical treatment.

Focal polymicrogyria
Focal PMGs are more common than generalized forms. They may

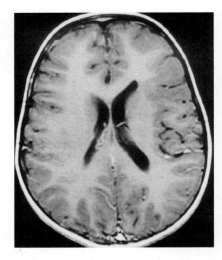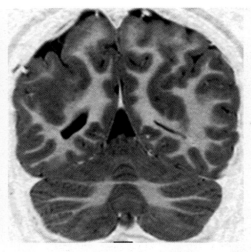

Fig. 2.23. Focal polymicrogyria. *(Left)* Large area of abnormal gyration involving the left frontal lobe. *(Right)* Bilateral sylvian syndrome: coronal cut showing microgyria around both sylvian fissures.

be either isolated or associated with schizencephaly (Barkovich et al. 2001a).

• *Focal PMGs without schizencephaly* (Fig. 2.23). These are common but their frequency in clinical practice is poorly known because many cases are only imaging diagnoses. Likewise, multiple processes can be responsible. Their clinical manifestations are nonspecific and depend on the extent of the microgyric areas, their location and the presence of associated malformations. Some small areas may not give rise to symptoms. Their major manifestation is *focal epilepsy*, often intractable (see below). Some cases of localized cortical dysplasia may be associated with relatively benign forms of epilepsy (Guerrini et al. 1996b). Whether areas of microgyria may be causally related to dyslexia, as suggested by Galaburda et al. (1985), remains uncertain. They are thus studied under the general heading of *focal cortical dysplasia*.

Most cases of focal PMG are sporadic. However, an increasing number of familial cases are being reported (Dobyns and Truwit 1995, Barkovich et al. 2001a, Guerrini and Filippi 2005). Some of these partial forms are part of syndromes of multiple, usually bilateral dysplasia (Barkovich et al. 1999), and some of these may be genetically determined and occur in families.

Bilateral cases of focal PMG include cases of *bilateral parasagittal parieto-occipital PMG* with complex partial seizures, often with a visual onset, reported by Guerrini et al. (1997); *bilateral frontal PMG* (Guerrini et al. 2000); and rare cases of *bilateral parieto-occipital PMG*. A familial form of *frontoparietal PMG* has been mapped to chromosome 16 in 10 families (Chang et al. 2004). It has been shown to be due to mutations in the *CPR56* gene (Piao et al. 2006); however, the syndrome appears to be genetically heterogeneous. Ferrie et al. (1995) described posterior cortical dysgenesis as a familial condition in two siblings. In most such cases, the actual histological nature of the disturbance is not known, even though the MR images are suggestive of pachygyria.

The *bilateral perisylvian syndrome* consists of a characteristic bilateral central rolandic and sylvian microgyria with thickened cortex that may be more or less symmetrical. PMGs, either four-layered or unlayered, have been demonstrated histologically in a few cases. Most patients have pseudobulbar palsy with dysarthria, dysphagia and limited ability to mimic facial expressions, and most have seizures (Kuzniecky and Andermann 1994, Kuzniecky et al. 1994). Such cases were also described as developmental Foix–Chavany–Marie syndrome. A wider spectrum of manifestations with both severe seizures including infantile spasms and milder cases presenting with language disorder (Saletti et al. 2007) has been reported in infants. Arthrogryposis of central origin is present in some patients (Hageman et al. 1994, Kuzniecky and Andermann 1994, Kuzniecky et al. 1994). *Genetic factors* are operative in some of these cases, with X-linked recessive, autosomal recessive or dominant inheritance (Guerreiro et al. 2000, Guerrrini and Filippi 2005).

• *PMGs associated with schizencephaly.* Schizencephaly (formerly termed 'true' porencephaly) (Friede 1989) represents an interesting and fairly common anomaly. It refers here only to clefts or cavities of developmental origin that extend through the full depth of the mantle from the ventricle to the subarachnoid space. It consists of clefts that may be virtual, their two walls being apposed to form a pia–arachnoid seam or widely open. Microgyria is almost consistently present in the immediate vicinity of schizencephalic defects. Areas of microgyria are lined on both sides of the cleft and extend down to the ventricle. Microgyria is often present on the contralateral side even in cases of unilateral cleft, particularly in the insular area. Microgyria may be associated with nodular heterotopia in the white matter (Friede 1989) or with other malformations such as agenesis of the corpus callosum. The presence of microgyria indicates that the clefts existed before the end of migration and prevented neurons from reaching their normal location. This does not imply that they represent failure

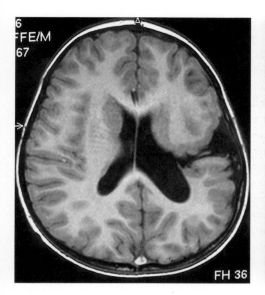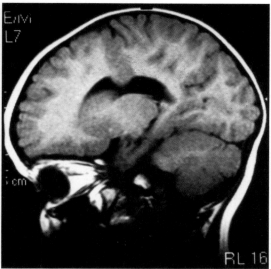

Fig. 2.24. Schizencephaly. *(Left)* Axial MRI showing wide cleft in central right hemisphere extending from the cortex to the ventricle. *(Right)* Sagittal cut in another case showing thick, microgyric cortex surrounding the cleft.

of the mantle to form, as implied by the term schizencephaly. The abnormality is more probably due to early destruction of the mantle, perhaps of circulatory origin, with faulty repair and interference with neuronal migration (Menezes et al. 1988, Battaglia and Granata 2003, Curry et al. 2005). Rare familiar cases are on record (Haverkamp et al. 1995). Granata et al. (1997) suggested that some cases are associated with mutations in the homeobox gene EMX 2 (Brunelli et al. 1996), and one familial case with the same mutation of this gene in two brothers is on record (Granata et al. 1997). However, this finding has been replicated in only a few cases (Kato and Dobyns 2003). Late cases with evidence of scarring and calcification are on record (Menezes et al. 1988). The clefts are most often located in the opercular area; they are frequently bilateral but often asymmetrical. In 75% of cases, the septum pellucidum is missing (Menezes et al. 1988, Barkovich and Norman 1988a). Absence of the septum pellucidum is strongly associated with a central, perisylvian location of the clefts (Raybaud et al. 2001). Even when schizencepahaly is unilateral, cortical dysplasia is often present in the opposite hemisphere. Large bilateral defects, so-called 'basket brain', constitute the most severe form of schizencephaly.

The clinical features of schizencephaly are extremely variable, and the severity of clinical features correlates with the importance of anatomical anomalies, being greater with open-lip clefts (Denis et al. 2000, Battaglia abd Granata 2003). Bilateral, open defects give rise to severe involvement (Barkovich and Kjos 1992, Guerrini and Filippi 2005). Some patients have quadriplegia and profound mental retardation. Unilateral clefts usually manifest with hemiplegia and/or focal epilepsy (Caraballo et al. 2004). With the use of neuroimaging it has been realized that many cases are much less severe, with mild retardation, congenital hemiplegia, a large head or even isolated partial seizures. The involvement of both sylvian and insular regions can be responsible for a biopercular syndrome with facial apraxia and speech difficulties (Becker

et al. 1989). Epilepsy is present in about 80% of patients (Granata et al. 1996).

The diagnosis is made by CT or MRI (Fig. 2.24), which not only shows the clefts but also demonstrates the presence of heterotopic grey matter alongside them, as well as cortical anomalies of the contralateral insular region in many apparently unilateral cases (Menezes et al. 1988, Aniskiewicz et al. 1990, Barkovich and Kjos 1992). Prenatal diagnosis is possible (Denis et al. 2001). Absence of the septum pellucidum may be the most obvious anomaly and should lead to careful search for narrow clefts or atypical gyration (Barkovich and Norman 1988a, Menezes et al. 1988).

Schizencephalies located to other brain areas – such as the ventral aspect of the brain, the orbital fissure, the posterior midline or the mesial occipital area (Granata et al. 1996) – are less common. Rare familial cases are on record (Haverkamp et al. 1995).

The diagnosis of schizencephaly is generally easy. However, large lesions may be difficult to distinguish from some cases of holoprosencephaly because of the depth and vertical location of the sylvian fissure, while minor lesions with septal agenesis may be difficult to separate from septo-optic dysplasia, especially as a double-contoured papilla has been reported (Menezes et al. 1988). Surgery with resection of the microgyric area is possible.

• *Focal cortical dysplasias* (see also Chapter 15). Although some focal dysplasias include areas of PMG, most are not usually PMGs from the histological point of view, and the non-committal term of focal cortical dysplasia, which can include both abnormalities of migration and of organization and, in some cases, disorders of proliferation and differentiation of neuroblasts, is thus preferable. A considerable number of reports have appeared in the epilepsy literature over the past 20 years (see Janota and Polkey 1992, Guerrini and Filippi 2005). Focal dysplasias can be

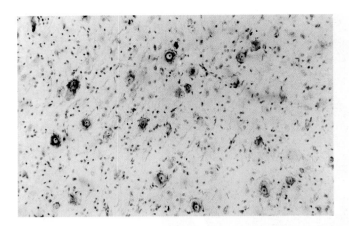

Fig. 2.25. Cortical biopsy of a child with focal dysplasia. Large neurons are irregularly located within cortex. Some neurons show characteristic peripheral condensation of chromatin. (Courtesy Dr B Harding, Institute of Neurology, Queen Square, London.)

TABLE 2.8
Classification of the cortical dysplasias*

Non-Taylor type cortical dysplasias
    Architectural dysplasias
        Disruption of cortical architecture (poor lamination, ectopic neurons
            in white matter, abnormal cell density in layer (1) without cellular
            abnormalities
    Cytoarchitectural dysplasias
        Disruption of cortical architecture as above
        Giant neurons
        Dysmorphic neurons

Taylor-type cortical dysplasias
    Same abnormalities as in previous types
    Balloon cells of large size staining both with glial (GFP) and neuronal
    (synaptophysin) markers, especially in deep cortical layers

*Modified from Tassi et al. (2002).

found in any cortical area. Opercular dysplasia is not rare (Ambrosetto 1992, Sébire et al. 1996). In fact, many cases of localized cortical dysplasia affect this area electively. In areas of cortical dysplasia, the cortex is firm and the gyri are enlarged. Histologically, the picture varies from simple disorganization of laminae or columns with subcortical heterotopic neurons, to more complex anomalies with giant neurons and 'balloon cells' as well as giant multinucleated astrocytes (Taylor et al. 1971, Tassi et al. 2002, Alonso-Nanclares et al. 2005) (Fig. 2.25).

Pathologically, there is still much discussion over the classification of these malformations (Palmini et al. 2004). At least two types are recognized, known as *Taylor* and *non-Taylor type cortical dysplasias*. A recent classification (Tassi et al. 2002) distinguishes three types: architectural dysplasia, in which cortical structure is disrupted but no giant neurons or abnormal cells are present; cyto-architectural dysplasia in which, in addition to abnormal cortical organization, giant and/or dysmorphic neurons are seen; and Taylor type dysplasia in which there are also 'balloon cells' that resemble those present in tuberous sclerosis lesions (Table 2.8). These cells stain with both neuronal and glial markers and result from an early disturbance of cell differentiation. Cor-

tical dysplasias may affect any part of the cortex and are a major cause of focal epilepsy, often intractable (Fig. 2.26). Taylor type lesions tend to predominate in the frontal and parietal lobes, whereas the other types are more often encountered in the temporal lobes (Kuzniecky et al. 1994). The major clinical manifestation is with focal seizures (Hamiwka et al. 2005, Fauser et al. 2006) often but not always refractory to drug treatment (see Chapter 15). Small areas of cortical dysplasia that were responsible for focal cortical myoclonus and focal motor seizures in four children have been reported (Kuzniecky et al. 1986). Similar lesions were found in a case of status epilepticus (Desbiens et al. 1993). Recent studies of the microanatomy, molecular pathogenesis and pathophysiology of these lesions have described their intimate structure and shown their intrinsic epileptogenic potential (Bentivoglio et al. 2003, Alonso-Nanclares et al. 2005, Crino 2005).

Imaging is basically by MRI, but detection (Chapter 15) may be difficult and advanced MR techniques may be necessary. Even so, a significant proportion of cases can escape recognition. Taylor-type dysplasias may have distinctive MR features, especially high signal in the white matter underlying the lesion, sometimes extending towards the ventricle, the so-called transmantle cortical dysplasia (Barkovich et al. 1997). Architectural and cyto-architectural dysplasias are more often marked by a thin cortex on MRI (Tassi et al. 2002). Focal cortical dysplasia may be associated with developmental tumours (gangliogliomas and developmental neuroepithelial tumours) in the same area of brain.

Surgical treatment for epilepsy due to focal dysplasia is possible in a significant proportion of cases and may control the seizures (Tassi et al. 2002; Cascino et al. 2004; Fauser et al. 2004, 2006; Hamiwka et al. 2005).

Most cases of cortical dysplasia appear to be sporadic but familial cases are on record (Kuzniecky et al. 1994).

Some *rare syndromes* feature pachygyria-like cortex in association with extracerebral abnormalities: congenital nephrosis in male siblings (Robain and Deonna 1983, Palm et al. 1986); familial lymphoedema and vermian agenesis (Hourihane et al. 1993); congenital short bowel (Nézelof et al. 1976); and familial pachygyria with disseminated brain calcification and ataxia (Harbord et al. 1990).

The major interest of focal cortical dysplasias is the surgical possibilities they may offer. These are discussed in Chapter 15.

• *Cortical microdysgenesis – minor cortical dysgenesis.* Minor anomalies of cortical arrangement (microdysgenesis) include persistence of the subpial or Ranke–Brun subpial layer (Evrard et al. 1989); presence of aggregates of large neurons in the plexiform zone; fragmented appearance of superficial neuronal layers; excess number of 'ectopic' neurons subcortically and throughout the cortex; and excess number of cells in the molecular layer. Such anomalies are frequently found in the brain of patients with epilepsy or mental retardation but they are also present in the cortex of normal individuals. Meencke and Veith (1992) have suggested that these could be the anatomical basis for cortical hyperexcitability in generalized epilepsy. Meencke and Veith found microdysgenesis in 32.7% of 591 brains of persons with epilepsy, as

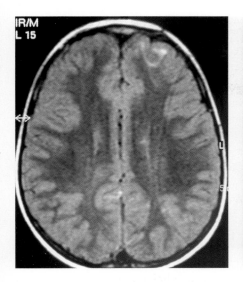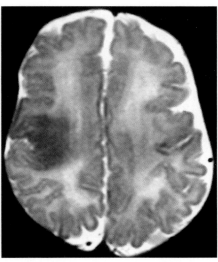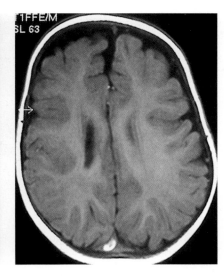

Fig. 2.26. *(Left)* Taylor-type cortical dysplasia confirmed histologically in a boy with intractable focal seizures. T$_2$-weighted MRI shows area of abnormal cortex in the right frontal lobe with high signal underlying the abnormal cortex. Resection of the abnormal cortex resulted in control of seizures. *(Middle)* MRI of another boy with seizures shows clearly the dysplastic area at 6 months of age, which became much less obvious at 18 months *(right)*.

against 6% of 7374 control brains, suggesting this anomaly plays a signficant role. Galaburda et al. (1985) found an excess of foci of cortical dysgenesis with a left temporal predominance in 4 brains of dyslexic subjects as compared with 10 control brains and thought they might play a role in the genesis of dyslexia. Cohen et al. (1989) attributed the dysphasia of their patient to bilateral minor dysgenesis involving the planum temporale and opercular area bilaterally. These provocative findings must await confirmation. Microdysgenesis is often associated with other epileptogenic lesions.

Other minor abnormalities of the cerebral hemispheres include abnormal synaptogenesis, and especially disturbances in the process of programmed cell death (apoptosis) that probably plays a major role in brain development but is currently poorly understood.

Other rare abnormalities include congenital Pick cell encephalopathy (De Léon et al. 1986), and localized dysgenesis (Tychsen and Hoyt 1985) resulting in hemianopsia or delayed operculation. Delayed early myelination may occur in cases with abnormal gestation, e.g. maternal diabetes mellitus or placental insufficiency, as well as in infants with severe prolonged asphyxia or other damaging factors (Dambska and Laure-Kaminowska 1990).

ABNORMALITIES OFTEN ASSOCIATED WITH DISORDERS OF CORTICAL DEVELOPMENT
Several deformities often coexist with migration disorders. However, they may also occur in isolation or in association with other malformations. They include agenesis of the corpus callosum, schizencephaly ('true' porencephaly), septo-optic dysplasia and colpocephaly.

Agenesis and dysgenesis of the corpus callosum
This may be complete or partial. In the latter case, the posterior part is usually missing because the corpus callosum develops in

an anteroposterior manner, although cases of anterior agenesis can also occur (Aicardi et al. 1987, Barkovich and Norman 1988b, Sztriha 2005). Atypical forms, difficult to separate from holoprosencephaly, may be encountered (Barkovich 1990). Callosal agenesis is relatively common. Its prevalence in the general population is estimated to be 3–7/1000 (Bedeschi et al. 2006). Its apparent frequency has risen with the introduction of CT and MRI. Jeret et al. (1987) found 33 cases in a series of 1447 CT scans. Even now, the diagnosis is made preferentially in patients with neurological manifestations, so that the true frequency is not known.

The absent callosal commissure is usually replaced by two longitudinal bundles, known as longitudinal corpora callosa or Probst bundles, that course on the inner aspect of the hemispheres (Fig. 2.27). Sulci on the internal aspect have a radial disposition, and enlargement of the occipital horn that maintains their fetal morphology, the so-called colpocephaly, is common (Noorani et al. 1988) (Fig. 2.27). Other associated abnormalities frequently include the formation of cysts dorsal to the third ventricle, communicating or noncommunicating (Yokota et al. 1984, Griebel et al. 1995, Barkovich et al. 2001b) cerebellar vermis and brainstem anomalies, and a miscellany of CNS malformations such as heterotopia, abnormalities of gyration, or cephaloceles (Jeret et al. 1987, Barkovich and Norman 1988b, Serur et al. 1988). Giant cysts may have a favourable outcome despite their impressive size (Lena et al. 1995, Haverkamp et al. 2002). CNS malformations were found in in 33% of patients with complete and 42% of those with partial agenesis in one series (Bedeschi et al. 2006). It is these associated anomalies that are responsible for the clinical manifestations. Lipoma of the corpus callosum (Fig. 2.28) is almost invariably associated with agenesis of the structure (Zee et al. 1981, Vade and Horowitz 1992). Peripheral malformations are common (Parrish et al. 1979). Eye abnormalities are especially frequent (Aicardi et al. 1987). Hypoplasia of the corpus

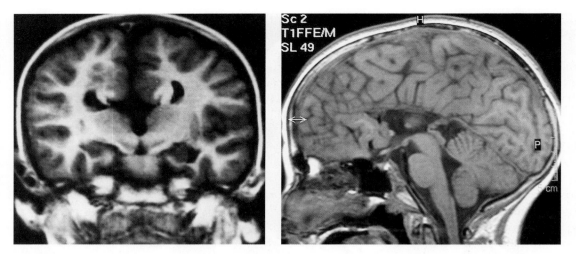

Fig. 2.27. Agenesis of the corpus callosum. *(Left)* MRI (inversion–recovery sequence) clearly shows longitudinal corpora callosa (Probst bundles) alongside inner aspects of ventricular bodies. *(Right)* Sagittal view showing complete absence of corpus callosum and radial distribution of the sulci of the internal aspect of hemisphere.

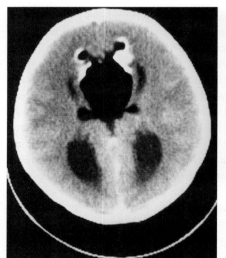

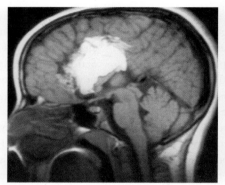

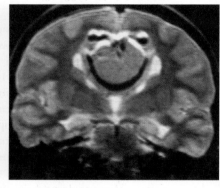

Fig. 2.28. Lipoma of the corpus callosum in an 8-year old girl with partial complex seizures but no neurodevelopmental abnormalities. *(Left)* CT scan showing large mass of fat density separating anterior horns of lateral ventricles, peripheral calcification and two small lateral expansions of the fatty mass. *(Middle)* MRI, sagittal cut showing replacement of corpus callosum by lipoma. *(Right)* MRI, T$_2$-weighted sequence showing complexity of mass and complete replacement of callosum by fatty tissue.

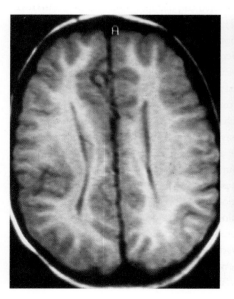

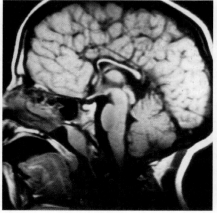

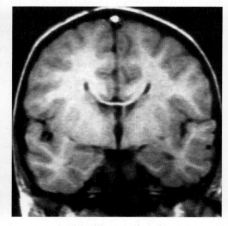

Fig. 2.29. Hypoplasia of the corpus callosum. *(Left)* MRI (axial cut) showing ventricular appearance consistent with callosal agenesis. *(Centre)* Sagittal cut showing complete callosum with genu and splenium, but short and thin. Note radial disposition of mesial gyri. *(Right)* Frontal cut showing wide separation of ventricular bodies by prolapsing limbic gyrus.

callosum (Bodensteiner et al. 1994) (Fig. 2.29) may be a minor form of callosal dysgenesis but is more often the consequence of cortical neuronal loss.

The *aetiology* is multiple. At least 46 malformation syndromes or metabolic disorders and 30 mutated genes have been identified (Kamnasaran 2005). In nonsyndromic forms, genetic transmission is rare although a few familial cases are on record with autosomal recessive (Finlay et al. 2000), X-linked recessive (Menkes et al. 1964, Kaplan 1983) and autosomal dominant inheritance (Aicardi et al. 1987). A large number of chromosomal defects, including trisomies 8, 13, 16 and 18, as well as a miscellany of less common chromosomal accidents have been found. Serur et al. (1988) reviewed 81 cases from the literature, of which 21 had trisomy 8, 14 had trisomy 13–15, and 18 involved abnormalities of chromosomes 17 or 18. Of 34 karyotypes they performed, 2 showed trisomy 8. Subtelomeric aberrations were found in 5% of the cases of Bedeschi et al. (2006). Environmental factors include the fetal alcohol syndrome. Several metabolic diseases, especially hyperglycinaemia (Dobyns 1989), pyruvate dehydrogenase deficiency (Bamforth et al. 1988, Raoul et al. 2003) and other metabolic disorders collectively account for up to 2% of cases of callosal agenesis. Most cases are of unknown origin.

The clinical manifestations of callosal agenesis can be described under two different headings: nonsyndromic and syndromic forms (Davila-Guttierez 2002).

Nonsyndromic forms are the most common (Jeret et al. 1987, Serur et al. 1988). An unknown proportion of cases remain completely asymptomatic or are discovered only because of a large head. Most patients have mental retardation, seizures and/or a large head (Aicardi et al. 1987). Hypertelorism is a frequent finding. Eighty-two per cent of the patients of Jeret et al. (1987) had mental retardation or delayed development, 43% had seizures, and 31% had cerebral palsy. However, a normal cognitive development was observed in 9 of 63 children (Bedeschi et al. 2006) and may be more frequent as asyptomatic cases are likely to be underdiagnosed. The seizures may be of any type, including infantile spasms, but more frequently are focal. Although a large head, sometimes as much as 5–7 SD above the mean, is common, indications for shunting should be extremely conservative as many of these cases of 'hydrocephalus' spontaneously stabilize without raising any problem. The macrocephaly may be due in part to the presence of giant cysts located dorsally to the third ventricle (Barkovich et al. 2001b). Specific disturbances of interhemispheric transfer are either totally lacking or only minimal (Jeeves and Temple 1987). However, subtle difficulties of interhemispheric communication and topographic memory have been reported. Endocrinological abnormalities may be present in rare cases (Paul et al. 2003).

Syndromic forms are listed in Table 2.9.

Aicardi syndrome (Chevrie and Aicardi 1986, Aicardi 2005) accounts for perhaps 1% of cases of infantile spasms and is probably due to an X-linked dominant mutation. It occurs almost exclusively in girls, although two cases in boys with an XXY chromosome complement have been reported. Only one familial case in two sisters is known (Molina et al. 1989). Characteristic features of the syndrome include infantile spasms and specific choroidal lacunae, often in association with coloboma of the optic disc. Vertebrocostal abnormalities are present in half the cases. The outcome is poor, with persistence of seizures and severe mental retardation. However, the spectrum of severity is wider than previously thought (Menezes et al. 1994). In rare cases, the corpus callosum may be present (Aicardi 1994, 1996). The choroidal lacunae and associated MRI abnormalities (periventricular heterotopia, dysplastic cortex, ependymal cysts) permit the diagnosis (Fig. 2.30). Pathologically, there are multiple areas of heterotopia and polymicrogyria of the unlayered type in the brain (Billette de Villemeur et al. 1992), while the so-called lacunae represent thinning of the pigment epithelium and choroid with loss of pigment granules. Ependymal cysts are frequently found around the third ventricle, and cysts or tumours of the choroid plexus may reach a large size (Aicardi 2005). They may permit prenatal diagnosis when found in association with callosal agenesis.

Other syndromic forms are rare or mostly restricted to certain ethnic groups.

A familial *syndrome of callosal agenesis with abnormal genitalia*, which may also feature microcephaly and other CNS anomalies, is a part of the much larger spectrum of disorders associated with mutations in the ARX gene on chromosome Xp22.3 (Hartmann et al. 2004).

Andermann syndrome was described in French Canadians in the Lake St John region (Andermann 1981) but a few cases have been reported outside Canada. The syndrome features involvement of the peripheral nervous system in addition to callosal agenesis or hypotrophy. Agenesis of the corpus callosum is often a part of oro-facio-digital syndrome type I.

The *syndrome of periodic hypothermia and diaphoresis* (Shapiro et al. 1969) can be treated effectively with clonidine, which was tried because of the discovery of an altered norepinephrine metabolism in this syndrome. However, half the cases are not accompanied by callosal agenesis (Sheth et al. 1994). Callosal agenesis with episodic hyperthermia ('reverse Shapiro syndrome') has been reported (Hirayama et al. 1994).

The diagnosis of callosal agenesis rests on neuroimaging. The diagnosis of complete agenesis is easy by ultrasonography, CT or MRI (Aicardi et al. 1987, Jeret et al. 1987, Serur et al. 1988). MRI is far superior for the diagnosis of partial agenesis. The diagnosis by imaging is generally easy, CT or MRI showing ascension of the third ventricle, and wide separation of the frontal horns with the classical image of 'bull horns' on frontal cuts. Diffusion tensor MR (Lee et al. 2005) allows visualization of the abnormally coursing tracts, especially the Probst bundles that run posteriorly alongside the ventricle and do not cross to the opposite side.

Prenatal diagnosis is possible from 22 weeks (Fig. 2.31) (Bennett et al. 1996, Simon et al. 2000a). A decision to terminate is difficult to take without reservation until more is known about the incidence of asymptomatic cases. Blum et al. (1990) reported that 6 of 12 infants in whom callosal agenesis had been diagnosed antenatally had a normal development at 2–8 years of age. Moutard et al. (2003) followed 17 cases of *isolated* agenesis

TABLE 2.9
Syndromic forms of corpus callosum agenesis

Syndrome	Clinical features	Genetics*	Associated malformations	References
Callosal agenesis constantly present[1]				
Aicardi syndrome	Infantile spasms and partial seizures, choroidoretinal lacunae and disc coloboma, severe mental retardation, vertebrocostal anomalies, 'split brain' EEG, ependymal cysts. Seen only in girls	XL dominant, lethal for males[2]	Periventricular heterotopia, cysts of choroid plexus, other intracranial cysts, microgyria, anomalies of posterior fossa	Chevrie and Aicardi (1986), Aicardi (2005)
Shapiro syndrome	Episodic hypothermia and diaphoresis	Nonfamilial	Hypothalamic lesion probably responsible for the syndrome that may occur with an intact callosum (Sheth et al. 1994)	Shapiro et al. (1969), Klein et al. (2001)
Reverse Shapiro syndrome	Hyperthermia, episodic		See Chapter 4	Hirayama et al. (1994)
Andermann syndrome	Neuropathy (mixed motor and sensory), peculiar facies	AR	See Chapter 20	Andermann (1981), Casaubon et al. (1996), Howard et al. (2002), Uyanik et al. (2006)
Acrocallosal syndrome	Mental retardation, dysmorphism	AR	Facial dysmorphism	Thyen et al. (1992)
X-linked lissencephaly	Ambiguous genitalia	XL	See text	Kitamura et al. (2002), Barth (2003a)
Mowat–Wilson syndrome	Callosal agenesis, mental retardation, facial dysmorphism, Hirschprung disease	AR (*2FXHB* mutations)[3]	Hypospadias, Hirschsprung disease	Ishihara et al. (2004), Sztriha et al. (2005)
Callosal agenesis inconstant feature				
Oro-facio-digital syndrome	Lingual hamartomas, abnormal buccal frenula, digital anomalies, sparse hair, mild mental retardation, limited to girls	XL dominant, lethal for males	Interhemispheric cysts, micropolygyria, dysplasia of cerebellum and pons	Towfighi et al. (1985), Leão and Ribeiro-Silva (1995)
Dandy–Walker syndrome	Vermian agenesis, hydrocephalus	Sporadic[4]	Abnormal inferior olive	Hirsch et al. (1984), Klein et al. (2003)
Lissencephaly	See text	Usually sporadic	Cortical malformation (see text)	Aicardi et al. (1987)
Apert syndrome	Acrocephalosyndactyly (see Chapter 6), callosal agenesis only occasional	AD	See Chapter 5	Chapter 5
Trisomy 8	See Chapter 5	Sporadic	See Chapter 5	Serur et al. (1988)
Meckel–Gruber syndrome	Callosal agenesis only occasional	AR (at least 3 different loci)	See text	Aicardi et al. (1987)
Di George syndrome	Facial dysmorphism, hypocalcaemia with neonatal seizures due to aplasia of parathyroid glands	Sporadic (rare cases dominant)	See Chapter 4	Conley et al. (1979), Phelan et al. (2001)
Goldenhar syndrome	Epibulbar dermoids, ear malformations, preauricular fibrochondromas	Sporadic	See Chapter 4	Wilson (1983)

*Where known. AD = autosomal dominant; AR = autosomal recessive; XL = X-linked.
[1]However, may be absent in Shapiro syndrome and in rare cases of Aicardi syndrome.
[2]Only one familial case known.
[3]Autosomal recessive inheritance demonstrated in only a few cases.
[4]Rare familial cases.

prenatally diagnosed with repeated IQ measurements. All had an IQ within normal limits at 6 years of age, with a trend towards low-normal levels. Nine children in the study by Bedeschi et al. (2006) had a normal development. However, 2 of 9 children diagnosed prenatally by MRI without associated anomalies were retarded (Volpe et al. 2006). Cases associated with other malformations or chromosomal anomalies invariably have a poor outcome. Fetal karyotyping and complete examination for associated malformations are therefore essential.

Septo-optic dysplasia
Septo-optic dysplasia consists of the association of optic nerve hypoplasia with absence of the septum pellucidum. Facial dysmorphism or endocrine abnormalities, especially growth hormone

TABLE 2.11
Some syndromes featuring genetic nonprogressive* cerebellar hypoplasia

Syndrome	Features	Genetics[1]	References
Joubert syndrome	Ataxia, hyperpnoea, mental retardation, abnormal eye movements	AR	Gleeson et al. (2004)
Congenital cerebellar hypoplasia (CCH)	Congenital ataxia, mental retardation	AR	Wichman et al. (1985)
		XD	Fenichel and Phillips (1989)
		XR	Renier et al. (1983)
	Less severe, no or only mild mental retardation	AD	Rivier and Echenne (1992)
Sutherland–Gillespie syndrome	Congenital ataxia, iris hypoplasia, mental retardation	AR	Nevin and Lim (1990)
Congenital cerebellar hypoplasia with hypogonadism	Ataxia, hypogonadism, retinopathy in some cases	AR	De Michele et al. (1990)
PEHO syndrome	Peripheral oedema, ataxia, hypsarrhythmia, optic atrophy	AR	Salonen et al. (1991)
Congenital cerebellar ataxia with retinopathy	Ataxia, mental retardation, visual problems	AR	Dooley et al. (1992)
Malamud–Cohen syndrome	Cerebellar ataxia	XR	Young et al. (1987)
Norman syndrome[2]	Ataxia and mental retardation (severe or mild)	AR	Pascual-Castroviejo et al. (1994)
Congenital cerebellar ataxia with endosteal sclerosis	Ataxia and mental retardation	AR	Charrow et al. (1991)
Cerebellar agenesis and diabetes insipidus	Ataxia (asymptomatic)	?	Zafeiriou et al. (2004)

*For some syndromes it may be impossible to decide whether they are static or very slowly progressive. Only cerebellar hypoplasia with ataxia is shown here. Syndromes without cerebellar signs such as Dandy–Walker or Walker–Warburg omitted.
[1]AR = autosomal recessive; AD = autosomal dominant; XD = X-linked dominant; XR = X-linked recessive.
[2]Regarded by some authors as a progressive degenerative disorder. Probably heterogeneous group.

molar tooth sign is not specific for Joubert syndrome and may be found in several conditions including the Dekaban–Arima (Kumada et al. 2004), Senior–Locken, COACH and orofacial type 6 syndromes, in some cases of cephalocele associated with cortical renal cysts (Satran et al. 1999, Gleeson et al. 2004) that are designated as Joubert-related syndromes, and in the case of pontine cap dysplasia recently reported by Barth et al. (2007). The major features of Joubert syndrome, especially the respiratory abnormalities, are accounted for by developmental defects of the brainstem (Harmant-Van Rijckevorsel et al. 1983).

The *outcome* is variable. Mental retardation is the rule but is of variable degree (Hodgkins et al. 2004). A normal intelligence may be preserved in some cases. Supportive treatment and physiotherapy and appropriate education are always justified.

• *Other rare syndromes of vermal agenesis* (Bordarier and Aicardi 1990) are shown in Table 2.10.

Aplasia and hypoplasia of the cerebellum (Table 2.11)
Major developmental defects of the cerebellum that affect predominantly the hemispheres (Robain et al. 1987) or about equally the hemispheres and vermis constitute a heterogeneous collection of rare anomalies with variable pathology and clinical manifestations (Sarnat and Alcala 1980, Robain et al. 1987, Altman et al. 1992). Cases of probable atrophy and of congenital pontocerebellar atrophies are discussed in Chapter 9. There is considerable diagnostic confusion as many apparent malformations are in fact acquired diseases due to destructive or metabolic processes (Sener 1995, Boltshauser 2004). Proper classification of developmental cerebellar defects is arduous. Friede (1989) argues that the classical separation into neocerebellar versus paleocerebellar

hypoplasia is artificial and that it may be wiser, in many cases, to talk of aplasia of the anterior or posterior cerebellar lobes.

Total cerebellar aplasia is exceptional (Glickstein 2004). Surprisingly, it is not always associated with clinical manifestations. In fact, cerebellar remnants are probably always present (Gardner 2001) and the terms 'hypoplasia' or 'atrophy' are more accurate than 'agenesis'. Cerebellar agenesis has been reported in association with diabetes insipidus (Zafeiriou et al. 2004). *Hypoplasia* is less uncommon and may be predominantly unilateral. In some cases it is restricted to specific structures such as the flocculus. Abnormalities of deep cerebellar and brainstem nuclei and dysplasia of the inferior olivary body are frequent concomitants. In some cases hydrocephalus is present (Friede 1989), and other anomalies such as callosal agenesis or arhinencephaly may occur.

Unilateral aplasia (Boltshauser et al. 1996, Kilickesmez et al. 2004) is less rare and is often asymptomatic. It may be associated with ipsilateral facial angioma and various abnormalities of cerebral and/or peripheral vessels in the PHACES syndrome (Pascual-Castroviejo et al. 2003, Bhattacharya et al. 2004) (see Chapter 3).

Clinical manifestations are extremely variable. They may be absent altogether or include ataxia, dysequilibrium and other cerebellar signs. Various degrees of mental retardation are common and may be the only feature. Some patients present as cases of ataxic cerebral palsy (Chapter 7). In most cases motor signs are prominent, but in some patients autistic features or microcephaly may be evident.

The diagnosis of cerebellar hypoplasia is mainly radiological (Fig. 2.33). Diffuse hypoplasia may be difficult to distinguish from Dandy–Walker variant by CT, and megacistern is frequently mistaken for cerebellar hypoplasia. Differential signs include visualization of the falx cerebelli, which is characteristic of

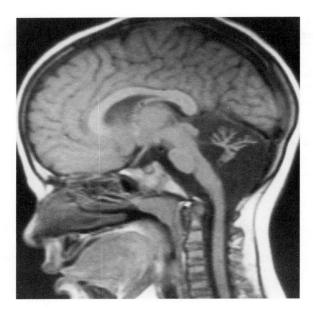

Fig. 2.33. Cerebellar atrophy of unknown origin in 8-year-old girl, affecting mostly the vermis. Part of the inferior vermis may be completely missing.

a cisternal image, and the presence of a complete vermis on sagittal MRI.

Some of the cases of cerebellar hypoplasia are part of genetic syndromes but these are far from being well-defined. Some feature isolated congenital ataxia with various modes of transmission, while additional features are present in others (Al Shahwan et al. 1995) (Table 2.11). An association with chromosomal aberration has been reported (de Azevedo-Moreira et al. 2005, Harper et al. 2007).

Other unusual cerebellar malformations
Tectocerebellar dysraphia (Mori et al. 1994, Dehdashti et al. 2004) is a complex anomaly that includes an inverted cerebellum developed inside the fourth ventricle, hypoplasia of the vermis and occipital cephalocele.

Rhombencephalosynapsis (Toelle et al. 2002) designates congenital fusion of the cerebellar hemispheres with fusion of the dentate nuclei on the midline and aqueductal atresia. Mild cases may be compatible with prolonged survival with only mild symptoms.

Complex malformation of the cerebellum in association with cephalocele may result from ischaemic destruction of a previously normally formed cerebellum as a consequence of arterial compression by a diverticulum of the fourth ventricle.

Dentato-olivary dysplasia responsible for neonatal tonic seizures reminiscent of Ohtahara syndrome has been found in a few patients (Harding and Boyd 1991, Robain and Dulac 1992). A genetic origin is likely (Harding and Copp 1997).

DISTURBANCES OF CEREBELLAR CORTICAL ORGANIZATION
Minor defects in microscopic organization of the cerebellar cortex

are extremely common. Rorke et al. (1968) found them in 84% of 147 cerebella. They have no clinical significance when not associated with other significant abnormalities. The so-called degeneration of the granular layer (Pascual-Castroviejo et al. 1994) is described in Chapter 9 even though its degenerative nature is far from certain.

Hypertrophy of the granular layer is probably a hamartomatous lesion intermediate between malformations and tumours. It is described in Chapter 13.

Cysts of the cerebellum, usually multiple, small and rounded, are found in many cases of the cobblestone group of migration disorders (see above).

PRENATAL DIAGNOSIS, TREATMENT AND PREVENTION OF BRAIN MALFORMATIONS

The possibilities for active treatment of brain malformations are limited. Those malformations that induce hydrocephalus can be effectively managed by ventriculo-peritoneal shunt or other shunting operations. Even in such cases, however, neurodevelopmental dysfunction may persist after successful operation because diffuse abnormalities are present in addition to hydrocephalus. The drug treatment of epilepsy has significantly progressed over the past decades, and surgery, especially for epileptogenic dysplasias (Chapter 15), has become a practical possibility in some cases and will continue to develop, being as yet under-utilized. For many patients, however, rehabilitation and physiotherapy are the major tools. Special education is needed in many cases, and institutionalization may be necessary for the most severe cases.

Prevention of CNS malformations is one of the major challenges for child neurology in the coming years. In the present state of knowledge, primary prevention is feasible for neural tube defects by administration of folic acid. Short of primary prevention, genetic counselling and prenatal diagnosis are the major preventive means available.

Genetic counselling requires that a precise diagnosis of fixed encephalopathies is made and that the rules of inheritance of the various types are known (Lie et al. 1994). Major advances in neuroimaging (D'Incerti 2003, Garel 2004, Gressens and Luton 2004) especially fetal MRI, have permitted visualization of important malformation syndromes like polymicrogyria and some 'minor' malformations that were very difficult or impossible to diagnose previously. Ideally, a diagnosis of CNS malformation should be not only precise but early if genetic counselling is to be effective.

The genetics of most of the common CNS malformations do not follow simple mendelian rules. Table 2.12 lists some of the main genetic malformations of the CNS and their mode of inheritance. However, an increasing number of malformations previously thought to be sporadic have proved to be sometimes genetically determined, and only a few malformation syndromes are firmly known to be nongenetic. This is the case for most nonsyndromic cases of agenesis of the corpus callosum, for Aicardi syndrome, Dandy–Walker syndrome and cortical dysplasias. Recognition of other syndromes of this type is obviously desirable.

TABLE 2.12
CNS malformations that may be genetically determined*

Malformation	Mode of inheritance[1]	Recurrence risk	Locus (gene)
Neural tube defects (anencephaly, spina bifida)	Multifactorial	1–5% (up to 10% if two family members are affected)	
Cephaloceles		<10%	
Meckel–Gruber syndrome	AR	25%	17q23 (MKS1) 11q13 (MKS2) 8q21.13–q22.1 (MKS3)
Holoprosencephaly	AD (AR or multifactorial in some cases)	6%[2]	7q36–qter (SHH) 13q32 (ZIC2) 2q21 (SIX3) 18p11.3 (TGIF) 9q22.3 (PTCH) (SHH receptor) 10q11.2 (DKK)
Kallmann syndrome	XR	50% of males	Xp22.3 (KAL1; FGFR1)
Microcephaly[3]	S, AR, AD	25% for AR cases	MCPH 1–6 (3 genes)
Subcortical laminar heterotopia	XD	<50% of males	Xq22.3–q23 (DCX)
Lissencephaly I	S, AR		17p13.3 (LIS1)
Cobblestone complex	AR	25%	
Walker–Warburg			3p32–34 (POMT1)
Muscle–eye–brain disease			1p32–34 (POMGnT1)
Fukuyama congenital muscular dystrophy			9q31 (FTCD)
Periventricular nodular heterotopia	XD	50% of males	Xq28 (FGN-A)
Joubert syndrome	AR	25%[4]	9q34.3 (JBTS1) 11p11.21 (JBTS2) 6q23 (JBTS3)
Agenesis of corpus callosum	S	Low	Variable chromosomal abnormalities in some cases
Sacral agenesis (Currarino syndrome)	AD	50%	7q36 (HLXB9)
Septo-optic dysplasia	S, AR	Low	3p21.1–p21.2 (HESX1, PAX3)

*Many malformations may be genetically determined. Only the best recognized types are listed. Non-genetic types may exist for all the malformations mentioned in the table.
[1]AR = autosomal recessive; AD = autosomal dominant; XR = X-linked recessive; XD = X-linked dominant; S = sporadic.
[2]Represents a mixture of sporadic cases and cases with various modes of transmission, hence little practical value.
[3]Heterogeneous conditions with many nongenetic cases. Several modes of inheritance.
[4]The risk is difficult to indicate with precision. An excess of males is frequent.

Unfortunately, it is more common for malformation syndromes to be either genetically or environmentally determined and, so far, we are not able to discriminate between the mechanisms. Chromosomal and MRI examination of parents, especially the mothers, can be helpful in some circumstances (see above).

Prenatal diagnosis of several brain malformations is feasible mainly by ultrasonography (American Academy of Pediatrics 1994, Aubry et al. 2003, Barnewolt and Estroff 2004). Improvement in techniques makes earlier and firmer recognition of many malformations possible. Fetal MRI is currently available in major centres and allows a more precise definition of the pathological features of the malformations (Garel 2004, Golja et al. 2004, Gressens and Luton 2004). It is indicated when sonographic diagnosis is uncertain or additional anatomic precision is re-

quired. With technical progress the diagnosis has become possible earlier in many conditions, but in others remains relatively late, with the consequence that only late termination is possible, which compares unfavourably with the earlier diagnosis of cases of metabolic diseases. Additionally, the reliability of ultrasonography depends heavily on the skill of examiners. A difficult ethical issue may be raised by some abnormalities such as the Dandy–Walker syndrome or agenesis of the corpus callosum as these may be unassociated with neurodevelopmental dysfunction in a significant proportion of cases.

For the diagnosis of chromosomal abnormalities, spina bifida and some metabolic disorders, amniocentesis or chorionic villus sampling may be required. These techniques are associated with a risk of fetal loss of approximately 0.5– 1% for amniocentesis

TABLE 2.13
CNS malformations that may be associated with metabolic disorders

Metabolic disorder	Malformation	References
Peroxisomal disorders		
Zellweger syndrome, neonatal adrenoleukodystrophy	Cortical migration disorders, pachygyria and microgyria	Powers (1995)
Trihydroxycholastanaemia	Cerebellar atrophy	Christensen et al. (1990)
Organic acid disorders		
Glutaric aciduria type I	Macrocephaly, pseudo-cysts of temporal lobes	Martinez-Lage et al. (1994)
Glutaric aciduria type II	Status verrucosus of cortex, vermal agenesis	Takanashi et al. (1999)
Nonketotic hyperglycinaemia	Agenesis of corpus callosum	Nissenkorn et al. (2001)
Mitochondrial disorders		
Pyruvate dehydrogenase complex deficiency	Agenesis of corpus callosum, migration disturbances, porencephaly	Matthews et al. (1993), Shevell et al. (1994)
Leigh disease	Abnormal gyration	Okumura et al. (2008)
Respiratory chain disorders	Migration disorder	Samson et al. (1994), Lincke et al. (1996), Del Giudice et al. (2000)
Abnormalities of folic acid metabolism	Neural tube defects	Volcik et al. (2003), Yerbi (2003)
Cholesterol metabolism disorders		
Smith–Lemli–Opitz syndrome	Microcephaly, abnormal gyration, holoprosencephaly	Tint et al. (1994), Nissenkorn et al. (2001)
Glycoprotein disorders	Pontocerebellar hypoplasia	Jaeken and Carchon (1993)
Carbohydrate-deficient glycoprotein (CDG) syndrome		
Adenylsuccinase deficiency	Vermis hypoplasia	Jaeken and Van den Berghe (1984)
Sphingosidoses		
Multiple sulfatase deficiency	Corpus callosum agenesis	Two personal cases
Mucopolysaccharidoses		
Hurler disease	Agenesis of corpus callosum	Jellinger et al. (1981)
Maternal metabolic disturbances		
Phenylketonuria	Microcephaly, callosal agenesis	Rouse et al. (2000)
Fetal alcohol syndrome	Excess neuronal migration, agenesis of corpus callosum, abnormal gyration, holoprosencephaly	Ronen and Andrews (1991), Autti-Rämö et al. (2002)
Maternal diabetes mellitus	Holoprosencephaly, sacral agenesis, septo-optic dysplasia	Anderson et al. (2005)

performed under ultrasound guidance (Seeds 2004) and of 3% for villus sampling (Caughey et al. 2006). The risk of of puncture injury of the fetus is very small but does exist (Mancini et al. 2001, Seeds et al. 2004).

Several developmental CNS anomalies may be associated with metabolic diseases. Some of these can be prevented by the control of the metabolic abnormality in the mother (e.g. phenylketonuria or diabetes) or by prevention of toxic effects of certain drugs or other toxic sustances like alcohol, and several can be detected prenatally (Table 2.13). Several *inborn errors of metabolism* are a cause of CNS malformations (Nissenkorn et al. 2001, Raoul et al. 2003). Nonketotic hyperglycinaemia, mitochondrial and peroxisomal disorders have been repeatedly indicted. Bamforth et al. (1988) found 8 cases of callosal agenesis in 50 patients with inherited diseases of metabolism. Some anomalies of cholesterol metabolism were more recently described (Haas et al. 2001; Chapter 8). A polymorphism in the gene coding for methylenetetrahydrofolate reductase may be a risk factor for spina bifida (van der Put et al. 1995).

Metabolic disturbances of environmental origin, whether due to maternal disease or to use of toxic substances during pregnancy, are a significant cause of fetal malformations. *Maternal diabetes mellitus* (Anderson et al. 2005) is one major metabolic disorder capable of increasing considerably the incidence of certain CNS malformations, especially holoprosencephaly. Moreover, the clear correlation that exists between high levels of glycosylated haemoglobin A1 in early pregnancy and the occurrence of severe defects in offspring supports the hypothesis that malformations in infants of diabetic mothers occur early during the first 7 weeks of gestation. Such findings indicate that strict control of maternal diabetes is essential.

Maternal phenylketonuria is another cause of CNS malformations (Chapter 8).

Maternal alcoholism is an important factor. Fetal effects including CNS malformations have been extensively reviewed and publicized, and the use of any quantity of alcohol during pregnancy is better avoided as no 'safe' level can be defined. Callosal agenesis and holoprosencephaly (Ronen and Andrews 1991) are on record.

Malformations resulting from cocaine use have been produced experimentally in mice (Nassogne et al. 1998). The situation in humans is less clear-cut, although the fetal effects of maternal addiction including disturbed head growth and behavioural effects are well recognized.

Careful monitoring of pregnancy is clearly important, and special attention should be given in cases involving higher risk factors such as maternal age over 35 years, multiple pregnancy, oligohydramnios or hydramnios, and to mothers with known disorders or who have previously given birth to a malformed infant. Fetuses that are small for gestational age are also at high risk. Khoury et al. (1988) found an incidence of malformation (of any type) of 8.0% in small for gestational age babies compared to 3.3% in infants appropriate for their gestational age. The discovery at ultrasonography of peripheral malformations, especially of cystic hygromas, is also an indication of high risk, and nuchal lucencies are an important clue to the diagnosis of Down syndrome and other abnormalities.

It is essential to inform future parents that even the best monitoring will miss a significant number of brain malformations whatever the technique used.

REFERENCES

Accardo P, Whitman B (1988) Severe microcephaly with normal non-verbal intelligence. *Pediatr Rev Commun* 3: 61–5.

Aghakhani Y, Kinay D, Gotman J, et al. (2005) The role of priventricular nodular heterotopia in epileptogenesis. *Brain* 128: 641–65.

Ahdab-Barmada M, Claassen D (1990) A distinctive triad of malformations of the central nervous system in the Meckel–Gruber syndrome. *J Neuropathol Exp Neurol* 49: 610–20.

Aicardi J (1991) The agyria–pachygyria complex: a spectrum of cortical malformations. *Brain Dev* 13: 1–8.

Aicardi J (1994) The place of neuronal migration abnormalities in child neurology. *Can J Neurol Sci* 21: 185–93.

Aicardi J (1996) Aicardi syndrome. In: Guerrini R, Andermann E, Canapicchi R, et al., eds. *Dysplasias of Cerebral Cortex and Epilepsy.* Philadelphia: Lippincott–Raven, pp. 211–6.

Aicardi J (2005) Aicardi syndrome. *Brain Dev* 27: 164–71.

Aicardi J, Chevrie JJ, Baraton J (1987) Agenesis of the corpus callosum. In: Vinken PJ, Bruyn GW, Klawans HL, eds. *Handbook of Clinical Neurology. Revised Series. Vol. 6. Brain Malformation.* Amsterdam: North Holland, pp. 149–73.

Aida N, Yagishita A, Takada K, et al. (1994) Cerebellar MR in Fukuyama-type congenital muscular dystrophy: polymicrogyria with cystic lesions. *AJNR* 15: 1755–9.

Albright AL, Gartner JC, Wiener ES (1989) Lumbar cutaneous hemangiomas as indicators of tethered spinal cord. *Pediatrics* 8: 977–80.

Albuisson J, Pécheux C, Carel JC, et al. (2005) Kalman syndrome: 14 novel mutations in KAL1 and FGFR1 (KAL2). *Hum Mutat* 25: 98–9.

Aleksic S, Budzilovich G, Greco MA, et al. (1983) Encephalocele (cerebellocele) in Goldenhar–Gorlin syndrome. *Eur J Pediatr* 140: 137–8.

Alexiev BH, Lin X, Son CC, Brenner DS (2006) Meckel–Gruber syndrome: pathologic manifestations, minimal diagnostic criteria, and differential diagnosis. *Arch Pathol Lab Med* 130: 1236–8.

Alfonso I, Vasconcellos E, Shuhaiber HH, et al. (2004) Bilateral decreased oxygenation during focal status epilepticus in a neonate with hemimegalencephaly. *J Child Neurol* 19: 394–6.

Alonso-Nanclares L, Garbelli R, Sola RG, et al. (2005) Microanatomy of the dysplastic cortex from epileptic patients. *Brain* 128: 158–73.

Al Shahwan SA, Bruyn GW, Al Deeb SM (1995) Non-progressive familial congenital cerebellar hypoplasia. *J Neurol Sci* 128: 71–7.

Altman NR, Altman DH (1987) MR imaging of spinal dysraphism. *AJNR* 8: 533–8.

Altman NR, Naidich TP, Braffman BH (1992) Posterior fossa malformations. *AJNR* 13: 691–724.

Amacher AL, Page LK (1971) Hydrocephalus due to membranous obstruction of the fourth ventricle. *J Neurosurg* 35: 672–6.

Ambrosetto G (1992) Unilateral opercular macrogyria and benign childhood epilepsy with centrotemporal (rolandic) spikes: report of a case. *Epilepsia* 33: 499–503.

American Academy of Pediatrics, Committee on Genetics (1994) Prenatal genetic diagnosis for pediatricians. *Pediatrics* 93: 1010–5.

Andermann E (1981) Sensorimotor neuronopathy with agenesis of the corpus callosum. In: Vinken PJ, Bruyn GW, eds. *Handbook of Clinical Neurology. Vol. 42. Neurogenetic Directory, Part I.* Amsterdam: North Holland, pp. 100–3.

Anderson JL, Walker DK, Camfield MA, et al. (2005) Maternal obesity, gestational diabetes and CNS birth defects. *Epidemiology* 16: 87–92.

Aniskiewicz AS, Frumkin NL, Brady DE, et al. (1990) Magnetic resonance imaging and neurobehavioral correlates in schizencephaly. *Arch Neurol* 47: 911–6.

Arai H, Sato K, Okuda O, et al. (2001) Surgical experience wih 120 patients with lumbosacral lipomas. *Acta Neurochir* 143: 857–64.

Arruda JA, Costa CM, Tella OI (2004) Results of the treatment of syringomyelia associated with Chiari malformation: analysis of 60 cases. *Arq Neuropsiquatr* 62: 341–52.

Ashley WW, Wright NM (2006) Resection of giant anterior sacral meningocele via an anterior approach: case report and review of literature. *Surg Neurol* 66: 89–93.

Aslan H, Ulker V, Gulcan EM, et al. (2002) Prenatal diagnosis of Joubert syndrome: a case report. *Prenat Diagn* 22: 13–6.

Assadi AH, Zhang G, Beffert U, et al. (2003) Interaction of reelin signaling and LIS1 in brain development. *Nat Genet* 35: 270–6.

Attal NA, Parker F, Tadie M, et al. (2004) Effects of surgery on sensory deficits of syringomyelia and predictors of outcome: a long-tem prospective study. *J Neurol Neurosurg Psychiatry* 75: 1025–30.

Aubry MC, Aubry JP, Dommergues M (2003) Sonographic prenatal diagnosis of central nervous system abnormalities. *Childs Nerv Syst* 19: 391–402.

Autti-Rämö I, Autti T, Korkman M, et al. (2002) MRI findings in children with school problems who had been exposed prenatally to alcohol. *Dev Med Child Neurol* 44: 98–106.

Autti-Rämö I, Fagerlund A, Ervalahti N, et al. (2006) Fetal alcohol spectrum disorders in Finland: clinical delineation of 77 older children and adolescents. *Am J Med Genet A* 140: 137–43.

Balci B, Uyanik G, Dincer P, et al. (2005) An autosomal recessive limb girdle muscular dystrophy (LGMD2) with mild mental retardation is allelic to Walker–Warburg syndrome (WWS) caused by a mutation of the POMT1 gene. *Neuromuscul Disord* 15: 271–5.

Bale JF, Bell WE, Dunn V, et al. (1986) Magnetic resonance imaging of the spine in children. *Arch Neurol* 43: 1253–6.

Ballarati L, Rossi E, Bonati MT, et al. (2007) 13q deletion and central nervous system anomalies: further insights from karyotype–phenotype analyses of 14 patients. *J Med Genet* 44: e60.

Bamforth F, Bamforth S, Poskitt K, et al. (1988) Abnormalities of corpus callosum in patients with inherited metabolic diseases. *Lancet* 2: 451.

Baraitser M, Burn J (1984) Brief clinical report: neural tube defects as an X-linked condition. *Am J Med Genet* 17: 383–5.

Baraitser M, Brett EM, Piesowicz AT (1983) Microcephaly and intracranial calcification in two brothers. *J Med Genet* 20: 210–2.

Barkovich AJ (1990) Apparent atypical callosal dysgenesis: analysis of MR findings in six cases and their relationship to holoprosencephaly. *AJNR* 11: 333–9.

Barkovich AJ (1998) Neuroimaging manifestations and classificaton of congenital muscular dystrophies. *AJNR* 98: 1389–96.

Barkovich AJ, Chuang SH (1990) Unilateral megalencephaly: correlation of MR imaging and pathologic characteristics. *AJNR* 11: 523–31.

Barkovich AJ, Kjos BO (1992) Schizencephaly: correlation of clinical findings with MR characteristics. *AJNR* 13: 85–94.

Barkovich AJ, Lindan CE (1994) Congenital cytomegalovirus infection of the brain: imaging analysis and embryologic considerations. *AJNR* 15: 703–15.

Barkovich AJ, Norman D (1988a) Absence of the septum pellucidum: a useful sign of the diagnosis of congenital brain malformations. *AJNR* 9: 1107–14.

Barkovich AJ, Norman D (1988b) Anomalies of the corpus callosum: correlation with further anomalies of the brain. *AJNR* 9: 493–501.

Barkovich AJ, Gressens P, Evrard P (1992) Formation, maturation, and disorders of brain neocortex. *AJNR* 13: 423–46.

Barkovich AJ, Guerrini R, Battaglia G, et al. (1994) Band heterotopia: correlation of outcome with magnetic resonance imaging parameters. *Ann Neurol* 36: 609–17.

Barkovich AJ, Kuzniecky RI, Dobyns WB, et al. (1996) A classification scheme for malformations of cortical development. *Neuropediatrics* 27: 59–63.

Barkovich AJ, Kuzniecky RI, Bollen AW, Grant PE (1997) Focal transmantle dysplasia: a specific malformation of cortical development? *Neurology* 49: 1148–52.

Barkovich AJ, Ferriero DM, Barr RM, et al. (1998) Microlissencephaly: a heterogeneous malformation of cortical development. *Neuropediatrics* 29: 113-9.

Barkovich AJ, Hevner R, Guerrini R (1999) Syndromes of bilateral symmetrical polymicrogyria. *AJNR* 20: 1814–21.

Barkovich AJ, Kuzniecky RI, Jackson MD, et al. (2001a) Classification system for malformations of cortical development: update 2001. *Neurology* 57: 2168–78.

Barkovich AJ, Simon EM, Walsh CA, et al. (2001b) Callosal agenesis with cysts. A better understanding and new classification. *Neurology* 56: 220–7.

Barkovich AJ, Miller KJ, Dobyns WB (2007) A developmental classification of malformations of the brainstem. *Ann Neurol* 62: 625–39.

Barnewolt CE, Estroff JA (2004) Sonography of the fetal central nervous system. *Neuroimaging Clin N Am* 14: 255–71, viii.

Barr M, Hanson JW, Currey K, et al. (1983) Holoprosencephaly in infants of diabetic mothers. *J Pediatr* 102: 565–8.

Barth PG, ed. (2003a) *Disorders of Neuronal Migration. International Review of Child Neurology Series.* London: Mac Keith Press for the International Child Neurology Association.

Barth PG (2003b) Fetal disruption as a cause of neuronal migration defects. In: Barth PG, ed: *Disorders of Neuronal Migration. International Review of Child Neurology Series.* London: Mac Keith Press for the International Child Neurology Association, pp. 182–94.

Barth PG, Majoie CB, Caan MW, et al. (2007) Pontine tegmental cap dysplasia: a novel brain malformation with a defect in axonal guidance. *Brain* 130: 2258–66.

Battaglia D, Di Rocco C, Iuvone L, et al. (1999) Neuro-cognitive development and epilepsy outcome in children with surgically treated hemimegalencephaly. *Neuropediatrics* 30: 307–13.

Battaglia G, Granata T (2003) Schizencephaly. In: Barth PG, ed. *Disorders of Neuronal Migration. International Review of Child Neurology Series.* London: Mac Keith Press for the International Child Neurology Association, pp. 127–34

Becker PS, Dixon AM, Troncosi JC (1989) Bilateral opercular polymicrogyria. *Ann Neurol* 25: 90–2.

Bedeschi MF, Bonaglia MC, Grasso R, et al. (2006) Agnenesis of the corpus callosum: clinical and genetic study in 63 young patients. *Pediatr Neurol* 34: 186–93.

Belhocine O, André C, Kalifa G, Adamsbaum C (2005) Does septal agenesis occur? A revew of 34 cases. *Pediatr Radiol* 35: 410–8.

Beltran-Valero de Bernabe D, Currier S, Steinbrecher A, et al. (2002) Mutations of the O-methyltransferase gene POMT1 give rise to the severe migration disorder Walker–Warburg syndrome. *Am J Hum Genet* 71: 1033–43.

Beltran-Valero de Bernabe D, Voit T, Longman C, et al. (2004) Mutations in the FKRP gene can cause muscle–eye–brain disease and Walker–Warburg syndrome. *J Med Genet* 41: e61.

Bennett GL, Bromley B, Benacerraf BR (1996) Agenesis of the corpus callosum: prenatal detection is not usually possible before 22 weeks of gestation. *Radiology* 199: 447–50.

Bentivoglio M, Tassi L, Pech E, et al. (2003) Cortical development and focal cortical dysplasia. *Epileptic Disord* 5 Suppl 2: S27–34.

Berry RJ, Li Z, Erickson JD, et al. (1999) Preventing neural tube defects with folic acid in China. *N Engl J Med* 341: 1485–90.

Berry-Kravis E, Israel J (1994) X-linked pachygyria and agenesis of the corpus callosum: evidence for an X chromosome lissencephaly locus. *Ann Neurol* 36: 229–33.

Berthet F, Caduff R, Schaad UB, et al. (1994) A syndrome of primary combined immunodeficiency with microcephaly, cerebellar hypoplasia, growth failure and progressive pancytopenia. *Eur J Pediatr* 153: 333–8.

Bhattacharya JJ, Luo CB, Alvarez H, et al. (2004) PHACES syndrome: a review of eight previously unreported cases, with late arterial occlusions. *Neuroradiology* 46: 227–33.

Biggio JR, Wenstrom KD, Owen J, et al. (2004) Fetal open spina bifida: a natural history of diease progression in utero. *Prenat Diagn* 24: 287–9.

Billette de Villemeur T, Chiron C, Robain O (1992) Unlayered polymicrogyria and agenesis of the corpus callosum: a relevant association? *Acta Neuropathol* 83: 265–70.

Bingham PM, Lynch D, McDonald-McGinn D, Zackai E (1998) Polymicrogyria in chromosome 22 deletion syndrome. *Neurology* 51: 1500–2.

Bingol N, Fuchs M, Diaz V, et al. (1987) Teratogenicity of cocaine in humans. *J Pediatr* 110: 93–6.

Bix GJ, Clark GD (1998) Platelet-activating factor receptor stimulation disrupts neuronal migration in vitro. *J Neurosci* 18: 307–18.

Blum A, André M, Droullé P, et al. (1990) Prenatal echographic diagnosis of corpus callosum agenesis. The Nancy experience 1982–1989. *Genet Couns* 1: 115–26.

Bodensteiner JB (1995) The saga of the septum pellucidum: a tale of unfunded clinical investigations. *J Child Neurol* 10: 227–31.

Bodensteiner JB, Gay CT (1990) Colpocephaly: pitfalls in the diagnosis of a pathologic entity utilizing neuroimaging techniques. *J Child Neurol* 5: 166–8.

Bodensteiner JB, Gay CT, Marks WA, et al. (1988) Macro cisterna magna: a marker for maldevelopment of the brain? *Pediatr Neurol* 4: 284–6.

Bodensteiner JB, Schaefer GB, Breeding L, Cowan L (1994) Hypoplasia of the corpus callosum: a study of 445 consecutive MRI scans. *J Child Neurol* 9: 47–9.

Boltshauser E (2004) Cerebellum–small brain but large confusion: a review of selected cerebellar malformations and disruptions. *Am J Med Genet A* 126: 376–85.

Boltshauser E, Steinlin M, Martin E, Deonna T (1996) Unilateral cerebellar aplasia. *Neuropediatrics* 27: 50–3.

Bordarier C, Aicardi J (1990) Dandy–Walker syndrome and agenesis of the cerebellar vermis: diagnostic problems and genetic counselling. *Dev Med Child Neurol* 32: 285–94.

Bordarier C, Aicardi J, Goutières F (1984) Congenital hydrocephalus and eye abnormalities with severe developmental brain defects: Warburg's syndrome. *Ann Neurol* 16: 60–5.

Borzyskowski M (1990) The conservative management of neuropathic vesico-urethral dysfunction. In: Borzyskowski M, Mundy AR, eds. *Neuropathic Bladder in Childhood. Clinics in Developmental Medicine No. 111.* London: Mac Keith Press, pp. 27–36.

Bosman C, Boldrini R, Dimitri L, et al. (1996) Hemimegalencephaly. Histological, immunohistochemical, ultrastructural and cytofluorimetric study of six patients. *Childs Nerv Syst* 12: 765–75.

Botto LD, Moore CA, Khoury MJ, Erikson JD (1999) Neural tube defects. *N Engl J Med* 341: 1509–19.

Botto LD, Olney RS, Erickson D, et al. (2004) Viatmin supplements and the risk of cogenital anomalies other than neural tube defects. *Am J Med Genet C Semin Med Genet* 125: 12–21.

Botto LD, Lisi A, Robert-Gnansia E, et al. (2005) International retrospective cohort study of neural tube defects in relation to folic acid recommendations: are the recommendations working? *BMJ* 330: 571.

Breningstall GN, Marker SM, Tubman DE (1992) Hydrosyringomyelia and diastematomyelia detected by MRI in myelomeningocele. *Pediatr Neurol* 8: 267–71.

Brismar J, Ozand PT (1995) CT and MR of the brain in glutaric acidemia type 1: a review of 59 published cases and a report of 5 new patients. *AJNR* 16: 675–83.

Brody BA, Kinney HC, Kloman AS, Gilles FH (1987) Sequence of central nervous system myelination in human infancy. 1: Autopsy study of myelination. *J Neuropathol* 46: 283–301.

Brown MS, Sheridan-Pereira M (1992) Outlook for the child with a cephalocele. *Pediatrics* 90: 914–9.

Brunelli S, Faiella A, Capra V, et al. (1996) Germline mutations in the homeobox gene EMX2 in patients with severe schizencephaly. *Nat Genet* 12: 94–6.

Bruner JP, Tulipan N, Reed G, et al. (2004) Intrauterine repair of spina bifida: preoperative predictors of shunt-dependent hydrocepahalus. *Am J Obstet Gynecol* 190: 1305–12.

Bulsara KR, Zomoroi AR, Villavicencio AT, et al. (2001) Clinical outcome differences for lipomyelomeningoceles, intraspinal lipomas and lipomas of the filum terminale. *Neurosurg Rev* 24: 192–4.

Bulsara KR, Zomorodi AR, Enterline DS, George TM (2004) The value of magnetic resonance imaging in the evaluation of fatty filum terminale. *Neurosurgery* 54: 375–9.

Burck U, Hayek HW, Zeidler U (1981) Holoprosencephaly in monozygotic twins—clinical and computer tomographic findings. *Am J Med Genet* 9: 13–7.

Burton BK (1981) Dominant inheritance of microcephaly with short stature. *Clin Genet* 20: 25–7.

Busis NA, Hochberg FH (1985) Familial syringomyelia. *J Neurol Neurosurg Psychiatry* 48: 936–8.

Bystron I, Molnar Z, Otellin V, Blakemore C (2005) Tangential networks of precocious neurons and early axonal outgrowth in the embryonic human forebrain. *J Neurosci* 16: 2781–92.

Calabrese P, Fink GR, Markowitsch HJ, et al. (1994) Left hemispheric neuronal heterotopia: a PET, MRI, EEG, and neuropsychological investigation of a university student. *Neurology* 44: 302–5.

Cama A, Tortori-Donati P, Piatelli GL, et al. (1995) Chiari complex in children – neuroradiological diagnosis, neurosurgical treatment and proposal of a new classification (312 cases). *Eur J Pediatr Surg* 5 Suppl 1 : 35–8.

Cantani A, Lucenti P, Ronzani GA, Santoro C (1990) Joubert syndrome. Review of the fifty-three cases so far published. *Ann Genet* 33: 96–8.

Caplan LR, Norohna AB, Amico LL (1990) Syringomyelia and arachnoiditis. *J Neurol Neurosurg Psychiatry* 53: 106–13.

Caraballo RH, Cersósimo GA, Pechacek TE (2004) Unilateral closed-lip schizencephaly and epilepsy: a comparison with cases of unilateral polymicrogyria. *Brain Dev* 26: 151–7.

Cardoso C, Leventer RJ, Matsumoto N, et al. (2000) The location and type of mutation predict malformation severity in isolated lissencephaly caused by abnormalities within the LIS1 gene. *Hum Mol Genet* 9: 3019–28.

Cascino GD, Bushhalter JR, Sirven JL, et al. (2004) Peri-ictal SPECT and surgical treatment for intractable epilepsy related to schizencephaly. *Neurology* 63: 2426–8.

Casaubon LK, Melanson M, Lopes-Cendes I, et al. (1996) The gene responsible for a severe form of peripheral neuropathy and agenesis of the corpus callosum maps to chromosome 15q. *Am J Hum Genet* 58: 28–34.

Caughey AB, Hopkins LM, Norton ME (2006) Chorionic villus sampling compared with amniocentesis and the difference in the rate of pregnancy loss. *Obstet Gynecol* 108: 612–6.

Caviness VS, Pinto-Lord MC, Evrard P (1981) The development of laminated pattern in the mammalian neocortex. In: Connelly TG, ed. *Morphogenesis and Pattern Formation*. New York: Raven Press, pp. 102–26.

Caviness VS, Takahashi T, Nowalowski RS (2003) Morphogenesis of the human cerebral cortex. In: Barth PG, ed. *Disorders of Neuronal Migration. International Review of Child Neurology Series*. London: Mac Keith Press for the International Child Neurology Association, pp. 1–23.

Chadduck WM, Glasier CM (1989) Megachoroid as a cause of isolated ventricle syndrome. *Pediatr Neurol* 5: 194–6.

Chang BS, Piao X, Bodell A, et al. (2004) Bilateral frontotemporal polymicrogyria: clinical and radiological features in 10 families with linkage to chromosome 16. *Ann Neurol* 53: 596–606.

Chao A, Wong AM, Hsueh C, et al. (2005) Integration of imaging and pathological studies in Meckel–Gruber syndrome. *Prenat Diagn* 25: 267–8.

Chapman PH, Swearingen B, Caviness VS (1989) Subtorcular occipital encephaloceles. Anatomical considerations relevant to operative management. *J Neurosurg* 71: 375–81.

Chard T, Macintosh M (1992) Antenatal diagnosis of congenital abnormalities. In: Chard T, Richards MPM, eds. *Obstetrics in the 1990s: Current Controversies. Clinics in Developmental Medicine No. 123/124*. London: Mac Keith Press, pp. 90–104.

Charrow J, Poznanski AK, Unger FM, Robinow M (1991) Autosomal recessive cerebellar hypoplasia and endosteal sclerosis: a newly recognized syndrome. *Am J Med Genet* 41: 464–8.

Chevrie JJ, Aicardi J (1986) The Aicardi syndrome. In: Pedley TA, Meldrum BS, eds. *Recent Advances in Epilepsy, vol. 3*. Edinburgh: Churchill Livingstone, pp. 189–210.

Christensen E, Van Eldere J, Brandt NJ, et al. (1990) A new peroxisomal disorder: di- and trihydroxycholestanaemia due to a presumed trihydroxycholestanoyl-CoA oxidase deficiency. *J Inherit Metab Dis* 13: 362–6.

Christian JC (1982) Kallmann syndrome (olfactogenital dysplasia). In: Vinken PJ, Bruyn GW, eds. *Handbook of Clinical Neurology. Vol. 43. Neurogenetic Directory, Part II*. Amsterdam: North Holland, pp. 418–9.

Chugani HT (1996) Functional imaging in cortical dysplasia: positron emission tomography. In: Guerrini R, Andermann F, Canapicchi R, et al., eds. *Dysplasias of Cerebral Cortex and Epilepsy*. New York: Lippincott–Raven, pp. 169–174.

Chulamorkodt NN, Estrada CR, Chaviano AH, et al. (2004) Continent urinary diversion: 10-year experience of Shriners Hospital for Children in Chicago. *J Spinal Cord Med* 27 Suppl 1: S84–7.

Clark GD (2004) The classification of cortical dysplasias through molecular genetics. *Brain Dev* 26: 351–62.

Cochrane B, Finley C, Kestle J, Steinbock P (2000) The pattern of late deterioration in patients with transitional lipomyelomeningocele. *Eur J Pediatr Surg* 10 Suppl 1: 13–7.

Cohen MM, Shiota K (2002) Teratogenesis of holoprosencephaly. *Am J Med Genet* 109: 1–15.

Cohen MM, Campbell R, Yaghmai F (1989) Neuropathological abnormalities in developmental dysphasia. *Ann Neurol* 25: 567–70.

Conley ME, Beckwith JB, Mancer JFK, Tenchkhoff L (1979) The spectrum of Di George syndrome. *J Pediatr* 94: 883–90.

Coppola G, Vojro P, De Virginis S, et al. (2002) Cerebellar vermis defect, oligophrenia, congenital ataxia and hepatic fibrosis without coloboma and renal anomalies: report of two cases. *Neuropediatrics* 33: 180–5.

Cordero JF (1994) Finding the causes of birth defects. *N Engl J Med* 331: 48–9.

Cormand B, Avela K, Pihko H, et al. (1999) Assignment of the muscle–eye–brain disease gene to 1p32–p34 by linkage analysis and homozygosity mapping. *Am J Hum Genet* 64: 126–35.

Cormand B, Pihko H, Santavuori P, et al. (2001) Clinical and genetic distinction between Walker–Warburg and muscle–eye–brain disease. *Neurology* 56: 1056–69.

Cornette L, Verpoorten C, Lagae L, et al. (1998) Closed spinal dysraphism: a review on diagnosis and treatment in infancy. *Eur J Paediatr Neurol* 2: 179–85.

Coupland SG, Sarnat HB (1990) Visual and auditory evoked potential correlates of cerebral malformations. *Brain Dev* 12: 466–72.

Cretolle C, Zerah M, Jaubert F, et al. (2006) New clinical and therapeutic perspectives in Currarino syndrome (a study of 29 cases). *J Pediatr Surg* 41: 126–31.

Crino P (2001) New RELN mutation associated with lissencephaly and epilepsy. *Epilepsy Curr* 1: 72.

Crino PB (2004) Malformations of cortical development: molecular pathogenesis and experimental strategies. *Adv Exp Med Biol* 548: 175–91.

Crino PB (2005) Molecular pathogenesis of focal cortical dysplasia and hemimegalencephaly. *J Child Neurol* 20: 330–6.

Croen LA, Shaw GM, Lammer EJ (1996) Holoprosencephaly: epidemiologic and clinical characteristics of a California population. *Am J Med Genet* 64: 465–72.

Currier SC, Lee CK, Chang BS, et al. (2005) Mutations of POMT1 are found in a minority of patients with Walker–Warburg syndrome. *Am J Med Genet A* 133: 53–7.

Curry CJ, Lammer EJ, Nelson V, Shaw GM (2005) Schizencephaly: heterogeneous etilogies in a population of 4 million California births. *Am J Med Genet A* 137: 181–9.

Czeizel AE, Dudás I (1992) Prevention of the first occurrence of neural-tube defects by periconceptional vitamin supplementation. *N Engl J Med* 327: 1832–5.

Dambska M, Laure-Kaminowska M (1990) Myelination as a parameter of normal and retarded brain maturation. *Brain Dev* 12: 214–20

Dambska M, Wisniewski KE, Sher JH (1986) Marginal glioneuronal heterotopias in nine cases with and without cortical abnormalities. *J Child Neurol* 1: 149–57.

D'Amico A, Tessa A, Bruno C, et al. (2006) Expanding the clinical spectrum of POMT1 phenotype. *Neurology* 66: 1564–7.

Danner R, Shewmon DA, Sherman RB (1985) Seizures in an atelencephalic infant: is the cortex essential for neonatal seizures? *Arch Neurol* 42: 1014–6.

Davila-Guttierez G (2002) Agenesis and dysgenesis of the corpus callosum. *Semin Pediatr Neurol* 9: 292–301.

Davis PC, Hoffman JC, Ball TI, et al. (1988) Spinal abnormalities in pediatric patients: MR imaging findings compared with clinical, myelographic, and surgical findings. *Radiology* 166: 679–85.

Day RE, Schutt WH (1979) Normal children with large heads—benign familial megalencephaly. *Arch Dis Child* 54: 512–7.

de Azevedo Moreira LM, Neri FB, et al. (2005) Multiple congenital malformations including severe eye anomalies and abnormal cerebellar development with Dandy–Walker malformation in a girl with partial trisomy 3q. *Ophthalmic Genet* 26: 37–43.

Dehdashti AR, Abouzeid H, Momjian S, et al. (2004) Occipital extra- and intracranial lipoencephalocele associated with tectocerebellar dysraphia. *Childs Nerv Syst* 20: 225–8.

De Léon GA, Breningstall G, Zaeri N (1986) Congenital Pick cell encephalopathy: a distinct disorder characterized by diffuse formation of Pick cells in the cerebral cortex. *Acta Neuropathol* 70: 235–42.

Del Giudice E, Gaetaniello L, Matrecano E, et al. (2000) Brain migration disorder and T-cell activation deficiency associated with abnormal signaling through TCR/CD3 complex and hyperactivity of Fyn tyrosine kinase. *Neuropediatrics* 31: 265–8.

De Michele G, Filla A, D'Armiento F, et al. (1990) Cerebellar ataxia and hypogonadism. A clinicopathological report. *Clin Neurol Neurosurg* 92: 67–70.

De Myer W (1972) Megalencephaly in children. Clinical syndromes, genetic patterns, and differential diagnosis from other causes of megalencephaly. *Neurology* 22: 634–43.

De Myer W (1987) Holoprosencephaly (cyclopia–arhinencephaly). In: Vinken PJ, Bruyn GW, eds. *Handbook of Clinical Neurology, Revised Series. Vol. 6. Brain Malformation.* Amsterdam: North Holland, pp. 225–244.

Denis D, Chateil JF, Brun M, et al. (2000) Schizencephaly: clinical and imaging features in 30 infantile cases. *Brain Dev* 22: 475–83.

Denis D, Maugey-Laulom B, Carles D, et al. (2001) Prenatal diagnosis of schizencephaly by fetal magnetic resonance imaging. *Fetal Diagn Ther* 16: 354–9.

Deray M, Duchowny M, Papazian O, et al. (1995) Sleep evaluation of respiratory abnormalities in children with Chiari II malformation. *Acta Neuropediatr* 1: 197–205.

de Rijk-van Andel JF, Arts WF, Barth PG, Loonen MC (1990) Diagnostic features and clinical signs of 21 patients with lissencephaly type I. *Dev Med Child Neurol* 32: 707–17.

de Rijk-van Andel JF, Arts WF, de Weerd AW (1992) EEG and evoked potentials in a series of 21 patients with lissencephaly type I. *Neuropediatrics* 23: 4–9.

Desbiens R, Berkovic SF, Dubeau F, et al. (1993) Life-threatening focal status epilepticus due to occult cortical dysplasia. *Arch Neurol* 50: 695–700.

des Portes JM, Pinard JM, Billuart P, et al. (1998) A novel CNS gene required for neuronal migration and involved in X-linked subcortical laminar heterotopia and lissencephaly syndrome. *Cell* 92: 51–61.

Devlin AM, Cross JH, Harkness W, et al. (2003) Clinical outcome of hemispherectomy for epilepsy in childhood and adolescence. *Brain* 126: 555–66.

Di Mario FJ, Cobb RJ, Ramsby GR, Leicher C (1993) Familial band heterotopias simulating tuberous sclerosis. *Neurology* 43: 1424–6.

D'Incerti L (2003) Morphological neuroimaging of malformations of cortical development. *Epileptic Disord* 5 Suppl 2: S59–66.

Di Rocco C (1996) Surgical treatment of hemimegalencephaly. In: Guerrini R, Andermann F, Canapicchi R, et al., eds. *Dysplasias of Cerebral Cortex and Epilepsy.* Philadelphia: Lippincott–Raven, pp. 295–304.

Dobyns WB (1989) Agenesis of the corpus callosum and gyral malformations are frequent manifestations of nonketotic hyperglycinemia. *Neurology* 39: 817–20.

Dobyns WB, Barkovich AJ (1999) Microcephaly with simplified gyral pattern (oligogyric microcephaly). *Neuropediatrics* 30: 104–6.

Dobyns WB, Leventer RJ (2003) Lissencephaly: the clinical and molecular genetic basis of diffuse malformations of neuronal migration. In: Barth PG, ed. *Disorders of Neuronal Migration. International Review of Child Neurology Series.* London: Mac Keith Press for the International Child Neurology Association, pp. 24–57.

Dobyns WB, Truwit CL (1995) Lissencephaly and other malformations of cortical development: 1995 update. *Neuropediatrics* 26: 132–47.

Dobyns WB, Stratton RF, Greenberg F (1984) Syndromes with lissencephaly. I. Miller–Dieker and Norman–Roberts syndromes and isolated lisssencephaly. *Am J Med Genet* 18: 509–26.

Dobyns WB, Kirkpatrick JB, Hittner HM, et al. (1985) Syndromes with lissencephaly. II. Walker–Warburg and cerebro-oculo-muscular syndromes and a new syndrome with type II lissencephaly. *Am J Med Genet* 22: 157–95.

Dobyns WB, Pagon RA, Armstrong D, et al. (1989) Diagnostic criteria for Walker–Warburg syndrome. *Am J Med Genet* 32: 195–210.

Dobyns WB, Patton MA, Stratton RF, et al. (1996) Cobblestone lissencephaly with normal eyes and muscle. *Neuropediatrics* 27: 70–5.

Dobyns WB, Guerrini R, Czapansky-Beilman DK, et al. (1997) Bilateral nodular heterotopia with mental retardation and syndactyly in boys: a new X-linked mental retardation syndrome. *Neurology* 49: 1042–47.

Dobyns WB, Berry-Kravis E, Havernick NJ, et al. (1999) X-linked lissencephaly with absent corpus callosum and ambiguous genitalia. *Am J Med Genet* 86: 331–7.

Dodson WE (1989) Deleterious effects of drugs on the developing nervous system. *Clin Perinatol* 16: 339–60.

Donat JF (1981) Septo-optic dysplasia in an infant of a diabetic mother. *Arch Neurol* 38: 590–1.

Dooley JM, LaRoche GR, Tremblay F, Riding M (1992) Autosomal recessive cerebellar hypoplasia and tapeto-retinal degeneration: a new syndrome. *Pediatr Neurol* 8: 232–4.

D'Orsi G, Tinuper P, Bisulli F, et al. (2004) Clinical features and long-term outcome of epilepsy and periventricular nodular heterotopia. Simple compared with plus forms. *J Neurol Neurosurg Psychiatry* 75: 873–8.

Dubeau F, Tampieri D, Lee N, et al. (1995) Periventricular and subcortical nodular heterotopia. A study of 33 patients. *Brain* 118: 1273–87.

Dvorak K, Feit J, Jurankova Z (1978) Experimentally induced focal microgyria and status verrucosus deformis in rats—pathogenesis and interrelation. Histological and autoradiographical study. *Acta Neuropathol* 44: 121–9.

Edwards BO, Fisher AQ, Flannery DB (1988) Joubert syndrome: early diagnosis by recognition of the behavioral phenotype and confirmation by cranial sonography. *J Child Neurol* 3: 247–9.

Emans PJ, Koostra G, Marcelis CL, et al. (2005) The Currarino triad: the variable expression. *J Pediatr Surg* 40: 1238–42.

Ersahin Y, Yurtseven T (2004) Ventral tethering of the spinal cord. *Pediatr Neurosurg* 40: 93–4.

Evrard P, Gadisseux JF, Lyon G (1984) [Prenatal development of the nervous system and its disturbances.] *Prog Neonatol* 4: 63–106 (French).

Evrard P, De Saint-Georges P, Kadhim H, Gadisseux JF (1989) Pathology of prenatal encephalopathies. In: French JH, Harel S, Casaer P, eds. *Child Neurology and Developmental Disabilities.* Baltimore: PH Brookes, pp. 153–76.

Fauser S, Schulze-Bonhage A, Honegger J, et al. (2004) Focal cortical dysplasias: surgical outcome in 67 patients in relation to histological subtypes and dual pathology. *Brain* 127: 2406–18.

Fauser S, Huppertz HJ, Bast T, et al. (2006) Clinical characteristics in focal cortical dysplasia: a retrospective evaluation in a series of 120 patients. *Brain* 129: 1907–16.

Fenichel GM, Phillips JA (1989) Familial aplasia of the cerebellar vermis—possible X-linked dominant inheritance. *Arch Neurol* 46: 582–3.

Fernandes ET, Reinberg Y, Vernier R, Gonzalez R (1994) Neurogenic bladder dysfunction in children: review of pathophysiology and current management. *J Pediatr* 124: 1–7.

Ferrer I (1984) A Golgi analysis of unlayered polymicrogyria. *Acta Neuropathol* 65: 69–76.

Ferrie CD, Jackson GD, Giannakodimos S, Panayiotopoulos CP (1995) Posterior agyria–pachygyria with polymicrogyria. Evidence for an inherited neuronal migration disorder. *Neurology* 45: 150–3.

Finlay DC, Peto T, Payling J, et al. (2000) A study of three cases of familial related agenesis of the corpus callosum. *J Clin Neuropsychol* 22: 731–42.

Finnell RH, Taylor LE, Bennett GD (1993) The impact of maternal hyperthermia on morphogenesis: clinical and experimental evidence for a fetal hyperthermia phenotype. *Dev Brain Dysfunc* 6: 199–209.

Flores-Sarnat L (2002) Hemimegalencephaly: part I. Genetic, clinical, and imaging aspects. *J Child Neurol* 17: 373–84.

Flores-Sarnat L, Sarnat HB, Davila-Gutierrez G, Alvarez A (2003) Hemimegalencephaly: part 2. Neuropathology suggests a disorder of cellular lineage. *J Child Neurol* 18: 776–85.

Forman MS, Squier W, Dobyns WB, Golden JA (2005) Genotypically defined lissencephalies show distinct pathologies. *J Neuropathol Exp Neurol* 64: 847–57.

Franzoni E, Benardi B, Marchiani V, et al. (1995) Band brain heterotopia. Case report and review of the literature. *Neuropediatrics* 26: 37–40.

Freeman JM, Nelson KB (1988) Intrapartum asphyxia and cerebral palsy. *Pediatrics* 82: 240–49.

Freeman MVR, Williams DW, Schimke RN, et al. (1974) The Roberts syndrome. *Clin Genet* 5: 1–16.

Friede RL (1989) *Developmental Neuropathology, 2nd edn.* Berlin: Springer.

Fusco L, Ferracuti S, Fariello G, et al. (1992) Hemimegalencephaly and normal intellectual development. *J Neurol Neurosurg Psychiatry* 55: 720–2.

Gage FH (2002) Neurogenesis in the adult brain. *J Neurosci* 22: 612–3.

Galaburda AM, Sherman GF, Rosen GD, et al. (1985) Developmental dyslexia: four consecutive patients with cortical anomalies. *Ann Neurol* 18: 222–33.

Gallucci M, Bozzao A, Curatolo P, et al. (1991) MR imaging of incomplete band heterotopia. *AJNR* 12: 701–2.

Gardner PA, Albright AL (2006) "Like mother, like son:" hereditary anterior sacral meningocele. Case report and review of the literature. *J Neurosurg* 104 (2 Suppl): 138–42

Gardner RJ, Coleman LT, Mitchell LA, et al. (2001) Near-total absence of the cerebellum. *Neuropediatrics* 32: 62–8.

Garel C (2004) The role of MRI in the evaluation of the fetal brain with an emphasis on biometry, gyration and parenchyma. *Pediatr Radiol* 34: 694–9.

Gaskill SJ (2004) Primary closure of open myelomeningocele. *Neurosurg Focus* 16: E3.

Gasser B, Lindner V, Dreyfus M, et al. (1998) Prenatal diagnosis of retinal detachment in Walker–Warburg syndrome. *Am J Med Genet* **28**: 610–24.

Gazioglu N, Vural M, Seckin MS, et al. (1998) Meckel–Gruber syndrome. *Childs Nerv Syst* **14**: 142–5.

Ghai S, Fong KW, Toi A (2006) Prenatal US and MR imaging findings of lissencephaly: review of fetal cerebral sulcal development. *Radiographics* **26**: 389–405.

Girard N, Ozanne A, Chaumoitre K, et al. (2003) [MRI and ventriculomegaly in utero.] *J Radiol* **84**: 1933–44 (French).

Giuliano F, David A, Edery P, et al. (2004) Macrocephaly–cutis marmorata telangiectatica congenita: seven cases including two with unusual cerebral manifestations. *Am J Med Genet A* **126**: 99–103.

Gleeson JG (2000) Classical lissencephaly and double cortex (subcortical band heterotopia): LIS1 and doublecortin. *Curr Opin Neurol* **13**: 121–5.

Gleeson JG, Minnerath S, Mills P, et al. (1999) Characterization of mutation in the gene DCX in patients with double cortex syndrome. *Ann Neurol* **45**: 146–53.

Gleeson JG, Luo RF, Grant PE, et al. (2000) Genetic and neuroradiological heterogeneity of double cortex syndrome. *Ann Neurol* **47**: 265–9.

Gleeson JG, Keeler LC, Parisi MA, et al. (2004) Molar tooth sign of the midbrain–hindbrain junction: occurrence in mutiple distinct syndromes. *Am J Med Genet A* **125**: 125–34.

Glickstein G (2004) Cerebellar agenesis. *Brain* **117**: 1209–12.

Goel A, Desai K (2000) Surgery for syringomyelia: an analysis based on 163 surgical cases. *Acta Neurochir* **142**: 293–301.

Golden JA, Chernoff GF (1995) Multiple sites of anterior neural tube closure in humans: evidence from anterior neural tube defects (anencephaly). *Pediatrics* **95**: 506–10.

Golja AM, Estroff JA, Robertson RL (2004) Fetal imaging of central nervous system abnormalities. *Neuroimaging Clin N Am* **14**: 293–306, viii.

Goodman SI, Frerman FE (1984) Glutaric acidaemia type II (multiple acyl-CoA dehydrogenation deficiency). *J Inherit Metab Dis* **7** Suppl 1: 33–7.

Gooskens RH, Willemse J, Faber JA, Verdonck AF (1989) Macrocephalies—a differentiated approach. *Neuropediatrics* **20**: 164–9.

Govaert P, de Vries LS (1997) *An Atlas of Neonatal Brain Sonography. Clinics in Developmental Medicine No. 141/142.* London: Mac Keith Press.

Gower DJ, Pollay M, Leech R (1994) Pediatric syringomyelia. *J Child Neurol* **9**: 14–21.

Granata T, Battaglia G, D'Incerti L, et al. (1996) Schizencephaly: neuroradiologic and epileptologic findings. *Epilepsia* **37**: 1185–93.

Granata T, Farina L, Faiella A, et al. (1997) Familial schizencephaly associated with EMX2 mutation. *Neurology* **48**: 1403–6.

Green NS (2002) Folic acid supplementation and prevention of birth defects. *J Nutr* **132** (8 Suppl): 2356–60.

Greenberg F, Stratton RF, Lockaart LH, et al. (1986) Familial Miller–Dieker syndrome associated with pericentric inversion of chromosome 17. *Am J Med Genet* **23**: 853–9.

Gressens P (2006) Pathogenesis of migration disorders. *Curr Opin Neurol* **19**: 135–40.

Gressens P, Luton D (2004) Fetal MRI: obstetrical and neurological perspectives. *Pediatr Radiol* **34**: 682–4.

Gressens P, Richelme C, Kadhim HJ, et al. (1992) The germinative zone produces the most cortical astrocytes after neuronal migration in the developing mammalian brain. *Biol Neonate* **61**: 4–24.

Griebel ML, Williams JP, Russell SS, et al. (1995) Clinical and developmental findings in children with giant interhemispheric cysts and dysgenesis of the corpus callosum. *Pediatr Neurol* **13**: 119–24.

Grinberg I, Northrup H, Ardinger H, et al. (2004) Heterozygous deletion of the linked genes ZIC1 and ZIC4 is involved in Dandy–Walker malformation. *Nat Genet* **36**: 1053–5.

Groeschel S, Brockmann K, Dechent P, et al. (2006) Magnetic resonance imaging and proton magnetic resonance spectroscopy of megalencephaly and dilated Virchow–Robin spaces. *Pediatr Neurol* **34**: 35–40.

Gross SJ, Oehler JM, Eckerman CO (1983) Head growth and developmental outcome in very-low-birth-weight infants. *Pediatrics* **71**: 70–5.

Guerreiro MM, Andermann E, Guerrini R, et al. (2000) Familial perisylvian polymicrogyria: a new familial syndrome of cortical maldevelopment. *Ann Neurol* **48**: 39–48.

Guerrini R, Dobyns WB (1998) Bilateral periventricular nodular heterotopia with mental retardation and frontonasal malformation. *Neurology* **51**: 499–503.

Guerrini R, Filippi T (2005) Neuronal migration disorders, genetics, and epileptogenesis. *J Child Neurol* **20**: 287–99.

Guerrini R, Dravet C, Bureau M, et al. (1996a) Diffuse and localized dysplasias of the cerebral cortex: clinical presentation, outcome, and proposal for a morphologic MRI classification based on a study of 90 patients. In: Guerrini R, Andermann F, Canapicchi R, et al., eds. *Dysplasias of Cerebral Cortex and Epilepsy.* Philadelphia: Lippincott–Raven, pp. 255–69.

Guerrini R, Parmeggiani A, Bureau M, et al. (1996b) Localized cortical dysplasia: good seizure outcome after sleep-related electrical status epilepticus. In: Guerrini R, Andermann F, Canapicchi R, et al., eds. *Dysplasias of Cerebral Cortex and Epilepsy.* Philadelphia: Lippincott–Raven, pp. 329–35.

Guerrini R, Dubeau F, Dulac O, et al. (1997) Bilateral parasagittal, parieto-occipital polymicrogyria and epilepsy. *Ann Neurol* **41**: 65–73.

Guerrini R, Barkovich A, Sztriha L, Dobyns WB (2000) Bilateral frontal polymicrogyria: a newly recognized brain malformation syndrome. *Neurology* **54**: 909–13.

Haas D, Kelley RI, Hoffmann GF (2001) Inherited disorders of cholesterol biosynthesis. *Neuropediatrics* **32**: 113–22.

Haberl H, Tallen G, Michael T, et al. (2004) Surgical aspects and outcome of delayed tethered cord release. *Zentralbl Neurochir* **65**: 161–7.

Hageman G, Hoogenraad TU, Prevo RL (1994) The association of cortical dysplasia and anterior horn arthrogryposis: a case report. *Brain Dev* **16**: 463–6.

Hahn JS, Plawner LL (2004) Evaluation and management of children with holoprosencephaly. *Pediatr Neurol* **31**: 79–88.

Haltia M, Leivo I, Somer H, et al. (1997) Muscle–eye–brain disease: a neuropathological study. *Ann Neurol* **41**: 173–89.

Hamdan AH, Walsh W, Bruner JP, Tulipan N (2004) Intrauterine myelomeningocele repair: effect on short-term complications of prematurity. *Fetal Diagn Ther* **19**: 83–6.

Hamiwka L, Jayakar P, Resnick T, et al. (2005) Surgery for epilepsy due to cortical malformations: ten-year follow-up. *Epilepsia* **46**: 556–60.

Hanefeld F (1999) Oligogyric microcephaly. *Neuropediatrics* **30**: 102–3.

Harbord MG, Lambert SR, Kriss A, et al. (1989) Autosomal recessive microcephaly, mental retardation with nonpigmentary retinopathy and a distinctive electroretinogram. *Neuropediatrics* **20**: 139–41.

Harbord MG, Boyd S, Hall-Crags MA, et al. (1990) Ataxia, developmental delay and an extensive neuronal migration abnormality in 2 siblings. *Neuropediatrics* **21**: 218–21.

Harding BN, Boyd SG (1991) Intractable seizures from infancy can be associated with dentato-olivary dysplasia. *J Neurol Sci* **104**: 157–65.

Harding BN, Copp JA (1997) Malformations. In: Graham DL, Lantos PL, eds. *Greenfield's Neuropathology, 6th edn.* London: Arnold, pp. 397–533.

Harmant-van Rijckevorsel G, Aubert-Tulkens G, Moulin D, Lyon G (1983) [Joubert syndrome. Clinical and anatomopathological study. Aetiopathogenic factors.] *Rev Neurol* **139**: 715–24 (French).

Harper T, Fordham LA, Wolfe HM (2007) The fetal Dandy–Walker complex: associated anomalies, perinatal outcome and postnatal imaging. *Fetal Diagn Ther* **22**: 277–81.

Harris CP, Townsend JJ, Klatt EC (1994a) Accessory brains (extracerebral heterotopias): unusual prenatal intracranial mass lesions. *J Child Neurol* **9**: 386–9.

Harris CP, Townsend JJ, Norman MG, et al. (1994b) Atelencephalic holoprosencephaly. *J Child Neurol* **9**: 412–6.

Harrison MJ, Mitnick RJ, Rosenblum BR, Rothman AS (1990) Leptomyelolipoma: analysis of 20 cases. *J Neurosurg* **73**: 360–7.

Hartley LM, Gordon I, Harkness W, et al. (2002) Correlation of SPECT with pathology and severe outcome in children undergoing epilepsy surgery. *Dev Med Child Neurol* **44**: 676–80.

Hartmann H, Uyanik G, Gross C, et al. (2004) Agenesis of the corpus callosum, abnormal genitalia and intractable epilepsy due to a novel familial mutation in the Aristaless-related homeobox gene. *Neuropediatrics* **35**: 157–60.

Has R, Ermis H, Yuksel A, et al. (2004) Dandy–Walker malformation: a review of 78 cases diagnosed by prenatal sonography. *Fetal Diagn Ther* **19**: 342–7.

Hasegawa Y, Hasegawa T, Yokoyama T, et al. (1990) Holoprosencephaly associated with diabetes insipidus and syndrome of inappropriate secretion of antidiuretic hormone. *J Pediatr* **117**: 756–8.

Hashimoto R, Seki T, Takuma Y, Suzuki N (1993) The 'double cortex' syndrome on MRI. *Brain Dev* **15**: 57–9.

Haslam R, Smith DW (1979) Autosomal dominant microcephaly. *J Pediatr* **95**: 701–5.

Haverkamp F, Zerres K, Ostertun B, et al. (1995) Familial schizencephaly: further delineation of a rare disorder. *J Med Genet* 32: 242–4.

Haverkamp F, Heep A, Woelfle J (2002) Psychomotor development in children with early diagnosed giant hemisphere cysts. *Dev Med Child Neurol* 44: 555–60.

Hays RM, Jordan RA, McLaughlin JF, et al. (1989) Central ventilatory dysfunction in myelodysplasia: an independent determinant of survival. *Dev Med Child Neurol* 31: 366–70.

Hayward JC, Titelbaum DS, Clancy RR, Zimmerman RA (1991) Lissencephaly–pachygyria associated with congenital cytomegalovirus infection. *J Child Neurol* 6: 109–14.

Hehr U, Gross C, Diebold U, et al. (2004) Wide phenotypic variability in families with holoprosencephly and a sonic hedgehog mutation. *Eur J Pediatr* 163: 347–52.

Hendrick EB, Hoffman HJ, Humphreys RP (1977) Tethered cord syndrome. In: McLaurin RL, ed. *Myelomeningocele*. New York: Grune & Stratton, pp. 369–73.

Hennekam RCM, Barth PG (2003) Syndromic cortical dysplasias: a review. In: Barth PG, ed. *Disorders of Neuronal Migration. International Review of Child Neurology Series*. London: Mac Keith Press for the International Child Neurology Association, pp. 135–69.

Henriques JG, Pianetti G, Henriques KS, et al. (2005) Minor skin lesions as markers of occult spinal dysraphisms—prospective study. *Surg Neurol* 63 Suppl 1: S8–12.

Herbert MR, Ziegler DA, Makris N, et al. (2004) Localization of white matter volume increase in autism and developmental language disorder. *Ann Neurol* 55: 530–40.

Hersh JH, Podruch PE, Rogers G, Weisskopf B (1985) Toluene embryopathy. *J Pediatr* 106: 922–7.

Hilal SK, Marton D, Pollack E (1974) Diastematomyelia in children: radiographic study of 34 cases. *Radiology* 112: 609–21.

Hirano S, Houdou S, Hasegawa M, et al. (1992) Clinicopathologic studies on leptomeningeal glioneuronal heterotopia in congenital anomalies. *Pediatr Neurol* 8: 441–4.

Hirayama K, Hoshino Y, Kumashiro M, Yamamoto T (1994) Reverse Shapiro's syndrome. A case of agenesis of the corpus callosum associated with periodic hyperthermia. *Arch Neurol* 51: 494–6.

Hirsch JF, Pierre-Kahn A (1988) Lumbosacral lipomas with spina bifida. *Childs Nerv Syst* 4: 354–60.

Hirsch JF, Pierre-Kahn A, Renier D, et al. (1984) The Dandy–Walker malformation. *J Neurosurg* 61: 515–22.

Hodgkins PR, Harris CL, Schawkat FS, et al. (2004) Joubert syndrome: long-term follow-up. *Dev Med Child Neurol* 46: 694–9.

Hoffman HJ, Neill J, Crone KR, et al. (1987) Hydrosyringomyelia and its management in childhood. *Neurosurgery* 21: 347–51.

Hoffmann GF, Trefz FK, Barth PG, et al. (1991) Macrocephaly: an important indication for organic acid analysis. *J Inherit Metab Dis* 14: 329–32.

Holtmann M, Woermann FG, Boenigk HE (2001) Multiple ptrerygium syndrome, bilateral periventricular nodular heterotopia and epileptic seizures—a syndrome? *Neuropediatrics* 32: 264–6.

Hong SE, Shugart YY, Huang DT, et al.(2000) Autosomal recessive lissencephaly with cerebellar hypoplasia is associated with human RELN mutations. *Nat Genet* 26: 93–6.

Hori A (1994) Tectocerebellar dysraphia with posterior encephalocele (Friede); report of the youngest case. Reappraisal of the condition uniting Cleland–Chiari (Arnold–Chiari) and Dandy–Walker syndromes. *Clin Neuropathol* 13: 216–20.

Hourihane JO, Bennett CP, Chaudhuri R, et al. (1993) A sibship with a neuronal migration defect, cerebellar hypoplasia and congenital lymphedema. *Neuropediatrics* 24: 43–6.

Howard HC, Mount DB, Rochefort D, et al. (2002) The K-Cl cotransporter KCC3 is mutant in a severe peripheral neuropathy associated with agenesis of the corpus callosum. *Nat Genet* 32: 384–92; erratum 681.

Hoyme HE, May PA, Kalberg WO, et al. (2005) A practical clinical approach to diagnosis of fetal alcohol spectrum disorders: clarification of the 1996 Institute of Medicine criteria. *Pediatrics* 115: 39–47.

Hughes HE, Miskin M (1986) Congenital microcephaly due to vascular disruption: in utero documentation. *Pediatrics* 78: 85–7.

Hunt GM (1990) Open spina bifida: outcome for a complete cohort treated unselectively and followed into adulthood. *Dev Med Child Neurol* 32: 108–18.

Huttenlocher PR, Taravath S, Mojtahedi S (1994) Periventricular heterotopia

and epilepsy. *Neurology* 44: 51–5.

Ianetti P, Raucci U, Basile LA, et al. (1993) Neuronal migrational disorders: diffuse cortical dysplasia or the "double cortex" syndrome. *Acta Paediatr* 82: 501–3.

Iida K, Hirano S, Takashima S, Miyahara S (1994) Developmental study of leptomeningeal glioneuronal heterotopia. *Pediatr Neurol* 10: 295–8.

Ishihara N, Yamada K, Yamada Y, et al. (2004) Clinical and molecular analysis of Mowat–Wilson syndrome associated with ZFHX1B mutations and deletions at 2q22-q24.1. *J Med Genet* 41: 387–93.

Izquierdo JM, Gil-Carcedo LM (1988) Recurrent meningitis and transethmoidal intranasal meningoencephalocele. *Dev Med Child Neurol* 30: 248–51.

Jaeken J, Carchon H (1993) The carbohydrate-deficient glycoprotein syndromes: an overview. *J Inherit Metab Dis* 16: 813–20.

Jaeken J, Van den Berghe G (1984) An infantile autistic syndrome characterized by the presence of succinyl purines in body fluids. *Lancet* 2: 958–1061.

James CCM, Lassman LP (1981) *Spina Bifida Occulta. Orthopedic, Radiological and Neurosurgical Aspects*. New York: Grune & Stratton.

Janota I, Polkey CE (1992) Cortical dysplasia in epilepsy—a study of material from surgical resections for intractable epilepsy. In: Pedley TR, Meldrum BS, eds. *Recent Advances in Epilepsy*. Edinburgh: Churchill Livingstone, pp. 37–49.

Jeeves MA, Temple CM (1987) A further study of language function in callosal agenesis. *Brain Lang* 32: 325–35.

Jellinger K, Gross K, Kaltenback E, Grisold W (1981) Holoprosencephaly and agenesis of the corpus callosum. Frequency of associated malformations. *Acta Neuropathol* 55: 1–10.

Jeret JS, Serur D, Wisniewski K, Lubin RA (1987) Clinicopathological findings associated with agenesis of the corpus callosum. *Brain Dev* 9: 255–64.

Jimenez D, Lopez-Mascaraque LM, Vaverde F, De Carlos JA (2002) Tangential migration in neocortical development. *Dev Biol* 244: 155–69.

Kamnasaran D (2005) Agensesis of the corpus callosum: lessons from humans and mice. *Clin Invest Med* 28: 267–82.

Kanatani S, Tabata H, Nakajima K (2005) Neuronal migration in cortical development. *J Child Neurol* 20: 274–9.

Kanev PM, Lemire RJ, Loeser JD, Berger MS (1990) Management and long-term follow-up review of children with lipomyelomeningocele, 1952–1987. *J Neurosurg* 73: 48–52.

Kaplan P (1983) X-linked recessive inheritance of agenesis of the corpus callosum. *J Med Genet* 20: 122–4.

Kaplowitz PB, Bodurtha J (1993) Congenital hypopituitarism and microphthalmia. Report of two cases. *Acta Paediatr* 82: 419–22.

Kato M, Dobyns WB (2003) Lissencephaly and the molecular basis of neuronal migration. *Hum Mol Genet* 12 Spec No 1: R89–96.

Kato M, Takizawa N, Yamada S, et al. (1999) Diffuse pachygyria with cerebellar hypoplasia: a milder form of microlissencephaly or a new genetic syndrome? *Ann Neurol* 46: 660–3.

Kato M, Das S, Petras K, et al. (2004) Mutations of ARX are associated with striking pleiotropy and consistent phenotype–genotype correlation. *Hum Mutat* 23: 147–59.

Kaufman BA (2004) Neural tube defects. *Pediatr Clin N Am* 51: 389–419.

Keefover R, Sam M, Bodensteiner J, Nicholson A (1995) Hypersomnolence and pure central sleep apnea associated with the Chiari I malformation. *J Child Neurol* 10: 65–7.

Kendall B, Kingsley D, Lambert SR, et al. (1990) Joubert syndrome: a clinico-radiological study. *Neuroradiology* 31: 502–6.

Khoury MJ, Erickson JD, Cordero JF, McCarthy BJ (1988) Congenital malformations and intrauterine growth retardation: a population study. *Pediatrics* 82: 83–90.

Kilickesmez O, Yavuz N, Hoca E (2004) Unilateral absence of cerebellar hemispheres: incidental diagnosis with magnetic resonance imaging. *Acta Radiol* 45: 876–7.

King JA, Gardner V, Chen H, Blackburn W (1995) Neu–Laxova syndrome: pathological evaluation of a fetus and review of the literature. *Pediatr Pathol Lab Med* 15: 57–9.

King MD, Dudgeon J, Stephenson JBP (1984) Joubert's syndrome with retinal dysplasia: neonatal tachypnoea as the clue to a genetic brain–eye malformation. *Arch Dis Child* 59: 709–18.

Kirk VG, Morielli A, Gozal D, et al. (2000) Treatment of sleep-disordered breathing in children with myelomeningocele. *Pediatr Pulmonol* 30: 445–52.

Kitamura K, Yanazawa M, Sugiyama N, et al. (2002) Mutation of ARX causes abnormal development of forebrain and testes in mice and X-linked lissencephaly with abnormal genitalia in humans. *Nat Genet* **32**: 359–69.

Klein CJ, Silber MH, Halliwill JR, et al. (2001) Basal forebrain malformation with hyperhidrosis and hypothermia: variant of Shapiro's syndrome. *Neurology* **56**: 254–6.

Klein O, Pierre-Kahn A, Boddaert N, et al. (2003) Dandy–Walker malformation: prenatal diagnosis and prognosis. *Childs Nerv Syst* **19**: 484–9.

Kobori JA, Herrick MK, Urich H (1987) Arhinencephaly: the spectrum of associated malformations. *Brain* **110**: 237–60.

Komagata M, Endo K, Nishiyama M, et al. (2004) Management of tight filum terminale. *Minim Invasive Neurosurg* **47**: 49–53.

Konkol RJ, Maister BH, Wells RG, Sty JR (1990) Hemimegalencephaly: clinical, EEG, neuroimaging, and IMP-SPECT correlation. *Pediatr Neurol* **6**: 414–8.

Kothari MJ, Kelly M, Darbey M, et al. (1995) Neurophysiologic assessment of urinary dysfunction in children with thoracic syringomyelia. *J Child Neurol* **10**: 451–4.

Kroon AA, Smit BJ, Barth PG, Hennekam RCM (1996) Lissencephaly with extreme cerebral and cerebellar hypoplasia. A magnetic resonance imaging study. *Neuropediatrics* **27**: 273–6.

Kumada S, Hayashi M, Arima K, et al. (2004) Renal disease in Arima syndrome is nephronophthisis as in other Joubert-related cerebello-oculo-renal syndromes. *Am J Med Genet A* **131**: 71–6.

Kuzniecky R (1994) Familial diffuse cortical dysplasia. *Arch Neurol* **51**: 307–10.

Kuzniecky R, Berkovic S, Andermann F, et al. (1986) Focal cortical myoclonus and rolandic cortical dysplasia: clarification by magnetic resonance imaging. *Ann Neurol* **23**: 317–25.

Kuzniecky R, Andermann F (1994) The congenital bilateral perisylvian syndrome: imaging findings in a multicenter study. CBPS Study Group. *AJNR* **15**: 139–44.

Kuzniecky R, Andermann F, Guerrini R (1994) The epileptic spectrum in the congenital bilateral perisylvian syndrome. CBPS Multicenter Collaborative Study. *Neurology* **44**: 379–85.

Lambert de Rouvroit C, Goffinet AM (2001) Neuronal migration. *Mech Dev* **105**: 47–56.

Lammer EJ, Chen DT, Hoar RM, et al. (1985) Retinoic acid embryopathy. *N Engl J Med* **313**: 837–41.

Lancet (2004) Indications for necessity of treatment in spina bifida cystica. *Lancet* **364**: 1883–95.

Larroche JC (1986) Fetal encephalopathies of circulatory origin. *Biol Neonate* **50**: 61–74.

Leão MJ, Ribeiro-Silva ML (1995) Orofaciodigital syndrome type I in a patient with severe CNS defects. *Pediatr Neurol* **13**: 247–51.

Leblanc E, Tampieri D, Robitaille Y, et al. (1991) Developmental anterobasal temporal encephalocele and temporal lobe epilepsy. *J Neurosurg* **74**: 933–9.

Lee BC, Zimmerman RD, Manning JJ, Deck MD (1985) MR imaging of syringomyelia and hydromyelia. *Am J Roentgenol* **144**: 1149–56.

Lee SK, Kim DI, Kim J, et al. (2005) Diffusion-tensor MR imaging and fiber tractography: a new method of describing aberrant fiber connections in develomental CNS anomalies. *Radiographics* **25**: 53–65.

Leech RW, Shuman RM (1986) Holoprosencephaly and related midline cerebral anomalies: a review. *J Child Neurol* **1**: 3–18.

Lena G, van Calenberg F, Genitori L, Choux M (1995) Supratentorial interhemispheric cysts associated with callosal agenesis: surgical treatment and outcome in 16 children. *Childs Nerv Syst* **11**: 568–73.

Lepinard C, Coutant R, Boussion F, et al. (2005) Prenatal diagnosis of absence of the septum pellucidum associated with septo-optic dysplasia. *Ultrasound Obstet Gynecol* **25**: 73–5.

Leventer RJ, Cardoso C, Ledbetter DH, Dobyns WB (2001) LIS1 missense mutations cause milder lissencephaly phenotypes including a child with normal IQ. *Neurology* **57**: 416–22.

Levine DN (2004) The pathogenesis of syringomyelia associated with lesions of the foramen magnum: a critical review of existing theories and proposal of a new hypothesis. *J Neurol Sci* **220**: 3–21.

Lewis AJ, Simon EM, Barkovich AJ, et al. (2002) Middle hemispheric variant of holoprosencephaly: a distinct cliniconeuroradiologic subtype. *Neurology* **59**: 1860–5.

Li LM, Dubeau F, Andermann F, et al. (1997) Periventricular nodular heterotopia and intractable temporal lobe epilepsy: poor outcome after temporal lobe resection. *Ann Neurol* **41**: 662–8.

Liang JS, Lee WT, Peng SS, et al. (2002) Schizencephaly: correlation between clinical and neuroimaging features. *Acta Paediatr Taiwan* **43**: 208–13.

Lie RT, Wilcox AJ, Skjaerven R (1994) A population-based study of the risk of recurrence of birth defects. *N Engl J Med* **331**: 1–4.

Lincke CR, van den Bogert C, Nijtmans LG, et al. (1996) Cerebellar hypoplasia in respiratory chain dysfunction. *Neuropediatrics* **27**: 216–8.

Lindhout D, Schmidt D (1986) In-utero exposure to valproate and neural tube defects. *Lancet* **1**: 1392–3.

Lindhout D, Barth PG, Valk J, Boen-Tan TN (1980) Joubert syndrome associated with bilateral chorioretinal coloboma. *Eur J Pediatr* **134**: 173–6.

Livingston JH, Aicardi J (1990) Unusual MRI appearance of diffuse subcortical heterotopia or 'double-cortex' in two children. *J Neurol Neurosurg Psychiatry* **53**: 617–20.

Lorber J (1975) Ethical problems in the management of myelomeningocele and hydrocephalus. The Milroy Lecture 1975. *J R Coll Physicians Lond* **10**: 47–60.

Lorber J, Priestley BL (1981) Children with large heads: a practical approach to diagnosis in 557 children with special reference to 109 children with megalencephaly. *Dev Med Child Neurol* **23**: 494–504.

Lorber J, Schofield JK (1979) The prognosis of occipital encephalocele. *Z Kinderchir Grenzgeb* **28**: 347–51.

Luciano R (1987) Epidemiology and etiology of neural tube defects: an updating. *J Pediatr Neurosci* **3**: 57–71.

Lyon G, Beaugerie A (1988) Congenital developmental malformations. In: Levene MI, Bennett MJ, Punt J, eds. *Fetal and Neonatal Neurology and Neurosugery.* Edinburgh: Churchill Livingstone, pp. 231–48.

Mahapatra AK, Agrawal D (2006) Anterior encephaloceles: a series of 103 cases over 32 years. *J Clin Neurosci* **13**: 536–9.

Malinger G, Lev D, Kidron D, et al. (2005) Differential diagnosis in fetuses with absent septum pellucidum. *Ultrasound Obstet Gynecol* **25**: 42–9.

Mancini J, Lethel V, Hugonenq C, Chabrol B (2001) Brain injuries in early fetal life: consequences for brain development. *Dev Med Child Neurol* **43**: 52–5.

Manning MA, Gunnef CM, Colby CE, et al. (2004) Neu–Laxova syndrome: detailed prenatal diagnostic and post-mortem findings and literature review. *Am J Med Genet* **125**: 240–8.

Mariani C, Cislaghi MG, Barbieri S, et al. (1991) The natural history and results of surgery in 50 cases of syringomyelia. *J Neurol* **238**: 433–8.

Marin-Padilla M (1991) Cephalic axial skeletal–neural dysraphic disorders: embryology and pathology. *Can J Neurol Sci* **18**: 153–69.

Marin-Padilla M (1999) Developmental neuropathology and impact of perinatal brain damage. III: Gray matter lesions of the neocortex. *J Neuropathol Exp Neurol* **58**: 407–29.

Marin-Padilla M (2000) Perinatal brain damage, cortical reorganization (acquired cortical dysplasias), and epilepsy. *Adv Neurol* **84**: 153–72.

Marques-Dias MJ, Harmant-Van Rijckevorsel G, Landrieu P, Lyon G (1984) Prenatal cytomegalovirus disease and cerebral microgyria: evidence for perfusion failure, not disturbance of histogenesis, as the major cause of fetal cytomegalovirus encephalopathy. *Neuropediatrics* **15**: 18–24.

Martinez-Lage JF, Casas C, Fernández MA, et al. (1994) Macrocephaly, dystonia, and bilateral temporal arachnoid cysts: glutaric aciduria type 1. *Childs Nerv Syst* **10**: 198–203.

Martinez-Lage JF, Esteban JA, Poza M, Casas C (1995) Congenital dermal sinus associated with an abscessed intramedullary epidermoid cyst in a child: case report and review of the literature. *Childs Nerv Syst* **11**: 301–5.

Martinez-Lage JF, Poza M, Sola J, et al. (1996) The child with a cephalocele: etiology, neuroimaging, and outcome. *Childs Nerv Syst* **12**: 540–50.

Masera N, Grant DB, Stanhope R, Preece MA (1994) Diabetes insipidus with impaired osmotic regulation in septo-optic dysplasia and agenesis of the corpus callosum. *Arch Dis Child* **70**: 51–3.

Matson DD (1969) *Neurosurgery of Infancy and Childhood, 2nd edn.* Springfield, IL: CC Thomas.

Matsunaga E, Shiota K (1987) Holoprosencephaly in human embryos: epidemiologic studies of 150 cases. *Brain Res* **400**: 239–46.

Matsuzaka T, Sakuragawa N, Nakayama H, et al. (1986) Cerebro-oculo-hepato-renal syndrome (Arima's syndrome): a distinct clinicopathological entity. *J Child Neurol* **1**: 338–46.

Matthews PM, Brown RM, Otero L, et al. (1993) Neurodevelopmental abnormalities and lactic acidosis in a girl with a 20-bp deletion in the X-linked pyruvate dehydrogenase E1a subunit gene. *Neurology* **43**: 2025–30.

McConnell SK (1992) Perspectives on early brain development and the epilepsies. *Epilepsy Res Suppl* **9**: 183–91.

McConnell S, Kaznowski CE (1991) Cell cycle dependence of laminar determination in developing neocortex. *Science* **254**: 282–5.

McLone DG, Dias MS (2003) The Chiari II malformation: cause and impact. *Childs Nerv Syst* 19: 540–50.

Meencke HJ, Veith G (1992) Migration disturbances in epilepsy. *Epilepsy Res Suppl* 12: 31–9.

Menezes AV, MacGregor DL, Buncic JR (1994) Aicardi syndrome: natural history and possible predictors of severity. *Pediatr Neurol* 11: 313–8.

Menezes L, Aicardi J, Goutières F (1988) Absence of the septum pellucidum with porencephalia: a neuroradiologic syndrome with variable clinical expression. *Arch Neurol* 45: 542–5.

Menkes JH, Philippart M, Clark DB (1964) Hereditary partial agenesis of the corpus callosum. *Arch Neurol* 11: 198–208.

Menzel O, Bekkeheien RC, Reymond A, et al. (2004) Knobloch syndrome: novel mutations in COL18A1, evidence for genetic heterogeneity, and a functionally impaired polymorphism in endostatin. *Hum Mutat* 23: 77–84.

Merello E, De Marco P, Mascelli S, et al. (2006) HLXB9 homeobox gene and caudal regression syndrome. *Birth Defects Res A Clin Mol Teratol* 76: 205–9; erratum 568.

Metry DW, Dowd CF, Barkovich AJ, Frieden IJ (2001) The many faces of PHACE syndrome. *J Pediatr* 139: 117–23; erratum 470.

Miki T, Wada J, Nakajima N, et al. (2005) Operative indications and neuro-endoscopic management of symptomatic cysts of the septum pellucidum. *Childs Nerv Syst* 21: 372–81.

Mikulis DJ, Diaz O, Egglin TK, Sanchez R (1992) Variance of the position of the cerebellar tonsils with age: preliminary report. *Radiology* 183: 725–8.

Ming JE, Muenke M (2002) Multiple hits during early embryonic development: digenic diseases and holoprosencephaly. *Am J Hum Genet* 71: 1017–32.

Mitchell LE, Adzick NS, Melchionne J, et al. (2004) Spina bifida. *Lancet* 364: 1885–95.

Mittermayer C, Lee A, Brugger IC (2004) Prenatal diagnosis of the Meckel–Gruber syndrome from 11th to 20th gestational week. *Ultraschall Med* 25: 275–9.

Moerman P, Fryns J-P, Vandenberghe K, Lauweryns JM (1992) Constrictive amniotic bands, amniotic adhesions, and limb–body wall complex: discrete disruption sequences with pathogenetic overlap. *Am J Med Genet* 42: 470–9.

Mohanty A, Biswas A, Satish S, et al. (2006) Treatment options for Dandy–Walker malformation. *J Neurosurg* 105 (5 Suppl): 348–56.

Molina JA, Mateos F, Merino M, et al. (1989) Aicardi syndrome in two sisters. *J Pediatr* 115: 282–3.

Moog U, Jones MC, Bird LM, Dobyns WB (2005) Oculocerebrocutaneous syndrome: the brain malformation defines a core phenotype. *J Med Genet* 42: 913–21; erratum 2006 43: 243.

Morgan NV, Bacchilli C, Gissen P, et al. (2002) A novel locus for Meckel–Gruber syndrome, MKS3, maps to chromosome 8q 24. *Hum Genet* 111: 456–61.

Mori K, Hashimoto T, Tayama M, et al. (1994) Serial EEG and sleep polygraphic studies on lissencephaly (agyria–pachygyria). *Brain Dev* 16: 365–73.

Morioka M, Marubayashi T, Masumitsu T, et al. (1995) Basal encephaloceles with morning glory syndrome, and progressive hormonal and visual disturbances: case report and review of the literature. *Brain Dev* 17: 196–201.

Morishima A, Aranov GS (1986) Syndrome of septo-optic dysplasia: the clinical spectrum. *Brain Dev* 8: 233–9.

Moutard MC, Kieffer V, Feingold J, et al. (2003) Agenesis of the corpus callosum: prenatal diagnosis and prognosis. *Childs Nerv Syst* 19: 1–6.

MRC Study Research Group (1991) Prevention of neural tube defects: results of the Medical Research Council vitamin study. *Lancet* 338: 131–7.

Murray JC, Johnson JA, Bird TD (1985) Dandy–Walker malformation: etiologic heterogeneity and empiric recurrence risks. *Clin Genet* 28: 272–83.

Naidich TP, McLone DG, Mutluer S (1983) A new understanding of dorsal dysraphism with lipoma (lipomyeloschisis): radiologic evaluation and surgical correction. *AJNR* 4: 103–16.

Naidich TP, Osbom RE, Bauer B, Naidich MJ (1990) Anterior basal encephalocele in the median cleft face syndrome. Comments on nosology and treatment. *Genet Couns* 1: 103–9.

Nanni l, Ming JE, Bocian M, et al. (1999) The mutational spectrum of the sonic hedgehog gene in holoprosencephaly: SHH mutations cause a significant proportion of autosomal dominant holoprosencephaly. *Hum Mol Genet* 8: 2479–88.

Nassogne MC, Evrard P, Courtoy PJ (1998) Selective direct toxicity of cocaine on fetal mouse neurons. Teratogenic implications of neurite and apoptotic neuronal loss. *Ann NY Acad Sci* 846: 51–68.

Natowicz M, Chatten J, Clancy R, et al. (1988) Genetic disorders and major extracardiac anomalies associated with the hypoplastic left heart syndrome. *Pediatrics* 82: 698–706.

Navarro R, Olavarria G, Seshadri R, et al. (2004) Surgical results of posterior fossa decompression for patients with Chiari 1 malformation. *Childs Nerv Syst* 20: 349–56.

Nelson MD, Maher K, Gilles FH (2004) A different approach to cysts in the posterior fossa. *Pediatr Radiol* 34: 720–32.

Nevin NC, Lim JH (1990) Syndrome of partial aniridia, cerebellar ataxia, and mental retardation—Gillespie syndrome. *Am J Med Genet* 35: 468–9.

Nézelof C, Jaubert F, Lyon G (1976) [Familial syndrome combining short small intestine, intestinal malrotation, pyloric hypertrophy and brain malformations. 3 anatomoclinical case reports.] *Ann Anat Pathol* 21: 401–12 (French).

Nievelstein RA, Valk J, Smit LM, Vermeij-Keers C (1994) MR of the caudal regression syndrome: embryologic implications. *AJNR* 15: 1021–9.

Nishikawa M, Ichiyama T, Hayashi T, Furukawa S (1997) A case of early myoclonic encephalopathy with the congenital nephrotic syndrome. *Brain Dev* 19: 144–7.

Nissenkorn A, Michelson M, Ben Zeev B, Lerman-Sagie T (2001) Inborn errors of metabolism: a cause of abnormal brain development. *Neurology* 56: 1265–72.

Noorani PA, Bodensteiner JB, Barnes PD (1988) Colpocephaly: frequency and associated findings. *J Child Neurol* 3: 100–4.

Nyberg DA, Mack LA, Bronstein A, et al. (1987) Holoprosencephaly: prenatal sonographic diagnosis. *AJNR* 149: 1051–8.

Oba H, Barkovich AJ (1995) Holoprosencephaly: an analysis of callosal formation and its relation to development of the interhemispheric fissure. *AJNR* 16: 453–60.

Okumura A, Kidokoro H, Itomi K, et al. (2008) Subacute encephalopathy: clinical features, laboratory data, neuroimaging, and outcomes. *Pediatr Neurol* 38: 111-7.

Olney RS, Mulinare J (2002) Trends in neural tube defect prevalence, folic acid fortification, and vitamin supplement use. *Semin Perinatol* 26: 277–85.

Opitz JM, Holt MC (1990) Microcephaly: general considerations and aids to nosology. *J Craniofac Genet Dev Biol* 10: 175–204.

Oren J, Kelly DH, Todres D, Shannon DC (1986) Respiratory complications in patients with myelodysplasia and Arnold–Chiari malformation. *Am J Dis Child* 140: 221–4.

Ouvrier R, Billson F (1986) Optic nerve hypoplasia: a review. *J Child Neurol* 1: 181–8.

Paetau A, Salonen R, Haltia M (1985) Brain pathology in the Meckel syndrome: a study of 59 cases. *Clin Neuropathol* 4: 56–62.

Paladin F, Chiron C, Dulac O, et al. (1989) Electroencephalographic aspects of hemimegalencephaly. *Dev Med Child Neurol* 31: 377–83.

Palm I, Hagerstrand I, Kristofferson U, et al. (1986) Nephrosis and disturbances of neuronal migration in male siblings. A new hereditary disorder. *Arch Dis Child* 61: 545–8.

Palmini A, Andermann F, Aicardi J, et al. (1991) Diffuse cortical dysplasia, or the 'double cortex' syndrome: the clinical and epileptic spectrum in 10 patients. *Neurology* 41: 1656–62.

Palmini A, Andermann F, de Grissac H, et al. (1993) Stages and patterns of centrifugal arrest of diffuse neuronal migration disorders. *Dev Med Child Neurol* 35: 331–9.

Palmini A, Gambardella A, Andermann F, et al. (1996) The human dysplastic cortex is intrinsically epileptogenic. In: Guerrini R, Andermann F, Canapicchi R, et al., eds. *Dysplasias of Cerebral Cortex and Epilepsy.* Philadelphia: Lippincott–Raven, pp. 43–52.

Palmini A, Najm I, Avanzini G, et al. (2004) Terminology and classification of the cortical dysplasias. *Neurology* 62 Suppl 3: 32–8.

Papasozomenos S, Roessmann U (1981) Respiratory distress and Arnold–Chiari malformation. *Neurology* 31: 97–100.

Parisi MA, Dobyns WB (2003) Human malformations of the midbrain and hindbrain: review and proposed classification scheme. *Mol Genet Metab* 80: 36–53.

Parmeggiani A, Santucci M, Ambrosetto P, et al. (1994) Interictal EEG findings in two cases with 'double cortex' syndrome. *Brain Dev* 16: 320–4.

Parrini E, Ramazzotti A, Dobyns WB, et al. (2006) Periventricular heterotopia: phenotypic heterogeneity and correlation with Filamin A mutations. *Brain* 129: 1892–906.

Parrish ML, Roessmann U, Levinsohn MW (1979) Agenesis of the corpus callosum: a study of the frequency of associated malformations. *Ann Neurol* 6: 349–54.

Pascual-Castroviejo I, Velez A, Pascual-Pascual SI, et al. (1991) Dandy–Walker malformation: analysis of 38 cases. *Childs Nerv Syst* 7: 88–97.

Pascual-Castroviejo I, Guttierez M, Morales C, et al. (1994) Primary degeneration of the granular layer of the cerebellum. A study of 14 patients and review of the literature. *Neuropediatrics* 25: 183–90.

Pascual-Castroviejo I, López-Gutiérrez JC, Pascual-Pascual SI, et al. (2003) [Cutaneous haemangiomas, vascular malformations and associated disorders. A new neurocutaneous syndrome.] *An Pediatr* 58: 339–49 (Spanish).

Pascual-Castroviejo I, Pascual-Pascual SI, Velázquez-Fragua R, Lapunzina P (2005) Oculocerebrocutaneous (Delleman) syndrome: report of two cases. *Neuropediatrics* 36: 50–4.

Patel S, Barkovich AJ (2002) Analysis and classification of cerebellar malformations. *AJNR* 24: 1074–87.

Paul LK, Van Lancker-Sidtis D, Schieffer B, et al. (2003) Communicative deficits in agenesis of the corpus callosum: nonliteral language and affective prosody. *Brain Lang* 85: 313–24.

Pelayo R, Barasch E, Kang H, et al. (1994) Progressively intractable seizures, focal alopecia, and hemimegalencephaly. *Neurology* 44: 969–71.

Peter JC, Fieggen G (1999) Congenital malformations of the brain—a neuroimaging perspective at the close of the 20th century. *Childs Nerv Syst* 15: 633–45.

Petersen MC, Wolraich M, Sherbondy A, Wagener J (1995) Abnormalities in control of ventilation in newborn infants with myelomeningocele. *J Pediatr* 126: 1011–5.

Phelan MC, Rogers RC, Saul RA, et al. (2001) 22q13 deletion syndrome. *Am J Hum Genet* 101: 91–9.

Piao X, Chang BS, Bodell A, et al. (2006) Genotype–phenotype analysis of human frontoparietal polymicrogyria syndromes. *Ann Neurol* 58: 680–7.

Pierre-Kahn A, Zerah M, Renier D, et al. (1997) Congenital lumbosacral lipomas. *Childs Nerv Syst* 13: 298–334.

Pierre-Kahn A, Schmit P, Zerah M, et al. (2003) Prenatal diagnosis of diastematomyelia. *Childs Nerv Syst* 19: 555–60.

Pihko H, Lappi M, Raitta C, et al. (1995) Ocular findings in muscle–eye–brain (MEB) disease: a follow-up study. *Brain Dev* 17: 57–61.

Pilz DT, Matsumoto N, Minnerath S, et al. (1998) LIS1 and XLIS (DCX) mutations cause most classical lissencephaly, but different patterns of malformation. *Hum Mol Genet* 7: 2029–37.

Pinard JM, Motte J, Chiron C, et al. (1994) Subcortical laminar heterotopia and lissencephaly in two families: a single X linked dominant gene. *J Neurol Neurosurg Psychiatry* 57: 914–20.

Polizzi A, Pavone P, Ianetti P, et al. (2006) Septo-optic dysplasia complex: a heterogeneous malformation complex. *Pediatr Neurol* 34: 66–71.

Poll-Thé BT, Aicardi J (1985) Pseudomonoventricle due to a malformation of the septum pellucidum. *Neuropediatrics* 16: 39–42.

Pou Serradell A, Mares Segura R (1988) [Clinico-morphological correlations based on MRI in syringomyelia: study of 22 cases.] *Rev Neurol* 144: 181–93 (French).

Powers M (1995) The pathology of peroxismal disorders with pathogenetic considerations. *J Neuropathol Exp Neurol* 28: 369–83.

Probst FP (1979) *The Prosencephalies.* Berlin: Springer.

Quirk JA, Kendall B, Kingsley DPE, et al. (1993) EEG features of cortical dysplasia in children. *Neuropediatrics* 24: 193–9.

Rainbow LA, Rees SA, Shaikh MG, et al. (2005) Mutation analysis of POUF-1, PROP-1 and HESX-1 show low frequency of mutations in children with sporadic forms of combined pituitary hormone deficiency and septo-optic dysplasia. *Clin Endocrinol* 62: 163–8.

Rakic P (1981) Developmental events leading to laminar and areal organization of the neocortex. In: Schmitt FO, Worden FG, Denis SG, eds. *The Organization of Cerebral Cortex.* Cambridge, MA: MIT Press, pp. 7–28.

Rakic S, Zecevic N (2003) Emerging complexity of layer I in human cortex. *Cereb Cortex* 13: 1072–83.

Raoul C, Hennekam M, Barth PG (2003) Syndromic cortical dysplasias: a review. In: Barth PG, ed. *Disorders of Neuronal Migration. International Review of Child Neurology Series.* London: Mac Keith Press for the International Child Neurology Association, pp. 135–69.

Ray JG, Meier C, Vermeulen MJ, et al. (2002) Association of neural tube defects and folic acid food fortification in Canada. *Lancet* 360: 2047–8.

Raybaud C, Girard N, Canto-Moreira N, Poncet M (1996) High-definition magnetic resonance imaging identification of cortical dysplasias: micropolygyria versus lissencephaly. In: Guerrini R, Andermann F, Canapicchi R, et al., eds. *Dysplasias of Cerebral Cortex and Epilepsy.* Philadelphia: Lippincott–Raven, pp. 131–43.

Raybaud C, Girard N, Levrier O, et al. (2001) Schizencephaly: correlation

between the lobar topography of the clefts and absence of the septum pellucidum. *Childs Nerv Syst* 17: 717–22.

Raymond AA, Fish DR, Stevens JM, et al. (1994) Subependymal heterotopia: a distinct neuronal migration disorder associated with epilepsy. *J Neurol Neurosurg Psychiatry* 57: 1195–202.

Rebhandl W, Rami B, Barcik U, et al. (1998) Neurenteric cyst mimicking pleurodynia: an unusual case of thoracic pain in a child. *Pediatr Neurol* 8: 272–4.

Renier WO, Gabreëls FJ, Hustins TW, et al. (1983) Cerebellar hypoplasia, communicating hydrocephalus and mental retardation in two brothers and a maternal uncle. *Brain Dev* 5: 41–5.

Rhodes RE, Hatten HP, Ellington KS (1992) Walker–Warburg syndrome. *AJNR* 13: 123–6.

Richaud J (1988) Spinal meningeal malformations in children without meningoceles and meningomyeloceles. *Childs Nerv Syst* 4: 79–87.

Rickwood AMK (1990) Investigations. In: Borzyskowski M, Mundy AR, eds. *Neuropathic Bladder in Childhood. Clinics in Developmental Medicine No. 111.* London: Mac Keith Press, pp. 10–26.

Rivier F, Echenne B (1992) Dominantly inherited hypoplasia of the vermis. *Neuropediatrics* 23: 206–8.

Robain O, Deonna T (1983) Pachygyria and congenital nephrosis: disorder of migration and neuronal orientation. *Acta Neuropathol* 60: 137–41.

Robain O, Dulac O (1992) Early epileptic encephalopathy with suppression bursts and olivary–dentate dysplasia. *Neuropediatrics* 23: 162–4.

Robain O, Dulac O, Lejeune J (1987) Cerebellar hemispheric agenesis. *Acta Neuropathol* 74: 202–6.

Robain O, Floquet C, Heldt N, Rozenberg F (1988) Hemimegalencephaly: a clinicopathological study of four cases. *Neuropathol Appl Neurobiol* 14: 125–35.

Robinson AJ, Russell S, Rimmer R, et al. (2005) The value of ultrasonic examination of the lumbar spine in infants with specific reference to cutaneous markers of occult spinal dysraphism. *Clin Radiol* 60: 72–7.

Rockel AJ, Hiorns RW, Powell TPS (1980) The basic uniformity in structure of the neocortex. *Brain* 103: 221–44.

Roelens FA, Barth PG, van der Harten JJ (1999) Subependymal nodular heterotopia in patients with encephalocele. *Eur J Paediatr Neurol* 3: 59–63.

Roessler E, Belloni E, Gaudenz K, et al. (1998) Mutations in the human Sonic Hedgehog gene cause holoprosencephaly. *Nat Genet* 14: 357–60.

Roessmann U, Horwitz SJ, Kennell JH (1990) Congenital absence of the corticospinal fibers: pathologic and clinical observations. *Neurology* 40: 538–41.

Romano S, Boddaert N, Desguerre I, et al. (2006) Molar tooth sign and superior vermian dysplasia: a radiological, clinical, and genetic study. *Neuropediatrics* 37: 42–5.

Ronen GM, Andrews WL (1991) Holoprosencephaly as a possible embryonic alcohol effect. *Am J Med Genet* 40: 151–4.

Rorke LB, Fogelson MH, Riggs HE (1968) Cerebellar heterotopia in infancy. *Dev Med Child Neurol* 10: 644–50.

Rosa FW (1991) Spina bifida in infants of women treated with carbamazepine during pregnancy. *N Engl J Med* 324: 674–7.

Ross GW, Miller JQ, Persing JA, Urich H (1989) Hemimegalencephaly, hemifacial hypertrophy and intracranial lipoma: a variant of neurofibromatosis. *Neurofibromatosis* 2: 69–77.

Ross ME, Swanson K, Dobyns WB (2001) Lissencephaly with cerebellar hypoplasia (LCH): a heterogeneous group of cortical malformations. *Neuropediatrics* 32: 256–63.

Rossi M, Guerrini R, Dobyns WB (2003) Characterization of brain malformations in the Baraitser–Winter syndrome and review of the literature. *Neuropediatrics* 34: 287–92.

Rouse B, Matalon R, Koch P, et al. (2000) Maternal phenylketonuria syndrome: congenital heart defects, microcephaly and developmental outcome. *J Pediatr* 136: 57–61.

Royo-Salvador MB, Sole-Llenas J, Domenech JM, Gonzalez-Adrio R (2005) Results of section of the filum terminale in 20 patients wth syringomyelia, scoliosis and Chiari malformation. *Acta Neurochir* 147: 515–23.

Sakai N, Nakakita N, Yamazaki Y, et al. (2002) Oral–facial–digital syndrome type II (Mohr syndrome): clinical and genetic manifestations. *J Craniofac Surg* 13: 321–6.

Salamon N, Andres M, Chute DJ, et al. (2006) Contralateral hemimicrencephaly and clinical–pathological correlations in children with hemimegalencephaly. *Brain* 129: 352–65.

Saletti V, Bulgheroni S, D'Incerti L, et al. (2007) Verbal and gestural communication in children with bilateral perisylvian polymicrogyria. *J Child Neurol* **22**: 1090–8.

Salonen R, Somer M, Haltia M, et al. (1991) Progressive encephalopathy with edema, hypsarrhythmia, and optic atrophy (PEHO syndrome). *Clin Genet* **39**: 287–93.

Samson JF, Barth PG, de Vries JI, et al. (1994) Familial mitochondrial encephalopathy with fetal ultrasonographic ventriculomegaly and intracerebral calcifications. *Eur J Pediatr* **153**: 510–6.

Santavuori P, Somer H, Sainio K, et al. (1989) Muscle–eye–brain disease (MEB). *Brain Dev* **11**: 147–53.

Santavuori P, Valanne L, Autti T, et al. (1998) Muscle–eye–brain disease: clinical features, visual evoked potentials and brain imaging in 20 patients. *Eur J Paediatr Neurol* **2**: 41–7.

Saraiva JM, Baraitser M (1992) Joubert syndrome: a review. *Am J Med Genet* **43**: 726–31.

Sarnat HB (1987) Disturbances of late neuronal migrations in the perinatal period. *Am J Dis Child* **141**: 969–80.

Sarnat HB, Alcala H (1980) Human cerebellar hypoplasia: a syndrome of diverse causes. *Arch Neurol* **37**: 300–5.

Sarnat HB, Flores-Sarnat L (2001a) A new classification of malformations of the nervous system: an integration of morphological and molecular genetic criteria as patterns of genetic expression. *Eur J Paediatr Neurol* **5**: 57–64.

Sarnat HB, Flores-Sarnat L (2001b) Etiological classification of CNS malformations: integration of molecular genetic and morphological criteria. *Epileptic Disord* **5** Suppl 2: S35–43.

Sarnat HB, Flores-Sarnat L (2002) Molecular genetic and morphologic interaction in malformations of the nervous system for etiologic classification. *Semin Pediatr Neurol* **9**: 335–44.

Sarnat HB, Flores-Sarnat L (2004) Integrative classification of morphology and molecular genetics in central nervous system malformations. *Am J Med Genet A* **126**: 386–92.

Sato N, Matsuishi T, Utsunomya H, et al. (1987) Aicardi syndrome with holoprosencephaly and cleft lip and palate. *Pediatr Neurol* **3**: 114–6.

Sato N, Katsumata N, Kagami M, et al. (2004) Clinical assessment and mutation analysis of Kallmann syndrome 1 (KAL1) and fibroblast growth factor receptor 1 (FGFR1, or KAL2) in five families and 18 sporadic patients. *J Clin Endocrinol Metab* **89**: 1079–88.

Satran D, Pierpont ME, Dobyns WB (1999) Cerebello-oculo-renal syndromes including Arima, Senior–Löken and COACH syndromes: more than just variants of Joubert syndrome. *Am J Med Genet* **86**: 459–69.

Schijman E (2003) Split spinal cord malformations: report of 22 cases and review of the literature. *Childs Nerv Syst* **19**: 104–5.

Schijman E, Steinbok P (2004) International survey on the management of the Chiari I malformation and of syringomyelia. *Childs Nerv Syst* **20**: 341–8.

Schoenle EJ, Haselbacher GK, Briner J, et al. (1982) Elevated concentration of IGF II in brain tissue from an infant with macrencephaly. *J Pediatr* **108**: 737–40.

Schwartz JF, O'Brien MS, Hoffman JC (1980) Hereditary spinal arachnoid cysts, distichiasis, and lymphedema. *Ann Neurol* **7**: 340–3.

Sébire G, Husson B, Dusser A, et al. (1996) Congenital unilateral perisylvian syndrome: radiological basis and clinical correlations. *J Neurol Neurosurg Psychiatry* **61**: 52–6.

Seeds JW (2004) Diagnostic mid trimester amniocentesis: how safe? *Am J Obstet Gynecol* **191**: 607–15.

Seemanova E, Passarge E, Beneskova D, et al. (1985) Familial microcephaly with normal intelligence, immunodeficiency and risk of lymphoreticular malignancies: a new autosomal recessive disorder. *Am J Med Genet* **20**: 639–48.

Seller MJ (1987) Neural tube defects and sex ratios. *Am J Med Genet* **26**: 699–707.

Sener NR (1995) Cerebellar agenesis versus vanishing cererebellum in Chiari II malformation. *Computer Med Imaging Graph* **19**: 491–4.

Serur D, Jeret JS, Wisniewski K (1988) Agenesis of the corpus callosum: clinical, neuroradiological and cytogenetic studies. *Neuropediatrics* **19**: 87–91.

Shanks DE, Wilson WG (1988) Lobar holoprosencephaly presenting as spastic diplegia. *Dev Med Child Neurol* **30**: 383–6.

Shapira SK, McGaskill C, Northrup H, et al. (1997) Chromosome 1p36 deletions: the clinical phenotype and molecular characterization of a common newly delineated syndrome. *Am J Hum Genet* **61**: 642–50.

Shapiro WR, Williams GH, Plum F (1969) Spontaneous recurrent hypothermia accompanying agenesis of the corpus callosum. *Brain* **92**: 423–36.

Sharma A, Sayal P, Badhe P, et al. (2004) Spinal intramedullary arachnoid cyst. *Indian J Pediatr* **71**: e 65–7.

Shaw CM, Alvord EC (1996) Global cerebral dysplasia due to dysplasia and hyperplasia of periventricular germinal cells. *J Child Neurol* **11**: 313–20.

Sher PK, Brown SB (1975a) A longitudinal study of head growth in pre-term infants. I. Normal rates of head growth. *Dev Med Child Neurol* **17**: 705–10.

Sher PK, Brown SB (1975b) A longitudinal study of head growth in pre-term infants. II. Differentiation between 'catch-up' growth and early infantile hydrocephalus. *Dev Med Child Neurol* **17**: 711–8.

Sheth RD, Barron TF, Hartlage PL (1994) Episodic spontaneous hypothermia with hyperhydrosis: implications for pathogenesis. *Pediatr Neurol* **10**: 58–60.

Shevell MI, Matthews PM, Scriver CR, et al. (1994) Cerebral dysgenesis and lactic acidemia: an MRI/MRS phenotype associated with pyruvate dehydrogenase deficiency. *Pediatr Neurol* **11**: 224–9.

Siffel C Wong LY, Olney RS, Correa A (2003) Survival of infants diagnosed with encephalocele in Atlanta, 1979–98. *Pediatr Perinat Epidemiol* **17**: 40–8.

Silengo M, Lerone M, Martinelli M, et al. (1992) Autosomal recessive microcephaly with early onset seizures and spasticity. *Clin Genet* **42**: 152–5.

Simon EM, Goldstein RB, Coakley FV, et al. (2000a) Fast MR imaging of fetal CNS anomalies in utero. *AJNR* **21**: 1688–90.

Simon EM, Hevner R, Pinter JD, et al. (2000b) Assessment of the deep gray nuclei in holoprosencephaly. *AJNR* **23**: 1955–61.

Simon EM, Hevner R, Pinter JD, et al. (2002) The middle hemispheric variant of holoprosencephaly. *AJNR* **23**: 151–6.

Simpson RK, Rose JE (1987) Cervical diastematomyelia: report of a case and review of a rare congenital anomaly. *Arch Neurol* **44**: 331–5.

Singh SK, Singh RD, Sharma A (2005) Caudal regression syndrome—case report and review of literature. *Pediatr Surg Int* **21**: 578–81.

Sisodiya SM, Free SL, Stevens JM, et al. (1995) Widespread cerebral structural changes in patients with cortical dysgenesis and epilepsy. *Brain* **118**: 1039–50.

Skjaerven R, Wilcox AJ, Lie RT et al. (1999) A population-based study of survival and childbearing among female subjects with birth defects and the risk of recurrence in their children. *N Engl J Med* **340**: 1057–62.

Smithells RW, Sheppard S, Schorah CJ, et al. (1981) Apparent prevention of neural tube defects by periconceptional vitamin supplementation. *Arch Dis Child* **56**: 911–8.

Snodgrass WT, Adams R (2004) Initial urologic management of myelomeningocele. *Urol Clin North Am* **31**: 427–34.

Sonigo PC, Rypens FF, Carteret M, et al. (1998) MR imaging of fetal cerebral anomalies. *Pediatr Radiol* **28**: 212–22.

Soto-Ares G, Vinchon M, Delmaire C, et al. (2001) Report of eight cases of occipital dermal sinus: an update, and MRI findings. *Neuropediatrics* **32**: 153–8.

Soufflet C, Bulteau C, Delalande O, et al. (2004) The nonmalformed hemisphere is secondarily impaired in young children with hemimegalencephaly: a pre- and postsurgery study with SPECT and EEG. *Epilepsia* **45**: 1375–82.

Stashinko EE, Clegg NJ, Kammann HA, et al. (2004) A retrospective survey of perinatal risk factors of 104 living children with holoprosencephaly. *Am J Med Genet A* **128**: 114–9.

Steinlin M, Zürrer M, Martin E, et al. (1991) Contribution of magnetic resonance imaging in the evaluation of microcephaly. *Neuropediatrics* **22**: 184–9.

Stephenson TP, Mundy AR (1990) Surgery of the neuropathic bladder. In: Borzyskowski M, Mundy AR, eds. *Neuropathic Bladder in Childhood. Clinics in Developmental Medicine No. 111*. London: Mac Keith Press, pp. 37–58.

Stevenson KL (2004) Chiari type II malformation: past, present, and future. *Neurosurg Focus* **16** (2): E5.

Stoll C, Dott B, Roth MP, Alembik Y (1988) [Etiological and epidemiological aspects of neural tube defects.] *Arch Fr Pediatr* **45**: 617–22 (French).

Stone DH (1987) The declining prevalence of anencephalus and spina bifida: its nature, causes and implications. *Dev Med Child Neurol* **29**: 541–6.

Stovner LJ, Cappelen J, Nilsen G, Sjaastad O (1992) The Chiari type I malformation in two monozygotic twins and first-degree relatives. *Ann Neurol* **31**: 220–2.

Sudo K, Doi S, Maruo Y, et al. (1990) Syringomyelia with spontaneous resolution. *J Neurol Neurosurg Psychiatry* **53**: 437–8.

Sugama S, Kusano K (1994) Monozygous twin with polymicrogyria and normal co-twin. *Pediatr Neurol* **11**: 62–3.

Sugimoto T, Yasuhara A, Nishida N, et al. (1993) MRI of the head in the evaluation of microcephaly. *Neuropediatrics* **24**: 4–7.

Suri M (2003) What's new in neurogenetics? Focus on "primary microcephaly". *Eur J Paediatr Neurol* **7**: 389–92.

Suri M (2005) The phenotypic spectrum of ARX mutations. *Dev Med Child Neurol* **47**: 133–7.

Sztriha L (2005) Spectrum of callosal agenesis. *Pediatr Neurol* **32**: 94–101.

Sztriha L, Dawodu A, Gururaj A, Johansen JG (2004) Microcephaly associated with abnormal gyral pattern. *Neuropediatrics* **35**: 346–52.

Sztriha L, Johansen JG, Al-Gazali LI (2005) Extreme microcephaly with agyria–pachygyria, partial agenesis of the corpus callosum, and pontocerebellar hypoplasia. *J Child Neurol* **20**: 170–2.

Takahashi T, Kinsman S, Makris N, et al. (2003) Semilobar holoprosencephaly with midline 'seam': a topologic and morphogenetic model based upon MRI analysis. *Cereb Cortex* **13**: 1299–1312.

Takanashi J, Fujii K, Sugita K, Kohno Y (1999) Neuroradiologic findings in glutaric aciduria type II. *Pediatr Neurol* **20**: 142–5.

Takashima S, Becker LE, Chan F, Takada S (1987) A Golgi study of the cerebral cortex in Fukuyama-type congenital muscular dystrophy, Walker-type "lissencephaly", and classical lissencephaly. *Brain Dev* **9**: 621–6.

Talwar D, Baldwin MA, Horbatt CI (1995) Epilepsy in children with meningomyelocele. *Pediatr Neurol* **13**: 29–32.

Tan EC, Takagi T, Karasawa K (1995) Posterior fossa cystic lesions—magnetic resonance imaging manifestations. *Brain Dev* **17**: 418–24.

Tashiro K, Fukazawa T, Morikawa F, et al. (1987) Syringomyelic syndrome: clinical features in 31 cases confirmed by CT myelography or magnetic resonance imaging. *J Neurol* **235**: 26–30.

Tassi L, Colombo N, Garbelli R, et al. (2002) Focal cortical dysplasia: neurophysiological subtypes, EEG, neuroimaging and surgical outcome. *Brain* **125**: 1719–32.

Tassi L, Colombo N, Cossu M, et al. (2005) Elecroclinical, MRI and neuropathological study of 10 patients with nodular heterotopia, with surgical outcomes. *Brain* **128**: 321–37.

Taylor DC, Falconer MA, Bruton CJ, Corsellis JA (1971) Focal dysplasia of the cerebral cortex in epilepsy. *J Neurol Neurosurg Psychiatry* **34**: 369–87.

Taylor MJ, Boor R, Keenan NK, et al. (1996) Brainstem auditory and visual evoked potentials in infants with myelomeningocele. *Brain Dev* **18**: 99–104.

ten Donkelaar HJ, Lammens M, Wesseling P, et al. (2003) Development and developmental disorders of the human cerebellum. *J Neurol* **250**: 1025–36.

Thyen U, Aksu F, Bartsch O, Herb E (1992) Acrocallosal syndrome: association with cystic malformation of the brain and neurodevelopmental aspects. *Neuropediatrics* **23**: 292–6.

Tint GS, Irons M, Elias ER, et al. (1994) Defective cholesterol biosynthesis associated with the Smith–Lemli–Opitz syndrome. *N Engl J Med* **330**: 107–13.

Toelle SP, Yalcinkaya C, Kocer T, et al. (2002) Rhombencephalosynapsis: clinical findings and neuroimaging in 9 children. *Neuropediatrics* **33**: 209–14.

Toi A, Lister WS, Fong KW (2004) How early are fetal cerebral sulci visible at prenatal ultrasound and what is the normal pattern of early fetal sulcal development? *Ultrasound Obstet Gynecol* **24**: 706–15.

Tolmie JL, McNay M, Stephenson JBP, et al. (1987) Microcephaly: genetic counselling and antenatal diagnosis after the birth of an affected child. *Am J Med Genet* **27**: 583–94.

Tortori-Donati P, Fondelli MP, Rossi A, Carini S (1996) Cystic malformations of the posterior cranial fossa originating from a defect of the posterior membranous area. Mega cisterna magna and persisting Blake's pouch: two separate entities. *Childs Nerv Syst* **12**: 307–8.

Towfighi J, Berlin CM, Ladda RL, et al. (1985) Neuropathology of oral–facial–digital syndromes. *Arch Pathol Lab Med* **109**: 642–6.

Truwit CL, Barkovich AJ, Grumbach MM, Martini JJ (1993) MR imaging of Kallmann syndrome, a genetic disorder of neuronal migration affecting the olfactory and genital system. *AJNR* **14**: 827–38.

Tsipouras P, Barabas G, Matthews WS (1986) Neurologic correlates of osteogenesis imperfecta. *Arch Neurol* **43**: 150–2.

Tubbs RS, Oakes WJ (2004) Treatment and management of the Chiari II malformation: an evidence-based review of the literature. *Childs Nerv Syst* **20**: 375–81.

Tubbs RS, McGirt MJ, Oakes WJ (2003a) Surgical experience in 130 pediatric patients with Chiari 1 malformation. *J Neurosurg* **99**: 291–6.

Tubbs RS, Wellons JC, Oakes WJ (2003b) Occipital encephalocele, lipomyelomeningocele, and Chiari I malformation: case report and review of the literature. *Childs Nerv Syst* **19**: 50–3.

Tulipan N (2004) Intrauterine closure of myelomeningocele: an update. *Neurosurg Focus* **16** (2): E2.

Tychsen L, Hoyt WF (1985) Occipital lobe dysplasia: magnetic resonance findings in two cases of isolated congenital hemianopsia. *Arch Ophthalmol* **103**: 680–2.

Urich H, Herrick MK (1985) The amniotic band syndrome as a cause of anencephaly. Report of a case. *Acta Neuropathol* **67**: 190–4.

Uyanik G, Aigner J, Martin P, et al. (2003) ARX mutation in X-linked lissencephaly with abnormal genitalia. *Neurology* **61**: 232–5.

Uyanik G, Elcioglu N, Penzien J, et al. (2006) Novel truncating and missense mutations of the KCC3 gene associated with Andermann syndrome. *Neurology* **66**: 1044–8; erratum **67**: 1528.

Vade A, Horowitz S (1992) Agenesis of corpus callosum and intraventricular lipomas. *Pediatr Neurol* **8**: 307–9.

Valanne L, Pihko H, Karevuo K, et al. (1994) MRI of the brain in muscle–eye–brain (MEB) disease. *Neuroradiology* **36**: 473–6.

Valente EM, Marsh SE, Castori M, et al. (2005) Distinguishing the four genetic causes of Joubert's syndrome-related disorders. *Ann Neurol* **57**: 513–9; erratum 934.

Valente EM, Brancati F, Silhavy JL, et al. (2006) AHI1 gene mutations cause specific forms of Joubert syndrome-related disorders. *Ann Neurol* **59**: 527–34.

Van den Hof MC, Nicolaides KH, Campbell J, Campbell S (1990) Evaluation of the lemon and banana signs in one hundred thirty fetuses with open spina bifida. *Am J Obstet Gynecol* **162**: 322–7.

Van der Knaap MJ, Smit LM, Barth PG (1997) Magnetic resonance imaging in classification of congenital muscular dystrophies with brain abnormalities. *Ann Neurol* **42**: 50–9.

van der Put NM, Steegers-Theunissen RP, Frosst P, et al. (1995) Mutated methylenetetrahydrofolate reductase as a risk factor for spina bifida. *Lancet* **346**: 1070–1.

van Hall MH, Beuls EA, Wilmink JT, et al. (1992) Magnetic resonance imaging of progressive hydrosyringomyelia in two patients with meningomyelocele. *Neuropediatrics* **23**: 276–80.

Verloes A, Lambotte C (1989) Further delineation of a syndrome of cerebellar vermis hypoplasia, oligophrenia, congenital ataxia, coloboma, and hepatic fibrosis. *Am J Med Genet* **32**: 227–32.

Vigevano F, Di Rocco C (1990) Effectiveness of hemispherectomy in hemimegalencephaly with intractable seizures. *Neuropediatrics* **21**: 222–3.

Vigevano F, Fusco L, Granata T, et al. (1996) Hemimegalencephaly: clinical and EEG characteristics. In: Guerrini R, Andermann F, Canapicchi R, et al., eds. *Dysplasias of Cerebral Cortex and Epilepsy.* Philadelphia: Lippincott–Raven, pp. 285–94.

Volcik KA, Shaw GM, Lamme EJ, et al. (2003) Evaluation of infant methylenetetrahydrofolate reductase genotype, maternal vitamin use, and risk of high versus low level spina bifida defects. *Birth Defects Res A Clin Mol Teratol* **67**: 154–7.

Volpe J (2001) *Neurology of the Newborn, 4th edn.* Philadelphia: WB Saunders.

Volpe P, Paladini D, Resta M, et al. (2006) Characteristics, associations and outcome of partial agenesis of the corpus callosum in the fetus. *Ultrasound Obstet Gynecol* **27**: 509–16.

Walsh CA (1995) Neuronal identity, neuronal migration, and epileptic disorders of the cerebral cortex. In: Schwartzkroin PA, Moshé SL, Noebels JL, Swaun JW, eds. *Brain Development and Epilepsy.* New York: Oxford University Press, pp. 122–43.

Walsh C, Cepko CL (1993) Clonal dispersion in proliferative layers of developing cerebral cortex. *Nature* **362**: 632–5.

Walsh DS, Adzick NS (2003) Fetal surgery for spina bifida. *Sem Neonatol* **8**: 197–205.

Ward M, Hutton J, McDonnell R, et al. (2004) Folic acid supplements to prevent neural tube defects: trends in East of Ireland. *Ir Med J* **97**: 274–6.

Ward SL, Jacobs RA, Gates EP, et al. (1986a) Abnormal ventilatory patterns during sleep in infants with myelomeningocele. *J Pediatr* **109**: 631–4.

Ward SL, Nickerson BG, van der Hal A, et al. (1986b) Absent hypoxic and hypercapneic arousal responses in children with meningomyelocele and apnea. *Pediatrics* **78**: 44–50.

Webby MC, O'Hollaren PS, Abtin K, et al. (2004) Occult filum terminale syndrome: results of surgical untethering. *Pediatr Neurosurg* **40**: 51–7.

White BJ, Rogol AD, Brown KS, et al. (1983) The syndrome of anosmia with hypogonadotropic hypogonadism: a genetic study of 18 new families and a review. *Am J Med Genet* **15**: 417–35.

Wichman A, Frank LM, Kelly TE (1985) Autosomal recessive congenital cerebellar hypoplasia. *Clin Genet* 27: 373–82.

Wieck G, Leventer RJ, Squier WM, et al. (2005) Periventricular nodular heterotopia with overlying polymicrogyria. *Brain* 128: 2811–21.

Williams J, Brodsky MC, Griebel M, et al. (1993) Septo-optic dysplasia: the clinical insignificance of an absent septum pellucidum. *Dev Med Child Neurol* 35: 490–501.

Williams RS, Caviness VS (1984) Normal and abnormal development of the brain. In: Tarter RE, Goldstein J, eds. *Advances in Clinical Neuropsychology, vol. 2.* New York: Plenum, pp. 1–62.

Williams RS, Swisher CN, Jennings M, et al. (1984) Cerebro-ocular dysgenesis (Walker–Warburg syndrome): neuropathologic and etiologic analysis. *Neurology* 34: 1531–41.

Wilmshurst JM, Kelly R, Borzyskowski M (1999) Presentation and outcome of sacral agenesis: 20 years' experience. *Dev Med Child Neurol* 41: 807–12.

Wilson GN (1983) Cranial defects in the Goldenhar syndrome. *Am J Med Genet* 14: 435–43.

Wiswell TE, Tuttle DJ, Northam RS, Simonds GR (1990) Major congenital neurologic malformations. A 17-year survey. *Am J Dis Child* 144: 61–7.

Worthington S, Turner A, Elber J, Andrews PI (2000) 22q11 deletion and polymicrogyria—cause or coincidence? *Clin Dysmorphol* 9: 193–7.

Wright RL (1971) Congenital dermal sinuses. *Prog Neurol Surg* 4: 175–89.

Wyldes M, Watkinson M (2004) Isolated mild fetal ventriculomegaly. *Arch Dis Child Fetal Neonatal Ed* 89: F9–13.

Yakovlev PI, Lecours AR (1967) The myelogenetic cycles of regional maturation of the brain. In: Minkowski A, ed. *Regional Development of the Brain in Early Life.* Oxford: Blackwell, pp. 3–10.

Yamaguchi E, Hayashi T, Kondoh H, et al. (1993) A case of Walker–Warburg syndrome with uncommon findings. Double cortical layer, temporal cyst and increased serum IgM. *Brain Dev* 15: 61–5.

Yerby MS (2003) Management issues for women with epilepsy: neural tube defects and folic acid supplementation. *Neurology* 61 (6 Suppl 2): S23–6.

Yglesias A, Narbona J, Vanaclocha V, Artieda J (1996) Chiari type 1 malformation, glossopharyngeal neuralgia and central sleep apnoea in a child. *Dev Med Child Neurol* 38: 1126–30.

Yokota A, Oota T, Matsukado Y, Okudera T (1984) Dorsal cyst malformations. Part II. Galenic dysgenesis and its embryological considerations. *Childs Brain* 11: 403–17.

Yokota A, Kajiwara H, Kohchi M, et al. (1988) Parietal cephalocele: clinical importance of its atretic form and associated malformations. *J Neurosurg* 69: 545–51.

Young ID, Moore JR, Tripp JH (1987) Sex-linked recessive congenital ataxia. *J Neurol Neurosurg Psychiatry* 50: 1230–2.

Younus M, Coode PE (1986) Nasal glioma and encephalocele: two separate entities. Report of two cases. *J Neurosurg* 64: 516–9.

Zafeiriou DI, Vargiami E, Boltshauser E (2004) Cerebellar agenesis and diabetes insipidus. *Neuropediatrics* 35: 364–7.

Zager EL, Ojemann RG, Poletti CE (1990) Acute presentations of syringomyelia. Report of three cases. *J Neurosurg* 72: 133–8.

Zambelli H, Barini R, Iscaife A, et al. (2007) Successful developmental outcome in intrauterine myelomeningocele repair. *Childs Nerv Syst* 23: 123–6.

Zaw W, Stone DG (2002) Caudal regression in twin pregnancy with type II diabetes. *J Perinatol* 22: 171–4.

Zee CS, McComb JG, Segall HD, et al. (1981) Lipomas of the corpus callosum associated with frontal dysraphism. *J Comput Assist Tomogr* 5: 201–5.

Zerah M (1999) [Syringomyelia in children.] *Neurochirurgie* 45 Suppl 1: 37–57 (French).

3
NEUROCUTANEOUS DISEASES AND SYNDROMES

Several diseases affect both the skin and the nervous system, which is probably a consequence of their common ectodermal origin. Most of these disorders are genetically determined and manifest early in life, although late manifestations are frequent as many of the neurocutaneous syndromes are evolutive conditions.

The group of the neurocutaneous disorders is highly heterogeneous and includes conditions completely unrelated pathophysiologically, studied together only because they feature clinically both cutaneous and neurological symptoms and signs, however different these can be. The term 'phakomatosis' is sometimes used as a synonym. However, it has come to be applied mainly to those neurocutaneous diseases in which an excessive growth potential, with frequent development of hamartomas or tumours, is present. This applies to neurofibromatosis, tuberous sclerosis, von Hippel–Lindau disease and some other conditions with a proliferative tendency such as the Proteus syndrome or the naevoid basal cell carcinoma syndrome. In this chapter, the term neurocutaneous syndrome is used for *all* diseases in which there is a nonfortuitous association of skin and nervous system abnormalities, including those in which the nervous system involvement consists of vascular abnormalities, even though the cutaneous manifestations may not be regularly present in all cases. The grouping used is clearly arbitrary, but it is justified from a clinical point of view as the association of cutaneous and neurological manifestations raises specific problems. Neurocutaneous diseases are much more pleiotropic than suggested by their name as they may involve viscera as well as skull and CNS. Most neurocutaneous diseases are genetically determined, all three major mendelian types of inheritance being possible. Sporadic syndromes may be due to somatic mutations or to other, unknown mechanisms.

NEUROFIBROMATOSIS

Neurofibromatosis is not a single disorder and includes a spectrum of disorders that share many features but clearly differ from one another. There is no agreement as to how many entities belong to the neurofibromatoses. Two distinct forms are generally recognized: type 1 (NF1), also termed von Recklinghausen's disease or peripheral type; and type 2 (NF2), also termed central neurofibromatosis. These two types are distinct diseases genetically and clinically. The gene of NF1 is located in the pericentric region of the long arm of chromosome 17 (17q11.2), while that of NF2 is on the long arm of chromosome 22 (22q11.2). Both genes act as tumour suppressor genes. The *NF1* gene codes for a protein, *neurofibromin*, that appears to be a GTPase-activating protein. GTPase converts the proto-oncogen p21-ras from active to inactive form, thus downregulating the production of oncogen and having a probable anti-oncogenic function (De Luca et al. 2005). Most NF1 cases with mental retardation are associated with large deletions of the gene. The *NF2* gene codes for merlin and also acts as a tumour suppressor; several mutations are known (Hamaratoglu et al. 2006). Interestingly, a loss of chromosome 22, and hence of the *NF2* gene, is commonly found in schwannomas and meningiomas that occur outside NF2. The clinical and pathological characteristics of these two diseases are also different (see below).

Other types of neurofibromatosis exist. Riccardi (1992) has proposed that seven distinct forms may be recognized. However, the individualization of some of these forms remains controversial.

The terms central and peripheral are better abandoned because both NF1 and NF2 produce CNS lesions, albeit of different types. Table 3.1 shows the criteria for the diagnosis of NF1 and NF2.

The basic disturbance in neurofibromatosis appears to be an abnormality in development of the neural crest cells with resulting tendency to abnormal, excessive growth of affected tissues and the development of multiple tumours.

NEUROFIBROMATOSIS TYPE 1

NF1 accounts for at least 85% of all cases of neurofibromatosis. The prevalence of the disease is about 1 in 3000 individuals. NF1 is inherited dominantly with a 98% penetrance but with a high degree of phenotypic variability. According to Huson et al. (1988) and North (1993), approximately half the cases have only minor manifestations. Paternal transmission is more common than maternal inheritance. Occasional occurrence of a paternal germline mosaicism may account for the rare occurrence of more than one affected offspring of clinically unaffected parents (Lázaro et al. 1994). About one third of cases are new mutations, and the mutation rate is approximately one mutation per 10,000 gametes per generation.

TABLE 3.1
Criteria for the diagnosis of the neurofibromatoses*

Neurofibromatosis type 1
1. Six or more café-au-lait spots >5 mm in diameter in prepubertal patients and >15 mm in postpubertal patients
2. Two or more neurofibromas (intracutaneous or subcutaneous) or one plexiform neurofibroma
3. Freckling in the axillary or inguinal region
4. Optic glioma
5. Two or more iris hamartomas (Lisch nodules)
6. Typical osseous lesion such as sphenoid dysplasia or tibial pseudarthrosis
7. One or more first-degree relative/s with NF1

NF1 may be diagnosed if two or more of above criteria are present

Neurofibromatosis type 2
1. Bilateral VIIIth nerve neurofibromas
2. Unilateral VIIIth nerve mass in association with any two of the following: meningioma, neurofibroma, schwannoma, juvenile posterior subcapsular cataracts
3. Unilateral VIIIth nerve tumour or other spinal or brain tumour as above in first-degree relative

NF2 may be diagnosed if one of the above criteria is present

*Modified from NIH Consensus Development Conference (1988).
Using these criteria a definite diagnosis can be made in 94% of patients.

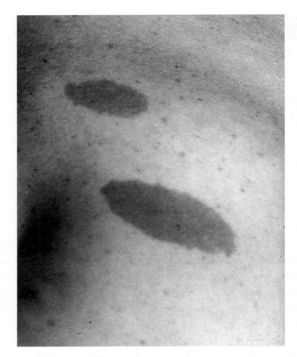

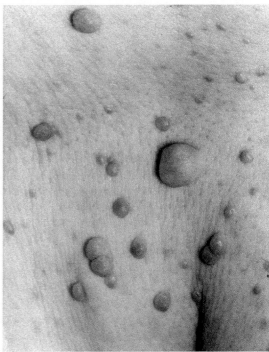

Fig. 3.1. Cutaneous manifestations of neurofibromatosis type I. *(Top)* Café-au-lait spots. *(Bottom)* Multiple neurofibromas.

CUTANEOUS MANIFESTATIONS
Skin features of NF1 consist of abnormalities of pigmentation and tumours (Fig. 3.1).

Café-au-lait spots are the hallmark of NF1 and are found in virtually all cases. Their size varies with age; they often are absent at birth but are present from an early age, although they are not as readily visible in infancy as they are later. Ordinarily, at least six spots 0.5–1.0 cm are apparent by 1 year of age but an occasional patient may have less. Of 46 children with such spots prospectively followed by Korf (1992), 27 had developed other signs of NF1 (in the majority, within three years), 6 had segmental neurofibromatosis, 3 received other diagnoses, and 8 remained without diagnosis. *Axillary freckling* was present in 84% of 200 children followed by North (1993), and inguinal freckling was found in about half these patients. Diffuse pigmentation may overlie a plexiform neuroma. Xanthomas and angiomas are less common features. *Neurofibromas* may be intracutaneous and are then of a violaceous colour and a soft consistency, or subcutaneous and presenting as firm tumours along the trunk of peripheral nerves. They vary from a few millimeters to 3–4 cm at their greatest diameter. Neurofibromas are sometimes found in children under 10 years old, but they increase steadily in number with age, especially around puberty (Riccardi 1992). They can lead to peripheral neuropathy when they affect larger nerves.

Plexiform neurofibromas combine cutaneous and subcutaneous elements to form tumours that may become huge and represent one of the most serious complications of NF1. They may be continuous with intracranial or intraspinal tumours. Plexiform tumours of the periorbital area, which occur in 5% of patients, can produce proptosis and visual compromise. Large plexiform neurofibromas occur in 25–32% of cases (Huson et al. 1988, North 1998) and tend to grow larger with age. The cosmetic burden may be considerable, and large cervical lesions may displace and com-press vascular and respiratory structures and be life threatening. Treatment is surgical but difficult so other methods are being studied (Packer and Rosser 2002). Plexiform neurofibromas of the limbs may be associated with partial gigantism. Involvement of the face is possible and may be associated with exophthalmos and rarely with unilateral megalencephaly (Cutting et al. 2002). Such lesions may be associated with bony abnormalities of the orbit; they require rapid treatment if the eyelid completely covers the eye, to avoid secondary amblyopia. Most plexiform neurofibromas appear before 2 years of age and some may be present at birth.

Involvement of the iris by pigmented hamartomas known as *Lisch nodules* is specific for NF1. Lisch nodules are found in 22–30% of NF1 patients by 6 years of age and in virtually all after age 12 years (Flueler et al. 1986, North 1998).

NEUROLOGICAL MANIFESTATIONS

Neurological manifestations of NF1 are protean and include mental retardation, specific learning difficulties, and symptoms and signs due to intracranial and intraspinal tumours (North, 1998, 2000; Evans et al. 1999; Friedman 2002).

Macrocephaly (>98th centile) is present in only 16–45% of children with NF1 (Huson et al. 1988, North 1997) and is not correlated with neurological or neuropsychological difficulties (Cutting et al. 2002). It is due to megalencephaly and is not accompanied by symptoms of increased intracranial pressure. Headache occurs in over half the patients and may be migraine-like.

Mental retardation and specific learning difficulties are well-known features of NF1 (Riccardi 1992). Mental retardation is relatively uncommon: Riccardi put the frequency at 8% but lower figures have been reported by other authors (North 1997, North et al. 2002). However, the IQ of NF1 patients is on average lower than that of affected siblings. Specific learning difficulties are a common problem, being present in 32% (Hofman et al. 1994) to 65% (North et al. 1998) if impaired academic performance is taken as the criterion. Depressed performance in verbal tasks and a high incidence of language deficits are particularly obvious, but all areas of cognition can be affected (Cutting et al. 2000). Attention deficit disorder without hyperactivity is common and may respond to amphetamine therapy. A significant association of cognitive deficits with the presence of T_2-intense areas on MRI has been found by several investigators (Denckla et al. 1996, Wang et al. 2000, Goh et al. 2004) but not by others (Moore et al. 1996, Rosenbaum et al. 1999) and requires further study. Social skills have been shown to be frequently affected with resulting difficulties in communication (Barton and North 2004). Behavioural difficulties are also common (Kayl and Moore 2000).

Epilepsy is more frequent in children with NF1 than in the general population, but available figures vary between 3.5% (North 1998), 4.2% (Kulkantrakorn and Geller 1998) and 7.3% (Huson et al. 1988). All types of seizures including infantile spasms (Motte et al. 1993, Fois et al. 1994) may occur.

Optic gliomas (see Chapter 13) are present in 15–20% of NF1 cases (North 1998). Histologically, they may differ from other optic gliomas by the presence of an arachnoidal gliomatosis surrounding the optic nerve (Seiff et al. 1987) but otherwise they are typical pilocytic astrocytomas. They may be limited to the optic nerve or involve the chiasm and the retrochiasmatic portion of the visual pathway. Between 10% and 60% of optic gliomas are associated with NF1. The proportion tends to increase in the case of gliomas of the optic nerve, and especially with bilateral gliomas, which are almost exclusively found in NF1 patients.

Clinical manifestations include proptosis and diminished visual acuity, but many gliomas are now discovered by systematic radiological evaluation of patients with known NF1 while they remain asymptomatic. Up to 39% of cases present with precocious puberty (Habiby et al. 1995). The proportion of symptomatic cases is 20–30%, and most symptomatic cases manifest early before age 6 and often by 2 years of age (Listernick et al. 1994). Optic gliomas in NF1 fall into two groups: those that remain stable, and those that are active, increase in size and threaten vision. Only 52% of patients whose optic gliomas were detected by MRI developed symptoms (Listernick et al. 1997). Emergence of symptoms after age 6 years is extremely rare, as is progression beyond age 10, although a few cases of late presentation or late progression are on record (Listernick et al. 2004). Even in symptomatic cases the outcome is often favourable, and this has to be taken into account for therapeutic indications and for those of repeated imaging. Guillamo et al. (2003) found a favourable outcome in a majority of 104 patients (88 of whom were children) with CNS tumours, including 88 optic gliomas, 55 of which were symptomatic. This high proportion of symptomatic cases is explained by the surgical origin of this study. Intraorbital gliomas only rarely spread intracranially. The evolution of optic gliomas in NF1 may be more benign than in isolated cases (Listernick et al. 1994) but there is no universal agreement in this regard. Tumours anterior to the chiasm frequently remain stable, whereas more posteriorly located gliomas are more often invasive. The diagnosis of optic glioma may be suggested by finding an enlarged optic foramen, although this sign is not specific as elongation of the optic nerve and dural ectasia can simulate a tumour (Riccardi 1992, North 1997).

Modern neuroimaging has transformed the conditions of diagnosis of optic pathway tumours in NF1 patients (Fig. 3.2). On CT, the tumours appear as irregular enlargements that may extend into the chiasm with bulging into or filling of the chiasmatic cistern. MRI better demonstrates the tumours. There is an ongoing controversy about the indications for imaging in NF1. All agree that symptomatic cases should be scanned. For asymptomatic cases, the NIH Consensus Development Conference (1988) did not advise systematic study as no treatment is usually indicated. Riccardi (1992) is of the opposite opinion, as some aggressive gliomas may progress silently for relatively long periods and may cause damage that could be prevented by early diagnosis. Monitoring of visual evoked potentials may permit early detection but there is a high level of false positives. It often indicates extension into the optic tract and radiations (Di Mario et al. 1993).

Treatment of optic glioma is still controversial (Riccardi 1992) (see Chapter 13). Most tumours that appear stable, especially if localized to the anterior optic pathways, should be watched carefully without surgical or other intervention. In a collaborative study, extension to the optic chiasm was seen in only four of 106 unilateral cases (Wilson 1998). For optic nerve gliomas that are growing and produce marked proptosis with complete unilateral loss of vision, surgical removal gives satisfactory results. For lesions that are not stable, radiotherapy is effective. However, irradiation with doses of 52 Gray, as usually required, is associated in children

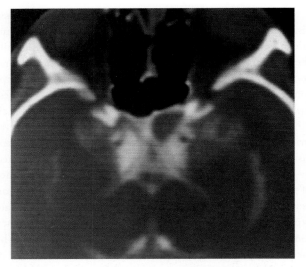

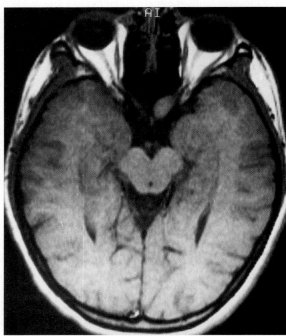

Fig. 3.2. NF1 in a 12-year-old girl. *(Top)* CT after lumbar injection of metrizamide contrast shows a small mass at the origin of the left optic nerve. *(Bottom)* T₁-weighted MRI clearly delineates a small optic glioma.

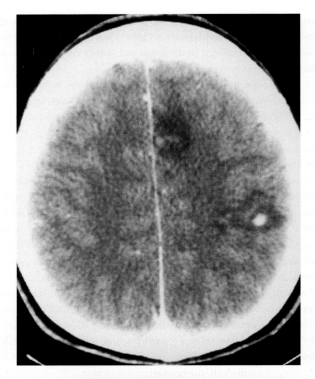

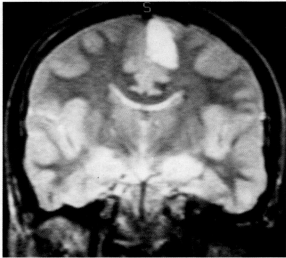

Fig. 3.3. 10-year-old girl with NF1 associated with right-sided partial motor seizures of recent onset. *(Top)* CT indicates two areas of decreased density in left hemisphere with central contrast enhancement in the posterior lesion. *(Bottom)* T₂-weighted MRI, coronal cut, shows intense signal from left frontomesial lesion. Two tumours (grade I–II astrocytomas) were subsequently removed at operation, with complete control of seizures for one year.

with mental retardation and with endocrinological sequelae in one third of cases. For patients under 5 years of age whose sensitivity to radiation is particularly high, chemotherapy tends to be substituted for radiotherapy. Combinations of vincristine and carbiplatin have been found effective and are often used (North 1997).

Other intracranial tumours are less common (Fig. 3.3). They are mostly astrocytomas that can involve the hemispheres, cerebellum, basal ganglia or brainstem. Brainstem tumours accounted for 21% of intracranial tumours in NF1 patients in the large series of Guillamo et al. (2003). These are of special interest because their prognosis is usually much better than that of brainstem

tumours unassociated with NF1. Molloy et al. (1995) studied 17 patients. In only 6 of these was there evidence of progression by imaging, and in only 3 was progression detectable clinically. The tumours involved the medulla in 14 cases. Fifteen of the patients were alive at follow-up after several years, although no treatment other than a shunt when required was given. The authors concluded that these lesions are intermediate between hamartomas and classical brainstem tumours, and that aggressive treatment is best withheld unless there is evidence of progression on monitoring. Pollack et al. (1996) came to similar conclusions in a study of 21 cases. Schmandt et al. (2000) reported spontaneous regression of some astrocytomas.

Multiple brain tumours are not uncommon (Hochstrasser et al. 1988). Intracranial calcification involving the central nuclei or the periventricular area is rare (Arts and Van Dongen 1986) and is not of tumoural origin. Peripheral nerve tumours are rare in children but do occur and can be malignant (Drouet et al. 2004).

Intraspinal tumours, comprising mainly astrocytomas, are uncommon. Intraspinal neurofibromas occur mainly in the cervicothoracic region. These tumours not uncommonly are both intra- and extraspinal and may be in continuity with a subcutaneous plexiform neurofibroma. Intramedullary tumours such as ependymomas and astrocytomas are not a feature of NF1. Rare cases of spinal neurofibromatosis with multiple symmetrical tumours are on record (Pascual-Castroviejo et al. 2007).

'Hamartomas' of the brain and cerebellum, so-called *'unidentified bright objects'* (UBOs) are hyperintense areas especially demonstrated by MRI, most frequently on T_2 sequences in the thalami, the pallidum, the cerebellar peduncles and hemispheres, but also in the hemispheral white matter in the optic tracts and radiations (Fig. 3.4). The significance of this finding is not fully understood. Such areas, in most cases, do not correspond to tumour extension, and may remain stable or disappear. They are frequent in patients without as well as those with optic pathway gliomas (Duffner et al. 1989, North 1998). North (1997) found high-intensity T_2 lesions in 32 of 50 systematically studied 8- to 16-year-old patients, 24 of whom had no tumour. The lesions were usually multiple, involved the optic tract in 20 patients, the basal ganglia in 24, the cerebellum in 8 and the brainstem in 6. Hyperintense lesions were seen in T_1-weighted sequences in 16 children, usually corresponding with T_2 abnormalities. As a result of improvement in MR techniques the frequency of these abnormalities has been even higher in recent series, and some authors have proposed them as a diagnostic criterion for NF1 (Curless et al. 1998, DeBella et al. 2000). They were present in 25 of the 29 cases of Rosenbaum et al. (1999) and in 89% of those of Raininko et al. (2001). The latter authors made a detailed study of these areas. They found them more commonly on proton density (80%) than on T_1 (50%) sequences and noted that they occasionally enhanced with gadolinium. In 5 of their cases they increased in size, with later regression and disappearance in 4. They often change with evolution, tending to disappear with age, although they may increase in number at adolescence, as also found by Kraut et al. (2004) who reported a biphasic evolution. They are not more common when an optic pathway tumour is present. Hyperintense areas tend to decrease and often disappear before adulhood (Sevick et al. 1992). Their histological nature is unknown. They are more common in children and adolescents than in adults. Those located in the optic tracts and the pallidum are larger than those found elsewhere and may give an abnormal signal, although a weak one, on T_1-weighted images (Inoue et al.

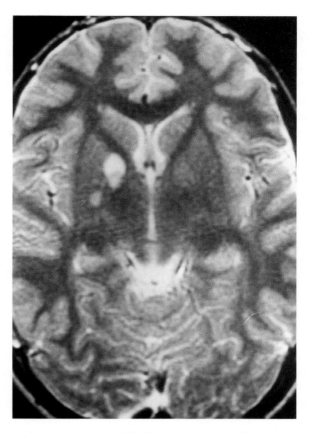

Fig. 3.4. NF1 in a 14-year-old girl. T_2-weighted MRI showing areas of increased signal ('hamartomas') in the right basal ganglia and in both thalami.

1997). The abnormally intense T_2 areas have been shown in a few cases to represent glial dysplasia or spongiotic changes rather than hamartomas (Di Paolo et al. 1995). Proton MRI of such lesions (Wang et al. 2000) showed initially an increase in choline and relatively normal N-acetylaspartate, later followed by a decrease in N-acetylaspartate, suggesting a secondary loss of neurons.

CNS malformations, especially disturbances of neuronal migration, are not common in NF1. However, *hemimegalencephaly* has been reported (Cusmai et al. 1990). Tumours of peripheral nerves may occur. One case of sudden death secondary to a neurofibroma of the Xth nerve is on record (Chow et al. 1993).

Hydrocephalus in a majority of cases is the result of aqueductal stenosis (Afifi et al. 1988, Riviello et al. 1988). It usually develops slowly and is recognized late. It is most commonly due to gliosis, diffuse or membranous, of the aqueduct. Small tumours of the peduncular region may be a cause, and MRI in the sagittal plane using both T_1- and T_2-weighted sequences should always be performed. An intense signal in T_2-weighted scans was present in 7 of 9 cases (Pou-Serradell and Ugarte-Elola 1989, Valentini et al. 1995). Other causes of ventriculomegaly in NF1 patients include Chiari I malformation (Afifi et al. 1988) and tumours of the posterior fossa.

Abnormalities of the skull are frequent in NF1. Craniofacial dysplasia can affect any portion of the cranial vault, most commonly the occipital regions along the lambdoid suture. Bones contributing to the orbit, especially the greater sphenoidal wing, are a site of election for dysplasia. The greater wing is missing in part, with resulting pulsating exophthalmos when the defect is large. The lesser wing and sella turcica are often involved in the dysplasia. *Dural ectasias* can produce bilateral enlargement of the auditory canal, which may suggest the diagnosis of NF2, but they are not associated with schwannoma of the VIIIth nerve (Inoue et al. 1997). Calvarial defects adjacent to the lambdoid suture are clinically asymptomatic. Scoliosis is present in 20% of cases and may be sufficiently severe to warrant surgical correction. It is occasionally associated with paraspinal neurofibromas. Vertebral abnormalities are frequent, and scalloping of the body of vertebrae is a common radiological finding in NF1, as is *scoliosis*. Lateral ectasia of the thinned dura through the intervertebral foramina (lateral meningoceles) is a rare complication of NF1 (Riccardi 1992). Tibial pseudoarthrosis is a common lesion (North 1997).

OTHER COMPLICATIONS OF NF1
These include *growth retardation*, which was reported in about 25% of patients by North (1998). Vassilopoulou-Sellin et al. (2000) found that 122 of 251 children were below the 25th percentile and 68 were below the 10th percentile for age. Eye disease, especially glaucoma and buphthalmos, osseous dysplasia and arachnoid cysts are classical findings, and EEG abnormalities are seen in 15% of patients (Riccardi 1992). *Vascular manifestations* (Tomsik et al. 1976) include systemic *hypertension* with or without renal artery stenosis, which should always be looked for, and, rarely, cerebrovascular accidents (Rosser et al. 2005). Multiple stenoses of carotid arteries with the development of a moyamoya pattern has been reported (Rizzo and Lessell 1994). Grill et al. (1999) observed that 13 of 69 children who received X-irradiation for glioma of the optic chiasma developed vascular stenosis of the intracranial carotid arteries. The incidence of *malignancies*, the most frequent of which are fibrosarcomas, is higher in persons with NF1 than in the rest of the population, but they are rare in childhood. Leukaemia, especially of chronic myelogenous type, can occur (Clark and Hutter 1982) and may be associated with the presence of cutaneous xanthomas. Visceral and endocrine tumours are relatively common in later life (Huson et al. 1988). Visceral autonomic localizations may be seen. In particular, *intestinal ganglioneuromatosis* with intestinal obstruction is recognized (Kim and Kim 1998).

COURSE
The course of NF1 is very variable and minor forms are common. However, many complications can occur and mortality is not negligible, especially when subcutaneous neurofibromas are present. Khosrotehrani et al. (2005) found 40 deaths in a 2.6 year follow-up of a series of 703 patients, 57.6% of whom were children. In this series, the presence of cutaneous neurofibromas was associated with a significantly higher mortality. In a 10 year follow-up study of 150 patients, Cnossen et al. (1998) showed that 41% of them developed complications during this period; 28% had one complication, 12% had two and 1.3% had three. All patients

should therefore be followed regularly, even in the absence of symptoms.

DIAGNOSIS
The diagnosis of NF1 is essentially clinical and by imaging (Table 3.1) and it is usually easy. Diagnostic criteria for NF1 and NF2 (Gutmann et al. 1997) are shown in. Histological study of pigmented spots could show abnormalities in melanosomes but is not usually justified. Molecular genetic diagnosis is possible (see above). Imaging diagnosis may be difficult, and MRI is the primary tool for the diagnosis of CNS abnormalitities.

MANAGEMENT
The management of patients with NF1 should start with assessment of the extent of the disease by a complete clinical, ophthalmological and radiological examination. A team approach, grouping specialists in the many different problems that are often associated with the condition, is important, as it has been shown that many patients are not appropriately diagnosed and treated for all their problems. A thorough search for neurological, visceral and bone abnormalities is essential. Careful clinical follow-up is mandatory. Huson (1999) thinks a consultation every two years is reasonable, but closer surveillance and complementary investigations are required when symptoms appear. Whether routine imaging studies of the CNS are required remains disputed, but generally they seem to be performed at least on the first examination. Repeat studies should be undertaken according to clinical indications. It is clearly necessary for those patients who have suspected brain tumours. For patients with known optic gliomas, at least an annual ophthalmological examination of visual acuity and fields should be performed, and MRI should be done if vision deteriorates.

There is no drug treatment for neurofibromatosis. Surgical treatment is indicated for invasive tumours but the results are often disappointing. Surgery is also indicated for visceral lesions, cosmetic deformities and orthopaedic problems that in many cases amount to a major problem (see below).

NEUROFIBROMATOSIS TYPE 2
NF2 is transmitted as a dominant autosomal trait. The gene has been mapped to chromosome 22 and several mutations have been found (Rouleau et al. 1993). Bilateral acoustic neuromas (schwannomas) are the essential feature, occurring in at least 90% of cases (Evans et al. 1992a). These tumours develop mainly in late adolescence and early adulthood, and NF2 is rarely found in children. Loss of hearing is the first symptom. Cutaneous manifestations are uncommon and most patients have no café-au-lait spots, or only a small number of them. Some of these are schwannomas. Histologically they differ from those in NF1; they are usually less than 2cm in diameter, slightly raised, well circumscribed, and may contain excess hair (MacCollin and Mautner 1998, Ruggieri et al. 2005). Lisch nodules are not found, but posterior subcapsular cataracts occur in 10% or more of patients (Ruggieri et al. 2004). Other intracranial tumours are frequent – especially *meningiomas*, often multiple – but optic nerve glioma has not been found in

NF2 patients. The occurrence of astrocytoma also seems to be exceptional.

Schwannomas of cranial nerves V to XII are common. They are frequently bilateral and multiple. Some authors indicate that atypical NF2 may occur sporadically and often presents with multiple cranial or spinal schwannomas (Purcell and Dixon 1989, Pou-Serradell 1991). MacCollin et al. (1996) proposed separating a subgroup of NF2 under the term 'schwannomatosis', manifested by peripheral painful nerve schwannomas and often by multiple spinal root tumours. Such cases may be difficult to distinguish from paediatric cases of NF2 in which peripheral tumours may long precede the appearance of acoustic schwannomas, and indeed have been shown to be a variant of NF2 (Evans et al. 1997).

Spinal cord tumours are of two types: schwannomas, which are of the same histological type as the acoustic neuroma, and ependymomas (Rubinstein 1986). The former may be multiple and lead to serious problems. Hamartomatous lesions resembling meningiomas, termed 'meningoangiomatosis' (Russell and Rubinstein 1977), may occur and be responsible for calcification, especially in the choroid plexus, at the periphery of one cerebellar hemisphere (Ruggieri et al. 2005), or as linear subependymal calcification (Arts and Van Dongen 1986), which may be associated with seizures. Involvement of peripheral nerves can occur. Presymptomatic diagnosis is possible with chromosome 22 markers (Ruttledge et al. 1993).

NF2 is a separate disorder from NF1 and there is only one known patient with both NF1 and NF2 inherited separately from each parent (Evans et al. 1992b). The disease may be mistaken for NF1 in the rare patient with bilateral auditory canal enlargement without tumour (Kitamura et al. 1989). The presence of bilateral acoustic neuromas in NF1 has, however, been reported (Pou Serradell 1991).

The management of NF2 should be supervised by a specialist team. It includes regular assessment, looking especially for acoustic nerve tumours. Surveillance for other tumours and ocular problems should also be regularly performed. Early assessment of siblings may allow effective treatment of ocular abnormalities and should be systematically offered. A first MRI of patients is indicated from 10–12 years of age (Evans et al. 2003).

OTHER FORMS OF NEUROFIBROMATOSIS
SEGMENTAL NEUROFIBROMATOSIS (NF5)
This form is closely related to NF1. NF5 is characterized by the unilateral occurrence of features that are typical of NF1 (café-au-lait spots and neurofibromas) in only one or in several dermal segments. The disorder is thought to result from a postzygotic mutation event, and any dermatome may be involved. Most cases are sporadic although familial transmission has been observed (Jung 1988). Although NF5 is said to be rare, Listernick et al. (2003) reported 39 cases from three centres. In 29 of these the disease was limited to pigmentary disorder with café-au-lait spots, isolated in 8 patients or associated with axillary freckling. Other abnormalities are rare but iris nodules or pseudarthrosis may be found in the affected segments (Ruggieri et al. 2005).

Roth et al. (1987) divide segmental neurofibromatosis into four subtypes, only one of which is genetically transmitted. The skin lesions are usually café-au-lait patches but neurofibromas may eventually develop. Other complications of neurofibromatosis do not occur. The prognosis is good.

OTHER POSSIBLE FORMS
Forms with only café-au-lait spots and other atypical forms are on record. Charrow et al. (1993) found suggestive evidence of non-linkage to the *NF1* locus, but Abeliovich et al. (1995) found close linkage to the *NF1* gene in a large pedigree. *Intestinal neurofibromatosis* may occur in isolation (Heimann et al. 1988) or form a part of syndromes related to neurofibromatosis and to the *multiple endocrine neoplasia disorders* (Fryns and Chrzanowska 1988, Griffiths et al. 1990). Type III or IIB multiple endocrine adenomatosis is characterized by a Marfan-like habitus, a lobulated tongue with multiple submucous neuromas, conjunctival nodules, thick lips, megacolon and multiple endocrine tumours.

A combination of NF1 with features of the Noonan phenotype (short stature, pectus carinatum, cardiac defect, ptosis and low intelligence) has long been known and has been termed *'neurofibromatosis–Noonan syndrome'* (Borochowitz et al. 1989). Baralle et al. (2003) found that 2 of 6 cases had novel mutations in the *NF1* exon and no mutation in the *PTPN11* gene, thus indicating that some cases belong to NF1. The frequency of NF1 mutation in such cases was recently confirmed (De Luca et al. 2005). However, Bertola et al. (2005) found in one patient the coexistence of *NF1* mutation and a *PTPN11* mutation known to cause Noonan syndrome. Watson syndrome (café-au-lait patches and pulmonic stenosis), which may include CNS involvement in the form of areas of increased T_2 signal (Leão and da Silva 1995), is probably allelic to NF1 (Tassabehji et al. 1993).

DIAGNOSIS AND MANAGEMENT OF THE NEUROFIBROMATOSES
The diagnosis of patients with neurofibromatosis is essentially clinical and is usually easy. Diagnostic criteria for NF1 and NF2 are shown in Table 3.1. Histological study of pigmented spots could show abnormalities in melanosomes (Martuza et al. 1985) but is not usually justified. Molecular genetic diagnosis is possible (see above).

The management of patients with neurofibromatoses should start with assessment of the extent of the disease by a complete clinical, ophthalmological and radiological investigation. A team approach, grouping specialists in the many different problems raised by the condition, is essential as it has been shown that many patients are not appropriately diagnosed and treated for all their problems. Careful clinical follow-up is mandatory, and the frequency of examinations has to be determined according to the abnormalities encountered. For NF2 suspected because of cutaneous or ocular abnormalities, special attention should be given to monitoring of hearing as acoustic neuromas usually occur relatively late. For NF1, yearly visits are probably indicated in the first years following diagnosis. Whether routine imaging studies are required remains disputed. It is clearly necessary for those patients in whom brain tumours are suspected.

There is currently no drug treatment for the neurofibromatoses. Surgical treatment is required only for invasive lesions as many tumours are either static or slowly growing. The same applies to radiotherapy, as sequelae are particularly prone to occur in young children. Surgery is also indicated for cosmetic deformities that in many cases amount to a major problem.

TUBEROUS SCLEROSIS

Tuberous sclerosis (TS) or tuberous sclerosis complex (TSC) is an autosomal dominantly transmitted disorder characterized by hamartomas that can affect many organs including the skin, brain, heart, kidneys and other sites, with a variable expression and a high incidence of new mutations in the order of 58–68% of recognized cases (Hunt and Lidenbaum 1984). The prevalence of the disease is imperfectly known because of the frequency of paucisymptomatic forms. Population surveys indicate a prevalence of 1 in 6000 to 1 in 10,000 (Kuntz 1988, Webb and Osborne 1995). Occurrence of affected siblings with apparently unaffected parents is rare. Two mutant genes are responsible for tuberous sclerosis. In about 25% of the families the gene maps to 9q34 (*TSC1*) and codes for the protein *hamartin*; in the remainder it is located on the short arm of chromosome 16 (*TSC2*) and encodes the protein *tuberin*. Sancak et al. (2005) in 490 cases found the *TSC2* gene responsible for TS in 78%, 3.4 times more often than *TSC1*. *TSC1* mutations account for 10–30% of affected families, whereas most cases of *TSC2* mutations are observed in sporadic cases. No mutation is detected in 15–20% of patients, who usually show a milder clinical disease. Both act probably as tumour-suppressor genes (Au et al. 2004) and are involved in neuronal specification and migration. *TSC2* mutations, often sporadic, tend to be more severe. The gene on 16p has been identified and has homology to the GTPase-activating protein GAP3 (Nellist et al. 1993).

The mechanism of the disease involves an abnormality of proliferation and differentiation of embryonic cells, with a tendency to hamartomatous proliferation, and a disturbance of the migrational process of CNS cells resulting from the disruption of either hamartin or tuberin. These proteins act as sensors for growth factors, linking the extracellular cues to the activity of mTOR, a major regulator of protein translation and cell growth. Growth factor receptors activate a cascade regulating a large number of cellular functions (Goh and Weiss 2006). Work in the past few years has considerably increased our understanding of the disorder, especially the role of reduced inhibition of the TOR activation factor (Crino et al. 2006).

PATHOLOGY AND PATHOGENESIS
The characteristic lesions found in the brain of patients with TS are cortical tubers, subependymal nodules and giant cell tumours. Tubers (Fig. 3.5) are hard nodules of variable size that show disruption of normal lamination, increased astrocytic nuclei and a reduction of the number of neurons, which are replaced by bizarre giant cells (Huttenlocher and Heydemann 1984, Yamanouchi et al. 1997) that take both glial and neuronal markers.

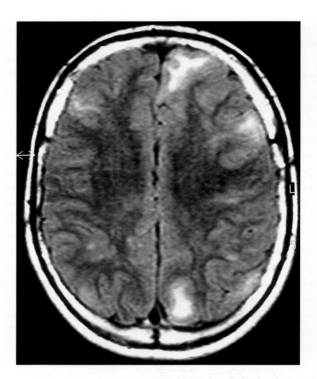

Fig. 3.5. Cortical tubers (hamartomas) in a patient with tuberous sclerosis complex – there are multiple tubers in the left hemisphere, and a few are visible in the right.

They may become calcified. Beneath the tubers, enlarged abnormal heterotopic neurons extend all the way to the ventricular walls. Subependymal nodules (Fig. 3.6a) are small excrescences on the ventricular walls that resemble solidified wax that has dripped down the side of a candle, hence the term 'candle guttering' that is traditionally used. They are composed of large round fusiform cells that are thought to be of astrocytic origin. Subependymal giant cell astrocytomas (Fig. 3.6b) are found in about 5% of cases (Gomez et al. 1988) and are consistently located to the region of the foramen of Monro. Unlike subependymal nodules, they tend to measure over 5 mm and to be less homogeneously dense; they sometimes grow to a large size but rarely, if ever, become malignant. The nature of the giant cells is still uncertain (Sharma et al. 2004).

Visceral tumours arise from various viscera. Rhabdomyomas are found in the heart of 40–50% of TS patients and are often multiple. Renal lesions include angiomyolipomas, which may be the only lesion of TS in some patients, and renal cysts (Robbins and Bernstein 1988). Retinal phakomas are benign astrocytic tumours that tend to calcify. Other hamartomatous lesions are seen less commonly (Gomez et al. 1988).

CLINICAL MANIFESTATIONS
The clinical manifestations of TS vary considerably with the extent of involvement and age of onset. Table 3.2 groups the findings into those that are highly suggestive and those that are less characteristic of the disease, according to the criteria proposed by Gomez et al. (1988) and revised by Roach et al. (1998). The

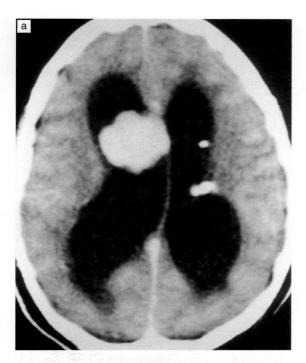

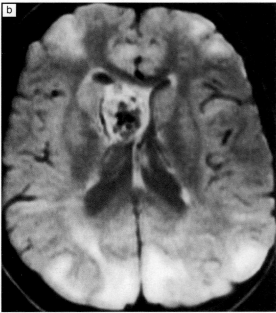

TABLE 3.2
Diagnostic criteria for tuberous sclerosis complex*

Major features
 Facial angiofibroma or forehead plaque
 Nontraumatic periungual fibroma[1]
 Three or more hypomelanotic macules
 Shagreen patch (connective tissue naevus)
 Retinal nodular hamartomas
 Cortical tuber[2]
 Subependymal giant cell astrocytoma
 Cardiac rhabdomyoma (single or multiple)
 Lymphangiomyomatosis[1]
 Renal angiolipoma

Minor features
 Multiple, randomly distributed pits in dental enamel
 Hamartomatous rectal polyps[1]
 Bone cysts
 Cerebral white matter radial migration lines[2]
 Gingival fibromas
 Nonrenal hamartoma
 Retinal achromic patch
 'Complete' skin lesions
 Multiple renal cysts

Definite tuberous sclerosis complex:
Either two major features or one major feature and two minor features

Probable tuberous sclerosis complex:
One major plus one minor feature

Possible tuberous sclerosis complex:
Either one major feature or two or more minor features

*Modified from Roach et al. (1998).
[1]Infrequent in childhood cases.
[2]If both cortical tubers and migration lines are present, they should be counted as one single feature.

Fig. 3.6. Tuberous sclerosis. *(a)* CT showing calcified subependymal nodules projecting into the lateral ventricles and a calcified giant cell astrocytoma obstructing the foramina of Monro with resulting hydrocephalus. *(b)* MRI of an 11-year-old boy with clinically isolated cutaneous manifestations, normal intelligence and no seizures. Heterogeneous mass in the right foramen of Monro corresponds to a giant cell astrocytoma. Multiple areas of increased signal in cortex represent tubers.

diagnosis now requires the presence of two major criteria or one major and two minor criteria. Because no feature is pathognomonic, involvement of two organ systems or at least two dissimilar lesions in the same organ is required for diagnosis (Roach and Sparagana 2004). The diagnosis is suspect if only one

suggestive feature is present, presumptive if two are present, and highly probable if one of the two features is a relative with TS.

SEIZURES
In infants and children, seizures are the most common presenting complaint, occurring in around 60% of patients. They are generalized in about 85% of cases. *Infantile spasms* (Gomez et al. 1988, Curatolo and Seri 2003) are the most common type in infancy. However, other types of seizure are not unusual, especially focal motor seizures. Tonic or atonic seizures are also frequently seen. Complex partial seizures were observed in 17 of 25 patients with TS who had initially had infantile spasms and in 11 of 15 children who had had other types of seizure (Yamamoto et al. 1987).

NEURODEVELOPMENTAL DIFFICULTIES
Mental retardation is the rule in hospital-based series and was present in 82% of children in one study (Monaghan et al. 1981). However, in the Mayo Clinic experience, only 47% of patients and their affected relatives were judged to have subnormal intelligence, while 44% had normal intelligence (Gomez et al. 1988). Webb et al. (1991) gave an even lower figure for mental retardation (40%) in a population study. Mental retardation is found only in patients who have had seizures, and especially where these had their onset before 2 years of age (Gomez et al. 1988). The prognosis of infantile spasms in TS patients is thus serious,

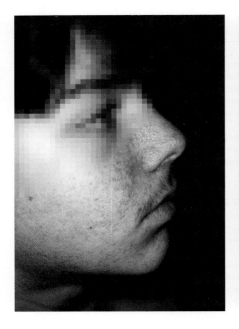
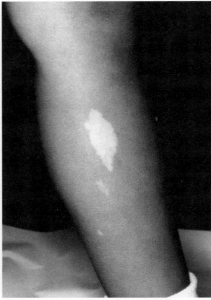
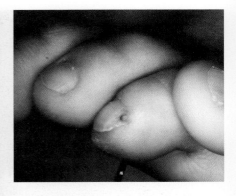

Fig. 3.7. Cutaneous manifestations of tuberous sclerosis. *(Left)* Facial angiofibromas (adenoma sebaceum). *(Centre)* Achromic naevus. *(Above)* Periungual fibroma. (Courtesy Dr D Teillac, Prof. Y de Prost, Hôpital des Enfants Malades, Paris.)

even though a proportion of these patients may develop a normal cognition (Rando et al. 2005). Riikonen and Simell (1990) found that infantile spasms due to TS have an especially poor prognosis, while Yamamoto et al. (1987) reported that the mental outcome in such patients was significantly better than that of patients with symptomatic spasms due to other causes. In addition to mental retardation other behavioural or cognitive abnormalities such as specific cognitive deficits and hyperkinesia are not infrequently found in TS patients (Hunt and Dennis 1987).

Autism is a frequent feature of TS, especially in those children who had infantile spasms (Bolton 2004). It is present in 25–50% of patients and TS may be responsible for 1–4% of cases seen in the population (Wiznitzer 2004). *Neurological deficits*, on the other hand, are rare, with the exception of increased intracranial pressure that occurs in less than 3% of cases and results from the development of intraventricular giant cell tumours and becomes symptomatic after the age of 5 years. These giant cell tumours may also be responsible for a hemiplegia.

CUTANEOUS MANIFESTATIONS (Fig. 3.7)
The classical cutaneous lesions of TS are present in 80% of cases. Classical angiofibromas (adenoma sebaceum) that occupy symmetrical areas over the cheeks, nasolabial folds and chin are red papular lesions, found in 50% of cases; they are rare in infants and generally appear between 3 and 15 years of age. Hypomelanotic macules (achromic patches or ash-leaf spots) are the earliest and most frequent cutaneous sign of TS and occur in 90% of cases (Fryer et al. 1990). They vary in number and size and are often present at birth, although they may become more visible and more numerous within a few months. They may be visible only under Wood's light in fair-skinned patients, especially infants. Isolated, small hypomelanotic spots are nonspecific. They are present in 0.8% of normal newborn infants (Alper and Holmes 1983). The association of white spots with seizures, es-

pecially infantile spasms, is characteristic of TS. A lock of depigmented hair may be an initial sign (McWilliam and Stephenson 1978). It results from the presence of a hypomelanotic spot on the scalp. Other cutaneous signs are seen later in life. They include fibrous plaques, usually on the forehead or scalp, that can occasionally be the sole manifestation of the disease; shagreen patches (20–40% of cases) that consist of a slightly elevated plaque of epidermis with a granular surface and sometimes a yellowish-brown discolouration and appear after a few years of life, commonly in the lumbar region; periungual fibromas that are a pathognomonic lesion but one that seldom occurs before puberty and then only in about 50% of patients; and molluscum pendulum in the cervical and lower facial region – not a specific lesion but quite unusual in childhood outside TS. Café-au-lait spots are not more frequent in TS than in the general population (Bell and McDonald 1985).

EYE ANOMALIES
Eye findings are represented by retinal astrocytomas (*phakomas*) (Fig. 3.8), which are found in half the cases and may be unique or multiple. They are round or oval in shape and become easy to diagnose when they calcify, assuming a typical mulberry appearance. Other ophthalmological findings in TS patients include depigmented retinal areas, hypopigmented iris spots, hyaline or cystic nodules, cataracts and iris coloboma.

OTHER FINDINGS
In some patients, the presenting manifestations are visceral rather than CNS ones (Franz 2004). A search for other localizations of TS is always indicated. Kidney tumours (angiolipomas), usually multiple and bilateral, are present in 60–75% of patients and may precede nervous system manifestations in infants, while hypertension may be the first feature in children (Robbins 1987). They are often highly vascular and can produce severe bleeding.

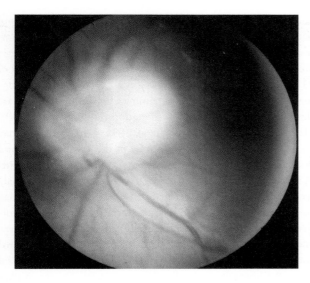

Fig. 3.8. Retinal phakoma in patient with tuberous sclerosis. Note tumour overlies retinal vessels.

Cardiac rhabdomyomas may be revealed by echography; they may occur prenatally or may only be revealed following administration of drugs such as carbamazepine. About half the cardiac rhabdomyomas are a manifestation of TS. Conversely, more than 50% of TS patients have cardiac tumours. Many are asymptomatic but some may manifest as cardiac failure, although arrhythmia is more common. Contrary to most other manifestations they have a marked tendency to disappear with time. They may be the cause of embolic strokes, although this is disputed by Gomez (1989).

Other visceral manifestations – especially pulmonary involvement frequent in adults – are rare in children. Partial gigantism has been reported (Franz 2004).

DIAGNOSIS

The diagnosis of TS is often clinically easy, but in infancy the most characteristic manifestations have not yet appeared. By far the most powerful diagnostic tool is neuroimaging by CT or MRI. CT is abnormal in 89% of patients. It shows subependymal calcified nodules, especially in the region of the foramen of Monro; cortical or subcortical areas of decreased attenuation that correspond to tubers and may be associated with widening of the adjacent gyrus; focal areas of increased attenuation corresponding to calcified tubers; in some cases ventricular dilatation or cortical atrophy or both; and occasionally cerebellar calcification. Gyriform calcification simulating that in Sturge–Weber syndrome may occur (Wilms et al. 1992). Contrast enhancement is useful if a giant cell astrocytoma is suspected as these take up contrast in 80% of cases.

MRI does not show the calcified lesions well, but does show cortical and subcortical tubers much better than CT. They present as high signal areas in T_2-weighted sequences. These areas are generally much more numerous than hypodense areas evidenced by CT and are located in the cortex (Roach et al. 1991). They vary in number and localization, and there is some relationship between the number and localization of tubers and mental development and neuropsychological findings (Shepherd et al. 1995, Goodman et al. 1997, Bozzao et al. 2003). Although there is no strict correlation between neurodevelopmental difficulties and the number or density of tubers detected by imaging, there is a trend for patients with more tubers to have more cognitive or behavioural disturbances, and frontal and parietal locations may be more closely related with autism and mental retardation (Curatolo 2003, Ridler et al. 2004). Deep white matter cystic abnormalities have been rarely reported (Canapicchi et al. 1996). Radial bands or wedge-shaped areas extending from ventricle to cortex or to a cortical tuber (Braffman et al. 1992) are composed of clusters of heterotopic cells and are indicative of a disorder of migration associated with abnormal cell differentiation. According to Gomez et al. (1988), a diagnosis of cerebral TS can probably be discarded if both CT and MRI are negative for cerebral abnormalities.

The EEG is of interest to better define the type of epilepsy associated with TS. Atypical hypsarrhythmia, often asymmetrical, is present in one third of cases. Focal signs are present in at least 40% of tracings (Yamamoto et al. 1987). In later childhood, focal paroxysms or bilateral slow spike–wave complexes may be found.

MANAGEMENT

Long-term follow-up of affected children should include monitoring of lesion growth with periodical imaging of the brain and abdomen, usually at least every three years. MRI of the brain is suggested on a yearly basis until 21 years of age (Crino et al. 2006).

There is no specific *treatment* for the disease itself, but several of its manifestations are amenable to therapy. Anticonvulsant drugs should be given for seizures, and infantile spasms may justify ACTH or steroid treatment. Vigabatrin seems to be particularly effective in the treatment of infantile spasms due to TS, and to a lesser extent for treatment of focal seizures (Curatolo and Seri 2003). Brain tumours should be removed surgically as far as possible, but in some cases palliative shunting may be necessary. Radiotherapy is not usually advised. Kidney angiolipomas can be embolized. Removal of a large tuber may be successful in controlling seizures in some patients. Determination of the existence of a single epileptogenic tuber is a prerequisite. This may be achieved by careful EEG and imaging studies (Lachwani et al. 2005). The use of alpha-methyltryptophan, which appears to fixate electively on active tubers, is promising (Chugani et al. 1998). It remains to be determined whether resection of an epileptogenic tuber may be associated with 'activation' of another lesion that could lead to persistence of seizures (Karefort et al. 2002). Careful assessment of learning ability of affected children is essential to ensure the best possible education. Surveillance of the patient is essential to detect early complications, especially a growing giant cell astrocytoma or a periperal complication. Disfiguring adenofibromas can be treated medically or surgically according to their nature. Recently, Franz et al. (2006) showed that rapamycin, an inhibitor of mTOR, can inhibit the growth of astrocytomas in TS.

Genetic counselling is an essential part of the management of TS patients and their parents. Careful examination of both parents including Wood's lamp inspection of the skin should be performed, especially clinical and ophthalmological assessment. If these are negative, imaging should be obtained initially and repeated as required clinically. Fryer et al. (1990) believe that CT is unlikely to help. Others systematically perform CT and/or MRI, but the latter may be difficult to interpret (Braffman et al. 1992) and may not show calcification well, although periventricular nodules can usually be made out easily. The nature of the disease should be explained in simple terms. In the usual case of an isolated patient without family history of the disease, a favourable genetic prognosis can be given with very few reservations, provided both parents have been carefully examined and have been found not to have any cutaneous, neurological or visceral features of the disease. Such an assessment includes, in addition to clinical examination and search for possible cases in families, ophthalmological examination, renal ultrasonography and CT. Even so, a small proportion of such cases (<1%) (Roach and Sparagna 2004) may be missed. Prenatal diagnosis can be suspected on the basis of a fetal ultrasound examination showing cardiac rhabdomyomas or polycystic kidneys. Molecular genetic diagnosis is difficult because of genetic heterogeneity. A mutation of the *TS2* gene has been identified (Vrtel et al. 1996).

LINEAR NAEVUS AND RELATED SYNDROMES

CLASSICAL LINEAR NAEVUS SYNDROME
In its complete form, this syndrome includes a cutaneous naevus with neurological and eye abnormalities. The skin lesion may be of several types. One typical appearance is that of the *sebaceous naevus of Jadassohn*. This lesion usually involves the head or face, and may be visible at birth or in infancy or become evident only after a few years (Clancy et al. 1985). It is a slightly raised, yellow-orange, smooth, linear plaque that abuts the midline of the forehead, nose or lips and often involves the scalp. It tends to become darker and verrucous as years pass. Early in life there is mainly acanthosis and little pigment, and sebaceous glands are often not prominent. Later, sebaceous glands proliferate, and apocrine glands may be located aberrantly throughout the thickness of the skin.

A second type of naevus is the *verrucous naevus*, which is formed of discrete papules, slightly darker than the surrounding skin, with a linear organization. Such naevi are more often located on the body and less on the face than the sebaceous naevus, and histologically there is only acanthosis and hyperkeratosis with abnormal dermis (Prensky 1987). It seems that either type of naevus may be associated with neurological abnormalities (Clancy et al. 1985), although most skin lesions are isolated. Associated cutaneous abnormalities such as ichthyosis, acanthosis nigricans, haemangiomas and café-au-lait spots are frequent, and linear naevus overlaps with other neurocutaneous syndromes with proliferative skin and subcutaneous tissue lesions (see below).

Neurological manifestations associated with both types of naevi (as in the *Feuerstein–Mims syndrome*) consist of mental retardation, seizures, cranial nerve palsies, hydrocephalus and asymmetrical macrocephaly (van de Warrenburg et al. 1998). Seizures are often partial, but infantile spasms have been observed in 4 of 11 patients in one series (Vigevano et al. 1984). From a pathological point of view, the most common brain abnormalities are disorders of proliferation and migration (Prayson et al. 1999). Hemimegalencephaly (Pavone et al. 1991) is frequent and may be associated with hemihypertrophy of the ipsilateral face and body. Hamartomatous tumours were present in several patients (Clancy et al. 1985). Destructive lesions such as porencephaly have also been found (Baker et al. 1987, Prensky 1987) and may be of vascular origin as arterial aneurysms, arteriovenous malformations and abnormal venous return have been reported (Dobyns and Garg 1991). Similar lesions have been found in the spinal cord. Other CNS abnormalities include arachnoid cysts, subtotal cerebellar agenesis, and callosal agenesis with Dandy–Walker malformation (Dodge and Dobyns 1995).

The most common eye abnormalities are dermoids or epidermoids of the conjunctiva and colobomas of the iris, choroid, retina or optic nerve. Enlargement of the orbit and of the greater wing of the sphenoid on the side of the naevus may be present. Familial cases are rare (Meschia et al. 1992).

The *diagnosis* may be difficult in early cases without visible naevus. The most common CT finding is hypertrophy of one hemisphere, usually on the same side as the naevus, with enlargement of the ipsilateral ventricle, and pachygyria with hypodense white matter (Kruse et al. 1998). Such an image is consistent with pathological reports of hemimegalencephaly or other migration disorders.

The EEG usually shows paroxysmal activity over the involved hemisphere, sometimes with a hypsarrhythmic pattern. The prognosis is usually serious but mild cases exist with only seizures or mild learning difficulties. The syndrome is probably sporadic and the cause is unknown. The relatively frequent ocurrence of tumours suggests a close relationship with the phakomatoses. Treatment is symptomatic. Removal of the cutaneous lesion is possible in some patients.

RELATED SYNDROMES WITH PROLIFERATIVE SKIN AND SUBCUTANEOUS TISSUE LESIONS
Encephalocraniocutaneous Lipomatosis (ECCL) and Oculocerebrocutaneous Syndrome (OCCS)
These are rare, closely related, apparently sporadic syndromes characterized by microcephaly, lipodermoids involving the conjunctiva, sclera or eyelids, and lipomatous swelling over the cranium or face. Convulsions and mental retardation may be present, and CT of the brain may show atrophy, cystic areas and intracranial calcification. In some studies (Fishman 1987) brain malformations in the form of porencephaly were present in all cases, eyelid excrescences in most, and iris abnormalities in 2. Moog et al. (2005) summarized the features of the brain malformation in 2 personal cases and 9 from the literature; these included predominantly frontal microgyria and periventricular heterotopias, callosal agenesis, giant tectum of the brainstem, and absence or

hypoplasia of the vermis or of the whole cerebellum. The condition may be related to the Delleman syndrome (Pascual-Castroviejo et al. 2005b), and to the Proteus syndrome (McCall et al. 1992).

PROTEUS SYNDROME

This term applies to a complex hamartomatous syndrome consisting of partial gigantism, asymmetry of the limbs, linear verrucous and intradermal naevi, shagreen patches, and variable combinations of lymphangiomas, haemangiomas, macrocephaly and hyperostoses. Plantar skin hyperplasia (the so-called 'mocassin lesion') is a frequent and useful diagnostic feature (Nguyen et al. 2004). Epibulbar dermoids, colobomas, glaucoma and retinal detachment can occur. Hemimegalencephaly is frequent (Griffiths et al. 1994). The deformities resulting from the syndrome can reach extreme proportions, as in the case of Joseph Merick, the so-called 'Elephant Man'. The disease is still commonly misdiagnosed as neurofibromatosis. As the name implies, the Proteus syndrome has a very variable expresssion. Most proven cases to date have been sporadic. Somatic mosaicism, lethal in the homozygous state, might account for most features of the syndrome but is not proved (Cohen 2005). Some of the cases are associated with mutations of the *PTEN* tumour suppressor gene (Thiffaut et al. 2004). Visceral tumours may occur (Gordon et al. 1995). The diagnosis is difficult as the limits of the syndrome are not well defined. Turner et al. (2004) found that among 205 cases published, only 97 (43%) met strict criteria. Cases that do not meet such criteria are sometimes termed 'Proteus-like syndrome' (Zhou et al. (2000).

OTHER SYNDROMES WITH TISSUE PROLIFERATION

Cowden syndrome is characterized by the association of various skin lesions especially facial teichilemomas and other cutaneous abnormalities, with other hamartomas that may include intestinal polyps. In childhood, clinical features include macrocephly, scrotal tongue and mild to moderate mental retardation, while cutaneous tumours and other characteristic features appear only later in life (Hanssen and Fryns 1995). The most striking neurological feature is the cerebellar hamartomatous cerebellar hyperplasia of Lhermitte–Duclos disease, also due to mutations in the *PTEN* gene, which in fact is part of the spectrum of Cowden syndrome (Perez-Nunez et al. 2004).

Bannayan–Riley–Ruvalcaba syndrome is associated with *PTEN* gene mutations in some cases (Hendricks et al. 2003). In its complete form it presents with macrocephaly, intestinal polyps, lipomas, angiomas, mucocutaneous pigmentation, and developmental delay or mental retardation.

NEUROCUTANEOUS SYNDROMES WITH PROMINENT VASCULAR COMPONENTS

Several syndromes are characterized by the association of cutaneous abnormalities and vascular malformations of the CNS. The type of vascular abnormalities is widely variable, and multiple associated anomalies are common.

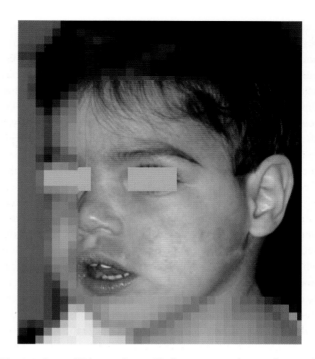

Fig. 3.9. Sturge–Weber syndrome. Flat haemangioma (naevus flammeus) on the left side of the face of a 5-year-old boy with focal seizures since the age of 5 months. The angioma involves the first and second divisions of the Vth nerve but resects the right side.

STURGE–WEBER SYNDROME

Sturge–Weber syndrome (SWS) is by far the most frequent of the disorders of this group. In its complete form it consists of a venous angioma of the leptomeninges, ipsilateral flat facial angiomatous naevus ('port-wine stain') (Fig. 3.9) and choroidal angioma. An identical pial angioma may be present in isolation or in association with choroidal angioma without facial naevus in up to 13% of cases (Gomez and Bebin 1987, Roach 1992, Pascual-Castroviejo et al. 1993). Such cases, for all practical purposes, should be regarded as belonging to the same syndrome. However, some of these cases may represent errors of diagnosis, e.g. cases of the syndrome of intracranial calcification with coeliac disease. On the other hand, cases of facial naevus without CNS involvement with or without glaucoma are common (Roach 1992).

CUTANEOUS MANIFESTATIONS

The naevus flammeus ('portwine stain') almost always lies above the level of the palpebral fissure involving the upper eyelid or frontal region or both. Frontal lesions close to the midline are more commonly associated with anteriorly located pial lesions and more external frontal involvement with the more frequent occipitoparietal angiomas, but the correlation between the extent and location of the naevus and that of the pial angioma is poor. In a survey of 310 patients, Tallman et al. (1991) found neurological or ophthalmological involvement in 6% of those with unilateral and 24% of those with bilateral naevi in the territory of the first two divisions of the trigeminal nerve (only 3 patients had isolated involvement of the second division). These figures are likely to be underestimates as no imaging was performed. Sujansky and Conradi (1995a,b) computed a frequency of between 8% and 33% from a review of the literature. Some children have bilateral naevi with unilateral pial involvement (Gomez and Bebin 1987). Bilateral meningeal angiomas may coexist with either unilateral or bilateral facial naevi. Pascual-Castroviejo et al. (1993) found 13 such cases in their 40 patients. In only 3 of these was the CNS angioma bilateral. Rare cases of angioma contralateral to the naevus flammeus are on record (Widdess-Walsh and Friedman 2003). Angiomas not uncommonly may extend beyond the face and involve the neck, trunk or limbs on one or both sides.

The intracranial angioma is limited to the pia mater that contains dilated and tortuous venules that may form several layers in the subarachnoid space but rarely enter the brain. The calcifications lie in the cortex underlying the angioma and subcortical white matter, tending to appear deeply at first and then extending toward the surface (Comi 2003, Thomas-Sohl et al. 2004). Localized or unilateral brain atrophy is virtually constant. In one severe case, four-layer microgyria was found underlying the angioma, indicating a prenatal origin of cortical damage (Simonati et al. 1994). Localized atrophy of prenatal origin (Portilla et al. 2002) also indicates the possible early repercussions of the angioma on cerebral development.

NEUROLOGICAL MANIFESTATIONS

Seizures are the major neurological manifestation of SWS, occurring in 75–90% of patients (Gomez and Bebin 1987, Sujansky and Conradi 1995b). They usually have their onset in the first months of life. They are generally partial motor in type and are often prolonged in episodes of status epilepticus. Generalized seizures and even myoclonic and atonic seizures or infantile spasms can occur (Chevrie et al. 1988, Arzimanoglou and Aicardi 1992). Many patients have frequent and repeated seizures (Oakes 1992) but some children have only an occasional seizure, and approximately half the patients in one series responded well to drug therapy (Arzimanoglou and Aicardi 1992). The EEG shows reduced background amplitude over the angioma in a majority of patients. Associated paroxysmal abnormalities are often found on the involved side, although this may be a late sign. Generalized bisynchronous discharges can be present in patients with unilateral pial lesions (Chevrie et al. 1988). Paradoxical predominance of the paroxysmal features on the normal side may be seen. According to Jansen et al. (2004), an abnormally small amplitude of the beta rhythm following administration of benzodiazepines may help to localize the area of parenchymal damage.

Hemiplegia occurs in at least one-half of cases and is localized to the side opposite the facial naevus, except in a very few patients who probably have bilateral disease (Terdjman et al. 1990). Hemiplegia usually first appears after an episode of seizures and may become more severe with the recurrence of seizures. *Hemianopia* is virtually constant, isolated or in association with hemiparesis.

Transient hemiplegias not following an epileptic attack and sometimes accompanied by migraine-like headache are observed in many cases of SWS (Arzimanoglou and Aicardi 1992, Jansen et al. 2004). These hemiplegic episodes are apparently not of epileptic nature and may be a consequence of vasomotor disturbances within and around the angioma (Terdjman et al. 1990). Migraine-like episodes can also occur in the absence of hemiplegia (Taddeucci et al. 2005).

Mental retardation is present in about 40% of the patients and in 75% of those with seizures. It does not occur in patients without epilepsy and is more common and more severe in bilateral forms (Gomez and Bebin 1987, Sujansky and Conradi 1995b). In many cases, there appears to be a definite regression of cognitive abilities parallel to the repetition and severity of the seizures.

Intracranial haemorrhage is not a feature of SWS. However, elevated spinal fluid protein is commonly found (Skoglund et al. 1978) and may correspond to minimal bleeding from the angioma. This interpretation is also consistent with the occasional occurrence of hydrocephalus (Fishman and Baram 1986), as observed also in a personal case, or with protein exudation from the angioma. Macrocephaly not due to hydrocephalus has also been reported (see Cohen 2003).

Glaucoma is present in 30–48% of SWS patients (Sujansky and Conradi 1995b), and 50% have choroidal angioma that may sometimes be visible with the ophthalmoscope. The glaucoma may be the consequence of overproduction of aqueous fluid by the choroidal angioma, or else exudate from the lesion may block the angle.

IMAGING FEATURES

Plain skull X-rays show the classical 'tramline' calcification most frequently in the parieto-occipital area. Although this has been occasionally detected in the neonatal period, it is often a late sign and may be absent even in adolescents. Angiography is not usually indicated. It does not show the angioma but demonstrates lack of superficial cortical veins, nonfilling of dural sinuses, and abnormal, tortuous veins that course toward the ventricle and vein of Galen system.

CT is a much more powerful tool for the detection of calcium and can often show its presence in infants of only a few months of age or even in neonates. CT also clearly demonstrates atrophy of the brain, enlargement of the choroid plexus on the side of the pial angioma, and abnormal veins draining into the deep venous circulation (Terdjman et al. 1990) (Fig. 3.10). MRI shows calcification less well than CT. Enhancement seen on CT may not represent opacification of the pial angioma but rather cortical injection similar to that occurring in postconvulsive hemiplegia, and it may disappear and reappear with the occurrence and disappearance of seizures (Terdjman et al. 1990, Shin et al. 2002). With gadolinium enhancement, the pial angioma can be clearly made out (Lipski et al. 1990, Sperner et al. 1990, Benedikt et al. 1993, Vogl et al. 1993). This may permit a preclinical diagnosis of the Sturge–Weber syndrome in patients with an apparently isolated facial naevus, and may indicate the extent of the angioma and the presence or absence of contralateral involvement (Fig. 3.11). High-resolution techniques of 3D MRA may show a blush at the site of the angioma, and MRI may demonstrate advanced myelination at this locus. Perfusion MRI may permit an earlier

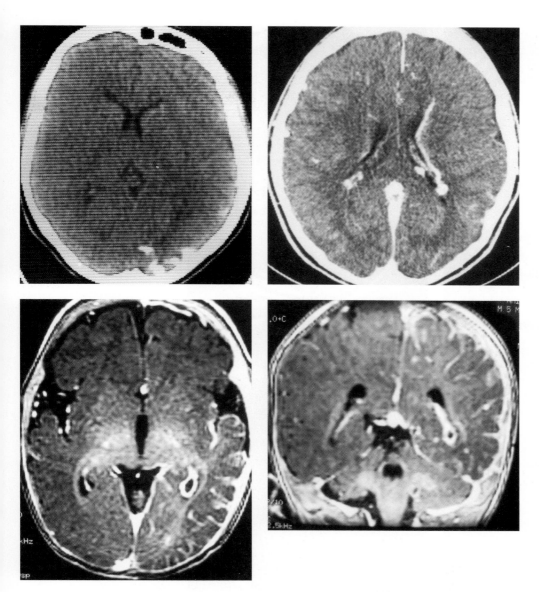

Fig. 3.10. Sturge–Weber syndrome. *(Top left)* CT showing typical occipital calcification. *(Top right)* Abnormal venous drainage along ventricular angle. *(Bottom)* MRI following gadolinium enhancement shows contrast uptake in the pial angioma in the posterior part of the left hemisphere on axial *(left)* and coronal *(right)* cuts. Note enlargement of the left choroid plexus glomus and presence of a vein draining into the anterior sagittal sinus.

diagnosis and more precise delineation of parenchymal abnormalities (Lin et al. 2003, Evans et al. 2006), and together with spectrosopy can determine the correlations with clinical symptoms and help surgery planning (Lin et al. 2006). A better definition of the venous abnormalities might also be obtained with BOLD MR venography (Mentzel et al. 2005).

Examination with PET or SPECT shows hypometabolism or marked underperfusion in the area of the pial angioma and may help to detect latent angioma (Chiron et al. 1989, Chugani et al. 1989). Ichinose et al. (2003) found in one case decreased blood flow and glucose hypometabolism of the involved hemisphere as shown by SPECT and fluorodeoxyglucose PET respectively on the one hand, and accumulation of 11C-methionine thought to result from gliosis on the other.

DIAGNOSIS

The diagnosis of Sturge–Weber syndrome is usually straightforward. However, in mild cases and in children who have not had seizures with a facial naevus that has been present from birth it may be very difficult to know whether a pial angioma is associated. MRI after enhancement with gadolinium or with water diffusion studies can answer this but whether it is justified is difficult to decide, as the frequency of cases of cutaneous angioma without seizures is not known. A few cases of tuberous sclerosis mimicking SWS with leptomeningeal enhancement and enlargement of the choroid plexus are on record (Kremer et al. 2005). The differential diagnosis includes other causes of cortical calcification and atrophy. The *syndrome of cortical calcification, epilepsy and coeliac disease* (Gobbi et al. 1988) is described below. Other

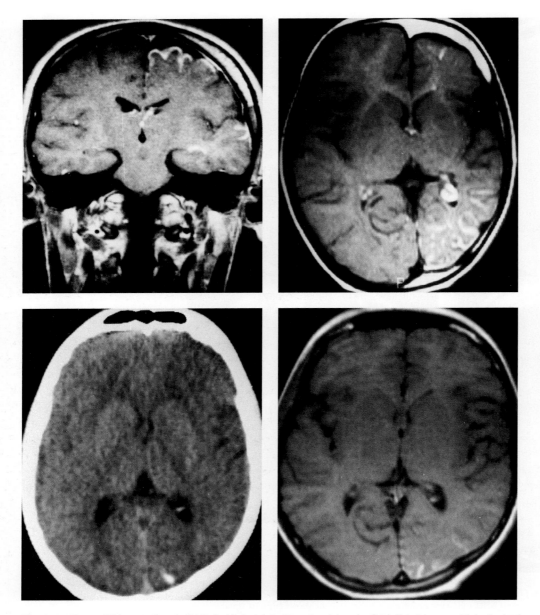

Fig. 3.11. Sturge–Weber syndrome. *(a)* Left-sided pial angioma involving the frontal and temporal lobe is clearly outlined following gadolinium enhancement in 6-year-old girl with left-sided facial angioma. *(b)* Left occipito-temporal angioma: gadolinium-enhanced MRI. Note considerable atrophy of the whole hemisphere, angioma of the left choroid plexus glomus and marked increase in skull thickness. *(c)* CT of 14-year-old boy who suffered two attacks, at 20 and 26 months of age, of right focal motor seizures associated with headache and vomiting. The small left occipital calcification had not been present on CT performed at 26 and 48 months. *(d)* T₁-weighted MRI after gadolinium injection shows small pial angioma over the occipital pole. This is isolated pial angiomatosis as the child had no facial angioma.

causes of calcification mimicking the 'tramline' type include neurofibromatosis and rare cases of tuberous sclerosis (Wilms et al. 1992).

The neurological defects seen in SWS are probably the consequence of blood stagnation, hypoxaemia and impaired neuronal metabolism (Comi 2003). The hypoxaemic effects are exaggerated by the increased metabolic rate resulting from epileptic seizures, and probably also by vasomotor changes and thrombotic phenomena that take place in and about the pial lesion (Aylett 1999). Such a mechanism may explain the progressive aggravation

of damage all too often observed in these patients. It would also account for the beneficial effect of early surgery, preventing this cascade of ill effects.

A common embryological origin from the neural crest of the vascular bed of the leptomeninges and optic cup probably explains the Sturge–Weber association. The disease is sporadic. Only a few, doubtful, familial cases are on record, and the genetic prognosis is good. However, Eerola et al. (2003) proposed that a susceptibility to the development of capillary angioma linked to a locus on chromosome 5q could play a predisposing role in some cases.

COURSE

The natural course of SWS depends on the presence, persistence and resistance to treatment of the seizures (Oakes 1992). In some patients, the disorder may remain static after marked atrophy has developed, and the seizures may subside or be relatively easily controlled. Onset of seizures before 1 year of age, a hypsarrhythmic EEG pattern, the occurrence of episodes of status and bilateral involvement predict an unfavourable spontaneous outcome. Cognitive and behavioural development is quite variable. It may be good, especially if control of the seizures is obtained. Intractable epilepsy is an indication for surgical treatment.

DIFFERENTIAL DIAGNOSIS

Children with epilepsy and intracranial calcification may have an incomplete form of SWS. However, Gobbi et al. (1988) have described a distinctive syndrome of epilepsy with intracranial calcification associated with coeliac disease different from SWS. The syndrome features unilateral images of calcification, similar to those in SWS, whose origin is not known. Calcification is often but not always occipital and is not necessarily bilateral. There is usually no detectable atrophy associated with the calcification and no abnormalities of the cortical veins or choroid plexus, but hypodensity of the white matter is often seen in the vicinity of calcified areas (Gobbi 2005). The pathology of the syndrome is poorly known. In a few cases, vascular abnormalities reminiscent of SWS in the form of foci of angiomatous venous dilatation were reported (Bye et al. 1993); they were not found in another case (Toti et al. 1996). The epilepsy is sometimes associated with progressive mental and epileptic deterioration (see Chapter 22). This syndrome may not be homogeneous. It is characterized by variable types of seizures that may have a severe course but may also occur infrequently and be controllable by drug therapy. The patients may have full-blown coeliac disease; more often, the disorder lacks digestive manifestations and the diagnosis then rests on jejunal biopsy showing typical mucosal atrophy. In some cases, the biopsy may give normal results, so the ultimate diagnostic criterion in such cases is the presence of antibodies against gliadin found in the blood. An immunological mechanism seems likely and is supported by the high incidence of certain HLA groups (HLA DQ2 and DQ8). Although calcification resembles that resulting from folic acid deficiency, administration of this compound has no positive effect. The treatment is suppression of gluten-containing foods, which has to be maintained throughout life. The effect of the diet on epilepsy is variable and may depend on the precocity of its use (Gobbi 2005). When early, there seems to be a positive effect on seizures.

A few rare vascular syndromes may be only variants of SWS. These include cases of SWS associated with macrocephaly and hydrocephalus (Fishman and Baram 1986), which have been attributed to abnormal venous drainage with resulting intracranial hypertension. A syndrome of bilateral facial naevi, macrocrania and anomalous venous return through superficial veins is regarded by some authors (Shapiro and Shulman 1976, Orr et al. 1978) as probably different from SWS. Association with bilateral lymphatic/venous malformation has been reported (Ramli et al. 2003). The Klippel–Trenaunay syndrome, which involves mainly the peripheral vascular system, may be associated with cranial anomalies (Williams et al. 1992).

TREATMENT

Treatment is mainly directed against the seizures, and an aggressive antiepileptic regimen should be established from the first seizure. Control can be obtained with drugs in about half the patients, even in those with early-onset seizures (Arzimanoglou and Aicardi 1992). Arrest of status epilepticus (Chapter 15) is of utmost importance, as hemiplegia is often postconvulsive. In uncontrollable cases, especially in infants, functional hemispherectomy, or classic occipital or parietal lobectomy or resection of the angiomatous area could render the patient seizure-free and possibly prevent mental deterioration. Hemispherotomy has also given very good results for the control of seizures (Schropp et al. 2006). It is indicated for uncontrollable seizures when fine hand movements are absent (Roach et al. 1994) although some authors have advocated it in nonparalytic severe cases (Kossef et al. 2002). Arzimanoglou et al. (2000) reported excellent control of seizures after hemispherectomy but less favourable results after lobar or incomplete resections. Kossef et al. (2002) reviewed 32 cases of hemispherectomy for SWS from the world literature; satisfactory control of seizures was obtained in about 26 of these patients without significant increase in hemiplegia. Even bilateral cases may be amenable to surgery provided the seizures consistently originate from one side as shown by clinical seizure features, repeated EEGs and possibly functional imaging techniques (Tuxhorn and Pannek 2002, Schropp et al. 2006). Clinical experience favours early intervention, preferably in the first year of life, if frequent seizures or status epilepticus occur. However, the results on neurodevelopment may be disappointing even with early control of epileptic activity. Given these results, the place of callosotomy (Rappaport 1988) proposed as an alternative to hemispherectomy seems to be limited.

The possibility of preventing the occurrence of seizures by early antiepileptic treatment has been studied by Ville et al. (2002). Although they found a significant, if slight, difference favouring the group treated with phenobarbitone over controls, the small number of patients and the heterogeneity of cases renders a conclusion difficult in view of the uncertainties about long-term side effects of such therapy.

Local treatment of the port-wine stain is psychologically important, and good results have been obtained with pulsed dye laser (Léauté-Lebrège et al. 2002).

OTHER NEUROCUTANEOUS SYNDROMES WITH PROMINENT VASCULAR COMPONENTS

SYNDROME OF HAEMANGIOMAS AND OTHER CARDIOVASCULAR DEFECTS (PHACES OR CASTROVIEJO II SYNDROME)

Several cases of cyst of the posterior fossa with partial cerebellar agenesis in association with facial angiomas have been reported. This association was expanded to other abnormalities, especially vascular, cardiac and ocular defects, and proposed to constitute a new neurocutaneous syndrome (Frieden et al. 1996) called *PHACE or PHACES syndrome* (posterior fossa malformation, *h*aemangiomas, *a*rterial abnormalities, *c*oarctation of the aorta, *e*ye abnormalities, and *s*ternal maldevelopment) or Pascual-Castroviejo syndrome II (Pascual-Castroviejo 1985; Pascual-Castroviejo et al. 1996, 2005a). This syndrome predominates in girls (90%) and has a wide spectrum of manifestations that can involve many organs throughout the body (Metry et al. 2001, 2006). Partial forms are probably common even though the criteria and limits of the syndrome are not completely defined (Rossi et al. 2001). The posterior fossa malformation usually resembles the Dandy–Walker syndrome but hypoplasia of the vermis or of the whole cerebellum and unilateral absence of a cerebellar hemisphere may be found. The angiomas are variably flat or tuberous, usually involve the face or neck, and may be multiple. They may appear only after birth. Rare cases have been familial. Diverse embryological abnormalities of the aortic arch and of cervical and especially extracranial and intracranial vessels, and variable degrees of uni- or bilateral cerebellar hypoplasia, or cortical dysplasia, are often found (Pascual-Castroviejo et al. 1996). Intracerebral haemangiomas and neuronal migration anomalies may be present (Poindexter et al. 2007). This syndrome may be related to facial hemiatrophy and to the velocardiofacial syndrome (Strenge et al. 1996).

Coarctation of the aorta and congenital heart disease, especially septal defects, are frequent. Abnormalities of the vessels, especially those derived from the first branchial arches, are common. They include persistence of the trigeminal artery, unilateral or bilateral carotid or vertebral hypoplasia, and/or absence of the minor branches. Variable eye defects may include proptosis, ptosis, cataracts and retinal anomalies (Kronenberg et al. 2005). Involvement of visceral vessels may occur. A malformed sternum is often found. Many patients have mental retardation or a borderline intellectual level. Vascular and cardiac complications may occur, and fatal cases are on record. Strokes are a possible manifestation (Drolet et al. 2006). Treatment of the haemangiomas with corticosteroids may be effective, and surgery may be required for correction of some of the congenital defects.

VON HIPPEL–LINDAU DISEASE
Although not a neurocutaneous disease in a majority of cases, cutaneous haemangiomas are known to occur in von Hippel–Lindau syndrome, which has many features in common with the phakomatoses, including a remarkable tendency to the development of nonvascular tumours. The disease consists of the association of cerebellar, retinal, spinal and cerebellar haemangioblastoma, pheochromocytoma, cysts of the pancreas and kidneys, renal cell carcinoma, and ependidymal cystadenoma (Joerger et al. 2005). Cutaneous involvement occurs in some cases. The condition is transmitted as a dominant trait with a penetrance of 80–90%. The gene (*VHL1*) has been mapped to chromosome 3p25–p26 and acts as a tumour suppressor gene (Glasker 2005).

The diagnosis is made in patients with more than one haemangioblastoma of the CNS or one isolated lesion in association with a visceral manifestation of the disease, or in patients with a known family history (Huson et al. 1986). Neumann et al. (1992) found that 44% of gene carriers had haemangioblastoma, multiple in 42%, and 44% of those with haemangioblastoma had retinal lesions. The retinal haemangioma has a characteristic appearance. About 20% of patients with retinal angioma develop neurological complications, and 40% of patients with cerebellar haemangioblastoma have von Hippel–Lindau disease (Huson et al. 1986). Polycythaemia is found in 10–20% of patients with a cerebellar tumour. The disease manifests usually after 10 years of age by acute eye complications, e.g. haemorrhage, or by a posterior fossa syndrome (Kreusel 2005). Pancreatic and renal cysts are asymptomatic and are detected by abdominal imaging in three quarters of cases. Renal carcinomas and phaeochromocytomas (Opocher et al. 2005) should be detected early if conservative treatment is to be contemplated.

Patients and at-risk relatives should have annual ophthalmological assessment from 5 years of age, urinary vanillylmandelic acid (VMA) and noradrenaline estimation from 10 years, annual or biennial brain imaging from 15 years, and abdominal imaging from 20 years. This protocol should be extended to all patients presenting with cerebellar or retinal haemangioblastoma (Huson et al. 1986).

Treatment is purely surgical (Vougioukas et al. 2006). The prognosis is dominated by the presence and size of tumours, both intracranial and intra-abdominal.

HEREDITARY HAEMORRHAGIC TELANGIECTASIA (RENDU–OSLER–WEBER SYNDROME)
Hereditary haemorrhagic telangiectasia is a familial disorder, transmitted as an autosomal dominant trait, characterized by the presence of multiple dermal, mucosal and visceral telangiectasias associated with recurrent bleeding (Mei-Zahav et al. 2006). The most common manifestations in children carrying a mutation include cutaneous and nasal telangiectasias, and pulmonary and hepatic arteriovenous malformations (AVMs); central nervous system AVMs or CNS ischaemic lesions complicating pulmonary AVMs were found in 12% of children with a mutation (Giordano et al. 2006). The most common complication is epistaxis, which, however, is rarely severe before age 35 years. Neurological involvement includes the complications of right-to-left shunt through pulmonary arteriovenous fistulas, responsible for brain abcesses, and thrombosis associated with polycythaemia. Vascular malformations of the brain, especially arteriovenous angiomas and fistulas (Weon et al. 2005), are a frequent complication. Spinal arteriovenous fistulas were found in infants and young children, whereas AVMs with a nidus were found only in adults in one large series (Krings et al. 2005). Recurrent alternating hemiplegia has been reported (Myles et al. 1970). Two major genetic subtypes are known (HTTI and HTT2) due respectively to mutations in the genes of endoglin (*ENG*) and *ALK1/ACVRL1*, each gene accounting for approximately half the cases (Bayrak-Toydemir et al. (2006). These genes code for

TABLE 3.3
Neurocutaneous syndromes with prominent vascular components

Syndrome	Clinical features	Genetics	References
Blue rubber bleb naevus syndrome	Subcutaneous and mucous angiomas. Rare cases of multiple cavernous angiomas of the CNS	S or AD	Kim (2000), Eiris-Puñal et al. (2002)
Rendu–Osler–Weber syndrome (hereditary haemorrhagic telangiectasia)	See text	AD[1]	Abdalla and Letarte (2006)
Klippel–Trenaunay syndrome	See text	S[2]	
Cobb syndrome	Cutaneous flat angioma and myelopathy due to spinal cord angioma in same metameric location	S	Baraitser and Shieff (1990)
Shapiro–Shulman syndrome	Bilateral facial naevi, abnormal venous damage of the brain, macrocephaly	S	Shapiro and Shulman (1976), Fishman and Baram (1986)
Banayan–Riley–Ruvalcaba syndrome	Macrocephaly, lipomatosis, cutaneous angiomas		Dobyns et al. (1987), Gorlin et al. (1992)
Sneddon syndrome	Livedo reticularis, generalized arterial occlusive disease that may affect the brain	S or A	Pettee et al. (1994), Lossos et al. (1995), Boesch et al. (2003), Szmyrka-Kaczmarek et al. (2005)
Divry–Van Bogaert syndrome	Livedo reticularis, noncalcifying leptomeningeal angiomatosis with progressive neurological impairment		Stone et al. (2001)
Macrocephaly–cutis marmorata telangiectatica	Livedo reticularis, dysmorphism, CNS malformations, mental retardation, macrocephaly syndrome	S ?	Garavelli et al. (2005), Lapunzina et al. (2005)
PHACES syndrome	See text	S	Reese et al. (1993)
Familial cavernous malformation of CNS and retina (Gass syndrome)	Cavernous angiomas of the brain, multiple in 50% of cases, retinal angiomas, occasional cutaneous involvement	AD	Gass (1971), Dobyns et al. (1987)
Wyburn–Mason syndrome (Dechaume–Blanc–Bonnet syndrome)	Retinal arteriovenous angioma, unilateral arteriovenous malformation extending from the retina along the visual pathways to the brainstem and sometimes the cerebellar hemisphere. Rupture of vessels frequent. Facial periorbital angioma	S	Gomez (1994), Lester et al. (2005)
Hereditary neurocutaneous angiomatosis	Cutaneous angiomas of skin, cerebral or cerebellar arteriovenous malformations	AD	Drigo et al. (1994), Leblanc et al. (1996)
Von Hippel–Lindau disease	See text (cutaneous involvement possible)	AD	Joerger et al. (2005)

[1]At least two subtypes due to different gene mutations are known.
[2]Various genetic factors are being studied but most cases are sporadic.

proteins that help maintain the integrity of vascular endothelium. Two minor genetic subtypes have been reported (Abdalla et al. 2005).

The cutaneous lesions may be hard to discover and should be looked for carefully, especially when pulmonary arteriovenous fistulas are present. Surgical removal or endovascular treatment of bleeding or otherwise functionally detrimental lesions is indicated, and regular surveillance for detection of tumours outside the CNS is essential. Treatment with antibodies antagonist of vascular endothelium growth factor (betacizumab) may be promising (Flieger et al. 2006).

RARE NEUROCUTANEOUS SYNDROMES WITH PROMINENT VASCULAR COMPONENT

Neurocutaneous syndromes of which vascular abnormalities are an important part are listed in Table 3.3. Several of these are genetically determined. Cutaneous involvement may not be a major feature, and neurological symptoms may be the presenting feature. In all cases of vascular abnormalities of the CNS it is important to make careful enquiries about possible other cases in the lineage. In cases with known genetic origin or where two cases of vascular malformation exist in the family, a thorough examination of all family members is in order. The exact nosological situation of several of these syndromes is unclear.

SNEDDON AND DIVRY–VAN BOGAERT SYNDROMES
Sneddon syndrome consists of the association of generalized *livedo reticularis* (livedo racemosa) with cerebrovascular accidents due to diffuse abnormalities of the small and middle arteries. Two subtypes are recognized: one where antiphospholipid antibodies are present with other features of inflammation (Szmyrka-Kacza-marek 2005), and an idiopathic type (Mascarenhas et al. 2003) that may be familial (Pettee et al. 1994, Lossos et al. 1995) The disorder is a cause of cerebrovascular accidents, mostly in young adults, with a few cases reported in children (Baxter et al. 1993, Wheeler et al. 1998). In Sneddon syndrome, which shares many features with the Divry–Van Bogaert syndrome (Stone et al. 2001), there is noncalcifying leptomeningeal and cortical angiomatosis with secondary white matter sclerosis. The two conditions appear to be closely related (Ellie et al. 1994).

Several of these syndromes feature vascular anomalies of a phakomatous type such as angiomas, ectatic veins or lymphangiectasias, in association with macrocephaly and/or CNS abnormalities. The syndrome of *cutis marmorata telangiectatica* is clearly heterogeneous and may be accompanied by neurological symptoms (Picascia and Esterly 1989) and the association of recurrent hemiplegias mimicking alternating hemiplegia has been reported (Baxter et al. 1993). The syndrome of *macrocephly–cutis marmorata congenita* is probably different and includes dysmorphism and brain malformations (Lapunzina et al. 2004, Nyberg et al. 2005). Several syndromes associate neurological abnormalities with proliferation of subcutaneous tissues, and in some there is a tendency to the development of tumours. The distinction between rare syndromes such as Riley–Smith, Bannayan–Zonana and Ruvalcaba–Myhre syndromes is difficult and may be to some extent artificial (Dvir et al. 1988, Gorlin et al. 1992).

Wyburn–Mason syndrome (also known as Bonnet–Dechaume–Blanc syndrome) consists of a complex vascular malformation including a retinal arteriovenous angioma associated with a unilateral arteriovenous malformation extending along the optic nerve and the optic tract all the way to the cerebral peduncles and sometimes as far as the ipsilateral cerebellar hemisphere (Gomez 1994, Lester et al. 2005). A facial periorbital angioma is often present. Rupture or thrombosis of the malformation is not rare, with ominous consequences (Rizzo et al. 2004).

ATAXIA–TELANGIECTASIA AND RELATED DISORDERS

Although the pathological features and course of ataxia–telangiectasia (AT) are more closely related to the heredodegenerative disorders, in particular the spinocerebellar degenerations of which this disease represents the second most common type after Friedreich ataxia, AT is discussed in this chapter because, from a purely clinical point of view, its presentation and diagnosis are mainly those of a neurocutaneous syndrome in a majority of cases, even though it can also be regarded as a degenerative genetic condition.

AT is a heredofamilial disease of DNA instability, characterized by progressive cerebellar ataxia and choreoathetosis, progressive oculocutaneous telangiectasias, immunodeficiency with susceptibility to sinopulmonary infections, impaired organ maturation, hypersensitivity to ionizing radiations and a high incidence of malignancies. It is a multisystem genetic disorder with an autosomal recessive inheritance. The responsible gene has been mapped to chromosome 11q22–23 in families (Shiloh 1995). Savitsky et al. (1995) isolated the gene that codes for a protein (ATM protein) with similarities to mammalian phosphatidylinositol-3′ kinases, and mutations in this gene have been found in all four complementation groups indicating that there is only one locus responsible for the condition. The ATM protein is a nuclear protein that plays a crucial role in the stability and repair of double-stranded DNA and thus in the control of the stability of the cell cycle and in the protection of the genome. Numerous mutations are known, most being null mutations (Gilad et al. 1996). Less severe mutations are encountered, giving rise to less severe clinical cases (Gilad et al. 1998, Taylor and Byrd 2005).

MECHANISMS AND PATHOLOGY

The *abnormal double-strand DNA maintenance* has widespread consequences. The ATM protein, a protein kinase, is thought to be essential for control of the cell cycle, in particular at the checkpoints G1 and G2/M. It plays a major role in signalling defects of double-stranded DNA and in blocking cell cycle (Lavin et al. 2005). Its failure thus allows *induced activation of the cell cycle*, which may be deviated towards apoptosis. One important consequence is the abnormal sensitivity of AT cells to ionizing radiation and certain radiomimetic chemicals but not to ultraviolet irradiation (Barlow et al. 1999). The cell might then incorporate damage into its DNA that leads to chromosome and chromatid breaks. The AT cell resumes DNA synthesis with undue speed after insults because of *defective control of systems of cell damage repair* (Chun and Gatti 2004). Mutations in the gene are heterogeneous, and the resulting different degrees of protein kinase activity are correlated to clinical severity with later onset and milder forms. A high proportion (10%) of chromosomal breaks is almost constant. Chromosomal breakpoints are randomly distributed, but nonrandom chromosome rearrangements affect selectively chromosomes 7 and 14 at sites that are concerned with T-cell receptors and heavy-chain immunoglobulin coding and with the development of haematological malignancies (Hecht and Hecht 1985, Aurias and Dutrillaux 1986). These sites include bands 7p14, 7p35, 14q2 and 14qter. Chromosomes 2 and 22 (at bands 2p11, 2p12 and 22q11) are also frequently involved (Gatti et al. 1985). In about 10% of cases, a clone of cells with a 14–14 translocation with breakpoint at 14q32 develops that may be related to the emergence of malignancies.

Such disturbances could account for the frequency of infections and neoplasias, especially of the lymphoid tissues, but they may have a more general effect on the stability of the genome increasing sensitivity to malignancies even in the heterozygous state. The mechanisms responsible for neurological disease, thymus aplasia, telangiectasias, growth retardation and impaired organ maturation have not been elucidated. There is a general disturbance in tissue differentiation that accounts for the frequent elevation of alpha-fetoprotein (AFP), a fetal serum protein of hepatic origin that indicates dedifferentiation of liver cells.

Considerable work suggests that AT may be associated with dysregulation of the immunoglobulin gene superfamily, which includes genes for T-cell receptors (Peterson and Funkhouser 1989). The normal switch from the production of IgM to IgG, IgA and IgE is defective, and the same may apply to the switch from immature T-cells that express the gamma/delta rather than the alpha/beta receptors (Carbonari et al. 1990). Conceivably, absence or mutation of a single protein coded for by chromosome 11 could explain the immunological and perhaps even the neurological features of the disease (Kastan 1995).

The major neuropathological lesion in the CNS is degeneration of Purkinje and granule cells in the cerebellum (De Léon et al. 1976, Paula-Barbosa et al. 1983). Usually, no vascular abnormalities are found except late degenerative gliovascular nodules in the white matter. Lesions of the basal ganglia are found only occasionally (Boder 1985). Degeneration of spinal tracts and anterior horn cells is often present in late cases. Nucleocytomegaly is a feature of several cell types throughout the body, notably in peripheral nerves (De Léon et al. 1976).

CLINICAL FEATURES

NEUROLOGICAL FINDINGS

The main neurological manifestations of AT are cerebellar ataxia and abnormal eye movements, in the form of ocular motor apraxia, which is present in most cases, and choreoathetosis that occurs in 25% of patients (Boder 1985). The *ataxia* has its onset in infancy, becoming evident when the child begins to walk. From this early stage, ataxia is associated with abnormal head movements, and affected children have a peculiar gait like 'little clowns' that is highly suggestive. However, ocular motor apraxia often appears only after some years. The ataxia is relentlessly progressive but the pace is variable even in the same sibship. Dysarthria of cerebellar type is the rule; intention tremor and myoclonus may be observed. Various movement disorders are often present. *Choreoathetosis* may be so marked in some patients as to overshadow or mask the ataxia. A dystonic component is possible and may seldom be prominent. Oropharyngeal dystonia may lead to aspiration (Lefton-Greif et al. 2000), and the relatively immobile face with a peculiar slow-spreading smile, which is a suggestive symptom, may be due to extrapyramidal involvement. Late pyramidal signs may be present. Ocular motor signs are diagnostically important because they may precede the appearance of telangiectasias. Saccades are slowly initiated and hypometric, so that fixation of a target is obtained by head rather than eye deviation, often in association with a head thrust or forced blinking as in Cogan's ocular motor apraxia (Baloh et al. 1978), but is present in both horizontal and vertical gaze. Eye deviation, when obtained, is saccadic and often halts midway, and optokinetic nystagmus is absent. Peripheral system involvement is a late feature first manifested by absence or weakness of the tendon jerks. The peculiar appearance of AT children is often striking, with a characteristic gait and posture, a dull facies at rest, and abnormal head movements due to oculomotor defect. About 30% of patients have mild mental retardation.

TELANGIECTASIAS AND OTHER CUTANEOUS ABNORMALITIES

Telangiectasias are first noticed after 3 years of age, sometimes not until adolescence. They may be absent even later in some cases (Chung et al. 1994). Dilated conjunctival vessels, first noticed in the angles of both eyes, spread horizontally in the equatorial region of the conjunctivae toward the corneal limb. They may involve the ears, eyelids, and cubital and popliteal fossae. In late childhood and adolescence, progeric skin changes may appear, as well as pigmentary changes and café-au-lait spots. The skin often has an unusual appearance with evidence of premature ageing, café-au-lait spots (Ortonne et al. 1980), and warts or molluscum pendulum. Multiple skin cancers may develop especially in areas of previous X-irradiation.

SENSITIVITY TO INFECTIONS

Patients with AT are unusually sensitive to infections, mostly bacterial but to a lesser extent viral, in part as a result of immune globulin abnormalities (Nowak-Wegrzyn et al. 2004) and of deficiency of cellular immunity (Schubert et al. 2002) with decreased numbers of B cell and of T4 and T8 lymphocytes. Nowak-Wegrzyn et al. (2004) found in 100 AT patients that lymphopenia was present in 71%, and that immunnoglobulin levels were lowered by 65% for Ig4, 63% for IgA, 48% for Ig2, 23% for IgE, and only 18% for IgG. Rare patients may have no immunodeficiency as a result of specific mutations (Toyoshima et al. 1998). The most common infections are those of the upper respiratory tract.

Repeated sinopulmonary infections were present in 48–81% of patients reviewed by Chung et al. (1994), but in the study of Nowak-Wegrzyn et al. (2004) only 15% of patients had pneumonia. Infections of viral origin in the latter series included warts, molluscum and herpes simplex, but none were severe. In a study by Chun and Gatti (2004), severe infection with progressive lung disease was present in one third of children, one third had sinopulmonary infection but not progressive lung disease, and the remaining third had only a normal incidence of infections. There was a good correlation betwen the occurrence of infections and immunodeficiency as assessed by laboratory tests. Such a correlation was not found in other series (Roifman and Gelfand 1985).

Retardation of somatic growth is found in most patients, and many do not achieve normal puberty. In girls, this may be related to absence of ovary differentiation that is found in some cases.

COURSE AND PROGNOSIS

The neurological features of AT are relentlessly progressive (Chun and Gatti 2004). In addition to the classical early features, older patients tend to develop other signs of spinocerebellar degeneration such as posterior cord involvement with loss of deep tendon reflexes and spinal muscular atrophy (Boder 1985, Kwast and Ignatowicz 1990). Most patients are wheelchair dependent by 10–15 years of age, but mild forms are not rare and can be related to specific mutations of the *AT* gene (Taylor and Byrd 2005). Early death is frequently due to pulmonary disease but *malignancies* are now the most common cause. The incidence is 60–300 times higher than in non-affected persons, and 49% of cases coming to autopsy had malignant tumours (Swift et al. 1991). The most common tumours are T-cell and B-cell lymphoreticular malignancies, especially non-Hodgkin lymphomas, lymphocytic leukaemia and Hodgkin lymphomas (Boder 1985), but other kinds of tumours also occur. Lymphoreticular neoplasms and leukaemia predominate in patients under 15 years of age, while epithelial tumours predominate in older patients. Malignancies are also thought to be more common in obligate heterozygotes for the mutant *AT* gene than in the general population (Swift et al. 1991). The frequency of cancers, especially breast carcinomas, is reported to be three to six times greater than in the general population (Thompson et al. 2005), and this information has to be included in genetic counselling, although it remains a disputed issue (Gumy-Pause et al. 2004, Tamimi et al. 2004). In older patients, insulin-resistant diabetes develops in half the cases but is not responsible for ketosis.

DIAGNOSIS AND LABORATORY MARKERS
The clinical diagnosis of AT is easy when both cardinal features are present. Before the appearance of telangiectasias, the diagnosis of ataxic cerebral palsy is often made. However, ocular motor abnormalities and the 'little clown' gait are suggestive of AT.

Laboratory markers are important for both diagnosis and prognosis. The most constant markers are *elevated levels of AFP* and carcinoembryonic antigen, and chromosomal abnormalities, especially inversions and translocations involving chromosomes 7 and 14 (Hecht and Hecht 1985), which are regarded as pathognomonic for AT. Neither of these abnormalities is always found, however, and their demonstration may require specific techniques available in only some centres.

The demonstration of humoral or cellular immunological defects may also suggest an early diagnosis, although such defects are nonspecific and less frequently present (Roifman and Gelfand 1985). The dysgammaglobulinaemia of AT includes absence or low level of IgA including secretory IgA, normal or low level of IgG, and elevated or normal level of IgM. A deficit in Ig2 and Ig4 subclasses has been demonstrated in several patients, and IgE may also be absent or low (Oxelius et al. 1982, Schubert et al. 2002). Defects of cellular immunity include a low lymphocyte count, a poor response to skin tests for common antigens, low T-lymphocyte proliferation in the presence of mitogens, and deficient antibody production to viral or bacterial antigens. Excessive T-cell suppressor activity and intrinsic B-cell defects have been described in some patients, suggesting disturbances of immunoregulatory mechanisms.

Chromosomal abnormalities, especially the increased incidence of breaks on certain chromosomes, remain of considerable practical value. Survival of cell colonies after exposure of cell cultures to ionizing radiation is of definitive diagnostic value (Chun and Gatti 2004) but not a routine procedure. These tests are being supplanted by molecular diagnosis, which is also considered for the prenatal diagnosis although this is difficult and not always possible. Most mutations of the *AT* gene are truncating or splicing mutations; only about 10% are missense mutations. Other investigations are of less importance. CT and MRI often show evidence of nonspecific cerebellar atrophy. Nerve conduction velocities may be slowed, and denervation of anterior horn cell type may be found in older patients (Dunn 1973).

ATYPICAL AND VARIANT FORMS OF
ATAXIA–TELANGIECTASIA
Patients with atypical forms of AT have recently attracted interest. Some cases are undoubtedly part of the spectrum of the disease,

with a slow course and prolonged survival and incomplete expression, e.g. absence of ocular motor signs (Trimis et al. 2004). Others include markedly abnormal features such as mental retardation and spasticity (Meshram et al. 1986), peripheral neuropathy as a predominant sign (Terenty et al. 1978), and absence of telangiectasia persisting into adulthood (Byrne et al. 1984). Some of these patients lack one or the other of the laboratory markers. They confirm the genetic heterogeneity of the disease, which has been demonstrated by molecular studies (Taylor and Byrd 2005).

MANAGEMENT
Although no specific treatment is available, several features of AT are accessible to active therapy. This applies especially to infections, and the life span of AT patients has been clearly prolonged by antibiotic treatment. Prevention of infections by regular injection of immunoglobulins is considered useful. Fetal thymus implants and stimulants of the immunological system have given inconclusive results.

Treatment of neurological manifestations is disappointing. Propanolol and sulpiride may improve fine motor coordination in a few cases. Rehabilitation and adequate educative support are always necessary. *The use of radiotherapy and chemotherapy in conventional doses is contraindicated in AT patients.* Reduced doses of X-rays or chemicals, avoiding bleomycin, actinomycin D and cyclophosphamide, have given favourable results in a few cases.

Regular surveillance of patients for the emergence of cancers and leukaemia should be strict. This also applies to heterozygotes and should probably be part of the family management.

DISORDERS RELATED TO
ATAXIA–TELANGIECTASIA
ATAXIA–TELANGIECTASIA-LIKE DISEASE (ATLD)
Some cases presenting with features that mimic AT are not associated with mutations in the *AT* gene. In such cases the disorder seems to be less severe. Increased sensitivity to ionizing radiation is present, as are chromosome breakages (Taylor et al. 2004). However, malignancies have not been reported (Delia et al. 2004). The gene responsible is *MRE11*, whose mutation seems to be responsible for absent activation of the *AT* gene, in conjunction with other genes such as *Nb1* (Fernet et al. 2005).

ATAXIA–OCULOMOTOR APRAXIA (AOA)
Although this disorder does not feature cutaneous abnormalities, it is mentioned in this chapter because of its striking resemblance to AT. Two distinct entities are recognized: AOA1 and AOA2 (see also Chapter 9).

AOA1 appears to occur predominanly in children, in contrast with AOA2, which is more frequent in adults (Le Ber et al. 2004). It is an autosomal recessive ataxia associated with ocular motor apraxia, hypoalbuminaemia and hypercholesterolaemia, with onset in childood and even in infancy (Ito et al. 2005). Chorea and peripheral neuropathy are frequent manifestations. AFP levels are normal (Aicardi et al. 1988, Gascon et al. 1995, Le Ber et al. 2003). The responsible gene, *APTX*, encodes the protein aprataxin, mapping to chromosome 9q13. It is probably important in single-strand DNA break repair. No telangiectasias are seen; there is no increased frequency of malignancies and no chromosome breakages are noted. The course is slowly progressive and may become static. MRI demonstrates marked cerebellar atrophy (Barbot et al. 2001, Shimazaki et al. 2002, Le Ber et al. 2003). The phenotype is variable, some cases having no oculomotor apraxia or presenting with a neuropathy.

In AOA2, the clinical features are similar, with a later onset in early teenage years. AFP is moderately elevated in three quarters of the cases (Le Ber et al. 2004). Oculomotor apraxia in inconstant (Le Ber et al. 2004, Duquette et al. 2005). The responsible gene (*SETX*) maps to chromosome 9q34 and codes for the protein senataxin whose role is not known.

The *Nijmegen breakage syndrome* (Seemanova et al. 1985) manifested by microcephaly, immunodeficiency and mental retardation, tends to be considered as a variant of AT, with a similar tendency to develop lymphoreticular malignancies, probably because they share defects of the DNA repair systems.

Other rare conditions that share some features with AT include the *dysequilibrium–diplegia syndrome* (Hagberg et al. 1970, Graham-Pole et al. 1975) in which immunodeficiency is a major feature. This syndrome is associated with purine nucleotide phosphorylase deficiency (Soutar and Day 1991). Patients with this disorder have normal immunoglobulins and pyramidal tract signs, and in one case heterotopia and cortical dysplasia were present (Soutar and Day 1991). Other syndromes with neurological features, especially microcephaly, in association with chromosomal instability may have some relationship to AT, especially the tendency to develop lymphoreticular malignancies.

NEUROCUTANEOUS SYNDROMES OF ABNORMAL PIGMENTATION

INCONTINENTIA PIGMENTI (BLOCH–SULZBERGER TYPE)

Bloch–Sulzberger syndrome is a rare genetic disorder, observed almost exclusively in girls, probably transmitted as an X-linked dominant trait prenatally lethal in males. The responsible gene, *NEMO*, a modulator of the activation of the NF-kappa B pathway (Fusco et al. 2004, Su et al. 2004), maps to Xq28.

SKIN FEATURES
The skin lesions are striking. They consist of three distinct but somewhat overlapping stages (Rosman 1992, Mangano and Barbagallo 1993). In the first stage, erythematous, papular, vesicular or bullous lesions are present at birth or during the first two weeks of life on the trunk and limbs. They are linear in distribution and last from days to months. In the second stage, between the second and the sixth weeks, the lesions are variably pustular, verrucous or keratotic. They may disappear without sequelae or are followed by the development of pigmentation, characteristic of the third stage of the disease. These pigmented lesions may be located outside the area of earlier lesions, and in 10% of cases are not preceded by them. The pigmentation persists into adulthood but tends to fade with the passing of time. Histologically

there is absent or decreased melanin in the basal epidermal cells with an accompanying excess in the dermis, thus suggesting a 'leakage' or 'incontinence' of the basal cells. In 50–80% of cases, noncutaneous abnormalities are present.

CNS INVOLVEMENT
CNS involvement occurs in one third to one half of the cases, although unbiased frequency in familial cases may not exceed 10% (Landy and Donnai 1993, Hadj-Rabia et al. 2003). Seizures may occur early (Pörksen et al. 2004) and be generalized, or focal often with secondary generalization. Infantile spasms have been reported. Destructive encephalopathies of apparently perinatal onset may occur in recurrent episodes suggestive of 'encephalomyelitis' (Brunquell 1987), with obtundation, hemiparesis and areas of low absorption in the brain white matter on CT, with subsequent atrophy (Avrahami et al. 1985). These are the most frequent neurological manifestations and appear to be the result of an arteritis that may be extensive and can be detected by angiography (Fiorillo et al. 2003, Hennel et al. 2003). Siemes et al. (1978), Shuper et al. (1990) and Hennel et al. (2003) found inflammatory lesions in all their cases. Other pathological lesions are possible. One patient had involvement of the anterior horn cells of the spinal cord (Larsen et al. 1987); in another case a migrational disorder was found (O'Doherty and Norman 1968). Prenatal molecular diagnosis has been made (Steffan et al. 2004).

EYE LESIONS
Various eye lesions are present in one third of cases, the most characteristic of which is a retrolental mass with detachment of a dysplastic retina (Rosenfeld and Smith 1983). This should be looked for systematically in affected infants, as early detection and therapy of the retinitis may protect vision (Wong et al. 2004). Dental abnormalities (peg-shaped teeth) occur in 70% of patients. Treatment is symptomatic and includes ophthalmological interventions, antiepileptic agents, physiotherapy and corticosteroids. Orthopaedic measures as well as educational support are vital. Genetic counselling is an important part of management. The outcome is not necessarily bad and a normal long-term outcome may be observed in some patients (Steffan et al. 2004).

Bloch–Sulzberger syndrome is probably different from the Naegeli type of incontinentia pigmenti rather than a subtype of the same disease (Rosman 1992). The latter occurs in boys and girls.

HYPOMELANOSIS OF ITO (INCONTINETIA PIGMENTI ACHROMIANS)

Another condition that should be distinguished from Bloch–Sulzberger disease is hypomelanosis of Ito or incontinentia pigmenti achromians. This disorder is characterized by hypopigmented areas with a peculiar streaked or whorled appearance, often unilateral or with a strong unilateral predominance along the Blaschko lines (Pascual-Castroviejo et al. 1988, Gordon 1994) (Fig. 3.12). The appearance is variable with the possibility of pigmented rather than achromic lesions and more commonly of an association of both. Associated abnormalities are described in

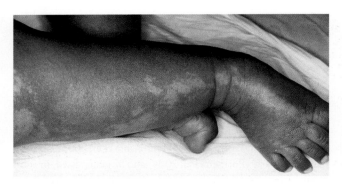

Fig. 3.12. Hypomelanosis of Ito. Note linear distribution of hypopigmented areas along axis of limb. (Courtesy Dr D Teillac, Prof. Y de Prost, Hôpital des Enfants Malades, Paris.)

33–94% of cases. CNS involvement is most common, thus justifying the term neurocutaneous syndrome (Steiner et al. 1996, Ruggieri and Pavone 2000). Only about one in four have average or above average IQ, and more than 50% have some degree of learning disability (IQ<70). Seizures are common (about half the group), and infantile spasms occur in about one in 10 individuals with typical skin changes. Macrocephalus is present in about one in seven cases. Ito disease is one of the causes of hemimegalencephaly (Pascual-Castroviejo et al. 1988, Auriemma et al. 2000). Glover et al. (1989) found psychomotor delay in 14 of their 19 patients, 9 had seizures, and 2 had severe sensorineural deafness. Recently, many cases of hypomelanosis of Ito associated with psychiatric disorder including symptoms compatible with the diagnoses of psychosis, autism, atypical autism and Asperger syndrome have been described (Åkefeldt and Gillberg 1991; Zappella 1993; Davalos et al. 2001; Pascual-Castroviejo et al. 1998, 2006). Most series have found a slightly higher rate of the condition in females.

Autism spectrum manifestations are known to occur (Åkefeldt and Gillberg 1996) in up to 10% of cases (Pascual-Castroviejo et al. 1988). Eye abnormalities (Rosenfeld and Smith 1983) include microphthalmia and related structural abnormalities, and were present in three of the patients of Glover et al. (1989). Hemihypertrophy and scoliosis are commonly present. There is also a wide spectrum of EEG abnormalities from normal records to multifocal paroxystic features. Fast rhythm may be associated with areas of pachygyria (Ogino et al. 1994). Seizures may be of several types including infantile spasms. CT may show bilateral or unilateral hemispheric atrophy or areas of low attenuation in white matter or cerebellar atrophy (Pini and Faulkner 1995). MRI has shown the presence of neuronal heterotopia (Glover et al. 1989, Malherbe et al. 1993), and Steiner et al. (1996) reported a wide specrum of major and minor imaging abnormalities. White matter signal abnormalities may be present, which is in agreement with the pathological findings of Fujino et al. (1995).

Most confirmed cases of Ito's disease are sporadic, although dominant transmission has been suggested but not demonstrated. Girls are much more commonly affected than boys. Mosaicism for miscellaneous chromosome aberrations appears to be a common but not a constant cause of the disease (Taibjee et al.

2004, Lambillo and Sybert 2005). Chromosome analysis should ideally be performed on keratinocyte cultures whereas lymphocyte and fibroblast cultures are usually negative. Prenatal diagnosis has been made (Steinberg Warren et al. 2001).

There is no treatment for the skin disorder, but cover-up make-up can be used if desired. Neurological, hearing and visual problems should be treated as indicated for those particular problems.

NEUROCUTANEOUS MELANOSIS
This rare nongenetic disorder is characterized by cutaneous pigmented naevi and variable involvement of the meninges and CNS (Makkar and Frieden 2004) (Fig. 3.13). The naevi are of the giant type, often in 'bathsuit topography' that covers the lower part of the trunk, the pelvis and the upper part of the lower limbs in two thirds of cases and multiple small lesions in one third. However, I have seen a child with biopsy-proven meningeal melanosis who had a single naevus of 5×5 cm on one arm, and a lesion of similar size was encountered by de Andrade et al. (2004). The naevi are heavily pigmented and hairy. More than half the patients with congenital hairy naevi develop early CNS involvement, in the form of progressive hydrocephalus, probably as a result of proliferation of meningeal melanocytes with consequent blockage of CSF reabsorption or circulation or of meningeal or CNS malignant tumours (Di Rocco et al. 2004). There is often cystic dilatation of the cisterna magna (Barkovich et al. 1994). Seizures are common, and variable neurological deficits may result from parenchymal tumoural proliferation of melanocytes (Rhodes et al. 1991), particularly at the base of the brain and brainstem.

The prognosis is poor in symptomatic cases, but hydrocephalus should be treated with a shunt (Di Rocco et al. 2004). An occasional patient survives many years but malignant degeneration of CNS lesions is extremely common.

OTHER NEUROCUTANEOUS SYNDROMES WITH ABNORMAL PIGMENTATION
Albinism refers to a group of inherited disorders in which there is a reduction or absence of melanin formation. Many types of albinism are known, and the main features of the condition are cutaneous and ocular rather than neurological. One remarkable finding is misrouting of the optic fibres, with an abnormally high proportion of crossed fibres and projection of only the most peripheral part of the temporal retina to the ipsilateral hemisphere, which may be demonstrated by study of the visual evoked potentials (Collewijn et al. 1985) and by appropriate MRI techniques (Hedera et al. 1994). Albino children also have a special pattern of cognitive function with a much higher score on verbal than on performance items (Cole et al. 1987).

Several rare syndromes of deficient pigmentation variably feature immunodeficiency (macrophagic activation syndrome) and/or neurological signs. *Chediak–Higashi syndrome* associates a peripheral neuropathy with immune and haematological abnormalities. Severe neurological problems affecting the CNS with seizures, mental retardation and motor deficits are prominent

pathology, and Immunology of a Degenerative Disease of Childhood. New York: Alan R Liss, pp. 273–85.

Rosenbaum T, Engelbrecht V, Krölls W, et al. (1999) MRI abnormalities in neurofibromatosis type 1 (NF1): a study of mice and men. *Brain Dev* 21: 268–73.

Rosenfeld SI, Smith ME (1983) Ocular findings in incontinentia pigmenti. *Ophthalmology* 90: 459–66.

Rosman NP (1992) Incontinentia pigmenti: presentations, pathology, pathogenesis and prognosis. In: Fukuyama Y, Suzuki Y, Kamoshita S, Casaer P, eds. *Fetal and Perinatal Neurology.* Basel: Karger, pp. 174–86.

Rosser TL, Vezina G, Packer RJ (2005) Cerebrovascular abnormalities in a population of children with neurofibromatosis 1. *Neurology* 64: 553–5.

Rossi A, Bava GL, Biancheri R, Tortori-Donati P (2001) Posterior fossa and arterial abnormalities in patients with facial capillary haemangioma: presumed incomplete phenotypic expression of PHACES syndrome. *Neuroradiology* 43: 934–40.

Roth RR, Martines R, James WD (1987) Segmental neurofibromatosis. *Arch Dermatol* 123: 917–20.

Rouleau GA, Merel P, Lutchman M, et al. (1993) Alteration in a new gene encoding a putative membrane-organizing protein causes neuro-fibromatosis type 2. *Nature* 363: 515–21.

Rubinstein LJ (1986) The malformative central nervous system lesions in the central and the peripheral forms of neurofibromatosis. *Ann NY Acad Sci* 486: 14–29.

Ruggieri M, Pavone L (2000) Hypomelanosis of Ito: clinical syndrome or just phenotype? *J Child Neurol* 15: 635–44.

Ruggieri M, Pavone P, Polizzi A, et al. (2004) Ophthalmological manifestations of segmental neurofibromatosis 1. *Br J Ophthalmol* 88: 1429–33.

Ruggieri M, Ianetti P, Polizzi A, et al. (2005) Earliest clinical manifestations and natural history of neurofibromatosis type 2 (NF2) in childhood : a study of 24 patients. *Neuropediatrics* 36: 21–3.

Russell DS, Rubinstein LJ (1977) *Pathology of Tumors of the Nervous System, 4th edn.* Baltimore: Williams & Wilkins.

Ruttledge MH, Narod SA, Dumanski JP, et al. (1993) Presymptomatic diagnosis for neurofibromatosis 2 with chromosome 22 markers. *Neurology* 43: 1753–60.

Sancak O, Nellist M, Goedbloed M, et al. (2005) Mutational analysis of the TSC1 and TSC2 genes in a diagnostic setting: genotype–phenotype correlations and comparisons of diagnostic DNA techniques in tuberous sclerosis complex. *Eur J Hum Genet* 13: 731–41.

Sarkozy A, Conti E, Digilio MC, et al. (2004) Clinical and molecular analysis of 30 patients with multiple lentigines LEOPARD syndrome. *J Med Genet* 41: e68.

Sevick RJ, Barkovich AJ, Edwards MS, et al. (1992) Evolution of white matter lesions in neurofibromatosis type 1: MR findings. *Am J Roentgenol* 159: 171–5.

Savitsky K, Bar-Shira A, Gilad S, et al. (1995) A single ataxia–telangiectasia gene with a product similar to P1-3 kinase. *Science* 268: 1749–53.

Scalais E, Verloes A, Sacre JP, et al. (1992) Sjögren–Larsson-like syndrome with bone dysplasia and normal fatty alcohol NAD+ oxidoreductase activity. *Pediatr Neurol* 8: 459–65.

Scheinfeld NS (2003) Syndromic albinism: a review of genetics and phenotypes. *Dermatol Online J* 9: 5.

Schmandt SM, Packer RJ, Vezina LG, Jane J (2000) Spontaneous regression of low-grade astrocytomas in childhood. *Pediatr Neurosurg* 32: 132–6.

Schievink WI, Michels VV, Mokri B, et al. (1995) A familial syndrome of arterial dissections with lentiginosis. *N Engl J Med* 332: 576–9.

Schropp C, Sörensen N, Krauss J (2006) Early periinsular hemispherotomy in children with Sturge–Weber syndrome and intractable epilepsy—outcome in eight patients. *Neuropediatrics* 37: 26–31.

Schubert R, Reichenbach J, Rose M, Zielen S (2002) Immunogenicity of the seven-valent pneumococcal conjugated vaccine in patients with ataxia–telangiectasia. *Pediatr Infect Dis* 23: 269–70.

Seemanova E, Passarge E, Beneskova D, et al. (1985) Familial microcephaly with normal intelligence, immunodeficiency, and risk for lymphoreticular malignancies. *Am J Med Genet* 20: 639–48.

Seiff SR, Brodsky MC, MacDonald G, et al. (1987) Orbital optic glioma in neurofibromatosis. Magnetic resonance diagnosis of perineural arachnoidal gliomatosis. *Arch Ophthalmol* 105: 1689–92.

Shanley S, Ratcliffe J, Hockey A, et al. (1994) Nevoid basal cell carcinoma syndrome: review of 118 affected individuals. *Am J Med Genet* 50: 282–90.

Shapiro U, Shulman K (1976) Facial nevi associated with anomalous venous return and hydrocephalus. *J Neurosurg* 45: 20–5.

Sharma MC, Ralte AM, Gackwad S, et al. (2004) Subependymal giant cell astrocytoma—a clinicopathological study of 23 cases with special emphasis on histogenesis. *Pathol Oncol Res* 10: 219–24.

Shepherd CW, Houser OW, Gomez MR (1995) MR findings in tuberous sclerosis complex and correlation with seizure development and mental impairment. *AJNR* 16: 149–55.

Shiloh Y (1995) Ataxia–telangiectasia: closer to unraveling the mystery. *Eur J Hum Genet* 3: 116–38.

Shimazaki H, Takiyama Y, Sakoe K, et al. (2002) Early-onset ataxia with ocular motor apraxia and hypoalbuminemia: the aprataxin gene mutations. *Neurology* 59: 590–5.

Shin RK, Moonis G, Imbese SG (2002) Transient focal leptomeningeal enhancement in Sturge–Weber syndrome. *J Neuroimaging* 12: 270–2.

Shuper A, Bryan RN, Singer HS (1990) Destructive encephalopathy in incontinentia pigmenti: a primary disorder? *Pediatr Neurol* 6: 137–40.

Siebert M, Markowitsch HJ, Bartel P (2003) Amygdala, affect and cognition: evidence from 10 patients with Urbach–Wiethe disease. *Brain* 126: 2627–37.

Siemes H, Schneider H, Dening D, Hanefeld F (1978) Encephalitis in two members of a family with incontinentia pigmenti (Bloch–Schulzberger syndrome). *Eur J Pediatr* 129: 103–15.

Simonati A, Colamaria V, Bricolo A, et al. (1994) Microgyria associated with Sturge–Weber angiomatosis. *Childs Nerv Syst* 10: 392–5.

Skoglund RR, Paa D, Lewis WJ (1978) Elevated spinal-fluid protein in Sturge–Weber syndrome. *Dev Med Child Neurol* 20: 99–102.

Soutar RL, Day RE (1991) Dysequilibrium/ataxic diplegia with immunodeficiency. *Arch Dis Child* 66: 982–3.

Sperner J, Schmauser I, Bittner R, et al. (1990) MR-imaging findings in children with Sturge–Weber syndrome. *Neuropediatrics* 21: 146–52.

Steffan J, Raclin V, Smahi A, et al. (2004) A novel PCR approach for prenatal detection of common NEMO rearrangement in incontinentia pigmenti. *Prenat Diagn* 24: 384–8.

Steinberg Warren N, Soukup S, King JL, St J Dignan P (2001) Prenatal diagnosis of trisomy 20 by chorionic villus sampling (CVS): a case report with long-term outcome. *Prenat Diagn* 21: 1111–1113.

Steiner J, Adamsbaum C, Desguerre I, et al. (1996) Hypomelanosis of Ito and brain abnormalities: MRI findings and literature review. *Pediatr Radiol* 26: 763–8.

Stewart RM, Tunell G, Ehle A (1981) Familial spastic paraplegia, peroneal neuropathy and crural hypopigmentation: a new neurocutaneous syndrome. *Neurology* 31: 754–7.

Stone J, Bhattacharya J, Wals TJ (2001) Divry–Van Bogaert syndrome in a female: relationship to Sneddon's syndrome and radiographic appearances. *Neuroradiology* 43: 562–4.

Strenge H, Cordes P, Sticherling M, Brossmann J (1996) Hemifacial atrophy: a neurocutaneous disorder with coup de sabre deformity, telangiectatic naevus, aneurysmatic malformation of the internal carotid artery and crossed hemiatrophy. *J Neurol* 243: 658–60.

Striano S, Ruosi P, Guzzetta V, et al. (1996) Cutis verticis gyrata–mental deficiency syndrome: a patient with drug-resistant epilepsy and polyneurogyria. *Epilepsia* 37: 284–6.

Su PH, Chen JY, Yu JS, et al. (2004) De novo incontinentia pigmenti in female twins. *Acta Paediatr Taiwan* 45: 178–80.

Sujansky E, Conradi S (1995a) Outcome of Sturge–Weber syndrome in 52 adults. *Am J Med Genet* 57: 35–45.

Sujansky E, Conradi S (1995b) Sturge–Weber syndrome: age of onset of seizures and glaucoma and the prognosis for affected children. *J Child Neurol* 10: 49–58.

Sunohara N, Sakuragawa N, Satoyoshi E, et al. (1986) A new syndrome of anosmia, ichthyosis, hypogonadism and various neurological manifestations with deficiency of steroid sulfatase and arylsulfatase C. *Ann Neurol* 19: 174–81.

Swift M, Morrell D, Massey RB, Chase CL (1991) Incidence of cancer in 161 families affected by ataxia–telangiectasia. *N Engl J Med* 325: 1831–6.

Szmyrka-Kaczmarek M, Daikeler T, Benz D, Koetter I (2005) Familial inflammatory Sneddon syndrome: case report and review of the literature. *Clin Rhumatol* 24: 79–82.

Taddeucci G, Boncelli A, Pollaco P (2005) Migraine-like attacks in a child with Sturge–Weber syndrome without facial nevus. *Pediatr Neurol* 32: 131–3.

Taibjee SM, Bennett DC, Moss CJ (2004) Abnormal pigmentation in hypomelanosis of Ito and pigmentary mosaicism: the role of pigmentary genes. *Br J Dermatol* 151: 269–82.

Tallman B, Tan OT, Morelli JG, et al. (1991) Location of port-wine stains and the likelihood of ophthalmic and/or central nervous system complications. *Pediatrics* **87**: 323–7.

Tamimi RM, Hankinson SE, Spiegelman D, et al. (2004) Common ataxia–telangiectasia mutation haplotypes and risk of breast cancer. *Breast Cancer Res* **6**: R416–22.

Tassabehji M, Strachan T, Sharland M, et al. (1993) Tandem duplication within a neurofibromatosis type 1 (NF1) gene exon in a family with features of Watson and Noonan syndromes. *Am J Hum Genet* **53**: 90–5.

Taylor AM, Byrd PJ (2005) Molecular pathology of ataxia–telangiectasia. *J Clin Pathol* **58**: 1009–15.

Taylor AM, Groom A, Byrd PJ (2004) Ataxia–telangiectasia-like disorder (ATLD) – its clinical presentation and molecular basis. *DNA Repair* **3**: 1219–25.

Taylor HM, Robinson R, Cox T (1997) Progressive facial hemiatrophy: MRI appearances. *Dev Med Child Neurol* **39**: 484–6.

Terdjman P, Aicardi J, Sainte-Rose C, Brunelle F (1990) Neuroradiological findings in Sturge–Weber syndrome (SWS) and isolated pial angiomatosis. *Neuropediatrics* **22**: 115–20.

Terenty TR, Robson P, Walton JN (1978) Presumed ataxia–telangiectasia in a man. *BMJ* **2**: 802.

Terstegge K, Kunath B, Felber S, et al. (1994) MR of brain involvement in progressive facial hemiatrophy (Romberg disease): reconsideration of a syndrome. *AJNR* **15**: 145–50.

Thiffault A, Swartz CE, Der Kaloustian V, Foulkes WD (2004) Mutation analysis of the tumor suppressor gene PTEN and the glypican 3 (CPG3 gene) in patients diagnosed with Proteus syndrome. *Am J Med Genet* **130**: 123–7.

Thomas-Sohl KA, Vaslow DF, Maria BL (2004) Sturge–Weber syndrome: a review. *Pediatr Neurol* **30**: 303–10.

Thompson D, Duedal S, Kirner J, et al. (2005) Cancer risks and mortality in heterozygous ATM mutation carriers. *J Natl Cancer Inst* **97**: 813–22.

Toelle SP, Valsangiacomo E, Boltshauser E (2001) Trichothiodystrophy with severe cardiac and neurological involvement in two sisters. *Eur J Pediatr* **160**: 728–31.

Tolmie JL, de Berker D, Dawber R, et al. (1994) Syndromes associated with trichothiodystrophy. *Clin Dysmorphol* **3**: 1–14.

Tomsik TA, Lukin RR, Chambers AA, Benton C (1976) Neurofibromatosis and intracranial arterial disease. *Neuroradiology* **11**: 229–34.

Toti P, Balestri P, Cano M, et al. (1996) Celiac disease with cerebral calcium and silica deposits: X-ray spectroscopic findings, an autopsy study. *Neurology* **46**: 1088–92.

Toyoshima M, Hara T, Zhang H, et al. (1998) Ataxia–telangiectasia without immunodeficiency: novel point mutation within and adjacent to the phophatidylinositol 3-kinase-like domain. *Am J Med Genet* **75**: 141–4.

Trimis GG, Athenassaki CK, Kanario MM, et al. (2002) Unusual absence of neurological symptoms in a six-year old girl with ataxia–telangiectasia. *J Postgrad Med* **50**: 270–1.

Turner JT, Cohen MML, Biesecker IG (2004) Reassessment of the Proteus syndrome literature: application of diagnostic criteria to published cases. *Am J Med Genet* **130**: 111–27.

Tuxhorn I, Panneck HW (2002) Epilepsy surgery in bilateral Sturge–Weber syndrome. *Pediar Neurol* **26**: 394–7.

Valentini L, Solero CL, Lasio G, et al. (1995) Triventricular hydrocephalus: review of 71 cases evaluated at the Istituto Neurologico "C. Besta" Milan over the last 10 years. *Childs Nerv Syst* **11**: 170–2.

van de Warrenburg BP, van Gulik S, Renier WO, et al. (1998) The linear naevus sebaceus syndrome. *Clin Neurol Neurosurg* **100**: 126–32.

Van Hale P (1988) Chediak–Higashi syndrome. In: Gomez MR, ed. *Neurocutaneous Diseases: a Practical Approach.* London: Butterworths, pp. 209–13.

Van Hougenhouk-Tulleken W, Chan I, Hamada T, et al. (2004) Clinical and molecular characterization of lipoid proteinosis in Nmaqualand, South Africa. *Br J Dermatol* **151**: 413–23.

Vassilopoulou-Sellin R, Klein MJ, Slopis JK (2000) Growth hormone deficiency in children with neurofibromatosis type 1 without suprasellar lesions. *Pediatr Neurol* **22**: 355–8.

Vigevano F, Aicardi J, Lini M, Pasquinelli A (1984) [The linear naevus sebaceous syndrome: presentation of a multicentric case study.] *Boll Liga Ital Epilessia* **45/46**: 59–63 (Italian).

Ville D, Enjolras O, Chiron C, Dulac O (2002) Prophylactic antiepileptic treatment in Sturge–Weber disease. *Seizure* **11**: 141–50.

Vogl TJ, Stemmler J, Bergman C, et al. (1993) MR and MR angiography of Sturge–Weber syndrome. *AJNR* **14**: 417–25.

Vougioukas VI, Glasker S, Hubbe U, et al. (2006) Surgical treatment of hemangioblastomas of the central nervous system in pediatric patients. *Childs Nerv Syst* **22**: 1149–53.

Vrtel R, Verhoef S, Bouman K, et al. (1996) Identification of a nonsense mutation at the 5′ end of the TSC2 gene in a family with a presumptive diagnosis of tuberous sclerosis complex. *J Med Genet* **33**: 47–51.

Wang PY, Kaufmann WE, Koth CW, et al. (2000) Thalamic involvement in neurofibromatosis type 1: evaluation with proton magnetic resonance spectroscopic imaging. *Ann Neurol* **47**: 477–84.

Webb DW, Osborne JP (1995) Tuberous sclerosis. *Arch Dis Child* **72**: 471–4.

Webb DW, Fryer AE, Osborne JP (1991) On the incidence of fits and mental retardation in tuberous sclerosis. *J Med Genet* **28**: 395–7.

Weon YC, Yoshida Y, Sachet M, et al (2005) Supratentorial cerebral arteriovenous fistulas (AVFs) in children: review of 41 cases with 63 non choroidal single-hole AVFs. *Acta Neurochir* **147**: 17–31.

Wheeler PG, Medina S, Dusick A, et al. (1998) Livedo reticularis, developmental delay and stroke-like episodes in a 7-year-old male. *Clin Dysmorphol* **7**: 69–74.

Widdess-Walsh P, Friedman NR (2003) Left-sided facial nevus with contralateral leptomeningeal angiomatosis in a child with Sturge–Weber syndrome: case report. *J Child Neurol* **18**: 304–5.

Willemsen MA, Ijlst L, Steijlan L, et al. (2001) Clinical, biochemical and molecular genetic characteristics of 19 patients with the Sjögren–Larsson syndrome. *Brain* **124**: 1426–37.

Willemsen MA, Van der Graaf M, Van der Knaap MS, et al. (2004) MR imaging and proton MR spectroscopic studies in Sjögren–Larsson syndrome: characterization of the leukoencephalopathy. *AJNR* **25**: 649–57.

Williams DM, Elster AD (1992) Cranial CT and MR in the Klippel–Trenaunay–Weber syndrome. *AJNR* **13**: 291–4.

Williams ML, Koch TK, O'Donnell JJ, et al. (1985) Ichthyosis and neutral lipid storage disease. *Am J Med Genet* **20**: 711–26.

Wilms G, Van Wijck E, Demaerel P, et al. (1992) Gyriform calcifications in tuberous sclerosis simulating the appearance of Sturge–Weber disease. *AJNR* **13**: 295–7.

Wilson WB (1998) The North American Study Group for Optic Glioma. *Neurofibromatosis* **1**: 199–200.

Wiznitzer M (2004) Autism in tuberous sclerosis. *J Child Neurol* **19**: 680–6.

Wong GA, Willoughby CE, Parslew R, Kaye SB (2004) The importance of screening for sight-threatening retinopathy in incontinentia pigmenti. *Pediatr Dermatol* **21**: 242–5.

Yamamoto N, Watanabe K, Negoro T, et al. (1987) Long-term prognosis of tuberous sclerosis with epilepsy in children. *Brain Dev* **9**: 292–5.

Yamanouchi H, Ho M, Jay V, Becker LE (1997) Giant cells in cortical tubers in tuberous sclerosis showing synaptophysin-immunoreactive halos. *Brain Dev* **19**: 21–4.

Yoon HK, Sargent MA, Prendiville JS, Poskitt KJ (2005) Cerebellar and cerebral atrophy in trichothiodystrophy. *Pediatr Radiol* **35**: 1019–23.

Zappella M (1993) Autism and hypomelanosis of Ito in twins. *Dev Med Child Neurol* **35**: 826–32.

Zhou XP, Marsh DJ, Hampel H, et al. (2000) Germline and germline mosaic PTEN mutations associated with a Proteus-like syndrome of hemihypertrophy, lower limb asymmetry, arteriovenous malformations and lipomatosis. *Hum Mol Genet* **22**: 765–68.

4

NEUROLOGICAL AND BEHAVIOURAL ASPECTS OF GENETIC ANOMALIES AND DYSMORPHIC SYNDROMES INCLUDING SOME 'BEHAVIOURAL PHENOTYPE SYNDROMES'

Christopher Gillberg, Jean Aicardi and Martin Bax

Neurological abnormalities, in particular impaired intellectual function, and behavioural problems are extremely common in patients with chromosomal anomalies. The frequency of chromosomal abnormalities, usually with major brain malformations, is greatly increased in aborted fetuses and stillborn infants. In one study (Gostason et al. 1991), chromosomal anomalies were found in 19.2% of individuals with mild mental retardation as opposed to 1.9% of controls. These figures are certainly underestimates, as more subtle chromosomal abnormalities such as small deletions or translocations may be detected only with modern more sophisticated techniques. Chromosomal abnormalities and mental retardation are not always related. Abnormalities of sex chromosomes and minor anomalies of autosomal chromosomes are often compatible with a normal intelligence, although that is not to say that such anomalies do not cause some degree of intellectual impairment and proclivity to developing behavioural problems.

In recent years it has become apparent that the classical chromosomal 'aberrations' are only the tip of the iceberg, and neurological/behavioural symptoms and signs are due to absent or faulty critical genes, detectable in the form of chromosomal deletions, insertions, duplications or other rearrangements. As a result, the traditional distinction between chromosomal and other syndromes (as used in the previous edition of this book) is now obsolete.

Over the past two decades it has become widely recognized that a number of disorders, usually of genetic origin, have a more or less distinctive behavioural phenotype. Several hundred syndromes associated with chromosomal abnormalities/specific gene disorders (ranging from single gene deletions/multiplications and uniparental disomies to multiply affected genes on a particular segment of a chromosome) have been reported, and their

description can be found in specialized texts (De Grouchy and Turleau 1984, Schinzel 1984, Jones 1988, O'Brien and Yule 1996). In some of these, such as Angelman syndrome, fragile X syndrome, Prader–Willi syndrome and Williams syndrome, the behaviours in themselves are often so characteristic as to arouse suspicion that the child might be suffering from a specific chromosomal/genetic abnormality. Oftentimes, the behaviours are more 'pathognomonic' than any of the physical symptoms or stigmata. A large number of dysmorphic syndromes in which, to date, underlying genetic or brain injury problems have not been identified, are also known, many of which feature mental retardation and/or neurological/behavioural symptoms or signs. Only some of the most common and neurologically/behaviourally important chromosomal/genetic abnormalities or dysmorphic syndromes will be reviewed in this chapter. For convenience, they will be listed in alphabetical order. Other, more rarely encountered syndromes are listed in Table 4.1.

Developmental delay and/or mental retardation, ranging in severity from mild to profound, feature in many of the behavioural phenotype syndromes. While general comments may apply to a particular syndrome, each child requires independent assessment and a programme of management related to their own abilities, taking into account the views of medical, social and educational authorities. For further discussion of these issues the reader is referred to Chapters 22 and 23.

ANGELMAN SYNDROME

Angelman syndrome (formerly known as 'happy puppet syndrome') encompasses jerky movements, unprovoked laughter and varying degrees of mental retardation, mostly severe or profound

TABLE 4.1
Some uncommon syndromes with prominent neurological and/or behavioural manifestations

Syndrome	Major features	Locus (gene/s)	References
Beckwith–Wiedemann syndrome	Macrosomia, omphalocele, microglossia, mild to moderate mental retardation, myoclonus, neonatal hypoglycaemia; Wilms tumour or other neoplasms in some cases	11p5.5 5q35	Cohen (2005)
Cat-eye syndrome	Mild mental retardation; coloboma of iris (bilateral)	22q11	Denavit et al. (2004)
Coffin–Lowry syndrome	Mental retardation, hypotonia, scoliosis, downslanting palpebral fissures, prominent brows and ears, tapering digits, cataplectic-like attacks	Xp22.2–p22.1	Delaunoy et al. (2006)
Coffin–Siris syndrome	Mental retardation, coarse facial features, feeding problems, infections, hypoplastic fifth fingernails and fifth distal phalanges	9p?	Fleck et al. (2001)
Cri du chat syndrome	Plaintive acute cry, microcephaly, moon-like face, severe mental retardation	5q12	Cerruti Mainardi et al. (2001)
Dubowitz syndrome	Intrauterine growth retardation, microcephaly, prominent epicanthus, short stature, short palpebral fissures with lateral telecanthus, eczema-like lesions on face and flexural areas, sparse hair, variable retardation, hoarse cry, stubbornness	?	Tsukuhara and Opitz (1996)
Freeman–Sheldon syndrome	Mask-like facies with small mouth, giving a 'whistling' appearance, broad nasal bridge, telecanthus, aberrant positioning of hands and face	17p13.1	Stevenson et al. (2006), Toydemir et al. (2006)
Gingival fibromatosis–hypertrophy–epilepsy syndrome	May simulate epilepsy treated with phenytoin	5q13–q22 2p22–p21	Anavi et al. (1969)
Marshall–Smith syndrome	Accelerated growth, shallow orbits, broad middle phalanges, respiratory difficulties, failure to thrive may suggest the diencephalic syndrome, unstable cranio-cervical junction	?	Adam et al. (2005)
Pallister–Hall syndrome	Hypothalamic hamartoma, imperforate anus, polydactyly or other digit anomalies, gelastic epilepsy	7p13	Minns et al. (1994), Kang et al. (1997)
Pallister–Killian syndrome	Coarse features, hypertelorism, sparse hair, mental retardation	Tetrasomy 12q, isochromosome 12q	Peltomaki et al. (1987)
Partial monosomy syndromes			
9p–	Trigonocephaly, mental retardation, hypoplastic supraorbital ridges, upslanting palpebral fissures		Su et al. (2005)
13q–	Microcephaly with high nasal bridge, thumb hypoplasia, mental retardation, eye defects, may include retinoblastoma		Araujo Junior et al. (2006)
18p–	Hypotonia, mental retardation, ptosis, epicanthal folds, holoprosencephaly in several cases		Maranda et al. (2006)
18q–	Severe lack of myelin in white matter, epilepsy, hypotonia, midfacial hypoplasia, prominent anthelix, hypoplasia of labia minora, long tapering fingers		Garcia-Cazorla et al. (2004), Hausler et al. (2005), Stephenson (2005)
Seckel syndrome ('bird-headed dwarfism')	Intrauterine growth retardation, marked dwarfism, severe microcephaly, mental retardation, single palmar crease, absence of 12th rib pair. Three subtypes are known	3q22–q24 (SCKL1) 18p11.31–q11.2 (SCKL2) 14q21–q22 (SCKL3)	Shanske et al. (1997)
Trisomy 9p	Growth deficiency, severe mental retardation, distal phalangeal hypoplasia, delayed closure of anterior fontanelle, ocular hypertelorism, Dandy–Walker malformation in a few cases		Chen et al. (2002), de Pater et al. (2002)
Trisomy 9 mosaic syndrome	Severe mental retardation, sloping narrow forehead, prominent nasal bridge, joint contractures, absent optic tract (occasional), self-injuring behaviour		Stoll et al. (1993)
Wolf–Hirschhorn syndrome (4p– syndrome)	Severe mental retardation, microcephaly, seizures, hypotonia, hypertelorism, strabismus, downturned mouth, small jaw, cleft lip/palate, cranial asymmetry	4p16.3	Battaglia et al. (1999), Battaglia and Carey (2005)

(Angelman 1965, Horsler and Oliver 2006). The population prevalence has been estimated at about 1 in 12,000 live births, with a 1:1 male:female ratio (Steffenburg et al. 1996). A comprehensive account of Angelman syndrome is currently in press (Dan 2008).

PATHOGENESIS

Angelman syndrome is caused in a majority of cases by a deletion of chromosome 15q11.2–12 that is similar, but not identical, to that found in children with Prader–Willi syndrome (Magenis et al. 1987, Knoll et al. 1989) and is maternally inherited (Knoll et al. 1989). The deletion includes a gene for the beta-3 subunit of GABA receptor (Saitoh et al. 1994). Sixty to 75 per cent of patients have deletions or rearrangements in the long arm of chromosome 15, and the deletion is always on the maternal chromosome. A small proportion of cases have paternal disomy for chromosome 15 (Malcolm et al. 1991, Prasad and Wagstaff 1997). However, at least 15% of affected persons have normal chromosomes and no evidence of disomy. In some of these cases, recurrence in relatives may be observed (Clayton-Smith 1992). Such cases may be due to a dominant mutation of the *UBE3A* gene (Kishino et al. 1997) at 15q11–13, resulting in an Angelman phenotype only when transmitted by females (Wagstaff et al. 1993). Differences in clinical presentation exist depending on the nature of the genetic defect (Lossie et al. 2001). Forms due to deletions are usually more severe than those due to single gene mutations or other genetic defects. Most cases are isolated but familial cases are on record.

DIAGNOSIS

Diagnosis is confirmed when the clinical phenotype coincides with a positive FISH test. The diagnosis is often difficult in infants (van Lierde et al. 1990, Yamada and Volpe 1990) even with the criteria proposed (Williams et al. 1995). The combination of mental retardation with autistic features, a cheerful demeanour, ataxia and epileptic attacks, often of a 'minor' character, is highly suggestive. Because of the apraxic gait, manual stereotypies and sometimes hyperventilation, the diagnosis of Rett syndrome can be wrongly entertained in girls. However, the early onset of seizures before 1 year of age, the cheerful mood and the dysmorphism should rule out that possibility.

CLINICAL FEATURES

The clinical features consist of severe mental retardation with especially severe speech deficit, ataxia, and a remarkable jerky movement disorder affecting the upper limbs and sometimes the trunk that has been shown to be a special type of cortical myoclonus (Guerrini et al. 1996, Beckung et al. 2004). Unmotivated bursts of laughter are characteristic but they may not be prominent, whereas a cheerful mood is constant (Williams and Frias 1982). Eighty-six per cent of affected children have seizures that are often repeated but of short duration and are more often atypical absences or tonic and atonic seizures than tonic–clonic ones (Dörries et al. 1988, Viani et al. 1995, Laan et al. 1997). The EEG pattern is often characteristic, showing runs of slow (3Hz)

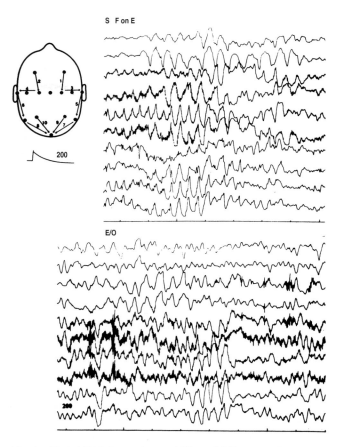

Fig. 4.1. Typical EEG features in two children of different ages (*upper trace*, 7 years; *lower trace*, 2 years) with Angelman syndrome. Note the calibration. In both examples, there is excess rhythmic theta activity mixed with runs of slower components seen particularly over the anterior half of the two hemispheres. In *upper trace*, runs of 3–4/s activity mixed with ill-defined sharp waves are seen over the posterior third of the head when the eyes are held shut by an attendant. S = shut; F on E = 'finger on eyes'; E/O = eyes open. (Courtesy Dr S Boyd, Great Ormond Street Hospital, London.)

waves, especially posteriorly, often notched and occasionally associated with actual spikes (Boyd et al. 1988) (Fig. 4.1). CT and MRI do not show any specific image, but mild dilatation of the ventricles and/or pericerebral spaces may be present (Dörries et al. 1988). Ambulation is acquired late, often after 5–6 years, and is very abnormal with the legs wide apart and with both ataxic and apraxic features (Sugimoto et al. 1992).

The dysmorphic syndrome is moderate and may be unnoticeable in young patients. Prognathism usually develops only after a few years of age.

Most cases are isolated but familial cases are on record.

Studies supporting the notion of a particular behavioural phenotype in this syndrome are only just being published, and it is too early to suggest details in this respect. One study of adolescents and young adults with Angelman syndrome (Clayton-Smith 1993) indicated that hyperactivity, often prominent in early childhood, usually gives way to more controllable behaviour in late childhood. Most studies to date suggest that muteness may be a constant feature, but that sign language may be acquired by some individuals. At one of our centres we have seen a young boy with Angelman syndrome and autism. Many children with Angelman syndrome have marked autistic features such as stubbornness, insistence on sameness and fascination with water (Steffenburg et al. 1996), while seeming happy and sociable in the sense that they may like the proximity of other people. However, contact is only accepted if it is on their own terms.

OUTCOME
The prognosis is poor, with severe mental retardation. Communicative language is not acquired (Beckung et al. 2004).

CORNELIA DE LANGE SYNDROME (BRACHMAN–DE LANGE SYNDROME, TYPUS DEGENERATIVUS AMSTELODAMENSIS)

Cornelia de Lange syndrome is a rare disorder first described by Brachman in 1916, but now bearing the name of the Dutch paediatrician de Lange. The syndrome is believed to be very rare, with a prevalence of only about 1 in 100,000 births (Beck 1976).

PATHOGENESIS
De Lange syndrome has been shown to be associated with mutations in the *NIPBL* gene on the short arm of chromosome 5 (Gillis et al. 2004, Krantz et al. 2004, Tonkin et al. 2004). Such mutations have recently been discovered to be a major aetiology for this syndrome, and have been detected in 27–56% of patients (Yan et al. 2006). However, various other chromosomal anomalies have also been found in individuals with de Lange syndrome (Jackson et al. 1993). Features suggestive of the syndrome are observed with partial trisomy of the distal portion of chromosome 3 (3q21–3ter) and other chromosome 3 rearrangements (DeScipio et al. 2005). The syndrome of chromosome 3q duplication [dup(3q) syndrome] at least superficially simulates de Lange syndrome (Holder et al. 1994). These findings, and those that connect the *MECP2* gene with Rett syndrome complex (see below), argue that some caution should still be observed when attributing full aetiological accountability to the *NIPBL* gene in de Lange syndrome.

De Lange syndrome may be dominantly inherited, virtually all cases being new mutations. A recurrence risk of 2–5% is quoted.

CLINICAL FEATURES
De Lange syndrome is a multisystem disorder featuring pre- and postnatal growth retardation, developmental delay, distinctive facial dysmorphism, limb malformations and multiple organ defects.

The phenotype is characterized by low birthweight, short stature, microcephaly, generalized hirsutism, and a curious facies, with synophrys (eyebrows growing together), low hairline on neck and forehead, long eyelashes, depressed bridge of nose, a long philtrum and upturned nostrils. The hands have a flat, spade-like

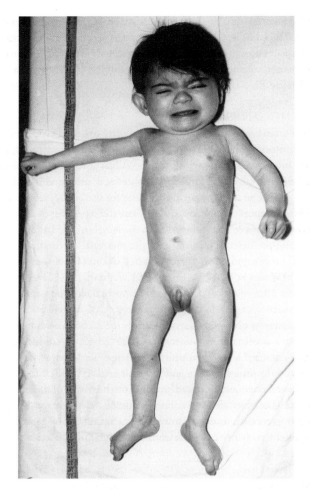

Fig. 4.2. Cornelia de Lange syndrome: depressed nasal bridge, low hairline, synophris (eyebrows meeting on the midline), short arms and flexed fingers and toes. (Courtesy Dr M Le Merrer, Hôpital des Enfants Malades, Paris.)

appearance and short, tapering fingers. There is clinodactyly of the fifth finger. The thumbs are proximally implanted and the thenar eminence is inconspicuous. More marked abnormalities of limbs may be present, including radial hypoplasia or reduction of finger number, often unilaterally. Micrognathia is usually present (Hawley et al. 1985, Opitz 1985) (Fig. 4.2). Optic atrophy, coloboma of the optic nerve, proptosis and choanal atresia have been reported. Gastrointestinal reflux, feeding difficulties, reduced lacrimation and other opthalmological problems are all extremely common.

In addition, there appears to be a rather characteristic behavioural phenotype with severe or profound learning disability in the majority (Horsler and Oliver 2006), often combined with self-injurious behaviours and social avoidance, quite often amounting to full syndromal autistic disorder (Gillberg and Coleman 2000, Arron et al. 2006, Bhuiyan et al. 2006). However, rare cases with borderline and even low-normal levels of intelligence have been reported. Two research groups have found significant differences between mutation-positive and mutation-negative patients in the severity or penetrance of some phenotypes (Yan et al. 2006,

Selicorni et al. 2007). Different clinical features have also been described among patients with missense versus truncating mutations. Mutation-positive patients tend to be more severely affected than mutation-negative individuals with respect to weight, height and mean head circumference at birth, facial dysmorphism and speech impairment.

OUTCOME
Severe cognitive and behavioural impairments will persist throughout life in the majority of cases. Mortality is increased, partly as an effect of the gastrointestinal problems, with regurgitation–vomiting–aspiration and fatal pneumonia as consequences in severe instances. A few individuals have been reported to live beyond their 40th birthday.

DI GEORGE SYNDROME (VELOCARDIOFACIAL SYNDROME, 22q11 DELETION SYNDROME)

Di George syndrome is due to a developmental defect of the third and fourth pharyngeal pouches and the fourth branchial arch. The syndrome is genetically heterogeneous, with partial monosomy of the proximal long arm of chromosome 22 detected microscopically in about one third of cases, and a higher frequency of deletion (88%) demonstrated by FISH studies (Driscoll et al. 1993). Uncommon cases have been associated with deletion of 17p and 10p (Levy-Mozziconacci et al. 1994).

The prevalence of 22q11deletion syndrome (22Q11DS) has been estimated at about 3 in 10,000 births (Oskarsdottir 2005), with a possibly slightly higher rate among females than among males (personal data, unpublished).

Most clinicians would now separate out 22Q11DS as the generally accepted syndrome within the Di George phenotype. Thus, diagnosis is reserved for those cases showing the 'CATCH-22 phenotype' [cardiac abnormality, anomalous face, thymus hypoplasia, cleft palate (including submucous only) and hypocalcaemia] and the typical FISH diagnosis of a deleted segment at 22q11.

CLINICAL FEATURES
The thymus and parathyroids are absent or ectopic, and the great vessels of the base of the heart are often malformed. Absence of the thymus may be associated with severe immunological deficiency, while that of the parathyroid glands may be responsible for severe hypocalcaemic convulsions in the neonatal period and later. Hypocalcaemia responds to parathyroid hormone. Cleft palate, micrognathia, low-set ears and hypertelorism are frequent (Conley et al. 1979). An overlapping phenotype, known as the velocardiofacial or *Schprintzen syndrome*, features similar cardiovascular abnormalities, facial dysmorphism, cleft palate and mental retardation, sometimes with late appearance of psychiatric disease, and is associated with the same 22q11 deletion. Cerebellar hypoplasia may be a feature (Devriendt et al. 1996).

22Q11DS is associated with a rather typical behavioural phenotype. Spoken language is delayed, but some verbal skills, in particular vocabulary, tend to be better than those associated with 'performance' from school age onwards. IQ is usually distributed around 70, with a few individuals testing above 100 and some (very few) under 40. Motor clumsiness is a typical feature of the disorder, and many individuals with 22Q11DS meet full criteria for developmental coordination disorder. There is a characteristic lack of energy in the majority from a very early age. It is as though they have to be manually 'wound up' in order to have the initiative to carry out any but the most simple activities (which contrasts with their relatively 'good' IQ – good, that is, when compared with other 'behavioural phenotype syndromes'). The vast majority have some degree of academic failure at school, even those few with IQs around 100 (Óskarsdóttir et al. 2005). Many meet criteria for attention deficit hyperactivity disorder (ADHD), particularly combined and inattentive subtypes. With age, more and more individuals 'move' from the combined to the inattentive subtype (Niklasson et al. 2005). Autistic features are common (Campbell et al. 2006), but classic autism is rare. There are often social and communication problems, even when criteria for an autism spectrum disorder are not met. These problems are often associated with the nasal 'drawl', articulation problems and poverty of facial movements common in 22Q11DS because of the velopharyngeal insufficiency encountered in so many cases. Depressed mood appears to be increasingly common from adolescence onwards. Psychosis may develop in late adolescence and early adult life, even in individuals who have shown a minimum of psychiatric problems in childhood (Sobin et al. 2005). ADHD and autism spectrum disorders in 22Q11DS may be the result of pathological brain abnormalities that include reduction of cortical grey matter, large caudate nuclei, and abnormal white matter in the frontal lobes and cerebellum. The risk of developing schizophrenia in adolescents or adults is increased (Niklasson et al. 2002).

INTERVENTIONS
As with other behavioural phenotype syndromes, the importance of early diagnosis and psychoeducation for the family cannot be stressed too much. ADHD can sometimes be successfully treated with stimulants and cognitive behaviourally oriented techniques plus special education measures. Serotonin or combined norepinephrine–serotonin reuptake inhibitors may be tried for longer periods of depressed mood or dysthymia. Psychosis, when it occurs, can be very difficult to treat, and typical and atypical neuroleptics, although effective in reducing psychotic symptoms, including auditory hallucinations in some cases, are often less helpful than in other young adult individuals with psychosis.

DOWN SYNDROME AND OTHER TRISOMY DISORDERS

DOWN SYNDROME (TRISOMY 21)
Trisomy 21 is the single most common cause of mental retardation. The condition occurs in about one in 650 births, although the frequency varies with maternal age, reaching one in 54 births in infants born to mothers aged 45 years or more. Advanced

paternal age has also been reported to be associated with a higher risk of Down syndrome in the offspring (Fisch et al. 2003), but the evidence in this respect is still equivocal. A high rate is also observed in infants of very young mothers (Smith and Berg 1976).

PATHOGENESIS

Down syndrome is caused by duplication of the genetic material localized on the long arm of chromosome 21 (Antonarakis 1993). Triplication of the 21q21–q22.3 region appears to be essential (Holtzman and Epstein 1992, Epstein 2006). Huret et al. (1987) found that a DNA fragment no larger than 3000 kb contains most of the genetic information involved in the pathogenesis of Down syndrome, and its presence in triplicate results in a similar phenotype.

The most common form, accounting for more than 90% of cases, is associated with the presence of an extra chromosome 21. Eight per cent of cases are due to a translocation of chromosome 21 to another chromosome, usually 14 or 21. Rare cases are mosaics of normal and trisomic cells (Uchida and Freeman 1985). Most translocations resulting in Down syndrome arise de novo and are not associated with a familial occurrence. In less than a quarter of the cases with a translocation, the carrier of the translocation was a parent, usually the mother (Antonarakis 1991, 1993). The recurrence rate for Down syndrome when a familial translocation is present varies between 5% and 15% depending on the type of translocation and whether the father or the mother is the carrier, as compared with approximately 1% in cases of nondisjunction. A higher risk exists for cases of 21q/21q translocation (Garver et al. 1982). Other mechanisms responsible for familial recurrence include parental mosaicism, found in 2.4% of cases (Uchida and Freeman 1985), and a familial tendency to nondisjunction despite a normal karyotype.

Very little is known about how the presence of excess genetic material from chromosome 21 is responsible for the clinical picture of Down syndrome.

Brain pathology is rather minor. The brain is small, correlating with the small head circumference of the patients. The cerebellum is especially atrophic. The disproportionately small cerebellum is easily detectable with MRI, which also shows a less marked volume reduction of the cerebrum (Becker et al. 1991, Golden and Hyman 1994). The first temporal gyrus is poorly developed and narrow. Microscopically, there is a reduction of granule cells in the cortex in some areas and curtailment of a specific cell type, probably the aspinous stellate cells (Ross et al. 1984, Wisniewski et al. 1985). The number of spines on apical dendrites may be reduced (Marin-Padilla 1976). Lamination of the superior temporal gyrus is delayed and disorganized, with increased cellular density in the upper layer (Golden and Hyman 1994). Histological abnormalities may be detectable as early as the 20th to 22nd week of intrauterine life (Wisniewski and Kida 1994).

CLINICAL FEATURES

About 20% of trisomy 21 fetuses are stillborn, and a trisomy 21 karyotype is found in 1 in 40 spontaneous abortions. Birthweight

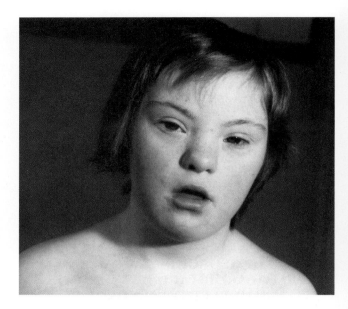

Fig. 4.3. Trisomy 21 (Down syndrome) in a 7-year-old-girl: classical features with upslanting palpebral fissures and epicanthus. (Courtesy Dr M-O Réthoré, Hôpital des Enfants Malades, Paris.)

of Down syndrome infants is usually low, about 20% of babies weighing <2500 g. Physical growth in height, weight and head circumference remains subnormal, although with large inter-individual variation (Gillberg and Söderström 2003).

The dysmorphic features of Down syndrome are very suggestive and the diagnosis is usually made at a glance even in newborn infants, although no individual dysmorphism is absolutely specific or constant (Fig. 4.3). Other malformations, especially atrioventricular canal and duodenal stenosis, are common. The palpebral fissures are oblique and there is a complete median epicanthal fold. Brushfield spots, accumulations of fibrous tissue in the superficial layer of the iris, are present in 85% of cases and differ from those observed in normal persons by their more central location. The external auditory meatus is narrow. The fifth finger is short and incurved, with a single flexion crease. A transverse palmar crease is seen in about half the cases, and dermatoglyphics are characteristic (Smith and Berg 1976).

Children with Down syndrome are more sensitive than controls to infections, and they have an increased risk of autoimmune diseases and leukaemia, in particular acute lymphoblastic and myeloid leukaemias (Krivit and Good 1957, Abildgaard et al. 2006, Whitlock 2006).

From the neurological point of view, individuals with trisomy 21 manifest considerable hypotonia, and independent ambulation is delayed to about the age of 2 years. The degree of mental retardation is variable, the average IQ being about 50 though tending to decrease with age (Smith and Berg 1976). Individuals with mosaicism may have higher IQ levels and better verbal–perceptual skills (Fishler et al. 1976). Epilepsy is present in 5–6% of patients (Stafstrom et al. 1991), a proportion lower than with most other causes of mental retardation in which 20–50% of affected persons have seizures. Infantile spasms are clearly abnormally frequent

(Pollack et al. 1978, Silva et al. 1996). Reflex seizures may be more common than in epilepsies of other causes (Guerrini et al. 1990). Hearing loss is a common problem in children with Down syndrome but is mainly conductive in type (Balkany et al. 1979). Calcification of the basal ganglia is frequently present (Takashima and Becker 1985). Stroke may be more frequent in Down syndrome patients than in the general population and occurs even in childhood. The development of moyamoya disease (see Chapter 14) has been reported (Aylett et al. 1996).

Instability of the cervical column is frequent and may be a contraindication to some athletic activities (Chapter 5).

Down syndrome, unlike other mental retardation syndromes, seems to be associated with a relatively low incidence of psychiatric disorder (Gillberg et al. 1986). Even though the stereotype of the happy, amiable and tractable personality is unsupported in many cases, and temper tantrums, irritability and stubbornness may be relatively common features in childhood, it seems clear that half or more of adolescents and young adults with Down syndrome do not have major psychiatric problems. There have been reports of a less persistent motivational orientation and over-reliance on social behaviours during cognitively challenging tasks in Down syndrome (Fidler et al. 2006). Behaviour problems can occur in Down syndrome, and even autism has been described in some cases. It seems that additional brain damage – or specific genetic influences on constitution – might be a prerequisite for the development of autism in Down syndrome and that the autistic symptoms are unassociated with the chromosomal abnormality as such. Most children with Down syndrome have IQs <50, and of the 10–20% who test higher, many are cases of mosaicism. Such cases comprise around 2–3% of all cases of Down syndrome. The cognitive profile in Down syndrome, in spite of a generally low level, shows considerable interindividual variation (Gillberg and Söderstrom 2003).

A remarkable feature of Down syndrome is the premature development of senile plaques and fibrillary tangles similar to those observed in Alzheimer disease. Such plaques are visible from age 30 years and correlate with the frequency of the development of dementia that occurs from 40 years of age in at least one third of people with Down syndrome (St Clair and Blackwood 1985, Wisniewski et al. 1985). Interestingly, the gene for amyloid precursor protein is located just outside the duplicated area critical for Down syndrome and is expressed about four times more than normal in affected individuals (Neve et al. 1988). This could conceivably lead to amyloid deposition, a hallmark of Alzheimer disease. The development of dementia after the age of 40 years in approximately two thirds of cases is the clinical correlate of the development of fibrillary bundles and plaques.

DIAGNOSIS AND MANAGEMENT
The diagnosis is usually made from birth on the basis of the dysmorphic syndrome. A karyotype is indicated in all cases to determine the type of trisomy present. If a translocation is present, the karyotype of the parents should be obtained.

Antenatal diagnosis can be made by amniotic fluid cell culture or by biopsy of the trophoblast. It is indicated for pregnant women over 35–37 years of age and for young mothers who have had an affected child.

Prenatal screening for trisomy 21 is systematic in many countries for pregnant women who would be aged 35 years or more at term, and is also indicated for young women who have had an affected child. Screening for low-risk pregnancies is possible during the second trimester. The so-called 'triple test' shows low maternal serum alpha-fetoprotein, decreased unconjugated oestriol and elevated chorionic gonadotrophins in maternal serum in more than 60% of cases of Down syndrome (Chard and Macintosh 1992). Ultrasound examination often shows short femora and cervical skin swelling. Amniocentesis is necessary to confirm the diagnosis by permitting demonstration of the trisomy. It is usually performed at 16 weeks gestational age. Early amniocentesis is possible but less effective. Chorionic villus biopsy, although it permits an earlier diagnosis, may be less reliable because of placental mosaicism (MRC 1991). Demonstration of abnormal numbers of gene copies in fetal cells by the polymerase chain reaction technique utilizing chromosome 21 markers is possible (Mansfield 1993) and may become a routine method of diagnosis.

The only effective treatments available in Down syndrome are for the management of infections and hearing deficit, and surgical treatment of correctable associated malformations. An adapted educational programme should be devised for each individual patient. Many children can be maintained within the family but the overall outlook for full autonomy is poor.

In recent years, several studies have indicated that with early intervention programmes, mainly focusing on physiotherapy and educating parents to train affected children (Spiker 1990, Connolly et al. 1993), IQ can be pushed up by 10–20 points and motor problems associated with hypotonia can be substantially reduced. Because in almost all cases the diagnosis of Down syndrome is made in the first few days of life, intensive intervention should start at once. For a detailed description of the training programme – which includes a language stimulation programme – the reader is referred to Rogers and Coleman (1992). In addition to the education programme, children with Down syndrome always require a medical work-up because major medical problems are frequently associated. Antisocial behaviour is relatively uncommon; indeed, social adjustment often tends to be ahead of that expected for the mental age.

Complications of Down syndrome may require complex treatment. Neurological complications related to the unstable cervico-occipital junction of patients with trisomy 21 are discussed in Chapter 5.

OUTCOME
The many medical complications of Down syndrome contribute to the much reduced survival rates. Cardiac problems may lead to death in early infancy or childhood, while the strong association with premature ageing and Alzheimer's disease may cause death around 50–65 years of age in many cases. The association with endocrine and malignant disorders accounts for sporadic cases of premature death at many different ages. Apart from the association with Alzheimer's disease, the behavioural phenotype

of Down syndrome, once established in early childhood, shows relatively little change over the years, i.e. those who are sociable tend to remain so, and those, relatively few (about one in ten), with autism still qualify for a diagnosis of autism in adulthood.

TRISOMY SYNDROMES OTHER THAN DOWN SYNDROME

Among the many other trisomy syndromes currently known (De Grouchy and Turleau 1984), only trisomy 13, trisomy 18 and trisomy 8 will be considered.

TRISOMY 13 (PATAU SYNDROME)

The frequency of trisomy 13 is probably between 1 in 4000 and 1 in 10,000 births. Elevated maternal age increases the risk. Average birthweight is 2600 g (De Grouchy and Turleau 1984). Affected children have profound mental retardation. The most characteristic features are hexadactyly, various types of facial clefts, most commonly bilateral cleft lip and palate, and microphthalmia. The feet are convex with protruding heels. Cryptorchidism and scrotal anomalies are the rule in boys, while bifid uterus and bifid vagina may be found in females. Visceral malformations are common. Heart disease is present in 80% of patients and renal abnormalities in 30–50%. Skin defects may occur, especially on the vertex. Eye abnormalities, in addition to microphthalmia, include cataracts, iris coloboma, retinal dysplasia and persistence of the primitive vitreous.

The major neurological abnormality is holoprosencephaly (see Chapter 2) (Gullotta et al. 1981), which is usually accompanied by several other anomalies, especially in the cerebellum (Norman 1966). Arhinencephaly was found in 40% of patients in the series of Gullotta et al. (1981). Severe neurological symptoms are present in most patients (Kunze 1980). Convulsions, often in the form of infantile spasms (Watanabe et al. 1976), are the rule. Most affected infants die before their first birthday. Rare exceptions are on record (Iliopoulos et al. 2006).

The diagnosis is suggested by the striking external abnormalities. From a neurological point of view, trisomy 13 should be sought in cases of holoprosencephaly associated with visceral and limb abnormalities. Isolated holoprosencephaly is only rarely due to trisomy 13 (Kobori et al. 1987). Partial trisomy 13 (De Grouchy and Turleau 1984) has a variable clinical expression depending on the triplicated segment.

TRISOMY 18 (EDWARDS SYNDROME)

The incidence of trisomy 18 is about one in 8000 births, and there is a 4:1 female preponderance. Increased maternal age increases the frequency of the condition. Average duration of pregnancy is 42 weeks, and hydramnios, a small placenta and a single umbilical artery are frequently found. Mean birthweight is 2240 g (De Grouchy and Turleau 1984). Affected children have a long narrow skull with prominent occiput. The bridge of the nose is protruding, the mandible is small and receding, and the ears are low set and imperfectly shaped. The index and fifth fingers cover the third and fourth fingers, and the fists are firmly closed. Cryptorchidism is constant in males. Visceral malformations include congenital heart disease (patent ductus arteriosus or ventricular septal defect) in 95% of cases. Meckel diverticulum, horseshoe kidneys, diaphragmatic hernia and hydronephrosis are also common (Cox 1999).

Mental retardation is severe and is associated with hypo- or hypertonia and weak sucking. Brain malformations (Gullotta et al. 1981) include partial agenesis of the corpus callosum, abnormalities of the cerebellum, especially the inferior olivary bodies, and variable types of cortical dysplasia. In half the cases no abnormalities are detectable.

The diagnosis is confirmed by a karyotype that shows a homogeneous free trisomy (80% of cases), a mosaic of trisomic and normal cells (10% of cases) or (in the remaining 10%) a translocation or complex abnormality (De Grouchy and Turleau 1984) such as a ring chromosome 18 (Amit et al. 1988).

TRISOMY 8

Trisomy 8 is less frequently recognized than trisomies 13 or 18 but its diagnosis may often be missed, as mental retardation is mild and dysmorphism is moderate. About one third of cases are not recognized before adulthood. The most suggestive facial feature is the thick and everted lower lip. Osteoarticular lesions such as brachydactyly, clinodactyly, club feet and joint contractures are extremely common (Riccardi 1977).

From a neurological point of view, the most remarkable abnormality is agenesis of the corpus callosum, which has been found in almost all cases in which it has been looked for (Aicardi et al. 1987). IQ is usually between 45 and 75.

The diagnosis should be systematically thought of in patients with callosal agenesis. Most cases are mosaics and all known cases have appeared de novo.

FRAGILE X AND OTHER SYNDROMES OF X-LINKED MENTAL RETARDATION

FRAGILE X SYNDROME

Fragile X syndrome (FXS) – sometimes referred to as FRAX-A, and occasionally as Martin–Bell syndrome – constitutes a combination of physical and behavioural characteristics associated with a fragile site (and a gene locus) on the long arm of the X chromosome at Xq27.3 that is apparent only when a medium deficient in folate is used for culture.

It is second only to Down syndrome as a cause of mental retardation, with IQ levels <50. It is the most common known cause of familial mental retardation, and it underlies a variety of behavioural problems including autism and hyperactivity syndromes (Percy et al. 1990, Reiss and Freund 1990, Hagerman and Hagerman 2002).

Many affected individuals have specific difficulties in speech, language, behaviour and social skills. 'Cluttered' speech is a suggestive feature (Hanson et al. 1986). Hyperactivity and attention deficit are common, and autism may be present in as many as 23% of cases (Bregman et al. 1987, Thake et al. 1987, Vieregge and Froster-Iskenius 1989). However, the behavioural phenotype is different from that of other causes of autism, and hyperactivity may be especially prominent (Baumgardner et al. 1995, Hagerman et al. 2005). Women carriers of the full mutation on one of their X chromosomes are usually phenotypically normal. Approximately 35% appear to have mental retardation, generally in the mild range, and 15% have borderline intelligence, learning disabilities or both (Kemper et al. 1986). FXS is thus an important cause of mild mental difficulties in women. In addition, about 10% of cognitively normal carriers may have psychiatric conditions, especially affective or schizoid disorders (Reiss and Freund 1990).

PATHOGENESIS
The syndrome is caused by an expansion of the 'normal' number of CGG repeats at Xq27.3 in the *FMR1* gene, which codes for the protein FMRP. When there are more than about 55 repeats (51–54 borderline) a premutation is said to occur, and a full mutation when the number exceeds 200. Transmission of the disease by asymptomatic males suggested the possibility of a premutation that is associated with expansion of the repeat to 55–200 copies. The premutation tends to remain stable during spermatogenesis but frequently expands to a full mutation during oogenesis, so that daughters of carrier males always carry only the premutation, while those of carrier females are often clinically affected. Males with a full mutation almost invariably have mental retardation, whereas only 30–50% of females do so, usually to a milder degree than males (Staley et al. 1993). Only 30–50% have a demonstrable fragile site. The presence of a full mutation prevents the traduction of the gene into a protein (as a result of methylation) (Knight et al. 1993). The same absence of FMRP has been reported in rare patients without trinucleotide expansion but with deletions or point mutations of the *FMR1* gene (Hirst et al. 1995). Rare cases of males with normal cognitive function in the presence of a full mutation are on record (Smeets et al. 1995). The FMRP is expressed in many tissues and is most abundant in neurons. It appears to be normal in persons with the premutation (Devys et al. 1993). The functions of the FMRP are still largely unknown.

Full-mutation forms of the gene can cause autism, learning disabilities, anxiety disorders and mental retardation. Evidence is mounting that autism also occurs in some young males who have premutation alleles. One recent study has found that approximately 30% of all individuals with FXS have autism; those with autism have lower cognitive abilities, and an increase in language problems and behavioural difficulties, compared to those with FXS alone. Other disorders associated with premutation forms of the gene include the 'tremor–ataxia syndrome' (FXTAS, see below) in older males and occasional females, and premature ovarian failure (Hagerman et al. 2005).

Metabotropic glutamate receptor 5 (mGluR5)-coupled pathways are dysregulated in individuals with FXS and this is thought to relate to the FXS phenotype.

PREVALENCE
FXS (full-mutation DNA diagnosis) is inferred to be present in around 1 per 4000 males and 1 per 8000 females, but, given that total population DNA studies have not been performed, it is impossible to determine whether these inferences are correct (Hagerman and Hagerman 2002a,b). Premutation carrier status is present in about 1 per 750–1000 males and 1 per 250–350 females. Considering that not all persons with FXS have IQ <70 and that there are carrier males and females with only slight or no learning problems, the true prevalence of FXS (full mutation and premutation cases with clinically significant problems combined) is likely to be higher. Most males affected by the full mutation appear to have moderate or severe problems, whereas most females are less severely affected, although about one third have IQ <70.

The prevalence of FXS among children with moderate to severe learning difficulties without specific dysmorphic features ranges from 2% to 10% (Slaney et al. 1995).

DIAGNOSIS
The diagnosis of FXS is suggested by the phenotype and is easy in postpubertal boys but can be difficult in prepubertal boys and in female carriers who lack typical physical findings. Conversely, even macroorchidism or large ears are frequently unassociated with a fragile site on the X chromosome (Hagerman 1987). A family history of mental retardation is an important feature but is found in only two thirds of cases (Simko et al. 1989).

DNA studies are now reliable and clearly cost-effective (Rousseau et al. 1991, 1994; Oostra et al. 1993; Wang et al. 1993; Hagerman and Hagerman 2002a). A rapid antibody test for the detection of the FMRP in lymphocytes has been proposed as a screening procedure for the full mutation (Willemsen et al. 1995).

Prenatal diagnosis of FXS is possible on cultured amniotic cells or chorionic villus cells and by DNA analysis. Highly difficult ethical problems arise, however, because only some carriers, especially among females, will be affected. Weaver and Sherman (1987) have computed the probability of retardation for offspring of affected carriers (Table 4.2) but precise counselling remains problematic.

CLINICAL FEATURES
The disorder is more easily recognizable in adolescents than in prepubertal children. The most important features are the absence of retarded physical growth that is commonly found with many causes of mental retardation, and especially a normal or increased head circumference; and a long face with prominent jaw and macroorchidism (Ho et al. 1989) (Fig. 4.4).

The classic facial features of a long, narrow face and prominent ears are often not obvious in the prepubertal period, although they are sometimes striking in the very young male with FXS. Adult females with the full mutation often have similar facial features, but many look much more 'normal' than adult males with the disorder. Macroorchidism is present in about one third of young boys with FXS, and in more than 90% of adult males. Other common physical features include hyperextensible finger joints, double-jointed thumbs, flat feet, soft skin, muscular hypotonia, a heart murmur or click (often associated with mitral valve prolapse or dilation of the aortic root), strabismus, and varying

TABLE 4.2
Probability of neurodevelopmental impairment in offspring of women carriers of the fragile Xq27 site and of normal transmitting males*

Offspring	Parent with fragile X			
	Normal woman	Mentally impaired woman	Normal transmitting man	Impaired man
Sons				
Mentally impaired	0.38	0.5	0	0
Asymptomatic carrier	0.12	0	0	0
Daughters				
Impaired carrier	0.16	0.28	0	>0.32[1]
Asymptomatic carrier	0.34	0.22	1.0	<0.68[1]

*Modified from Weaver and Sherman (1987).
[1]Estimates based on a known penetrance of 32% of fragile X in females.

TABLE 4.3
Clinical features of fragile X syndrome

Anthropometry	Normal weight and size Normal or large head (>75th centile) (>90th centile in 10%)
Facial features	Long face High-arched palate Prominent jaw Epicanthal folds Mildly coarse facial features Strabismus
Genitalia	Macroorchidism (more common in, but not exclusive to, postpubertal boys)
Others	Hyperextensible fingers and other joints Hyperelastic skin Large floppy ears
Neurodevelopmental manifestations	Mental retardation (IQ<70) Autistic features Hyperactivity Poor coordination

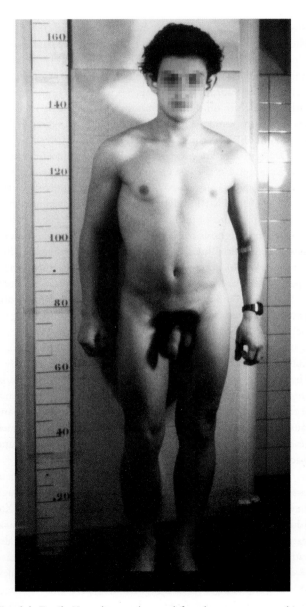

Fig. 4.4. Fragile X syndrome: elongated face, large ears, prognathism. General body development is good but the testicles are enlarged. (Courtesy Dr M-O Réthoré, Hôpital des Enfants Malades, Paris.)

degrees of high-arched palate. Recurrent otitis media is extremely common in childhood and much overrepresented as compared to non-affected siblings and children in the general population.

In prepubertal children, only a large head, large ears and high-arched palate are present. Joint hyperextensibility and floppy ears may be of diagnostic help. Despite the lack of prominence of macroorchidism in young patients, 15–40% of them have some degree of testicular enlargement (Simko et al. 1989).

The common physical manifestations of FXS are listed in Table 4.3.

Mental retardation in FXS is usually in the mild to moderate range but tends to become more severe in adolescence and adulthood (Borghgraef et al. 1987; Hagerman 1987, 1989; Wisniewski et al. 1989). Most males test below IQ 70 (the most common level of cognitive functioning seems to be 35–40) on standard IQ tests, but a proportion have IQs in the normal or low-normal range. Verbal abilities are usually superior to performance and visuospatial skills.

Epilepsy is a relatively common phenomenon, occurring in 15–25% of cases (Hagerman and Hagerman 2002a,b). They are often of the complex partial variant, and have typically been reported to be relatively benign with a tendency to resolve at adolescence, even though severe and complex cases of epilepsy do occur in a few cases. It has been hypothesized that the seizure activity might be related to cerebellar vermal abnormalities noted in FXS.

There is clear evidence of social dysfunction in a vast majority of male cases. Almost all males exhibit 'autistic' features, but only a minority exhibit the full syndrome of autism, with or without mental retardation. The fragile X abnormality is the most common of the known causes of autism. Hyperkinetic syndromes, with and without autism, usually with many autistic features, are common and occur in about half or more of all boys with the full mutation (Sullivan et al. 2006). The cognitive test profile in FXS is different from that ordinarily seen in low-functioning autism, but is quite commonly encountered in high-functioning autism cases and Asperger syndrome. Several authors have described the concurrence of Asperger syndrome and the fragile X chromosome abnormality (see Hagerman 1989).

Some of the behaviours most often encountered in males with FXS are: gaze avoidance, tactile defensiveness and social withdrawal (age 0–2 years); gaze avoidance, avoidant greeting behaviour (turning away with head and body on greeting other people), shyness, motor stereotypies of various kinds and hyperactivity (3–4 years); echolalia, cluttered speech, 'nervous fidgetiness', hand flapping, stereotypic waving of things, wrist or knuckle biting, and gaze avoidance and avoidant greeting behaviour in spite of signs that there is a drive for social 'proximity' and interest in other humans (5–8 years); continuing shyness, gaze avoidance and 'nervousness', and often also a preoccupation with certain objects or human beings in the general setting of moderate mental retardation, with fast, cluttered echolalic speech (very often used in a half whispering, half 'nervously' laughing manner) (9–12 years); continuing difficulties of the same type, often aggravated by various problems associated with onset of puberty, including cross-dressing, over-arousability, self-injurious behaviours and clothing problems (because of large genital size) (13–20 years). Often there is cognitive stagnation, or even setback, around the time of puberty.

The same picture is occasionally seen in affected females, but the majority of girls have less severe problems. A small proportion have full-blown autism, and shyness and gaze avoidance appear to be rather common phenomena even in the relatively large group with no major difficulties. Various kinds of learning problems appear to affect one third to one half of all fragile-X-positive females. These range from dyslexia to mild/moderate mental retardation. There have been occasional reports of the development of schizoaffective psychosis in some young women with the fragile X chromosome abnormality (see Hagerman 1989). Some of these have had relatively minor learning problems before the onset of psychosis, but have otherwise, at least outwardly, appeared to be doing well.

The fragile X phenotype is also associated with a 'tremor–ataxia syndrome' (FXTAS) that consists of tremor, ataxia, peripheral neuropathy and cognitive deficits. Significant brain atrophy and white-matter disease are usually seen. FXTAS develops after adolescence in males (and occasional females) with premutations. It is believed to be related to elevated levels of abnormal FMR1 mRNA. Current findings, coupled with recent evidence linking the degree of neuropathology (numbers of intranuclear inclusions) to the size of the premutation allele, provide evidence that the neurodegenerative phenotype in FXTAS is a consequence of the CGG repeat expansion (Cohen et al. 2006).

Convincing evidence now relates the FMR1 premutation to altered ovarian function and loss of fertility (Wittenberger et al. 2007). An FMR1 mRNA gain-of-function toxicity may underlie this altered ovarian function. Women with premature ovarian failure are at increased risk of having an FMR1 premutation and should be informed of the availability of fragile X testing. Specialists in reproductive medicine can provide a supportive environ-

ment in which to explain the implications of FMR1 premutation testing, facilitate access to testing, and make appropriate referral to genetic counsellors.

INTERVENTION

As yet, there is no specific treatment for fragile X syndrome (see Hagerman 1989). Folic acid (0.5–1.5 mg/kg b.i.d.) has been used by several clinicians, but its efficacy is in doubt. Some reports have suggested a beneficial effect of folic acid on autistic symptoms, at least if given from the preschool period, but no or even a slightly negative effect if given after puberty. Many authors have used stimulants to counter excessive hyperactivity (in doses recommended for children with severe ADHD regardless of aetiology) and reported fair or good results (Hagerman and Hagerman 2002a,b). Serotonin reuptake inhibitors may be helpful for anxiety, depressed mood and irritability, but should always be carefully monitored for possible increases in impulsivity and violent behaviours.

OTHER SYNDROMES OF X-LINKED MENTAL RETARDATION

FXS accounts for only 50% of the excess of boys with mental retardation. Many other more or less well-defined syndromes of X-linked mental retardation have been described (Opitz et al. 1986). Some individuals with sex chromosome aneuploidies have learning disability and other neuropsychiatric problems. They are reported under a separate heading later in this chapter.

FRAX-E

A second fragile X syndrome (FRAX-E) caused by an expanded GCC trinucleotide repeat in Xq28, 600kb down from the FMR1 gene, has been found in several cases (Flynn et al. 1993). Mental retardation is usually mild and is absent altogether in many cases.

FRAX-F

A third fragile X site (FRAX-F) that is also due to an expanded repeat and may be associated with mental retardation and seizures has been reported (Hirst et al. 1993).

RENPENNING SYNDROME

Renpenning syndrome, initially believed to constitute one clinical presentation of FXS, is characterized by moderate to severe mental retardation, mild microcephaly, short stature and normal chromosomes (Archidiacono et al. 1987).

JUBERG–MARSIDI SYNDROME

This rare syndrome includes a number of features including growth retardation, deafness and microgenitalism (Juberg and Marsidi 1980).

OTHER VARIANTS OF X-LINKED RECESSIVE MENTAL RETARDATION SYNDROMES

X-linked recessive mental retardation has also been reported in association with bodily overgrowth (Golabi and Rusen 1984), coarse features, short stature and macroorchidism (Atkin et al.

1985), and progressive complex neurological disorders (Schimke et al. 1984, Pfeiffer and Steffann 1985). Male relatives of patients with X-linked aqueductal stenosis may have moderate to severe mental retardation without hydrocephalus (Willems et al. 1987), sometimes in association with paraplegia, adducted thumbs and language disturbances (mental retardation–aphasia–shuffling gait–adducted thumbs syndrome or MASA). X-linked nerve deafness, optic nerve atrophy and dementia may constitute a specific X-linked recessive syndrome (Jensen 1981; see also Chapter 18).

GOLDENHAR SYNDROME

Goldenhar syndrome – which commonly involves the eyes (e.g. conjunctival dermoid tumours), the external ears (preauricular skin tags and malformation of the ears) and the vertebrae – is now generally believed to be part of a broader spectrum of syndromes referred to as oculo-auriculo-vertebral (OAV) dysplasia. It shows occasional association with mild/moderate mental retardation. A small proportion of cases appear to be familial. It is too early to decide whether there might be a more specific behavioural phenotype in this syndrome, but a recent study (Strömland et al. 2007) has documented the occurrence of some patients with OAV who have a smiling (occasionally hemimicrosomic) face, generally happy predisposition, slightly subnormal intelligence and many autistic features. Occasionally, there is more cognitive impairment and full DSM-IV criteria for autistic disorder may be met.

HYPOMELANOSIS OF ITO (see also Chapter 3)

Hypomelanosis of Ito was once – probably erroneously – referred to as incontinentia pigmenti achromians. It is possibly a relatively common condition, whose prevalence has never been rigorously studied. It appears to be considerably more common among females.

PATHOGENESIS
Chromosomal mosaicism and sporadic mutations are the causes, but the identity of a specific gene has not been confirmed. Probably, several gene abnormalities cause the phenotype that is recognized as hypomelanosis of Ito. For this reason, some authors believe that it constitutes a symptom rather than a distinct disease. Xp21.2 has been proposed as the most likely region of interest for the genetic abnormality causing this 'symptom'. X-linked familial cases are rare.

CLINICAL FEATURES
Apart from the diagnostic skin changes there is a variable degree of involvement of other organs including the brain. Only about one in four affected individuals have average or above average IQ, and more than 50% have some degree of learning disability (IQ <70). Seizures are common (about half the group), and infantile spasms occur in about 10% of individuals with typical skin changes. Macrocephaly is present in about one in seven cases. Ito syndrome may be a cause of hemimegalencephaly. Cleft palate and hearing and visual problems are not uncommon. Recently,

many cases of hypomelanosis of Ito associated with psychiatric disorder including symptoms compatible with the diagnoses of psychosis, autism, atypical autism and Asperger syndrome have been described (Åkefeldt and Gillberg 1991; Zappella 1992; Pascual-Castroviejo et al. 1998, 2006; Davalos et al. 2001). Most series have found a slightly higher rate of the condition in females.

MANAGEMENT
There is no treatment for the skin disorder, but cover-up make-up can be used if desired. Neurological, hearing and visual problems should be treated as indicated for those particular problems.

KLEINE–LEVIN SYNDROME

Originally described in the 1930s, the Kleine–Levin syndrome has received attention in paediatrics and child psychiatry only in recent years (see Gillberg 1987). It occurs mostly in adolescent boys (population prevalence unknown), and presents with the combination of intense hunger or specific craving for certain foods, increased need for sleep (somnolence and withdrawal or fugue-like states may be difficult to distinguish from each other) and a variety of emotional/behavioural/neuropsychiatric problems. This symptom constellation appears abruptly and is present for a few days to a few weeks, whereafter symptoms subside. Weeks to months later a new episode occurs and follows a similar pattern, albeit quite often of more limited duration. New episodes can occur for a period of one to several years. Gradually, however, relapses tend to occur less often and the episodes become shorter and shorter.

PATHOGENESIS
Hypothalamic–diencephalic dysfunction may account for the symptomatology because: (a) the appetite and sleep symptoms implicate hypothalamic systems; (b) the syndrome occurs mostly in the teenage period; (c) it affects mostly boys and its episodic nature could be seen as a counterpart to variable behaviour in connection with onset of menarche in girls; and (d) EEG and SPECT findings are compatible with hypothalamic–diencephalic dysfunction, particularly during hypersomniac episodes (Hong et al. 2006, Huang et al. 2006).

INVESTIGATIONS
The work-up should include a neuropsychiatric assessment. If the history and symptoms are typical there is no need for further investigations, but in case of doubt, neurological and laboratory work-up to exclude other neurological disorders and metabolic problems may be essential. A urine and/or blood screen for narcotics and other drugs might also be appropriate in some cases. The EEG sometimes shows mild to moderate increase of low-frequency activity and there may be subtle signs of damage to the CSF blood–brain barrier.

TREATMENT
Management need often consist only of assessment and a proper diagnosis. In severe cases affecting school attendance over long

periods, a trial of stimulants (e.g. dexamphetamine, two or three doses of 5–15 mg given at 3- to 4-hour intervals) might be indicated (Lishman 1978). In most cases, however, information given to the affected child/teenager and to his/her parents and teachers will suffice. Because of similarities between Kleine–Levin syndrome and certain mood disorders, lithium and carbamazepine may be prescribed. Responses to treatment have often been limited. This disorder needs to be differentiated from cyclic reoccurrence of sleepiness during the premenstrual period in teenage girls that may be controlled with birth control pills.

OUTCOME

Long-term outcome is good, although a year or two of school work may be wasted and there is quite often the need to repeat a form (grade), and most affected individuals do well by early adult life. The behaviour problems encountered are extremely variable and are often associated with some degree of somnolence and clouded consciousness. All sorts of psychiatric diagnoses may be discussed before a correct diagnosis is established. These may range from depression or manic depression to schizophrenia and drug abuse. Encephalitis is commonly suspected if the family seeks help during the first episode. The episodic nature of the disorder might not be evident until three or more episodes have occurred. There is also commonly partial or total amnesia for the episodes.

MILLER–DIEKER SYNDROME (17p– SYNDROME)

Miller–Dieker syndrome is a dysmorphic syndrome, usually with severe or profound learning disability, which features a distinctive facies with bitemporal hollowing, prominent forehead often with vertical furrows, upturned nares, a long philtrum with a thin vermilion border and a small jaw. Digital deformities, mainly camptodactyly and clinodactyly, are common (Dobyns et al. 1984). The most important pathological feature is the presence of type I lissencephaly (Chapter 2). There is deletion at the critical region of 17p13.3, detectable cytogenetically or by DNA analysis, and apparently of paternal origin. Although most cases occur de novo, familial recurrence is possible in cases with parental translocation (Dobyns et al. 1984, Goutières et al. 1987) and as an X-linked trait (Chapter 2). The neurological features are those of type I lissencephaly.

NOONAN SYNDROME

In 1968, Jacqueline Noonan reported a syndrome occurring in both males and females that bore many similarities to Turner syndrome (see below).

PREVALENCE

Most authors cite prevalence figures of 1 in 1,000–2,500 live births. However, these estimates have not been based on a population study. Fetal loss occurs for Noonan syndrome so disease incidence is higher than prevalence, but no estimate of the magnitude of this discrepancy is available.

CLINICAL FEATURES AND CLINICAL DIAGNOSIS

The diagnosis of Noonan syndrome is made on clinical grounds, by observation of key features. Despite a lack of defined diagnostic criteria, the cardinal features are well delineated (Allanson 1987, Fragale et al. 2004): short stature, broad or webbed neck similar to that seen in Turner syndrome, heart defects (and a variety of coagulation defects and lymphatic dysplasias), unusual chest shape with superior pectus carinatum and inferior pectus excavatum, seemingly low-set nipples, cryptorchidism in males and a characteristic face. The facial appearance shows considerable change with age, being most striking in the newborn period and middle childhood, and most subtle in the adult (Allanson 1987). Key features found irrespective of age include low-set, posteriorly rotated ears with fleshy helices; vivid blue or blue-green irides; and eyes that are often wide-spaced, with epicanthal folds and thick or droopy eyelids.

There is often some degree of learning disability (severe learning disability is rare). Mean IQ is probably in the order of 85 (and possibly with bell-shaped distribution of IQ around this mean). Performance IQ tends to be slightly higher than verbal IQ. Motor coordination problems are very common and about half of all cases present with many features of developmental coordination disorder. There is no consistent 'behavioural phenotype' (Lee DA et al. 2005).

GENETIC DIAGNOSIS AND PATHOGENESIS

Three genes are known to be associated with Noonan syndrome: *PTPN11* mutations are observed in about 50% of cases (Allanson 2002); *KRAS* mutations are seen in about 5–10% of individuals with the syndrome who do not have mutations in *PTPN11* (Schubert et al. 2006); and *SOS1* mutations can be detected in about 10–20% of all cases not showing either of the other two gene abnormalities (Lee JS et al. 2005). It is presumed that additional loci may be identified. Molecular genetic clinical testing is available (usually with sequence analysis), including for prenatal diagnosis.

Both the *PTPN11* and *KRAS* genes are on chromosome 12 (albeit at widely separated sites). *PTPN11* encodes a tyrosine protein phosphatase, a widely expressed extracellular protein that has a key role in the cellular response to growth factors and cell adhesion molecules, and in modulating cellular proliferation, differentiation, migration and apoptosis (Fragale et al. 2004). The abnormal KRAS protein induces hypersensitivity of primary hematopoietic progenitor cells to growth factors and deregulates signal transduction in a cell lineage-specific manner. Strong gain-of-function *KRAS* mutations may be incompatible with life. Missense mutations in the *SOS1* gene will lead to disturbances in the encoding of a RAS-specific guanine nucleotide exchange factor and may be responsible for the syndrome in approximately 20% of cases.

PARTIAL MONOSOMY 1p36

Deletion of the telomeric portion of the p-arm of chromosome 1 is one of the most common chromosomal/genetic deletion syndromes with a rather characteristic phenotype (Knight-Jones et al. 2000) and the best-defined example of the new category of abnormalities of the subtelomeric segment of chromosomes that may be responsible for a significant number of the dysmorphic/behavioural syndromes.

PREVALENCE

Current estimates of the prevalence of partial monosomy 1p36 range from about 1 in 5000 to 1 in 10,000 births (Heilstedt et al. 2003). However, knowledge about the syndrome is growing at a fast pace, and it is possible that these estimates will have to be revised in the near future.

PATHOGENESIS

The syndrome is caused by a deletion of the terminal locus of the short arm of chromosome 1. It is estimated that about 80% of all cases involve the 1p36 deletion only, but that the remainder may have other chromosomal regions affected. This sometimes occurs when the child has inherited a translocated chromosome from one of the parents. The partial monosomy may then be associated with extra material from another chromosome. The deleted region contains several genes that are important for fetal and child development. It is believed that the symptoms of the 'core' disorder arise when there is only one copy of these genes in the 1p36 (deleted) region. A contiguous gene syndrome sometimes arises when the adjacent region of 1p36 is also deleted. Parents of the translocation cases (who themselves may have balanced translocations) are reported to be at 10–15% risk of having another affected baby at their next pregnancy.

DIAGNOSIS

The clinical picture (Battaglia 2005a) is usually suggestive of the diagnosis, which can be confirmed at chromosomal analysis, but more specifically by DNA analysis (FISH or MLPA).

CLINICAL FEATURES

Mild, moderate, severe or profound learning disability appears to be a universal phenomenon and there may be some association between severity and the size of the deleted segment of the chromosome. Behaviour problems are extremely common, perhaps particularly behaviours that lead to self-injury. Language is more affected than motor development.

Epilepsy occurs in at least 70% of affected children. It can be of any type, has its onset in infancy or early childhood, and sometimes resolves by adolescence. The so-called *KCNAB2* gene, one of the documented epilepsy susceptibility genes, is located in the 1p36 area, and studies have shown that those affected by early onset and more severe epilepsies have a deletion of this gene.

Most children with partial monosomy 1p36 have growth abnormalities, and some have microcephaly. Cardiac abnormalities (ductus arteriosus persistens, septal defects, Fallot tetralogy, and dilated cardiomyopathy) are found in almost 50% of cases. Hydrocephalus and brain atrophy are relatively common also. One third of the group have cleft lip/palate syndromes of varying severity. Hypothyroidism occurs in about one in five cases, and

a small number of children have additional problems resembling Prader–Willi syndrome (see below).

Half of all affected children have a major hearing problem, and visual problems (cataracts, strabismus, refraction errors and optic nerve atrophy) are very common also.

The majority of affected children have a rather typical physical appearance with a small bracycephalic head, frontal bossing, straight uncurved eyebrows, flat nasal ridge, deep-set eyes, small middle portion of face, low-seated ears, small mouth with down-turning corners and a pointed chin. The whole face is often somewhat asymmetrical. The large fontanelle is often extremely large, and synostosis may be much delayed.

INTERVENTION

Because of the complexity of the syndrome, affected children and their families are in need of early diagnosis and long-term follow-up (into adult life) and support provided by an expert team. There is, as yet, no specific treatment available for any of the many impairing symptoms of the disorder, but a multidisciplinary approach is always needed.

PARTIAL TETRASOMY 15

The chromosome region 15q11q13 is particularly unstable, and many rearrangements can occur in this imprinted segment. To date, reports have occurred regarding deletions associated with either Angelman or Prader–Willi syndrome, according to parental origin; translocations; inversions; and supernumerary marker chromosomes formed by the inverted duplication of proximal chromosome 15. Inv dup (15) constitutes the most common of the heterogeneous group of the extra structurally abnormal chromosomes, and their presence results in tetrasomy 15p and partial tetrasomy 15q.

The general population frequency of partial tetrasomy 15 is not known.

CLINICAL FEATURES

The syndrome comprises mental retardation (often severe), autistic and hyperkinetic behaviours and, often, skeletal abnormalities (a characteristic facies, high arched palate, kyphosis and short stature) and epilepsy (Gillberg et al. 1991). Clinicians should suspect this syndrome in any infant/child with early central hypotonia, minor dysmorphic features, autism or an autistic-like condition, and who subsequently develops hard to control seizures/epilepsy (Battaglia 2005b). There is delayed development early on, and a spectrum of behaviour and communication problems (Cohen et al. 2007) that usually, but not always fits the diagnosis of autistic disorder or atypical autism. Hand stereotypies in the midline are common, as is a characteristic 'high-strung' oversensitivity to environmental stimuli.

The typical partial tetrasomy syndrome is associated with two extra copies of the q11–13 portion of chromosome 15. These copies are usually maternally derived and are located in an extra 'marker' chromosome, visible at ordinary karyotyping, but the diagnosis can be made with greater precision using FISH analysis.

Management should be geared to alleviating, if possible, the behavioural problems and to the treatment of epilepsy (often of the minor motor type).

PRADER–WILLI SYNDROME

Prader–Willi syndrome (PWS) is characterized by overeating, overweight, and a number of other characteristic physical and behavioural features. It occurs at a rate of about 1 per 7000 children surviving the first year of life (Åkefeldt et al. 1991). The male to female ratio is about equal.

PATHOGENESIS
PWS is caused by an absence of paternal DNA at the chromosome l5q11 locus. The paternally derived gene may be deleted or there may be maternal disomy. Preconception exposure to benzene in the fathers has been documented in one study (Åkefeldt et al. 1995). The syndrome is associated, in approximately half the patients, with an interstitial deletion of chromosome 15q11–13 (Ledbetter et al. 1982, Mattei et al. 1983, Caldwell and Taylor 1988). The deletion, in virtually all cases, is of paternal origin (Butler et al. 1986, Knoll et al. 1989). Approximately 40% of cases without cytogenetic deletion have deletions detectable by DNA studies, and 60% have maternal disomy for all or part of chromosome 15 (Mascari et al. 1992). PWS and Angelman syndrome (see above) are classical examples of *imprinting* (i.e. the different expression of a gene according to the sex of the transmitting parent). A gene for PWS was shown to be exclusively expressed when of paternal origin (Wevrick et al. 1994). Cases without chromosome 15 anomalies should be clinically reassessed and other conditions, such as the Smith–Magenis syndrome, considered (Greenberg et al. 1991). Patients with a deletion may be more typical than those without (Mattei et al. 1983), although atypical forms have been seen in patients with a demonstrated 15q deletion (Pauli et al. 1983, Schwartz et al. 1985, Miike et al. 1988). Butler et al. (1986) compared 21 children with deletion to 18 others with normal high-resolution karyotype. The differences between the two groups were only minor. Just over half the deletion patients (11/21) walked by 24 months, as compared to two thirds of the non-deletion cases. Deletion patients were also blonder than nondeletion children and all were blue-eyed as compared to only 13/18 nondeletion patients (Lee et al. 1994).

DIAGNOSIS
The clinical diagnosis of PWS is corroborated by typical DNA findings at FISH analysis for the Prader–Willi gene on chromosome 15.

Diagnosis in the neonatal period should be considered in infants with low birthweight, marked hypotonia, swallowing difficulties requiring tube feeding, and dysmorphism. In older patients, obesity and an abnormal facies are suggestive. The differential diagnosis of PWS includes neuromuscular diseases and hypotonia due to cerebral disorders. Congenital muscular dystrophy, neonatal myotonic dystrophy and congenital myopathies

are serious considerations. The dysmorphism, however, favours PWS, as does the prominent place of sucking and swallowing difficulties without significant respiratory impairment. Other causes of hypotonia of cerebral origin can raise a problem in older patients. Muscle biopsy (which should be avoided), serum creatine-kinase level and EMG are all normal.

Cohen syndrome (Norio et al. 1984) may mimic PWS and is transmitted as an autosomal recessive trait. Ophthalmological signs (choroidoretinal dystrophy, optic atrophy when present) are of great diagnostic significance. Teeth abnormalities may be suggestive.

There may be relatively wide clinical variation across cases, including milder forms. Many children may not have a severe learning disorder. This means that the diagnosis of PWS should be considered for all 'extremely fat and hungry' children who show features of the behavioural phenotype.

CLINICAL FEATURES
The clinical features of the syndrome are highly suggestive, especially in the neonatal period, and in patients seen later, typical neonatal history is extremely useful for the diagnosis. Newborn infants with PWS are generally born at term but are small for gestational age. Thirty per cent are born by the breech. They demonstrate from birth a profound muscular hypotonia, so that a diagnosis of muscle disease is often entertained. Swallowing difficulties necessitate tube feeding for two to five weeks. The dysmorphic appearance is sufficient for a karyotype to be requested in virtually all cases (Stephenson 1980). Later on, the clinical picture changes. The most striking feature is the hyperphagia and obesity that develop in most children towards the end of the second year of life. At a late stage, there is marked obesity, persistent hypotonia and often proximal weakness and relatively mild mental retardation, with an average IQ of 65 (Butler et al. 1986), although up to 10% of adult patients may have an IQ within the normal range (Clarke et al. 1989, Greenswag 1987). Hypogenitalism, often with cryptorchidism, and short stature and notable smallness of the face, nose, ears, hands and feet are also frequent features (Holm et al. 1993). There is often a characteristic facies with a small, 'round' head and almond-shaped eyes.

Adults with PWS are short, overweight, cognitively impaired and emotionally labile. Many have kyphosis, scoliosis and osteoporosis. They have poor motor skills and hyperphagia (Greenswag 1987, Lee 2002), and a peculiar behavioural phenotype including 'skin-picking' and other obsessive–compulsive behaviours (Åkefeldt et al. 1991).

Atypical patients may have severe mental retardation (3%) or be cognitively normal. Occasional patients may not be obese, and in rare cases emaciation has been reported (Miike et al. 1988).

Recent studies have shown that mental retardation is not an invariable feature (Clarke et al. 1989) and that there are cases with microdeletions at 15q11 with all the characteristics of the syndrome except for mental retardation, short stature and small hands and feet (Åkefeldt et al. 1991). It now seems that PWS as originally described may be part of a wider phenotype involving a particular behavioural profile with onset in the first year of life.

As the child in the second or third year of life begins to grow fat, many parents often apply for help. By this time the child may be unusually docile and placid but have occasional episodes of irritability, and extremely severe and destructive temper tantrums. The tantrums are usually immediately followed by the 'baseline' hypoactivity and remorse. Recent studies have suggested that the obsessive–compulsive behaviours are sometimes strikingly reminiscent of autism spectrum disorders, but controlled studies have failed to document a higher than expected rate of diagnosable autism spectrum disorder when the level of overall learning disability is taken into account (Descheemaeker et al. 2006).

The majority of children with PWS exhibit the strange habit of picking their skin and inflicting wounds, bruises and scratches. Most children with the syndrome are bulimic during exacerbations. They will go to any ends to gain access to food in the fridge, freezer or pantry. Almost all parents have had to install lock mechanisms to limit the amount of food otherwise bolted by the child. Even in scientific investigations, their inability to stop eating (in an experimental setting) has been amply demonstrated.

MANAGEMENT

Parents need to be informed about the nature of their child's condition. Oral and written information is essential in all cases. The parents have frequently been blamed by doctors, dietitians and psychologists (and by themselves) for the child's extreme obesity. The associated behavioural problems often lead to referral to a child psychiatric service. Without a proper diagnosis there is a great risk that counselling may focus on child-rearing practices, with the underlying implication that they might be at the root of the child's problems. Informing the parents about the almost identical behaviour problems encountered in other children with PWS often has very positive psychological consequences. For the family to belong to a national or local Prader–Willi support group is almost always valuable.

The parents may need to be advised (although most will have already found out for themselves) about locking fridges, cupboards, etc. With a very strict attitude on the part of parents and staff at school, it is sometimes feasible to make the child lose weight and even to achieve normal weight. However, maintaining this strict regime is by no means easy and the family who cannot cope with all the restrictions is not to be blamed. Various diets and drug treatments including fenfluramine have been tried in PWS in attempts to reduce weight (and the unusually high level of cerebrospinal fluid serotonin), but the long-term effects, if any, remain to be demonstrated.

For the past 10 years, growth hormone therapy has been launched as an essential component of a comprehensive intervention programme for children and adults with PWS. It leads to increased growth and possibly to some improvement in various mental capacities. However, concerns have been raised that there might be important (and sometimes dangerous) side effects in some individuals, meaning that growth hormone therapy should be prescribed and followed-up only by expert clinicians working in the field.

TABLE 4.4
Diagnostic criteria for Rett syndrome*

Necessary criteria

Apparently normal prenatal and perinatal period

Apparently normal psychomotor development through the first 6 months[1]

Normal head circumference at birth

Deceleration of head growth between ages 5 months and 4 years

Loss of acquired purposeful hand skills between ages 6 and 30 months, temporally associated with communication dysfunction and social withdrawal

Development of severely impaired expressive and receptive language, and presence of severe psychomotor retardation

Stereotypic hand movements such as hand wringing/squeezing, clapping/tapping, mouthing and 'washing'/rubbing automatisms appearing after loss of purposeful hand use

Mouthing and buccal stereotypies (tooth grinding)

Appearance of gait apraxia and truncal apraxia/ataxia between 1 and 4 years of age

Diagnosis tentative until 2–5 years of age[2]

Supportive criteria

Breathing dysfunction

EEG abnormalities

Seizures

Spasticity often associated with development of muscle wasting and dystonia

Peripheral vasomotor disturbances

Kyphoscoliosis

Growth retardation

Hypotrophic small feet

Exclusion criteria

Evidence of intrauterine growth retardation

Organomegaly or other signs of storage disease

Retinopathy or optic atrophy

Microcephaly at birth

Evidence of perinatally acquired brain damage

Existence of identifiable progressive disorder

Acquired neurological disorders due to infection or trauma

*From the Rett Syndrome Diagnostic Criteria Work Group (1988).
[1]Development may appear slightly slow from birth.
[2]Early diagnosis may be possible (<1 year in some cases).

RETT SYNDROME COMPLEX

Rett syndrome is a curious disorder of neurodevelopment that shows features that would suggest either autism or a neurodegenerative disorder, but in fact is neither. Rett syndrome is a characteristic cluster of clinical manifestations that includes early psychomotor regression with autistic features, purposeful use of the hands which is replaced by stereotypic activity, ataxia and apraxia of gait, and acquired microcephaly (Hagberg 1989). Table 4.4 shows the internationally accepted criteria for the diagnosis (Rett Syndrome Diagnostic Criteria Work Group 1988, Trevathan and Naidu 1988). The syndrome is observed almost exclusively in girls, with few exceptions (Zoghbi 1988, Hagberg 1989).

PREVALENCE

The prevalence of Rett syndrome as reported in Sweden and in western Scotland is 1 in 10,000 to 1 in 18,000 girls (Kerr and Stephenson 1985, Hagberg 1993, Bienvenu et al. 2006).

PATHOGENESIS

Rett syndrome is associated with a mutation of the *MECP2* gene in about 80% of cases, and it has long been assumed that this mutated gene is *the* cause of Rett syndrome. However, the phenotypic spectrum of *MECP2* mutations is broad and includes mental retardation with or without seizures, Angelman syndrome-like phenotype, and autism (Zoghbi 2005). At least a second gene (*CDKL5*) is associated with the convulsive variant (see below). The *MECP2* gene is a transcription factor inhibitor that can silence several genes that may be important in brain development and also acts on overall body development as it is expressed in many cell types and organs. Therefore, it seems possible that the *MECP2* gene mutation in Rett syndrome is part of a cascade of events involved in a number of neurodevelopmental X-linked disorders.

Rett syndrome now appears to be a developmental rather than a degenerative disorder (Naidu 1997). Structural brain abnormalities are mild, including a small brain with densely packed neurons and a decrease in cell processes. It is not, in the vast majority of cases, an hereditary condition even though the exclusive involvement of girls suggests a genetic origin.

CLINICAL FEATURES

The course of Rett syndrome is remarkable. The disorder initially presents as a progressive condition with a more or less rapid deterioration with loss of previously acquired skills.

The course can be divided into four stages (Table 4.5). The onset of clinical manifestations is between 6 months and 3 years, most cases becoming manifest before 18 months of age. Initial development may be entirely normal but affected girls are often somewhat hypotonic from birth and have a mildly slowed development (Einspieler et al. 2005).

Most girls with Rett syndrome show normal or near-normal development up to the age of 6–16 months. Mild hypotonia and minor developmental delay are often noted retrospectively. Acquisition of purposeful use of the hands is a prerequisite for the diagnosis. Many then stagnate or rapidly begin to lose skills (social smile, interaction and some language skills might be lost). Loss of hand use is a major feature. It is often rapid over a few weeks and may be 'explosive' in a few days. Some, but not all, become aloof, emotionally detached and are described as 'autistic'. Others slowly develop an emotionally stunted style of social interaction that may eventually also be described as autistic. A few are affected with attacks of rage, anxiety, confusion and chaotic hyperactivity. If there is an autistic or autistic-like phase, this may last from one month to several years. Usually by school age – or at least by puberty – the autistic symptoms begin to subside, although this does not happen in all cases. The available evidence shows that the same type of development applies in most people with autism almost regardless of underlying cause.

Girls with Rett syndrome show a variety of hand stereotypies, most of which involve 'midline procedures', i.e. both hands are 'washed' or clapped in the midline, put together into the mouth, or used to slap the forehead or neck in the midline. At an early stage some patients may show more typical 'autism-type' hand-flapping stereotypies.

TABLE 4.5
Rett syndrome: staging*

Stage	Clinical features
Early onset deceleration stage	
Onset 6–18 months	Developmental stagnation
Duration: months	Deceleration of head growth
	Disinterest in play
	Hypotonia
Rapid 'destructive' stage	
Onset: 1–3 years	Rapid regression with irritability
Duration: weeks to months	Loss of purposeful hand use
	Hand stereotypies
	Autistic manifestations
	Loss of language
Pseudostationary stage	
Onset: 2–10 years	Severe mental retardation
Duration: years	Improvement of autistic features
	Seizures
	Hand stereotypies
	Ataxia/apraxia
	Scoliosis
	Respiratory disturbances
Late motor deterioration	
Onset: after 10 years	Combined upper and lower
Duration: years	motor neuron signs
	Progressive scoliosis
	Decreasing mobility, eventually
	wheelchair-dependent
	Trophic disturbances of feet and hands
	Reduced seizure frequency

*Adapted from Hagberg and Witt-Engerström (1986).

Some affected girls are reported to laugh in the middle of the night. This occurs in a number of neurometabolic/neurological disorders affecting the brain (e.g. the Sanfilippo variant of mucopolysaccharidosis) and in many girls with autism who do not have Rett syndrome.

Bruxism and hyperventilation are common features in Rett syndrome and are sometimes interpreted as signs of extreme anxiety, a notion for which there is generally no empirical support.

The third stage of the disease is marked by the slow appearance of neurological signs such as pyramidal tract signs. Epileptic seizures appear in two thirds to three quarters of cases at this stage. They are often preceded by EEG abnormalities that include a suggestive rhythmic fronto-central theta activity, paroxysmal features (spikes or spike–waves) often posteriorly located, bursts of slow spike–waves especially during sleep, and a progressive slowing and deterioration of background tracing (Niedermeyer et al. 1986, Glaze et al. 1987).

Hyperventilation with intervening respiratory pauses is a frequent finding and it may be responsible for episodes of syncope often mistaken for epileptic seizures. Between two thirds and three quarters of patients do not acquire independent ambulation, and with the progression of the fourth stage of the disease ambulation is ultimately lost in most patients (Hagberg 1989). Growth failure is present in most cases (Fig. 4.5). Kyphoscoliosis is extremely common and is one of the major complications of the syndrome. No consistent laboratory marker has been found. The hyperammonaemia initially reported is found only in rare cases

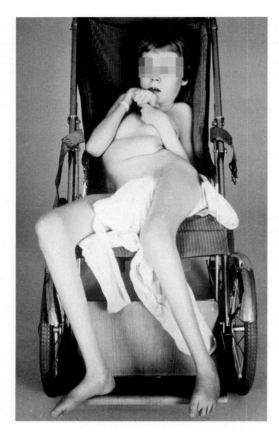

Fig. 4.5. Rett syndrome in a 15-year-old girl. Note characteristic hand stereotypies, marked scoliosis and atrophy of lower limbs. (Courtesy Prof. B Hagberg, Östrasjukhuset, Göteborg.)

and usually due to external factors such as valproate treatment.

MRI shows a diminished cerebral volume, predominantly at the expense of white matter, reduced volume of the caudate and midbrain and a normal gyration (Reiss et al. 1993).

RETT SYNDROME VARIANTS
The phenotype of girls with Rett syndrome is broad, from the congenital form with almost complete absence of neurodevelopment to mild forms that can be compatible with ambulation or even speech (Huppke et al. 2003). Hagberg and Skjeldal (1994) recognize: 'formes frustes' with mild but typical features; a severe congenital form in which almost no neurodevelopment is observed; milder forms with late childhood regression; formes frustes with a broad range of manifestations; and preserved speech variants. In this last form, the girls may have a vocabulary of from 20 to several hundred words, and some speak in long – usually echolalic – sentences (Zappella et al. 1998, 2001). A form presenting many features of Angelman syndrome is also described (Hitchins et al. 2004). The *convulsive variant* is characterized by an early onset of seizures in the form of infantile spasms that may be preceded by other types of tonic or focal seizures and are resistant to treatment. This form has been shown to be due to mutations in the *CDKL5* gene (Weaving et al. 2004). However, mutations in this gene are not consistently found in such cases;

conversely, not all cases of CDKL5 mutations exhibit Rett-like features. These were present in only 1 out of 7 patients with this mutation, all with infantile spasms and severe retardation (Archer et al. 2006). Rare cases of typical Rett syndrome in boys are on record (Matsuyama et al. 2005). Boys carrying the mutation more often present with neonatal encephalopathy without typical features (Moog et al. 2006).

DIAGNOSIS
The diagnosis of Rett syndrome is still made on history and clinical grounds, but the demonstration of the presence of a mutated *MECP2* gene is seen as corroborating evidence in many cases (Huppke and Gartner 2005).

The diagnostic criteria of Rett syndrome are detailed in Table 4.4. Many girls with Rett syndrome in the early stages of the disorder show several autistic features without clear-cut neurological signs. Therefore, the diagnosis of autism is commonly made in patients under 3 years of age. The diagnosis of Rett syndrome should be considered in all very young girls presenting with autistic symptoms. In one study, 80% of girls with Rett syndrome had initially been suspected of suffering from autism or autistic features (Witt-Engerström and Gillberg 1987), and on the basis of available prevalence estimates for Rett syndrome and autism it was estimated that of all girls presenting in the first few years of life with autistic symptoms, one third to one half will eventually turn out to have Rett syndrome. An occasional child with Rett syndrome runs an unusually slow course. In such cases, the diagnosis of 'pure autism' with severe/moderate mental retardation can be retained for many years.

In the frequent atypical forms (Goutières and Aicardi 1985), the lack of a reliable marker should prevent definite inclusion in many cases. The possible coexistence of Rett syndrome and mental retardation in siblings suggests the possibility of a wide spectrum of manifestations, but confirmation by a definitive test is required (Huppke et al. 2003). Hagberg and Skjeldal (1994) have presented tentative diagnostic criteria for such Rett syndrome variant cases (Table 4.6).

DIFFERENTIAL DIAGNOSIS
The main differential diagnosis is with the autism syndromes (Chapter 24). The infantile type of ceroid–lipofuscinosis with the 'knitting hand movements' described by Santavuori and colleagues may resemble Rett syndrome but is rare outside Finland (Santavuori et al. 1973, Santavuori 1988). Ornithine transcarbamylase deficiency has also been mistaken for Rett syndrome. Angelman syndrome may resemble Rett syndrome because of the jerky ataxia observed in both conditions in addition to autistic features, mental retardation and seizures. Chromosomal studies permit differentiation in difficult cases.

Children who show symptoms in the borderland of Rett syndrome and autism (Gillberg 1989) including the so-called 'forme fruste' and 'preserved speech' variants (Hagberg and Rasmussen 1986) show many of the features of classical Rett syndrome but do not fulfil all the criteria; they usually also meet most, or all, of the criteria for autistic disorder (or infantile autism). Some girls

TABLE 4.6
Diagnostic* and exclusion** criteria for Rett syndrome (RS) variant cases

Inclusion criteria

A girl of at least 10 years of age with mental retardation of unexplained origin and with at least three of the six following primary criteria:

A1 Loss of (partial or subtotal) acquired fine finger skill in late infancy/early childhood

A2 Loss of acquired single words/phrases/modulated babble

A3 RS hand stereotypies, hands together or apart

A4 Early deviant communicative ability

A5 Deceleration of head growth of 2 SD (even when still within normal limits)

A6 The RS disease profile: a regression period (stage II) followed by a certain recovery of contact and communication (stage III) in contrast to slow neuromotor regression through school age and adolescence

and, in addition, at least 5 of the following 11 supportive manifestations:

B1 Breathing irregularities (hyperventilation and/or breath-holding)

B2 Bloating/marked air swallowing

B3 Characteristic RS teeth grinding

B4 Gait dyspraxia

B5 Neurogenic scoliosis or high kyphosis (ambulant girls)

B6 Development of abnormal lower limb neurology

B7 Small blue/cold impaired feet, autonomic/trophic dysfunction

B8 Characteristic RS EEG development

B9 Unprompted sudden laughing/screaming spells

B10 Impaired/delayed nociception

B11 Intensive eye communication, 'eye pointing'

Exclusion criteria

Evidence of intrauterine growth retardation

Organomegaly or other signs of storage disease

Retinopathy or optic atrophy

Microcephaly at birth

Evidence of perinatally acquired brain damage

Existence of identifiable metabolic or other progressive neurological disorder

Acquired neurological disorders resulting from severe infections or head trauma

*Hagberg and Skjeldal (1994).
**Rett Syndrome Diagnostic Criteria Work Group (1988).

---

show the classical symptoms of autism only after a prolonged premorbid (or stage I) period of the disorder. Rett-like symptoms also occur in conjunction with other neurological disorders such as Moebius syndrome (Gillberg and Steffenburg 1989) and mucopolysaccharidosis.

TREATMENT AND MANAGEMENT

Treatment of Rett syndrome is unsatisfactory. Bromocriptine and naloxone have been tried without convincing results. Physical therapy and careful attention to details of everyday life are essential.

Stimulation should be provided to affected girls who respond well following the early period of withdrawal. Orthopaedic management to avoid or limit the development of scoliosis is a major part of the care of Rett patients.

Management of the behavioural/psychiatric problems encountered in Rett syndrome requires knowledge of the natural course of the disorder so that symptoms such as autism and night laughter are not inappropriately interpreted as signalling specific psychological or interactional problems. The degree of language comprehension is extremely low in Rett syndrome. Communication should be achieved by other means such as through eye gaze and manual prompting. Some degree of hand function can often be maintained if both hands are trained separately for long periods of time every day.

Pharmacologically, some worthwhile results with bromocriptine (20 mg/kg/day) have been reported (Zappella et al. 1990), but confirmatory double-blind placebo-controlled studies are needed. Naloxone has also been tried, with conflicting results.

OUTCOME

The ultimate course of Rett syndrome is only partially known. The life span is relatively preserved, some individuals reaching the age of 80 or more. The vast majority of patients – possibly all – become extremely mentally and/or neurologically impaired and remain dependent on other people for virtually all matters in everyday life. Epilepsy, constipation, scoliosis, progressive motor (and vasomotor) control problems complicate the clinical picture in a majority of cases. The psychiatric/behavioural problems can be frustrating through childhood and, sometimes, adolescence, but usually cause less concern in the adult age group.

RUBINSTEIN–TAYBI SYNDROME

Rubinstein–Taybi is a contiguous gene syndrome with a variable clinical expression. It is due in most cases to an interstitial deletion of 16p13.3. The deletion involves the 3′ end of the *CREB* gene, an activator of the CREB-binding protein. In addition to the dysmorphism, this results in failure to thrive and abnormal sensitivity to infections (Bartsch et al. 2006).

The syndrome is mainly characterized by the presence of broad thumbs and great toes, short stature, a peculiar facies, microcephaly and mental retardation. IQs range from 17 to 86 (Jones 1988). The palpebral fissures slant downwards, the maxilla is hypoplastic, and the nose is beaked with a nasal septum extending below the alae nasi. Epicanthal folds, strabismus and refractive errors are frequent (Fig. 4.6). There is an excess dermal ridge patterning in thenar and first interdigital areas of the palm. Pulmonary stenosis, large foramen magnum, vertebral anomalies and parietal foramina have been reported. There is a wide range of variability among affected individuals (Padfield et al. 1968). The incidence of this syndrome is probably underestimated (Sammito et al. 1988). Most cases are sporadic. Dominant transmission has been reported, and several sets of concordant monozygotic twins are on record. Breuning et al. (1993) found submicroscopic deletions of 16p13 in 25% of cases.

SEX CHROMOSOME ANEUPLOIDIES

Most cases of sex chromosome aneuploidies (which occur in about 0.3% of all live births) have an increased risk of psychiatric disorders. Conversely, sex chromosome aneuploidies are relatively common in child psychiatric clinic attenders. In one study (Crandall et al. 1972), 1.6% of children referred to a child psychiatry clinic had sex chromosome aneuploidies.

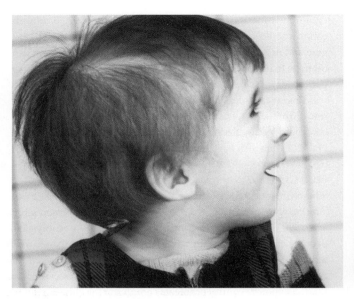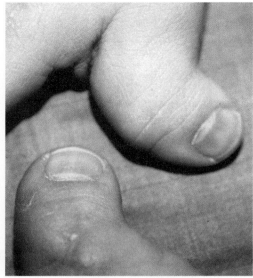

Fig. 4.6. Rubinstein–Taybi syndrome: *(left)* typical facies; *(right)* broad, abnormally oriented thumbs. (Courtesy Dr M Le Merrer, Hôpital des Enfants Malades, Paris.)

These abnormalities are associated with a slightly increased risk of mental retardation. For example, Ratcliffe et al. (1994) found an XXY chromosome complement in 5.4 per 1000 phenotypic boys in institutions for people with mental retardation and that the mean IQ of such children was slightly lower than that of controls. The mean IQ of girls with three X chromosomes was 86.8, that of XXY boys 91.4, and that of XYY boys 101.7, all significantly lower than IQs of controls (109.1 and 115.8 for girls and boys respectively). They also found that head circumference was smaller in the group with excess sex chromosomes, even at birth, implying an effect of extra gonosomes on brain growth pre- and postnatally. An XXX complement has been found in 4.3 per 1000 institutionalized phenotypic girls (Pennington et al. 1980). The mean IQ of XO (Turner syndrome) girls is normal, but many XO females do exhibit right–left disorientation and defects in perceptual organization, and their verbal IQ tends to be higher than the performance IQ but with considerable interindividual variation (Temple and Carney 1993).

More severe mental retardation is probably more common in patients with more complex anomalies such as phenotypic males with three or more X chromosomes (Zaleski et al. 1966), or with duplication of both X and Y chromosomes (Schlegel et al. 1965). However, the main abnormalities encountered in such children are learning and perceptual disorders and behavioural difficulties (Bender et al. 1983, Ratcliffe et al. 1994).

XYY SYNDROME
Boys with an extra Y chromosome (about 0.1% in the general male population) are at much increased risk of delay and other problems in language development and of temper tantrums and aggressiveness. They also often show hypotonia, and early-onset attention deficits and hyperactivity. Temper tantrums are frequent in early childhood. Poor sociability is a common feature, and the

risk of autism appears to be increased (Hagerman 1989). IQ is usually in the normal range, but learning disorders are very common and the incidence of mental retardation is possibly increased as compared with the general male population. A slightly increased tendency to aggressiveness and features of sadism in sexual orientation in adult life is suggested by at least one unbiased prospective study (Schiavi et al. 1988). The majority are tall and proportionate with regard to leg and head size. Affected individuals are usually at least 13 cm taller than their fathers. There is a need to consider XYY in all tall boys with behavioural and learning disorders.

XXY SYNDROME (KLINEFELTER SYNDROME)
Boys with one or more extra X chromosomes (around 0.1–0.2% of all live-born males) are collectively referred to as having Klinefelter syndrome (Lanfranco et al. 2004). About two thirds of all cases are 47,XXY. Height, weight and head circumference are small at birth. From about 2–4 years of age there is increased growth velocity, particularly with regard to leg length. Mean adult height is on average 13 cm more than paternal height. Head size does not show catch-up. It appears that the extra X chromosome inhibits brain growth in utero. Boys with Klinefelter syndrome usually have a relatively low verbal IQ even though full-scale IQ is often in the normal (or slightly subnormal) range (IQs are usually reported to be in the 60–130 range). Speech and language is delayed, and the vast majority receive speech and language therapy long before a chromosomal diagnosis has been made. Affected boys are often described as clumsy and show many of the problems typical of children with DAMP (deficits in attention, motor control and perception), sometimes with a tendency towards hypoactivity. These problems may be enhanced by abnormal body build and neuromotor performance. Reading and writing disorders are often severe and out of keeping with the general IQ

level. Brain imaging findings (MRI) of preferentially affected frontal, temporal and motor regions and relative sparing of parietal regions are consistent with observed cognitive and behavioural strengths and weaknesses in XXY subjects (Giedd et al. 2007).

From middle childhood the legs of affected individuals tend to be long, and arm span often exceeds height. The penis may or may not be small, and the testicles are almost always small with failed sperm production. Many develop breast enlargement, and the incidence of breast cancer is increased as compared with normal males. They are often described as timid and with poor self-confidence. Most have mild/moderate social interaction problems, and tend to withdraw from group activities. A small number have autism. One prospective study suggests that in adult life they may be less sexually active and more submissive in sexual orientation than other men (Schiavi et al. 1988).

Testosterone treatment should be started in pre-puberty and monitored by endocrine specialists with expertise in Klinefelter syndrome. Intracytoplasmic sperm injection offers an opportunity for procreation even when there are no spermatozoa in the ejaculate. In a substantial number of azoospermic patients, spermatozoa can be extracted from testicular biopsy samples, and pregnancies and livebirths have been achieved (Lanfranco et al. 2004).

X0 SYNDROME (45X0 SYNDROME, TURNER SYNDROME)

The majority of 45X0 individuals may be recognized at birth because of the characteristic oedema of the dorsum of their hands and feet and the webbing of the neck. In addition, they are often born preterm with low birthweight and short stature. Girls with this syndrome have a low rate of psychiatric disorder. IQ is usually normal, but performance IQ shows a downward shift. About 10% have some degree of mental retardation. Visuospatial skills are often particularly poor, and this tends to affect mathematical skills. On the WISC-R, the results on the Block Design and Object Assembly subtests are usually poor. Many individuals with XO syndrome are hyperactive in early childhood but tend to be hypoactive from adolescence (Swillen et al. 1993). An association of X0 syndrome with anorexia nervosa (particularly in X0 mosaicism) has been suggested, but a recent systematic chromosome study including a population sample did not support this (Råstam et al. 1991). After adolescence, subjects are of short stature and have infantile external and internal genitalia. Replacement therapy with oestrogen is essential but there is, as yet, no consensus as to the optimal age to initiate such treatment. Many women with Turner syndrome marry and lead well-adjusted lives in adulthood. Individuals with Turner syndrome who have inherited their X chromosome from their mother tend to have more social interaction problems than those whose X chromosome is paternally derived (Skuse et al. 1997).

XXX SYNDROME

Girls with triple X syndrome constitute 0.1% of all live-born females. They are at much increased risk of language and learning disorders (with a need for special education in most cases, and IQs in the low-normal range); however, reading and writing disorders tend to correspond to the general level of IQ), shyness, immaturity and conduct problems of various kinds (Linden et al. 1988). They are tall and have poorly coordinated movements. This, in connection with their odd behaviour and conduct problems, leads to a high rate of referral for institutional treatment.

SMITH–LEMLI–OPITZ SYNDROME

This uncommon disorder has recently come to the forefront of neurologists' and psychiatrists' attention because of its striking association with autistic features. It is possibly the genetic disorder with the strongest link of all to autistic symptomatology (see below).

Smith–Lemli–Opitz syndrome (SLOS) has been reported to occur in about 1 in 70,000 live births. There is a high perinatal mortality and stillbirth rate. Among survivors, at least 80% have severe impairments, while the remainder have a much milder phenotype.

SLOS is still diagnosed on the basis of the typical clinical presentation of the disorder. However, it is caused by an inborn error of post-squalene cholesterol biosynthesis. Deficient cholesterol synthesis in SLOS is caused by inherited mutations of the 3–β-hydroxysterol-δ-7 reductase gene (*DHCR7*). DHCR7 deficiency impairs both cholesterol and desmosterol production, resulting in elevated 7DHC/8DHC levels, typically decreased cholesterol levels and, importantly, developmental dysmorphology. The discovery of SLOS has led to new questions regarding the role of the cholesterol biosynthesis pathway in human development. To date, a total of 121 different mutations have been identified in over 250 patients with SLOS who represent a continuum of clinical severity. Two genetic mouse models have been generated which recapitulate some of the developmental abnormalities of SLOS and have been useful in elucidating the pathogenesis.

The most striking features of the syndrome, in addition to mental retardation, autism and other behavioural impairments, and marked hypotonia, are a peculiar facies with a high, square forehead, anteverted nostrils and micrognathia, and genital abnormalities in males including cryptorchidism and/or hypospadias and, in extreme instances, a complete failure of development of male genitalia despite a normal XY karyotype (Scarbrough et al. 1986). Other features include abnormal auricles, ptosis of the eyelids, inner epicanthal folds, transverse palmar crease, and various limb and visceral abnormalities (Opitz et al. 1994).

Seizures are present in some patients, and feeding problems may be considerable. Mortality is high during the first year of life. Brain abnormalities may include micrencephaly, hypoplasia of the frontal lobes, abnormal gyration and cerebellar hypoplasia. The most severely affected cases are sometimes separated from the rest as type II SLOS (Curry et al. 1987).

The syndrome is inherited as an autosomal recessive trait. The apparently increased frequency in males is probably related to the fact that diagnosis is easier in males because of the obvious genital abnormalities.

Plasma cholesterol concentrations are very low, while 7-dehydrocholesterol is raised, suggesting a defect in the enzyme that reduces the C-7,8 double bond in the latter compound (Tint et al. 1994). Survival correlates strongly with higher plasma cholesterol levels (Tint et al. 1995). Prenatal diagnosis by measurement of 7-dehydrocholesterol in amniotic fluid is possible (Dallaire et al. 1995). A high-cholesterol regime can normalize the level of cholesterol but is not necessarily clinically effective (Ullrich et al. 1996).

Autism spectrum disorders have consistently been reported to be common in SLOS (Gillberg and Coleman 2000, Tierney et al. 2001, Sikora et al. 2006). These findings and the report of low levels of cholesterol in a relatively large sample of cases of familial autism suggest that disorders of sterol metabolism may be important in a subset of individuals with the behavioural syndrome of autism, and that, at least theoretically, cholesterol 'therapy' might be indicated in cases with autism and low cholesterol levels.

SMITH–MAGENIS SYNDROME

This rare syndrome presents with a highly characteristic behavioural phenotype. It is caused by an interstitial deletion of chromosome 17p11.2 (Greenberg et al. 1991, 1996). Rare cases without deletion are associated with de novo mutations in the *RAI1* gene (Slager et al. 2003, Girirajan et al. 2005, Bi et al. 2006). Affected individuals are delayed in overall development and usually test in the moderately mentally retarded range (although some are only mildly mentally retarded). The majority have brachycephaly, midface hypoplasia, ear malformations and brachydactyly. Otolaryngological abnormalities are present in almost all patients, and eye abnormalities in 85%; other visceral anomalies may also occur (Greenberg et al. 1996). Sleep is reduced in three quarters of patients, with an inversion of the circadian rhythm of melatonin secretion (De Leersnyder et al. 2001a) raising a major problem. There are major behaviour problems in most cases, with aggressive and self-mutilatory symptoms (including onychotillomania and insertion of foreign objects into various body orifices). Head banging, hand biting and another stereotypic behaviour, unusual in other conditions, of hand or arm clasping, now sometimes referred to as 'spasmodic upper body squeeze' or 'self-hugging' (Finucane et al. 1994), are all characteristic of the syndrome. This behaviour, a major clinical clue to the diagnosis, and one which should prompt chromosomal analysis, is often elicited in a familiar setting when the patient is relaxed and in a good mood. The history is important in that it is quite uncommon for this type of behaviour to be readily observable in a clinic setting. Most affected individuals are affectionate and have a positive affective tone in spite of the outbursts of aggression and self-mutilation.

Sleep problems and behaviour in Smith–Magenis syndrome were found to be improved in nine patients with the use of beta-1 adrenergic antagonists (De Leersnyder et al. 2001b).

SOTOS SYNDROME

This disorder is characterized by cerebral gigantism and rapid body growth. The vast majority of patients have behaviour and learning disorders (Tatton-Brown et al. 2005).

Sotos syndrome is uncommon, but so far there have been no reliable estimates of incidence. It may not be very rare in children who present with behaviour and learning problems and who, in addition, have large body size.

Cole and Hughes (1991) have presented the following diagnostic criteria: (a) a distinctive facies with macrocephalus, a prominent jaw, antimongoloid slant and hypertelorism; (b) a period of accelerated growth in early childhood; (c) advanced bone age during development; and (d) early developmental delay. At adolescence, growth rate may be normal.

Cases of Sotos syndrome are almost always sporadic, although there is evidence for dominant transmission in several cases (Bale et al. 1985). Under this hypothesis, most cases would represent new mutations. The mechanism of excessive growth is thought to be centrally determined but no precise data are available. Other abnormalities such as deletion 10p13–14 or 17p13 have also been observed (Punnett and Zakai 1990).

The syndrome commonly features mental retardation (83%), the IQ of affected individuals varying from 18 to 119 with a mean of 72 (Jones 1988, Cole and Hughes 1994). The most striking feature is the excessively rapid somatic growth that begins before birth and is associated with advanced osseous maturation and with features reminiscent of acromegaly in adults (Sotos et al. 1977). Growth is especially fast during the first two or three years of life but then slows down so that the ultimate size may not always be outside the normal range (Cole and Hughes 1994). Even patients with a normal mental level usually have delay in expressive language and motor development (Bale et al. 1985). Low frustration tolerance, irritability, impulsive and violent behaviours, destructiveness and poor peer relationships are common problems. ADHD is present in about one third of all young children (Finegan et al. 1994), and autistic disorder appears to be overrepresented (Morrow et al. 1990, Zappella 1990).

Neurological features may include seizures and strabismus. There is macrocephaly with mild dilatation of the lateral ventricles. Pigmentary abnormalities and intestinal polyps have been reported (Ruvalcaba et al. 1980) but may indicate a different syndrome.

TUBEROUS SCLEROSIS COMPLEX (TSC)

There are at least two variants of tuberous sclerosis complex (once referred to as Bourneville's disease), corresponding to genetic defects on chromosome 16 (the most common variant) and chromosome 9. The condition is described in Chapter 3 and only the neuropsychiatric manifestations are briefly mentioned here.

At least half of all children with tuberous sclerosis diagnosed before age 3 years have autism and the majority of these also meet full diagnostic criteria for impairing ADHD (of the combined type). Patients with tuberous sclerosis presenting with major symptoms before age 2 years have autism or autistic features with severe hyperactivity (Hunt and Dennis 1987, Ahlsén et al. 1994). The triad of mental retardation, epilepsy and autism – rather than

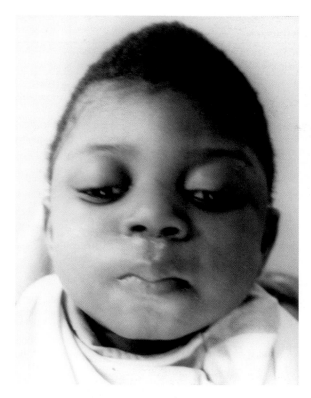

Fig. 5.4. Oxycephaly resulting from premature closure of both the coronal and sagittal sutures. (Courtesy Dr D Renier, Prof. J-F Hirsch, Hôpital des Enfants Malades, Paris.)

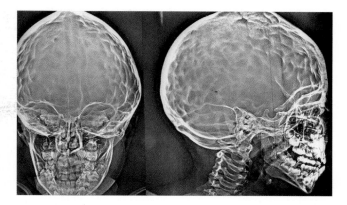

Fig. 5.5. Microcephalic synostosis (X-rays). All sutures are closed. Bones of the cranial vault are thin and digital markings are prominent. Venous sinuses are deeply grooved in bone. (7-year-old boy with intracranial hypertension and papilloedema. Two siblings were simultaneously affected. All had normal intelligence.)

DIAGNOSIS

The radiological signs of craniosynostoses (Aviv et al. 2004) include markedly increased digital markings that are especially prominent in cases with several sutures obliterated (Fig. 5.5). In sagittal synostosis, digital markings usually predominate in the frontal area bilaterally. Venous sinus grooves are deep and abnormally visible. The sella turcica may be greatly enlarged with erosion of the dorsum sellae. Such signs, which are present to some extent even in asymptomatic patients, indicate the presence of long-standing high ICP that can be confirmed by direct measurement. The sutures are not visible, and hyperostosis is present along their normal course. At an early stage, however, the suture lines may remain visible in part or in totality. In such cases, the diagnosis is suggested by the narrow and straight appearance of the affected suture lines and the densification of their margins.

The *differential diagnosis* of nonsyndromic craniosynostosis is usually easy as the skull deformities are fairly characteristic. Similarly misshapen skulls can exist in the absence of craniosynostosis, e.g. in secondary plagiocephaly due to positional stress in preterm or immobilized infants. In such cases no ridge is palpable over the involved sutures, and X-rays of the skull do not show digital markings or hyperdense or closed sutures. Plagiocephaly due to synostosis of one side of the coronal or lambdoid suture can be differentiated from that resulting from prolonged posturing by absence of the supraorbital ridge and obliquity of the eyebrow (Kane et al. 1996).

The diagnosis of hydrocephalus is sometimes wrongly suggested in patients with sagittal craniosynostosis because of the large head circumference.

Conversely, cases of primary microcephaly are not infrequently referred with a suggestion of craniosynostosis that is easily dismissed because of the usual presence of mental retardation and lack of radiological evidence of craniosynostosis.

The *prenatal diagnosis* of craniosynostosis is mainly by ultrasonography and determination of the overall shape of the head, and measurements especially of the skull diameters allow recognition of many types of synostosis. A list of signs specifically designed to facilitate sonographic recognition of several forms of synostosis is available (Petersen and Chitty 2004). In a search of the computerized database of the UCLH, those authors found that only a small minority of dubious cases (11 of 297) actually had a craniosynostosis. In families at risk, for whom a definite type has been diagnosed, invasive testing based on DNA analysis of villus samples or amniotic fluid is possible in a number of instances.

SYNDROMIC CRANIOSYNOSTOSES

Approximately 15–20% of the craniosynostoses occur in various syndromes, most of which are genetically determined. Comprehensive reviews of the syndromic craniosynostoses are available (Cohen 1986, 1988), and their clinical and genetic aspects have been reviewed in detail (Britto and Reardon 2004, Thompson and Britto 2004). Some of the most common syndromes are listed in Table 5.2. Such syndromes consist of multiple anomalies only one of which is the craniosynostosis. Within the same syndrome, the type of craniosynostosis present is not always the same nor the most important management consideration; abnormalities of the viscerocranium may be of more concern because of the respiratory, feeding or eye problems. The diagnosis should not rely mainly on determination of the sutures involved.

Crouzon syndrome and Apert syndrome each account for roughly one third of cases of syndromic craniosynostosis. The last

TABLE 5.2
Main syndromes with craniosynostosis

Syndrome	Main features	Proportion of cases with craniosynostosis	Genetics (gene location)	Reference
Crouzon	Hypoplasia of maxilla, shallow orbits, proptosis	Almost all	AD (10q25–q26, *FGFR2*)	Kreiborg (1981), Thompson and Britto (2004)
Apert type I acrocephalosyndactyly	Midface deficiency, proptosis, downslanting palpebral fissures, complete symmetrical syndactyly of hands and feet (digits II–IV)	Almost all; wide calvarial defect from root of nose to posterior fontanelle in infants	AD (10q25–q26, *FGFR2*) (most cases new mutations)	Cohen and Kreiborg (1990), Thompson and Britto (2004)
Pfeiffer (type V acrocephalosyndactyly)	Strabismus, proptosis, hypertelorism, broad thumbs and great toes, mild variable cutaneous anomalies, syndactyly of fingers and toes	All cases (coronal)	AD (8p11–12; *FGFR1* 10q25–26, *FGFR2*)	Cohen (1993a)
Saethre–Chotzen (type III acrocephalosyndactyly)	Facial asymmetry, low-set frontal hairline, ptosis, deviated nasal septum, variable syndactyly (esp. digits II–III); normal thumbs and great toes; parietal foramina	All cases (complex)	AD (7p21; *TWIST*)	Reardon and Winter (1994)
Carpenter (type V acrocephalosyndactyly)	Preaxial polydactyly of the feet, obesity, short stature, congenital heart defect, soft tissue syndactyly, brachymetaphalangy; mental retardation frequent	All cases (complex)	AR	Cohen et al. (1987), Taravath and Tonsgard (1993)
Baller–Gerold	Radial aplasia, radiohumeral synostosis, hypoplastic carpal bones	Common (coronal, lambdoid or metopic)	AR, AD (*TWIST*)	Gripp et al. (1999), Seto et al. (2001)
Cranio-fronto-nasal dysplasia	Brachycephaly, ocular hypertelorism, clefting of nasal tip, skeletal abnormalities, hand and foot involvement, median cleft in some; normal intelligence	Common (coronal)	AD or XD (10p11, ?Xpter-p22)	Slover and Sujansky (1979)
Chromosomal abnormalities and other rare syndromes	Variable		S (sometimes dominant)	

third consists of a miscellany of rare syndromes, some of them not yet definitely classified (Le Merrer et al. 1988, Lajeunie et al. 1995).

CROUZON SYNDROME

Crouzon syndrome follows an autosomal dominant mode of transmission. More than half of the 61 cases studied by Kreiborg (1981) represented new mutations, and the syndrome accounted for 3% of the 370 craniosynostosis patients of Hunter and Rudd (1977). Cohen and Kreiborg (1990) estimated that Crouzon and Apert syndomes account respectively for 4.8% and 4.5% of the cases of craniosynostosis at birth. The phenotype is variable even in the same lineage; mild cases are frequent, and the appearance of affected adults may be deceptively normal. Looking at early photographs of the parents may help recognize minimal involvement. The gene for Crouzon syndrome has been mapped to 10q25–q26 (Preston et al. 1994) and shown to code for fibroblast growth factor receptor 2 (FGFR2) (Jabs et al. 1994). Several mutations have been demonstrated (Reardon et al. 1994, Oldridge et al. 1995).

Hypoplasia of the maxilla with shallow orbit and proptosis are essential components of the syndrome. Craniosynostosis is constant, begins in the first year of life, and most frequently affects first the coronal sutures. Eventually, all sutures become involved, but the shape of the skull is variable from cloverleaf skull (Rohatgi 1991) to scaphocephaly. Protuberance of the skull in the region of the closed anterior fontanelle is frequent. A high degree of variability is found among Crouzon patients. Conductive hearing loss is common and should be tested for. No consistent abnormalities of viscera or extremities are present, but nasopharyngeal obstruction may lead to chronic respiratory insufficiency and cor pulmonale (Moore 1993). Seizures occurred in 12% of patients in Kreiborg's series, but mental retardation is rare (3%). Hydrocephalus is also rare (Marchac and Renier 1982), but high ICP is found in 37% of cases and chronic tonsillar herniation has been reported (Cinalli et al. 1995). Anomalies of the metacarpal and carpal bones reminiscent of those in Pfeiffer syndrome are frequent. Surgical treatment taking into account the multiple problems of the face, airway obstruction and feeding, gives favourable results if undertaken early.

APERT SYNDROME

Apert syndrome virtually always results from a new dominant mutation. The disorder is allelic to Crouzon disease and due to different mutations of the *FGFR2* gene (Wilkie et al. 1995). It is characterized by craniosynostosis, midfacial malformations and symmetrical syndactyly of the hands and feet, involving at least the second, third and fourth digits (Cohen 1986) (Fig. 5.6).

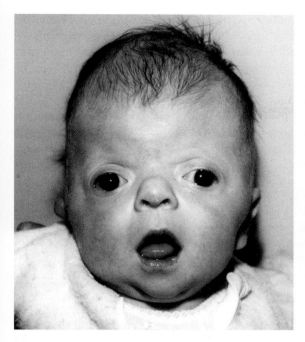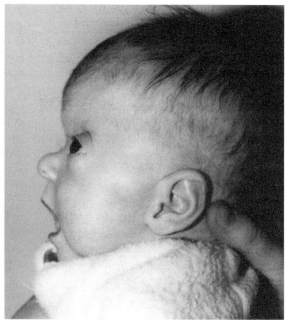

Fig. 5.6. Apert syndrome. There is hypoplasia of the maxillary bone, absence of supraorbital ridge and exophthalmos. (Courtesy Dr D Renier, Prof. J-F Hirsch, Hôpital des Enfants Malades, Paris.)

The coronal suture is usually affected early, resulting in a brachycephalic high skull, but the synostosis pattern is variable. A wide open calvarial defect extends from the root of the nose to the posterior fontanelle in infants, and closes before age 3 years with bulging of the skull. The anterior cranial fossa is short and the orbits are shallow. The intracranial volume is considerably greater than that of controls. Cleft palate is common. Mental retardation is very frequent and often severe. However, only half the patients in the series of Patton et al. (1988) were mentally retarded. Hydrocephalus is fairly common, and abnormalities, especially partial agenesis of the corpus callosum, are present in 12% of cases (Cohen and Kreiborg 1990). Fusion of the fifth and sixth cervical vertebrae is present in 70% of cases, and deafness and optic atrophy are frequent. Approximately 10% of patients have visceral abnormalities. The prognosis is poor even with modern reconstructive techniques, and may be even more severe when associated malformations such as cardiac abnormalities, scoliosis or microphthalmia are present.

OTHER SYNDROMIC CRANIOSYNOSTOSES (Table 5.2)
Saethre–Chotzen syndrome (de Heer et al. 2005) and *Pfeiffer syndrome* (Vanek and Losan 1982, Zankl et al. 2004) come next in frequency. The cognitive prognosis is often favourable but there is marked variability of both neurological and morphological features, at times with severe deformity.

In Saethre–Chotzen syndrome, a bicoronal craniosynostosis, frequently asymmetrical, is most common (Reardon and Winter 1994). Abnormalities of the face, eye (ptosis), external ears and fingers remain of a mild degree. The syndrome is predominantly familial with frequent minimal forms (Chun et al. 2002).

Pfeiffer syndrome, also an autosomal dominant disease, consists of the association of craniosynostosis (predominantly of the coronal suture) with characteristic limb abnormalities. These include broad, short thumbs and great toes, symphalangism of the fingers, and partial soft tissue syndactylies of the fingers and thumbs. Mild to moderate conductive hearing loss is frequent. Intelligence is usually normal. Three subgoups of different severity have been described (Cohen 1993b).

Many *minor craniosynostosis syndromes* have been described (Thompson and Britto 2004); currently at least 67 syndromes with craniosynostosis have been defined (Cohen 1986), and probably several more await delineation. Genetic counselling in such cases is obviously less precise, but 7 of 11 undiagnosed syndromic craniosynostoses reported by Le Merrer et al. (1988) had a positive family history, so that a high recurrence rate is likely.

MOLECULAR AND DEVELOPMENTAL ASPECTS OF SYNDROMIC CRANIOSYNOSTOSES
The genetic aspects of the syndromic craniosynostoses have received considerable attention in the past few years (Superti-Furga et al. 2001). Apert, Crouzon and Pfeiffer syndromes are all associated with mutations of the *FGFR2* gene. Pfeiffer syndrome may also be associated with mutation in the *FGFR1* gene. In all, 30 of the syndromic cranosynostosis syndromes are considered to be monogenic disorders (Britto and Reardon 2004). Nonsyndromic syndromes, especially coronal synostosis, may also be related to mutations in *FGFR1* (Lajeunie et al. 1995).

The reasons for different phenotypes for mutations in a single gene are not well understood. A large number of different mutations in the *FGFR* genes are known (Kannu and Aftimos

2007) and some correlation exists between genotype and phenotype, but other factors are certainly operative including epigenetic factors and environmental factors. Responsible mutations are mostly missense ones and appear to function as 'gain-of-function' factors, with the exception of the *TWIST* gene on chromosome 7 associated with the Saethre–Chotzen syndrome whose haploinsufficiency is responsible for the syndrome.

TREATMENT
The treatment of craniosynostosis has progressed considerably over the past decade. The multiple aspects of management cannot be dealt with at any length in this book and the reader is referred to the recent exhaustive book on the topic edited by Hayward et al. (2004). The cosmetic results are quite satisfactory in cases of sagittal and unilateral coronal synostosis and in many cases of bilateral coronal and complex synostosis. The best results are obtained by early operation before the age of 6 months, but significant correction can be achieved later. Various complex procedures have been described (Marchac and Renier 1982, Marsh and Schwartz 1983) and all are major surgical operations. There is agreement that surgical treatment is indicated in the presence of ICP and/or incipient optic atrophy. For some types, such as sagittal synostosis or plagiocephaly, there is little if any risk of neurological complication, and intervention aims only at correcting skull appearance. With current techniques, surgical risk is very small for isolated synostosis, and indications for surgery tend to be extended even to relatively benign cases such as sagittal synostosis because the cosmetic appearance would be likely to generate significant embarassment and relational difficulties at school age or later. However, a recent study of 30 cases found that unoperated individuals were doing well intellectually and psychologically at the end of the first decade (9.25 years), thus questioning systematic intervention (Boltshauser et al. 2004). The aims of the procedure should be clearly explained to parents. Syndromic synostoses may raise very difficult problems because of involvement of the viscerocranium and of multiple skeletal and neurological defects. These require specialized multidisciplinary teams familiar with the specific challenges presented. The important aspects of hearing, speech and language, feeding and psychological issues need careful attention (Hayward et al. 2004). It is important to realize that management of the craniosynostoses is not limited to surgery. Ophthamological aspects are essential. If the frequency of optic atrophy has decreased as a result of earlier and better surgery, visual impairment remains frequent; it was bilateral in 35.5% of cases and unilateral in 9.1%, due to strabismus, astigmatism, hypermetropia or anisometropia, which require specialist attention and correction (Tay et al. 2006). Otolaryngological advice is often essential in complex cases as respiratory obstruction is common.

OTHER SKULL DYSPLASIAS

A large number of osseous dysplasias involve the skull, especially the base of the skull, and can be responsible for neurological disturbances (Lachman 1997). Some of these conditions are listed in Table 5.3.

In such cases, CNS involvement may be due to various mechanisms, the most common being compression of the spinal cord or cranial nerves in the basal foramina, and intracranial hypertension as a result of encroachment of thickened bone on intracranial volume or of venous hypertension (Chapter 6). Other mechanisms include associated brain malformations and processes of obscure origin such as intracerebral calcification. Aplasia of the greater wing of the sphenoid is associated with neurofibromatosis type 1 in some cases. It may be responsible for pulsatile exophthalmos (Chapter 3).

INVOLVEMENT OF CRANIAL NERVES
The IInd and VIIIth cranial nerves are those most frequently affected in patients with skull dysplasias. The facial nerve is also commonly involved. Cranial nerves V and IX–XII and the oculomotor nerves are less frequently interfered with.

Compression of the optic nerves generally results in primary optic atrophy that may develop very rapidly and can lead to complete blindness, as is often the case in osteopetrosis (Lehman et al. 1977). Secondary optic atrophy following episodes of high ICP with papilloedema may also occur, perhaps as a result of venous obstruction. Episodes of high ICP with vomiting, fundal venous congestion and oedema sometimes respond dramatically to corticosteroid treatment, as I have observed in a patient with craniometaphyseal dysplasia.

Hearing loss is usually due to compression of the VIIIth nerve in its bony canal. However, involvement of the cochlea by thickening and densification of the petrous bone may also be a factor. Deafness is often progressive as are palsies of other lower cranial nerves.

Hyperostosis cranialis interna is a recently described hereditary syndrome with multiple cranial nerve involvement (Manni et al. 1990).

OTHER MECHANISMS OF NEURAL INVOLVEMENT
Other mechanisms of neural involvement are at play in some cases, even though compression by bony overgrowth is the most common. This applies especially to two diseases: osteopetrosis and carbonic anhydrase II deficiency. Osteopetrosis designates a group of disorders of bone modeling that can be due to at least three different mutations that result in defective acidification of bone (Tolar et al. 2004).

In the *severe form of osteopetrosis* (Lehman et al. 1977), a progressive neurological disorder and choroidoretinal degeneration (Ruben et al. 1990) can evolve in addition to cranial nerve palsies. Gerritsen et al. (1994) reviewed 33 cases, half of which had optic nerve involvement. Three had associated retinal degeneration and two a progressive neurodegenerative disease. Five patients had histological evidence of ceroid-lipofuscinosis storage in neurons and may represent a separate subgroup of the disease (Ambler et al. 1983). Hydrocephalus is present in some cases but cannot explain the progressive deterioration that is seen in some patients with Albers–Schoenberg disease and includes cognitive regression and pyramidal tract signs.

be spontaneous, traumatic or inflammatory. Taggard et al. (2000) found it in 15 of 36 children with Down syndrome and craniovertebral instability. Neurological symptoms such as pain or torticollis were common: signs included ataxia, found in all 36 children, diffuse hyperreflexia (24), and quadriparesis of variable severity (13). Uncomplicated surgical correction was successfully achieved in 24 patients. Such complications are facilitated by the ligamentous hyperlaxity that is present in persons with Down syndrome, especially girls (Davidson 1988).

Cervical *vertebral blocks* occur with several syndromes, the commonest being Klippel–Feil syndrome (McGaughran et al. 2003). Mirror movements can be present (Farmer et al. 1990), although their mechanism is unclear (see Chapter 9). Various associated defects, in particular deafness, spina bifida and hemivertebrae, can be present.

CLINICAL FEATURES

Several clinical syndromes can obtain in patients with cervicooccipital abnormalities. Each clinical syndrome is not necessarily related to a specific type of osteoarticular anomaly even though definite preferential associations exist. For instance, basilar impression tends to be associated with a chronic, late-onset neurological picture, whereas atlantoaxial dislocation is mainly associated with acute complications, and some of the most severe neurological complications of achondroplasia are due to narrowing of the foramen magnum (Ryken and Menezes 1994).

CHRONIC, LATE-ONSET NEUROLOGICAL SYNDROME ASSOCIATED WITH BASILAR IMPRESSION

Children with basilar impression have usually no neurological symptoms or signs until adolescence even though the deformity is present from birth. However, many of these children have a low hairline, a head tilt or torticollis and limitation of head motion. Neurological symptoms may include vertiginous sensations, unsteady walking and occipital pain. Swallowing difficulties are usually a late symptom. Typical features include ataxia of lower limbs, bilateral pyramidal tract signs, loss of proprioception in the upper limbs, nystagmus and involvement of cranial nerves V to XII. Hydrocephalus is common and can occur in association with syringomyelia with or without Chiari 1 malformation, which may be manifested early only by *scoliosis* despite impressive cavitation demonstrated by MRI (Chapter 2). Radiological landmarks of the region, especially for the odontoid process, have been reported (Stovner et al. 1992, 1993) and are useful for diagnosis. Brainstem auditory evoked potentials are frequently abnormal. Sood et al. (1992) found them to be significantly more often abnormal in 22 patients with basilar impression than in 7 with atlanto-axial dislocation. Barnet et al. (1993) found an abnormal N20 component of somatosensory evoked potentials from stimulation of the median nerve in 11 of 16 children with a Chiari malformation, often in association with clinical symptoms of brainstem involvement. CT and (preferably) MRI, using 3D technique when necessary (Tsitouridis et al. 2002) now permit accurate assessment of both osseous and neural abnormalities, thus allowing optimal planning of treatment (Koenigsberg et al. 2005).

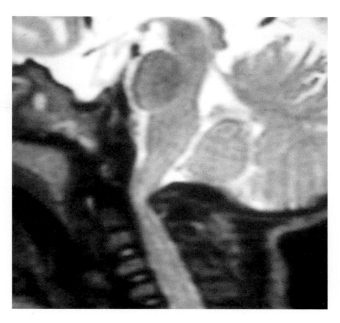

Fig. 5.7. Stenosis of the foramen magnum in a boy with achondroplasia. Sagittal MRI showing severe compression of the bulbospinal junction by the posterior rim of the occipital bone. The neural axis is pushed forward and angulated.

NEUROLOGICAL COMPLICATIONS OF ACHONDROPLASIA (Fig. 5.7)

Achondroplasia can induce a neurological disorder through several mechanisms.

Cervical cord and brainstem compression can occur through a variety of causes. The most usual is compression of the upper cervical cord and medulla by narrowing of the foramen magnum. The cord may also be compressed by stenosis of the cervical spinal canal and anteriorly by an abnormal odontoid process (Gordon 2000). Syringomyelia has only rarely been encountered (Hecht and Butler 1990). Compression myelopathy may produce overt quadriplegia or paraplegia. Insidious neurological signs are more common than overt quadriplegia: ankle clonus, extensor plantar responses and hyperreflexia are indications of spinal involvement, whereas hypotonia, although frequent and marked, is an unreliable sign as it is commonly observed in achondroplastic patients with ligament laxity (Reid et al. 1987). Such signs may precede respiratory failure or sudden death (Colamaria et al. 1991) and are an indication for surgery or careful surveillance of these children. Surgical decompression of the posterior fossa is indicated when neurological symptoms and signs have occurred. The results are usually satisfactory. However, there is no agreement about surgical indications in the absence of definite neurological signs or symptoms or when these remain static.

Respiratory insufficiency can give rise to chronic hypoxaemia, sometimes with bradycardia, to obstructive or central apnoea (Reid et al. 1987, Nelson et al. 1988, Pauli et al. 1995, Gordon 2000) or even to sudden death (Bland and Emery 1982), mostly in children with achondroplasia under 4 years of age, especially when hypoxia is marked. Developmental delay, especially of muscle tone, is relatively frequent. Intellectual development may also be affected with 10–16% of patients having an IQ <80 (Hecht and Butler 1990). This may be related to respiratory insufficiency.

Apnoea may be the sole manifestation of myelopathy in some patients (Fremion et al. 1984). Complete assessment of achondroplastic children with apnoea or other respiratory difficulties should include blood gas measurements, electrocardiography and polygraphic sleep recording (Botelho et al. 2003). Tasker et al. (1998) assessed 17 children with achondroplasia and respiratory symptoms often associated with hydrocephalus and a small foramen magnum. In 5 of these the disorder was severe, all having developed chronic cor pulmonale. Ultrasonography and MRI are essential investigations in such cases, as additional factors like upper airway obstruction and gastrointestinal reflux can play a role and need evaluation and treatment of their own. A *narrow foramen magnum* or spinal canal and, especially, absence of both anterior and posterior perispinal subarachnoid spaces and an abnormal T_2 signal on MRI of the upper spinal cord seem to be the best indicators of imminent danger and should lead to consideration of the need for surgical treatment by decompression of the posterior fossa and cervical cord (Pauli et al. 1995). Rimoin (1995) observed that MR criteria are not sufficient arguments for surgery as children with the same imaging findings may remain well, although he agrees that surgery is indicated in selected cases. Surgery can prevent immediate and late complications including syringomyelia (Hecht et al. 1984) but is not without risk, and the decision must be taken only after thorough consideration of all factors by a specialized team.

Other neurological complications of achondroplasia include *macrocephaly*, which is usually associated with ventricular dilatation. The degree of *hydrocephalus* is usually mild to moderate, and there is also *external hydrocephalus*. Only rarely has obstructing hydrocephalus been reported (Gordon 2000). This communicating hydrocephalus is probably related to increased venous pressure due to stenosis of the basal jugular foramina (Chapter 6). Other mechanisms have been discussed (Hecht and Butler 1990). Shunting is only uncommonly indicated. Surgery to relieve venous flow (Lundar et al. 1990) may be justified if obstruction is confirmed. The use of gated cine phase contrast and MR venography may be useful in defining the pathology of brainstem compression and hydrocephalus (Rollins et al. 2001).

Vertebral canal stenosis in the lumbar region is a classical complication of achondroplasia and can produce root or spinal cord compression. Any deterioration in bladder or bowel function should lead to suspicion of spinal compression. Motor and sensory signs may also be found (Nelson et al. 1988). Lumbosacral lordosis may be at the origin of minor trauma to the cord and be associated with claudication of the cauda equina or conus medullaris (Hecht and Butler 1990).

Nerve root compression can affect the lower or upper limbs. Occipital neuralgia is not uncommon and can be treated by occipital neurectomy provided significant craniocervical junction compression has been excluded. The diagnosis of achondroplasia can now be easily confirmed by demonstration of mutation in the *FGFR3* gene (Stoilov et al. 1995), making the differential diagnosis with related conditions easy (Hall 1995).

ATLANTOAXIAL DISLOCATION
Atlantoaxial dislocation results from either incompetence of the transverse ligament or from abnormalities of the dens itself (Stevens et al. 1994). It can occur following cervical trauma, infection and inflammation of the pharynx, or rheumatoid arthritis. It is favoured by congenital abnormalities such as Morquio disease and by Down syndrome, owing to marked ligament laxity (Pueschel et al. 1987, Pueschel 1988). Dislocation can produce quadriplegia with incontinence or paraplegia that may have a sudden onset but is often preceded by such manifestations as head tilt, abnormal staggering gait and the emergence of neurological signs. Hemiplegia is occasionally seen (Coria et al. 1983b). Diagnosis is confirmed by radiography that shows a distance of more than 5 mm between the anterior aspect of the odontoid and the atlas, and by MRI or CT that also show the rotation and lateral displacement of the dens (Chaudry et al. 1987).

Down syndrome is an important cause of atlantoaxial instability. The problem is to distinguish between simple asymptomatic atlantoaxial instability, which occurs in 19–31% of patients with Down syndrome (Pueschel et al. 1987, Pueschel 1988), and dangerous subluxation and dislocation (Chaudry et al. 1987) that is found in 1–2% of cases. Atlantoaxial dislocation is defined radiologically by an atlanto-dens interval ≥5 mm. CT may show additional abnormalities such as rotatory subluxation of C1–C2, an os odontoideum, atlanto-occipital fusion, or narrowing (<16 mm) of the cervical canal. Patients with atlantoaxial dislocation who are at risk of developing symptoms usually have a wide atlanto-dens interval (>7 mm) and may have mild pyramidal tract signs and gait disturbance. Their sensory evoked potentials from the wrist, especially the latency of N19 potential minus Erb latency, may be increased. Such children should not be allowed to practice somersaulting, trampolining or similar activities. For symptomatic cases, vertebral fusion is the preferred surgical method, whereas posterior decompression that produces further vertebral instability is contraindicated.

REFERENCES

Ambler MW, Trice J, Grauerholz J, O'Shea PA (1983) Infantile osteopetrosis and neuronal storage disease. *Neurology* 33: 437–41.

Aviv RI, Armstrong D, Chong WK (2004) Imaging the patient with craniosynostosis. In: Hayward R, Jones B, Dunaway D, Evans R, eds. *The Clinical Management of Craniosynostosis. Clinics in Developmental Medicine No. 163.* London: Mac Keith Press, pp. 98–115.

Azevedo AC, Schwartz IV, Kakakun L, et al. (2004) Clinical and biochemical study of 28 patients with mucopolysaccharidosis type VI. *Clin Genet* 66: 208–13.

Baraitser M (1990) *The Genetics of Neurological Disorders, 2nd edn. Oxford Monographs on Medical Genetics No. 18.* Oxford: Oxford University Press.

Barnet AB, Weiss IP, Shaer C (1993) Evoked potentials in infant brainstem syndrome associated with Arnold–Chiari malformation. *Dev Med Child Neurol* 35: 42–8.

Bland JP, Emery JL (1982) Unexpected death of children with achondroplasia after the perinatal period. *Dev Med Child Neurol* 24: 489–92.

Boltshauser E, Ludwig S, Dietrich F, Landolt MA (2004) Sagittal craniosynostosis: cognitive development, behaviour, and quality of life in unoperated children. *Neuropediatrics* 34: 293–300.

Botelho RV, Bittencourt LR, Rotta JM, Tufik S (2003) A prospective controlled study of sleep respiratory events in patients with craniovertebral junction malformations. *J Neurosurg* 99: 1004–9.

Braakhekke JP, Gabreëls FJM, Renier WO, et al. (1985) Craniovertebral pathology in Down syndrome. *Clin Neurol Neurosurg* 87: 173–9.

Britto J, Reardon W (2004) Syndromic craniofacial dysostosis: molecular and developmental aspects. In; Hayward R, Jones B, Dunaway D, Evans R, eds. *The Clinical Management of Craniosynostosis. Clinics in Developmental Medicine No. 163.* London: Mac Keith Press, pp. 45–71.

Brockmeyer D (1999) Down syndrome and craniovertebral instability. Topic review and treatment recommendations. *Pediatr Neurosurg* 31: 71–7.

Charnas LR, Marini JC (1993) Communicating hydrocephalus, basilar invagination, and other neurologic features in osteogenesis imperfecta. *Neurology* 43: 2603–8.

Chaudry V, Sturgeon C, Gates AJ, Myers G (1987) Symptomatic atlantoaxial dislocation in Down's syndrome. *Ann Neurol* 21: 606–9.

Chen CP, Chem SR, Shih JC, et al. (2001) Prenatal diagnosis and genetic analysis of type I and type II thanatophoric dysplasia. *Prenat Diagn* 21: 59–95.

Chun K, Teubi AS, Jung JH, et al. (2002) Genetic analysis of patients with the Saethre–Chotzen phenotype. *Am J Hum Genet* 110: 136–43.

Cinalli G, Renier D, Sebag G, et al. (1995) Chronic tonsillar herniation in Crouzon's and Apert's syndromes: the role of premature synostosis of the lambdoid suture. *J Neurosurg* 83: 575–82.

Cohen DM, Green JG, Miller J, et al. (1987) Acrocephalopolysyndactyly type II—Carpenter syndrome: clinical spectrum and an attempt at unification with Goodman and Summit syndromes. *Am J Med Genet* 28: 311–24.

Cohen MM (1979) Craniosynostosis and syndromes with craniosynostosis: incidence, genetics, penetrance, variability, and new syndromes updating. *Birth Defects Orig Artic Ser* 15: 13–63.

Cohen MM (1986) Syndromes with craniosynostosis. In: Cohen MM, ed. *Craniosynostosis: Diagnosis, Evaluation and Management.* New York: Raven Press, pp. 413–590.

Cohen MM (1988) Craniosynostosis update 1987. *Am J Med Genet Suppl* 4: 99–148.

Cohen MM (1993a) Pfeiffer syndrome update, clinical subtypes, and guidelines for differential diagnosis. *Am J Med Genet* 45: 300–307.

Cohen MM (1993b) Sutural biology and the correlates of craniosynostosis. *Am J Med Genet* 47: 581–616.

Cohen MM, Kreiborg S (1990) The central nervous system in the Apert syndrome. *Am J Med Genet* 35: 36–45.

Cohen MM, Rollnick BR, Kaye CI (1989) Oculoauriculovertebral spectrum: an updated critique. *Cleft Palate J* 26: 276–86.

Colamaria V, Mazza C, Beltramello A, et al. (1991) Irreversible respiratory failure in an achondroplastic child: the importance of an early cervicomedullary decompression and a review of the literature. *Brain Dev* 13: 270–9.

Coria F, Quintana F, Rebollo M, et al. (1983a) Occipital dysplasia and Chiari type I deformity in a family. Clinical and radiological study of three generations. *J Neurol Sci* 62: 147–58.

Coria, F, Quintana, F, Villalba M, et al. (1983b) Craniocervical abnormalities in Down's syndrome. *Dev Med Child Neurol* 25: 252–5.

Cotter M, Connell T, Colhoun E, et al. (2005) Carbonic anhydrase II deficiency: a rare autosomal recessive disorder of osteopetrosis, renal tubular acidosis, and cerebral calcification. *J Pediatr Hematol Oncol* 27: 115–7.

Davidson RG (1988) Atlantoaxial instability in individuals with Down syndrome: a fresh look at the evidence. *Pediatrics* 81: 857–65.

de Heer LM, de Klein A, van der Ouweland AM, et al. (2005) Clinical and genetic analysis of patients with Saethre–Chotzen syndrome. *Plastic Reconstruct Surg* 115: 1894–902.

Duc G, Largo RH (1986) Anterior fontanel: size and closure in term and preterm infants. *Pediatrics* 78: 904–8.

Dunaway D (2004) Craniofacial growth and development: a clinical perspective. In: Hayward R, Jones B, Dunaway D, Evans R, eds. *The Clinical Management of Craniosynostosis. Clinics in Developmental Medicine No. 163.* London: Mac Keith Press, pp. 1–11.

Farmer SF, Ingram DA, Stephens DA, Stephens JA (1990) Mirror movements studied in a patient with Klippel–Feil syndrome. *J Physiol* 428: 467–84.

Fremion AS, Garg BP, Kalsbeck J (1984) Apnea as the sole manifestation of cord compression in achondroplasia. *J Pediatr* 104: 398–401.

Frost M, Huffer WE, Sze CI, et al. (1999) Cervical spine abnormalities in Down syndrome. *Clin Neuropathol* 18: 250–9.

Fryburg JS, Hwang V, Lin KY (1995) Recurrent lambdoid synostosis within two families. *Am J Med Genet* 58: 262–6.

Gerritsen EJA, Vossen JM, van Loo IHG, et al. (1994) Autosomal recessive osteopetrosis: variability of findings at diagnosis and during the natural course. *Pediatrics* 93: 247–53.

Goel A, Bhatjiwhile M, Desai K (1998) Basilar invagination: a study based on 190 surgically treated patients. *J Neurosurg* 88: 962–8.

Golan I, Baumert U, Held P, et al. (2002) Radiological findings and molecular genetic confirmation of cleidocranial dysplasia. *Clin Radiol* 57: 525–9.

Gordon N (2000) The neurological complications of achondroplasia. *Brain Dev* 22: 3–7.

Goutières F, Aicardi J, Farkas–Bargeton E (1971) [An unusual cerebral malformation associated with thanatophoric dwarfism.] *Rev Neurol* 125: 435–40 (French).

Graham JM, Badura RJ, Smith DW (1980) Coronal craniostenosis: fetal head constraint as one possible cause. *Pediatrics* 65: 995–9.

Greenberg AD (1968) Atlanto-axial dislocations. *Brain* 91: 655–84.

Gripp KW, Stolle CA, Celle L, et al. (1999) TWIST gene mutation in a patient with radial aplasia and craniosynostosis: further evidence for heterogeneity of Baller–Gerold syndrome. *Am J Med Genet* 82: 170–6.

Hall JG (1995) Information update on achondroplasia. *Pediatrics* 95: 620 (letter).

Hayward R, Jones B, Dunaway D, Evans R, eds. (2004) *The Clinical Management of Craniosynostosis. Clinics in Developmental Medicine No. 163.* London: Mac Keith Press.

Hecht JT, Butler IJ (1990) Neurologic morbidity associated with achondroplasia. *J Child Neurol* 5: 84–97.

Hecht JT, Butler JJ, Scott CI (1984) Long-term neurologic sequelae in achondroplasia. *Eur J Pediatr* 143: 58–60.

Hecht JT, Nelson FW, Butler IJ, et al. (1985) Computerized tomography of the foramen magnum: achondroplastic values compared to normal standards. *Am J Med Genet* 20: 355–60.

Hernandez-Cassis C, Vogel CK, Hernandez TP, et al. (2003) Autosomal dominant hyperostosis/osteosclerosis with high serum alkaline phosphatase activity. *J Clin Endocrinol Metab* 88: 2650–5.

Hevner RF (2005) The cerebral cortex malformation in thanathophoric dysplasia: neuropathology and pathogenesis. *Acta Neuropathol* 110: 208–21.

Higginbottom MC, Jones KL, James HE (1980) Intrauterine constraint and craniosynostosis. *Neurosurgery* 6: 39–44.

Hirano A, Akita S, Fujii T (1995) Craniofacial deformities associated with juvenile hyperthyroidism. *Cleft Palate Craniofac J* 32: 328–33.

Hirsch JF, Renier D, Sainte-Rose C (1982) Intracranial pressure in craniostenosis. *Monogr Paediatr* 15: 114–8.

Hunter AGW, Rudd NL (1976) Craniosynostosis. I. Sagittal synostosis: its genetics and associated clinical findings in 214 patients who lacked involvement of the coronal suture(s). *Teratology* 14: 185–93.

Hunter AGW, Rudd NL (1977) Craniosynostosis. II. Coronal synostosis: its familial characteristics and associated clinical findings in 109 patients lacking bilateral polysyndactyly or syndactyly. *Teratology* 15: 301–10.

Iughetti P, Alonso LG, Wilcox W, et al. (2000) Mapping of the autosomal recessive (AR) craniometaphyseal dysplasia locus to chromosome region 6q21-22 and confirmation of genetic heterogeneity for mild AR spondylocostal dysplasia. *Am J Med Genet* 95: 482–91.

Jabs EW, Li X, Scott AF, et al. (1994) Jackson–Weiss and Crouzon syndromes are allelic with mutations in fibroblast growth factor receptor 2. *Nat Genet* 8: 275–9.

Janus GE, Engelbert RH, Beek E, et al. (2003) Osteogenesis imperfecta in childhood: MR imaging and basilar impression. *Eur J Radiol* 47: 19–24.

Kane AA, Mitchell LE, Craven KP, Marsh JL (1996) Observations on a recent increase in plagiocephaly without synostosis. *Pediatrics* 97: 877–85.

Kannu P, Aftimos S (2007) FGFR3 mutations and medial temporal lobe dysgenesis. *J Child Neurol* 22: 211–3.

Keeney G, Gebarski SS, Brunberg JA (1992) CT of inner ear anomalies including aplasia, in a case of Wildervanck syndrome. *AJNR* 13: 201–2.

Koenigsberg RA, Vakil N Hong TA, et al. (2005) Evaluation of platybasia with MR imaging. *AJNR* 26: 89–92.

Kreiborg S (1981) Crouzon syndrome. A clinical and roentgencephalometric study. *Scand J Plast Reconstr Surg Suppl* 18: 1–198.

Lachman RS (1997) Neurological abnormalities in the skeletal dysplasias: a clinical and radiological perspective. *Am J Med Genet* 69: 33–43.

Lajeunie E, Le Merrer M, Bonaiti-Pellie C, et al. (1995) Genetic study of nonsyndromic coronal craniosynostosis. *Am J Med Genet* 55: 500–4.

Lajeunie E, Le Merrer M, Bonaiti-Pellie C, et al. (1996) Genetic study of scaphocephaly. *Am J Med Genet* 62: 282–5.

Lajeunie E, LeMerrer M, Marchac D, Renier D (1998) Syndromal and non-syndromal primary trigonocephaly: analysis of a series of 237 patients. *Am J Med Genet* 75: 211–5.

Lajeunie E, El Ghouzzi V, Le Merrer M, et al. (1999) Sex related expressivity of the phenotype in coronal craniosynostosis caused by the recurrent P250R FGFR3 mutation. *J Med Genet* 36: 9–13.

Lajeunie E, Barcik U, Thorne JA, et al. (2001) Craniosynostosis and fetal exposure to sodium valproate. *J Neurosurg* 95: 778–82.

Leão MJ, Ribeiro-Silva ML (1995) Orofaciodigital syndrome type I in a patient with severe CNS defects. *Pediatr Neurol* 13: 247–51.

Le Merrer M, Ledinot V, Renier D, et al. (1988) [Genetic counselling in craniostenosis. Results of a prospective study performed with a group of studies on craniofacial malformations.] *J Genet Hum* 36: 295–306.

Littlefield TR, Kelly KM, Pomatto JK, Beals SP (1999) Multiple birth infants at higher risk for the development of plagiocephaly. *Pediatrics* 103: 565–9.

Lundar T, Bakke SJ, Nornes H (1990) Hydrocephalus in an achondroplastic child treated by venous decompression at the jugular foramen. Case report. *J Neurosurg* 73: 138–40.

Manni JJ, Scaf JJ, Huygen PLM, et al. (1990) Hyperostosis cranialis interna. A new hereditary syndrome with cranial nerve entrapment. *N Engl J Med* 322: 450–4.

Marchac D, Renier D (1982) *Craniofacial Surgery for Craniosynostosis.* Boston: Little Brown.

Marsh JL, Schwartz HG (1983) The surgical correction of coronal and metopic craniosynostoses. *J Neurosurg* 59: 245–51.

McGaughran JM, Oates A, Donnai A, et al. (2003) Mutations in PAX1 may be associated with Klippel–Feil syndrome. *Eur J Hum Genet* 11: 468–74.

Menezes AH, VanGilder JC, Graf CJ, McDonnell DE (1980) Craniocervical abnormalities. A comprehensive surgical approach. *J Neurosurg* 53: 444–55.

Moloney DM, Wall SA, Ashworth GJ, et al. (1997) Prevalence of Pro250Arg mutation of fibroblast growth factor receptor 3 in coronal craniosynostosis. *Lancet* 349: 1059–62.

Moore MH (1993) Upper airway obstruction in the syndromal craniosynostoses. *Br J Plast Surg* 46: 355–62.

Morgan DF, Williams B (1992) Syringobulbia: a surgical appraisal. *J Neurol Neurosurg Psychiatry* 55: 1132–41.

Nelson FN, Hecht JT, Horton WA, et al. (1988) Neurological basis of respiratory complications in achondroplasia. *Ann Neurol* 24: 89–93.

Ohaegbulam C, Woodard EJ, Proctor M (2005) Occipitocondylar hyperplasia: an unusual craniovertebral junction anomaly causing myelopathy. Case report. *J Neurosurg* 103 (4 Suppl): 379–381.

Oldridge M, Wilkie AOM, Slaney SF, et al. (1995) Mutations in the third immunoglobulin domain of the fibroblast growth factor receptor-2 gene in Crouzon syndrome. *Hum Mol Genet* 4: 1077–82.

Patton MA, Goodship J, Hayward R, Lansdown R (1988) Intellectual development in Apert's syndrome: a long term follow up of 29 patients. *J Med Genet* 25: 164–7.

Pauli RM, Horton VK, Glinski LP, Reiser CA (1995) Prospective assessment of risks for cervicomedullary-junction compression in infants with achondroplasia. *Am J Hum Genet* 56: 732–44.

Petersen OB, Chitty LS (2004) Prenatal diagnosis of craniosynstosis. In: Hayward R, Jones B, Dunaway D, Evans R, eds. *The Clinical Management of Craniosynostosis. Clinics in Developmental Medicine No. 163.* London: Mac Keith Press, pp. 85–97.

Preston RA, Post JC, Keats BJB, et al. (1994) A gene for Crouzon craniofacial dysostosis maps to the long arm of chromosome 10. *Nat Genet* 7: 149–53.

Pueschel SM (1988) Atlantoaxial instability and Down syndrome. *Pediatrics* 81: 879–80.

Pueschel SM, Findley TW, Furia J, et al. (1987) Atlantoidal instability in persons with Down syndrome: roentgenographic, neurologic and somatosensory evoked potential studies. *J Pediatr* 110: 515–21.

Reardon W, Winter RM (1994) Saethre–Chotzen syndrome. *J Med Genet* 31: 393–96.

Reardon W, Winter RM, Rutland P, et al. (1994) Mutations in the fibroblast growth factor receptor 2 gene cause Crouzon syndrome. *Nat Genet* 8: 98–103.

Reichenberger E, Tiziani V, Watanabe S, et al. (2001) Autosomal dominant craniometaphyseal dysplasia is caused by mutation in the transmembrane protein ANK. *Am J Hum Genet* 68: 1321–6.

Reid CS, Pyeritz RE, Kopits SE, et al. (1987) Cervicomedullary compression in young patients with achondroplasia: value of comprehensive neurologic and respiratory evaluation. *J Pediatr* 110: 522–30.

Ricci D, Vasco G, Baranello G, et al (2007) Visual function in infants with non-syndromic craniosynostosis. *Dev Med Child Neurol* 49: 574–6.

Rimoin DL (1995) Cervicomedullary junction compression in infants with achondroplasia: when to perform neurosurgical decompression. *Am J Hum Genet* 56: 824–7.

Rohatgi M (1991) Cloverleaf skull—a severe form of Crouzon's syndrome: a new concept in aetiology. *Acta Neurochir* 108: 45–52.

Rollins N, Booth T, Shapiro K (2001) The use of gated cine phase contrast and MR venography in achondroplasia. *Childs Nerv Syst* 16: 569–75.

Ruben JB, Morris RJ, Judisch GF (1990) Chorioretinal degeneration in infantile malignant osteopetrosis. *Am J Ophthalmol* 110: 1–5.

Ryken TC, Menezes AH (1994) Cervicomedullary compressioin in achondroplasia. *J Neurosurg* 81: 43–8.

Sakai N, Nakakita N, Yamazaki Y, Uchinuma E (2002) Oral–facial–digital syndrome type II (Mohr syndrome): clinical and genetic manifestations. *J Craniofac Surg* 13: 321–6.

Saltzman CL, Hensinger RN, Blane CE, Phillips WA (1991) Familial cervical dysplasia. *J Bone Joint Surg* 73: 163–71.

Santos de Oliveira R, Lajeunie E, Arnaud E, Renier D (2006) Fetal exposure to sodium valproate associated with Baller–Gerold syndrome: case report and review of the literature. *Childs Nerv Syst* 22: 90–4.

Schrander-Strumpel T, de Die-Smulders CE, Hennekam RC, et al. (1992) Oculoauriculovertebral spectrum and cerebral anomalies. *J Med Genet* 29: 326–31.

Seto ML, Lee SJ, Sze RW, Cunningham ML (2001) Another TWIST on Baller–Gerold syndrome. *Am J Med Genet* 104: 323–30.

Singer S, Bower C, Southall P, Goldblatt J (1999) Craniosynostosis in Australia, 1980–1994: a population-based study. *Am J Med Genet* 83: 382–7.

Sly WS, Whyte MP, Sundaram V, et al. (1985) Carbonic anhydrase II deficiency in 12 families with the autosomal recessive syndromes of osteopetrosis with renal tubular acidosis and cerebral calcification. *N Engl J Med* 313: 139–45.

Sood S, Mahapatra AK, Bhatia B (1992) Somatosensory and brainstem auditory evoked potential in congenital craniovertebral anomaly; effect of surgical management. *J Neurol Neurosurg Psychiatry* 55: 609–12.

Stevens JM, Chong WK, Barber C, et al. (1994) A new appraisal of abnormalities of the odontoid process associated with atlanto-axial subluxation and neurological disability. *Brain* 117: 133–48.

Steward CG (2003) Neurological aspects of osteopetrosis. *Neuropathol Appl Neurobiol* 29: 87–97.

Stoilov I, Kilpatrick MW, Tsipouras P (1995) A common FGFR3 gene mutation is present in achondroplasia but not in hypochondroplasia. *Am J Med Genet* 55: 127–33.

Stoll C, Sauvage P (2002) Long-term follow-up of a girl with oro-facio-digital syndrome type 1 due to a mutation of the OFD1 gene. *Ann Genet* 45: 59–62.

Stovner LJ, Cappelen J, Nilsen G, Sjaastad O (1992) The Chiari type I malformation in two monozygotic twins and first-degree relatives. *Ann Neurol* 31: 220–2.

Stovner LJ, Bergan U, Nilsen G, Sjaastad O (1993) Posterior cranial fossa dimensions in the Chiari 1 malformation: relation to pathogenesis and clinical presentation. *Neuroradiology* 35: 113–8.

Superti-Furga A, Bonafé L, Rimoin DL (2001) Molecular–pathogenetic classification of genetic disorders of the skeleton. *Am J Med Genet* 106: 282–93.

Taggard DA, Menezes AH, Ryken TC (2000) Treatment of Down syndrome-associated craniovertebral junction abnormalities. *J Neurosurg* 92 (Suppl 2): 205–13.

Taravath S, Tonsgard JH (1993) Cerebral malformation in Carpenter syndrome. *Pediatr Neurol* 9: 230–4.

Tasker RC, Dundas I, Laverty A, et al. (1998) Distinct patterns of respiratory difficulty in young children with achondroplasia: a clinical, sleep, and lung function study. *Arch Dis Child* 79: 99–108.

Tay T, Martin F, Rowe N, et al. (2006) Prevalence and causes of visual impairment in craniosynostotic syndromes. *Clin Experiment Ophthamol* 34: 434–40.

Thompson DNP, Harkness W, Jones B, Gonsalez S, et al. (1995) Subdural intracranial pressure monitoring in craniosynostosis: its role in surgical management. *Childs Nerv Syst* 11: 269–75.

Thompson DNP, Britto J (2004) Classification and clinical diagnosis. In: Hayward R, Jones B, Dunaway D, Evans R, eds. *The Clinical Management of Craniosynostosis. Clinics in Developmental Medicine No. 163.* London: Mac Keith Press, pp. 12–44.

Tolar J, Teitelbaum SL, Orchard D (2004) Osteopetrosis. *N Engl J Med* **351**: 2839–49.

Tracy MR, Dormans JP, Kusumi K (2004) Klippel–Feil syndrome: clinical features and current understanding of etiology. *Clin Orthop Relat Res* July (424): 183–90.

Tsipouras P, Barabas G, Matthews WS (1986) Neurologic correlates of osteogenesis imperfecta. *Arch Neurol* **43**: 150–2.

Tsitouridis I, Goutsaridou F, Morichovitou A, et al. (2002) Malformations of the craniocervical junction: 3D-CT evaluation. *Stud Health Technol Inform* **91**: 320–1.

Vanek J, Losan F (1982) Pfeiffer's type of acrocephalosyndactyly in two families. *J Med Genet* **19**: 289–92.

Van Hul W, Vanhoenacker F, Balemans W, et al. (2001) Molecular and radiological diagnosis of sclerosing bone dysplasias. *Eur J Radiol* **40**: 198–207.

Weinzweig J, Kirschner RE, Farley A, et al. (2003) Metopic synostosis: Defining the temporal sequence of normal suture fusion and differentiating it from synostosis on the basis of computed tomography images. *Plastic Reconstr Surg* **112**: 1211–8.

Wieacker P, Wieland I (2005) Clinical and genetic aspects of craniofrontonasal syndrome: towards resolving a genetic paradox. *Mol Genet Metab* **86**: 110–6.

Wieland I, Reardon W, Jakubiczka S, et al. (2005) Twenty-six novel EFNB1 mutations in familial and sporadic craniofrontonasal syndrome (CFNS). *Hum Mutat* **26**: 113–8.

Wilkie AOM (2000) Epidemiology and genetics of craniosynostosis. *Am J Med Genet* **90**: 82–4.

Wilkie AOM, Slaney SF, Oldridge M (1995) Apert syndrome results from localized mutations of FGFR2 and is allelic with Crouzon syndrome. *Nat Genet* **9**: 165–72.

Wilson LC (2004) Incidence and epidemiology of craniosynostosis. In: Hayward R, Jones B, Dunaway D, Evans R, eds. *The Clinical Management of Craniosynostosis. Clinics in Developmental Medicine No. 163*. London: Mac Keith Press, pp. 72–84.

Wilson LC, Hall CM (2002) Albright's hereditary osteodystrophy and pseudohypoparathyroidism. *Semin Musculoskelet Radiol* **6**: 273–83.

Young R, Kleinman G, Ojemann RG, et al. (1980) Compressive myelopathy in Maroteaux–Lamy syndrome: clinical and pathological findings. *Ann Neurol* **8**: 336–40.

Zankl A, Jaeger G, Bonafe C, et al. (2004) Novel mutation of the tyrosine-kinase domain of FGRF2 in a patient with Pfeiffer syndrome. *Am J Med Genet A* **131**: 299–300.

PART III

NEUROLOGICAL CONSEQUENCES OF PRENATAL, PERINATAL AND EARLY POSTNATAL INTERFERENCE WITH BRAIN DEVELOPMENT: HYDROCEPHALUS, CEREBRAL PALSY

6

HYDROCEPHALUS AND NONTRAUMATIC PERICEREBRAL COLLECTIONS

HYDROCEPHALUS

Hydrocephalus is one of the possible consequences of some of the brain malformations or lesions described in the preceding chapters. It may also be acquired later in life as a result of tumours, infections or other causes. For convenience, all types of hydrocephalus of whatever cause in children of any age are studied in this chapter.

DEFINITION AND MECHANISMS

Hydrocephalus means an excess of fluid within the cranium. However, it is customary to reserve the term for the condition in which the volume of cerebrospinal fluid (CSF) is increased in all or part of the intracranial fluid spaces, and in which that increased volume is not the result of primary atrophy or dysgenesis of the brain. The abnormal accumulation of CSF results from an excessive pressure, at least in the initial stages of the disorder.

The greater part of the CSF is secreted actively by the choroid plexuses. Experiments in animals indicate that 35–70% of CSF, depending on species, may come from extraplexic sources. In humans, it is estimated that 70–90% of the fluid originates from the choroid plexuses (McComb 1983), the remainder originating in brain parenchyma as a result of exchanges with cerebral extracellular spaces. The daily formation of CSF in children and adults is about 500 mL. The night and day rhythm of secretion is relatively stable and amounts to 0.35 mL/min in adults. The total volume of CSF in the head of an adult is about 120 mL, and the average ventricular volume is around 25 mL, although individual variations occur. In the neonate, CSF volume is about 50 mL.

The hydrostatic pressure of the CSF (synonymous with intracranial pressure) originates from the CSF secretion pressure and from the resistances to its circulation and resorption. Secretion of CSF seems to result from a two-step process. The first step is the formation, by hydrostatic pressure, of a plasma ultrafiltrate through the choroidal capillary endothelium, which is devoid of tight junctions. The second step transforms the ultrafiltrate by an active metabolic process within the choroidal epithelium.

The rate of CSF formation is relatively independent of pressure. The rate of CSF resorption depends on CSF pressure and is relatively linear over the range of physiological pressures (McComb 1983).

CSF flows from the lateral ventricles through the lateral and third ventricles and reaches the fourth through the aqueduct of Sylvius. Passage through the aqueduct is fast, and its pulsatile nature has been demonstrated by dynamic MRI techniques (Badhelia et al. 1997). Although these pulsations probably play a significant role in CSF circulation, they have not yet been shown to play a role in the pathophysiology of hydrocephalus (Czosnyka et al. 2004). CSF then flows through the foramina of Magendie and Luschka through the lateral and third ventricles into the posterior fossa and then the basal cisterns. CSF flow then divides; most of the CSF passes upward through the incisura and reaches the parasagittal arachnoid villi via the ambient cisterns, the sylvian fissures and the convexity cisterns. About 20% of the fluid flows downward through the foramen magnum along the spinal subarachnoid space to the arachnoid villi along the nerve root sleeves. This flow is maintained by continuous entry of newly secreted CSF into the ventricles.

Most of the CSF is resorbed passively, through the arachnoid granulations along the superior sagittal sinus, into the sinus blood flow. The CSF pressure is normally greater than venous blood pressure. A pressure gradient of 20–50 mmH$_2$O is necessary for allowing resorption into the venous sinuses through the arachnoid villi and granulations, although the development of these structures in infancy is still disputed. Thus, the mean CSF pressure normally depends on several factors, constituting on the one hand *pressure secretion* of the fluid, and on the other *yield pressure* (venous blood pressure, resistance of CSF pathways including cisterns and granulations, and distensibility of the walls of CSF spaces, i.e. brain parenchyma, meninges and skull), the latter being important mainly in pathological situations (Naidich 1989). A significant amount of CSF may be resorbed via cervical lymph vessels (McComb et al. 1983) and this pathway may be of importance in hydrocephalus. Absorption of CSF by the brain in pathological circumstances (transependymal resorption) is suggested by CT or MRI (see below). However, the presence of subependymal CSF over the cortex is no proof of its normal circulation or resorption as the fluid may simply move through the parenchyma to the pericerebral spaces (James et al. 1974).

This classical concept remains essential for the understanding of the causes and clinical features of hydrocephalus. However, more recent work has shown that it has to be substantially modified to account for multiple aspects of the condition (see Sato et al. 1994, Czosnyka et al. 2004). In particular, extrachoroidal sources of fluid, especially within the brain parenchyma, are of great importance; resorption is not exclusively through the granulations of Pacchioni but also into the brain extracellular space; and factors other than resistance to absorption such as pulsation of the brain arteries are significant in the circulation of CSF.

Normal intracranial (or CSF) pressure at the level of the foramen of Monro is 100–150 mmH$_2$O in children and adolescents at rest in the lying position. In the newborn, CSF pressure is lower, around 40–50 mmH$_2$O.

Except in the rare cases of CSF hypersecretion, hydrocephalus is virtually always due to an increase in the resistance of CSF circulation pathways resulting in an increase in CSF pressure. Increased resistance may be located within the ventricular system, in the posterior fossa, in the cisterns or subarachnoid spaces or at the sites of resorption. CSF flow is a function of the difference between CSF and venous sinus pressures, divided by the resistance of pathways. As CSF production is stable over a relatively wide range or pressures, an *increase in CSF pressure* is inevitable to allow evacuation of newly formed CSF.

The magnitude of the effects of this increase in pressure will depend largely on the yield pressure or compliance of the brain and skull. When the brain and envelopes are distensible (low yield pressure), there is rapid ventricular enlargement, large final ventricular size, rapid decline in intraventricular pressure (IVP) and relatively low final pressure after compensation. This is the situation in newborn babies and infants. In contrast, with low compliance (high yield pressure), ventricular enlargement is slow, final ventricular size is relatively small, IVP remains high for long periods, and final pressure after compensation remains high. This situation obtains in older children and in adolescents, and also in fetuses, in which pressure from the uterine wall limits ventricular enlargement (Oi et al. 1990). In such cases, severe hydrocephalus with high pressure can develop with deceptively little ventricular dilatation (Jones 1987).

In addition to increase in mean intracranial pressure (ICP), *CSF pulse pressure* probably plays an important role in the determination of some aspects of hydrocephalus. It has been shown that flow through the aqueduct is synchronous with the systolic contraction (Marks et al. 1992). CSF pulse pressure designates the systolic–diastolic variations in CSF pressure that result from those of arterial blood pressure transmitted by arterial wall pulsations to the CSF. The amplitude of the CSF pulse pressure varies with the mean ICP and rises sharply with increasing mean CSF pressure. Pulse pressure also depends on ventricular compliance and on the rapidity with which outflow of venous blood and CSF can compensate for the instantaneous pressure rise. CSF pulse

pressure has a significant role in determination of ventricular size. An experimental threefold increase in the pulse amplitude causes hydrocephalus in animals (Avezaat et al. 1979). Conversely, removal of one plexus is associated with decrease of pulse pressure and of size of the corresponding ventricle, and the same mechanism is probably responsible for the smaller size of shunted lateral ventricles. Pressure measurements have confirmed that in such cases, the pulse pressure is decreased in the ventricle where the tip of the catheter lies, probably as a result of damping of CSF pulsations by CSF outflow into the shunt.

Later effects of increased ICP and dilatation of the CSF spaces include the progressive development of cerebral atrophy that predominantly affects white matter and, in turn, facilitates further ventricular dilatation. There is splitting of the ependymal lining, spongy dissociation of nerve fibres and, eventually, development of astrocytosis (Da Silva 2004). The grey matter, on the contrary, is long preserved. Reduction of cerebral blood flow, in particular in the anterior cerebral arteries, may play a role by inducing ischaemic injury to the cerebral hemispheres (Hill and Volpe 1982).

The *eventual course of hydrocephalus* will depend on the achievement of a new balance between CSF production, preservation of residual absorption capacity and development of alternative resorption pathways. If and when resorption and secretion of CSF equalize under a stable regime of pressure, stabilization of hydrocephalus occurs but at the expense of a variable degree of stable or slowly diminishing ventricular dilatation.

Differentiating hydrocephalus that is stabilized or arrested from that which is slowly evolutive may be extremely difficult or even impossible, especially as several variables are at play at the same time. These include: skull compliance; CSF pressure, which fluctuates with plateau waves occurring especially during REM sleep (Rosner and Becker 1983); and the development of new resorption pathways. It seems, however, that true arrest – or compensation – of hydrocephalus does occur in a small proportion of children (10–20%) as shown by radionuclide clearing studies (Johnston et al. 1984).

The effects of hydrocephalus will also vary with the age of first development of the disorder. In addition to the differences resulting from the diverse yield pressures, one may observe modifications in the shape of the skull, which may expand frontally with aqueductal stenosis, whereas a fourth ventricle cyst, as in Dandy–Walker malformation, may impede caudal migration of the tentorium, which inserts on the parietal bones in an abnormally high situation. Similar mechanisms may be responsible for the skull changes that are present in hydrocephalus associated with spina bifida (Britton et al. 1988).

EPIDEMIOLOGY
The incidence of hydrocephalus is imperfectly known. The figure of 3 per 1000 live births that is commonly quoted applies only to congenital (or early onset) hydrocephalus. Moreover, the practice of antenatal diagnosis of malformations and systematic ultrasonographic examination during pregnancy has modified our knowledge of both the incidence and the distribution of causes

TABLE 6.1
TABLE 6.1
Main mechanisms of hydrocephalus

Mechanism	Main causes
Overproduction of CSF	Papilloma of choroid plexuses[1]
Obstruction of CSF pathways	
Intraventricular block[2]	
Foramen of Monro	Tumours (e.g. giant cell astrocytoma)
Third ventricle	Tumours (e.g. craniopharyngioma, colloid cyst, suprasellar arachnoid cyst[3])
Aqueduct of Sylvius	Tumours of the quadrigeminal plate, pineal region tumours, malformations (forking, membrane, gliosis), infections (e.g. toxoplasmosis, meningitis, mumps), posthaemorrhagic ependymitis
Fourth ventricle	Tumours, retrocerebellar cyst, Dandy–Walker syndrome, membranous obstruction of the foramina of Magendie and Luschka[2], Chiari malformation types I and II
Extraventricular block[2]	
Basilar block	Symphysis of basal cisterns of post-haemorrhagic or postinfectious origin, malignancy of meninges, tumours (e.g. craniopharyngioma, chiasmatic), suprasellar arachnoid cysts[3], mucopolysaccharidosis (Hurler syndrome)
Convexity block	Organization and symphysis of areas of CSF resorption
Absence of block but increased resistance to circulation or resorption of CSF into the venous sinuses	Sinus or jugular vein obstruction
Blockage or absence/paucity of granulations of Pacchioni	Exceptional, unknown
Venous hypertension suppressing the pressure differential between CSF and sinus blood	Compression or thrombosis of sinuses within cranium or basal skull foramina or superior vena cava
Unknown or multiple mechanisms	Spinal cord tumours

[1]Mechanism uncertain; bleeding may also play a role.
[2]Both intra- and extraventricular blocks may coexist.
[3]Suprasellar and incisural cysts can block both the aqueduct and the basal cisterns.

of congenital hydrocephalus. For the period 1958–1981, Lorber (1984) found an incidence of 0.6 per 1000 live births. Later studies in Sweden (Fernell et al. 1986) found a mean prevalence of hydrocephalus manifesting during the first year of life of 0.53 per 1000 during the years 1967–1982, with a slightly increasing trend from 0.48 in 1967–1970 to 0.63 in 1979–1982 (cases of tumours and of neural tube defects were not included). Of the 202 infants studied, 30% were born preterm. The increase did not continue after 1982 (Fernell et al. 1994). The increased prevalence was entirely ascribable to cases occurring in preterm infants, in whom it rose from 0.13 to 0.30 per 1000 during the study period. The origin of the hydrocephalus differed between term and preterm infants. Among term infants the origin was considered to be prenatal in 70%, perinatal in 25% and postnatal in 5%, whereas among infants born preterm the corresponding proportions were 40%, 60% and less than 1% respectively (Fernell et al. 1986, 1994).

CLASSIFICATION AND DIAGNOSIS
Hydrocephalus comprises a highly heterogeneous group of conditions that have little in common aside from the dilatation of the CSF spaces. Several systems of classification can be used. One early approach separated 'communicating' hydrocephalus (i.e. those cases in which intraventricularly introduced dye was recovered in the lumbar cul-de-sac after a few minutes) from 'noncommunicating' or 'blocked' hydrocephalus in which dye could not be detected by lumbar puncture. Such terms are now obsolete, and recent classifications are based on age of occurrence, aetiology and suspected mechanisms (Mori et al. 1995, Oi 2004).

The major *mechanisms and causes* are shown in Table 6.1. More detailed descriptions will be given in paragraphs dedicated to aetiological diagnosis in different *age categories* because age of occurrence has a major influence not only on prognosis and management but also on the likely causes of hydrocephalus (Table 6.2) as the causes, clinical manifestations and therapeutic decisions differ considerably with the age of onset and diagnosis. In the series reported by Mori et al. (1995), 68 cases were of fetal onset, 316 were associated with myelomeningocele, 332 were congenital of other causes, 152 were of posthaemorrhagic and 103 of postmeningitic origin.

Classification according to the site of the obstacle to CSF circulation is clearly essential as the distinction of obstructive versus non-obstuctive hydrocephalus has major therapeutic consequences. Classification of cases of hydrocephalus as *acute* and *chronic* is also important because the circumstances of diagnosis, outcome and treatment differ profoundly depending on this criterion. However, hydrocephalus is an evolutive condition and the rate of progression can change completely over time. Many

TABLE 6.2
Main causes of hydrocephalus in relation to age

Fetal hydrocephalus
  Malformations[1]
    Involving the CSF pathways
      Atresia, stenosis or membrous diaphragms of aqueduct
      Forking of aqueduct
      Stenosis of foramen of Monro
      Chiari II malformation
      Membranous obstruction of 4th ventricle foramina
      Maldevelopment of Pacchioni granulations (exceptional)
      Dandy–Walker syndrome[2]
    Involving more extensively the brain
      Holoprosencephaly (especially alobar type)
      Hydranencephaly
      Walker–Warburg syndome and related malformations[3]
  Abnormal events during pregnancy
    Intrauterine viral infections (toxoplasmosis, cytomegalovirus,
      parvovirus B19, lymphocytic choriomeningitis)
    Intrauterine bacterial infections
    Prenatal haemorrhage (intra- or periventricular)
    Trauma

Infantile hydrocephalus
  Late manifestation or recognition of prenatal cause
  Perinatal intracranial haemorrhage, especially severe intraventricular
  Intraventricular haemorrhage (grade III, IV)
  Bacterial meningitis
  Chemical meningitis (fissuring of craniopharyngioma or dermoid cyst)
  Parasitic infections, especially cysticercosis
  Aneurysm of vein of Galen or other vascular anomalies, e.g. venous
    compression or thrombosis
  Mucopolysaccharidosis (Hurler syndrome)
  Dandy–Walker syndrome[2]

Childhood hydrocephalus
  Posterior fossa tumours, including periaqueductal tumours
  Suprasellar and sellar tumours (craniopharyngiomas, optic gliomas,
    pinealomas)
  Suprasellar and incisural arachnoid cysts
  Infections and haemorrhages
  Cysticercosis and other parasitic infestations
  Late revelation of aqueductal stenosis (until adulthood)
  Late manifestation of Dandy–Walker malformation
  Late reactivation of toxoplasmosis

[1]Malformations may be genetically determined, of unknown origin, or may be secondary to acquired pathology (see text).
[2]The malformation is present during gestation but hydrocephalus develops mostly in the first year of life.
[3]Maldevelopment of meninges around the brainstem and convexity plays an important role.

cases have an acute onset that may be followed by a more chronic course, while chronic hydrocephalus may suffer acute exacerbations that may require dramatic changes in the therapeutic approach.

FETAL AND NEONATAL HYDROCEPHALUS
The development of imaging techniques of ultrasonography and MRI have made prenatal diagnosis of hydrocephalus possible, but the therapeutic problems are not easily solved and therapeutic attitudes remain disputed.

AETIOLOGY
Fetal hydrocephalus can be due to malformations or to diseases acquired during embryo-fetal development. *Malformations* are the most common causes of antenatal hydrocephalus (Table 6.2).

They may involve only the CSF pathways – e.g. atresia of the foramen of Monro, aqueductal stenosis, maldevelopment of arachnoid granulations – or may be associated with more extensive CNS defects such as hydranencephaly, holoprosencephaly, dysraphism, Dandy–Walker syndrome, Chiari malformation, lissencephaly, or arachnoid cysts (Oi et al. 1996).

Some malformations, whether affecting only the CSF pathways or more diffusely the CNS, are known to be genetically determined, and the genes may be known in some such cases (e.g. X-linked aqueductal stenosis, Walker–Warburg syndrome, some cases of holoprosencephaly). In other cases, genetic factors are probably at play, based on the familial clustering of cases. Many malformations are not genetically determined. It is important to realize that the same type of malformation can be due to either genetic or acquired factors, that this cannot often be determined for a particular case, and that no aetiological specificity exists. Therefore, no genetic classification is universally applicable. Whilst it is believed that malformations tend to occur early, the lack of glial response to insults in the first half of gestation can make scar lesions acquired early in pregnancy indistinguishable from primary genetic errors.

A significant proportion of cases of congenital hydrocephalus result from *disorders or accidents incurred during fetal life*, including infections usually of maternal origin such as toxoplasmosis, prenatal haemorrhage and congenital tumour (Fernell et al. 1994). These are termed 'secondary fetal hydrocephalus' (Oi et al. 1996). They can be diagnosed during pregnancy but often are recognized late. Myelomeningoceles and Dandy–Walker malformations may be a cause, but hydrocephalus usually develops later (postnatally) in such cases.

A small subgroup of fetuses with hydrocephalus without obvious cause and without associated malformation or chromosomal abnormalities might be candidates for fetal hydrocephalus surgery (Davis 2003). The feasibility and results of such operations are still under study and no consensus has yet been reached regarding their indications.

Most causes of fetal hydrocephalus are also major causes of infantile hydrocephalus and are described below as they commonly become manifest only after birth. Several causes of antenatal hydrocephalus are responsible for neonatal or very early death. These include complex malformation syndromes such as the hydrolethalus syndrome (Salonen et al. 1981, Herva and Seppäinen 1984), which features microphthalmia, polydactyly, and heart and lung malformations; the Meckel–Gruber and Walker–Warburg syndromes (see Chapter 2); the 'VACTERL' association (Evans et al. 1989, Faivre et al. 2005); and trisomies 13 and 18. Many of these are genetically determined (see below).

DIAGNOSIS
Ultrasonography
Ultrasonography is the first imaging method used when there is a possibility of fetal CNS malformation or a suspicious finding on routine sonography. Hydrocephalus can be suspected sometimes as early as the 13th week (Hudgins et al. 1988), usually by the 16th week, and can be confirmed between the 20th and

22nd weeks. It is always difficult and should always be confirmed by an experienced observer.

The diagnosis is made by determining the ratio of the width of the lateral ventricles to that of the whole brain (Chervenak et al. 1984). The shape of the ventricles, an asymmetry of the choroid plexus, or abnormalities of the size and shape of the fourth ventricle may support diagnosis.

Magnetic resonance imaging
MRI can better demonstrate the ventricular system as well as the rest of the CNS. MRI is not a routine technique but is increasingly used. It requires either fetal immobilization or rapid MRI techniques. It is thus indicated for cases with abnormalities detected by sonography and not clearly diagnosed by this sole investigation (Oi et al. 1998). Differential diagnosis includes agenesis of the corpus callosum with dilatation of the posterior horns, cysts of the choroid plexus that are usually transient and insignificant, holoprosencephaly, and especially non-evolutive ventriculomegaly. The presence of ventriculomegaly cannot be equated with a diagnosis of hydrocephalus. Cases of isolated ventriculomegaly without other abnormalities (21 of 47 in the series of Hudgins et al. 1988) may resolve before birth and be compatible with normal development (Serlo et al. 1986). Conversely, a few cases are on record in which fetal ultrasonography did not reveal ventricular dilatation until the 24th week of gestation (Kelley et al. 1988, Ko et al. 1994, Brewer et al. 1996). Goldstein et al. (2005) found that 26 of 34 infants in whom ventricular width at the level of the atrium was <10–15 mm were normal at age 2 years. Gaglioti et al. (2005) followed 176 infants with mild (10–12 mm), moderate (12.1–14.9 mm) and severe (≥15 mm) dilatation. The proportions of children with normal development in the three groups were respectively 93%, 75% and 62.5%. Parilla et al. (2006) found that mild prenatal ventricular dilatation disappeared in 41% of their cases, remained stable in 43%, and progessed in only 16%. It thus appears that mild dilatation has an excellent prognosis in fetuses without detectable malformations and a normal karyotype, and often disappears as gestation progresses. Asymmetrical mild/moderate dilatation may have a similarly good outcome (Durfee et al. 2001).

The *search for associated anomalies* is of extreme diagnostic importance. A careful search for facial, limb, renal, cardiac and other intracranial abnormalities must be part of the examination. Associated abnormalities may also also of grave prognostic significance: in the series of Nyberg et al. (1987) they were present in 85% of 61 fetuses with prenatal hydrocephalus, and the mortality rate for these was 66%. Similarly, associated malformations herald a poor prognosis in cases of apparently stable ventriculomegaly (Drugan et al. 1989).

When fetal hydrocephalus is suspected on sonographic examination, a complete investigation including karyotype, determination of alpha-fetoprotein and search for specific infectious agents by serology or by fetal blood sampling, as indicated, is in order.

OUTCOME AND MANAGEMENT
The overall *prognosis* of fetal hydrocephalus is poor. In many cases,

spontaneous abortion or stillbirth results. The outcome of intra-uterine shunting operations is at best uncertain, and most centres do not use the procedure (Bruner et al. 2006). In one series (Futagi et al. 2002), only 3 of 58 fetuses survived and developed reasonably. Termination of pregnancy is often performed for hydrocephalus of very early onset or with associated malformations and/or chromosome abnormalities (Serlo et al. 1986). In cases with a relatively thick mantle and slow progression, when parents decide to go on with pregnancy, delivery will usually be by caesarian section.

The outcome of *'secondary fetal hydrocephalus'* tends to be worse than that of later onset postnatal cases although there are marked differences in various series. Differences in evaluation depend, to a large extent, on the diagnostic criteria. Renier et al. (1988) included in their study only patients with head circumference at birth >2 SD above the mean. The survival rate of their 108 patients was 62% at 10 years. Only 21 of the 75 survivors had an IQ ≥80, and 16 were of borderline intelligence. Kirkinen et al. (1996) found that 7 of 25 infants diagnosed during pregnancy (excluding cases with associated malformations and/or lethal syndromes) were severely disabled, and 6 had intermediate disability. They consider that termination should be considered if there are associated anomalies or chromosomal disorder, and if rapidly increasing ventricular dilatation is found on repeated echography.

HYDROCEPHALUS IN CHILDREN UNDER 2 YEARS OF AGE
AETIOLOGY
The aetiological diagnosis of hydrocephalus is essential, especially as the prognosis depends largely on the causal mechanism. In most cases a cause can be identified. However, the cause remained undetermined in 14% of the series of 719 patients reported by Sainte-Rose et al. (1989). In the same series, malformations accounted for 38.6% of cases, tumours or other space-occupying processes for 20.4%, haemorrhages for 15.6%, meningitides for 7.4%, and several miscellaneous other causes for 4.4% of patients, with the cause being undetermined in the remaining 13.6%. It should be noted that the distinction between malformations and acquired causes is by no means absolute from an aetiological viewpoint. Some malformations may be due to inflammatory processes that are not recognizable because no glial reponse to aggressions develops ruring the first half of gestation. There is some evidence, in mice and humans, that aqueductal stenosis may be a secondary phenomenon, resulting from compression of the aqueduct by the cerebral hemispheres, dilated because of some other cause of hydrocephalus (Landrieu et al. 1979) or from inflammation due to viruses such as mumps virus. Lymphocytic choriomeningitis is a rare and often forgotten cause of congenital hydrocephalus (Wright et al. 1997, Barton and Mets 2001).

The same cause can produce hydrocephalus by different mechanisms. Haemorrhage and infections can produce either stenosis of the aqueduct as a result of organization of blood clots in its lumen or granular ependymitis or blockage of the basilar cisterns or of the CSF resorption areas. It is therefore difficult to

TABLE 6.3
Hydrocephalus of genetic origin

Type or syndrome	Main features	Genetics* (gene, locus)	References
Aqueductal stenosis (Bickers–Adams syndrome, MASA syndrome, CRASH syndrome)	Triventricular hydrocephalus, flexion–adduction of thumbs, mental retardation, paraplegia, agenesis of corpus callosum, gyration anomalies	XR (LICAM, Xq28)	Graf et al. (1998), Senat et al. (2001)
X-linked hydrocephalus without aqueductal stenosis	Mental retardation, clasped thumbs, spastic paraplegia	XR	Willems et al. (1987), Castro-Gago et al. (1996)
Non-X linked hydrocephalus[1]	No special features	AR	Hamada et al. (2000)
Walker–Warburg syndrome	Lissencephaly, severe mental and neurological abnormalities, eye anomalies, cerebellar malformations and cortical cysts, encephalocele in some cases	AR (POMT1, POMT2, 14q24.3)	Currier et al. (2005), van Reeuwijk et al. (2005)
Cobblestone complex with muscular dystrophy (COMS[2], muscle–eye–brain disease), Fukuyama congenital dystrophy	Similar brain malformations as in Walker–Warburg syndrome; associated congenital muscular dystrophy. Several types	AR	See Chapter 2
VACTERL[3] association	Imperforate anus, short or missing upper-limb bones; Fanconi anaemia in some cases	AR, XR (10q23–31)	Lomas et al. (1999), Faivre et al. (2005)
Hydrolethalus syndrome[1]	Microphthlamia, polydactyly, external hydrocephalus, congenital heart disease, pulmonary hypoplasia, early death	AR (HYLS1, 11q23–25)	Salonen et al. (1981), Visapaa et al. (1999), Mee et al. (2005)
Waaler–Aarskog syndrome[1]	Costovertebral dysplasias, Sprengel deformity, communicating hydrocephalus	AD?	Waaler and Aarskog (1980)
Metabolic disorders that may generate hydrocephalus	Include the mucopolysaccharidoses, cases of pyruvate dehydrogenase deficiency, cases of nonketotic hyperglycinaemia	Mostly AR, some XR	See Chapters 8, 9

*XR = X-linked recessive, AR = autosomal recessive.
[1]Rare syndromes.
[2]COMS = cerebro-oculo-muscular syndrome.
[3]VACTERL = (vertebral anomalies and atresia, cardiac malformation, tracheo-oesophageal fistula, renal anomalies, limb anomalies) with hydrocephalus.

predict which site of CSF obstruction will follow such events, and this may have therapeutic consequences.

Fetal infectious causes include toxoplasmosis, most often due to aqueductal stenosis, and cytomegalovirus infection that is rarely responsible for prenatal aqueductal stenosis. Acute obstructive hydrocephalus has also been reported with Epstein–Barr virus infection (Yanofsky et al. 1981, Cotton et al. 1997). Lymphocytic choriomeningitis is another rare infection that can produce hydrocephalus with retinal abnormalities mimicking toxoplasmosis (Wright et al. 1997, Barton and Mets 2001). Genetic causes of hydrocephalus are relatively uncommon but are important for genetic counselling (Table 6.3).

Malformations
• *Chiari malformations*, especially type II (Fig. 6.1) (see also Chapter 2) formerly accounted for over 20% or more of cases of hydrocephalus although the frequency of this cause is now declining. Hydrocephalus associated with Chiari II malformation and myelomeningocele may develop prenatally, and sonographic examination has shown that ventricular dilatation develops early before surgical closure (Chapter 2). The mechanisms of hydrocephalus are probably multiple. Descent of the brainstem results

in crowding of the posterior fossa with obstruction of the fourth ventricle orifices and difficult circulation of CSF around the brainstem in the region of the foramen magnum. Prevention of hindbrain herniation is one of the reasons that might support prenatal surgery for hydrocephalus due to myelomeningocele (Tulipan et al. 1998, Sutton et al. 1999). Aqueductal stenosis is associated in one third of cases. Alternative mechanisms may include atresia of the foramina of the fourth ventricle or ascending infection. As indicated in Chapter 2, hydrocephalus associated with the Chiari II malformation is not infrequently accompanied by involvement of lower cranial nerves, and respiratory or swallowing difficulties that in some cases can be alleviated by treatment of the hydrocephalus alone. Chiari type I malformation is commonly associated with hydrocephalus in adults without myelomeningocele but with basilar osseous abnormalities (Levy et al. 1983). Such cases are rare in children.

• *Stenosis or atresia of the aqueduct* can either be due to malformations, some of them genetically determined, or be acquired as a result of infection, haemorrhage or other mechanisms (Landrieu et al. 1979). The pathology is variable. It includes simple stenosis; forking characterized by division of the aqueduct into two or

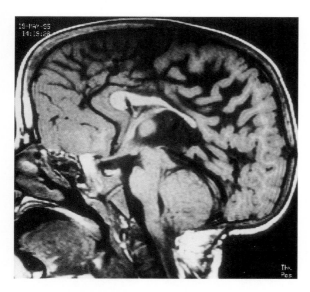

Fig. 6.1. Chiari II malformation. The brainstem is elongated and the medulla descends below the foramen magnum with kinking on the dorsal aspect of the cervical spinal cord. The 4th ventricle is very small. Note 'beaking' of the quadrigeminal plate, large interthalamic commissure and dysplastic corpus callosum.

several channels, most of them ending blindly; glial membrane located at the intercollicular sulcus level, which seems to have a special relationship to neurofibromatosis type 1; and simple gliosis surrounding the stenosed aqueduct. In some cases there is wide dilatation of the upper part of the aqueduct. Such anomalies do not need to represent a primary abnormality but can be a consequence of acquired events either prenatally of after birth following intraventicular haemorrhage or bacterial meningitis.

Malformative stenosis may be associated with neighbouring anomalies such as 'beaking' of the collicular plate, suggesting that they may represent a mild form of dysraphism. With the use of MRI it has become clear that many cases of the so-called 'idiopathic' aqueductal stenosis were in fact due to lesions encroaching on the aqueduct (Fig. 6.2), especially slow growing tumours of the quadrigeminal plate or periaqueductal and 'pencil' brainstem tumours. In a series of 71 cases of triventricular hydrocephalus (Valentini et al. 1995), MRI revealed such lesions in 15 of the 25 cases studied. A number of these tumours were associated with neurofibromatosis. None was progressive after 1–5 years follow-up, but regular examination is clearly indicated.

Aqueductal stenosis may occur as a familial X-linked condition, the Bickers–Adams syndrome, affecting only boys. Patients usually have severe mental retardation. Most have a flexed and adducted thumb deformity, but this is neither constant nor specific. It may occur as an isolated defect and has also been observed in the Walker–Warburg syndrome (Bordarier et al. 1984). Male relatives of patients with the Bickers–Adams syndrome may have severe mental retardation without hydrocephalus (Willems et al. 1987). Other types of hydrocephalus without aqueductal stenosis may have a similar X-linked transmission (Willems et al. 1987). This is due to multiple mutations at the

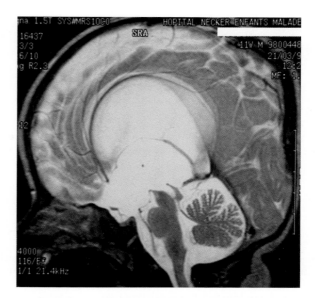

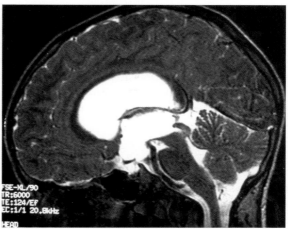

Fig. 6.2. Stenosis of the aqueduct. *(Top)* Congenital stenosis due to membranous diaphragm. *(Bottom)* Stenosis due to a small tumour of the quadrigeminal plate obstructing the initial part of the aqueduct.

L1-cell adhesion molecules gene locus at Xq28. The abnormal cell adhesion molecules that form thereby, apparently determine an anomaly of brainstem cell migration (Jouet et al. 1994, Jouet 1995). Mutations of the same gene can be expressed as X-linked spastic paraplegia without hydrocephalus (SPG1) or as the *MASA syndrome* (mental retardation, aphasia, shuffling gait, adduction of the thumbs), which may coexist with X-linked hydrocephalus in the same lineages (Jouet et al. 1994). The spectrum of conditions related to mutations in this gene has been broadened to form the so-called CRASH syndrome (corpus callosum agenesis, retardation, adducted thumbs, spastic paraplegia and hydrocephalus) (Fransen et al. 1995, Silan et al. 2005). The syndrome is highly heterogeneous within the same family and may present with isolated individual syndromes (MASA, spastic paraplegia or X-linked hydrocephalus) in different individuals or in a complete form. X-linked hydrocephalus can be diagnosed prenatally in most cases. Difficulties may arise, however, because of late onset

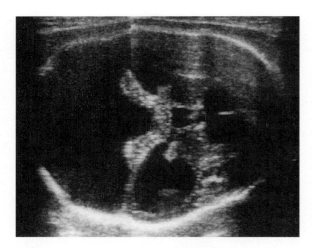

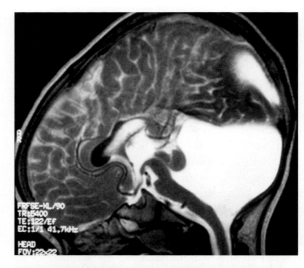

Fig. 6.3. Dandy–Walker malformation. Prenatal diagnosis by ultrasound scan at 33 weeks of amenorrhoea. Absence of cerebellar vermis and massive dilatation of posterior fossa (left side of picture) are clearly visible. (Courtesy Dr M-C Aubry, Maternité Port Royal, Paris.)

of ventricular dilatation (see above) and of features suggestive of a destructive process such as gross ventricular asymmetry (Brewer et al. 1996). A few cases of autosomal recessive congenital stenosis of the aqueduct have been reported (Barros-Nuñes and Rivas 1993), so a careful family history should be taken of all relatives when giving genetic counselling.

• *Dandy–Walker malformation* is an uncommon cause of hydrocephalus, accounting for less than 2% of cases (Hirsch et al. 1984). Prenatal diagnosis is possible because of absence of the cerebellar vermis (Fig. 6.3). In most cases, hydrocephalus is not present at birth but develops during the first year of life (Hirsch et al. 1984). The shape of the head, with a posterior bulge, may be suggestive, but the diagnosis rests on neuroimaging examination (Hanigan et al. 1985–86) (Fig. 6.4). The condition is not usually familial although some cases are due to chromosomal aberrations, and great care should be taken not to confuse the Dandy–Walker syndrome proper with other causes of agenesis or hypogenesis of the cerebellar vermis, which often belong to genetic syndromes (Bordarier and Aicardi 1990; see Chapter 2).

• *Walker–Warburg syndrome* comprises type II lissencephaly, congenital hydrocephalus, severe neurological dysfunction from the first days of life, retinal dysplasia, microphthalmia and abnormalities of the anterior chamber of the eye (Chapter 2). The association of eye anomalies and hydrocephalus may wrongly suggest a fetal infection but the condition is familial with a 25% recurrence risk. The presence of Peters' anomaly, retinal detachment or falciform fold of the retina should always raise the possibility of this syndrome, which may also include an abnormal posterior fossa reminiscent of the Dandy–Walker syndrome (Bordarier et al. 1984).

• *Other malformations associated with hydrocephalus* include encephaloceles, which are approximately as common as the

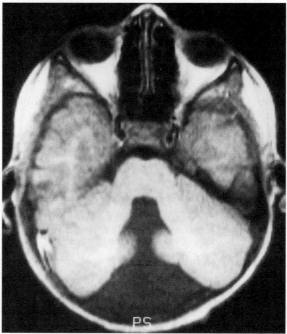

Fig. 6.4. Dandy–Walker malformation. *(Top)* Sagittal MRI: large cyst of the posterior fossa pushing forward the brainstem with hydrocephalus. Note the excessive posterior development of the skull. Partial agenesis of the corpus callosum is associated with radial distribution of sulci of the inner aspect of the hemisphere. *(Bottom)* Axial view of another child showing absence of cerebellar vermis and communication of the fourth ventricle with the cyst.

Dandy–Walker malformation, as well as a miscellany of malformation syndromes, some of which are of chromosomal origin (Chapter 4), and some are genetically determined (Waaler and Aarskog 1980, Herva and Seppainen 1984). Agenesis of the corpus callosum is often associated with marked ventricular dilatation and a large head (Chapter 2). Although virtually nothing is known about the hydrodynamics of such cases, experience indicates that many of these eventually stabilize, so that shunting should be resorted to only in the face of evident progression in patients with callosal agenesis. Agenesis of the granulations of Pacchioni and arachnoid villi is exceptional.

• *Tumours* other than those obstructing the aqueduct are not a common cause of hydrocephalus in infants, in contrast to their high frequency in older patients. They generate hydrocephalus through variable mechanisms including blockage of CSF pathways by dissemination or compression. Congenital tumours may be associated with hydrocephalus (Chapter 13), although macrocephaly in such cases may also be due to the bulk of the tumour itself. Craniopharyngiomas and optic nerve gliomas usually manifest later. Aqueductal tumours that may be difficult to distinguish from simple aqueductal stenosis (Raffel et al. 1988) have been described above. Meningeal leukaemia (Ricevuti et al. 1986) or gliomatosis (Civitello et al. 1988), as well as meningeal dissemination of primary brain tumours can produce hydrocephalus through basilar obstruction or blockage of arachnoid cisterns of the convexity. Some mucopolysaccharidoses, especially *Hurler syndrome*, commonly cause moderate hydrocephalus associated with extreme dilatation of the Virchow–Robin spaces, due to infiltration of the meninges by mucopolysaccharides.

• *Cysts of the meninges and other space-occupying lesions* in contrast to tumours are not uncommon. Posterior fossa cysts (Di Rocco et al. 1981, Barkovich et al. 1989), paramesencephalic arachnoid cysts (Grollmus et al. 1976) and suprasellar cysts (Pierre-Kahn et al. 1990) can all produce hydrocephalus. Suprasellar cysts are often responsible, in addition, for a special endocrinological syndrome (Brauner et al. 1987). Other space-occupying lesions, e.g. retrocerebellar subdural cyst or haematoma, can rarely cause hydrocephalus.

• *Haemorrhages* can be the cause of acquired hydrocephalus by two distinct mechanisms. In the acute stage of an intraventricular or subarachnoid haemorrhage, the presence of a blood clot in the aqueduct or the cisterna magna, or the increased resistance resulting from the augmented viscosity of the CSF by admixture of blood, will induce ventricular dilatation. After the acute stage is over, the hydrocephalus may stabilize or regress. However, the development of meningeal adhesions in the fourth ventricle outlets, basal CSF cisterns or granular ependymitis in the aqueduct can be responsible for the persistence or increase of chronic hydrocephalus, necessitating the placement of a permanent shunt.

The main causes of haemorrhage are preterm birth with peri-intraventricular haemorrhage (PIVH), trauma with subarachnoid or subdural bleeding, or bleeding from vascular malformations. PIVH was responsible for the rising incidence of hydrocephalus in preterm infants in the decades from 1970 to 1980 (Fernell et al. 1986). Camfield et al. (1981) suggested that the incidence might be as high as 22% in infants <1500g birthweight. More recently the incidence of PIVH has decreased significantly (Chapter 1). Prospective studies have shown that progressive post-haemorrhagic hydrocephalus is less common than nonprogressive or regressive ventricular dilatation following PIVH in preterm infants. Dykes et al. (1989) found that hydro-

cephalus developed in 53 of 409 infants with PIVH. In a majority of the cases progressive hydrocephalus remained asymptomatic. Hydrocephalus either regressed or was arrested in 35 of these 53 infants, only 18 having progressive hydrocephalus. Progressive hydrocephalus mainly follows grade III and IV haemorrhage. Hydrocephalus following grade II haemorrhage is uncommonly persistent and has a relatively favourable neurodevelopmental outcome (Krishnamoorthy et al. 1984; see also Chapter 1). However, late hydrocephalus may develop after arrest and resolution of neonatal posthaemorrhagic hydrocephalus, so regular follow-up is essential (Perlman et al. 1990). The long-term prognosis of post-haemorrhagic hydrocephalus is more dependent on the presence of parenchymal lesions due to the haemorrhage than to the hydrocephalus itself (Futagi et al. 2005).

Infections
• *Bacterial infections* are an important cause of hydrocephalus as a result of adhesive arachnoiditis or granulations that may develop following the bacteriological cure of acute meningitis or in the course of a subacute or chronic meningitis, especially tuberculous meningitis. In the latter case, ventricular dilatation is often the result of both brain atrophy and increased CSF pressure. CT or MRI show evidence of active arachnoiditis in the form of contrast enhancement of the meninges in the posterior fossa and basal cisterns (Chapter 10). Hydrocephalus may result from chemical meningitis due to fissuration of a dermoid cyst of the posterior fossa or spinal canal. The resulting arachnoiditis may also be due in part to added infection. Fungal infections include cryptococcosis and *Candida* meningitis, and occur especially in small preterm infants or immunosuppressed patients (Ciurea et al. 2004; see also Chapter 10).

• *Toxoplasmosis* is a common cause of aqueductal stenosis (Fig. 6.5) that usually is recognized shortly after birth (Couvreur and Desmonts 1988). In exceptional cases, a late flare-up of an old periaqueductal cystic lesion has produced aqueductal stenosis in adolescents.

• *Neurocysticercosis* in its racemose type can result in obstruction of the aqueduct or the cavities of the third and fourth ventricles or basal cisterns, thus provoking acute hydrocephalus (Cavalheiro et al. 2004).

• *Viral infections* are only exceptionally a cause of aqueductal stenosis. A few cases following mumps infection are on record (Ogata et al. 1992, Lahat et al. 1993), and cases of cerebellar swelling have been reported associated with varicella (Chapter 10), with Epstein–Barr virus infection (Roulet Perez et al. 1993), with prenatal lymphocytic choriomeningitis, and with human T lymphotrophic virus 1 (HTLV-1) infection (Tohyama et al. 1992).

Rare causes of hydrocephalus due to different mechanisms
Among the rare causes of hydrocephalus in infants, special interest attaches to *venous causes*.

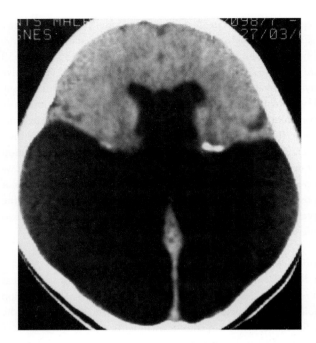

Fig. 6.5. Hydrocephalus due to toxoplasmic aqueductal stenosis. There is complete destruction of temporal, parietal and occipital cortex on both sides. Note also periventricular calcification.

TABLE 6.4
Frequency of major clinical features of progressive hydrocephalus in 51 non-shunted patients*

Symptoms		
Asymptomatic	25	(49%)
Irritability or headache	17	(33%)
Vomiting	8	(16%)
Jitteriness		
Anorexia, drowsiness	}	(5–10%)
Signs		
Abnormally increased head circumference	39	(76%)
Tense anterior fontanelle	33	(65%)
Splayed sutures	20	(39%)
Scalp vein distension	17	(33%)
Sunsetting or loss of upward gaze	11	(22%)
Neck retraction or rigidity	7	(14%)
Decreased consciousness level		
Pupillary changes		
Decerebration	}	(5–10%)
Papilloedema		

*Data from Kirkpatrick et al. (1989).

• *Obstruction within veins and sinuses* or compression of these structures has long been held responsible for hydrocephalus due to deficient resorption of CSF although experimental ligation of veins is usually well tolerated in animals. It has been postulated that an increase in sinus blood pressure can be the cause either of the syndrome of benign intracranial hypertension (or pseudotumour cerebri) or of hydrocephalus, depending on the compliance of the skull. In infants with high compliance, hydrocephalus will result, whereas pseudotumour will obtain if the brain is rigidly encased in a virtually inextensible skull (Rosman and Shands 1978). In fact, diminished compliance of the brain is essential and is probably due to increased volume of the blood compartment of the skull thus augmenting the resistance (Karahalios et al. 1996). Abnormal increases in sinus pressure may result from an anatomical obstacle or from functional factors. The former includes stenosis of the venous foramina at the base of the skull, such as occurs with *achondroplasia* (Pierre-Kahn et al. 1980), certain types of craniostenosis (Sainte-Rose et al. 1984), tumours compressing or invading the sinuses (Kinal 1966), and thrombosis of jugular veins or superior vena cava (Haar and Miller 1975) as a result of catheterization (Newman et al. 1980) or surgical operations. Such cases may potentially be improved by surgically widening the basal foramina (Lundar et al. 1990).

Functional abnormalities resulting in high venous sinus pressure are mostly due to high-flow arteriovenous malformations (Chapter 14), especially of the vein of Galen, which may also act through direct compression of the aqueduct. Rarely, a more distant arteriovenous shunt, such as produced by anastomosis of the right pulmonary artery to the superior vena cava in the treatment of congenital heart disease, can produce a similar increase in intra-cranial venous pressure (Rosman and Shands 1978). Hydrocephalus produced by high venous pressure is generally of mild to moderate severity, although shunting has been necessary in a few cases (Haar and Miller 1975). Venous bypass between intracranial and extracranial circulations can also correct the hydrocephalus (Sainte-Rose et al. 1984), as does cure of an arteriovenous malformation.

• *Hypersecretion of CSF* is observed in *choroid plexus papilloma* or carcinoma (Pascual-Castroviejo et al. 1983). In this case, haemorrhage from the tumour and mechanical impairment of CSF circulation from the bulk of the intraventricular mass may also play a major role in the development of hydrocephalus. The diagnosis of such lesions is easy with CT or MRI, and removal of the tumour may cure the hydrocephalus, although complementary shunting is often necessary.

• *Hydrocephalus of unknown cause* may be due to unnoticed haemorrhage or infection or may be the late manifestation of a silent malformation.

DIAGNOSIS
The diagnosis of hydrocephalus is usually easy in this age group.

The main symptoms and signs are listed in Table 6.4. However, the first manifestations before the head growth is obvious can go unrecognized for long periods in slowly progressive cases such as with congenital aqueductal stenosis.

Abnormally rapid development of skull volume is the major and most striking manifestation. It is sometimes associated with irritability and unexplained vomiting. In rapidly evolutive cases, vomiting, irritability, anorexia and drowsiness may be observed (Table 6.4). Not infrequently there is a delay in passing milestones, and this may be the first sign of alarm if the macrocephaly is moderate and has not drawn the attention of the family. The skull volume is evaluated by measurement of the occipitofrontal head circumference. Repeated measurements are especially important because the rapidity of growth gives some idea of the degree of severity of hydrocephalus. Comparison of the values obtained (preferably using a steel tape and ensuring that the maximum circumference has been obtained) should be displayed on an adequate head-growth chart (e.g. Raymond and Holmes 1994). A head circumference that crosses one or more grid lines over a period of a few weeks is evidence of definite abnormality in term infants, regardless of the absolute value, and any break in the normal slope of the curve is an absolute indication for further investigation. Interpretation of head growth may be difficult in preterm infants as ventricular size may increase without corresponding head enlargement. In such cases, comparison of ultrasound measurement with reference values for ventricular area (Saliba et al. 1990) is extremely useful.

Macrocephaly (i.e. a head circumference >98th centile or >2 SD above the mean for age) is usually symmetrical. It contrasts with the normal development of the face, lending an inverted triangular appearance to the head. The anterior fontanelle is usually large and tense or full in the sitting position. Splaying of the sutures of the cranial vault may be palpable. The scalp may appear abnormally thin and its veins are dilated, strikingly so when the infant cries. This dilatation is the result of diversion of the intracranial venous drainage through emissary veins as a result of increased venous sinus pressure (Sainte-Rose et al. 1984).

Ocular manifestations are useful for the diagnosis. The 'setting sun' phenomenon is a downward conjugate deviation of gaze such that the iris is partially covered by the lower lid while the sclera is exposed above the upper rim of the iris. The latter is due in part to retraction of the upper eyelid. The mechanism of the setting sun phenomenon is probably compression of the mesencephalic tectum, but it is not specific for hydrocephalus as it has been observed in children with subdural haematomas (Fig. 6.6). Moreover, retraction of the upper eyelids is occasionally present in otherwise normal infants at rest and can be regularly induced in neonates by sudden change from a vertical to a supine horizontal position or by removal of a bright light that had been placed in front of the eyes (Cernerud 1975). External strabismus is common and is probably related to involvement of the optic radiations rather than to VIth nerve paralysis. Optic atrophy is found in advanced cases, but papilloedema is rare unless the hydrocephalus is evolving rapidly such as occurs with papilloma of the choroid plexus (Pascual-Castroviejo et al. 1983). Seizures are a common manifestation of hydrocephalus. They may be due to the effects of hydrocephalus itself, with brain ischaemia resulting from increased ICP, to associated brain malformation, or to complications such as infections. They were observed in almost half the cases of Noetzel and Blake (1992). However, some of them may be tonic seizures resulting from intracranial hypertension. In most children, functional symptoms are not obvious and enlargement of the head is the major feature.

It is of note that a complete absence of symptoms is frequent in infants with hydrocephalus (49% of cases in the series of Kirkpatrick et al. 1989). That series also points to the rare occurrence

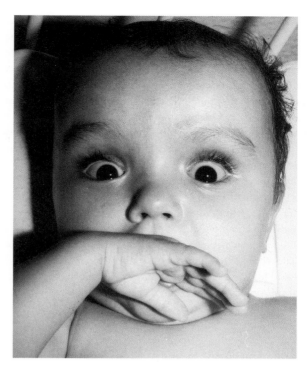

Fig. 6.6. 'Setting sun' phenomenon in boy with subdural haematoma, illustrating the fact that the phenomenon is not specific for hydrocephalus. Note retraction of upper eyelid and lowering of the globes, the iris being partly covered by the lower eyelid.

of atypical features such as profuse sweating, neurogenic pulmonary oedema and stridor (Chapter 2). An interesting presentation is the *bobble-head doll syndrome*, which is caused by dilatation of the third ventricle or by suprasellar cysts and consists of 2–3 Hz oscillatory movements of the head, usually in association with developmental delay. A slow tremor in patients with hydrocephalus has been regarded as a possible equivalent of the bobble-head doll phenomenon (Battacharyya et al. 2003).

UNUSUAL PRESENTATIONS OF INFANTILE HYDROCEPHALUS

Acute hydrocephalus
Acute hydrocephalus is less common in infants than in older patients because of the low yield pressure of the skull and brain (Jones 1987). It is marked by intense symptoms, especially lethargy and stupor, vomiting, and signs such as ocular motor palsies, extreme tension of the fontanelle, rigidity of decerebration or other signs of brainstem affectation. Parkinsonism is uncommon in children; it is probably related to compression of the negrostriatal pathways (Racette et al. 2004). Papilloedema may be present but is rare. Rapid dilatation of the ventricular cavities may be the cause of secondary haemorrhage. Such patients require immediate surgical attention.

Late chronic hydrocephalus
The late picture of chronic (non-shunted) hydrocephalus has now become uncommon. It features a special neuropsychological

profile with fluent speech but a low performance IQ, resulting in what Hagberg and Sjögren (1966) have termed the 'cocktail party syndrome' because patients are extremely talkative even though the semantic content of their language is rather limited. The syndrome also includes motor disturbances. Cerebellar ataxia was present in 41 of the 63 patients of Hagberg and Sjögren, and bilateral spasticity was found in 7 of these. The picture of ataxic diplegia is suggestive of hydrocephalus (Chapter 7). Hypothalamic and pituitary disturbances may also be a part of this syndrome (Brauner et al. 1987). Short stature and obesity are frequent. Precocious puberty (before 10 years of age in girls and before 11 in boys) is frequent (15% of patients in the series of Fernell et al. 1987). It is not related to a specific cause of hydrocephalus, although it is common with suprasellar cysts (Pierre-Kahn et al. 1990). Late sequelae may also include specific learning disorders (Billard et al. 1987) and memory difficulties (Cull and Wyke 1984). This clinical syndrome may be seen in cases of arrested or of still slowly progressive hydrocephalus. It may also be seen as a sequela in late shunted cases.

Very slowly progressive hydrocephalus
Very slowly progressive hydrocephalus, also termed 'occult' hydrocephalus (Di Rocco et al. 1989), is more frequent than acute forms in certain aetiologies, e.g. aqueductal stenosis. In such cases, the diagnosis may be made only by systematic serial measurements of head circumference or because of stagnation or regression of psychomotor development. In some cases, when hydrocephalus develops as a consequence of a previously known disease such as spina bifida, the occurrence of hydrocephalus is specifically looked for and, indeed, ventriculomegaly is usually detected by sonography or CT before symptoms or increase of head circumference are present (Chapters 1, 2). The problem then is to detect which of these cases of ventriculomegaly will result in progressive hydrocephalus. In cases of intraventricular haemorrhage or purulent meningitis, a significant proportion (up to 50% of cases) will not. Such cases may be termed 'arrested' hydrocephalus but the distinction can be made only by follow-up examinations.

Localized forms of hydrocephalus
These can result from *obstruction of one foramen of Monro* by a tumour or, rarely, by post-ependymitis adhesions. Congenital atresia has also been reported (Wilberger et al. 1983). Even rarer is *entrapment of the temporal horn* resulting in focal obstructive hydrocephalus that can mimic an arachnoid cyst or an expansive porencephaly (Maurice-Williams and Choksey 1986). Reversible diencephalic dysfunction as a result of a trapped third ventricle has been reported (Darnell and Arbit 1993). *Multiloculated hydrocephalus* (Albanese et al. 1981) was rarely recognized before the era of modern imaging. Its incidence remains unknown; it has been thought to occur in 20% of patients under 3 years of age (Cipri and Gambardella 2001). It is mainly observed following intraventricular haemorrhage or neonatal meningitis but repeated shunt infection may be a cause (Spennato et al. 2004). The diagnosis is made by MRI. The symptoms vary with the distribution of lesions, from a picture of intracranial hyperten-

sion suggestive of a dysfunctioning shunt to posterior fossa compression syndrome due to a trapped fourth ventricle (Coker and Anderson 1989) or to a mass effect as in trapped temporal horn (Hirsch and Hoppe-Hirsch 1988). Blockage may also be present at an orifice of Monro with resultant dilatation of the ipsilateral ventricle. Treatment has been considerably improved by the advent of neuroendoscopic surgery.

HYDROCEPHALUS IN OLDER CHILDREN
Aetiology
The aetiological diagnosis of late hydrocephalus in older children and adolescents is dominated by tumours and other space-occupying lesions and by congenital stenoses of the aqueduct.

Tumours of the posterior fossa are the commonest cause (Chapter 13). Aqueductal stenosis can decompensate very late, even in adulthood. Such patients often have headaches and mild neurological signs such as pyramidal or cerebellar dysfunction. They frequently have optic atrophy attesting to the long-standing hypertension. Their heads are usually moderately enlarged, and skull X-rays show marked digital markings and ballooning of the sella turcica. Small periaqueductal tumours or slowly growing brainstem gliomas should be sought by careful neuroradiological examination, including MRI (Raffel et al. 1988, Valentini et al. 1995). Neurofibromatosis type 1 may be associated with a diaphragm of the aqueduct or with periaqueductal gliosis or tumour (Balestrazzi et al. 1989, Valentini et al. 1995).

Hydrocephalus may occur in the absence of intracranial lesions in children with *spinal cord tumours* or associated with a diaphragm of the aqueduct or with periaqueductal gliosis or tumour (Cinalli et al. 1995). Gelabert et al. (1990) reviewed 23 published cases and added one of their own, and a complete review of the literature was presented by Maroulis et al. (2004). Onset was between 4 months and 16 years. Astrocytomas and ependymomas were most common, and the most frequent location of masses was thoracolumbar. High protein levels in CSF are regularly found and, together with compression of CSF outflow, have been thought to play a role in their mechanism. In five cases seen at our institution imaging showed evidence of basilar arachnoiditis similar to tuberculous meningitis, and seeding of the basilar meninges was demonstrated. This is a significant cause of apparently idiopathic hydrocephalus, and in such cases CT or MRI of the cord is indicated.

Hydrocephalus can be associated with spinal dermoid cysts and dermal sinuses, probably as a result of chronic infection or chemical meningitis (Martinez-Lage et al. 2006).

Diagnosis
The symptoms of hydrocephalus in older children with a rigid skull may be acute, with symptoms developing over 1–4 weeks in cases of rapidly developing intracranial masses or increase in CSF volume; subacute, appearing in less than 6 months; or chronic, when CSF compartment increases slowly over long periods.

Acute cases are marked by headache, nausea, vomiting, visual disturbances and progressive disturbances in vigilance. The diagnosis is by intracranial hypertension with symptoms and signs of high ICP, with headache, lethargy, strabismus and papilloedema (Kirkpatrick et al. 1989; see Chapter 13).

Chronic cases of slowly evolving hydrocephalus (e.g. aqueductal stenosis) may manifest with moderate macrocrania and progressive neurological signs such as disturbances of behaviour, neuropsychological regression, ataxia and pyramidal tract signs. Abnormal movements may result from decreased basal ganglia blood flow (Shahar et al. 1988). Ocular features are of diagnostic importance. The most characteristic is paresis of upward gaze (*Parinaud syndrome*), at times associated with deficient convergence and pupillary abnormalities. Ocular signs, especially paralysis of elevation of gaze with better preservation of accommodative than to light responses, are a major feature of the *sylvian aqueduct syndrome* (Chattha and De Long 1975) that also features in its complete form convergenge spasm, nystagmus retractorius on attempted upward gaze and upper lid retraction. This syndrome is due to severe deformation of the periaqueductal region compressing the rostral interstitial nucleus and the medial longitudinal fasciculus (Cinalli et al. 1999). It may evolve to global rostral midbrain dysfunction with parkinsonism, spastic quadriparesis, alteration in consciousness, and eventually decreased vigilance and coma (Barrer et al. 1980). MRI shows a hyperintense T_2 signal in the area probably due to oedema (Cinalli 2004). It is also observed in children with previously shunted hydrocephalus with shunt dysfunction, of which it may be the revealing manifestation. In such cases, it may not include at onset any significant ventricular dilatation. Simultaneous pressure measurements in both the posterior fossa and the lateral ventricles have shown the presence of a marked pressure gradient (C Sainte-Rose, personal communication 2005).

NEUROIMAGING AND ANCILLARY INVESTIGATIONS IN HYDROCEPHALUS

Modern progress in neuroimaging has radically modified the practice of neurology and neurosurgery and thus has transformed the evaluation and diagnostic methods for patients with hydrocephalus.

Ultrasonographic examination through the anterior fontanelle is safe and simple as long as the fontanelle is open. It is particularly well suited for repeated follow-up examinations. Measurements of ventricular span and surface can be obtained, and the sonographic characteristics of the ventricular walls and the presence of pericerebral effusions (if not located too high) can be verified (Fig. 6.7). Ultrasonography is better associated with another imaging technique (CT or MRI) to permit the continuation of follow-up after closure of the fontanelle and to try to determine the cause of ventricular dilatation.

Computed tomography allows for assessment of ventricular dilatation and for some rough quantification: measurement of the ventricular surface and of the ventricular surface index (ventricular surface/total surface on the same cut), and of Evan's index (distance between the two caudate nuclei/total width of brain). CT also explores the parenchyma, and the presence of periventricular hypodensities, especially around the anterior and, to a

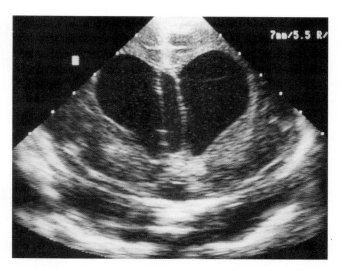

Fig. 6.7. Moderate hydrocephalus due to basilar block (transfontanelle ultrasonography): note presence of cyst in septum pellucidum.

lesser extent, the posterior horns, indicates transependymal CSF absorption and is a good index of progression (Fig. 6.8). CT with contrast may help demonstrate the presence of tumours, arachnoiditis or other aetiological abnormalities.

Magnetic resonance imaging is more precise than CT, and the possibility of obtaining multiplanar cuts allows for a detailed study of intracranial anatomy (Britton et al. 1988). Transependymal resorption is shown as areas of low T_1 and intense T_2 signal, and the status of myelination can be assessed. MRI can permit measurement of CSF volume in the various compartments of the CNS (Condon et al. 1986, Brunelle 2004) and also an evaluation of movements of fluid within the head.

New techniques have been developed for studying the volume of CSF and the dynamics of CSF flow. MRI can reliably measure the volume of the various CSF compartments. CSF flow can be demonstrated using specially designed sequences. Aqueductal CSF flow can be seen in the foramina of Monro, fourth ventricle and aqueduct of Sylvius (Nitz et al. 1992, Quencer 1992, Curless et al. 1992). In the aqueduct, downward flow can clearly be seen to be synchronous with the cardiac systole and reversed upward flow with diastole, illustrating the importance of arterial pulsations in CSF circulation. Semiquantitative methods are being developed (Brunelle 2004). Such techniques are of great theoretical interest and are already practically useful for precise assessment of aqueductal function. They are also used to assess the functioning of therapeutic ventriculocisternostomies.

Measurement of CSF pressure can be through the open fontanelle (Plandsoen et al. 1986, Bunegin et al. 1987), but intracranial determination is more reliable, if invasive, and may be resorted to when other means of determining the progression of hydrocephalus have failed (Fig. 6.9). In some centres, it has become a routine part of the management, although it can certainly be dispensed with in most cases. Normal pressure in reclining patients is 50–120 mmH$_2$O at the level of the foramen of Monro. In the standing position it becomes negative (average

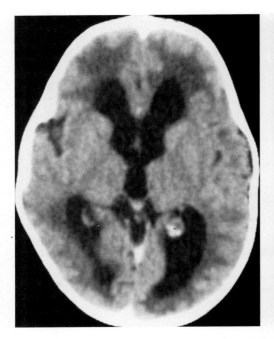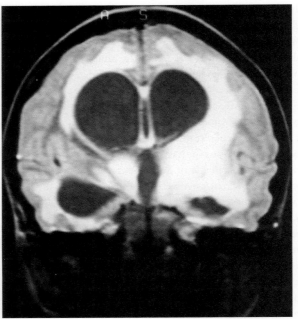

Fig. 6.8. Transependymal CSF resorption in active hydrôcephalus. *(Left)* Axial CT showing areas of decreased attenuation, most prominent around anterior and posterior ventricular horns. *(Right)* MRI, frontal cut, T_2-weighted image: areas of transependymal absorption give an intense signal.

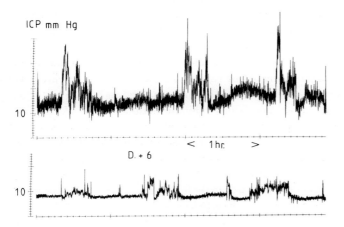

Fig. 6.9. Intracranial pressure curve in chronic hydrocephalus. Upper trace (preoperative) shows mild elevation of CSF pressure above 10 mmHg and very high peaks up to 40–50 mmHg, synchronous with phases of REM sleep. Lower trace (postoperative) shows normalization of basal pressure and low plateau waves. (Courtesy Prof. C Sainte-Rose, Hôpital des Enfants Malades, Paris.)

–50 mmH₂O). It fluctuates during the sleep–waking cycle, with plateau waves of about 100 mmH₂O every 50–75 minutes during REM sleep (Miller 1991), and it appears that high plateau waves even with a normal resting pressure indicate that hydrocephalus is not arrested (Allen 1986). The practical significance of these waves is not yet clear (Czosnyka et al. 2004)

Assessment of blood flow velocity, which varies in inverse relationship to ICP (Goh and Minns 1993), is of interest as it is indicative of brain vascularization.

The *EEG* may be normal or slowed, and with high ICP may show runs of anterior delta waves, irrespective of the cause.

Auditory brainstem potentials are frequently abnormal, perhaps indicating a special sensitivity of this part of the brain to increased pressure.

DIFFERENTIAL DIAGNOSIS OF HYDROCEPHALUS
The diagnosis of hydrocephalus has been considerably simplified by the availability of neuroimaging, especially sonography in fetuses and young infants and CT/MRI at all ages.

In older children with symptoms and signs of increased ICP, the diagnostic evaluation is similar to that for tumour suspects (Chapter 13).

In infants and younger children, the problem is usually that of a large or enlarging head, often without symptoms. Causes of macrocephaly, aside from hydrocephalus and pericerebral collections, have been discussed in Chapter 2 (see Table 2.5, p. 64) and are easily diagnosed by neuroimaging. Agenesis of the corpus callosum is often associated with a large head. This may result from the presence of associated interhemispheric cysts; ventricular enlargement, especially of the occipital and temporal horns, may present, suggesting hydrocephalus. MRI shows incomplete development of the hippocampus (Baker and Barkovitch 1992). The cause of ventriculomegaly in such cases is not clear but clinical experience shows that they are often well tolerated and it seems that only when there is progression should surgical therapy be considered.

Pericerebral collections are discussed later in this chapter. Such collections may be associated with some degree of ventricular dilatation thought to be secondary to the compression of the subarachnoid space. This secondary hydrocephalus usually disappears after treatment of the subdural effusion. The imaging appearance permits an easy differentiation.

The same applies to the *rapid head growth* that is often observed in preterm or small for gestional age infants, usually starting between 30 and 40 days of age. It is therefore important to use appropriate tables (Raymond and Holmes 1994). When in doubt, sonography provides a rapid and precise answer. A similar phenomenon is sometimes observed in older infants up to 2–3 years of age when rapid 'catch-up' growth follows a prolonged period of caloric deprivation. Rapid growth can be associated with an increase in width of the pericerebral fluid spaces, and separation of the sutures may occur. *Large congenital tumours* can give rise to a large head mimicking hydrocephalus but imaging is totally different (Chapter 13).

In fact, real difficulties arise in only three sets of circumstances. The first is represented by some cases of *brain atrophy*. Although, in principle, the head should be small in such cases, this does not universally apply and the head circumference can be normal or even mildly increased. Whether this is related to a previous period of high CSF pressure cannot be determined in many cases. Pressure measurements in some such children have given normal figures. Moreover, brain imaging indicates that the distension of the ventricular system predominates in the frontal horns, whereas in true hydrocephalus dilatation is virtually always more marked in the temporal and occipital horns, at least early on. A combination of true hydrocephalus and atrophy may be seen in some patients. In such cases a marked dilatation of the anterior part of the lateral ventricles should lead one to suspect an associated destructive lesion process.

The second circumstance in which serious diagnostic difficulties may arise is in infants who have had an *intracranial haemorrhage* or in infants or children following the acute state of *bacterial meningitis*. Repeated sonographic or CT examinations may be necessary before it can be decided whether one is dealing with acute temporary ventricular distension or progressive hydrocephalus. It should be noted that a considerable degree of ventricular dilatation can take place in preterm infants with obstructive hydrocephalus before any increase in head circumference is detectable.

A third difficulty is in distinguishing between 'arrested' and slowly progressive hydrocephalus. Serial examinations, repeat neuroimaging studies and, in some cases, ICP monitoring can all be necessary to reach a decision that may never be definitive. In infants, the ICP may be relatively normal even in the presence of progressive hydrocephalus because of the high compliance of the soft brain and unfused skull sutures. Continuous ICP recording in such cases may show relatively normal basal pressure with abnormally high plateau waves (Di Rocco et al. 1975) especially during REM sleep. Therefore, many cases of hydrocephalus at this age are cases of 'normal pressure hydrocephalus', but. Although cases resembling those in adults have been reported in older children and adolescents (Bret and Chazal 1995) the concept as it applies to adults with disturbances of sphincter control and ambulation and progressive dementia, is not applicable to infants.

TREATMENT OF HYDROCEPHALUS
MEDICAL TREATMENT
There is no satisfactory drug for hydrocephalus. Acetazolamide (up to 100 mg/kg/day) and furosemide (1 mg/kg/day) can reduce CSF production in humans by about 30% (Libenson et al. 1999). Isosorbide also increases osmotic resorption of CSF. These drugs are mainly used as a temporizing measure, especially in cases in which a decision about surgical intervention is uncertain and can be postponed.

SURGICAL TREATMENT
Surgical treatment of hydrocephalus has been radically modified by the introduction of extracranial shunting procedures. A striking evolution has been the development of alternative treatments to shunts, especially *endoscopic procedures* that are now preferred whenever possible to shunts because of the many problems these pose. Although shunts are still the more common form of treatment they are no longer the first surgical possibility to consider in many cases. Treatment of the cause of hydrocephalus, alternative types of derivation are also to be discussed before considering shunts. There is some indication that internal derivations such as ventriculocisternostomy might be effective even for postmeningitis or posthaemorrhagic cases.

INDICATIONS FOR TREATMENT
Medical treatment is rarely considered except in slowly progressive hydrocephalus and in the specific case of posthaemorrhagic hydrocephalus in preterm infants (see below).

As discussed previously, the decision to operate on a patient with hydrocephalus may not be easy because 'arrested hydrocephalus', or 'compensated hydrocephalus', even though it is rare, does exist and because complications of treatment are far from negligible. It seems reasonable to defer operation in children over 3 years of age with apparently arrested hydrocephalus when intellectual performance is within normal limits and seems stable (McLone and Aronyk 1993). In younger children, the trend is to place a shunt because of the danger for normal development posed by persistent hydrocephalus.

The borderline between hydrocephalus and acute ventricular dilatation following haemorrhage or meningitis is difficult to draw, and various medical treatments such as drugs or repeated lumbar punctures have been used in such situations (Chapter 1).

The *treatment of hydrocephalus in preterm infants* following neonatal intraventricular haemorrhage poses a difficult problem. Surgery in the smallest infants is risky. Shunts in such infants are technically difficult to place, and dysfunction and infection are frequent, especially when the CSF has a high protein content (Hislop et al. 1988). In addition, nonprogressive hydrocephalus is frequent and the course is unpredictable (Dykes et al. 1989). The applicability of endoscopic surgery for these situations is now seriously considered.

For these reasons, alternative forms of treatment, especially repeated lumbar punctures (Ventriculomegaly Trial Group 1994) and external drainage, have been tried in infants with progressive hydrocephalus as shown by weekly ultrasound examination and/or enlarging head (>2 cm/week). The results of repeated lumbar punctures have been generally disappointing. Ninety per cent of children had poor mental development and the infection rate was 7% in the Ventriculomegaly Trial Group study. External drainage usually does not remove the need for an internal shunt, and the risk of infection is not negligible. The combination of acetazolamide and furosemide seems the best recourse in such infants (Hansen and Snyder 1998) as it may allow a delay in the placing of a shunt until the medical condition of the infant is less precarious (see also Chapter 1).

The decision for surgical treatment may also be difficult in patients with long-standing hydrocephalus, spastic diplegia and neurodevelopmental problems. The degree of reversibility of such abnormalities is not known. On the other hand, insidious deterioration certainly occurs in many cases, and surgical treatment is indicated whenever there is doubt about the progression of the disorder.

TREATMENT OF THE CAUSE

This applies to hydrocephalus secondary to space-occupying processes. Removal of a brain tumour will re-establish a normal CSF circulation. However, postoperative bleeding and aseptic meningitis may lead to the development of adhesions that will maintain active hydrocephalus. Although some neurosurgeons advise shunting preliminary to tumour removal, the majority prefer to shunt only postoperatively when necessary. Excision or shunting of an arachnoid cyst is also a form of aetiological treatment but will be considered with shunting techniques.

Surgical treatment over the last three decades has been mainly by CSF derivation by shunts. More recently, however, major improvements in surgical techniques and the realization that shunts were the source of multiple and often severe complications that might occur many years after surgery (see below) has led to an increased use of internal derivation techniques especially ventriculocisternostomy, which tends now to be regarded as the intervention of choice whenever it is possible.

Ventriculocisternostomy

Any form of hydrocephalus that is purely obstructive in nature, with one of multiple sites of obstruction located between the third ventricle and the peripontine cistern, can be cured by endoscopic third ventriculostomy (Cinalli 2004). The main types amenable to ventriculocisternostomy are indicated below.

Primary aqueductal stenosis due to forking, glial stenosis, membrane or other congenital anomaly is the best candidate for the operation. A satisfactory circulation of CSF can be restored by establishing a patent communication between the anterior recess of the third ventricle and the chiasmatic cistern, as the CSF pathways below the aqueduct are patent. The operation consists in perforating the floor of the third ventricle anterior to the mamillary bodies under endoscopic control, usually with a semi-rigid stylet neuroendoscope behind the posterior clinoid.

Tumoural hydrocephalus is also amenable to ventriculocisternostomy in some tectal gliomas and in pineal tumours (Ferrer et al. 1997, Oi et al. 2001, Mizoguchi et al. 2000, Pople et al.

2001). It is also used as preoperative prevention of postoperative hydrocephalus in tumours of the posterior fossa. Sainte-Rose et al. (2001) performed it preoperatively in 4 patients and postoperatively in 6 cases with satisfactory results.

Hydrocephalus of other causes in which ventriculostomy has been used include obstructive tetraventicular hydrocephalus due to obstruction of the fourth ventricle foramina (Cinalli 2004), some cases of vein of Galen malformation, and cases of post-infectious aqueductal stenosis due to toxoplasmosis and mumps encephalomyelitis. Some investigators have used it as a first therapeutic attempt in cases of post-haemorrhagic hydrocephalus, when it is not indicated in principle because of the possibility of basal cistern blockage, and found it effective in a significant proportion of cases.

Cysts associated with hydrocephalus, especially suprasellar cysts (Pierre-Kahn et al. 1990; see Chapter 13) and incisural cysts, can be treated by ventriculocystostomy, a procedure similar in its principle to ventriculocisternostomy whereby a communication is established between the third ventricle and the cysts. In such cases, the operation may avoid a pressure dysequilibrium between the ventricular system and the cyst that can be responsible for postoperative dilatation of either cavity.

Hydrocephalus in shunt malfunction has also been treated by ventriculostomy, when feasible (Punt 2004), and was successful in 23 of 30 cases in one series (Cinalli et al. 1998) allowing control without shunt.

The *success rate of ventriculostomy* reported in the literature ranges widely, with a mean of 68% (Cinalli 2004). The variable results are mainly due to the heterogeneity of the operated cases. If only triventricular hydrocephalus cases are considered, the average success rate is above 60%. Ventriculocisternostomy is effective in reducing intracranial hypertension but usually leaves a persistent dilatation of the ventricles (Hirsch 1982, Cinalli 2004). The decrease in ventricular size is less than with shunting operations. Volume reduction of the order of 30–50% is expected unless there is parenchymal atrophy in long-standing cases. This less marked decrease avoids the problem sometimes seen of ventricular collapse with post-shunt pericerebral collections in patients with a large skull. Symptoms and signs of intracranial hypertension disappear promptly, and intracranial pressure should return to normal within 10 days. In case of persistence, shunting becomes necessary.

Complications of ventriculostomy include intraoperative complications such as bradycardia, asystole and haemorrhage, and also damage to the fornices that usually has minimal consequences. Hypothalamic damage may produce severe consequences (Teo 2004). Vascular damage to the basilar artery can be life threatening but is rare. Failure to control the hydrocephalus is frequent in young infants. Most of these complications should be avoided by correct technique (Navarro et al. 2006). However, success rate decreased with increasing age to less than 50%, even when taking into account aetiology (Koch-Wiewrodt and Wagner 2006). Late failure of the venticulostomy does occur, sometimes years after the procedure. It may result from glial scarring stenosing or obstructing the orifice but may also occur in the face of an open stoma. This is a dangerous complication that may result in acute midbrain syndrome. Therefore, patients should be informed and followed closely. Failure of the ventriculostomy seems not to occur after the five years following operation (Cinalli 2004).

Shunting operations

These techniques aim at diverting the CSF that cannot reach its normal areas of resorption towards another site of drainage. This is achieved by inserting a unidirectional valve system with a specified level of opening pressure between a proximal catheter placed in the ventricular system (or other fluid-containing cavity) and a distal catheter that carries the outflow of the valve to the draining site.

Under special circumstances, for instance when there is infection of the CSF or the fluid is haemorrhagic and might obstruct the system, the distal catheter may be temporarily drained into a sterile pouch, external to the patient. External drainage is limited by the risk of infection and the consequent necessity to maintain the patient in strict aseptic conditions.

Internal shunts have become the standard treatment in the vast majority of cases of hydrocephalus. Numerous catheters and valve systems are available with different mechanisms and hydrodynamic characteristics. Residual ICP after shunting will depend on the opening pressure of the valve or the pressure within the drainage cavity and on the resistance of the shunt. Available valves are classified into low-pressure (opening pressure 20–50 mmH$_2$0), mid-pressure (50–80 mmH$_2$0) and high-pressure valves (80–120 mmH$_2$0). The flow once the valve is open will be determined by the ratio of the differential pressure between the two extremities of the system to its resistance. Most systems have a constant resistance so that the standing position inevitably produces overdrainage. Variable resistance systems have been proposed (reviewed by Sainte-Rose et al. 1987) in order to avoid such problems.

Currently, drainage is generally into the peritoneal cavity (ventriculoperitoneal shunt), because this form of shunt is easier to insert and does not need lengthening with growth of the patient since a considerable length of catheter may be left within the peritoneum without serious problems (Vinchon and Dhellemes 2004). Ventriculoatrial shunts are now used only when the peritoneum does not absorb enough fluid or in cases of peritoneal or intraperitoneal infection.

In some patients, for instance those with the Dandy–Walker syndrome, the proximal shunt may be placed in the fourth ventricle rather than in the lateral ventricle.

Most systems include an inbuilt reservoir, placed subcutaneously over the skull, which theoretically allows shunt functioning to be assessed by pumping the reservoir. In fact, the correlation between response to pumping and functioning of the shunt is poor. According to Piatt (1992) only 18–20% of blocked shunts cannot be pumped, and the ability to pump indicates shunt patency in only 65–81% of cases. There is thus no simple manoeuvre for assessing shunt functioning. For this reason, some surgeons always use a separate fluid reservoir for pressure measurement and fluid collection (Leggate et al. 1988).

TABLE 6.5
Main complications of ventricular shunts

Infection
Septicaemia (only with ventriculoatrial shunts)
Meningitis
Peritonitis
Shunt nephritis (only with ventriculoatrial shunts)
Wound infection

Primary misplacement
Intracranial
Intra-abdominal
Intravascular
Puncture porencephaly

Blockage and underdrainage
Proximal obstruction by choroid plexus, brain tissue, meninges, ependyma,
    pathological tissue or foreign material
Distal obstruction of abdominal or atrial catheter; development of
    intra-abdominal cyst; CSF ascites

Fractures of catheter or connectors

Migration of catheter
In hollow viscera (intestine, bladder, stomach)
In inguinal canal with hydrocele; coiling around intestine with intestinal
    obstruction

Isolated ventricles—especially trapped 4th ventricles with secondary stenosis
    of the sylvian aqueduct

Overdrainage
Intracranial hypotension
Shunt dependency
Post-shunt pericerebral collections
Slit ventricle syndrome
Post-shunt craniostenosis
Stenosis of the spinal canal

Epilepsy

Lumboperitoneal and other shunts are now only rarely used. Some surgeons employ them for the treatment of pseudotumour cerebri. The catheter is introduced into the lumbar subarachnoid space and anchored to the lumbar fascia. The tube is then fed through a subcutaneous tunnel to exit through a small incision in the loin. Then, with or without interposition of a valve, the catheter is fed into another subcutaneous tunnel to the paraumbilical area where it is introduced into the peritoneal cavity as a ventriculoperitoneal catheter.

In spite of considerable progress in the development and techniques of use of CSF shunts, numerous *complications* can and do occur (Hirsch and Hoppe-Hirsch 1988, Sainte-Rose et al. 1989, Di Rocco et al. 1994). They are more common in infancy and following operation for aqueductal stenosis (Di Rocco et al. 1994). Table 6.5 lists the main complications of shunts. The major complications are infection and shunt failure, and associated incidents such as fracture and migration of catheters.

Infection remains a serious complication of shunt procedures. Its incidence varies between 4% and 8% in published series (Renier et al. 1984, Ammirati and Raimondi 1987, Hirsch and Hoppe-Hirsch 1988, Di Rocco et al. 1994) but the lower figure now seems to be generally accepted. The rate is higher in infants under 6 months of age. The infecting organism is *Staphylococcus epidermidis* in half the cases, *S. aureus* in a quarter, and gram-negative organisms in about a fifth (Bayston 1994). Rare pathogens may colonize shunts (Chapter 10). Infection is usually an early complication but can occur months or years after operation. Meningitis is the dominant infection (almost two thirds of cases), while peritonitis occurs in about 20% and wound infection in over 10%. The clinical picture is often insidious, especially when *S. epidermidis* is the cause, and the diagnosis may be difficult, especially when eosinophilia is the prominent CSF anomaly (Vinchon et al. 1992). Death is possible, especially with gram-negative meningitis. Localized peritoneal infection can lead to ulceration of the bowel with exteriorization of the catheter through the anus. Septicaemia has become rare since ventriculoatrial shunt is now uncommon. The same applies to shunt nephritis (Wald and McLaurin 1978) and to cor pulmonale (Sleigh et al. 1993).

Prevention of infection by strict aseptic measures is essential (Hirsch and Hoppe-Hirsch 1988). Prophylactic antibiotics seem to reduce shunt infections and should be given on the day of operation and the following day. Treatment of established infection includes aggressive antibiotic therapy for 10–20 days on average after removal of the shunt. The shunt is reinserted when CSF cultures are sterile and CSF glucose back to normal. Some authors advocate initial antibiotic treatment for 5–6 days before removal, and immediate replacement of the shunt. Antibiotics are then continued for 2–3 weeks (Hirsch and Hoppe-Hirsch 1988). In an occasional case antibiotic treatment with injections into the shunt may sterilize the CSF (Bayston 1994). Removal of the shunt seems to give the lowest mortality. On the other hand, the incidental ocurrence of *Haemophilus influenzae* meningitis in a shunted child can often be successfully treated without removing the shunt (Rennels and Wald 1980). Peritonitis is usually cured by antibiotic therapy and removal of the infected catheter. Surgery is rarely necessary. Low-grade infection with formation of intraperitoneal cysts can be detected with the help of sonography.

Shunt failure can result from primary misplacement of the shunt. In such cases, parenchymal haemorrhage, traumatic puncture of the internal capsule or *puncture porencephaly* can be responsible for hemiplegic sequelae (Boltshauser et al. 1980).

Most commonly, shunt failure occurs in correctly placed shunts. In the series of Sainte-Rose et al. (1989), 81% of 1620 shunts had failed by 12 years after insertion. The risk of failure was highest, at 30%, in the first postoperative year. Disappointingly, the risk was 7–14% for each subsequent year and there was no indication of a trend toward improvement with time. Blockage of the shunt was the cause of failure in half the cases, most frequently at the ventricular end. Fracture, migration and disconnection were next in frequency, being observed in 14% of cases.

Migration of catheters following rupture of connectors may be particularly difficult to diagnose as CSF often continues to flow along the subcutaneous fibrous tunnel for prolonged periods. Cortical visual impairment is a complication of shunt dysfunction. It is probably due to compression of the posterior cerebral arteries by the tentorium, when there is a sudden increase of ventricular size with resultant downward displacement of the brain. CT shows bilateral occipital infarcts (Arroyo et al. 1985).

Sainte-Rose et al. (1989) reported a *mortality related to shunt failures* of 1%, and the incidence of subsequent epilepsy and of recurrent shunt failure was significantly increased. The symptoms and signs of obstruction may be overt or insidious. Parents should be advised to report immediately bouts of headaches or vomiting, lethargy, or the development of diplopia or other neurological signs. In other patients, only vague symptoms and behavioural changes are present such as decreased spontaneity or poor school performance, perhaps in association with mild headaches. Still other children have intermittent shunt obstruction. Sudden death can occur (Hayden et al. 1983), hence the need for rapid hospitalization. Non-functioning shunts need not be symptomatic. In the experience of Hayden et al., 23% of 307 patients with non-functional shunts remained asymptomatic for an average of 27 months.

It seems that about 85% of shunted patients will have to keep a shunt in place indefinitely if no complications supervene, and there is no simple means of determining in which patients the shunt can be removed despite the fact that various techniques have been proposed (Hayden et al. 1983). The diagnosis of blocked shunt is often difficult, and various techniques of assessment have been proposed, such as measurement of the Doppler pulsatility index (Pople et al. 1991) and MR flow study (Frank et al. 1990). Watkins et al. (1994) showed that a normal CT scan does not exclude blockage; percutaneous manometry in 26 cases gave no false positives or negatives but the results were equivocal in five children. In fact, all shunts are bound to stop functioning with time, as the annual rate of failure remains constant over the years (Sainte-Rose et al. 1991). This is due mostly to fibrous changes and calcification around the catheters. However, the diagnosis of non-functioning shunt is quite difficult and no method of recognition is consistently successful. This gives rise to discussions about removal of uncomplicated but probably nonfunctional shunts. There is no reason to remove a shunt in asymptomatic patients, even if it is thought to be non-functional, as this can result in intracranial hypertension.

It is hoped that the development of new material can lead to prevention of the formation of biofilms and may reduce inflammatory or other tissue reactions, thus avoiding the two most common shunt complications, failure and calcification.

Overdrainage is a frequent complication of ventriculoperitoneal shunts because of the 'siphon effect' that occurs in the upright position, due to the height of the hydrostatic column between the inlet and the outlet of the shunt. In standing patients, the draining capacity of the shunt exceeds the ventricular CSF secretion rate and overdrainage is constant. Overdrainage is more important with low-resistance valves (spring-ball type or silicone rubber diaphragm type) than with high-resistance valves (silicone rubber slit types).

Complications of overdrainage include subdural effusions, slit ventricle syndrome, orthostatic CSF hypotension, craniosynostosis and shunt dependency (Serlo et al. 1985, Epstein et al. 1988). Overdrainage is also an important factor in the mechanism of trapped ventricles. A trapped fourth ventricle can behave as any space-occupying posterior fossa lesion and requires placement

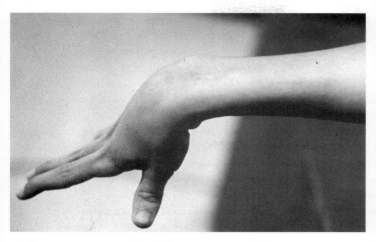

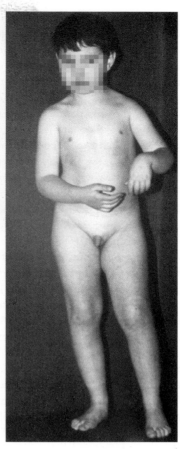

Fig. 7.6. Congenital hemiplegia. *(Right)* 7-year-old boy with left hemiplegia predominating markedly in upper limb. *(Above)* Typical attitude of hand in patient with right hemiplegia. (Courtesy Dr J-P Padovani, Hôpital des Enfants Malades, Paris.)

graphy is good, but some change in the appearance of the lesions can be observed after several years so that it may not always be possible retrospectively to diagnose their time of occurrence and exact type.

The various types of brain lesion, as indicated by neuro-imaging studies, have some prognostic value. Generally, lesions involving the cortex, such as cystic softening, are associated with a higher frequency of epilepsy and cognitive deficit than mainly subcortical lesions (Kotlarek et al. 1981, Taudorf et al. 1984, Molteni et al. 1987). However, individual prediction on the basis of CT is unreliable.

Clinical features
Unilateral paresis and spasticity are the characteristic features of hemiplegia. Weakness usually predominates in the distal part of limbs. Hemiplegia is rarely diagnosed at birth. Indeed, hemisyndromes of unilateral motor deficit observed during the neonatal period generally disappear without hemiparetic sequelae. A free interval is present in more than 90% of cases and lasts until the age of 4–9 months. That this period is really symptom-free has been demonstrated by repeatedly normal neurological examination in the face of known extensive hemispheric lesions in several patients (Bouza et al. 1994a). The first manifestations become apparent by 4–5 months in a majority of cases, when attempts at reaching are always on the same side. An early 'hand preference' should lead one to suspect congenital hemiplegia. Fisting

and an abnormal posture of the arm with flexion at the elbow are usually present. However, diagnosis is often very late. It was established by 10 months of age in only 53% of the cases of Uvebrant (1988) and by 18 months in only 67% of the cases of Goutières et al. (1972). In severe cases, there is delay in passing milestones but approximately half the affected children walk at the average age. Involvement of the lower limb often becomes apparent only with ambulation.

Prehension of hemiplegic children is characteristic: there is excessive abduction of the arm, flexion at the wrist and hyperextension of the fingers, which are spread apart (Fig. 7.6). No pincer grasp develops in many patients (Brown et al. 1987).

The upper limb is usually much more involved than the leg (Crothers and Paine 1959; Ingram 1964, 1966; Brown et al. 1987). However, Uvebrant (1988) found that the lower limb was predominantly affected in about half his patients, and Bouza et al. (1994a) also found some evidence for predominant lower limb involvement in preterm infants. This may be due to the increased survival of very preterm infants, in whom the predominant lesion is hydrocephalus or periventricular leukomalacia, which preferentially involve the periventricular pyramidal fibres that control the lower limb. The face is not affected or there is only a mild deficit predominantly involving the lower VIIth nerve, in contrast to the marked facial palsy usually seen with acquired hemiplegia (Goutières et al. 1972, Brown et al. 1987). Growth of the affected side of the body is usually less than that of the opposite side. This dwarfism predominantly involves the hand and upper limb. It may also be observed in acquired hemiplegia incurred before the end of the growth period. Associated movements are prominent and tend to persist indefinitely. Physical signs include 'pyramidal' type spasticity, increased tendon reflexes, and Babinski and Rossolimo signs (Lin et al. 1994). Weakness is usually mild, overshadowed by spasticity and associated movements. Frank choreoathetosis is not rare (Dooling and Adams 1975), and in some cases the term hemidystonia is more appropriate than hemiplegia (Nardocci et al. 1996). Motor deficit is rarely severe: fewer than 2% of patients in the population-based series of Uvebrant (1988) did not walk at the age of 5 years; more than half could walk without much restriction; and 30% had a moderate and 10% a severe limp. Contractures tend to develop if appropriate measures are not taken.

Cortical sensory abnormalities were present in 68% of the patients examined by Tizard et al. (1954), and 25% of them had a visual field defect sparing the macula. Brown et al. (1987) indicated that sensory abnormalities are difficult to test and may be less common than previously suggested. Mercuri et al. (1996) found that visual field defects, decreased visual acuity or deficient stereopsis were present in 11 of 14 children studied.

The severity of hemiplegia can be graded functionally (Claeys et al. 1983). In mild cases, there is a pincer grasp and individual finger movements are possible. In moderate hemiplegia, the hand can be used globally, while in severe cases it is not used at all. In such cases there is usually relatively severe involvement of the lower limb. Secondary motor problems with contractures are mainly seen in the paretic foot with equinus posture; hip subluxation is not a frequent problem. Hypotrophy of the affected limbs is often seen. Correction of leg length is seldomly necessary.

Strabismus is frequent, and optic atrophy is occasionally observed (Brett 1997). Congenital cataract has been reported in assocation with congenital hemiplegia. Severe cerebral visual problems are rare, reported mainly in term-born children (around 5% of cases). Hemianopsia is probably often overlooked as it is well compensated for by the children and only recognized when specifically looked for; neuroimaging may be suggestive.

Epilepsy is a major complication of congenital hemiplegia. It was present in 27% (Diebler and Dulac 1987), 34% (Uvebrant 1988) and 44% of cases (Goutières et al. 1972), the frequency depending mainly on the type of referral to any particular centre. Epilepsy may be focal or secondarily generalized. It is not necessarily intractable, and approximately 80% of cases are successfully treated medically (Uvebrant 1988). Rare cases of benign rolandic epilepsy have been reported in patients with congenital hemiplegia (Santanelli et al. 1989). Startle epilepsy (Chauvel et al. 1992) is a frequent type and should always lead to a careful search for mild pyramidal signs or body hemiatrophy as it is commonly seen in patients with minimal hemiparesis.

Mental retardation is present in 18–50% of cases. The prevalence of mental retardation is strongly correlated to the presence of epilepsy (Aicardi 1990). Epilepsy is five times more common in patients with mental retardation than in those without (Uvebrant 1988), and 71.4% of children with epilepsy in the series

of Goutières et al. (1972) had mental retardation as against 28.6% of nonepileptic children with hemiplegia. Vargha-Khadem et al. (1992) have shown that epileptogenic lesions of similar extent and location have a significantly more deleterious effect on intelligence and language than those unassociated with seizures. The prevalence of mental retardation is also correlated with the severity of hemiplegia. Thus, there is a strong tendency for cases of hemiplegia to separate into two subgroups: severe cases with multiple disabilities and a poor outlook for social and professional integration, and mild cases that interfere relatively little with everyday life.

Unilateral spastic CP – a model to study neuroplasticity
• *Language.* There is no gross difference in language with the hemisphere affected (Aram et al. 1985, Carlsson et al. 1994, Staudt et al. 2002b, Lidzba and Krägeloh-Mann 2005), although children with left hemisphere lesions are reported to be slower in language development (Chilosi et al. 2001), which may indicate that reorganization of language to the right hemisphere 'takes some time' but can well be achieved. However, this may be at the expense of originally right hemispheric functions, as visuospatial functions can be shown to be mildly deficient, which seems to be correlated to the degree of right hemispheric language reorganization and not to the overall lesion size (see Lidzba et al. 2006). This supports the concept of 'crowding' initially proposed by Teuber (Teuber 1974, Lidzba and Krägeloh-Mann 2005). Although there is no gross difference in language with the hemisphere affected, impairment of both verbal and nonverbal IQ is greater in children with left hemisphere lesions, while visuospatial functions are equally affected with lesions of either side (Vargha-Khadem et al. 1985, Carlsson et al. 1994). Speech and language defects are also related to the severity of mental retardation.

• *Motor function.* The compensatory potential of the young nervous system following brain injury is considered to be superior to that of the adult brain (Kennard principle; Kennard 1936). The malformations and lesions, which are characterizing pathogenic events at different times during early brain development, offer a proper model to study compensatory mechanisms of the developing brain. The healthy hemisphere plays an important role after unilateral lesions within the central motor system. In smaller lesions, not disrupting the motor tracts, an enlarged motor network involves also the healthy hemisphere (Staudt et al. 2002a). However, this is also described in adult patients following stroke (Weiller et al. 1993). In larger lesions, disrupting the motor tracts, abnormal fast conducting corticospinal projections from the healthy hemisphere exert the primary motor control. Such ipsilateral projections are physiological in the neonate; they do not mature and can no longer be elicited in later normal development (Eyre et al. 2001). They can apparently be maintained under pathological conditions, e.g. when the contralateral projections are severed (Farmer et al. 1991, Carr et al. 1993). However, their functional role seems to decrease already during late gestation, as Staudt et al. (2004) found evidence that hand function

that share with CP some weakness or hypotonia. The correct diagnosis of CP is highly dependent on knowledge of normal development and its variants. It is relatively easy to exclude the diagnosis of CP early if the developmental pattern of a suspected infant is normal. Early diagnosis is important: Prechtl et al. (1997) developed an early diagnostic system for the diagnosis of CP that evaluates video-documents of spontaneous neonatal and early infantile movements. A repeatedly documented occurrence of writhing movements and the lack of development of fidgety movements during the first three months are reported to be a highly sensitive and specific sign for the development of CP. It cannot, however, differentiate between the different subtypes of CP.

DIFFERENTIAL DIAGNOSIS OF CP IN GENERAL
The differential diagnosis of specific types of CP has already been discussed. Only problems common to most types of CP are reviewed here.

An essential diagnostic consideration is the differentiation of progressive vs static neurological disorders, especially treatable ones, from CP. Spinal cord tumour in the cervical region and slow growing brain tumours should always be excluded (Haslam 1975).

Many metabolic or heredodegenerative diseases run a slow course and their clinical manifestations can mimic all types of CP. The leukodystrophies, for example, may be initally impossible to distinguish from spastic diplegia, and ataxia–telangiectasia has features indistinguishable from those of many nonprogressive ataxias (Aicardi et al. 1988). Some cases of dopa-sensitive dystonia may simulate diplegia or athetoid CP, and a trial of L-dopa is indicated when history and examination make this a realistic possibility. Leigh disease (Fryer et al. 1994), organic acidaemias (Gascon et al. 1994), mitochondrial diseases (Tsao et al. 1994) and carbohydrate-deficient glycoprotein syndrome (Jaeken and Carchon 1993, Stibler et al. 1993) can also mimic any type of CP, and differentiation of fixed from progressive metabolic disorders is becoming increasingly difficult, so that indications for investigations may need to be reviewed.

The diagnosis of progressive neurological diseases can be helped by laboratory tests (Chapters 8, 9). However, these should be used only in cases selected on a clinical basis. In some cases, laboratory tests may be misleading. One patient with paraplegia due to a congenital spinal tumour (Aicardi, personal case) had for several years a diagnosis of metachromatic leukodystrophy, on the basis of pseudodeficiency of aryl sulfatase A.

Patients with mental retardation without motor abnormalities are often given a diagnosis of CP because, in both situations, normal milestones are attained late. Yet it is essential not to consider children with CP as being mentally retarded on this basis.

Hypotonia is a feature common to most early cases of CP but also to different diseases that are not infrequently misdiagnosed as CP. Prader–Willi syndrome is especially likely to be confused with CP because of the mental retardation, difficulties with swallowing, respiratory depression and frequent low birthweight (Wharton and Bresman 1989). The same applies to congenital myotonic dystrophy (Chapter 21), which indeed often coexists with actual hypoxic encephalopathy due to early asphyxia resulting from respiratory muscle involvement (Rutherford et al. 1989).

Hypertonia, which is a common early feature of several forms of CP, may also occur in infants with other problems or in otherwise normal infants (PeBenito et al. 1989). Neck extensor hypertonia in particular is often a precursor of CP (Amiel-Tison et al. 1977, Ellenberg and Nelson 1981). Touwen and Hadders-Algra (1983) found this to apply only when other abnormalities were associated with hyperextension of the neck and trunk. The marked hypertonia observed in hyperekplexia (Chapter 16) may simulate diplegia or tetraplegia, but there is progressive improvement, and touch stimuli frequently produce a considerable hypertonic response with apnoea. Georgieff and coworkers have emphasized increased muscle trunk tone as a marker of development in low-birthweight infants, not followed by CP (Georgieff and Bernbaum 1986, Georgieff et al. 1986).

DIAGNOSTIC DIFFICULTIES THAT AND EARLY DIAGNOSIS
As discussed above, the diagnosis of CP is a clinical one. Consequently, because the typical clinical picture becomes clear only over time, early diagnosis may be difficult. Abnormal neurological signs may be transient, so asymmetries of posture and tone, hyperexcitability and hyper- or hypotonia may be found in infants in whom no brain abnormality can be demonstrated. Such features are transitory in over 90% of cases (Michaelis et al. 1993). Transient dystonia occurs in some apparently normal infants during the first year of life (Willemse 1986, Deonna et al. 1991). It usually affects one or more limbs, does not involve the trunk or neck, presents after 4 months of age and interferes relatively little with the child's activities. The limb posturing may be intermittent or permanent and disappears after weeks or months (Chapter 9). Such transient anomalies may be the cause of overdiagnosis of CP and be responsible for the description of children who 'outgrow CP' (Nelson and Ellenberg 1982, Taudorf et al. 1984). However, we are not aware of any positively documented case in which clear neurological signs and/or MR findings as described above were associated with normal outcome. Niemann et al. (1996) found no abnormal MRI features in 6 children initially diagnosed as having spastic hemiplegia, who on re-examination no longer showed signs of hemiplegia but were neurologically normal. In the population-based study on bilateral spastic CP (Krägeloh-Mann et al. 1993), 20 children described in the medical records as having bilateral spastic CP were found not to have spastic CP at the time of re-examination (age 5 years and more). Ten who proved to be normal had been thought to have mild diplegia because of tiptoe walking after ambulation had been acquired. The others proved to have severe mental retardation with also severe motor delay but without clear neurological signs. Such figures indicate how much the diagnosis can err if infants are not followed up and how one should be careful in evaluating the 'effect' of early intervention. For this reason, it is generally agreed that the diagnosis of CP should be tentative before the age of 3 years and that CP registers should definitively

accept CP children when the diagnosis is confirmed at the age of 5 years. Modern imaging techniques can contribute to an early diagnosis. In one series (Truwit et al. 1992) 37 of 40 CP patients had an abnormal MRI, and in another (Candy et al. 1993) 17 of 22 infants with apparently isolated motor delay had MRI anomalies suggestive of CP. Of course, there are clear individual situations, especially when the aetiology is known, where the diagnosis can be established earlier.

The changing clinical picture or features of CP can also be a source of diagnostic problems, especially in choreoathetotic and ataxic CP, in which hypotonia is often an early sign. Dyskinetic CP may be wrongly diagnosed in children who are hypotonic and have stereotyped movements. Infants who later prove to have mental retardation without CP, and who have early neurological signs such as truncal hypotonia, hyperexcitability and decreased variability of motor patterns, can be misdiagnosed with spastic CP. In most infants with hemiplegia, asymmetry of movement usually becomes evident only after 4–6 months, even when the lesion is known.

The diagnosis of CP can be delayed in children with variants of normal development. Robson and Mac Keith (1971) showed that the diagnosis of spastic diplegia was significantly delayed in 'shufflers' with hypotonia of the lower limbs and axial muscles. Hand function, for example, cannot be judged before hand function develops, and milder changes become clear only with the development of more sophisticated fine motor skills.

Finally, it should be emphasized that a history of abnormal factors in pregnancy, birth or the neonatal period should never be a basis for the diagnosis of CP in the absence of objective evidence, even though it may be supportive of the diagnosis of CP.

MANAGEMENT

Rosenbaum et al. (2007) have proposed a classification of CP that no longer sees it as being exclusively a motor syndrome but recognizes also associated or indeed dominant other signs and symptoms that may occur in individual cases. Since these include practically any manifestation of activity of the central nervous system it means that it is necessary when considering issues of management to think about a very wide range of functions including vision, hearing, speech and language development and intellectual status. All these are the subjects of other chapters in this book and here we largely restrict ourselves to some general principles and a look at current developments in the management of CP.

While not affecting the motor system directly, associated features such as visual disorders may have an impact on motor function. For instance, the dorsal visual stream in the mammalian visual cortex is concerned with visual motor guidance and activity; its role in affecting movement in the damaged brain has not been fully assessed but is likely to be significant (Milner and Goodale 2006).

Equally, our understanding of the physiology of the gross motor system and of walking in man emphasizes the role of spinal generators. It may be that the primary role of the cortex

in motor function is an executive, controlling one of turning on the lower motor systems to achieve walking (Dietz 2002). Meanwhile, clinically in the last decade emphasis has been on the development of reliable testing instruments for gross and fine motor function (Himmelman et al. 2006). Measures of fine motor function include the Assisting Hand Assessment (Krundlinde-Sundholm and Eliasson 2003). The Gross Motor Function Measure (GMFM; Russell et al. 2002) has been widely developed and used. It has led to the development of prediction bands with which levels of gross motor function in children with CP can be predicted very accurately from the age of 2–3 years (Palisano et al. 1997, Rosenbaum et al. 2002). The implication of these prediction bands is that treatment or management is not in fact going to change the overall outcome for movement in the child with CP. Many people would feel that while neglect of any management of the motor system in the child with CP may lead to undesirable secondary effects such as contractures, effective management will not play a part in improving motor function beyond that which can be identified or predicted around the age of 2–3 years. Perhaps this has had some bearing on the stress on early treatment of the motor disorder and indeed often now on the presentation of the child from the neonatal unit. This raises parental hopes/expectations that early intervention will improve the long-term prognosis for their child. There is a continuing debate about how much early 'treatment' can affect the outcome (Palmer 1988). While there is some increase in mortality in CP, most children will not only survive but live for the full life span, and it is therefore important to consider a plan for health and service needs from infancy through to adulthood.

CP is defined as a nonprogressive disorder but also as a not unchanging disorder. Unfortunately there are still few studies of the natural history of CP throughout childhood, although the work of Rosenbaum and his colleagues is now producing longer-term follow-up of populations, albeit with particular emphasis on the motor findings (Palisano et al. 1997, Rosenbaum et al. 2002, Russell et al. 2002). Reports on many populations are cross-sectional. In one classic text, Crothers and Payne (1959) recounted their experiences in a clinic they had run together. While this did look in rather general terms at the outcomes and produce some life expectancy tables, the accounts were somewhat anecdotal and this applies to a number of other studies. Some cross-sectional studies have looked at CP in older individuals. One such study by Thomas et al. (1989) found a generally poor outcome in adult life. It is difficult to know whether these findings showing sometimes apparent deterioration in early adult life, which are beginning to be replicated, are a consequence of the original static encephalopathy or represent an inadequate level of care. It is clear that the level of care for young people with CP tends to drop in most developed countries when they leave school. While occasional individuals with athetoid CP have been reported to have a degenerating genetic disease in early adult life, equally anyone who sees young adults with CP is aware of a deterioration not accompanied by a degenerating condition. For example, it is not uncommon to find people who have been able to feed themselves losing this ability in early adult life. Certainly the movement disorder has secondary consequences such as osteoarthritis, which is more prevalent in this population than in others. In planning services, therefore, problems of providing community care are significant.

A diagnosis of CP has implications not only for the health services but also for education and social services. The associated visual and social problems impact on the child's functioning within school. In most studies at least half the children with CP have moderate or severe learning disability, but even those with cognitive levels in the normal range may have specific problems in school such as reading difficulties. In the past in developing countries children with CP were often educated in special schools provided specifically for such children or more generally for those with motor disabilities. In the 1990s the emphasis shifted toward integration ('mainstreaming' in America – Butler 1996), and inclusive education is demanded by some parents, although more recently others have again begun to press for special education. The debate is unresolved but the clinician will often be involved in discussing with parents what they perceive as the best option for their child.

The child with CP as with other children with chronic neurodisability benefits from a good preschool facility where educational needs may be assessed and planned. A period of observation in a nursery school may be extremely helpful, and it is important to have the input of speech, physio- and occupational therapists to that assessment, together with a psychological assessment as the child gets older.

MEETING THE NEEDS OF THE DISABLED CHILD
It has been felt appropriate to place this section here but the general implications are pertinent to any child with neurodisability.

The child needs: (1) diagnosis, (2) assessment, (3) treatment, (4) management, (5) care, (6) counselling, and (7) periodic diagnostic review and reassessment. In most developed countries now assessments will be carried out in an assessment centre, maybe within a hospital setting although sometimes in separate facilities. The organization of such a service has been well described by Robards (1994). The diagnosis of CP has been discussed earlier in this chapter; because it is to some extent one of exclusion this will often mean that there is a painful pause for the parents while it is being confirmed. Blood tests may need to be carried out to exclude progressive diseases such as some metabolic disorders. Genetic testing may also be important at this time, but often events during the pregnancy will mean that the brain damage has been clearly identified and a diagnosis has to be conveyed to the parents. Disclosure of a diagnosis of chronic illness in their child is obviously deeply disturbing to the family and the process needs to be carried out sensitively. Good guidelines about disclosure are contained in a booklet provided by the UK charity Scope (Leonard 1999).

ASSESSMENT
Any child with CP needs regular assessment of their general health status. Upper respiratory tract infections are just as common, or may be more common, in children with CP as in the

TABLE 7.3
Prediction of future ambulation at age 2 years*

1. Physical signs
The child is unlikely to walk if there is:
Persistence of: Extensor thrust ①
Asymmetrical tonic neck reflex ③
Moro reflex ④
Neck-righting response ⑤
Failure to develop a parachute reaction ②

2. Type of cerebral palsy

Hemiplegia	All walk
Spastic diplegia	~90% walk
Spastic quadriplegia	? Probably around 50% walk
Athetosis	? ~70% walk
Ataxia	All walk

3. Developmental assessment at around 2 years
The child is likely to walk if the following milestones are achieved by this age:
Arm propping (parachutes)
Sitting from prone
Reciprocal crawling
Maintaining sitting

*Adapted from Sala and Grant (1995).
At around 2 years of age, three factors enable one to predict future walking ability; *first*, physical signs (figures in circles represent significance of signs); *second*, type of cerebral palsy; and *third*, developmental status.

normal population, but poor swallowing, perhaps a weakened cough reflex and other factors may influence the child's physical health. As suggested earlier, some development may be delayed and some milestones may or may not be achieved, for example walking. Apart from these motor problems, which will be discussed later, another common health problem is the delay of bowel and bladder control, and some children with CP have a neuropathic bladder (Borzyskowski and Mundy 1990, Reid and Borzyskowski 1993). This problem will need appropriate investigation and management (Borzyskowski 1996).

While a diagnostic label such as 'spastic diplegia' or 'hemiplegia' will give a broad indication of the nature of the child's motor problems, to plan a management programme it is necessary to know what the child is actually able to do. Assessment of the child involves comparing functions of all aspects of development with the expected norms for the age (Bax et al. 1990). The child with CP will commonly have delayed development as well as abnormal development. For example, in children with hemiplegia, 90% of whom will walk, walking will often be delayed (Scrutton et al. 2004). Children with learning disability will have an uneven developmental profile but commonly some delay in motor development as well. There is sometimes a problem as to whether to give a child of 2–3 years a primary diagnosis of CP or learning disability (mental retardation). This depends partly on whom the child has seen, but by the age of 2–3 years future ambulatory ability can be predicted as stated above with around a 90% accuracy. Table 7.3 briefly summarizes the situation in CP but the far larger studies of Russell et al. (2002) in their book *Gross Motor Function Measure* provide much more detail on the predictions that can be made from motor assessments. The availability of

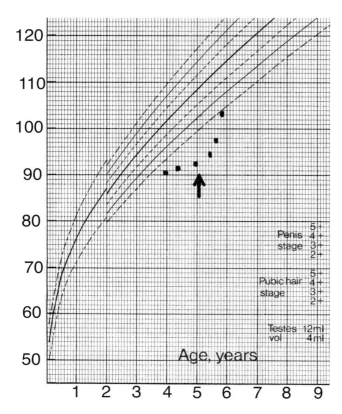

Fig. 7.8. Height chart from a child, showing return to 3rd centile within nine months of commencement of vigorous dietary supplementation *(arrowed)*. His weight followed rather more slowly.

cult to treat (Bax 1992, Blasco and Allaire 1992). Various drugs have been tried, of which scopolamine patches are probably the most useful (Lewis et al. 1994). Benzhexol and glycopyrrolate have also been used (Lewis et al. 1994, Blasco and Stansbury 1996). Redirection of the salivary ducts and removal of the salivary glands is another possibility that has good rates of success in experienced hands (Burton 1991).

The assessment of epilepsy in children with CP presents particular problems. The EEG is often disorganized and unusual movements are not uncommon, so the decision as to whether or not the child is having a epileptic episode can be difficult. Equally, epilepsy in brain-damaged children is often persistent, and its management and treatment are an integral part of the components of care for the child with CP (Arzimanoglou et al. 2004). The use of video-recording by parents is often helpful in coming to some decision about the nature of the phenomenon, but telemetric recording in hospital may be necessary to determine the nature and regularity of the seizures. The subject of epilepsy is discussed more fully in Chapter 15.

Another technique that has been developed over the last two to three decades to help in assessing a child with a motor problem is the gait laboratory. Here a videotape, EMG and force plates allow one to study objectively the origins of the child's abnormal gait. Sutherland and coworkers made standardized measures of normal gait in children (Sutherland 1984, Sutherland et al. 1988) and these have been very helpful in identifying abnormal gait in children with CP. In developing countries where such high-tech equipment is not available, simple ways of measuring and recording gait have been used (Law and Minns 1987). Standard measures of development formulated for use in normal children such as the Griffiths Scale or the Bailey Scale are often used in CP. These scales have not been assessed in relation to a CP population and in consequence findings have to be interpreted cautiously.

TREATMENT

When a health professional talks about treatment, the patient and their family may assume that the health professional is talking about a cure. In the early years they may be under the misapprehension that 'normality' can be achieved. The parents may believe that the child will become 'normal'. While as indicated below some aspects of the child's condition can be effectively managed there are many others where problems will persist. Spectacles may deal with visual problems and a squint and in this case one may talk of a 'cure'. However, in CP all that can be offered is a management programme that ameliorates the condition and allows the child to develop the best possible function. In perhaps 50% of patients with associated epilepsy, treatment may in time lead to the cessation of seizures. Such 'treatments' go some way to allow the child to function at an optimal level. However, even with excellent function the underlying neurological problem can usually be identified.

The prevention of contractures and of congenital dislocation of the hip are important management activities but they are not curative. Positional deformities that develop due to the child's

standardized measures of gross and fine motor development in the last decade has been extremely helpful.

Apart from gross and fine motor function it is important to look at other aspects of the child's physical development. Children with CP often experience disturbances in growth; for instance, the child with hemiplegia may develop shortening of both upper and lower limbs but predominantly the latter, while in spastic diplegic there is bilateral diminished growth in the lower limbs. Most of this delay will probably occur in the first two years of life.

Another feature of growth in these children is that many have feeding difficulties and every care has to be taken to maintain adequate nutrition bearing in mind that their basal metabolic rates may be different to those of children without disabilities (Sullivan and Rosenbloom 1996). Malnutrition can lead to growth failure and it is difficult to be certain what causes such suppression of growth. It is important to remember that the developing brain too needs adequate nutrition. Figure 7.8 shows a height chart from a child whose failure to grow was thought to be an intrinsic part of his condition until more vigorous dietary supplements were introduced when it was shown that this was not the case. It is noteworthy that height responded more rapidly than weight to supplementation.

A particular problem in CP is drooling, which may occur in as many as 50% of cases. It is a very unpleasant problem and diffi-

inability to move normally range from windblown hips to scoliosis. These are fully discussed by Fulford and Brown (1976) and Brown et al. (1982).

MANAGEMENT OF MOTOR DISORDERS

Numerous ways have been tried to moderate the abnormalities found in the different varieties of CP. The protean nature of the condition attracts enthusiasts who believe there must be some way of reversing the inevitable consequences of the damage in the motor areas of the brain. Sometimes in association with a medical centre, but more often not, many unorthodox treatments have been tried. In the following sections discussion will be limited to physiotherapy, surgical (largely orthopaedic) management, and drug treatments. In general, most of the treatments relate to the spastic form of the disorder; athetoid problems are mentioned separately. While the cause of the disorder is central, it is clear the effects are peripheral and it is important to have an understanding of the neurophysiology of movement and the qualities of muscles. This subject has been well reviewed by Walsh (1993).

Physiotherapy

Until very recently, therapists have used particular systems of therapy to treat (or manage) the child. The best known (and probably the best thought out) are the techniques developed by the Bobaths (Semens 1967, Bobath 1980, Bobath and Bobath 1984) but there are many other systems of therapy including those of Vojta (1984) and the Peto School (Hári and Ákos 1971). A danger with some of these systems of therapy (such as those advocated by Doman and Delacato – see Cummins 1988) is the great strains they place on the family, disrupting the normal pattern of family life (McConachie et al. 1997). In recent years the American Academy of Cerebral Palsy and Development Medicine has had working parties reviewing many of these systems and published reports on them. In general, these have failed to find that these systems of therapy are effective, and despite the enthusiasm their use is diminishing with the emphasis being on evidence-based methods being used. Thus the Butler and Darrah (2001) report on the NDT (neurodevelopmental treatment, based on the Bobath method) cast doubt on the value of this method of treatment. However, it should be noted that while orthodox medicine has in recent years been largely converted to the importance of evidence-based medicine, many physical therapy approaches are still widely promoted and parents may still embrace claims that the child can be 'cured'. The emphasis now is on the prevention of contractures and deformities and on efforts to see that practical functions such as standing, walking and eating are developed. The therapist will therefore look at the child together with the parents and other members of the team and produce a programme aimed at preventing abnormal patterns of behaviour developing and providing a management programme that will help the child to achieve their optimal development.

We give here one example of such a programme, developed to deal with an abnormal pattern of behaviour emerging in a child described by Scrutton (2004):

Problem: Consistent preferred head turning (PHT) and asymmetric tonic neck response (ATNR) in an infant with quadriplegic cerebral palsy—probably rigid/dystonic.
Consideration: We cannot treat the ATNR as such—it will diminish or remain depending on factors within the child. We can usually prevent the PHT and ATNR from being perfected through practice—leading to unnecessarily retained asymmetry long after the response has disappeared—and so reduce the effect this has on gross movement and posture.
Aim: To encourage head turning to the opposite side and movements and postures against the asymmetric response.
Action:
(1) Parents to approach, play, and feed the child from the opposite side.
(2) Use a foam cut-out to hold his head to the neutral or opposite side when supine or in a 'baby relax'.
(3) Use a prone wedge: some infants lose all preferred head turning in a supported prone position, others spontaneously turn to the opposite side.
(4) Corner seat: placed high in the room (on a table) to encourage looking down and positioned so that the preferred side is to a blank wall. Preferred head turning is often less in sitting than supine.
(5) Supported sitting propping on an extended 'occipital' arm.
(6) Creeping: facilitating jaw-side leg flexion and abduction followed by symmetrical creeping facilitated through shoulder girdle or head/neck.
(7) Jaw-side upper limb exploring face, sucking fingers, *etc.*
(8) Any symmetrical activity.

Curiously enough the simplest form of help for the child with CP has been ignored until recently and that is the use of basic exercise patterns that are used in normal children with the aim of strengthening the child's physical abilities. Because the limbs were felt to be stiff it used to be assumed that strengthening exercises would in fact make the spasticity worse ('never strengthen spasticity'). By 2004 there were significant studies in the literature to show that strengthening the muscles in CP was achievable (Damiano et al. 2002, Damiano 2004). Before discussing the evidence for this new approach to therapy it is important to draw attention to one other feature of management of the child with CP that has changed in recent years and that is the emphasis on the value and importance of helping the child's mobility and access to the environment. An initial study in this regard was that of Butler (1986) but others including Bottos (2001) have emphasized the importance of stimulating the child whose movement capacity limits his/her ability to explore the environment. All the data recently well reviewed by Damiano (2004) herald a long overdue positive approach to the strengthening of the child's motor system in CP and the abandonment of older theories of therapies attempting to change the basic neurological pattern.

The role of the physiotherapist is as a physical exercise trainer. Views on CP have therefore changed dramatically in recent years and it is an exciting field at the moment.

Constraint-based therapy

Another recent development in approaches to the management

of the motor disorder in CP has been constraint-based therapy. This has been developed in adult stroke patients where the unaffected limb is constrained, requiring the patient to attempt to use their partially inactive limb. It has proved effective for these patients and its use has been extended to children, particularly those with hemiplegia.

Studies have shown that even in children who have had other treatments and are of school age, functional improvement can be observed. There are various theoretical suggestions about how this is achieved. The first is the notion of some plasticity in the central nervous system, whereby function might be taken over by the contralateral hemisphere. On the other hand, functional MRI studies have suggested that constraint therapy in some way stimulates those cells inactivated by the stroke to become active again (Eliasson et al. 2005).

Orthopaedic management
It has already been mentioned that many contractures and the abnormal growth of muscles and hence joints may be prevented by early postural management, helped by splinting to maintain joints in their neutral position. The management of this will be the responsibility of both the orthopaedic surgeon and a physical therapist. For whatever reason, however, preventive treatment even in the best of hands may not be effective with problems particularly in the development of the lower limbs. The hips need regular assessment and standard ways of doing this are described (Banta and Scrutton 2003). Probably the commonest orthopaedic procedures are carried out around the ankle to address problems such as tightening of the Achilles tendon, which may mean that a child who has been walking 'goes off his feet' because he simply trips up as he attempts to walk. The development of gait analysis (Gage 1991, 2004) has led to careful assessments of what the orthopaedic surgeon can contribute to the care of the child with CP (Horstman and Bleck 2007). Scoliosis may be a particular problem and is very difficult to treat in CP. While surgery on the upper limbs is less commonly carried out it can be helpful. Thus with an over-flexed wrist the surgeon may transplant a wrist flexor onto the dorsum of the hand to increase extension. Interestingly, transferred muscle will adapt to a new role.

Other surgical approaches
Dorsal rhizotomies were considered in the 1970s but were not performed for many years until Peacock and Arans (1982) initiated the use of this form of therapy again. Functional improvement has been demonstrated as much as 20 years later. As with many approaches to CP, the procedure is probably more effective when a clinician has a particular interest, and at the time of writing it is probably less commonly used than it was in the 1990s. McLaughlin et al. (2002) compared patients treated by dorsal rhizotomy with others treated by physiotherapy (combined in some cases with botulinum toxin injections) and found little difference in the outcome between the two patient groups.

Drug therapy
The two most commonly used drugs in CP are botulinum toxin and baclofen. The background to the use of botulinum toxin goes back to the work of Tardieu et al. (1972) who reported that alcohol or phenol injections into spastic muscles decreased spasticity by blocking the release of acetylcholine at the neuromuscular junction. Long-term results were, however, debatable. With the introduction of botulinum toxin there has been a great increase in attempts to reduce spasticity by this means. Although the number of controlled studies of any length is still quite small, the early papers of Cosgrove et al. (1994) and Corry et al. (1997) with reasonable trials in both upper and lower limbs have lent quite powerful support to its use as an adjunct to other forms of management of the motor disorder. Now botulinum toxin is very widely used and there are frequent papers on it (e.g. Graham et al. 2000, Ade-Hall and Moore 2002). However, the effects are transitory and with continued use it becomes less effective. Results from long-term follow-up studies (e.g. Gough et al. 2005) have led to some people being less enthusiastic than others about using this treatment because of the possible long-term effect on muscle architecture. It would be interesting to see papers comparing the effects of activity training combined with the use of botulinum toxin, but at the time of writing we are not aware of such studies.

Baclofen has been used in CP for a long time and it can be an effective muscle relaxant. It often has to be used in relatively high doses, and the consequent side effects, particularly of sleepiness, may be significant. A more recent development has been the use of baclofen intrathecally, giving the drug by continuous infusion or in boluses (Armstrong et al. 1997). It is not effective in spastic diplegia but its use in quadriplegia, where stiffness may make it difficult for the child to be nursed and managed, is more common. While there are several reports of its usefulness in this context, its management clearly requires a team of people familiar with its use; regular review of the intrathecal pump and the necessity for top ups of intrathecal baclofen mean that it is a programme that is hard to implement without access to a good paediatric neurology or neurodevelopmental centre.

OTHER ASPECTS OF THE MOTOR DISORDER
The above discussion about management of the motor disorder largely relates to the spastic forms of CP. In patients with athetoid CP, contractures and fixed deformities are not usually a problem (although they do occur). The main difficulties relate to the involuntary movements. Sometimes these can be very powerful and extremely difficult to interrupt, making all purposeful movement impossible. Again various drugs have been tried with no great success. Small quantities of alcohol are reported by some adult patients to be useful. Motor training using bio-feedback has been tried and again can be effective but requires specialized units.

FEEDING
It is curious that older textbooks on CP (Crowthers and Paine 1959, Ingram 1964) make no mention of feeding problems in the child. In fact a very large proportion of children with CP have feeding difficulties. These often persist through into adult life. In moderate to severe CP something like 15% of young adults may

have a gastrostomy (Eltumi and Sullivan 1997). Difficulties occur early and need to be recognized so that the child does not suffer from inadequate nutrition, which may have an effect on the developing brain. A child with CP may never develop beyond the suck–swallow pattern of feeding and never be able to chew. CP clinics and child development centres now have specialist feeding clinics with dieticians, speech therapists and physicians as part of a team trying to maintain adequate nutrition and a satisfactory feeding pattern. It is important to remember that apart from a nutritional role, mealtimes are significant social occasions in most societies and it is desirable that the child should not be isolated by being fed away from the rest of the family (Sullivan and Rosenbloom 1996).

COMMUNICATION AND LEARNING DISORDERS

In a recent study of some 300 children with CP (Bax et al. 2006) communication problems were identified in just under 40% of the children with hemiplegia or diplegia and in nearly 89% in those with quadriplegia. Problems in the latter group were often profound, whereas most of the children with hemi- or diplegia had some communication. Children with athetosis may have dysarthric problems with speech or they may have phonological problems in producing effective language. As with physiotherapy, evidence for the effectiveness of time spent with a speech and language therapist to try to improve speech or language function is not very firm. On the other hand, children and adults with CP will benefit from communication aids with either low- or high-tech equipment (Decoste and Glennen 1997). The child with dysarthria in particular has speech problems making him/her incomprehensible but the quality of speech synthesizers has developed greatly in recent years. Assessment of the child or young adult with communication problems needs to be an ongoing and regular activity (for a review of the subject, see Carroll and Reilly 1996). The child who has deficits in language is likely to go on to have a learning disorder, and roughly 50% of children with CP have some degree of intellectual difficulty. They may have global retardation, commonest in the quadriplegic group, or they may have specific language disorders such as reading difficulties and psychological and educational assessment of the child is essential as school age approaches. However, whatever the nature of the learning disorder, efforts must be made to try to assess the child's level of function as early as possible and to provide appropriate educational support. Sometimes remarkable intellectual function remains intact despite very severe motor and communication difficulties (see for example Christie Brown's example of himself in *My Left Foot*). However, such instances are the exception rather than the rule, and usually one has the responsibility of helping the parents to understand that their child is not just physically disabled but also has learning difficulties. Assessment too cannot be 'one-off': it is necessary to see how the child progresses over time, and reassessment should be carried out at regular intervals.

BEHAVIOURAL DIFFICULTIES

Rutter et al. (1970) established that the child who has CNS damage is much more likely than a normal child to have behavioural problems. Early studies showed that behaviour problems were five or six times as common in children with CP than in the normal population. While in some instances brain damage will cause a specific behavioural abnormality associated with the part of the brain that was damaged, in general the pattern of behaviour disorders tends to be the same as that found in normal children. Family psychopathology may play a part in generating such problems. It may be possible to plan potential rehabilitation within the family. However, the family with a disabled child may find it hard to accept that they have a role in the child's behavioural difficulties. Psychiatric referral to a centre that uses a family therapy approach to problems may initially prove helpful. There are certain specific studies of different subgroups of children with CP. For example, children with hemiplegia have been very carefully studied by Goodman and Yude (1996). They noted a number of behaviours specific to that particular group of children. They noted that many of the children had fears and worries and felt miserable at times. Difficult behaviours were common, as also were inattention and overactivity. While autism spectrum disorders such as infantile autism and Asperger syndrome affected only 3% of the population studied, the authors became aware that many of the children had aspects of behaviours seen in autistic children. They noted, for example, preoccupations with an unusual topic such as washing machines, lawnmowers or yoghurt pots and that these preoccupations were associated with impoverished pretend play. They also observed social difficulties in the children's relationships with other children.

For the families with children with learning and behaviour disorders it is perhaps good to be aware of 'crisis points', although these occur also in normal children. There are special difficulties when the question of schooling comes up. In recent years there has been tremendous emphasis on 'inclusion', i.e. seeing children with all kinds of disabilities educated alongside their peers in 'normal' schools. While enthusiasm for this kind of approach remains high in many developed countries there is also beginning to be a realization that some types of behaviour (such as autistic behaviour and overactivity) are extremely difficult to maintain in a classroom with normal children. Unless very adequate assistance is provided in the class such children may prove to be uncontainable. Equally, some parents find that 'special' schooling is what they want and feel is best for their child. Another crisis point is when the child moves on from primary to secondary education – round about the age of 11 in most countries – when the parents have to confront the level of learning difficulties their child has; further crisis points arise at school leaving and puberty. Work has been done on the psychosexual problems of young disabled adults (Blackburn 2002). Awareness and sensitivity to these issues in disabled young adults is not always widespread.

ADOLESCENCE AND ADULT LIFE

It is beyond the scope of this book to discuss the issues that arise as the child with a disability gets older. Often services that have been provided by paediatricians or paediatric neurologists fall away and young people find themselves in the community without a dedicated health service (Thomas et al. 1989). The tasks for the adolescent include the achievement of independence, self-image and identity, the expression of sexuality and vocation. The word vocation rather than work is used deliberately because for many of these young people open employment may be difficult to find. The situation may have to be faced that the young person is not going to have a job but nevertheless needs to have a purposeful life plan. For the family this is often a difficult period. The parents/carers are becoming older and if their child is severely disabled they may begin to realize that the care that they have formerly lavished on the child may not be possible in the future. Plans for where a severely disabled young person is going to spend adult life vary considerably from country to country and are often unsatisfactory. It is important to realize that after the first three or four years the expectation of life for people with CP is not substantially lower than that for the normal population.

CONCLUSION

The World Health Organization (WHO) in 1980 issued its first attempt to define disability. They used the word 'impairment' to describe the actual pathology or lesion the individual has, 'disability', to describe the functional effect of that, and 'handicap' to describe the practical consequences. However, this definition has been called into question, particularly by adults with disability, and a revision of the WHO definition was produced in 2001 (see Chapter 23). The emphasis is now on 'impairment' and 'participation', and it sees the difficulties that the person with disabilities may have as being as much the responsibility of the community as anything to do with the biological difficulties that the disabled person may have. The quality of life of children with CP has recently been assessed (Colver 2006), and somewhat to the surprise of most people the findings were that 8- to 12-year-olds had as good a view about the quality of their life as did their normal peers. Therefore perceptions of disability and how it affects people and the community are changing and will continue to change, but the neurologist will be left with the task of trying to assess to what extent difficulties presenting in the child may be directly related to neurological phenomena.

REFERENCES

Abuelo DN, Barsel-Bowers G, Tutschka G, et al. (1981) Symmetrical infantile thalamic degeneration in two sibs. *J Med Genet* 18: 448–50.

Ade-Hall RA, Moore AP (2000) Botulinum toxin type A in the treatment of lower limb spasticity in cerebral palsy. *Cochrane Database Syst Rev* 2000 (2): CD001408.

Ahdab-Barmada M, Moossy J (1984) The neuropathology of kernicterus in the premature neonate: diagnostic problems. *J Neuropathol Exp Neurol* 43: 45–56.

Ahdab-Barmada M, Painter M (1980) Pontosubicular necrosis and hyperoxemia. *Pediatrics* 66: 840–7.

Aicardi J (1990) Epilepsy in brain-injured children. A review. *Dev Med Child Neurol* 32: 191–202.

Aicardi J (1994) *Epilepsy in Children, 2nd edn.* New York: Raven Press.

Aicardi J, Chevrie JJ (1983) Consequences of status epilepticus in infants and children. *Adv Neurol* 34: 115–25.

Aicardi J, Amsili J, Chevrie JJ (1969) Acute hemiplegia in infancy and childhood. *Dev Med Child Neurol* 11: 162–73.

Aicardi J, Barbosa C, Andermann E, et al. (1988) Ataxia–ocular motor apraxia: a syndrome mimicking ataxia–telangiectasia. *Ann Neurol* 24: 497–502.

Al Otaibi SF, Blaser L, McGregor DL (2005) Neurological complications of kernicterus. *Can J Neurol Sci* 32: 273–4.

Amato M, Hüppi P, Herschkowitz N, Huber P (1991) Prenatal stroke suggested by intrauterine ultrasound and confirmed by magnetic resonance imaging. *Neuropediatrics* 22: 100–2.

Ambler M, O'Neill W (1975) Symmetrical infantile thalamic degeneration with focal cytoplasmic calcification. *Acta Neuropathol* 33: 1–8.

Amiel-Tison C, Korobkin R, Esque-Vaucouloux MT (1977) Neck extensor hypertonia: a clinical sign of insult to the central nervous system of the newborn. *Early Hum Dev* 1: 181–90.

Angelini L, Rumi V, Lamperti E, Nardocci N (1988) Transient paroxysmal dystonia in infancy. *Neuropediatrics* 19: 171–4.

Aram DM, Ekelman BL, Rose DF, Whitaker HA (1985) Verbal and cognitive sequelae following unilateral lesions acquired in early childhood. *J Clin Exp Neuropsychol* 7: 55–78.

Armstrong RW, Steinbok P, Cochrane DD, et al. (1997) Intrathecal baclofen for treatment of children with spasticity of cerebral origin. *J Neurosurg* 87: 409–14.

Arzimanoglou A, Guerrini G, Aicardi J (2004) Epilepsy as a presenting manifestation of structural brain lesions. In: *Aicardi's Epilepsy in Children, 3rd edn.* Philadephia: Lippincott, Williams & Wilkins, pp. 284–311.

Ashwal S, Russman BS, Blasco BA, et al. (2004) Practice parameter: diagnostic assessment of the child with cerebral palsy: report of the Quality Standards Subcommittee of the American Academy of Neurology and the Practice Committee of the Child Neurology Society. *Neurology* 62: 851–63.

Asindi AA, Stephenson JBP, Young DG (1988) Spastic hemiparesis and presumed prenatal embolisation. *Arch Dis Child* 63: 68–9.

Baenziger O, Martin E, Steinlin M, et al. (1993) Early pattern recognition in severe neonatal asphyxia: a prospective MRI study. *Neuroradiology* 35: 437–42.

Banta J, Scrutton D, eds. (2003) *Hip Disorders in Childhood. Clinics in Developmental Medicine no. 160.* London: Mac Keith Press.

Barkovich AJ, Truwit CL (1990) Brain damage from perinatal asphyxia: correlation of MR findings with gestational age. *AJNR* 11: 1087–96.

Barkovich AJ, Westmark K, Partridge C, et al. (1995) Perinatal asphyxia: MR findings in the first 10 days. *AJNR* 16: 427–38.

Barkovich AJ, Kuzniecky RI, Dobyns WB, et al. (1996) A classification scheme for malformations of cortical development. *Neuropediatrics* 27: 59–63.

Barkovich AJ, Kuzniecky RI, Jackson GD, et al. (2001) Classification system for malformations of cortical development. *Neurology* 57: 2168–78.

Baumann RJ, Carr WA, Shuman RM (1987) Patterns of cerebral arterial injury in children with neurological disabilities. *J Child Neurol* 2: 298–306.

Bax MCO (1992) Drooling. *Dev Med Child Neurol* 34: 847–8 (editorial; republished in *The Collected Editorials of Martin C.O. Bax from Developmental Medicine and Child Neurology 1961–2003.* London: Mac Keith Press, 2004, p. 165).

Bax MCO, Hart H, Jenkins SM (1990) *Child Development and Child Health. The Preschool Years.* Oxford: Blackwell Scientific.

Bax M, Goldstein M, Rosenbaum P, et al. (2005) Proposed definition and classification of cerebral palsy. *Dev Med Child Neurol* 47: 571–6.

Bax M, Tydeman C, Flodmark O, et al. (2006) Clinical and MRI correlates of ccerebral palsy: the European CP study. *JAMA* 296: 1603–8.

Bax M, Flodmark O, Tydeman C (2007) From syndrome toward disease. *Dev Med Child Neurol Suppl* 109: 39–41.

Beckung E, Hagberg G (2001) Correlation between ICDIH handicap code and Gross Motor Function Classification System in children with cerebral palsy. *Dev Med Child Neurol* 42: 669–73.

Beltran RS, Coker SB (1995) Transient dystonia of infancy, a result of intrauterine cocaine exposure? *Pediatr Neurol* 12: 354–6.

Benecke R, Meyer BU, Freund HJ (1991) Reorganisation of descending motor pathways in patients after hemispherectomy and severe hemispheric lesions demonstrated by magnetic brain stimulation. *Exp Brain Res* 83: 419–426.

Bennett FC, Chandler LS, Robinson NM, Sells CJ (1981) Spastic diplegia in premature infants. Etiologic and diagnostic considerations. *Am J Dis Child* 135: 732–7.

Berg RA, Aleck KA, Kaplan AM (1983) Familial porencephaly. *Arch Neurol* 40: 567–9.

Bhatt MH, Obeso JA, Marsden CD (1993) Time course of postanoxic akinetic–rigid and dystonic syndromes. *Neurology* 43: 314–7.

Billard C, Dulac O, Boulloche J, et al. (1989) Encephalopathy with calcification of the basal ganglia in children. A reappraisal of Fahr's syndrome with respect to 14 new cases. *Neuropediatrics* **20**: 12–9.

Bjerre JV, Ebbesen F (2006) [Incidence of kernicterus in newborn infants in Denmark.] *Ugeskr Laeger* **168**: 686–91 (Danish).

Blackburn M (2002) *Sexuality and Disability.* London: Butterworth-Heinemann.

Blasco PA, Allaire JH (1992) Drooling in the developmentally disabled: management practices and recommendations. Consortium on Drooling. *Dev Med Child Neurol* **34**: 849–62.

Blasco PA, Stansbury JC (1996) Glycopyrrolate treatment of chronic drooling. *Arch Paediatr Adolesc Med* **150**: 932–5.

Blumel J, Evans EB, Eggers GWN (1960) A combination of congenital cataract and cerebral palsy in a brother and a sister. *Arch Ophthalmol* **63**: 246–53.

Bobath K (1980) *A Neurophysiological Basis for the Treatment of Cerebral Palsy. Clinics in Developmental Medicine No. 75.* London: Spastics International Medical Publications.

Bobath K, Bobath B (1984) The neuro-developmental treatment. In: Scrutton D, ed. *Management of the Motor Disorders of Children with Cerebral Palsy. Clinics in Developmental Medicine No. 90.* London: Spastics International Medical Publications, pp. 6–18.

Bordarier C, Aicardi J (1990) Dandy–Walker syndrome and agenesis of the cerebellar vermis: diagnostic problems and genetic counselling. A review. *Dev Med Child Neurol* **32**: 285–94.

Borzyskowski M (1996) An update on the investigation of the child with a neuropathic bladder. *Dev Med Child Neurol* **38**: 744–8.

Borzyskowski M, Mundy AR, eds. (1990) *Neuropathic Bladder in Childhood. Clinics in Developmental Medicine No. 111.* London: Mac Keith Press.

Bottos M, Bolcati C, Sciuto L, et al. (2001) Powered wheelchairs and independence in children with tetraplegia. *Dev Med Child Neurol* **43**: 769–77.

Bouza H, Dubowitz LMS, Cowan F, Pennock JM (1994a) Late magnetic resonance imaging and clinical findings in neonates with unilateral lesions on cranial ultrasound. *Dev Med Child Neurol* **36**: 951–64.

Bouza H, Dubowitz LMS, Rutherford M, Pennock JM (1994b) Prediction of outcome in children with congenital hemiplegia: a magnetic resonance imaging study. *Neuropediatrics* **25**: 60–6.

Bouza H, Rutherford M, Acolet D, et al. (1994c) Evolution of early hemiplegic signs in full-term infants with unilateral brain lesions in the neonatal period: a prospective study. *Neuropediatrics* **25**: 201–7.

Breedveld G, de Coo IF, Lequin MH, et al. (2006) Novel mutations in three families confirm a major role of COL4A1 in hereditary porencephaly. *J Med Genet* **43**: 490–5.

Brett EM, ed. (1997) *Pediatric Neurology, 3rd edn.* Edinburgh: Churchill Livingstone.

Brown C (1954) *My Left Foot.* London: Secker & Warburg.

Brown JK, Bell E, Fulford GE (1982) Mechanism of deformity in children with cerebral palsy – with special reference to positional deformity. *Paediatr Fortbild Praxis* **53**: 78–94.

Brown JK, Van Rensburg F, Walsh G, et al. (1987) A neurological study of hand function of hemiplegic children. *Dev Med Child Neurol* **29**: 287–304.

Bundey S (1992) *Genetics in Neurology, 2nd edn.* Edinburgh: Churchill Livingstone.

Burke RE, Fahn S, Gold AP (1980) Delayed onset dystonia in patients with 'static' encephalopathy. *J Neurol Neurosurg Psychiatry* **43**: 789–97.

Burton MJ (1991) The surgical management of drooling. *Dev Med Child Neurol* **33**: 1110–6.

Butler C (1986) Effects of powered mobility on self-initiated behaviors of very young children with locomotor disability. *Dev Med Child Neurol* **28**: 325–32.

Butler C (1996) Mainstreaming experience in the United States: is it the appropriate educational placement for every disabled child? *Dev Med Child Neurol* **38**: 861–6.

Butler C, Darrah J (2001) Effects of neurodevelopmental treatment (NDT) for cerebral palsy: an AACPDM evidence report. *Dev Med Child Neurol* **43**: 778–90.

Candy EJ, Hoon AH, Capute AJ, Bryan RN (1993) MRI in motor delay: important adjunct to classification of cerebral palsy. *Pediatr Neurol* **9**: 421–9.

Carlsson G, Uvebrant P, Hugdahi K, et al. (1994) Verbal and non-verbal function of children with right- versus left-hemiplegic cerebral palsy of pre- and perinatal origin. *Dev Med Child Neurol* **36**: 503–12.

Carr LJ, Harrison LM, Evans AL, Stephens JA (1993) Patterns of central motor reorganization in hemiplegic cerebral palsy. *Brain* **116**: 1223–47.

Carroll L, Reilly S (1996) The therapeutic approach to the child with feeding difficulty: II. Management and treatment. In: Sullivan PB, Rosenbloom L, eds. *Feeding the Disabled Child. Clinics in Developmental Medicine No. 140.* London: Mac Keith Press, pp. 117–31.

Chauvel P, Trottier S, Wignal JP, Bancaud J (1992) Somatomotor seizures of frontal lobe origin. In: Chauvel P, Delgado–Escueta AV, Halgren E, Bancaud J, eds. *Frontal Lobe Seizures and Epilepsies.* New York: Raven Press, pp. 185–232.

Chilosi AM, Cipriani CP, Bertuccelli P (2001) Early cognitive and communication development in children with focal brain lesions. *J Child Neurol* **16**: 309–16.

Christen HJ, Hanefeld F, Kruse F, et al. (2000) Foix–Chavany–Marie (anterior opercular) syndrome in childhood: a reappraisal of Worster-Drought syndrome. *Dev Med Child Neurol* **42**: 122–32.

Christensen E, Melchior J (1967) *Cerebral Palsy—a Clinical and Neuropathological Study. Clinics in Developmental Medicine No. 25.* London: Spastics International Medical Publications.

Chugani HT, Miller RA, Chugani DC (1996) Functional brain reorganization in children. *Brain Dev* **18**: 347–56.

Chutorian AM, Michener RC, Defendini R, et al. (1979) Neonatal polycystic encephalomalacia: four new cases and review of the literature. *J Neurol Neurosurg Psychiatry* **42**: 154–60.

Cioni G, Fazzi B, Ipata AE, et al. (1996) Correlation between cerebral visual impairment and magnetic resonance imaging in children with neonatal encephalopathy. *Dev Med Child Neurol* **38**: 120–32.

Cioni G, Sales B, Paolicelli PB, et al. (1999) MRI and clinical characteristics of children with hemiplegic cerebral palsy. *Neuropediatrics* **30**: 249–55.

Claeys V, Deonna T, Chrzanowski R (1983) Congenital hemiparesis: the spectrum of lesions. A clinical and computerized tomographic study of 37 cases. *Helv Paediatr Acta* **38**: 439–55.

Clancy RR, Sladky JT, Rorke LB (1989) Hypoxic–ischemic spinal cord injury following perinatal asphyxia. *Ann Neurol* **25**: 185–9.

Clark M, Carr L, Reilly N, Neville BG (2000) Worster-Drought syndrome, a mild tetraplegic perisylvian cerebral palsy. Review of 47 cases. *Brain* **123**: 2160–70.

Clement MC, Briard ML, Ponsot G, Arthuis M (1984) [Non-progressive congenital cerebellar ataxia.] *Arch Fr Pediatr* **41**: 685–700 (French).

Coker SB, Beltran RS, Myers TF, Hmura L (1988) Neonatal stroke: description of patients and investigation into pathogenesis. *Pediatr Neurol* **4**: 219–23.

Colamaria V, Curatolo P, Cusmai R, Dalla Bernardina B (1988) Symmetrical bithalamic hyperdensities in asphyxiated full-term newborns: an early indicator of status marmoratus. *Brain Dev* **10**: 57–9.

Colver A (2006) Study protocol: SPARCLE – a multicentre European Study of the relationship of environment to participation and quality of life in children with cerebral palsy. *BMC Public Health* **6**: 105.

Colver A, Sethumadhavan T (2003) The term diplegia should be abandoned. *Arch Dis Child* **88**: 286–90.

Cooke RWI (1987) Early and late cranial ultrasonographic appearances and outcome in very low birthweight infants. *Arch Dis Child* **62**: 931–7.

Corry IS, Cosgrove AP, Walsh EG, et al. (1997) Botulinum toxin A in the hemiplegic upper limb: a double-blind trial. *Dev Med Child Neurol* **39**: 185–93.

Cosgrove AP, Corry IS, Graham HK (1994) Botulinum toxin in the management of the lower limb in cerebral palsy. *Dev Med Child Neurol* **36**: 386–96.

Cowan F, Rutherford M, Groenendaal F, et al. (2003) Origin and timing of brain lesions in term infants with neonatal encephalopathy. *Lancet* **361**: 713–4.

Crothers B, Paine RS (1959) *The Natural History of Cerebral Palsy.* (Reprinted 1988 as *Classics in Developmental Medicine No. 2.* London: Mac Keith Press.)

Cummins RA (1988) *The Neurologically Impaired Child: Doman–Delacato Techniques Reappraised.* London: Croom Helm.

Damiano D (2004) Physiotherapy management in cerebral palsy: moving beyond philosophies. In: Scrutton D, Damiano D, Mayston M, eds. *Management of the Motor Disorders of Children with Cerebral Palsy, 2nd edn. Clinics in Developmental Medicine No. 161.* London: Mac Keith Press, pp. 161–9.

Damiano DL, Dodd K, Taylor NF (2002) Should we be testing and training muscle strength in cerebral palsy? *Dev Med Child Neurol* **44**: 68–72.

Decoste DC, Glennen SL, eds. (1997) *The Handbook of Augmentative and Alternative Communication.* San Diego: Singular Publishing.

Deonna TW, Ziegler AL, Nielsen J (1991) Transient idiopathic dystonia in infancy. *Neuropediatrics* **22**: 220–4.

D'Eugenio DB, Slagle TA, Mettelman BB, Gross SJ (1993) Developmental outcome of preterm infants with transient neuromotor abnormalities. *Am J Dis Child* 147: 570–4.

de Vries LS, Eken P, Groenendaal F, et al. (1993) Correlation between the degree of periventricular leukomalacia diagnosed using cranial ultrasound and MRI later in infancy in children with cerebral palsy. *Neuropediatrics* 24: 263–8.

de Vries LS (1996) Neurological assessment of the preterm infant. *Acta Paediatr* 85: 765–71.

de Vries LS, Groenendaal F, Eken P, van Haastert IC, et al. (1997) Infarcts in the vascular distribution of the middle cerebral artery in preterm and full-term infants. *Neuropediatrics* 28: 88–96.

Diebler C, Dulac O (1987) *Pediatric Neurology and Neuroradiology.* Berlin: Springer.

Dietz V (2002) Do human bipeds use quadrupedal coordination? *Trends Neurosci* 25: 462–7.

Dommergues MA, Patkai J, Renauld JC, et al. (2000) Proinflammatory cytokines and interleukin-9 exacerbate excitotoxic lesions of the newborn murine neopallium. *Ann Neurol* 47: 54–63.

Dooling EC, Adams RD (1975) The pathological anatomy of post-hemiplegic athetosis. *Brain* 98: 29–48.

Doyle LW, Betheras FR, Ford GW, et al. (2000) Survival, cranial ultrasound and cerebral palsy in very low birthweight infants: 1980s versus 1990s. *J Paediatr Child Health* 36: 7–12.

Drillien CM (1964) *The Growth and Development of the Prematurely Born Infant.* Edinburgh: Churchill Livingstone.

Duggan PJ, Maalouf EF, Watts TL, et al. (2001) Intrauterine T-cell activation and increased proinflammatory cytokine concentrations in preterm infants with cerebral lesions. *Lancet* 358: 1699–700.

Edebol-Tysk K (1989) Epidemiology of spastic tetraplegic cerebral palsy in Sweden. I. Impairments and disabilities. *Neuropediatrics* 20: 41–5.

Edebol-Tysk K, Hagberg B, Hagberg G (1989) Epidemiology of spastic tetraplegic cerebral palsy in Sweden. II. Prevalance, birth data and origin. *Neuropediatrics* 20: 46–52.

Edwards AD, Tan S (2006) Perinatal infections, prematurity and brain injury. *Curr Opin Pediatr* 18: 119–24.

Eliasson AC, Krumlinde-Sundholm L, Rösblad B, et al. (2006) The Manual Ability Classification System (MACS) for children with cerebral palsy: scale development and evidence of validity and reliability. *Dev Med Child Neurol* 48: 549–54.

Eliasson AC, Krumlinde-Sundholm L, Shaw K, Wang C (2005) Effects of constraint-induced movement therapy in young children with hemiplegic cerebral palsy: an adapted model. *Dev Med Child Neurol* 47: 266–75.

Ellenberg JH, Nelson KB (1981) Early recognition of infants at high risk for cerebral palsy: examination at age four months. *Dev Med Child Neurol* 23: 705–16.

Eltumi M, Sullivan PB (1997) Nutritional management of the disabled child: the role of percutaneous endoscopic gastrostomy. *Dev Med Child Neurol* 39: 66–8.

Esscher F, Flodmark O, Hagberg B (1996) Non-progressive ataxia: origins, brain pathology, and impairments in 78 Swedish children. *Dev Med Child Neurol* 38: 285–6.

Evrard P, Caviness VS (1974) Extensive developmental defect of the cerebellum associated with posterior fossa ventriculocele. *J Neuropathol Exp Neurol* 33: 385–90.

Evrard P, Miladi N, Bonnier C, Gressens P (1992) Normal and abnormal development of the brain. In: Rapin I, Segalowitz SJ, eds. *Handbook of Neuropsychology, vol. 6. Section 10: Child Neuropsychology (Part 1).* Amsterdam: Elsevier, pp. 11–44.

Eyre JA, Taylor JP, Villagra F, et al. (2001) Evidence of activity-dependent withdrawal of corticospinal projections during human development. *Neurology* 57: 1543–54.

Farmer SF, Harrison LM, Ingram DA, Stephens JA (1991) Plasticity of central motor pathways in children with hemiplegic cerebral palsy. *Neurology* 41: 1505–10.

Fedrizzi E, Inverno M, Bruzzone MG, et al. (1996) MRI features of cerebral lesions and cognitive functions in preterm spastic diplegic children. *Pediatr Neurol* 15: 207–12.

Fenichel GM, Phillips JA (1989) Familial aplasia of the cerebellar vermis. Possible X-linked dominant inheritance. *Arch Neurol* 46: 582–3.

Fletcher NA, Marsden CD (1996) Dyskinetic cerebral palsy: a clinical and genetic study. *Dev Med Child Neurol* 38: 873–80.

Flodmark O, Lupton B, Li D, et al. (1989) MR imaging of periventricular leukomalacia in childhood. *Am J Roentgenol* 152: 583–90.

Foley J (1992) Dyskinetic and dystonic cerebral palsy and birth. *Acta Paediatr* 81: 57–60.

Friede RL (1989) *Developmental Neuropathology, 2nd edn.* Berlin: Springer.

Fryer A, Appleton R, Sweeney MG, et al. (1994) Mitochondrial DNA 8993 (NARP) mutation presenting with a heterogeneous phenotype including 'cerebral palsy'. *Arch Dis Child* 71: 419–22.

Fulford GE, Brown JK (1976) Position as a cause of deformity in children with cerebral palsy. *Dev Med Child Neurol* 18: 305–14.

Furman JM, Baloh RW, Chugani H, et al. (1985) Infantile cerebellar atrophy. *Ann Neurol* 17: 399–402.

Gage JR (1991) *Gait Analysis in Cerebral Palsy. Clinics in Developmental Medicine No. 121.* London: Mac Keith Press.

Gage JR (2004) *The Treatment of Gait Problems in Cerebral Palsy. Clinics in Developmental Medicine No. 164–5.* London: Mac Keith Press.

Gascon GG, Ozand PT, Brismar J (1994) Movement disorders in childhood organic acidurias—clinical, neuroimaging and biochemical correlations. *Brain Dev* 16 (Suppl): 94–103.

Gastaut H, Poirier F, Payan H, et al. (1960) H.H.E. syndrome; hemiconvulsions, hemiplegia, epilepsy. *Epilepsia* 1: 418–47.

Georgieff MK, Bernbaum JC (1986) Abnormal shoulder girdle muscle tone in premature infants during their first 18 months of life. *Pediatrics* 77: 664–9.

Georgieff MK, Bernbaum JC, Hoffman-Williamson M, Daft A (1986) Abnormal truncal muscle tone as a useful early marker for developmental delay in low birth weight infants. *Pediatrics* 77: 659–63.

Goodman R, Yude C (1996) IQ and its predictors in childhood hemiplegia. *Dev Med Child Neurol* 38: 881–90.

Gough M, Fairhurst C, Shortland AP (2005) Botulinum toxin and cerebral palsy: time for reflection? *Dev Med Child Neurol* 47: 709–12.

Goutières F, Challamel MJ, Aicardi J, Gilly R (1972) [Congenital hemiplegia; semiology, aetiology and pronosis.] *Arch Fr Pediatr* 29: 839–51.

Govaert P, de Vries LS (1997) *An Atlas of Neonatal Brain Sonography. Clinics in Developmental Medicine No. 141/142.* London: Mac Keith Press.

Govaert P, Matthys E, Zecic A, et al. (2000) Perinatal cortical infarction within middle cerebral artery trunks. *Arch Dis Child Fetal Neonatal Ed* 82: F59–63.

Graham HK, Aoki KR, Autti-Rämö I, et al. (2000) Recommendations for the use of botulinum toxin type A in the management of cerebral palsy. *Gait Posture* 11: 67–79.

Graziani LJ, Pasto M, Stanley C, et al. (1986) Neonatal neurosonographic correlates of cerebral palsy in preterm infants. *Pediatrics* 78: 88–95.

Gubbay SS (1985) Clumsiness. In: Vinken PJ, Bruyn GW, Klawans HL, eds. *Handbook of Clinical Neurology. Revised Series, vol. 2. Neurobehavioral Disorders.* Amsterdam: Elsevier, pp. 159–67.

Guzzetta F, Shackelford GD, Volpe S, et al. (1986) Periventricular intraparenchymal echodensities in the premature newborn: critical determinant of neurologic outcome. *Pediatrics* 78: 995–1006.

Guzzetta F, Mercuri E, Bonanno S, et al. (1993) Autosomal recessive congenital cerebellar atrophy. A clinical and neuropsychological study. *Brain Dev* 15: 439–45.

Haar F, Dyken P (1977) Hereditary nonprogressive athetotic hemiplegia: a new syndrome. *Neurology* 27: 849–54.

Hadders-Algra M, Bos AF, Martin A, Prechtl HFR (1994) Infantile chorea in an infant with severe bronchopulmonary dysplasia: an EMG study. *Dev Med Child Neurol* 36: 177–82.

Hagberg B, Hagberg G (1989) The changing panorama of infantile hydrocephalus and cerebral palsy over forty years—a Swedish survey. *Brain Dev* 11: 368–73.

Hagberg B, Hagberg G (1993) The origins of cerebral palsy. In: David TJ, ed. *Recent Advances in Paediatrics, vol.11.* London: Churchill Livingstone, pp. 67–83.

Hagberg B, Hagberg G, Olow I (1975a) The changing panorama of cerebral palsy in Sweden 1954–1970. I. Analysis of general changes. *Acta Paeditr Scand* 64: 187–92.

Hagberg B, Hagberg G, Olow I (1975b) The changing panorama of cerebral palsy in Sweden 1954–1970. II. Analysis of the various syndromes. *Acta Paediatr Scand* 64: 193–200.

Hagberg B, Hagberg G, Olow I, von Wendt, L. (1989a) The changing panorama of cerebral palsy in Sweden. V. The birth year period 1979–1982. *Acta Paediatr Scand* 78: 283–90.

Hagberg B, Hagberg G, Zetterström R (1989b) Decreasing perinatal mortality: increase in cerebral palsy morbidity. *Acta Paediatr Scand* 78: 664–70.

Hagberg B, Hagberg G, Olow I (1993) The changing panorama of cerebral palsy in Sweden. VI. Prevalence and origin during the birth year period 1983–86. *Acta Paediatr Scand* 82: 387–93.

Hagberg B, Hagberg G, Olow I, von Wendt L (1996) The changing panorama of cerebral palsy in Sweden. VII. Prevalence and origin in the birth year period 1987–90. *Acta Paediatr* 85: 954–60.

Hagberg G, Sjögren I (1966) The chronic brain syndrome of infantile hydrocephalus. A follow-up study of 63 spontaneously arrested cases. *Am J Dis Child* 112: 189–96.

Hagberg G, Sanner G, Steen M (1972) The dysequilibrium syndrome in cerebral palsy. Clinical aspects and treatment. *Acta Paediatr Scand Suppl* 226: 1–63.

Hagberg H, Mallard C (2005) Effects of inflammation on central nervous system development and vulnerability. *Curr Opin Neurol* 18: 117–23.

Hagberg H, Peebles D, Mallard C (2002) Models of white matter injury: comparison of infectious, hypoxic–ischemic, and excitotoxic insults. *Ment Retard Dev Disabil Res Rev* 8: 30–8.

Hansen TW (2002) Kernicterus: an international perspective. *Semin Neonatol* 7: 103–9.

Harbord MG, Kobayashi JS (1991) Fever producing ballismus in patients with choreoathetosis. *J Child Neurol* 6: 49–52.

Hári M, Ákos K (1971; translated 1988) *Conductive Education*. London: Routledge.

Harris SR, Purdy AH (1987) Drooling and its management in cerebral palsy. *Dev Med Child Neurol* 29: 805–14.

Harrison A (1988) Spastic cerebral palsy: possible spinal interneuronal contributions. *Dev Med Child Neurol* 30: 769–80.

Haslam RHA (1975) 'Progressive cerebral palsy' or spinal cord tumour? Two cases of mistaken identity. *Dev Med Child Neurol* 17: 232–7.

Himmelmann K, Hagberg G, Beckung E, et al. (2005) The changing panorama of cerebral palsy in Sweden. IX. Prevalence and origin in the bith-year period 1995–1998. *Acta Paediatr* 94: 287–94.

Himmelmann K, Beckung E, Hagberg G, Uvebrant P (2006) Gross and fine motor function and accompanying impairments in cerebral palsy. *Dev Med Child Neurol* 48: 417–23.

Hoffmann GF, Charpentier C, Mayatepek E, et al. (1993) Clinical and biochemical phenotype in 11 patients with mevalonic aciduria. *Pediatrics* 91: 915–921.

Horstman HM, Bleck EE (2007) *Orthopaedic Management in Cerebral Palsy, 2nd edn. Clinics in Developmental Medicine No. 173/174*. London: Mac Keith Press.

Iida K, Takashima S, Takeuchi Y, et al. (1993) Neuropathologic study of newborns with prenatal-onset leukomalacia. *Pediatr Neurol* 9: 45–8.

Ingram TTS (1964) *Paediatric Aspects of Cerebral Palsy*. Edinburgh & London: ES Livingstone (reprinted 2005, Department of Child Life and Health, The University of Edinburgh).

Ingram TTS (1966) The neurology of cerebral palsy. *Arch Dis Child* 41: 337–57.

Isler W (1971) *Acute Hemiplegias and Hemisyndromes in Childhood. Clinics in Developmental Medicine No. 41/42*. London: Spastics International Medical Publications.

Jaeken J, Carchon H (1993) The carbohydrate-deficient glycoprotein syndromes: an overview. *J Inherit Metab Dis* 16: 813–20.

Johnston MV, Trescher WH, Ishida A, Nakajima W (2001) Neurobiology of hypoxic–ischemic injury in the developing brain. *Pediatr Res* 49: 735–41.

Jung J, Graham JM, Schultz N, Smith DW (1984) Congenital hydranencephaly/porencephaly due to vascular disruption in monozygotic twins. *Pediatrics* 73: 467–9.

Kanda T, Ashida HM, Fukase H (1988) Electromyography in spastic diplegia. *Brain Dev* 10: 120–4.

Kataoka K, Okuno T, Mikawa H, Hojo H (1988) Cranial computed tomographic and electroencephalographic abnormalities in children with posthemiconvulsive hemiplegia. *Eur Neurol* 28: 279–84.

Kato M, Dobyns WB (2003) Lissencephaly and the molecular basis of neuronal migration. *Hum Mol Genet* 12 Spec No 1: R89–96.

Keeney SE, Adcock EW, McArdle CB (1991) Prospective observations of 100 high-risk neonates by high-field (1.5 Tesla) magnetic resonance imaging of the central nervous system. II. Lesions associated with hypoxic–ischemic encephalopathy. *Pediatrics* 87: 431–7.

Kennard MA (1936) Age and other factors in motor recovery from precentral lesions in monkeys. *Am J Physiol* 115: 137–46.

Koeda T, Takeshita K (1992) Visuo-perceptual impairment and cerebral lesions in spastic diplegia with preterm birth. *Brain Dev* 14: 239–44.

Koeda T, Takeshita K, Kisa T (1995) Bilateral opercular syndrome: an unusual complication of perinatal difficulties. *Brain Dev* 17: 193–5.

Koelfen W, Freund M, Varnholt V (1995) Neonatal stroke involving the middle cerebral artery in term infants: clinical presentation, EEG and imaging studies, and outcome. *Dev Med Child Neurol* 37: 204–12.

Konishi Y, Kuriyama M, Hayakawa K, et al. (1991) Magnetic resonance imaging in preterm infants. *Pediatr Neurol* 7: 191–5.

Kotlarek F, Rodewig R, Brüll D, Zeumer H (1981) Computed tomographic findings in congenital hemiparesis in childhood and their relation to etiology and prognosis. *Neuropediatrics* 12: 101–9.

Krägeloh-Mann I (2004) Imaging of early brain injury and cortical plasticity. *Exp Neurol* 190: 84–90.

Krägeloh-Mann I , Horber V (2007) The role of magnetic resonance imaging in elucidating the pathogenesis of cerebral palsy: a systematic review. *Dev Med Child Neurol* 49: 144–51.

Krägeloh-Mann I, Hagberg B, Petersen D, et al. (1992) Bilateral spastic cerebral palsy—pathogenetic aspects from MRI. *Neuropediatrics* 23: 46–8.

Krägeloh-Mann I, Hagberg G, Meisner C, et al. (1993) Bilateral spastic palsy—a comparative study between South-west Germany and West Sweden. I. Clinical patterns and disabilities. *Dev Med Child Neurol* 35: 1037–47.

Krägeloh-Mann I, Hagberg G, Meisner C, et al. (1994) Bilateral spastic cerebral palsy—a comparative study between South-west Germany and West Sweden. II. Epidemiology. *Dev Med Child Neurol* 36: 473–83.

Krägeloh-Mann I, Hagberg G, Meisner C, et al. (1995a) Bilateral spastic cerebral palsy—a collaborative study between South-west Germany and West Sweden. III. Etiology. *Dev Med Child Neurol* 37: 191–203.

Krägeloh-Mann I, Peterson D, Hagberg G, et al. (1995b) Bilateral spastic cerebral palsy—MRI pathology and origin. Analysis from a representative series of 56 cases. *Dev Med Child Neurol* 37: 379–97.

Krägeloh-Mann I, Toft P, Lundig J, et al. (1999) Brain lesions in preterms: origin, consequences and compensation. *Acta Paediatr* 88: 897–908.

Krägeloh-Mann I, Helber A, Mader I, et al. (2002) Bilateral lesions of the thalamus and basal ganglia: origin and outcome. *Dev Med Child Neurol* 44: 477–84.

Krundlinde-Sundholm L, Eliasson AC (2003) Development of the Assisting Hand Assessment: a Rasch build measure intended for children with unilateral upper limb impairments. *Scand J Occup Ther* 10: 16–26.

Kurihara M, Kumagi K, Yagishita S, et al. (1993) Adrenomyeloneuropathy presenting as cerebellar ataxia in a young child: a probable variant of adrenoleukodystrophy. *Brain Dev* 15: 377–80.

Kvistad PH, Dahl A, Skre H (1985) Autosomal recessive nonprogressive ataxia with an early childhood debut. *Acta Neurol Scand* 71: 295–302.

Kyllerman M (1977) Dyskinetic cerebral palsy. An analysis of 115 Swedish cases. *Neuropädiatrie* 8 (Suppl): S28–32.

Kyllerman M (1981) Dyskinetic cerebral palsy. MD thesis, Department of Pediatrics, University of Göteborg.

Kyllerman M (1983) Reduced optimality in pre- and perinatal conditions in dyskinetic cerebral palsy—distribution and comparison to controls. *Neuropediatrics* 14: 29–36.

Kyllerman M (1989) The epidemiology of chronic neurologic diseases of children in Sweden. In: French JH, Harel S, Casaer P, eds. *Child Neurology and Developmental Disabilities*. Baltimore: Paul Brookes, pp. 137–43.

Larroche JC (1986) Fetal encephalopathies of circulatory origin. *Biol Neonate* 50: 61–74.

Law HT, Minns RA (1987) Assessment of abnormalities of gait in children from measurements of instantaneous foot velocities during the swing phase. *Child: Care Health Dev* 13: 311–27.

Leonard A (1999) *Right From the Start*. London: Scope.

Levy SR, Abrams IF, Marshall PC, Rosquette EE (1985) Seizures and cerebral infarction in the fullterm newborn. *Ann Neurol* 17: 366–70.

Lewis DW, Fontana C, Mehallick LK, Everett Y (1994) Transdermal scopolamine for reduction of drooling in developmentally delayed children. *Dev Med Child Neurol* 36: 484–6.

Lidzba K, Krägeloh-Mann I (2005) Development and lateralization of language in the presence of early brain lesions. *Dev Med Child Neurol* 47: 724.

Lidzba K, Staudt M, Wilke M, Krägeloh-Mann I (2006) Visuospatial deficits in patients with early left-hemispheric lesions and functional reorganization of language: consequence of lesion or reorganization? *Neuropsychologia* 44: 1088–94.

Lin J-P, Brown JK, Brotherstone R (1994) Assessment of spasticity in hemiplegic cerebral palsy. II: Distal lower-limb reflex excitability and function. *Dev Med Child Neurol* 36: 290–303.

Lyen KR, Lingam S, Butterfill AM, et al. (1981) Multicystic encephalomalacia due to fetal viral encephalitis. *Eur J Pediatr* **137**: 11–6.

Lyon G, Robain O (1967) [Comparative study of prenatal and perinatal circulatory encephalopathies (hydranencephalies, porencephalies and cystic encephalomalacias of the white matter).] *Acta Neuropathologica* **9**: 79–98 (French).

Mancini GM, de Coo IT, Lequin MH, Arts WF (2004) Hereditary porencephaly: clinical and MRI findings in two Dutch families. *Eur J Paediatr Neurol* **8**: 45–54.

Mathews KD, Afifi AK, Hanson JW (1989) Autosomal recessive cerebellar hypoplasia. *J Child Neurol* **4**: 189–94.

McConachie H, Smyth D, Bax M (1997) Services for children with disabilities in European countries. *Dev Med Child Neurol Suppl* **76**: 1–72.

McKusick VA (1988) *Mendelian Inheritance in Man, 7th edn.* Baltimore: Johns Hopkins University Press.

McLaughlin J, Bjornson K, Temkin N, et al. (2002) Selective dorsal rhizotomy: meta-analysis of three randomized controlled trials. *Dev Med Child Neurol* **44**: 17–25.

Mercuri E, Spanò M, Bruccini G, et al. (1996) Visual outcome in children with congenital hemiplegia: correlation with MRI findings. *Neuropediatrics* **27**: 184–8.

Mercuri E, Rutherford M, Barnett A et al. (2002) MRI lesions and infants with neonatal encephalopathy: is the Apgar score predictive? *Neuropediatrics* **33**: 150–6.

Michaelis R, Rooschütz B, Dopfer R (1980) Prenatal origin of congenital spastic hemiparesis. *Early Hum Dev* **4**: 243–55.

Michaelis R, Asenbauer C, Buchwald-Saal M, et al. (1993) Transitory neurological findings in a population of high risk infants. *Early Hum Dev* **43**: 143–53.

Miller G, Cala LA (1989) Ataxic cerebral palsy—clinico-radiologic correlations. *Neuropediatrics* **20**: 84–9.

Milner D, Goodale MA (2006) *The Visual Brain in Action, 2nd edn. Oxford Psychology Series No. 27.* Oxford: Oxford University Press.

Minear WL (1956) A classification of cerebral palsy. *Pediatrics* **18**: 841–52.

Molteni B, Oleari G, Fedrizzi E, Bracchi M (1987) Relation between CT patterns, clinical findings and etiological factors in children born at term, affected by congenital hemiparesis. *Neuropediatrics* **18**: 75–80.

Morton RE, Bonas R, Fourie B, Minford J (1993) Videofluoroscopy in the assessment of feeding disorders of children with neurological problems. *Dev Med Child Neurol* **35**: 388–95.

Mulligan JC, Painter MJ, O'Donoghue PA, et al. (1980) Neonatal asphyxia. II. Neonatal mortality and long-term sequelae. *J Pediatr* **96**: 903–7.

Mutch L, Alberman E, Hagberg B, et al. (1992) Cerebral palsy epidemiology: where are we now and where are we going? *Dev Med Child Neurol* **34**: 547–55.

Myers RE (1972) Two patterns of brain damage and their conditions of occurrence. *Am J Obstet Gynecol* **112**: 246–76.

Nardocci N, Zorzi G, Grisoli M, et al. (1996) Acquired hemidystonia in childhood: a clinical and neuroradiological study of thirteen patients. *Pediatr Neurol* **15**: 108–13.

Nass R (1985) Mirror movement asymmetries in congenital hemiparesis: the inhibition hypothesis revisited. *Neurology* **35**: 1059–62.

Nelson KB, Ellenberg J (1982) Children who "outgrew" cerebral palsy. *Pediatrics* **69**: 529–36.

Newman CJ, Ziegler AL, Jeannot PY, et al. (2006) Transient dystonic toe-walking: differentiation from cerebral palsy and a rare explanation for some unexplained cases of toe-walking. *Dev Med Child Neurol* **48**: 96–102.

Niemann G, Wakat JP, Krägeloh-Mann I, et al. (1994) Congenital hemiparesis and periventricular leukomalacia: pathogenetic aspects on magnetic resonance imaging. *Dev Med Child Neurol* **36**: 943–50.

Niemann G, Grodd W, Schöning M (1996) Late remission of congenital hemiparesis: the value of MRI. *Neuropediatrics* **27**: 197–201.

Nygaard TG, Waran SP, Levine RA, et al. (1994) Dopa-responsive dystonia simulating cerebral palsy. *Pediatr Neurol* **11**: 236–40.

O'Dwyer NJ, Neilson PD (1988) Voluntary muscle control in normal and athetoid dysarthric speakers. *Brain* **111**: 877–99.

Okuno T (1994) Acute hemiplegia syndrome in childhood. *Brain Dev* **16**: 16–22.

Olsén P, Vainionpää L, Pääkkö E, et al. (1998) Psychological findings in preterm children related to neurological status and magnetic resonance imaging. *Pediatrics* **102**: 329–36.

Ong BY, Ellison PH, Browning C (1983) Intrauterine stroke in the neonate. *Arch Neurol* **40**: 55–6.

Palisano R, Rosenbaum P, Walter S, et al. (1997) Development and reliability of a system to classify gross motor function in children with cerebral palsy. *Dev Med Child Neurol* **39**: 214–23.

Palmer FB, Shapiro BK, Wachtel RC, et al. (1988) The effect of physical therapy on cerebral palsy. *N Engl J Med* **318**: 803–8.

Papile L-A, Munsick-Bruno G, Schaefer A (1983) Relationship of cerebral intraventricular hemorrhage and early childhood neurologic handicaps. *J Pediatr* **103**: 273–7.

Parisi JE, Collins GH, Kim RC, Crosley CJ (1983) Prenatal symmetrical thalamic degeneration with flexion spasticity at birth. *Ann Neurol* **13**: 94–7.

Pascual-Castroviejo I, Guttierez M, Morales C, et al. (1994) Primary degeneration of the granular layer of the cerebellum. A study of 14 patients and review of the literature. *Neuropediatrics* **25**: 183–90.

Pasternak JF (1987) Parasagittal infarction in neonatal asphyxia. *Ann Neurol* **21**: 202–4.

Peacock WJ, Arens LJ (1982) Selective posterior rhizotomy for relief of spasticity in cerebral palsy. *South Afr Med J* **62**: 119–24.

PeBenito R, Santello MD, Faxas TA, et al. (1989) Residual developmental disabilities in children with transient hypertonicity in infancy. *Pediatr Neurol* **5**: 154–60.

Perlman JM, Volpe JJ (1989) Movement disorder of premature infants with severe bronchopulmonary dysplasia: a new syndrome. *Pediatrics* **84**: 215–8.

Perlstein MA (1960) The late clinical syndrome of post-icteric encephalopathy. *Pediatr Clin North Am* **7**: 665–87.

Pharoah PO, Cooke T, Cooke RW, Rosenbloom L (1990) Birthweight specific trends in cerebral palsy. *Arch Dis Child* **65**: 602–6.

Piper MC, Mazer B, Silver KM, Ramsay M (1988) Resolution of neurological symptoms in high-risk infants during the first two years of life. *Dev Med Child Neurol* **30**: 26–35.

Platt MJ, Cans C, Johnson A, et al. (2007) Trends in cerebral palsy among infants of very low birthweight (<1500 g) or born prematurely (<32 weeks) in 16 European centres: a database study. *Lancet* **369**: 43–50.

Powell TG, Pharoah POD, Cooke RWI, Rosenbloom L (1988a) Cerebral palsy in low birthweight infants. I. Spastic hemiplegia: associations with intrapartum stress. *Dev Med Child Neurol* **36**: 11–8.

Powell TG, Pharoah POD, Cooke RWI, Rosenbloom L (1988b) Cerebral palsy in low-birthweight infants. II. Spastic diplegia: associations with fetal immaturity. *Dev Med Child Neurol* **30**: 19–25.

Prechtl HFR (1980) The optimality concept. *Early Hum Dev* **4**: 201–5.

Prechtl HFR, Stemmer CJ (1962) The choreiform syndrome in children. *Dev Med Child Neurol* **4**: 119–27.

Prechtl HF, Einspieler C, Cioni G, et al. (1997) An early marker for neurological deficits after perinatal brain lesions. *Lancet* **349**: 1361–3.

Rademakers RP, van der Knaap MS, Verbeeten B, et al. (1995) Central cortico-subcortical involvement: a distinct pattern of brain damage caused by perinatal and postnatal asphyxia in term infants. *J Comput Assist Tomogr* **19**: 256–63.

Rapin I (1995) Acquired aphasia in children. *J Child Neurol* **10**: 267–70.

Rasmussen A, Ravn P (2004) High frequency of congenital thrombophilia in women with pathological pregnancies? *Acta Obstet Gynecol Scand* **83**: 808–17.

Reid CJD, Borzyskowski M (1993) Lower urinary tract dysfunction in cerebral palsy. *Arch Dis Child* **68**: 739–42.

Robards MF (1994) *Running a Team for Disabled Children and Their Families. Clinics in Developmental Medicine No. 130.* London: Mac Keith Press.

Robson P, Mac Keith RC (1971) Shufflers with spastic cerebral palsy: a confusing clinical picture. *Dev Med Child Neurol* **13**: 651–9.

Roland EH, Hill A, Norman MG, et al. (1988) Selective brainstem injury in an asphyxiated newborn. *Ann Neurol* **23**: 89–92.

Rorke LB, Zimmerman RA (1992) Prematurity, postmaturity, and destructive lesions in utero. *AJNR* **13**: 517–36.

Rosebaum D, Walter SD, Hanna SE, et al. (2002) Prognosis for gross motor function in cerebral palsy: creation of motor development curves. *JAMA* **288**: 1357–63.

Rosenbaum P, Paneth N, Leviton A, et al. (2007) A report: the definition and classification of cerebral palsy. April 2006. *Dev Med Child Neurol Suppl* **109**: 8–14; erratum *Dev Med Child Neurol* **49**: 480.

Rosenbloom L (1994) Dyskinetic cerebral palsy and birth asphyxia. *Dev Med Child Neurol* **36**: 285–9.

Russell DJ, Rosenbaum PL, Avery LM, Lane M (2002) *Gross Motor Function Measure (GMFM-66 and GMFM-88) User's Manual. Clinics in Developmental Medicine No. 159.* London: Mac Keith Press.

Rutherford MA, Heckmatt JZ, Dubowitz V (1989) Congenital myotonic dystrophy: respiratory function at birth determines survival. *Arch Dis Child* **64**: 191–5.

Rutherford MA, Pennock JM, Murdoch-Eaton DM, et al. (1992) Athetoid cerebral palsy with cysts in the putamen after hypoxic–ischaemic encephalopathy. *Arch Dis Child* **67**: 846–50.

Rutherford MA, Pennock JM, Dubowitz LMS (1994) Cranial ultrasound and magnetic resonance imaging in hypoxic–ischaemic encephalopathy: a comparison with outcome. *Dev Med Child Neurol* **36**: 813–25.

Rutherford MA, Pennock JM, Shwieso JE, et al. (1995) Hypoxic–ischaemic encephalopathy: early magnetic resonance imaging findings and their evolution. *Neuropediatrics* **26**: 183–91.

Rutter M, Graham P, Yule W (1970) *A Neuropsychiatric Study in Childhood. Clinics in Developmental Medicine No. 35/36.* London: Spastics International Medical Publications.

Saint-Hilaire MH, Burke RE, Bressman SB, et al. (1991) Delayed-onset dystonia due to perinatal or early childhood asphyxia. *Neurology* **41**: 216–22.

Sala DA, Grant AD (1995) Prognosis for ambulation in cerebral palsy. *Dev Med Child Neurol* **37**: 1020–6.

Sanger TD, Delgado MR, Gaebler-Spira D, et al. (2003) Classification and definition of disorders causing hypertonia in childhood. *Pediatrics* **111**: e89–97.

Sanner G (1973) The dysequilibrium syndrome. A genetic study. *Neuropädiatrie* **4**: 403–13.

Sanner G (1979) Pathogenetic and preventive aspects of non-progressive ataxic syndromes. *Dev Med Child Neurol* **21**: 663–71.

Sanner G, Hagberg B (1974) 188 cases of non-progressive ataxic syndromes in childhood. Aspects of etiology and classification. *Neuropädiatrie* **5**: 224–35.

Santanelli P, Bureau M, Magaudda A, et al. (1989) Benign partial epilepsy with centrotemporal (or rolandic) spikes and brain lesion. *Epilepsia* **30**: 182–8.

Schachat WS, Wallace HM, Palmer M, Slater B (1957) Ophthalmological findings in children with cerebral palsy. *Pediatrics* **19**: 623–8.

Schenk-Rootlieb AJF, van Nieuwenhuizen O, van Waes PFGM, van der Graaf Y (1994) Cerebral visual impairment in cerebral palsy: relation to structural abnormalities of the cerebrum. *Neuropediatrics* **25**: 68–72.

Scher MS, Dobson V, Carpenter NA, Guthrie RD (1989) Visual and neurological outcome of infants with periventricular leukomalacia. *Dev Med Child Neurol* **31**: 353–65.

Scheuerle AE, McVie R, Beaudet AL, Shapira SK (1993) Arginase deficiency presenting as cerebral palsy. *Pediatrics* **91**: 995–6.

Schiffmann R, Moller JR, Trapp BD, et al. (1994) Childhood ataxia with diffuse central nervous system hypomyelination. *Ann Neurol* **35**: 331–40.

SCPE (2000) Surveillance of Cerebral Palsy in Europe: a collaboration of cerebral palsy surveys and registers. *Dev Med Child Neurol* **42**: 816–24.

SCPE (2002) Prevalence and characteristics of children with cerebral palsy in Europe. *Dev Med Child Neurol* **44**: 633–40.

Scrutton D, Damiano D, Mayston M, eds. (2004) *Management of the Motor Disorders of Children with Cerebral Palsy, 2nd edn. Clinics in Developmental Medicine No. 161.* London: Mac Keith Press.

Semens S (1967) The Bobath concept in the treatment of neurological disorders. *Am J Phys Med* **46**: 732–85.

Sibon I, Coupry I, Menegon P, et al. (2007) COL4A1 mutation in Axenfeld–Rieger anomaly with leukoencephalopathy and stroke. *Ann Neurol* **62**: 177–84.

Sie LT, van der Knaap MS, Oosting J, et al. (2000) MR patterns of hypoxic–ischemic brain damage after prenatal, perinatal or postnatal asphyxia. *Neuropediatrics* **31**: 128–36.

Silverstein AM, Hirsh DK, Trobe JD, Gebarski SS (1990) MR imaging of the brain in five members of a family with Pelizaeus–Merzbacher disease. *AJNR* **11**: 495–9.

Sinha SK, D'Souza SW, Rivlin E, Chiswick ML (1990) Ischaemic brain lesions diagnosed at birth in preterm infants: clinical events and developmental outcome. *Arch Dis Child* **65**: 1017–20.

Skranes JS, Nilsen G, Smevik O, et al. (1992) Cerebral magnetic resonance imaging (MRI) of very low birth weight infants at one year of corrected age. *Pediatr Radiol* **22**: 406–9.

Sladky JT, Rorke LB (1986) Perinatal hypoxic/ischemic spinal cord injury. *Pediatr Pathol* **6**: 87–101.

Stanley FJ, Blair E, Hockey A, et al. (1993) Spastic quadriplegia in Western Australia: a genetic epidemiological study. I: Case population and perinatal risk factors. *Dev Med Child Neurol* **35**: 191–201.

Stanley FJ, Blair E, Alberman E (2000) *Cerebral Palsies: Epidemiology and Causal Pathways. Clinics in Developmental Medicine No. 151.* London: Mac Keith Press.

Staudt M, Nieman G, Grodd W, et al. (2000) The pyramidal tract in congenital hemiparesis: relationship between morphology and function in perinatal lesions. *Neuropediatrics* **31**: 257–64.

Staudt MB, Grodd W, Gerloff C, et al. (2002a) Two types of ipsilateral reorganization in congenital hemiparesis: a TMS and fMRI study. *Brain* **125**: 2222–37.

Staudt MB, Lidzba K, Grodd W, et al. (2002b) Right–left hemispheric reorganization of language following early left-sided lesions: functional MRI and topography. *Neuroimaging* **16**: 954–67.

Staudt M, Pavlova M, Bohm S, et al. (2003) Pyramidal tract damage correlates with motor dysfunction in bilateral periventricular leukomalacia (PVL). *Neuropediatrics* **34**: 182–8.

Staudt M, Gerloff C, Grodd W, et al. (2004) Reorganization in congenital hemiparesis acquired at different ages. *Ann Neurol* **56**: 854–63.

Staudt M, Krägeloh-Mann I, Grodd W (2005) Ipsilateral corticospinal pathways in congenital hemiparesis on routine magnetic resonance imaging. *Pediatr Neurol* **32**: 37–9.

Steinlin M, Good M, Martin E, et al. (1993) Congenital hemiplegia: morphology of cerebral lesions and pathogenetic aspects from MRI. *Neuropediatrics* **24**: 224–9.

Steinlin M, Zangger B, Boltshauser E (1998) Non-progressive congenital ataxia with or without cerebellar hypoplasia: a review of 34 subjects. *Dev Med Child Neurol* **40**: 148–54.

Stewart AL, Rifkin L, Amess PN, et al. (1999) Brain structure and neurocognitive and behavioural function in adolescents who were born very preterm. *Lancet* **353**: 1653–7.

Stibler H, Westerberg B, Hanefeld F, Hagberg B (1993) Carbohydrate-deficient glycoprotein (CDG) syndrome—a new variant, type III. *Neuropediatrics* **24**: 51–2.

Sullivan PB, Rosenbloom L (1996) *Feeding the Disabled Child. Clinics in Developmental Medicine No. 140.* London: Mac Keith Press.

Surman G, Newdick H, Johnson A (2003) Cerebral palsy rates among low-birthweight infants fell in the 1990s. *Dev Med Child Neurol* **45**: 456–62.

Sutherland DH (1984) *Gait Disorders in Childhood and Adolescence.* Baltimore: Williams & Wilkins.

Sutherland DH, Olshen RA, Biden EN, Wyatt MP (1988) *The Development of Mature Walking. Clinics in Developmental Medicine No. 104/105.* London: Mac Keith Press.

Tang-Wai R, Webster RJ, Shevell MI (2006) A clinical and etiologic profile of spastic diplegia. *Pediatr Neurol* **34**: 212–8.

Tardieu G, Tardieu T, Hariga J (1972) Selective partial denervation by alcohol injections and their results in spasticity. *Reconstr Surg Traumatol* **13**: 18–36.

Tardieu M, Evrard P, Lyon G (1981) Progressive expanding congenital porencephalies: a treatable cause of progressive encephalopathy. *Pediatrics* **68**: 198–202.

Taudorf K, Melchior JC, Pederson H (1984) CT findings in spastic cerebral palsy. Clinical, aetiological and prognostic aspects. *Neuropediatrics* **15**: 120–4.

Teuber HL (1974) Why two brains? In: Schmitt FO, Worden FG, eds. *The Neurosciences: Third Study Program.* Cambridge: MIT Press, pp. 71–4.

Tharp BR, Scher MS, Clancy RR (1989) Serial EEGs in normal and abnormal infants with birthweights less than 1200 grams. A prospective study with long-term follow-up. *Neuropediatrics* **20**: 64–72.

Thomas AP, Bax MCO, Smyth DPL (1989) *The Health and Social Needs of Young Adults with Physical Disabilities. Clinics in Developmental Medicine No. 106.* London: Mac Keith Press.

Tizard JPM, Paine RS, Crothers B (1954) Disturbances of sensation in children with hemiplegia. *JAMA* **155**: 628–32.

Tomiwa K, Baraitser M, Wilson J (1987) Dominantly inherited congenital cerebellar ataxia with atrophy of the vermis. *Pediatr Neurol* **3**: 360–2.

Topp M, Uldall P, Greisen G (2001) Cerebral palsy births in eastern Denmark, 1987–90: implications for neonatal care. *Paediatr Perinat Epidemiol* **15**: 271–7.

Touwen BCL, Hadders-Algra M (1983) Hyperextension of neck and trunk and shoulder retraction in infancy. A prognostic study. *Neuropediatrics* **14**: 202–5.

Truwit CL, Barkovich AJ, Koch TK, Ferriero DM (1992) Cerebral palsy: MR findings in 40 patients. *AJNR* **13**: 67–78.

Tsao CY, Wright FS, Boesel CP, Luquette M (1994) Partial NADH dehydrogenase defect presenting as spastic cerebral palsy. *Brain Dev* **16**: 393–5.

Turkel SB, Guttenberg ME, Moynes DR, Hodgman JE (1980) Lack of identifiable risk factors for kernicterus. *Pediatrics* **66**: 502–6.

Uvebrant P (1988) Hemiplegic cerebral palsy. Aetiology and outcome. *Acta Paediatr Scand Suppl* **345**: 1–100.

van Bogaert P, Baleriaux D, Christophe C, Szliwowski HB (1992) MRI of patients with cerebral palsy and normal CT scan. *Neuroradiology* **34**: 52–6.

Van de Bor M, Verloove-Vanhorick SP, Baerts W, et al. (1988) Outcome of periventricular–intraventricular hemorrhage at 2 years of age in 484 very preterm infants admitted to 6 neonatal intensive care units in the Netherlands. *Neuropediatrics* **19**: 183–5.

Van de Bor M, van Zeben-van der Aa TM, Verloove-Vanhorick SP, et al. (1989) Hyperbilirubinemia in preterm infants and neurodevelopmental outcome at 2 years of age: results of a national collaborative survey. *Pediatrics* **83**: 915–20.

van der Knaap MS, Smit LM, Barkhof F, et al. (2006) Neonatal porencephaly and adult stroke related to mutations in collagen 1V A1. *Ann Neurol* **59**: 504–11.

Van Nieuwenhuizen O, Willemse J (1984) CT-scanning in children with cerebral visual disturbance and its possible relation to hypoxia and ischaemia. *Behav Brain Res* **14**: 143–5.

Van Nieuwenhuizen O (1987) *Cerebral Visual Disturbance in Infantile Encephalopathy.* Dordrecht: Martinus Nijhoff.

Vargha-Khadem F, O'Gorman AM, Watters GV (1985) Aphasia and handedness in relation to hemispheric side, age at injury and severity of cerebral lesion during childhood. *Brain* **108**: 677–96.

Vargha-Khadem F, Isaacs E, van der Werf S, et al. (1992) Development of intelligence and memory in children with hemiplegic cerebral palsy. The deleterious consequences of early seizures. *Brain* **115**: 315–29.

Veelken N, Hagberg B, Hagberg G, Olow I (1983) Diplegic cerebral palsy in Swedish term and preterm children. Differences in reduced optimality, relations to neurology and pathogenetic factors. *Neuropediatrics* **14**: 20–8.

Vojta V (1984) The basic element of treatment according to Vojta. In: Scrutton D, ed. *Management of the Motor Disorders of Children with Cerebral Palsy. Clinics in Developmental Medicine No. 90.* London: Spastics International Medical Publications, pp. 75–85.

Volpe JJ, Hershkovich P, Perlman JM, et al. (1985) Positron emission tomography in the asphyxiated term newborn: parasagittal impairment of cerebral blood flow. *Ann Neurol* **17**: 287–96.

Volpe JJ (1997) Brain injury in the premature infant – from pathogenesis to prevention. *Brain Dev* **19**: 519–34

Volpe JJ (2001) *Neurology of the Newborn, 4th edn.* Philadelphia: WB Saunders.

Walsh EG (1993) *Muscles, Masses and Motion. The Physiology of Normality, Hypotonicity, Spasticity and Rigidity. Clinics in Developmental Medicine*

No. 125. London: Mac Keith Press.

Watanabe K (1992) The neonatal electroencephalogram and sleep cycle patterns. In: Eyre JA, ed. *The Neurophysiological Examination of the Newborn Infant. Clinics in Developmental Medicine No. 120.* London: Mac Keith Press, pp. 11–47.

Watson L, Stanley F, Blair E (1999) *Report of the Western Australia CP Register.* Perth: Western Australia CP Register.

Weiller C, Ramsay SC, Wise RJ, et al. (1993) Individual patterns of functional reorganization in the human cerebral cortex after capsular infarction. *Ann Neurol* **33**: 181–9.

Wennberg RP, Alfors CE, Bhutani VK, et al. (2006) Toward understanding kernicterus: a challenge to improve the management of jaundiced newborns. *Pediatrics* **117**: 474–83.

Wharton RH, Bresman MJ (1989) Neonatal respiratory depression and delay in diagnosis in Prader–Willi syndrome. *Dev Med Child Neurol* **31**: 231–6.

WHO (1980) *International Classification of Impairments, Disabilities and Handicaps.* Geneva: World Health Organization.

WHO (2001) *International Classification of Functioning, Disability and Health.* Geneva: World Health Organization.

Wichman A, Frank LM, Kelly TE (1985) Autosomal recessive congenital cerebellar hypoplasia. *Clin Genet* **27**: 373–82.

Wiklund LM, Uvebrant P, Flodmark O (1990) Morphology of cerebral lesions in children with congenital hemiplegia: a study with computed tomography. *Neuroradiology* **32**: 179–86.

Willemse J (1986) Benign idiopathic dystonia with onset in the first year of life. *Dev Med Child Neurol* **28**: 355–63.

Worster-Drought C (1974) Suprabulbar paresis. Congenital suprabulbar paresis and its differential diagnosis with special reference to acquired suprabulbar paresis. *Dev Med Child Neurol Suppl* **30**: 1–33.

Wüllner U, Klockgether T, Petersen D, et al. (1993) Magnetic resonance imaging in hereditary and idiopathic ataxia. *Neurology* **43**: 318–25.

Wu YW, Lindan CE, Henning LH, et al. (2006) Neuroimaging abnormalities in infants with congenital hemiparesis. *Pediatr Neurol* **35**: 191–6.

Yokochi K, Horie M, Inukai K, et al. (1989) Computed tomographic findings in children with spastic diplegia: correlation with the severity of their motor abnormality. *Brain Dev* **11**: 236–40.

Yokochi K, Aiba K, Kodama M, Fujimoto S (1991) Magnetic resonance imaging in athetotic cerebral palsied children. *Acta Paediatr Scand* **80**: 818–23.

Young ID, Moore JR, Tripp JH (1987) Sex-linked recessive congenital ataxia. *J Neurol Neurosurg Psychiatry* **50**: 1230–2.

Zonana J, Adornato BT, Glass ST, Webb MJ (1986) Familial porencephaly and congenital hemiplegia. *J Pediatr* **109**: 671–4.

PART IV

METABOLIC AND HEREDODEGENERATIVE DISORDERS OF THE CENTRAL NERVOUS SYSTEM

Diseases due to inborn errors of metabolism account for a large proportion of CNS disorders. Several hundred genetic diseases are currently known and the list is rapidly growing as a result of progress in biochemistry and molecular biology.

Metabolic and heredodegenerative CNS disorders have been traditionally divided into three groups. The first includes those diseases for which a definite enzymatic defect has been demonstrated, thus allowing for a firm and usually also a prenatal diagnosis as well as some understanding of the mechanisms. The second group consists of those diseases in which accumulation of storage material within neural cells clearly indicates the presence of a catabolic defect and is also of practical use for the diagnosis. The third group comprises a heterogeneous collection of progressive neurological diseases, usually genetically determined, that may have a clinical presentation similar to that of the first two groups but for which no biochemical or molecular error has been identified or suggested by the presence of storage products. These are usually referred to as *neurodegenerative diseases*.

This distinction has now become obsolete, as the vast majority, if not all, of these diseases have been shown to result from metabolic errors or are highly likely to be due to such disturbances. The error is usually the result of a DNA mutation, but other genetic processes, especially epigenetic ones such as alternative splicing, transduction errors, etc., might affect substances with an enzymatic action then resulting in 'classical' metabolic diseases. Similar genetic disorders can involve structural proteins (e.g. glial acidic protein in Alexander disease) or other proteins or peptides, due to errors involving their cellular location, addressing or transport, their intracellular traffic, processing (e.g. by Golgi apparatus), catabolism or other functions essential for survival or function of the cell, and large number of disorders have been demonstrated – or are strongly suspected – to be due to or associated with such abnormalities. Some of these diseases can be associated with the presence of intracellular cytoplasmic or intranuclear inclusions as in Huntingdon disease or some types of spinocerebellar degeneration. Unfortunately, too little is known about the mechanisms involved to allow a rational classification of these conditions. We shall thus assume in the following chapters that most if not all of the neurodegenerative diseases are due to genetically determined errors of metabolism involving not only enzymatic processes but also the synthesis and processing of proteins, and to a lesser degree, other substances by a number of known, or most often unknown, mechanisms.

Recent advances in molecular genetics have allowed mapping of the responsible genes for many of these diseases, and cloning has been performed for a substantial proportion of them. The proteins coded for by these genes are of many types, including cytoskeletal and signalling proteins, regulatory and growth factors, and membrane receptors. The exact nature of the proteins is currently an essential theme of research. Despite cloning of the abnormal gene and determination of the protein structure, the mechanisms of most disorders remain unknown, although these discoveries permit a precise classification and sometimes the diagnosis – including in some cases prenatal diagnosis – of these disorders, through direct testing for abnormal DNA or protein or through linkage studies.

For metabolic and degenerative diseases, an early diagnosis is of more than academic interest, as in some cases a specific therapy is available, for many a prenatal diagnosis is feasible, and, for all, prognosis and genetic counselling critically depend on a correct recognition. In some cases, it has become possible to detect not only actual diseases but also individual susceptibility to certain diseases by determining the genotype of individuals (e.g. susceptibility to vascular thrombosis in heterozygotes for homocystinuria, increased liability to some cancers in carriers of certain genes, such as *BCRA* genes for breast cancer, or in heterozygotes for the gene of ataxia–telangiectasia), thus opening a completely new domain whose limits and medical, ethical and sociological consequences are currently difficult to predict.

This part is divided into two chapters. Chapter 8 deals with defined inborn errors of metabolism. The main subgroups of neurological importance are disorders of amino acid and organic acid intermediary metabolism, lysosomal diseases, the peroxisomal disorders, and errors in energy metabolism, especially the mitochondrial diseases, but many other defects can also involve the CNS. Chapter 8 is concerned with storage disorders without known biochemical error and Chapter 9 with 'neurodegenerative diseases' in which the metabolic basis – if any – is yet undetermined. A biochemical error, although not necessarily affecting catabolism, has now been recognized in an increasing proportion of these conditions and the distinction between the various groups is becoming increasingly blurred and is bound ultimately to disappear when molecular mechanisms are discovered. As a result, the clinical presentation is still taken into account, e.g. the leukodystrophies are described in Chapter 9 even when a metabolic defect has been discovered. Some rare diseases that may have completely different mechanisms are included for convenience even though in a few cases their progressive nature may not be established.

Virtually all metabolic and degenerative CNS diseases are genetically determined, and they are generally transmitted as autosomal recessive traits, less commonly as autosomal dominant or X-linked ones. In recent years, other modalities of genetic transmission have been uncovered, such as trinucleotide repeats, often with anticipation, imprinting or uniparental disomy, and this knowledge makes genetic counselling more precise. For diseases with specific biochemical defects a variety of tests are available, and many can be diagnosed before birth by study of cultured amniotic cells or chorionic villus biopsy. A few can even be detected in germinal cells allowing preimplantation diagnosis after selection of unaffected cells thus eliminating the risk of an affected offspring.

The diagnostic consequences of these methods are enormous. Prenatal diagnosis is now possible for an increasing number of conditions in which specific DNA abnormalities can be demonstrated. Systematic screening techniques are available for some disorders whose frequency is high enough, especially those for which prevention is feasible. However, the diagnosis of heredodegenerative diseases without known molecular or metabolic errors raises special problems as it may rest exclusively on clinical grounds, if clinical medicine is broadly defined as "an intellectual process whereby data from all sources, whether strictly clinical (in the restricted sense) or from the laboratory and other technical tools, is integrated and shaped into a meaningful profile" (Aicardi 1987). In many instances, there is no technical tool capable of providing the clinician with a yes-or-no answer. Even determination of genotypic abnormalities may not be totally reliable because of genetic heterogeneity and variable expression of many genes depending on interactions of mutant genes with the rest of the genome, epigenetic factors and environmental factors.

The most important clinical feature of a large majority of the

TABLE IV.1
Investigations in children with suspected metabolic or neurodegenerative diseases

Neuroimaging
Ultrasound may be useful in some infants mainly to exclude structural lesions
CT with and without enhancement
MRI using T_1, T_2, FLAIR sequences. In some cases diffusion-weighted MR or tractography
Magnetic resonance angiography (MRA) in rare cases
Functional imaging, especially MR spectroscopy (MRS) in some cases

Neurophysiological investigations
EEG including sleep tracings and slow photic stimulation routinely, polygraphic recordings in selected cases
Electroretinogram (ERG)
Evoked potentials (visual, auditory, somatosensory) in selected patients
Electromyography and conduction velocity studies for detection of peripheral nervous sytem involvement

Haematology, microbiology, immunology
Search for abnormal blood cells
Marrow examination in selected cases
Protein assay including electrophoresis for determination of protein profile
CSF studies

Biochemical studies
pH determination, search for ketone bodies, aminoacids and organic acids
Glucose in blood and CSF
Lactate in blood and CSF
Very long chain fatty acids
Enzyme studies in blood
Molecular genetic investigations when appropriate
Liver function tests

Tissue examination
Skin, conjuntival, rectal nerve biosy as appropriate for morphological and enzyme studies, especially if mitochondrial disease suspected
Brain biopsy exceptionally
Muscle biopsy
Fibroblast or other tissue culture for possible further investigations

Genetic studies
(when specific diagnosis suspected on reasonable basis)

More complex studies are often indicated *in selected cases.*
(Always keep urine, blood and tissue samples when available for further more sophisticated studies.)

metabolic and heredodegenerative CNS diseases is their progressive character. A progressive encephalopathy marked by cognitive and/or developmental regression in a child is, prima facie for all practical purposes, a genetic disease, even though no precise diagnostic tag can be affixed, provided a subacute or chronic inflammatory disorder can be ruled out (the commonest of these being infectious – e.g. AIDS – or inflammatory disorders). The progressive character is not always easily affirmed.

Two essential arguments are drawn from history: (1) the notion of a free interval during which development had been normal; (2) the loss of already acquired skills. These features may be obvious in late-onset disease with abrupt or rapid deterioration. They may be difficult to discern in diseases of very early (or neonatal) onset, in those in which deterioration sets in insidiously, and in those in which the initial development had never been normal. The associated occurrence of epileptic attacks, heavy drug treatment or other intervening pathological events may further compound the problem.

The appearance of new neurological signs should not necessarily be interpreted as indicating progression as it is commonly observed in the first two or three years of life in children with various types of cerebral palsy.

Some forms of actual deterioration do not indicate a relentlessly destructive process in the brain. Loss of acquired skills does occur with epilepsy, especially with West and Lennox–Gastaut syndromes, but the deterioration stops after a few months or years and resumption of progress can be observed. Similarly, the regression associated with some cases of autism is different from the degenerative diseases as there is apparently no progressive brain pathology.

In all cases, deterioration of known cause, metabolic or otherwise, must be ruled out if an effective treatment may be available. Such include inflammatory diseases, some cases of brain tumours, obstructive hydrocephalus, vascular disorders such as moyamoya disease or sickle cell disease with repeated strokes, and arteriovenous malformations responsible for deterioration as a result of blood 'steal' through the malformation with consequent neighbouring ischaemia.

In the past few years, it has become clear that a genetic cause of CNS disease is not excluded by the apparent lack of clinical progression. It is now well established that genetic degenerative conditions can be very difficult to separate from fixed encephalopathies caused by malformations or prenatally acquired insults. Barth (1992) has drawn attention to the progressive disorders of the fetal brain present at birth, often in the form of an apparently static encephalopathy. An increasing number of such slowly progressive congenital conditions are known, including peroxisomal diseases (Shimozawa et al. 2005, Wanders and Waterham 2005), mitochondrial disorders (Zeviani 2004, DiMauro and Davidzon 2005, Di Mauro and Hirano 2005, Taylor and Turnbull 2005), lactic acidosis and other organic acid diseases (De Meirleir 2002), and cholesterol biosynthesis defects (Hennemann 2005), and some of these conditions are responsible for true CNS (and peripheral) malformations, thus blurring the limits between domains classically considered separate. This may result in the temptation to investigate extensively a vast number of cases with a view to recognizing genetic diseases. The cost of such a policy, not only in economic but also in human terms (e.g. pain, hospitalization, anxiety generated) is an obvious limiting factor, but the 'reasonable' indications and limitations are impossible to define precisely, and physicians have to rely heavily on common sense and clinical acumen. A history of neurological disorders in relatives may be an essential argument in favour of a metabolic or neurodegenerative disease.

For a number of neurodegenerative disorders, MRI techniques especially spectroscopy, allow some insight into the chemical composition of the brain, its energy metabolism (Tzika et al. 1993) and brain neurotransmitters (Novotny et al. 2003). Morphological tissue diagnosis remains important and in many cases may be feasible using peripheral rather than brain biopsy.

Skin and conjunctival biopsy and, less commonly, other biopsies (e.g. gingival) are sufficient for most diagnoses. Brain biopsy is seldom indicated, except when an inflammatory disease is a serious consideration because in this case practical conclusions may result. The development of new, minimally invasive stereotactic techniques may widen the use of brain biopsy in conditions such as tumours or neurodegenerative disorders because of their ease of use and relative innocuity (Linskey 2004). However, this is still uncommonly the case with degenerative diseases, as a suspected diagnosis of genetic disease may not be possible to exclude in some cases by a negative biopsy (e.g. because of possible sampling error), whereas a positive biopsy does not add much to the genetic counselling because recessive autosomal inheritance is very likely if the progressive character of the disease is established.

Molecular genetic techniques are essential to formally confirm the diagnosis of many disorders. However, it should be remembered that, whilst the presence of an abnormal mutant gene is clearly of great importance for diagnosis, it is not sufficient as some common genetic abnormalities may not be the cause of the disease affecting a particular patient. In addition, it does not necessarily provide the information necessary to predict the course and make a prognosis, or to anticipate the many practical problems that are of major importance to the patient and their family.

Investigations that may be indicated in children suspected of progressive disorders of the CNS are shown in Table IV.1. The choice of tests used is heavily dependent on the clinical features, and the number of tests performed should be kept to a minimum (Stephenson and King 1989). The specificity and reliability of the tests is variable (see later chapters); for instance, an extinguished ERG is of considerable value for the diagnosis of ceroid–lipofuscinosis or of peroxisomal diseases, whereas in some patients with these disorders the ERG may be normal. Even enzymatic tests are fallible, with both false positive (arylsulfatase pseudo-deficiency) and false negative tests. Close clinical supervision and control of interpretation of laboratory examination is essential in all cases.

REFERENCES

Aicardi J (1987) The future of clinical child neurology. *J Child Neurol* 2: 152–9.
Barth PG (1992) Inherited progressive disorders of the fetal brain: a field in need of recognition. In: Fukuyama Y, Suzuki Y, Kamoshita S, Casaer P, eds. *Fetal and Perinatal Neurology*. Basel: Karger, pp. 299–313.
De Meirleir L (2002) Defects of pyruvate metabolism and the Krebs cycle. *J Child Neurol* 17 Suppl 3: 3S26–33; discussion 3S33–4.
Di Mauro S, Davidzon G (2005) Mitochondrial DNA and disease. *Ann Med* 37: 222–32.
Di Mauro S, Hirano M (2005) Mitochondrial encephalomyopathies: an update. *Neuromuscul Disord* 15: 2876–86.
Hennemann PC (2005) Congenital brain anomalies in distal cholesterol biosynthesis defects. *J Inherit Metab Dis* 28: 369–83.
Linskey ME (2004) The changing role of stereotaxis in surgical neuro-oncology. *J Neurooncol* 69: 1–18.
Novotny EJ, Fulbright RK, Pearl PL, et al. (2003) Magnetic resonance spectroscopy of neurotransmitters in human brain. *Ann Neurol* 54 Suppl 6: S25–31.
Shimozawa N, Nagase T, Takemoto Y, et al. (2005) Molecular and neurologic findings of peroxisomal biogenesis disorders. *J Child Neurol* 20: 326–9.
Stephenson JB, King MD (1989) *Handbook of Neurological Investigations in Children*. London: Wright.

Taylor RW, Turnbull DM (2005) Mitochondrial DNA mutations in human disease. *Nat Rev Genet* **6**: 389–402.

Tzika AA, Ball WS, Vigneron DB, et al. (1993) Clinical proton MR spectroscopy of neurodegenerative disease in childhood. *AJNR* **14**: 1267–81.

Wanders RJ, Waterham HR (2005) Peroxisomal disorders I: biochemistry and genetics of peroxisomal disorders. *Clin Genet* **67**: 107–33.

Zeviani M (2004) Mitochondrial disorders. *Suppl Clin Neurophysiol* **57**: 304–12.

8
METABOLIC DISEASES

Hélène Ogier, Folker Hanefeld and Jean Aicardi

Metabolic diseases of the nervous system comprise a vast group of heterogeneous conditions that have in common only the presence of a known metabolic deficit at their origin but that differ enormously in pathology, clinical presentation and diagnostic problems.

Several broad subgroups of metabolic diseases will be considered successively:

(1) *Disorders involving subcellular organelles.* These include diseases of lysosomes, the Golgi and pre-Golgi apparatus and peroxisomes. The classical example is that of lysosomal disorders that are due to lack of lysosomal enzymes and result in storage disorders. In such cases, an enzymatic block produces accumulation of storage substances that may interfere with the function and/or survival of neural cells. The metabolic block may also act by inducing deficiency of metabolites normally produced beyond the block or by interfering with other metabolic pathways as a result of deviation from normal to accessory or normally unused pathways. However, some disorders of subcellular organelles (e.g. peroxisomal diseases) do not produce accumulation of storage substances but interfere in various ways with essential metabolic processes.

(2) *Disorders of intermediary metabolism.* These diseases are extremely diverse but here the metabolic blocks do not generate storage. Interference with numerous metabolic pathways leads to disturbances of energy production, amino acid and organic acid catabolism with endogenous intoxication, and interference with neurotransmitter synthesis.

(3) *Disorders of lipid metabolism* other than those in lysosomes or other organelles (e.g. cholesterol).

(4) *Disorders of neurotransmitter metabolism.*

(5) *Disorders of metal, especially copper, metabolism.*

(6) *Miscellaneous metabolic diseases.*

Progressive metabolic CNS disorders are individually rare. However, their prevalence in Sweden was found to be 0.58 per 1000 live births, a frequency similar to that of neural tube defects or congenital hemiplegia (Uvebrant et al. 1992).

A number of metabolic diseases involve only occasionally or secondarily the nervous system and will only be alluded to.

Several disorders of carbohydrate metabolism can affect the CNS indirectly by inducing hypoglycaemia, e.g. various types of glycogenosis, especially type I, and fructose intolerance. Fructose-1-6-diphosphate deficiency can be associated with severe ventricular dilatation and hypoplasia of the vermis and cerebellar hemispheres, and alpha-ketoglutarate dehydrogenase deficiency and pyruvate dehydrogenase deficiency are often responsible also for basal ganglia abnormalities (Brismar and Ozand 1994a,b). Isolated hypoglycorrhachia caused by deficit of specific glucose carrier is described in Chapter 1. The effects on the brain can be prevented by a ketogenic diet.

Galactosaemia resulting from deficit of galactose-uridyltransferase or rarely of epimerase is associated with CNS toxicity and growth failure, in addition to cataracts (Segal 1993). The gene is located to chromosome 9q13 and several mutations are known, which in 90% of cases result in complete absence of enzymatic activity. Even in cases correctly treated by low galactose diet, significant visual–perceptual deficits and EEG abnormalities are found in one third to one half of the patients. This may be due to the continuing endogenous formation of toxic galactose-1-phosphate from glucose-1-phosphate through the action of epimerase. A few patients have more definite neurological signs, including cerebellar or extrapyramidal features that can be progressive (Bohu et al. 1995). Waggoner and Buist (1993) found that 18% of 175 patients had cerebellar signs. Cognitive deficits are frequent and may be progressive. Verbal dyspraxia with disturbances of speech rhythm without receptive deficit usually of a severe degree is frequent even in patients treated in the neonatal period (Hansen et al. 1996, Robertson et al. 2000). Pseudotumour cerebri (Huttenlocher et al. 1970) and skeletal muscle nvolvement (Bresolin et al. 1993) have been reported. In contrast, galactokinase deficiency is associated with cataracts but does not generate neurodevelopmental deficits.

Cystinosis primarily affects the kidney with progressive renal insufficiency. However, with successful management of renal disease neurological manifestations may become apparent. An encephalopathy with cerebellar and pyramidal signs and progressive deterioration may develop (Broyer et al. 1996) and may be associated with cerebral atrophy and multifocal calcification of the internal capsules and periventricular white matter (Fink et al. 1989). A distal vacuolar myopathy may develop in the late stages of the disease (Vester et al. 2000). Preventive treatment with cysteamine may be effective.

Lowe syndrome features congenital cataracts, hypotonia, absent deep tendon reflexes, mental retardation, generalized aminoaciduria and renal tubular acidosis with hypophosphataemia. Although 12 of 47 patients studied by Kenworthy et al. (1993)

had an IQ >70, tantrums and irritability were frequent. MRI may show periventricular lesions (Schneider et al. 2001, Sener 2004). The oculocerebrorenal syndrome is a sex-linked genetic disease mapping to Xq26.1 affecting only males. Female carriers can be detected by the presence of multiple fine lens opacities. The gene *OCRL1* codes for a 105 kD protein that may be related to the Golgi complex (Olivos-Glander et al. 1995) and plays a role in the metabolism of phosphoinositol. Prenatal diagnosis is possible. Although clearly a metabolic disorder, Lowe syndrome is currently difficult to classify.

DISORDERS OF SUBCELLULAR ORGANELLES

LYSOSOMAL DISEASES

Lysosome function is to hydrolyse a large number of complex molecules. When this function fails, storage disorders within the lysosomes result. Most lysosomal diseases are due to a genetic defect of one of the lysosomal enzymes involved in the degradation of a specific substance. However, some diseases, including mucolipidoses II and III, result from post-traductional abnormalities affecting normally synthesized proenzymes. Others (e.g. Salla disease and cystinosis) are due to defective transport of substrates across lysosomal membrane.

All lysosomal diseases are inherited as recessive – mostly autosomal recessive – traits. New diseases (e.g. infantile ceroid–lipofuscinosis) are still being added to the list.

The clinical presentation is variable with the defective enzyme. Even for the same enzyme deficit, the phenotypic manifestations are variable, reflecting the possible existence of multiple different abnormalities of the same gene and/or occurrence of joint effects of other genes, alternative messenger RNA splicing, or post-traductional modifications. These, in turn, result in absence or in different abnormalities of proteins, with variable activity and therefore different clinical features.

SPHINGOLIPIDOSES

The sphingolipidoses are lysosomal diseases with absent or imperfect degradation of the sphingolipids, which are essential components of CNS membranes. The major steps of sphingolipid catabolism and the corresponding enzymes and enzymatic blocks are represented in Figure 8.1.

Gangliosidoses

These are important diseases that result from enzymatic blocks involving the removal of N-acetylgalactose from the complex ganglioside molecules. Gangliosides are found mainly in nuclear areas of grey matter and not, in any great amount, in myelin. Their normal functions are incompletely understood. Although many gangliosides have been isolated from the brain, four major components, GM1 to GM4, account for over 90% of the total ganglioside fraction. Hopes of effective therapy are raised by the use of imino sugar inhibitors of glycosyl ceramide transferase that are effective in Gaucher disease (see below) and are being tried in other glycosphingolipid disorders (Aerts et al. 2006).

• *GM2 gangliosidoses* are the commonest diseases of this group. Several varieties are known depending on the nature of the enzyme defect. Three isoenzymes of hexosaminidase have been recognized. *Hexosaminidase A* is composed of one alpha and two beta subunits (A1, B2), *hexosaminidase B* solely of B units (B2, B2) and hexosaminidase S only of A units (A2). In classical Tay–Sachs disease or B variant, hexosaminidase A (HexA) and S are inoperative as a result of a mutation at the alpha locus on chromosome 15 (15q22–q25.1). Hexosaminidase B is normal but unable to hydrolyse gangliosides in vivo. Different mutations at the alpha locus are known. Thus GM2 gangliosidosis in French Canadians (Palomaki et al. 1995) may be due to a different DNA defect (deletion of intron 1 and promoter region) to that in Ashkenazi Jews, which in 73% of cases comprises a four-base insertion in exon 11. However, some French Canadians have the same mutation as Ashkenazi Jews and, within a single population, different mutations can be observed. B1 mutation results in an altered substrate specificity of HexA. In this variant, the mutated enzyme displays essentially normal activity when tested with conventional methylumbelliferyl substrates but is unable to hydrolyse GM2 or sulfated methyl-umbelliferyl synthetic substrate. The O variant (Sandhoff disease) is characterized by deficiency of both beta-hexosaminidase isoenzymes A and B due to a mutation at the beta locus on chromosome 5q13. Variant AB is caused by the deficiency of an activator protein (saponin) required for the interaction of HexA with its natural substrate (Cordeiro et al. 2000). There is, thus, a considerable clinical and biochemical heterogeneity among the GM2 gangliosidoses (Lyon et al. 2006).

The pathological changes in the CNS are common to all forms of gangliosidosis, with some variations related to the length of the course and undefined factors. The main finding is the presence in neurons of lipid-soluble material within the cytoplasm, with later disappearance of many neurons and the development of extensive gliosis. Purkinje cells and neurons in brainstem nuclei, and neurons in visceral plexus, are also affected. Inflammatory signs are promininent and coincide with the presence of clinical symptoms, suggesting that they play a role in the mechanism of brain lesions (Jeyakumar et al. 2003). Visceral involvement, especially of the kidney, is marked in Sandhoff disease, in which a large accumulation of globoside is characteristic.

Electron microscopy shows multiple membranous cytoplasmic bodies (Terry bodies) composed essentially of lipids with 10% protein. The processes of involved neurons are massively expanded, and this excess of probably excitable membranes may be responsible for abnormal neuronal function.

Tay–Sachs disease is by far the most frequent form of gangliosidosis, affecting 1 in 2000 persons among Ashkenazi Jewish populations of eastern European background. The gene frequency is estimated to be 1 in 27 among Ashkenazi Jews and 1 in 380 in non-Jews.

The onset is between 3 and 9 months, with loss of acquired milestones and of muscle tone following an essentially normal initial development. Acoustic startles may precede all other symptoms and persist for several months. Neurological symptoms

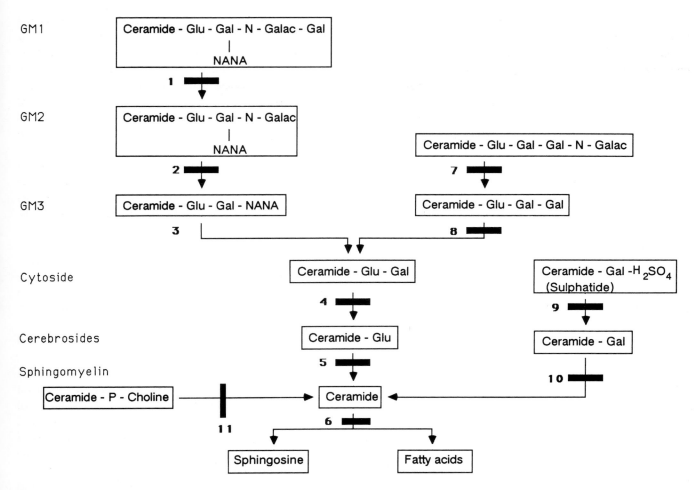

Fig. 8.1. Metabolism of the sphingolipids.

Key: Gal = galactose. Glu = glucose. N-Galac = *N*-acetylgalactosamine. NANA = neuraminic acid (*N*-acetylneuraminic acid).

1 = β-galactosidase. 2 = β-hexosaminidase A (Tay–Sachs disease) and other GM2 gangliosidoses. 3 = GM3 sialidase. 4 = lactosylceramidase (lactosylceramidosis). 5 = β-glucosidase (glucocerebrosidase) (Gaucher disease). 6 = ceramidase (Farber disease). 7 = β-hexosaminidase B (Sandhoff disease and other O variants of GM2 gangliosidosis). 8 = ceramide-trihexosidase/α-galactosidase (Fabry disease). 9 = cerebroside sulfatase/arylsulfatase* (metachromatic leukodystrophy). 10 = β-galactosidase/β-galactocerebrosidase (Krabbe disease). 11 = sphingomyelinase (Niemann–Pick disease A and B).

*Activity measured on artificial substrates, not always parallel to cerebroside sulfatase activity.

rapidly progress. Initial hypotonia is replaced by spastic tetraparesis, and epileptic seizures may appear late in the course. After the first year of life, the infants are helpless, blind and unresponsive and often develop a progressive macrocephaly. MRI in the early stages of the disease shows increased T_2 signal from the basal ganglia. The caudate nuclei often protrude into the lateral ventricles. Later, T_2 signal is increased throughout the white matter (Grosso et al. 2003).

Death usually occurs before 3 years of age. From early in the course, a *cherry-red spot* is present in both macular areas, surrounded by a zone of milky whitish retina. This whitish zone is due to lipid storage in the retinal ganglion cells that are especially dense in the posterior pole, whereas the red spot represents the normal macula, which is devoid of ganglion cells and appears abnormally red by contrast with the surrounding retina. Although characteristic of Tay–Sachs disease, the cherry-red spot may also be seen in other types of gangliosidosis, in sialidosis, in

Niemann–Pick disease, in infantile Gaucher disease and in rare cases of metachromatic leukodystrophy and of Krabbe disease (Naidu et al. 1988).

Sandhoff disease (type O gangliosidosis) is clinically indistinguishable from classical Tay–Sachs but represents only 7% of cases of GM2 gangliosidosis.

The diagnosis of Tay–Sachs disease is easily confirmed by absence of Hex A or of both Hex A and Hex B in serum or leukocytes. Patients with a B1 mutation have intermediate levels of Hex A activity when tested with a nonsulfated umbilliferyl substrate. For them the use of sulfated 4-Mu-gal-N-Ac-6-sulfate (4-MUG) substrate is necessary for diagnosis (Matsuzawa et al. 2003). Prenatal diagnosis by Hex A assay is possible in the second trimester of gestation.

Carrier detection using blood is possible and has been automated for mass screening surveys (Kaback et al. 1993, Leib et al. 2005). Fibroblast testing is required if the woman is pregnant, or if either partner is diabetic, has had a myocardial infarct or has hepatitis. Pseudodeficiency of Hex A occurs in compound heterozygotes who carry one common disease-causing mutation on one allele and one of two benign mutations on the second allele. Such individuals are clinically normal although they cannot hydrolyse synthetic 4-MUG substrates. These benign mutations have significant implications for heterozygote screeening programmes and for prenatal diagnosis. Their frequency was found to be respectively 3% and 38% in Ashkenazi Jewish and non-Jewish enzyme-defined carriers (Cao et al. 1993).

Juvenile GM2 gangliosidosis is rare. Onset is between 2 and 6 years by gait instability and often speech disturbances, followed by ataxia and pyramidal tract signs. Intellectual deterioration is present at end stage (Hendriksz et al. 2004). Ataxia and dysarthria may be the first manifestation. Seizures may occur and dystonia and choreoathetotic movements have been reported (Nardocci et al. 1992). There is no racial predilection.

Late-onset GM2 gangliosidosis (Neudorfer et al. 2005) is also termed chronic GM2 gangliosidosis or 'adult form', although the onset is before 10 years in 35% of cases. Onset is with a special form of dysarthria followed by gait difficulties, pyramidal tract signs, ataxia and lower motor neuron involvement. Psychiatric disturbances occur later in half the cases. Dystonia is present in some patients, and supranuclear ophthalmoplegia has been reported (Rucker et al. 2004).

Atypical forms may present as anterior horn cell disease of juvenile onset (Navon et al. 1995, Drory et al. 2003), as isolated dystonia, or as atypical spinocerebellar degeneration. An unusual presentation mimicking a brainstem tumour is on record (Nassogne et al. 2003). Myoclonic seizures were observed in a case of AB variant (Sakuraba et al. 1999).

A clinical picture of Tay–Sachs disease may be seen in patients with normal amounts of Hex A and B (AB variant) (Cordeiro et al. 2000, Lyon et al. 2006) and is difficult to diagnose as it requires direct study of labelled natural gangliosides catabolism. The B1 variants usually present as infantile disease but may also be found in patients with juvenile and chronic forms (Grosso et al. 2003), although in the latter type an AB variant may be less rare.

No effective therapy for the GM2 gangliosidoses is yet available. Substrate reduction therapy with the ceramide synthesis inhibitor miglustat has been shown in animals to be partially effective (Andersson et al. 2004, Cox 2005) (see below). The process of ganglioside accumulation and consequent brain degeneration is already well established by the midtrimester of fetal life, so the prospects for enzyme replacement therapy are not favourable.

• *GM1 gangliosidoses.* This group of disorders is caused by deficiency of acid beta-galactosidase, whose gene is located on 3pter–3p21 (see Fig. 8.1). In addition to lipid storage closely similar to that in the GM2 gangliosidoses, the stored material also includes vacuolar inclusions with accumulation of numerous mannose-containing oligosaccharides, resulting from defective terminal beta-galactose residue removal during glycoprotein catabolism. Several beta-galactosidase isoenzymes are recognized.

The three isoenzymes (A1, A2, A3) are defective in all forms of GM1 gangliosidosis, and the various phenotypes are probably explained by different mutations resulting in proteins with different residual substrate specificities (Suzuki et al. 1991, Lyon et al. 2006), although there is no necessary correlation between mutation, residual protein activity and clinical severity. Pathological evidence of inflammation is present in the brain, as in GM2 gangliosisosis, and probably plays a role in clinical manifestations (Jeyakumar et al. 2003).

GM1 gangliosidosis type 1 (pseudo-Hurler disease, Landing disease) is a rare autosomal recessive disease, clinically present at birth or even prenatally (Tasso et al. 1996). Affected infants are markedly hypotonic, suck poorly, fail to thrive and do not make any psychomotor progress. They have frontal bossing, coarse facial features, macroglossia and hirsutism. Half of them have a retinal cherry-red spot, and hepatosplenomegaly is usually evident. The skeletal deformities are similar to those of Hurler syndrome. The course is severe. Blindness, quadriplegia and epileptic seizures appear, and death usually supervenes before 2 years of age.

GM1 gangliosidosis type 2 has a later onset between 6 months and 3 years of age. No marked skeletal abnormalities are present, although the first or second lumbar vertebrae are abnormally shaped, so that the presentation is one of progressive neurological deterioration with spasticity, and cerebellar and extrapyramidal signs such as dystonia (Nardocci et al. 1993). Optic atrophy and a cherry-red spot may be present, and acoustic startles occur in half the cases although usually late in the course. The gene is the same as for infantile type 1 but there is heterozygosity for two separate mutations, one of which is that commonly found in homozygous form in type 1.

GM1 gangliosidosis type 3 (so-called adult type) is uncommon. Onset may be in childhood or adolescence with abnormal gait and worsening speech (Tanaka et al. 1995, Muthane et al. 2004). The presentation is variable; dystonia and parkinsonism are frequent (Roze et al. 2005). A picture of spinocerebellar degeneration is possible. Variants include a dystonic form (Tanaka et al. 1995) and atypical cases, e.g. with myopathy and cardiomyopathy (Charrow and Hvizd 1986). Intellectual deterioration may be late or absent in such forms. Low T_1 signal from the pallidum and putamen has been reported (Tanaka et al. 1995), and a leukoencephalopathy is present (van der Voorn et al. 2004).

The diagnosis of GM1 gangliosidosis can be helped by the absence of urinary excretion of mucopolysaccharides, by the presence of bony abnormalities, especially of the lumbar vertebrae, and by the presence of foamy cells in the bone marrow. It is confirmed by the absence or marked reduction of beta-galactosidase activity in leukocytes or fibroblasts. In the late (type 3) forms, beta-galactosidase deficiency is partial (5–20% normal). Prenatal diagnosis can be made on cultured amniotic cells or trophoblasts.

Beta-galactosidase is also deficient in *Morquio type B disease* (p. 255), which is a skeletal disorder without neurological involvement, and in galactosialidosis, which is described with the sialidoses (p. 256).

• *GM3 gangliosidosis* is an exceptional condition characterized by poor physical development, abnormal facies, rapid neurological deterioration and early death. The existence and nosological situation of this disease remains unsettled.

• *Deficiency in lysosomal alpha-N-acetylgalactosaminidase* (Chapter 9) may pathologically resemble neuroaxonal dystrophy.

Gaucher disease

Gaucher disease is a relatively frequent recessive disease affecting 1 in 40,000 to 1 in 200,000 persons and 1 in 400 to 1 in 2000 persons among Ashkenazi Jews. It is due to deficiency of beta-glucocerebrosidase (see Fig. 8.1). The gene coding for beta-gluco-cerebrosidase is located on chromosome 1q21–q31. The different types may correspond to allelic mutations at this locus, although other factors are operative as shown by phenotypic differences even for the same mutations (Goker-Alpan 2005, Ron and Horowitz et al. 2005). Over 150 mutations are currently known, some with neurological manifestations. It has been proposed that phenotypic variations may be due to compound heterozygosity, which is frequent, or to post-transcriptional abnormalities. Homoallelism is common in types 3 and 2 but not in type 1. Three main phenotypes are encountered: chronic adult form, neuropathic infantile form and juvenile type.

• *Type 1 Gaucher disease* is the most common type but is only occasionally observed in children. It is mainly marked by hepatosplenomegaly, bone abnormalities, and sometimes hypersplenism and pulmonary manifestations. There is no involvement of the CNS except in rare cases (Filocamo et al. 2004). However, there is some evidence that subclinical neurological involvement may be detected, e.g. by study of saccadic eye movements (Accardo et al. 2005). Glucocerebrosides accumulate throughout the reticuloendothelial system. The major marker is the Gaucher cell that has a lacy, striated cytoplasm and is found in the bone marrow, spleen, liver and lymph nodes. Electron microscopy shows inclusion bodies containing tubular elements (Kaye et al. 1986). Increased acid phosphatase is a constant finding of some diagnostic value.

• *Type 2 Gaucher disease (acute infantile Gaucher disease or neur-onopathic type)* is also due to glucosyl ceramide beta-glucosidase deficiency. There is some suggestion of heterogeneity as the glycolipid content of the liver is variable and the composition of the glycolipids may also be variable. The clinical onset is at 3–5 months of age with muscle hypotonia and loss of interest in surroundings. Spasticity gradually sets in. Neck retraction and bulbar signs are often prominent and result in marked feeding difficulties. Splenomegaly is usually pronounced but, in one personal patient, it was hardly detectable clinically. Cherry-red spots are sometimes present. Convulsions may occur at age 6–12 months. Death usually occurs before 2 years of age.

The pathological changes in the CNS include foci of cell loss and neuronophagia (Kaye et al. 1986). A few perivascular Gaucher cells may be present but there is usually no marked degree of cytoplasmic storage in this form. An even more severe neonatal form, associated with congenital ichthyosis, has been reported (Ince et al. 1995).

• *Type 3 Gaucher disease (juvenile Gaucher disease)* becomes apparent during the first decade of life, the major features at this period being slowly progressive hepatosplenomegaly, rapidly associated with intellectual deficiency. Cerebellar ataxia and extrapyramidal signs frequently develop. The most suggestive features include supranuclear horizontal ophthalmoplegia that may be the initial feature, and in some myoclonic epilepsy (Verghese et al. 2000, Frei and Schiffmann 2002). Audiometric studies show that involvement of the auditory pathways is frequent (Bamiou et al. 2001). Moderate bony changes such as widening of humeral and femoral diaphyses may be present.

A phenotypic variant of type 3, known as the Norrbottnian type, is frequently encountered in northern Sweden. The onset is early, around 1 year of age, with progressive hepatosplenomegaly and hypersplenism. Mental deterioration, ataxia and spastic tetraplegia evolve slowly after age 3 years. Splenectomy often precipitates appearance or aggravation of neurological signs. This type is regularly associated with a homozygous 444 mutation. Some investigators separate type IIIa with progressive neurological disease and mild systemic manifestations, and type IIIb with severe systemic disease.

A type IIIc with onset of oculomotor apraxia, splenomegaly, cardiac valve anomalies and corneal opacities has been described (Mistry 1995).

In fact, the neurological features are quite variable. Some patients have early features such as ophthalmoplegia starting in the first few years and may keep a normal intellect to adulthood with only extrapyramidal signs without epilepsy or deterioration, and many intermediate forms exist (Lyon et al. 2006).

Pathologically, intraneuronal storage disease is obvious and glucosylceramide is detected chemically.

Treatment of non-neuronopathic Gaucher disease has been transformed in the past few years. Enzyme replacement therapy (Grabowski 2005) is highly effective for type 1 and the systemic manifestations in type 3. It does not improve neurological signs because the enzyme does not cross the blood–brain barrier, although some improvement might occur in the long term. It is also ineffective in acute type II cases. Substrate reduction therapy with imino sugar inhibitors of glycosyl ceramide glucosyl transferase, especially N-butyl deoxygalactonojirimycin (miglustat), the key enzyme in synthesis of glycosyl sphingolipids, has been shown to be effective against the visceral manifestations of the disease, resulting in decrease in size of the spleen and correction of haematological abnormalities (Pastores et al. 2005). Its effect is probably less complete than with enzyme replacement. In addition to its substrate reduction effect (Cox 2005), it may also produce a chaperone-mediated stabilization of mutant beta-galactosidase enzyme. Neurotoxic side effects of this agent have been mentioned, but decreased cognitive efficiency has not been confirmed (Elstein et al. 2005, Pastores et al. 2005). Splenectomy is contraindicated in type III cases.

Lactosyl ceramidosis

This is an exceptional disease caused by deficient ceramide lactosyl beta-galactosidase. There is cognitive and motor regression from 1 or 2 years of age with associated hepatosplenomegaly and a rapidly lethal course (Watts and Gibbs 1986).

Niemann–Pick disease A and B

Niemann–Pick disease comprises a heterogeneous group of disorders linked by an accumulation of sphingomyelin in the reticuloendothelial system. Of the three main types A, B and C, types A and B are due to a deficiency of acid sphingomyelinase and constitute type I, while other forms without sphingomyelinase deficit form group II in the classification proposed by Schuchman and Desnick (1995). Type C will be studied with disorders of cholesterol metabolism (pp. 307–8).

• *Niemann–Pick disease type A (neurovisceral type, type 1)* is transmitted as an autosomal recessive character and occurs especially in Ashkenazi Jews. The gene maps to 11p15, and multiple mutations are known. Some correlation is found between certain mutations and the phenotype. Three mutations account for 92% of cases in Ashkenazi Jews (Schuchman 1995). The pathological hallmark of the condition is the presence in the reticuloendothelial system of large vacuolated cells. Foam cells and ballooned ganglion cells are found in the CNS. Biochemically, there is a marked storage of sphingomyelin, a major component of normal myelin, in association with cholesterol in the spleen, liver and kidney. Storage is also present in the brain, although usually at moderate level.

The clinical onset of the disease is during the first year of life, with hepatosplenomegaly and poor physical and cognitive development. Jaundice, diarrhoea and pulmonary infiltrates are common. Neurological features are prominent in approximately one third of infants and appear eventually in most. Myoclonic seizures, spasticity and blindness are the major manifestations. One quarter of the patients have retinal cherry-red spots. A peripheral neuropathy occurs in 10% of cases, with slowing of conduction velocities. Death occurs before age 5 years.

The diagnosis is suggested by the presence of vacuolated cells in the bone marrow. Sphingomyelinase deficiency in leukocytes or fibroblasts is definitive confirmation of the diagnosis.

• *Niemann–Pick disease type B (visceral type)* is characterized by visceral involvement without neurological features and occurs mainly in older children and adults. An occasional patient may develop neurological signs.

In fact, the distinction between types A and B is not always clear-cut. Protracted neurovisceral forms with a course extending over periods of years are recognized and intermediate forms were the most common type in a recent large series, being observed in 12 of 25 patients (Pavlu-Pereira et al. 2005). Trials of miglustat therapy are being conducted.

Fabry disease

This rare, sex-linked disorder is due to a deficiency (absence, low activity or fast catabolism) of the A isoenzyme of alpha-galactosidase (ceramide trihexosidase) caused by several mutations of the GLA gene, mapping at Xq22. As a result, large amounts of trihexoside accumulate in various organs, especially the kidneys. Foam cells with vacuolated cytoplasm are found in smooth and striated muscle, in marrow and renal glomeruli. In the CNS, storage is confined to walls of the blood vessels and, to a lesser extent, to the autonomic nervous system. MRI may show periventricular high signal and discrete lesions suggestive of demyelination.

Clinical manifestations of the disease usually begin in childhood. Skin abnormalities may be the presenting feature, in the form of punctate angiectatic lesions (*angiokeratoma corporis diffusum*) that are commonly found on the genitalia or umbilicus or about the hips, but may rarely involve the face. Episodes of pain or dysaesthesia in the limbs and sometimes in the abdomen are often the first symptoms. Pain is deep, of a burning character and occurs in episodes lasting from hours to weeks. These are often associated with unexplained fever. Cornea verticillata is seen by slit lamp examination and is often present in heterozygotes (Watts and Gibbs 1986). Peripheral neuropathy involving small fibres has been reported and anhidrosis is frequent. Approximately 30% of patients have cardiac defects including mitral valve prolapse and cardiomyopathy, and transient ischaemic attacks commonly occur (Ries et al. 2005).

The disease runs a progressive course, and CNS and visceral vascular accidents often occur with focal neurological signs, hypertension or myocardial infarcts. Renal involvement is the usual cause of death. Women carriers usually display late and milder symptoms.

The diagnosis is confirmed early by determination of alpha-galactosidase in plasma, leukocytes or fibroblasts. Antenatal diagnosis and carrier detection are possible.

Treatment includes prevention of painful episodes, which can usually be achieved with carbamazepine, gabapentin or phenytoin, and therapy for renal insufficiency. Renal transplants have little effect on the CNS lesions, although sensory symptoms and renal function may be improved. Enzyme replacement therapy has changed the evolution of the disease. Large controlled studies in affected males have shown the safety and efficacy of recombinant enzyme preparations, which decrease pain and stabililize renal function (Clarke and Iwanochko 2005, Schaefer et al. 2005). The quality of life of patients is significally improved (Hoffmann et al. 2005). Preventive treatment for nonsymptomatic female carriers is not generally advised. Antibodies agains the enzyme have been found to develop (Linthorst et al. 2004) but their clinical significance is not yet clear.

Ceramidosis (lipogranulomatosis, Farber disease)

This rare disease is due to deficient activity of lysosomal ceramidase and is transmitted as an autosomal recessive character. The onset is during the first weeks of life, with irritability, a hoarse cry and the appearance of nodular erythematous swellings around the wrists and other joints (Kim et al. 2007). Severe motor and mental retardation is frequent and convulsions are common.

TABLE 8.1
Main characteristics of the mucopolysaccharidoses

Type	Eponym	Osseous visceral abnormalities	Neurological features	Urinary excretion of MPS[1]	Mode of inheritance[2]	Enzyme deficiency (gene location)
IH	Hurler	Marked. Severe dwarfism	Severe	DS + HS	AR	α-L-iduronidase (4p16)
IS or V	Scheie	Mild[3]	Mild	DS + HS	AR	α-L-iduronidase (4p16)
II	Hunter	Marked. Severe dwarfism	Mild or moderate	HS	XR	Iduronosulfate-sulfatase (Xq28)
III	Sanfilippo	Mild. May be lacking at onset	Severe with progressive mental deterioration and seizures	HS	AR	A: Heparan-N-sulfamidase B: α-N-glucosamine-N-acetylglucosaminidase C: α-glucosamine-N-acetyl transferase D: N-acetyl-α-glucosaminido-6-sulfatase (12q14)
IV	Morquio (B milder)	Marked osseous anomalies	Absent (except as complication of bony lesions)	KS	AR	A: N-acetylgalactosamine-6-sulfatase (3p21–p14) B: β-galactosidase (16q24)
VI	Maroteaux–Lamy	Severe dwarfism and bony abnormalities	Absent (except as complication of meningeal involvement)	DS	AR	N-acetylgalactosamine-4-sulfatase (5p11–5q13)
VII	Sly	Mild to severe	Absent to severe	DS + HS	AR	β-glucuronidase (7q21–q22)

[1]DS = dermatan sulfate; HS = heparan sulfate; KS = keratan sulfate.
[2]AR = autosomal recessive; XR = X-linked recessive.
[3]Limited to carpal tunnel syndrome.

Cardiac valvular lesions may be present. Death occurs before 2–3 years of age although a mild form may allow survival for several years. Prenatal onset marked by hydrops fetalis has been reported (Kattner et al. 1997).

The basic lesion is a granuloma that forms around mesenchymal cells containing large amounts of ceramide. Neurons and glial cells are swollen by storage material.

Sulfatidosis (see also Chapter 9)
• *Metachromatic leukodystrophy* is an autosomal recessive disease due to deficiency of cerebroside sulfatase. Diffuse demyelination and accumulation of metachromatic material (metachromasia), caused by the presence of sulfatides, produces an unusual staining with the use of certain dyes when they combine with storage material. Sulfatides are stored in the CNS and in many peripheral tissues including skin and gall bladder. The gene for cerebroside sulfatase maps to 22q13–22qter. A mutation on exon 2 (459.1G) is responsible for most cases of the late infantile form, whereas a mutation on exon 8 (P426L) is commonly found in a later onset form (Barth et al. 1994), but the phenotype/genotype correspondence is imperfect. Complex arylsulfatase A alleles can cause various types of metachromatic leukodystrophy (Kappler et al. 1994). Compound heterozygosity seems to be responsible for juvenile forms (Gieselmann 2003). Metachromatic leukodystrophy is further described in Chapter 9.

• *Mucosulfatidosis (multiple sulfatase deficiency, Austin disease)* is a rare disease characterized by absence of arylsulfatase A, B and C and of mucopolysaccharide sulfatase activity due to mutations in the formyl glycine generating enzyme (Cosma et al. 2004, Lyon et al. 2006). As a result, patients accumulate sulfatides, mucopolysaccharides and cholesterol sulfate in CNS and viscera and there is increased excretion of heparan sulfate in urine. Ichthyosis is a suggestive manifestation.

Globoid cell leukodystrophy (Krabbe disease)
This disease results from deficiency of beta-galactocerebrosidase and is transmitted as an autosomal recessive trait. The gene maps to 14q24–q32 (Cannizzaro et al. 1994) and a number of molecular defects have been identified (Tatsumi et al. 1995). Several forms are known (Hagberg 1984): the infantile form is most common, but rare juvenile, late infantile and adult forms have been observed. An infantile case due to the absence of saponin, an activator of galactocerebrosidase, has been recently reported (Spiegel et al. 2005). Krabbe disease is further described in Chapter 9.

MUCOPOLYSACCHARIDOSES (MPS) (Table 8.1)
The mucopolysaccharidoses are inborn errors of metabolism due to deficiency of a lysosomal glucosidase or sulfatase that leads to the accumulation of mucopolysaccharides or glycosaminoglycans in the lysosomes. Table 8.1 indicates the main characteristics of the diseases of this group. These disorders will be dealt with only briefly as the neurological manifestations are often overshadowed by the dysmorphic and visceral features. Details can be found in specialized books.

Hurler and Scheie diseases (MPS IH and I-H/S)
In Hurler disease, visceral alterations are widespread and muco-

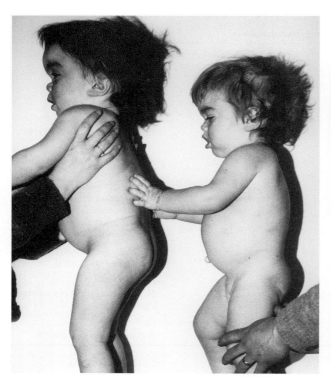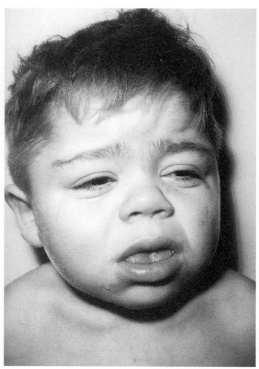

Fig. 8.2. Type I mucopolysaccharidosis (Hurler disease). *(Left)* Two sisters aged 7 and 3 years, demonstrating enlarged head with scaphocephaly, typical profile, umbilical hernia, and short hands with broad, partially flexed fingers. *(Right)* 12-year-old boy with typical facies. (Courtesy Dr P Maroteaux, Hôpital des Enfants Malades, Paris.)

polysaccharide-containing cells are present in the reticuloendothelial system and connective tissue. The CNS is severely affected with infiltration of the meninges, leading to hydrocephalus. Neurons are distended by inclusions that on electron microscopy appear as 'zebra bodies'. The stored material in the brain is mainly composed of GM2 and GM3 gangliosides, whereas, in peripheral tissues, the stored material is mainly formed of dermatan and heparan sulfates, which are also excreted in the urine in large quantities.

Hurler disease is an autosomal recessive disorder that occurs in 1 in 100,000 births. Affected infants appear normal at birth but develop slowly with bony changes becoming apparent between 6 months and 2 years of age. Hepatosplenomegaly, nasal discharge and umbilical hernia are evident. Characteristic skeletal deformities set in progressively, together with coarsening of facial features, kyphoscoliosis, articular contractures and intellectual deterioration. Corneal opacities are seen, and marked dwarfism is consistently present. The head is large, often dolichocephalic (Fig. 8.2). CT and MRI show ventricular dilatation and hypodensity of hemispheral white matter (Zarifi et al. 2001, Matheus et al. 2004). Cystic arachnoiditis is often found in the hypothalamic region and is responsible for hydrocephalus. Dilation of the Virchow–Robin spaces on MRI is often striking. Death supervenes before 20 years of age.

The diagnosis can be confirmed by *L-iduronidase assay*. The presence of azurophilic granules in granulocytes, Reilly granules, vacuolated lymphocytes (Gasser I cells) and basophilic cells in the bone marrow (Gasser II cells) is a strong argument for the diagnosis. Prenatal diagnosis is possible. The gene is located at 4p16.3. Multiple mutations are known, two of them being responsible for 80% of cases.

The treatment of Hurler disease is currently based on enzyme replacement therapy by L-iduronidase; this has largely replaced bone marrow transplantation, which was the first therapy to be used with partial success. Enzyme replacement has proved well tolerated and efficacious for the visceral manifestations of the disease. Corneal clouding disappears, and effects on growth and development are at least partial. Early treatment is essential before definitive abnormalities have set in. Improvement of neurological manifestations has not been demonstrated although anecdotal reports mention increased activity and responsiveness in some children treated early (Wraith 2005). These limited results are explained by the inability of the enzyme to cross the blood–brain barrier. Attempts at circumventing the barrier with haematopoietic cells by bone marrow or hematopoietic stem cell transplantation are under study (Grewal et al. 2005, Lücke et al. 2007). In general, enzyme replacement therapy tends to replace bone marrow transplantation not only in the mucopolysaccharidoses but also for several other lysosomal storage disorders (Germain 2005, Hoffmann and Mayatepek 2005). These therapies are used mainly for the severe conditions that generally feature CNS involvement, especially mucopolysaccharidoses I, II, III and VI. Many problems remain to be solved, a major one being the difficulty for large enzymatic molecules to cross the blood–brain barrier. Other techniques are also being explored, e.g. gene therapy.

In *Hurler–Scheie disease (MPS1-H/S)*, formerly known as MPS type V, a clinical picture analogous to that in Hurler disease obtains and dysmorphism may be marked (Schmidt et al. 1987), but neurological involvement is limited to a high incidence of the carpal tunnel syndrome and mentation is unaffected. Some patients develop hydrocephalus.

Hunter disease (MPS type II)

This disorder is due to deficit in iduronate-2-sulfatase (Kato et al. 2005) and is transmitted as an X-linked trait. It is about five times less frequent than MPS I. Depending on the presence or absence of mental retardation, a mild and a severe form are recognized. Neurological abnormalities in the mild type may include sensorineural deafness, retinitis pigmentosa and moderate hydrocephalus (Froissart et al. 2002). Nerve entrapment syndromes are common as a result of thickening of connective tissue. Enzyme assay permits antenatal and postnatal diagnosis. The gene is located to Xq28 and a deletion is found in 30% of cases. Therapy with bone marrow transplantation may be used in severe cases.

Sanfilippo disease (MPS III)

Sanfilippo disease is a genetically heterogeneous disorder of which four types resulting in four chemical defects are known (Table 8.1). The clinical presentation is that of a progressive neurological and mental retardation beginning between 2 and 6 years of age. Corneal opacities are absent, and abnormally coarse features and thick hair, although present early, are superseded by the neurological disturbances. Epilepsy is frequent.

The course is inexorably progressive and most patients die before the age of 20 years.

The diagnosis is often difficult initially because of the predominantly neurological and psychiatric manifestations. Urine screening for excretion of mucopolysaccharides is routinely indicated in patients with unexplained regression. Enzyme assay permits differentiation of four types that are phenotypically indistinguishable. Antenatal diagnosis is feasible. Therapeutic attempts have been made with bone marrow and stem cell transplantation and with gene therapy but results are at best equivocal.

Morquio disease (MPS IV)

Morquio disease has two types due to different genetic and enzymatic defects (Table 8.1). The clinical manifestations are predominantly bony abnormalities and corneal opacities without mental retardation. In type A, hypoplasia of the odontoid process is regularly present and bulbospinal compression may occur (Montano et al. 2003). Meningeal and neuronal involvement is possible. In the mild or B form, neurological features are absent. Atlantoaxial instability is frequent and may be responsible for spinal compression. Orthopaedic and neurological surveillance and treatment are essential.

Maroteaux–Lamy disease (MPS VI)

This disorder has a variable severity with diverse degrees of dwarfism and visceral involvement. Intellectual dysfunction is mild or absent. The main neurological complication is spinal compression, usually at cervical level, that may produce quadriplegia. This complication results from thickening of the meninges due to deposition of MPS and is difficult to treat surgically. Trials of enzyme replacement therapy have been reported (Karageorgos et al. 2004).

Sly disease (MPS VII)

Sly disease is a very rare disorder that may present with a wide range of phenotypic manifestations from nonimmune hydrops fetalis to cases mimicking Hurler disease with severe neurodevelopmental delay, to cases with limited expression without neurological features (Bernsen et al. 1987, Saxonhouse et al. 2003).

Other forms of MPS

Atypical and unclassified types occur in rare cases. Maroteaux (1973) described a new type in which prominent athetosis is associated with the excretion of keratan sulfate.

MUCOLIPIDOSES, SIALOSIDOSES AND DISORDERS OF GLYCOPROTEIN METABOLISM

MUCOLIPIDOSES

The mucolipidoses are rare disorders that have features of both the mucopolysaccharidoses and the lipidoses. Four types are described (Table 8.2), although types 2 and 3 may be regarded as two degrees (severe and mild) of the same disease. They are transmitted as autosomal recessive characters.

Sialidosis I (cherry-red spot myoclonus syndrome)

Sialidosis I has a juvenile or adult onset and produces a rather pure intention and action myoclonus with a slow progression and no or only mild intellectual deterioration (Rapin et al. 1978, Young et al. 1987). Minor dysmorphic features may appear at late stages.

Mucolipidosis IV

This is a rare disease that affects mainly but not exclusively Ashkenazi Jews. Onset may vary from birth to adolescence, with clinically severe, moderate and mild forms. It is caused by mutations in the *MCOLN1* gene, which encodes a transmembrane protein called mucolipin 1. In the early-onset form, failing vision and intellectual delay develop simultaneously following a normal neonatal period (Amir et al. 1987), and neurological signs such as dystonia are often present. Corneal opacities may be absent despite poor vision in the first months of life. Milder forms may variously combine ophthalmological features with various degrees of cognitive delay and neurological signs (Bargal et al. 2002).

DISORDERS OF GLYCOPROTEIN METABOLISM

These conditions (Fig. 8.3) overlap with the mucolipidoses. Sialidoses I and II belong to both groups. Three main conditions are described.

Mannosidosis

Mannosidosis is due to deficiency of alpha-mannosidase A and

TABLE 8.2
The mucolipidoses (ML) and sialidoses

Type	Age of onset	Clinical features	Enzyme deficiency (gene location)	References
Sialidosis I (cherry-red spot –myoclonus syndrome)	Late childhood to adulthood	Action and intention myoclonus, retinal cherry-red spot, normal intelligence, no dysmorphism	Sialidase (α-neuraminidase) (6p21)	Rapin et al. (1978), Lukong et al. (2000)
Sialidosis II or ML II	Congenital to second decade	Facial dysmorphism, gingival hyperplasia, hepatosplenomegaly, severe mental retardation, macular cherry red spot, renal failure	Sialidase (α-neuraminidase) (6p21)	Lukong et al. (2000), Kudo et al. (2006)
ML II (I-cell disease)	First year of life	Dysmorphism, gingival hyperplasia, severe neurodevelopmental deterioration	N-acetylglucosamine-1-phosphotransferase (12q23.3)[1]	Ben-Yoseph et al. (1987)
ML III (pseudo-Hurler polydystrophy)	Early childhood	Moderate mental retardation in 50% of cases, Hurler-like or Morquio-like skeletal dysplasia	N-acetylglucosamine-1-phosphotransferase (12q23.3)[1]	Kudo et al. (2006)
ML IV	Early childhood but may be later, even into adulthood (male form)	Severe mental retardation, corneal clouding, no bony or visceral involvement, self-mutilation	Mucolipin I (MCOLN1 at 19p13.2–13.3)	Casteels et al. (1992), Bach (2001), Slaugenhaupt (2002)

[1]Same enzyme deficient in some but not all types.

B, caused by several mutations in the gene for alpha-mannosidase (Beccari et al. 2003) resulting in neuronal storage of mannose-rich oligosaccharides. A severe type (type I) has an infantile onset and is characterized by a Hurler-like appearance, mental retardation, hearing loss and hepatosplenomegaly. Type II has a juvenile onset and a milder course, but there is considerable overlap between the two forms (Bennet et al. 1995). Cognitive deficit is variable and usually not progressive (Noll et al. 1989).

Fucosidosis

Fucosidosis is caused by deficiency of the enzyme fucosidase – encoded by the *FUCA1* gene, in which many mutations have been characterized (Lin et al. 2007) – responsible for storage of fucose in tissues. Three types have been described: type 1 or severe type with early infantile onset, type 2 with onset around 18 months of age, and a rare type 3 with onset in adolescence. Type 2 is most common and has a slower course. Clinically the condition presents with skeletal anomalies, cutaneous manifestations (angiokeratoma corporis diffusum involving preferentially the genitalia and gingiva) and neurological symptoms often in the form of dystonia (Gordon et al. 1995). Intermediate forms are common (Willems et al. 1991). Treatment with medullary transplant has been performed.

Galactosialidosis

Galactosialidosis results from a combined deficiency of neuraminidase and beta-galactosidase due to the absence of a protective protein that prevents proteolysis of the active enzyme. The disorder is genetically heterogeneous (Suzuki et al. 1988).

The onset of the *juvenile form* is between 5 and 10 years of age with cerebellar and extrapyramidal signs. Myoclonic seizures and action myoclonus usually develop after several years, and cognitive deterioration is late. There are no bony changes except for the frequent wedging of the first lumbar vertebrae. Coarse features progressively develop. An *infantile form* can closely resemble type 1 gangliosidosis (Galjaard et al. 1984).

Disorders related to the mucolipidoses and MPS

Salla disease is a disorder of the transport of sialic acid across lysosomal membranes. As a result lysosomes store a large quantity of free sialic acid (Renlund et al. 1986). Clinical manifestations include psychomotor retardation of early onset during the first year of life, later followed by slowly progressive cerebellar and extrapyramidal dysfunction with severe intellectual deterioration. Involvement of the peripheral nervous system is evidenced by the decrease in nerve conduction velocity (Varho et al. 2000). The disease is frequent in Finland but cases also occur in other populations (Robinson et al. 1997). Dysmorphic features appear only at a later stage. Diagnosis can be helped by finding vacuolated lymphocytes in blood and vacuolated cells in skin and conjunctival biopy samples, and confirmed by demonstration of high levels of sialic acid in urine. Prenatal diagnosis is possible by determination of sialic acid in amnioic fluid. Several mutations are known (Myall et al. 2007).

Other disorders of sialic acid metabolism include *infantile sialuria* without evidence of lysosome storage (Wilcken et al. 1987), *French-type sialuria* and *infantile sialic acid storage disease*, in which there is marked storage in lysosomes with fetal hydrops, severe retardation and bone defects (Froissart et al. 2005). The clinical presentation of these patients varies from progressive deterioration with death in early childhood to a mild disease with a normal life span. In the severe forms, renal disease may be

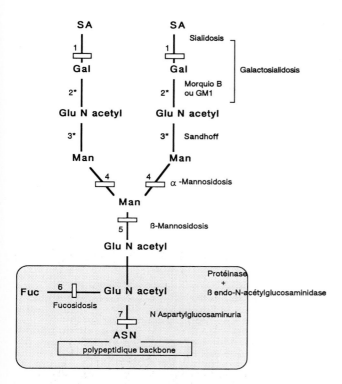

Fig. 8.3. Oligosaccharidoses: catabolism of glycoproteins. The two parts of the chain are degraded after the action of proteinases and β-endo-N-acetylglucosaminidase.

Key: 1 = sialidase = α-neuraminidase. 2* = β-galactosidase (see Fig. 9.1: sphingolipid catabolism = GM1 gangliosidosis). 1+2 = galactosialidosis. 3* = hexosaminidase A or B (see Fig. 9.1: sphingolipid catabolism = Sandhoff disease). 4 = α-mannosidase. 5 = β-mannosidase. 6 = α-fucosidase. 7 = N-aspartylglucosaminidase.

associated. Prenatal diagnosis is possible (Aula and Aula 2006).

Aspartylglucosaminuria consequent to a deficit of aspartyl glucosaminidase is also frequent in Finland. It is marked by mental retardation that begins in childhood or adolescence, lenticular opacities, bony changes reminiscent of the mucopolysaccharidoses, and mitral valve insufficiency (Arvio et al. 1993). Increased excretion of glycoasparagines can be detected by chromatography.

Storage of glucosyl-ribose-5- phosphate has been reported in one patient with progressive neurological deterioration, facial dysmorphism and renal failure, possibly transmitted as an X-linked recessive trait (Williams et al. 1984)

CONGENITAL DISORDERS OF GLYCOSYLATION

Glycosylation of proteins is an essential step in the cotranslational maturation of nascent polypeptides. This process is essential for viability and normal development. It concerns most extracellular proteins such as serum proteins (transferrin, α_1-antitrypsine, α_1-antichimotrypsine, some clotting factors, apolipoprotein C-III), most membrane proteins such as receptors in specialized cells, and several intracellular proteins such as lysosomal enzymes. Congenital disorders of glycosylation (CDGs) have been subdivided into disorders of N- and of O-glycosylation. Disorders due to

defects in mannose-α-O-glycosylation are associated with Walker–Warburg syndrome and different forms of muscular dystrophies such as muscle–eye–brain disease, Fukuyama congenital dystrophy and related myopathies (these are described elsewhere) (Muntoni et al. 2004, Martin 2005). Disorders of N-glycosylation result in multisystemic abnormalities that usually include the central nervous system. This group is subdivided into two types. Type I CDGs are characterized by a defective elongation of the glycan, while type II CDGs are due to defects in the processing pathway (for reviews, see Leroy 2006, Sparks 2006).

BIOCHEMICAL BACKGROUND AND PATHOGENESIS
Glycosylation of proteins is a very complex process that involves numerous enzymes and transporters.

The build-up of the required oligosaccharide (OS), also called glycan, takes place in the endoplasmic reticulum (ER). The various sugar donors are activated as nucleotide-linked sugars and as dolichyl-phosphate monosaccharides on the cytoplasmic side of the ER. OS synthesis is initiated by the attachment of two N-acetyl-glucosamine-phosphate units to a lipid carrier (dolichol phosphate) required for the OS elongation process. Subsequently, a stepwise elongation occurs with further attachments of mannose and glucose residues. Each step is catalysed by specific transferases that are encoded by corresponding *ALG* genes. In the last step, the OS is transferred to the nascent protein by an oligosaccharide protein glycosyl transferase (OST). The various congenital defects in this pathway are responsible for CDG type I (Fig. 8.4a).

After the OST-mediated transfer, the process ensues in the Golgi apparatus by removal of glucose and mannose residues through catalytic activities of specific glucosidases and mannosidases. At that point, two pathways diverge. One serves the lysosomal phosphorylation, defects of which result in mucolipidosis type II (I-cell disease) and type III (pseudo-Hurler syndrome). The second pathway serves the specific orientation of proteins to their site of function, e.g. within the plasma membrane or for secretion in the intercellular space. This pathway, also called the trimming pathway, comprises removal of mannose residues via specific mannosidases and attachment of two N-acetyl-glucosamine units via specific transferases. One fucose, two sialic acid and two galactose units are added sequentially. This maturation requires specific fucose and sialic acid transporters and a galactosyltransferase respectively. Defects in this trimming pathway are responsible for type II CDGs (Fig. 8.4b). Two other type II CDGs caused by defects in the conserved oligomeric golgi (COG) have been described. COG is a protein complex embedded in the Golgi membrane and involved in the maintenance of the Golgi apparatus and its functions.

DIAGNOSIS
Diagnosis of CDGs is usually performed by isoelectric focusing of serum transferrin. The patterns are divided into two types. Type 1 is characterized by elevated disialo- and asialotransferrin bands together with a decrease of tetrasialotransferrin. Type 2 is characterized by increase of trisialo- and monosialotransferrin bands.

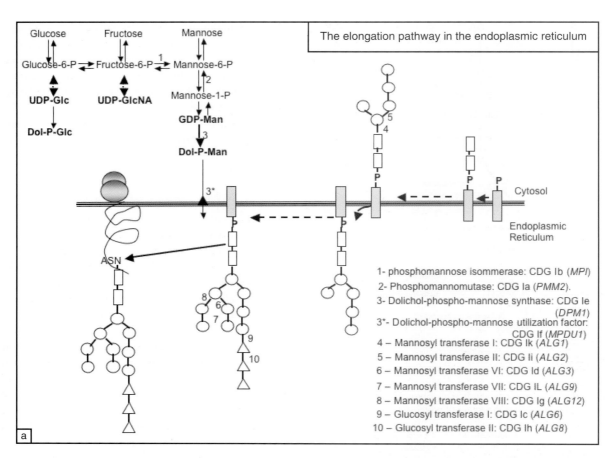

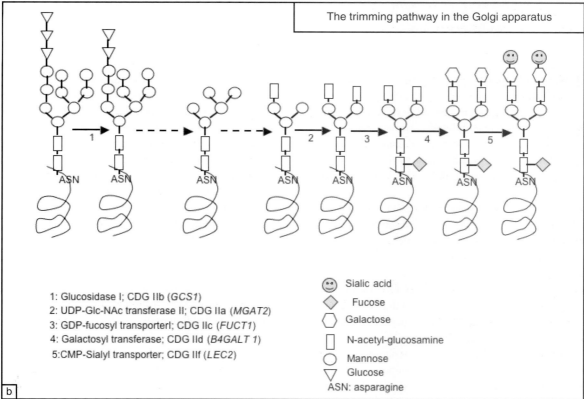

Fig. 8.4. Schematic representations of the glycosylation process indicating the sites of defects in, respectively, CDG types I and II: *(a)* the elongation pathway in the endoplasmic reticulum; *(b)* the trimming pathway in the Golgi apparatus.

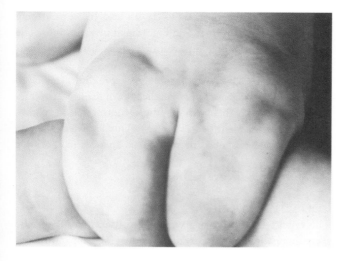

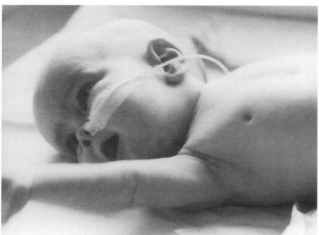

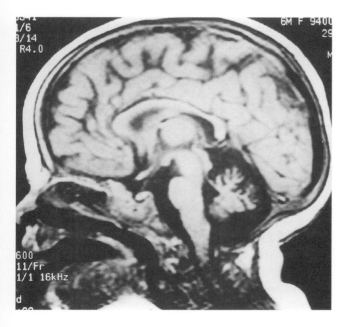

Fig. 8.5. Carbohydrate-deficient glycoprotein syndrome type 1. *(Top)* Abnormal fat pads on the buttocks *(Centre)* Inverted nipples; note also feeding difficulties (tube feeding). *(Bottom)* MRI, sagittal cut, showing marked cerebellar atrophy and relatively thin brainstem. (Courtesy Prof. Billette de Villemeur, Hôpital Trousseau, Paris.)

In addition to the isofocusing of transferrin, isofocusing of other serum sialylated proteins improves the diagnosis (Fang et al. 2004). Apolipoprotein C-III (ApoC-III) isoelectric focusing is used to screen for O-glycosylation defect either in isolation or in association with N-glycosylation defects. Three types of isoforms are recognized: ApoC-III$_0$, ApoC-III$_1$ and ApoC-III$_2$, depending on the number of sialic acid residues attached to the glycoprotein (Wopereis et al. 2007).

TYPE 1 CDGs
CDG type 1a (CDG-Ia)
CDG-Ia is the most common and the best-known CDG disease, with an incidence of around 1 in 50,000. In the classical forms the manifestations are progressive with three stages representing the evolution with age (Hagberg et al. 1993, Stibler et al. 1994).

The infantile stage is dominated by an alarming multisytemic involvement that progresses from the neonatal period through late infancy. It is characterized by poor feeding, failure to thrive and floppiness. Early psychomotor retardation is present in all patients, with severe gross motor delay, pronounced axial hypotonia, muscular weakness and later signs of dysequilibrium or of true cerebellar ataxia. A normal head circumference at birth can progress to acquired microcephaly. Tendon reflexes are initially weak, and areflexia appears within the first 2–3 years of life. Visual inattention, roving eye movements and internal strabismus are frequent. Congenital cataracts have been noted in a few cases. The majority of patients have some facial dysmorphism, inverted nipples, and peculiar body morphology with limb joint restrictions, thorax deformity and unusual lipodystrophy with fat pads above the buttocks (Fig. 8.5), over parts of the perineal region and/or on the fingers. Lipoatrophic streaks or patches on the lower limbs are frequently present. Mild hepatomegaly is associated with hepatic fibrosis or giant cell hepatitis. Enlarged kidneys and proteinuria have been noted. In many cases, alarming episodes of multiple organ system failure may occur: these include severe infections, hepatic failure, cardiac effusion with tamponade, and stupor occasionally associated with seizures and intracerebral haemorrhage. These acute episodes of deterioration are responsible for the high infantile mortality (15–20%).

The childhood stage is dominated by a nonprogressive mental retardation of variable degree. Most patients have DQ/IQ around 50. Cerebellar ataxia and peripheral neuropathy, responsible for muscular atrophy, prevent independent ambulation in most cases. Recurrent episodes of dyskinetic or choreoathetotic movements may occur. Strabismus and retinitis pigmentosa regularly develop. Stroke-like episodes, related to partial cerebrovascular thrombosis, occur in half the patients after the age of 4–5 years with coma, seizures and transient blindness. About one half of patients develop epilepsy.

During adolescence and adulthood the condition is static. Most patients achieve some social functioning but remain dependent.

This clinical course applies to the majority of patients, although mild and unusual phenotypes have been described (Neumann et al. 2003, Coman et al. 2005, Noelle et al. 2005).

Mildly elevated CSF protein levels can be present in the early stages. EEG patterns are nonspecific. ERGs are abnormal with progressive decrease of rod responses (Andréasson et al. 1991). Visual, auditory brainstem and somatosensory evoked potential studies may be abnormal. Nerve conduction velocities are reduced in both motor and sensory nerves, with gradual slowing until adolescence.

Neuroimaging of the brain shows rapidly progressive cerebellar and brainstem hypoplasia in most patients during the first year of life. Supratentorial structures are usually normal, although one third of patients have central and/or cortical atrophy. Nearly all cases exhibit olivopontocerebellar atrophy (OPCA) and myelin-like lysosomal storage (Eyskens et al. 1994). In two twins who died at ages 4 months and 6 years the atrophy was more marked in the longer surviving brother, suggesting a progressive degenerative process. Localized cerebral infarction suggests vascular occlusion. Microscopy reveals a complete loss of Purkinje cells, a subtotal loss of granular cells throughout the cerebellar cortex, and gliosis of pontine nuclei (Stromme et al. 1991). Sural nerve biopsies have shown abnormal myelin sheaths (Nordborg et al. 1991), and lysosomal storage has been found in anterior horn cells (Eyskens et al. 1994) and also in hepatocytes, indicating a change in myelin turnover.

Other type 1 CDGs
Eleven more deficiencies in the OS elongation pathway have been identified. They are termed alphabetically (Ia–Il) following the order of descriptions. Abnormal CNS development and functions are involved in all but one disorder (CDG-Ib). CDG-Ic is the second most common disease with a clinical phenotype that resembles a mild form of CDG-Ia. The other clinical phenotypes are poorly defined due to the small number of affected patients in each category. Some have mild to moderate developmental delay with hypotonia, ataxia, strabismus, nystagmus, and seizures ranging from febrile episodes to epilepsy. Most have neonatal severe encephalopathy with a constellation of signs reminiscent of CDG-Ia. Some patients have sensorineural deafness, blindness, coloboma of the iris and eventually cataracts. Among the extra-neurological signs frequently associated are failure to thrive, dysmorphism, skeletal involvement, cardiomyopathy or pericardial effusion, liver fibrosis or cirrhosis, and renal failure. Some neonates present with hydrops fetalis. Cerebral MRI may be normal or reveal cortical or subcortical atrophy, hypoplasia of corpus callosum, or hypomyelination. Cerebellar hypolasia has been described but is far from being a rule.

Type 1 CDGs may alter various serum glycoproteins, analyses of which may help the diagnosis. Low clotting factors and inhibitors (factor XI, antithrombin III, protein C, protein S, heparin cofactor) could explain the stroke-like episodes. Due to nonspecific leakage to serum, several lysosomal enzymes (e.g. arylsulfatase A, beta-hexosaminidase) and non-lysosomal enzymes (e.g. transaminases) are elevated. Many transport proteins (e.g. apoprotein B), glycoprotein hormones (e.g. IGF1) and complement factors are involved as well. Final CDG-I diagnosis is documented by the presence of a type 1 serum transferrin isoforms profile. At that point, the most common CDG-Ia, Ib and Ic are routinely searched for using enzymatic and molecular investigations. The other types are diagnosed on a research basis when the previous approach has failed.

The type 1 CDGs are autosomal recessive disorders due to a defective step in OS assembly. All the known defective enzymes or transporters have their corresponding genes located and pathogenic mutations identified (Fig. 8.4). This knowledge allows reliable prenatal diagnosis by mutational analyses in chorionic DNA.

There is no effective treatment.

CDG TYPE 2 (CDG-II)
The type 2 CDGs are a group of disorders that affect the trimming pathway of glycosylation in the Golgi apparatus.

CDG type 2a (CDG-IIa)
CDG-IIa was the first described disorder in this group. The few affected patients had very severe developmental delay, no peripheral neuropathy and a normal cerebellum on MRI. They had hypotonia from infancy, generalized seizures from childhood, and abnormal behaviour with stereotypic handwashing movements, tongue thrusting and head banging. They all had small stature, skeletal deformities, hypogonadism and mild liver dysfunction. Biochemically, the carbohydrate deficiency of transferrin is marked with a type 2 transferrin isoforms pattern. The patients' bleeding tendency was explained by decreased clotting factor XI. The defective UDP-Glc-NAc transferase II activity is due to mutations in the *MGAT2* gene located on chromosome 14q21 (Cormier-Daire et al. 2000).

Other type 2 CDGs
Four other types have been described due to defective activity of glucosidase (IIb), galactosyl transferase (IId) and fucose or sialic acid transporters (IIc, IIf) (Fig. 8.4). Each was represented by a few or even single patients. Neurological symptoms have been prominent in types IIb and IId with early and severe encephalopathy, intractable seizures and normal cerebral MRI (IIb) or with moderate developmental delay, muscular weakness and Dandy–Walker malformation on brain imaging (IId). Severe haematological symptoms have been associated in IIc and IIf. The transferrin isoelectric focusing profiles are normal in all but one type; CDG-IIf is associated with an ApoC-III$_1$ profile (Wopereis et al. 2007).

Three other defects are linked to abnormalities in the COG complex: CDG-IIe/COG7, CDG-IIg/COG1 and CDG-IIh/COG8. The plasma transferrin isoelectric focusing type 2 profile and the ApoC-IIIo profile were indicative of altered N- and O-glycosylation. The first disease has been described in two sibling neonates affected with a lethal multisystemic failure and intractable seizures. The COG1 defect has been recognized in a single child with dysmorphic features, some developmental delay and mild cerebral and cerebellar atrophy on brain imaging at 2 years of age. The patient with COG8 deficiency had a severe encephalopathy (Kranz et al. 2007).

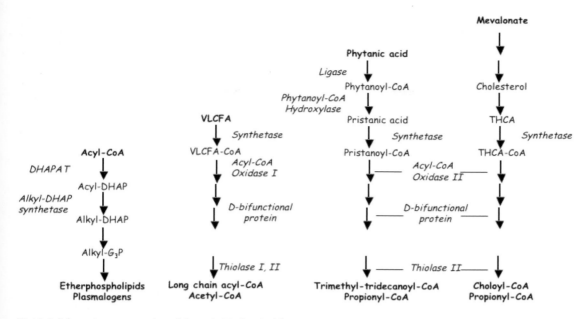

Fig. 8.6. Schematic representation of the main biochemical functions in peroxisomes.
Key: DHAPAT = dihydroxyacetone phosphate acyltransferase; DHAP = dihydroxyacetone phosphate; Alkyl-G3P = alkyl-glycerol-3-phosphate; VLCFA = very long chain fatty acids; THCA = trihydroxycholestanoic acid.

Oral administration of fucose may have improved the haematological signs in patients affected with CDG-IIc without improvement of the neurological status (Leroy 2006). There is no specific treatment in the other types.

It is clear that this group of disorders remains far from being completely investigated and that phenotypic variability among already described types as well as additional forms will probably be delineated when all enzymes and their corresponding genes implicated in the complex processing of glycosylation are known.

PEROXISOMAL DISORDERS
The peroxisomal disorders are a group of diseases caused by inherited defects of peroxisomal biogenesis that result in generalized peroxisomal enzyme defects, or by dysfunction of either a single or multiple peroxisomal enzyme(s). These disorders may present with a wide range of phenotypes. The prototypes are Zellweger syndrome, rhizomelic chondrodysplasia punctata, X-linked adrenoleukodystrophy and Refsum disease, which combine all characteristic symptoms. Besides these 'classical' syndromes, many patients present with variant forms that lack one or more characteristic clinical signs and may be more difficult to diagnose without adequate biochemical screening (for extensive reviews, see Wanders 2004, Poll-Thé et al. 2006).

PEROXISOMES AND THEIR METABOLIC FUNCTIONS
Peroxisomes are ubiquitous organelles containing integral membrane proteins, membrane-associated proteins and more than 50 matrix enzymes that participate in multiple metabolic processes. Peroxisomes are more numerous in cells that specialize in the metabolism of complex lipids (very-long-chain fatty acids

and plasmalogens) and in the developing nervous system than they are in mature cells, suggesting that they serve important physiological functions in the CNS.

Biochemical peroxisomal pathways
Peroxisomal disorders are characterized by a build-up of metabolites normally degraded by peroxisomal enzymes or by decreased amounts of metabolites normally synthesized by peroxisomes, depending on the specific enzyme defects involved. Only those that are of direct diagnostic relevance are described.

Peroxisomal beta-oxidation
Peroxisomal beta-oxidation is a major metabolic route along which several inborn errors can occur. The main substrates oxidized in peroxisomes are saturated very-long-chain fatty acids (VLCFAs), di- and trihydroxycholestanoic acids (DHCA, THCA) that are intermediate substrates in bile acid synthesis from cholesterol, pristanic acid and the long-chain dicarboxylic acids. The peroxisomal beta-oxidation system of VLCFAs, THCA and pristanic acid includes three main steps. The first step, leading to the formation of CoA-substrates, is mediated by three distinct acyl-CoA synthetases. The second step is catalysed by two specific peroxisomal oxidases. The subsequent oxidation of VLCFAs, THCA and pristanic acid proceeds via the same D-bifunctional protein, whereas two thiolases are required for the last step (Fig. 8.6). Absence of peroxisomes is responsible for generalized beta-oxidation impairment (Zellweger syndrome, neonatal adrenoleukodystrophy, infantile Refsum disease), while isolated defects may involve each step of this peroxisomal beta-oxidation system with specific biochemical abnormalities.

TABLE 8.3
Classification of human peroxisomal disorders

Disorders	Peroxisomes in liver	Peroxisomal enzyme defects
Group I: Peroxisomal biogenesis defects		
Zellweger syndrome	Absent	
Neonatal adrenoleukodystrophy	Scarce/Absent	Generalized defects
Infantile Refsum disease	Scarce/Absent	
Rhizomelic chondrodysplasia punctata	Present and abnormal	Plasmalogens synthesis, phytanic oxidase, unprocessed thiolase
Zellweger-like syndrome	Present and normal	VLCFA oxidation, bile acid synthesis, plasmalogen synthesis
Group II: Single peroxisomal enzyme deficiencies involving β-oxidation defects		
X-linked adrenoleukodysrophy	Present and normal	ALD protein
Pseudo-neonatal adrenoleukodystrophy	Present and abnormal	Acyl-CoA oxidase
Pseudo-Zellweger	Present and abnormal	Thiolase
Bifunctional enzyme deficiency	Present and normal	Bifunctional protein
Group III: Single peroxisomal enzyme deficiencies without β-oxidation involvement		
Refsum disease	Unknown	Phytanic acid oxidase
Pseudo-rhizomelic chondrodysplasia	Unknown	Plasmalogen synthesis
Di-(tri-)hydroxycholestanoic acidaemia	Unknown	Bile acid synthesis
Mevalonic aciduria	Unknown	Cholesterol synthesis

Plasmalogen biosynthesis

Plasmalogens are a special class of ether phospholipids. Their role is unknown, but they are especially abundant in the CNS. The first two steps in plasmalogen synthesis are catalysed by peroxisomal dihydroxyacetone phosphate acyltransferase and alkyl-dihydroxyacetone phosphate synthase. Their deficient activity is responsible for low plasmalogen synthesis in patients affected with either peroxisomal biogenesis defects or isolated deficiency of one of these enzymes.

Phytanic oxidation

Phytanic acid is a branched-chain fatty acid derived from dietary sources. Its degradation is via an alpha-oxidative pathway to yield pristanic acid. Further oxidation occurs via peroxisomal beta-oxidation. Due to defective phytanic and pristanic oxidation, both derivatives accumulate with several peroxisomal disorders. Both alpha- and beta-oxidation of phytanic acid are located in the peroxisome.

Pipecolic catabolism

L-pipecolate oxidase is a peroxisomal enzyme that catalyses the hydrogenation of L-pipecolate. Its deficiency explains high levels of pipecolic acid in plasma, CSF and urine of patients with Zellweger syndrome.

Molecular and genetic background

The peroxisomal disorders can be subdivided into two main groups (Table 8.3) (Gärtner 2000, Wanders 2004). The first group is characterized by loss of multiple peroxisomal enzyme activities often associated with morphological abnormalities of the organelle (Roels et al. 1988). In this group nearly all peroxisomal matrix proteins are synthesized but mislocated in the cytosol, a characteristic due to a defective import machinery for peroxisomal proteins. Both peroxisomal and matrix proteins are synthesized on free ribosomes and directed to peroxisomes through distinct peroxisomal targeting sequences (PTS1, PTS2). These targeted proteins are recognized by cytosolic PTS1- and PTS2-receptors, which are encoded by *PEX5* and *PEX7* genes respectively. The proteins are then delivered to the translocation machinery. Complementation studies using patient fibroblasts have defined at least 16 complementation groups. They are caused by mutations in different *PEX* genes encoding peroxins, proteins involved in peroxisomal biogenesis and proliferation. Complementation group 1 is the largest group, including more than half of all peroxisome biogenesis defect patients. Mutations in *PEX1* are responsible for this group. Regarding the clinical syndromes, complementation groups have no clear relationship with clinical phenotypes with the exception of the 11th one, which correlates with the rhizomelic chondrodysplasia punctata type I, and is due to mutations in *PEX7*. All generalized peroxisomal disorders are autosomal recessive diseases with an aggregate incidence of approximately 1 in 50,000 live births.

In the second group, the structure of the organelle is intact and the defects involve only one peroxisomal enzyme activity. Each disorder represents a complementation group. The gene of X-linked adrenoleukodystrophy (X-ALD) has been cloned and mapped to the X chromosome (Xq28). The gene encodes an integral membrane protein that is one of the ATP-binding cassette (ABC) transporters in the peroxisomal membrane. These transporters import CoA derivatives of VLCFAs for peroxisomal beta-oxidation. Different mutations in the *X-ALD* gene impair this import function. About 500 mutations have been identified, most of them being private mutations in each of the affected families (Aubourg 2007). Except for X-ALD, all these single peroxisomal enzyme deficiencies are inherited in an autosomal recessive manner.

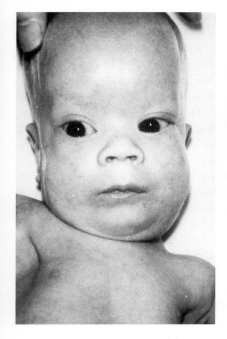
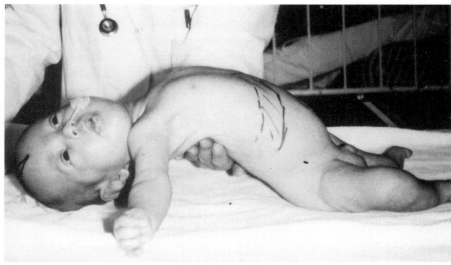

Fig. 8.7. Zellweger syndrome. *(Left)* Note high forehead, epicanthus, slanting palpebral fissures. *(Above)* Marked hypotonia, hepatomegaly and swallowing difficulties (nasal feeding tube). (Courtesy Dr B-T Poll-Thé, Academisch Ziekenhuis, Utrecht.)

All peroxisomal disorders can be prenatally detected on chorionic villi or amniocytes using tests similar to those described for postnatal diagnosis. VLCFA assays in plasma and/or fibroblasts can identify almost 80% of the *X-ALD* female carriers, while molecular biology would allow more accurate identification (Moser et al. 1999).

CLINICAL CONSEQUENCES OF PEROXISOMAL DYSFUNCTION

Group I: disorders with multiple peroxisomal enzyme defects
This group derives from errors in peroxisomal biogenesis. Zellweger syndrome, neonatal adrenoleukodystrophy, and infantile Refsum disease belong to this group. They share several clinical, biochemical and genetic abnormalities and are grouped together as Zellweger spectrum. Rhizomelic chondrodysplasia punctata is the fourth disorder in this group. It has a peculiar clinical phenotype and genetic cause (Table 8.3).

• *The cerebrohepatorenal syndrome of Zellweger (ZS).* ZS, the most severe of the group I disorders, presents in the newborn infant with typical facial dysmorphism including high forehead, widely patent fontanelles and sutures, shallow orbital ridges, low and broad nasal bridge, epicanthus, external ear deformity, micrognathia and redundant neck skin folds (Fig. 8.7). Neurological manifestations are dominated by severe hypotonia with depressed or absent tendon reflexes and poor sucking and swallowing. Generalized seizures frequently start during the first days of life. Absence of psychomotor development, failure to thrive and retinal degeneration with extinguished ERG are constant findings. Optic atrophy, cataracts or glaucoma may occur. Hepatomegaly and liver dysfunction are always present, and polycystic kidneys are frequent. Stippled calcifications of the epiphyses may result in

skeletal deformities and joint contractures. A biological adrenal insufficiency is frequently observed. The EEG is always abnormal with multifocal paroxysmal activity, and evoked potentials are grossly disturbed. Nerve conduction velocities and EMG are normal. Cerebral imaging shows severe gyral abnormalities, especially extensive pachygyria, low density of the white matter and, in some cases, vermian hypoplasia. Death usually occurs within the first year of life. Post-mortem studies of the brain show a striking and characteristic disorder of neuronal migration. A sudanophilic leukodystrophy of variable severity may be associated. Variable organ involvement is the rule, including hepatic cirrhosis/fibrosis, renal cysts, and striated adrenal cells similar to those found in X-ALD (Chapter 9). Absence of demonstrable peroxisomes or presence of peroxisomal membrane 'ghosts' in liver and other tissues with generalized biochemical peroxisomal impairment characterize this disorder.

• *Neonatal adrenoleukodystrophy (NALD).* NALD is a less severe form. Craniofacial dysmorphism is absent or mild, and patients may show some developmental progress before progressive deterioration and death, which occurs within the first decade of life. The main clinical features include developmental delay or deterioration, hypotonia, seizures, sensorineural deafness, and poor vision usually due to retinal degeneration, sometimes associated with cataracts or optic atrophy. Failure to thrive is frequent, as are subclinical adrenal insufficiency and liver dysfunction. CT and MRI of the brain may show contrast enhancement around hypodense areas of the white matter as described in X-ALD (Chapter 9). The main neuropathological findings are demyelination (cerebral hemispheres, cerebellum and brainstem), neuronal migration disturbances less consistent and less marked than in ZS (polymicrogyria and neuronal heterotopias), perivascular lymphocytic infiltrates, and PAS-positive macrophages. Ultrastructurally, these macrophages contain bilamellar inclusions similar to those found in other tissues, especially in adrenal cortex. Patients with NALD also have biochemical evidence of multiple peroxisomal dysfunctions resembling that found in ZS.

• *Infantile Refsum disease (IRD).* First described as a phytanic acid storage disorder, IRD has subsequently proved to be the mildest form of peroxisomal disease with absence of identifiable liver peroxisomes. The clinical course is characterized by a normal neonatal period followed by a few months of nonspecific features, with digestive signs resembling a malabsorption syndrome, hepatomegaly with impaired liver function, low plasma levels of cholesterol and apolipoproteins, and mild facial dysmorphism. Developmental delay with hypotonia and ataxic gait, choroido-retinopathy and sensorineural hearing loss becomes evident by the age of 1–3 years. Patients may survive until the second decade of life with severe cognitive dysfunction. Milder forms of the disorder, with normal intellectual progress, seem possible (Poll-Thé et al. 2004a). Cerebral imaging shows moderate atrophy without signs of cortical malformation or hypodense lesions. Post-mortem study in one case has revealed micronodular liver cirrhosis, adrenal hypoplasia, and absence of macroscopic brain malformation but a severe cerebellar granular layer hypoplasia with ectopic Purkinje cells in the molecular layer (Moser 1989). Hepatic peroxisomes are morphologically absent, and patients display multiple peroxisomal dysfunction.

ZS, NALD and IRD are phenotypic variants resulting from mutations in various *PEX* genes. Many other phenotypic variants have been described that are difficult to classify. However, variable developmental delay, liver disease, retinopathy, sensorineural deafness and onset in early infancy are major common signs. Similarly, clinical course is highly variable, and whatever the disease, a significant number of patients have prolonged survival with variable disability (Poll-Thé et al. 2004a).

• *Rhizomelic chondrodysplasia punctata (RCDP).* RCDP type 1 is characterized by rhizomelic dwarfism, facial dysmorphism, cataracts, mental retardation and spasticity. Stippled epiphyseal and extra-epiphyseal calcifications present during infancy, and may disappear after the age of 2 years leaving skeletal deformities. Some patients have hepatomegaly and ichthyosis. There is remarkable clinical heterogeneity, and variant forms with eventually lack of the rhizomelic shortening and mild developmental delay may have typical biochemical abnormalities. In the severe phenotype, cerebral MRI displays delayed myelination and signal abnormalities in supratentorial white matter and progressive cerebral and cerebellar atrophy. In the mild phenotype, MRI is normal (Bams-Mengerink et al. 2006). This entity results from mutations in the *PEX7* gene blocking PTS2 protein import. Deficient plasmalogens in erythrocytes is the most reliable marker of this disorder. It is usually associated with raised plasma phytanic acid levels.

These peroxisome biogenesis disorders are associated with either generalized or multiple loss of peroxisomal functions. Increased plasma levels of VLCFAs, notably C26:0 (hexacosanoic acid), is the most useful diagnostic test in ZS, NALD, and IRD. These results are confirmed by studies in cultured fibroblasts, in which oxidation of VLCFAs is severely impaired. Elevated plasma levels of bile acid intermediates (DHCA and THCA) are due to defective beta-oxidation of bile acids. Elevated blood levels of phytanic and pristanic acids are due to their impaired alpha- and beta-oxidations respectively. However, plasma phytanic acid accumulation is much less marked than in adult Refsum disease. High pipecolate levels in plasma and CSF are present in nearly all patients. Decreased plasmalogen content in red blood cells and in cultured fibroblasts, and defective dihydroxyacetone phosphate acyltransferase activity in fibroblasts, leukocytes or thrombocytes are major features in these disorders. In contrast, the biochemical abnormalities of RCDP include low erythrocyte levels of plasmalogens due to impaired biosynthesis, accumulation of phytanic acid, and normal plasma levels of VLCFAs.

Group II: disorders involving a single peroxisomal enzyme
• *X-linked adrenoleukodystrophy* (see also Chapter 9). X-ALD (Moser HW et al. 1995) is a relatively common disease that features combined involvement of the CNS and adrenals. Adrenal involvement is clinically manifest in only a minority of cases. Over half the patients have the childhood form of the disorder, approximately 25% have a late-onset presentation with adrenomyeloneuropathy, and 10% have isolated Addison disease. In some studies, adrenomyeloneuropathy is the most common phenotype (van Geel et al. 1997). One of the remarkable features of X-ALD is the intensity of the CNS inflammatory reaction. The cause is unclear but is probably related to the presence of abnormal lipids. This reaction may play an important role in the pathogenesis of the disease. It is absent in patients with adrenomyeloneuropathy. The disorder is described in Chapter 9 with the leukodystrophies.

• *Other isolated peroxisomal beta-oxidation defects.* Several cases resembling NALD or ZS have been described with isolated deficiency of one of the specific enzymes involved in the peroxisomal beta-oxidation system (see Fig. 8.6). *Acyl-CoA oxidase 1 deficiency* has been described in a few patients with signs resembling NALD. *Defective D-bifunctional protein* is responsible for a severe neonatal encephalopathy, dysmorphia and abnormal neuronal migration reminiscent of ZS. Most patients have died within the first two years, with a few having a longer survival with severe cognitive impairment, visual and hearing failure, and eventually peripheral neuropathy (Ferdinandusse et al. 2006). Whatever the site of the defect, patients all have high plasma levels of VLCFAs, while other peroxisomal functions are normal. In the latter two conditions, THCA and DHCA accumulations coexist with high levels of VLCFAs. Within this group an apparently restricted biochemical defect leads to multiorgan involvement analagous to that observed in the disorders of peroxisome biogenesis, suggesting that defects in the peroxisomal beta-oxidation system can cause profound developmental disturbances. In addition, *2-methylacylCoA racemose deficiency* has been found in two adult patients suffering from an adult-onset neuropathy similar to those encountered in adult X-ALD and in Refsum patients. The biochemical profile was characterized by 2-methyl branched-chain fatty acid, THCA and DHCA accumulation.

• *Isolated peroxisomal enzyme defects other than beta-oxidation.* Classical Refsum disease (see also Chapter 20) is characterized by accumulation of phytanic acid in tissue and body fluids due to phytanic oxidation defect. Other peroxisomal functions are intact. Final diagnosis requires enzymatic measurement and mutation analysis, as a subset of patients with normal phytanoyl oxidase activity have *PEX7* mutations (Wills et al. 2001, van den Brink et al. 2003).

Two types of RCDP due to isolated enzyme deficiencies of either dihydroxyacetone phosphate acyltransferase (DHAPAT, RCDP type 2) or alkyl-dihydroxyacetone phosphate synthase (ADHAPS, RCDP type 3) have been described. In severe forms, the patients have a clinical phenotype similar to that of the 'classical' RCDP syndrome. These cases underline the potential pathophysiological role of plasmalogens in CNS abnormalities. Some milder forms have also been described with a partial clinical phenotype, and especially with mild dysmorphia and mild neurological impairment (Bams-Mengerink et al. 2006).

TREATMENT
For classical Refsum disease, dietary restriction of phytanic acid, with or without with plasmapheresis, can prevent further progression of the disease (Wills et al. 2001). Therapeutic options for patients with disorders of peroxisomal biogenesis are limited by severe abnormalities already present in utero, and no specific therapy is presently available. Supplementation of docosahexaenoic acid may have improved patients with milder or atypical forms of peroxisomal biogenesis defects and isolated beta-oxidation defects (Martinez 1996, Martinez and Vazquez 1998).

In X-ALD, dietary treatment with a mixture of glycerol esters of oleic and erucic acids (Lorenzo's oil) is effective in normalizing VLCFA levels (Korenke et al. 1995). However, the clinical efficacy of the diet is uncertain and it has not prevented aggravation of the condition, although some suggestion to the contrary has been offered. The possibility of preventing deterioration in boys treated at the presymptomatic stage remains to be explored (Mahmood et al. 2005, Aubourg 2007). Erucic acid does not enter the brain, which probably explains these limited results (Aubourg et al. 1993). Bone marrow transplantation has occasionally given spectacular results (Aubourg et al. 1990), and improvement has been observed in 7 of 52 boys treated. Mortality is high if no compatible donor is available. It may be indicated in the absence of clinical symptoms when early MRI abnormalities appear in the internal capsules or corpus callosum (Aubourg et al. 1992, Moser HW et al. 1995). A different approach, currently being tried, is with anti-inflammatory agents (beta-interferon and thalidomide) in an effort to suppress the intense inflammatory response that may be responsible for at least some of the clinical manifestations of the disease.

DISORDERS OF AMINO ACID AND ORGANIC ACID CATABOLISM

PHENYLKETONURIA AND HYPERPHENYLALANINAEMIA
Hyperphenylalaninaemia (HPA) is defined as elevated fasting levels of phenylalanine in blood as compared with values obtained from healthy subjects of identical age. The HPAs represent a group of disorders, among which phenylalanine-hydroxylase (PAH) deficiency is the most common. A small number are due to defects in the biopterin cofactor system (for a review, see Burgard et al. 2000).

BIOCHEMICAL AND GENETIC BACKGROUND
The metabolic derangement
Hydroxylation of phenylalanine to tyrosine requires three enzymes – PAH, carbinolamine dehydratase (PCD) and dihydropterin reductase (DHPR) – and two cofactors – tetradihydrobiopterin (TBH) and reduced NAD (Fig. 8.8). Based on plasma phenylalanine levels and residual PAH activity in liver, three different inherited phenotypes of HPA due to PAH defiency are described: classical phenylketonuria (PKU), atypical PKU, and non-PKU HPA (Table 8.4). Defects in THB synthesis and recycling are responsible for both HPA and neurotransmitter disorders (see p. 277).

Genetics
HPA is one of the most prevalent disorders of amino acid metabolism in the White population, occurring in approximately 1 in 10,000 live births. This autosomal recessively inherited disorder is caused by more than 500 mutations at the *PAH* locus. Different groups of mutations predominate in a given ethnic population, allowing prenatal diagnosis, carrier detection, and the prediction of the PKU phenotype linked with a particular haplotype. Some *PAH* mutations result in PAH deficiency with a residual enzymatic activity that is enhanced with TBH. In such cases, pharmacological dose of TBH results in, at least, a 30% decrease of blood phenylalanine levels (Fiori et al. 2005).

Pathogenesis
The clinical manifestations of HPA are thought to result from phenylalanine accumulation and its secondary effects on brain chemistry. The fact that PKU is most often accompanied by mental retardation whilst non-PKU HPA is not, suggests that there is a threshold level of phenylalanine in extracellular fluids above which persistent postnatal (or fetal) HPA causes irreversible brain damage. If the threshold value is exceeded only later in life, after diet discontinuation in the early-treated PKU patients, reversible chemical changes appear that may affect neuropsychological function.

Patients with PKU exhibit a reduction of amine neurotransmitter synthesis when plasma phenylalanine levels are high. Defective neurotransmitter synthesis may be due both to a competitive inhibition of transport of large aminoacids (tyrosine, tryptophane and branched chain aminoacids) into the brain

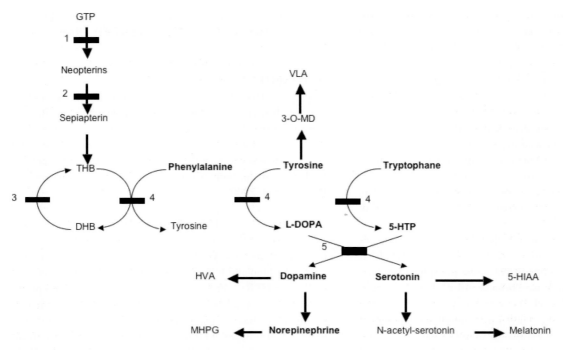

Fig. 8.8. Synthesis and catabolism of pterins and monoamines.
Key: 1 = GTPcyclohydrolase; 2 = biopterin synthetase; 3 = dihydropteridine reductase; 4 = phenylalanine-, tyrosine-, tryptophane hydroxylases; 5 = aromatic L-amino acid decarboxylase (pyridoxal phosphate dependent).
GTP = guanosine triphosphate; THB = 5,6,7,8-tetrahydrobiopterin; DHB = 7,8-dihydrobiopterin; 3-O-MD = 3-O-methyldopa; VLA = vanillactic acid; HVA = homovanillic acid; MHPG = methoxy-hydroxy-phenylglycol.

TABLE 8.4
The different hyperphenylalaninaemia (HPA) phenotypes due to phenylalanine hydroxylase (PAH) deficiency

	Residual PAH activity	Blood phenylalanine
HPA type I (classical PKU)	<1%	>1200 µmol/L
HPA type II ('atypical PKU')	1–5%	600–1200 µmol/L
HPA type III (mild HPA, non-PKU HPA)	>5%	<600 µmol/L

PKU = phenylketonuria.

across the blood–brain barrier and from the CSF back into blood – resulting in low tyrosine and tryptophane concentrations in the brain of PKU patients despite high levels in the CSF – and to a possible direct or competitive inhibition of hydroxylation of tyrosine by high levels of phenylalanine. The prefrontal dysfunction (executive function deficit) described in PKU patients support the hypothesis that dopaminergic synthesis is impaired by high phenylalanine levels.

Abnormal myelination, reduction of brain weight and decreased myelin content are found in brain of untreated older PKU patients. These detrimental effects have been confirmed using the HPH-5 mouse model. Current and previous observations have led to the hypothesis that myelin reduction is due to inhibition of an oligodendroglial cell-specific ATP-sulfurylase that results in low content of sulfatides in myelin that in turn is exposed to pro-

teolytic degradation. Consequently, neuronal loss and decreased interneuronal connections occur, as has been demonstrated by quantitative evaluation of neurotransmitter receptor density. If the results obtained in animals can be extrapolated to humans, special involvement of hippocampus and occipital area of the cortex could explain some of the neurophysiological disturbances observed in non- or poorly treated PKU patients.

Abnormal brain protein synthesis due to polysome disaggregation and reduced rate of polypeptide chain elongation may result in low brain weight. Polysome disaggregation also occurs in heart and brain of fetal rats exposed to maternal HPA, a finding that has a bearing on the fetopathy associated with human maternal HPA.

Decreased DNA content and synthesis in neurons exposed to high levels of phenylalanine can also account for decreased proliferation of neurons, neuronal loss and impaired brain growth.

CLINICAL FINDINGS
Untreated PKU
The clinical features of untreated PKU include mental retardation, neurological abnormalities and extraneural symptoms (although the timing varies from patient to patient). Retarded intellectual development is often associated with microcephaly. Abnormal EEGs are frequent (78–95% of cases), but only 25% of patients have seizures, most often of grand mal type. Psychotic behaviour with hyperactivity, destructiveness, self-injury, impulsiveness, and uncontrolled behaviour with episodes of

excitement is not infrequent. The majority of patients present with lightly pigmented or eczematous skin. A peculiar musty odour has been repeatedly mentioned. The general physical development is usually good.

This clinical phenotype is largely a matter of historical interest because the disease is now prevented by early diagnosis and treatment. However, patients with HPA continue to be missed in the neonatal period because testing is not done or false negative results are obtained.

Early-treated PKU
Children with PKU detected by routine neonatal screening and started on a phenylalanine-controlled diet soon after birth generally have intelligence levels within the normal range (Hanley 2004). However, retrospective studies indicate that even with the most favourable treatment characteristics, children tend to have an IQ below those of their first-degree relatives and an educational performance inferior to their siblings and age-matched controls. Subclinical neuropsychological and neurophysiological (evoked potentials and nerve velocities) disturbances are frequent, especially in those patients who do not strictly adhere to the diet. Frequency of an abnormal EEG increases with age despite early and strict dietary control, and MRI studies indicate that dysmyelination is almost universal in older patients affected with both classical and atypical PKU. The MRI changes involve the occipital–parietal regions and extend into the frontal and temporal lobes in the most severe cases. They have no clear relationship with the clinical or the neuropsychological status nor with the phenylalanine control in early childhood but are correlated with the blood phenylalanine level at the time of imaging and are partially reversible by reducing blood phenylalanine concentrations.

TREATMENT
In patients with classical and atypical PKU, a phenylalanine-restricted diet must be initiated shortly after birth to prevent irreversible brain damage. Daily treatment with oral TBH could be an alternative to the diet in patients with the TBH-responsive form of atypical PKU (Muntau et al. 2002). In order to prevent intellectual, neurological and neuropsychological degradation after diet relaxation, treatment for life is a universal policy. In patients with persistent non-PKU HPA (serum phenylalanine levels <600mmol/L), outcome is not impaired and dietary treatment is not necessary.

With treatment initiated later in childhood, some improvement in behaviour can occur, but follow-up of these patients suggests that they are more susceptible to develop behavioural changes after withdrawal of the diet than are early-treated patients.

MATERNAL PKU
Maternal PKU syndrome is a fetopathy that occurs in children of women with untreated PKU, despite the fact, as is usually the case, that the children themselves do not have PKU (Lee et al. 2005).

Phenotype
The syndrome is characterized by microcephaly, low birthweight, dysmorphism, congenital defects and further developmental retardation. There is evidence that an increased risk is directly correlated to maternal phenylalanine level during pregnancy without obvious threshold in effect. When maternal plasma phenylalanine concentrations are above 1200µmol/L (classical PKU), the incidence of fetal pathology is high: 92% have mental retardation, 73% microcephaly, 40% intrauterine growth delay, and 12% congenital heart malformation. Children born to women with atypical PKU (blood phenylalanine levels 600–1200µmol/L) also have increased incidence of microcephaly, mental retardation, and other congenital anomalies such as cardiac defects (Lenke and Levy 1980). When maternal HPA is below 900µmol/L congenital abnormalities are uncommon but risks for microcephaly and mental retardation remain high. Microcephaly is the most constant clinical finding, thus its presence must always suggest maternal HPA even when the mother is of normal intelligence. MRI studies have revealed abnormal development of the corpus callosum without the white matter changes noted in children with PKU (Levy et al. 1996). Children of women with mild-HPA (160–600µmol/L) have normal early IQs. However, head size, birthweight and intelligence scores may be inversely correlated to the maternal phenylalanine concentrations, a finding suggesting the absence of a threshold for adverse effects of PA on the fetal brain.

Pathogenesis
Fetal damage and postnatal PKU probably have a similar pathogenesis in which phenylalanine is the initiator of harm. In all species, fetal amino acid concentrations are higher than maternal levels (average ratio = 1.48). Thus a 'safe' maternal phenylalanine level could lead to an 'unsafe' level in the fetus.

Phenylalanine probably competes with other neutral amino acids for placental and brain transport, which may contribute to decreased fetal growth and abnormal CNS maturation. Tyrosine and tryptophan deficiencies may have a central role in this process as the pattern of congenital abnormalities seen in maternal PKU is characteristic of damage to neural crest derivatives (heart, aortic arch and face). It seems possible that failure of normal crest migration and development is associated with insufficient neurotransmitter fetal biosynthesis from tyrosine and tryptophan (Kudo and Boyd 1996).

Prevention
There is good evidence that, provided maternal blood phenylalanine levels can be controlled both before conception and during the course of pregnancy, the outcome for the fetus is good. Recommended levels at which the maternal blood phenylalanine must be kept are between 250 and 360µmol/L. Therefore, prevention requires high compliance to a strict low-phenylalanine diet along with adequate calorie and micronutrient provision.

TYROSINAEMIA TYPE I
Hereditary tyrosinaemia type I (HT1) is characterized by pro-

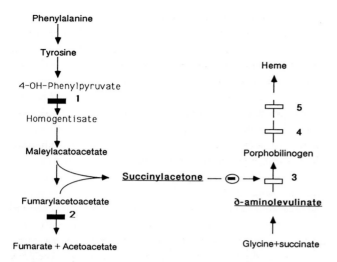

Fig. 8.9. Tyrosine metabolism and its relationship to haem synthesis.
Key: 1 = para-OH-phenylpyruvate dioxygenase (the site of NTBC inhibition); 2 = fumarylacetoacetase; 3 = δ-aminolaevulinate dehydratase; 4 = acute intermittent porphyria; 5 = other porphyrias.

gressive hepatorenal dysfunction and accumulation of tyrosine and its metabolites. In both acute and chronic forms, most un-treated patients die from liver failure or hepatoma. However, in infants and children recurrent acute peripheral neuropathy may be responsible for death independently from liver failure. This neuropathy, mainly described among patients from Quebec, may arise whatever the ethnic origin of patients (Ashorn et al. 2006).

BIOCHEMICAL AND GENETIC ASPECTS
HT1 is an autosomal recessive disorder caused by a deficiency of fumarylacetoacetase, the final enzyme in the catabolic pathway of tyrosine (Fig. 8.9). Maleylacetoacetate and fumarylacetoacetate accumulate and are metabolized to succinylacetone. Succinyl-acetone inhibits delta-aminolaevulinate dehydratase (ALDH) activity and is responsible for abnormally high urinary excretion of delta-aminolaevulinic acid (δ-ALA). Accumulation of suc-cinylacetone and δ-ALA in plasma and urine permits the diag-nosis, which is confirmed by the measurement of fumarylaceto-acetase activity in lymphocytes or fibroblasts or by molecular analysis. Antenatal diagnosis relies on similar determinations in amniotic fluid or in chorionic villus samples. HT1 is now con-sidered a disease that fulfils the criteria for newborn screening (Magera et al. 2006).

PATHOGENESIS
The pathogenesis is not fully understood. For unexplained rea-sons, not all patients experience neurological crises. Comparison with other pathological conditions in which δ-ALA is increased, such as acute intermittent porphyria, hereditary ALDH defi-ciency (Jaffe and Stith 2007) and lead poisoning, suggests that the recurrent onset of neuropathy is linked to δ-ALA accumula-tion and/or hepatic haem deficiency (*Lancet* 1990). Liver trans-plantation and treatment with nitisinone (NTBC), which both

correct the δ-ALA accumulation, prevent neurological crises (Mitchell et al. 1990, Gibbs et al. 1993).

CLINICAL FEATURES
Symptoms may start within a few weeks (acute forms) or months (subacute forms) after birth, or in the following years (chronic forms). Patients present with signs of hepatic and tubular dys-function (Debré–de Toni–Fanconi syndrome). In acute and sub-acute forms, liver dysfunction may be prominent and tubulopa-thy only biologically expressed. If untreated, death from liver failure occurs within a few months. In chronic forms, liver dis-ease is milder, and renal involvement is expressed as a tubulopa-thy with hypophosphataemic rickets. Hepatoma and end-stage renal failure are late complications.

Neurological crises, described as porphyria-like symptoms, may arise, along with intercurrent infections, in patients affected with either the acute or subacute forms. Features include rapid progression of diffuse pain, mainly localized in legs and abdomen, associated with vomiting, irritability, hypertonia, painful attacks of opisthotonic posturing and brisk tendon reflexes. A rapidly ascending paralysis associated with areflexia may follow and results in respiratory insufficiency and death in the absence of assisted ventilation. Throughout this course patients are con-scious. Oral self-mutilation, such as tongue-biting, and grinding and avulsion of the teeth, is observed especially during the initial phase.

Seizures secondary to metabolic disturbances (hypona-traemia, hypoxia) and sustained hypertension may occur. Dura-tion of recovery varies greatly from one crisis to another. A full recovery is most often noted, but multiple recurrences lead to chronic and disabling peripheral neuropathy with amyotrophy. EEG and CSF are normal. Sequential motor and sensory nerve conduction studies have shown progressive alteration in motor action potentials and nerve conduction velocities with histopatho-logical axonal degeneration and demyelination (Mitchell et al. 1990, Gibbs et al. 1993).

Two young patients are described with abnormal myelination of the white matter on brain MRI at the time of diagnosis. One of them had two abnormal peaks on proton MR spectroscopy from these lesions, probably linked to tyrosine molecule. Years later, the second patient affected with a chronic form displayed high bilateral changes in globus pallidus without other lesion in the brain (Sener 2005a,b).

TREATMENT
Nitisinone is a powerful inhibitor of the para-hydroxyphenyl-pyruvate dioxygenase activity, the second step of tyrosine catab-olism (see Fig. 8.9). Its administration to tyrosinaemic patients prevents toxic metabolite accumulation with further increase in tyrosinaemia. The latter is avoided by a phenylalanine/tyrosine-restricted diet. Such a regimen has clear beneficial effects. It normalizes liver and renal function and prevents neurological crises. More data, however, are required to confirm that long-term use of nitisinone is not harmful and that it is effective to prevent hepatocarcinoma (Koelink et al. 2006, McKiernan 2006).

DISORDERS OF BRANCHED-CHAIN AMINO ACIDS (BCAAS)

Maple syrup urine disease (MSUD), methylmalonic aciduria, propionic aciduria, isovaleric aciduria and other organic acidurias secondary to BCAA catabolism defects collectively comprise the most commonly encountered inborn errors of amino acid metabolism. They have many symptoms in common and usually present with one of three clinical types: severe neonatal form, intermittent late-onset form and chronic progressive form. Recurrent coma, the main feature of these disorders, appears to be due to direct toxicity of the accumulated metabolites, while chronic accumulation may interfere with CNS development or cerebral metabolism leading to developmental delay (Morton et al. 2002, Deodato et al. 2006, Vockley and Ensenauer 2006).

BIOCHEMICAL AND GENETIC BACKGROUND
These diseases result from defects of enzymes involved in the catabolism of leucine, valine and isoleucine (Fig. 8.10). The three neutral BCAAs are initially metabolized through a common pathway: a transamination is followed by a thiamine-dependent decarboxylation, which is deficient in MSUD (step 1). The decarboxylation defect is responsible for accumulation of BCAAs and their corresponding keto acids. Subsequently the catabolic pathways of the BCAAs diverge. Leucine is further metabolized to acetoacetate and acetyl-CoA. Specific enzyme deficiencies may occur at every step. Isovaleryl-CoA dehydrogenase deficiency is responsible for isovaleric aciduria (step 2), isovalerate being a highly toxic substrate. Deficiency of 3-methylcrotonyl-CoA carboxylase, a biotin-dependent enzyme, (step 3) produces 3-methyl-crotonyl-glycinuria, as a result of either apoenzyme decarboxylase mutation or abnormal biotin metabolism (see pp. 287–9). 3-methylglutaconic aciduria type I (step 4) is another rare disease due to defective leucine catabolism (Ly et al. 2003). The catabolism of valine and isoleucine produces propionyl-CoA and methylmalonyl-CoA. Methionine and threonine, fatty acids with odd-number carbons and the side-chain of cholesterol, are other precursors of propionyl-CoA. Propionyl-CoA forms methylmalonyl-CoA through a biotin-dependent decarboxylase (step 5) whose deficiency is due to apoenzyme decarboxylase mutation (propionic aciduria) or to abnormal biotin metabolism. Methylmalonyl-CoA is converted to succinyl-CoA in two consecutive steps by the methyl-CoA epimerase (Dobson et al. 2006) and then by the B_{12}-dependent methylmalonyl-CoA mutase (step 6). Deficient activity of each enzyme leads to methylmalonic aciduria. Abnormal B_{12} metabolism is responsible for variant forms of methylmalonic aciduria. Prior to the propionyl-CoA junction, defects have been described at each step of the isoleucine and valine catabolism that are responsible for various neurometabolic disorders (Nguyen et al. 2002, Matern et al. 2003, Poll-Thé et al. 2004b, Salomons et al. 2007). Many of the intramitochondrial CoA metabolites accumulated are substrates for carnitine esterification, a process that results in accumulation of specific acylcarnitines detectable in whole blood by tandem mass spectroscopy. Consequently, most of these disorders are amenable to neonatal mass screening (Tarini 2007).

All but one of the disorders of this group are inherited in an autosomal recessive manner; *2-methyl-3-hydroxybutyryl CoA dehydrogenase deficiency* is an X-linked disorder. Antenatal diagnosis can be performed through the measurement of metabolites in amniotic fluid, specific enzyme activity in chorionic villus samples or amniotic cells, and/or the determination of pathogenic mutations. Newborn infant screening programmes coupled with mutation studies have revealed that a number of patients screened with either isovaleric aciduria or 3-methylcrotonylglycinuria have mild or even asymptomatic phenotypes.

NEUROPATHOLOGY
Available autopsy studies indicate cerebral atrophy and a variety of histological changes. Spongiform degeneration of the white matter is a nonspecific lesion observed in neonates. Mainly described in patients affected with methylmalonic or propionic acidurias, degeneration of basal ganglia is a remarkable sign in older children with pallidal necrosis, spongiosis and cystic cavitation. Cerebral and cerebellar grey matter and the dentate nucleus can be altered by a diffuse vacuolization around neurons and within neuropils (Feliz et al. 2003). A subcortical brain oedema during acute metabolic decompensations is often the cause of death in MSUD patients. A few cases of cerebellar haemorrhage are described.

PATHOGENESIS
The pathogenesis of cerebral involvement in BCAA disorders is poorly understood. In acutely ill patients, accumulation of toxic metabolites can be responsible for energy deprivation due to inhibition of certain enzymes involved in the pyruvate oxidation, in the Krebs cycle or in the mitochondrial respiratory chain. Susceptibility of basal ganglia to energy deprivation may explain their particular involvement along the course of all these diseases especially in methylmalonic and propionic acidurias. In MSUD patients, high leucine levels may result in defective catecholamine synthesis secondary to defective brain uptake of the neutral amino acids tyrosine and tryptophan. Similarly, interference of methylmalonic acid with succinate may reduce gamma-amino-butyric acid (GABA) synthesis. Irreversible changes may be the result of interaction with myelin synthesis due to defective transport of all the neutral amino acids (Schwab et al. 2006). In addition, accumulated propionyl-CoA and methylmalonyl-CoA are precursors of the synthesis of odd-numbered and methyl-branched long-chain fatty acids. Their incorporation into lipid layers may be responsible for abnormal lipid membrane synthesis in the CNS.

CLINICAL FEATURES
Severe neonatal forms
A typical clinical presentation is with relentless deterioration without apparent cause in newborn infants following an initial symptom-free period of a few days. The first signs are poor sucking and difficulty feeding, followed by unexplained and progressive coma. In comatose state most patients have axial hypotonia with peripheral dystonia, choreoathetosis, episodes

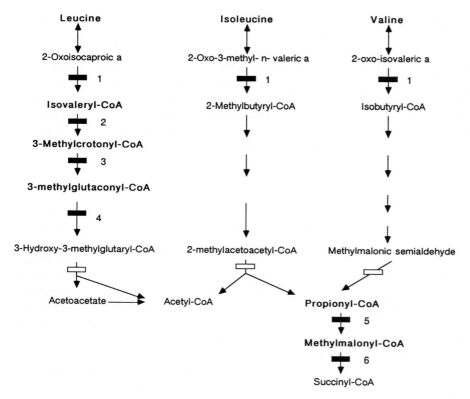

Fig. 8.10. Metabolism of branched-chain amino acids, indicating origin of some known inherited metabolic disorders.

Key: 1 = BCAA decarboxylase (maple syrup urine disease); 2 = isovaleryl-CoA dehydrogenase (isovaleric aciduria); 3 = 3-methylcrotonyl-CoA carboxylase (3-methylcrotonylglycinuria); 4 = 3-methyl-glutaconyl-CoA hydratase (3-methylglutaconic aciduria type I); 5 = propionyl-CoA carboxylase (propionic aciduria); 6 = methylmalonyl-CoA mutase (methylmalonic aciduria).

of opisthotonus, and boxing and bicycling movements of the limbs. Convulsions may inconsistently occur later in the course. Affected babies may have cerebral oedema with bulging fontanelle, arousing suspicion of CNS infection. EEGs often show a burst–suppression pattern. Biochemical abnormalities include metabolic acidosis and ketonuria associated with hyperammonaemia and hyperlactacidaemia. The overall short-term prognosis is improving. Later, despite the treatment, acute life-threatening intercurrent episodes often occur, with clinical manifestations resembling those of late intermittent forms.

Intermittent late-onset forms
In approximatively one third of patients, BCAA disorders present in childhood, or even in adolescence or adulthood. Recurrent attacks are frequent, though in between these the patient may seem entirely normal. The onset in most cases is precipitated by conditions that enhance protein catabolism (infection, trauma, etc.) or by excessive protein intake, but may occur without overt cause. Recurrent attacks of coma or lethargy with ataxia are the main presentations. Most often, coma is not accompanied by other abnormal neurological signs. Ketoacidosis and various glycaemic abnormalities indicate a metabolic origin. A few patients, however, may present with acute hemiplegia and hemi-

anopia, or signs and symptoms of cerebral oedema mimicking a cerebrovascular accident or CNS tumour.

Abnormal EEGs with slow delta waves, loss of normal alpha rhythm, mild nonspecific irregularities or grossly aberrant patterns are often encountered. Focal activity, when present, is usually localized in the temporal regions.

Patients may die during these episodes. Severe cerebral oedema with brainstem compression has been reported in several MSUD patients. It appears to be a reversible cytotoxic oedema as judged on the results of diffusion-weighting imaging and MR spectroscopy studies. This complication, which is worsened by intemperate rehydration, may, however, be a major cause of death in all BCAA patients presenting with acute decompensation. Some recover without sequelae. Many children who survive severe, prolonged or recurrent metabolic disturbances are left with brain damage. Seizures are a common sequela. In infancy and early childhood they tend to be generalized, often myoclonic in type. During later childhood, tonic–clonic or atypical absence seizures are common. Neuroimaging usually shows cerebral atrophy and some delay in myelination. In untreated or poorly treated MSUD, cerebral oedema may persist. The most commonly affected areas are the brainstem, basal ganglia, and occipital periventricular and cerebellar white matter. An increasing number

and methoxy-hydroxy-phenylglycol (MHPG), the end-products of the dopamine pathway, contrasting with normal 5-HIAA and 3-O-methyl-dopa, the end-products of serotonin and epinephrine pathways respectively. When serum prolactin has been assayed, raised levels have been found. Phenylalanine, tyrosine and pterin levels are all normal.

Treatment with dopa substitution is often poorly tolerated. Even low doses may result in side effects. However, with progressive increase from 2 to 6 mg/kg/day over weeks or months some improvement can be obtained.

AROMATIC L-AMINO ACID DECARBOXYLASE (AADC) DEFICIENCY

AADC deficiency leads to a combined deficiency of catecholamines and serotonin as described in THB deficiency (Pons et al. 2004). Affected neonates may have feeding difficulties, autonomic dysfunction and hypotonia. However, they usually develop the characteristic signs during the first year of life with a progressive delay in motor acquisitions, oculogyric crises and a movement disorder with diurnal fluctuations, all of which are due to dopamine deficiency and resemble those described in THB and TH deficiencies. In addition, serotonin deficiency may be responsible for temperature instability, sleep disturbances, and irritability that can be linked to defective synthesis of melatonin from serotonin.

CSF metabolites are characterized by reduced levels of HVA and 5-HIAA and increased level of 3-O-methyldopa. Pterin profiles, phenylalanine and tyrosine are normal. The presence of vanillactic acid on urinary organic acids analysis can suggest the diagnosis. Decreased AADC activity in plasma and gene analyses confirm the diagnosis (Pons et al. 2004, Abdenur et al. 2006).

Therapeutic approaches including dopamine receptor agonists, monoamine oxidase inhibitors, antiepileptics and serotoninergic agents give modest or transient improvement in many patients, while side effects with dystonic and dyskinesic reactions are frequent (Swoboda et al. 2003). However, early treatment has resulted in better outcome in young patients (Pons et al. 2004).

PYRIDOX(AM)INE 5'-PHOSPHATE OXIDASE (PNPO) DEFICIENCY (see also Chapter 22)

In humans vitamin B_6 is present in various forms of which pyridoxal 5'-phosphate is the cofactor for numerous enzymes including AADC, glycine cleavage enzyme and threonine dehydratase. In tissues, the conversion of pyridoxine to the active form of vitamin B_6 requires PNPO. In a few neonates and infants, a pyridoxine-resistant epileptic encephalopathy that is cured with pyridoxal phosphate administration has recently been described. This condition is due to an autosomal recessive defect in PNPO (Clayton et al. 2003, Hoffmann et al. 2007). CSF and urine analyses show evidence of secondary deficiencies of the several PLP-dependent enzymes. The CSF concentrations of dopamine and serotonin metabolites are similar to those described in AADC deficiency. In addition, CSF amino acid analysis reveals raised levels of glycine and threonine due to reduced activity of glycine cleavage system and threonine dehydratase. In addition, CSF

levels of histidine and taurine are also elevated. When it has been looked for, the CSF concentration of pyridoxal phosphate is low. Treatment is not yet clearly codified. However, it would be logical to systematically test oral administration of pyridoxal phosphate (50 mg/day) in addition to pyridoxine in all neonates and infants with epileptic encephalopathy as soon as sufficient CSF samples have been properly frozen for further analysis.

NONKETOTIC HYPERGLYCINAEMIA (NKH)

NKH or glycine encephalopathy is an inborn error of amino acid catabolism in which large amounts of glycine accumulate in body fluids. The classical phenotype is a life-threatening illness that develops in the neonatal period, during which most patients die. Survivors are severely mentally retarded and usually have seizures. Atypical variants with variable age of onset and clinical manifestations have less severe prognosis. Rare patients may present a transient neonatal form characterized by biological normalization (Applegarth and Toone 2001, Hoover-Fong et al. 2004, Pearl et al. 2005).

Biochemical basis

Glycine is implicated in numerous biochemical reactions, among which glycine–serine interconversion appears to be the most important for maintaining glycine homeostasis. This reaction involves two reversible enzymatic steps, one subserved by serine hydromethyltransferase, the other by the glycine cleavage system. This last step serving the catabolism is defective in NKH.

$$\text{Serine} + \text{THF} \rightleftharpoons \text{Glycine} + \text{CH}_2\text{THF};$$
$$\text{Glycine} + \text{THF} + \text{H}_2\text{O} \rightleftharpoons \text{CH}_2\text{THF} + \text{CO}_2 + \text{NH}_3.^*$$

The glycine cleavage system localized in kidney and brain includes four protein components named P (pyridoxal phosphate-dependent decarboxylase, GLDC), T (tetrahydrofolate requiring aminomethyltransferase, AMT), H (glycine cleavage system hydrogen carrier protein, GCSH) and L (lipoamide dehydrogenase). The majority of NKH patients (75–80%) have a defect in P-protein; most of the remainder have a T-protein defect; H-protein deficiency is rare. L-protein is not implicated in this disorder (Applegarth and Toone 2001, 2004).

Genetic background

Whatever the protein defect involved, NKH is an inherited autosomal recessive disorder. The three genes *GLDC*, *AMT* and *GCSH* have been cloned and various mutations have been identified. With the exception of three common mutations in the *GLDC* gene among Finnish patients, most unrelated patients are compound heterozygotes and the majority of the mutations are found in single cases. Antenatal diagnosis can be performed using direct enzymatic assay from fresh chorionic villus. However, false-negative and false-positive results have been reported. DNA analysis will provide a reliable result in families where both mutations in the proband are identified. Measurement of glycine/serine ratio in amniotic fluid is unreliable (Applegarth and

*THF = tetrahydrofolate; CH_2THF = methylenetetrahydrofolate.

Toone 2001, 2004). Newborn screening by tandem mass spectrometry is not beneficial for NKH (Tan et al. 2007).

Neuropathology

The most striking feature is lack of myelination, frequently associated with abnormal brain morphology. Ten out of 16 brains studied by Dobyns (1989) showed an abnormal gyral pattern, hypoplasia, agenesis of the corpus callosum, colpocephaly or cerebellar hypoplasia. A severe spongy leukodystrophy is present. These descriptions are concordant with the brain malformations observed in a transgenic mouse model for NKH (Applegarth and Toone 2001).

Pathogenesis

Although the mechanism underlying the neurological dysfunction is not fully understood, glycine itself has an important role in the pathogenesis. Glycine is an inhibitory neurotransmitter whose receptors are mainly located in the spinal cord and brainstem. These glycine receptors are specifically antagonized by strychnine and competitively inhibited by benzodiazepines. This inhibitory neurotransmission can explain hypotonia and apnoea. Another, strychnine-insensitive, site associated with the NMDA receptor plays a major role in excitatory transmission in the cortex and diencephalon. NMDA-mediated neurotoxicity is markedly potentiated by glycine, and excessive activation of NMDA receptors may directly result in neurotoxicity (Hoover-Fong et al. 2004).

Brain dysmyelination could also result from the defective glycine–serine interconversion with decreased production of one-carbon units, a metabolism that has higher activity in the period of myelination (Hayasaka et al. 1987).

Clinical features

• *Classical early-onset phenotype.* This is the most frequently occurring type of NKH. Symptoms may appear from hours postpartum to the first few days of life. Lethargy and muscular weakness appear first. Shallow breathing follows and rapidly yields to apnoeic spells. Affected infants are flaccid and unresponsive to stimuli but often present with erratic myoclonias and subtle partial seizures. The burst–suppression pattern on the EEG (Fig. 8.17), though nonspecific, is an important diagnostic feature.

A majority of patients die in this early period. For some infants, episodes of apnoea and respiratory depression are transient difficulties, and they may survive. However, no effective treatment is known, and early survivors invariably develop a severe epileptic encephalopathy and die within the first years of life. They display spastic cerebral palsy, associated in most cases with infantile spasms or less often with partial convulsions. The periodic EEG pattern most often disappears after a few months and changes to atypical hypsarrhythmia or multifocal epileptic discharges.

CT and MRI show progressive cerebral atrophy and delayed myelination of the supratentorial white matter. Agenesis or hypoplasia of corpus callosum is a frequent sign. The high peak of glycine individualized on proton MR spectroscopy allows non-

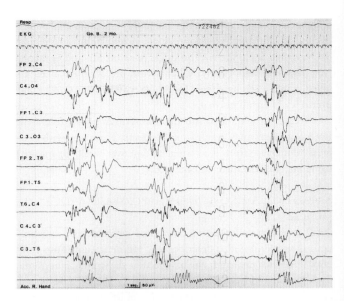

Fig. 8.17. Glycine encephalopathy (nonketotic hyperglycinaemia): typical suppression–burst EEG tracing in 2-month-old boy. Note myoclonic jerks of right hand synchronous with EEG bursts *(lower trace)*. (By permission of John Libbey Eurotext, London.)

invasive measurement of glycine concentration in the brain in classical NKH (Huisman et al. 2002, Korman et al. 2004, Dinopoulos et al. 2005).

• *Atypical cases.* There are three major types: neonatal, infantile, and late onset (Dinopoulos et al. 2005). The presentation of the neonatal type is similar to that of classical NKH but the subsequent psychomotor development is significantly better.

The infantile type is the most frequent presentation of atypical NKH. It can be easily misdiagnosed as static encephalopathy. After a neonatal period that may be uneventful, these children have developmental delay that can progress to moderate or profound intellectual disability (60% of cases). Most have some upper motor neuron signs, poor fine motor coordination, expressive speech deficit, hyperactivity and aggressive behaviour (Steiner et al. 1996). About 50% develop seizures of any type. An acute deterioration induced by intercurrent febrile illness or trauma has been described in some patients with lethargy, hypotonia, ataxia, and seizures that are often difficult to control, or unusual symptoms such as myoclonic jerks, abnormal twitching movements, agitated delirium, chorea, ataxia and vertical gaze palsy.

The late-onset form is very rare and more heterogeneous. The presentation is after the second year of life and even in adulthood, mainly with mild cognitive decline and behavioural problems. In a few cases, spinocerebellar degeneration with optic atrophy and neuropathy has been described. The cause of the hyperglycinaemia in these late-onset cases is uncertain, since they all lack enzymatic or genetic confirmation.

• *Transient forms* clinically and biologically resemble the classical

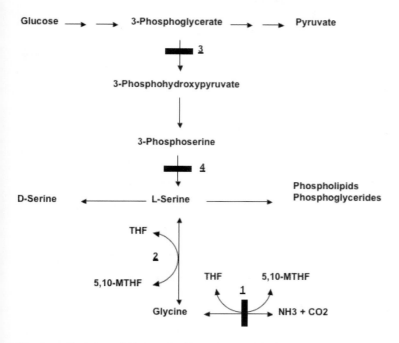

Fig. 8.18. Glycine metabolism, serine biosynthesis and utilization.
　　Key: 1 = glycine cleavage system; 2 = serine hydromethyltransferase; 3 = 3-phosphoglycerate dehydrogenase; 4: 3-Phophoserine phosphatase; THF = tetrahydrofolate; 5,10-MTHF = 5,10-methylenetetrahydrofolate.

type; however, the biochemical abnormalities resolve within weeks. Long-term clinical outcome is uncertain. This type has been reported in association with mutation conferring significant residual enzymatic activity (Applegarth and Toone 2004).

Diagnosis
The diagnosis is confirmed by demonstration of elevated plasma and CSF glycine levels, with a high glycine CSF/plasma ratio, which is the most specific abnormality. Secondary hyperglycinaemia with inhibition of the glycine cleavage system is due to accumulation of several metabolites (e.g. organic acids, valproate). The clinical setting and a rapid screening of urine organic acids and blood acylcarnitine profile would exclude most other metabolic disorders. Definitive diagnosis relies on enzymatic studies on liver or transformed lymphoblasts in classical forms without residual activity. Atypical and transient forms may have normal activity in lymphoblasts and should have their enzymatic activity measured in liver and/or extensive molecular analysis for diagnosis (Applegarth and Toone 2001, 2004).

Treatment
There is no known effective therapy. Strychnine is aimed at inhibiting peripheral glycine receptors. Treatment with high-dosage sodium benzoate is directed toward reducing plasma and CSF glycine levels. Dextromethorphan, ketamine and tryptophan would antagonize the excitatory effect of glycine on NMDA receptors. They all have been used in isolation or in combination without consistent improvement (Dinopoulos et al. 2005, Korman et al. 2006).

Another disease associated with disorder of the neurotransmitter glycine is hyperekplexia (or startle disease, Chapter 16), which is linked to mutations on the $\alpha 1$ or β subunits of the glycine receptor (Rees et al. 2002).

SERINE DEFICIENCY SYNDROMES
Serine deficiency syndromes are rare autosomal recessive disorders due to defective synthesis of the amino acid L-serine. So far two disorders have been described: *3-phosphoglycerate dehydrogenase (3-PGDH) deficiency* and *3-phosphoserine phosphatase (3-PSP) deficiency*. Both result in a severe encephalopathy but are potentially treatable (de Koning et al. 2000, de Koning and Klomp 2004, Pearl et al. 2005, de Koning 2006).

BIOCHEMICAL BASIS
L-serine can be derived from different sources. However, its biosynthesis from 3-phosphoglycerate is a predominant route notably in the central nervous system. In the L-serine synthetic pathway, 3-phosphoglycerate is converted to L-serine in three consecutive steps. The two disorders described here concern the first and third steps (Fig. 8.18) and result in important defective brain metabolism. In situ, L-serine is the precursor for the synthesis of the neurotransmitter L-glycine and the neuromodulator D-serine. The folate metabolite 5,10-methylene tetrahydrofolate, which is generated along with glycine, is a key metabolite especially for purine and pyrimidine synthesis, and for various methylation reactions. Finally, L-serine is a precursor for the synthesis of phosphoglycerides, sphingolipids and glycolipids.

GENETIC BACKGROUND

3-PGDH deficiency is an autosomal recessive disorder. The *3-PGDH* gene is located on chromosome 1q12, and two homozygote missence mutations have been identified in six patients. These mutations result in an enzymatic defect with high residual activity. Nul mutation without residual enzymatic activity might be lethal in utero. Molecular investigation is the only tool for prenatal diagnosis in the absence of enzymatic data in chorionic villi and amniocytes. 3-PSP deficiency was found in a unique patient whose molecular investigations have not been completed.

PATHOGENESIS

L-serine deficiency is thought to reduce cell proliferation. This hypothesis is sustained by the 3-PGDH knockout mouse model that shows a lethal developmental defect with severe brain atrophy. From the experience with prenatal follow-up and treatment of one patient, it seems that the onset of symptoms occurs after the 27th week of gestation. Within this period, the brain development is marked by glial cell proliferation, neuronal differentiation, dendritogenesis and apoptosis. These late pathological consequences may explain the therapeutic effectiveness with serine supplement.

CLINICAL FEATURES

3-PGDH deficiency mainly affects the central nervous system. Patients present with congenital microcephaly. Severe psychomotor delay develops in the first months of life followed by the onset of intractable epilepsy. Seizures can be tonic–clonic in type or flexor spasms in infants. In older children, tonic, atonic, myoclonic, absence and gelastic seizures have been observed. EEGs register patterns of either hypsarrhythmia or severe multifocal epileptic abnormalities with poor background. Other neurological signs include hyperexcitability, generalized hypertonia, spastic quadriplegia and nystagmus. In 4 patients the pre-treatment MRI showed severe hypomyelination, a thin and short corpus callosum, and enlarged subarachnoid spaces and ventricles in the presence of microcephaly. In some patients, adducted thumbs, cataract, hypogonadism and megaloblastic anaemia were additional features.

DIAGNOSIS

Low concentrations of serine and, to a variable degree, of glycine in plasma and CSF are the biochemical hallmark of the disease. In plasma, the abnormality can be missed if it has been sampled after the patient has eaten. In contrast, serine levels in CSF are not influenced by meals. Therefore, CSF amino acid analysis is preferable over plasma analysis. Amino acid analysis in urine is not informative. Besides deficiency of serine and glycine in CSF, low levels of folate have also been observed with normal neurotransmitter amines. The diagnosis is further confirmed by measurement of enzymatic activity in fibroblasts and by molecular analysis.

TREATMENT

Oral L-serine supplementation has been effective to control seizures and to improve spasticity, well-being and behaviour of

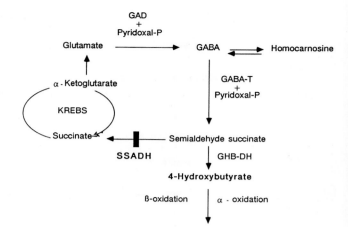

Fig. 8.19. Metabolism of γ-aminobutyric acid (GABA). Key: GAD = glutamic acid decarboxylase; GABA-T = GABA-transaminase; SSADH = succinic semialdehyde dehydrogenase; GHB-DH = γ-hydroxybutyric acid dehydrogenase.

these patients. High dosages up to 600 mg/kg/day in four or six divided doses are required to normalize the biological abnormalities. If seizures are not controlled, glycine can be added at a dose of 200–300 mg/kg/day. In patients treated after their first year of life, little or no progress in psychomotor development was observed. In some patients, a marked increase in the white matter volume and progression of myelination was observed in MRI follow-up.

A girl diagnosed prenatally was treated in utero with oral L-serine supplementation given to the mother from the 27th week of gestation. This normalized the fetal head growth and with subsequent postnatal therapy this 3-year-old girl had normal development.

INBORN ERRORS OF GABA METABOLISM

Gamma-aminobutyric acid (4-aminobutyric acid), a major inhibitory neurotransmitter amino acid, is synthesized from glutamic acid via glutamate decarboxylase. The catabolic steps comprise transamination, which yields succinate semialdehyde, and an oxidation to succinate, which finally enters the Krebs cycle. Pyridoxal phosphate is a coenzyme for all these three reactions. A secondary route, catalysed by a dehydrogenase, converts succinate semialdehyde to gamma-hydroxybutyrate, which is further oxidized (Fig. 8.19). In addition, the major precursor of glutamate in neurons is glutamine, which is synthesized in glial cells via glutamine synthetase. Glutamine is then transported to neurons, where glutamate and then GABA are metabolized. This GABA shuttle between neurons and glial cells allows the maintenance of this system. Homocarnosine is the dipeptide form of GABA. The most frequent defect in GABA metabolism is succinic semialdehyde dehydrogenase. GABA transaminase deficiency and homocarnosinosis are very rare disorders (Table 8.7) (Pearl et al. 2005). Defective glutamine synthesis is a newly described disorder in neonates with severe brain malformation (Häberle et al. 2005).

young patients the second period is not observed, and they deteriorate abruptly following an acute event such as generalized tonic–clonic seizures. In adolescence and adulthood, many signs are similar to the late stage described above, except that most patients have normal development before the onset, the first sign being rapid mental deterioration and in a very few patients signs of schizophrenia. Less commonly, cerebrovascular complications may reveal the disorder. Biological investigations reveal mild homocystinuria and hypomethioninaemia in association with low to normal folate levels. Low CSF neurotransmitter levels have been reported (Haworth et al. 1993). CT and MRI reveal non-specific cortical and subcortical atrophy and periventricular demyelination. Results of neurophysiological investigations are all in accordance with a diffuse process of demyelination (Ogier de Baulny et al. 1998). Hydrocephalus internus has been a revealing sign in two newborns (Baethmann et al. 2000).

The pathological changes in autopsied young infants include dilated cerebral ventricles, internal hydrocephalus, microgyria, demyelination and gliosis (Beckman et al. 1987). In some cases, vascular changes resemble those described in 'classic' homocystinuria (Kanwar et al. 1976, Wendel et al. 1983). In children, the presence of classical findings of subacute combined degeneration of the cord supports the hypothesis of methionine and adenosylmethionine deficiencies in the genesis of neurological changes (Surtees 1998).

Hereditary folate malabsorption

Congenital folate malabsorption presents in infants by 2 months of age with severe megaloblastic anaemia, diarrhoea, failure to thrive, skin rashes, mucositis, recurrent infections due to unusual organisms, and progressive neurological deterioration with convulsions. The diagnosis is based on low levels of folate in serum, red blood cells and CSF, with undetectable amounts of CH_3THF. There is loss of the normal CSF to serum folate ratio of 3:1, indicative of failure to transport folates across the choroid plexus (Geller et al. 2002). Oral or intramuscular folic acid, folinic acid or methylfolate supplementation usually leads to haematological and general improvement, with normalization of serum folate content. However, methyltetrahydrofolate in red blood cells and in CSF remains low. Supplementation with betaine or methionine may prevent neurological deterioration. We have treated a 2-month-old patient with oral and intramuscular folinic acid and betaine. At 5 years of age he has developed normally and has normal brain MRI (personal case). Conversely, some patients have remained mentally retarded with variously combined neurological signs such as recurrent seizures, ataxia, athetosis and peripheral neuropathy. Calcification affecting the parietal cortex and basal ganglia has been reported (Geller et al. 2002).

Glutamate formiminotransferase deficiency

The clinical expression of this disorder is variable (Whitehead 2006). In type I, mental retardation, hypotonia, abnormal EEG and cortical atrophy are reported in half the cases, in association with folate-responsive megaloblastic anaemia. These features appear between the ages of 2 weeks and 18 months. In type II,

mental retardation is mild with only a speech defect. There is no evidence of folate deficiency, and the biochemical hallmark is spontaneously high excretion of FIGLU. Mutations in the formiminotransferase cyclodeaminasen (FTCD) gene have been identified in 3 children with the mild phenotype.

TREATMENT
Supplementation with different forms of folate must be systematically tested with either oral or intramuscular administration. Addition of methionine or betaine may benefit patients whose CSF abnormalities are not normalized by folate supplementation. Their administration may be the only available means to correct methionine levels in CNS and to prevent further neurological deterioration (Surtees 1998, Whitehead 2006).

RESPIRATORY CHAIN DISORDERS

The respiratory chain is the main biochemical system used to yield aerobic energy in all eukaryotic organisms. In humans, its dysfunction is responsible for numerous and highly variable mitochondrial diseases that all have in common the defective ATP production along with insufficient energy provision in one or several tissues or organs. This effect may vary from one tissue to another according to their dependence on phosphorylative oxidation. Muscle tissue in general is particularly sensitive to diminished ATP supply, resulting in various symptoms such as ptosis, ophthalmoplegia, muscle weakness, exercise intolerance, and cardiomyopathy. The central nervous system is also highly susceptible, resulting in encephalopathy, sensorineural signs and peripheral neuropathies. Other tissues may also be affected depending on the extent and severity of the defect. Kidney, liver, pancreas and gastrointestinal tissues are the most often implicated organs. Clinically, mitochondrial disorders are extremely heterogeneous. They may affect a single organ or tissue but most often cause multisystemic disorders, among which syndromic conditions have been described for years (Zeviani and Di Donato 2004, DiMauro and Hirano 2005).

FUNCTIONAL ORGANIZATION OF THE RESPIRATORY CHAIN

The mitochondrial respiratory chain (RC) is a group of five enzyme complexes embedded in the inner mitochondrial membrane. Each complex is composed of multiple polypeptide subunits and prosthetic groups (Table 8.9). In addition, the RC contains two electron carriers, coenzyme Q10 and cytochrome c. The RC is especially organized to accept electrons from the NADH and $FADH_2$, the reducing factors generated from the intermediary metabolism (Fig. 8.25). These electrons flow down the RC to molecular oxygen to produce water. Simultaneously, the energy liberated during this flux is used by complexes I, III and IV to pump protons (H^+) out of the mitochondrial matrix into the intermembrane space. Complex V allows protons to flow back into the mitochondrial matrix and uses the released energy to synthesize ATP from ADP and inorganic phosphate (Chinnery and Schon 2003, DiMauro and Schon 2003).

TABLE 8.9
Composition and genetic control of the mitochondrial respiratory chain

Respiratory chain complex	Polypeptide subunits and prosthetic groups*	Number of mt-DNA encoded subunits
NADH coenzyme Q reductase (complex I)	42 8 iron-sulfur proteins FMN	7 (ND 1, 2, 3, 4, 4L, 5, 6)
Succinate coenzyme Q (complex II)	4–5 Few iron-sulfur proteins FAD	0
Ubiquinol cytochrome c (cyt-c) reductase (complex III)	11 (cyt-b, cyt-c1) 2 iron-sulfur proteins	1 (cyt-b)
Cyt-c reductase (complex IV)	13 (cyt-a, cyt-a3)	3 (CoI, II, III)
ATP synthase (complex V)	12–14 (adenine)	2 (ATP 6, 8)

*FMN = flavine mononucleotide; FAD = flavine adenine nucleotide.

GENETIC BACKGROUND

The approximately 90 protein subunits that constitute the five complexes are under a unique dual genetic control with proteins encoded by either the nuclear DNA (nDNA) or the mitochondrial DNA (mtDNA) with the exception of complex II, which is entirely derived from nDNA. Human mtDNA contains the genes for 13 OXPHOS (aka respiratory chain, electron transport chain) subunits, as well as for the 22 transfer RNAs (tRNAs) and the two ribosomal RNAs (rRNAs) required for the intra-mitochondrial synthesis. The remaining structural proteins are encoded by nDNA. nDNA also encodes hundreds of additional factors required for subunit protein expression, transport and assembly as well as for mtDNA synthesis, expression and stabilization. In addition, mitochondria are not static organelles and other nuclear encoded factors govern their mobility, fission and fusion. In total, it is estimated that respiratory chain functions require about 1000 separate proteins, mostly encoded by nDNA, with mutations potentially responsible for mendelian inherited diseases.

In consequence, mitochondrial diseases may be caused by mutations in genes from either mtDNA or nDNA. However, clinically indistinguishable disorders may be caused by separate mutations in different genes on different genomes. Conversely, one specific mutation may result in a number of distinct clinical symptoms in different individuals.

MUTATIONS IN mtDNA

These include point mutations and large-scale rearrangements. Point mutations were first described in genes encoding various tRNAs resulting in wide spread impairment of protein synthesis. They usually are heteroplasmic, maternally inherited and associated with a striking variety of multisystem disorders. Disease-causing point mutations in the 12S rRNA gene have been described.

Point mutations in protein-coding genes affect one of the mitochondrial encoded subunits in complex I (ND), complex III (Cytb), complex IV (COX) or complex V (ATPase6). The affected patients tend to suffer a muscle-specific disorder rather than a multisystem disorder and have no maternal inheritance. However,

ND5, which encodes the subunit 5 of complex I, is the site of numerous point mutations associated with various multisystem disorders.

Large-scale rearrangements consist of a unique deletion/duplication in mtDNA. They differ in size from one patient to another but always delete several protein-coding and t-RNA genes. They tend to arise spontaneously and are heteroplasmic. However, some cases may be maternally inherited with variable phenotypic expression between the affected female and her offspring.

MUTATIONS IN NUCLEAR GENES

These include mutations in genes that encode complex subunits, ancillary proteins, protein factors required for intergenomic signalling, and protein factors necessary for membrane maintenance and for mobility of mitochondrion. These mutations are responsible for mendelian autosomal recessive, dominant or X-linked inherited diseases.

Mutations in genes encoding RC subunits are increasingly recognized. Various mutations in genes encoding subunits of complex I (NDUFS and NDUFV) and complex II (SDHA) are mainly responsible for Leigh or Leigh-like syndromes. Mutations in genes (APTX, PDSS2, COQ2) encoding enzymes implicated in the biosynthetic pathway of CoQ10 have been identified (Lopez et al. 2006).

The only known nuclear gene (BCS1L) involved in complex III deficiency codes for an ancillary protein required for the subunits' assembly. Mutations are responsible for an early and severe multisystem disorder first described in Turkish patients and also called GRACILE syndrome (growth retardation, aminoaciduria, cholestasis, iron overload, lactic acidosis and early death) in Finland, where it has a high incidence. Mutations in the COX-assembly gene SURF1 are frequently associated with Leigh syndrome due to complex IV deficiency. Other mutations in four more COX-assembly genes (SCO1, SCO2, COX10, COX15) have been described in patients affected with Leigh-like encephalopathy and other visceral involvement. A distinct form

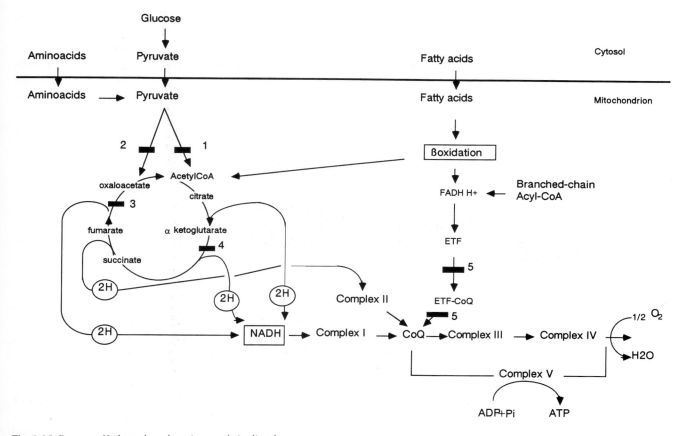

Fig. 8.25. Pyruvate, Krebs cycle and respiratory chain disorders.

Key: 1 = pyruvate dehydrogenase; 2 = pyruvate carboxylase; 3 = fumarase; 4 = α-ketoglutarate dehydrogenase; 5 = electron transfer factor (ETF) and ETF-CoQ dehydrogenase.

of COX-deficient Leigh syndrome due to mutations in the *LRPPRC* gene has been described in French Canadian families. Patients with muscle COX deficiency and ethylmalonic aciduria have mutations in the *ETHE1* gene. Finally, mutations in the *ATP12* gene impair the assembly of complex V and are responsible for a lethal encephalomyopathy.

MUTATIONS IN GENES ENCODING FACTORS FOR INTERGENOMIC SIGNALLING

These mendelian disorders with qualitative (deletions) or quantitative (depletion) alterations in mtDNA result from an imbalanced supply of deoxyribonucleotides to the mitochondrion (Alberio et al. 2007). Five genes have so far been implicated in the pathogenesis of mitochondrial depletion syndromes (MDS) namely, the thymidine kinase (*TK2*) gene in myopathic forms, the β-subunit of the ADP-forming succinyl-CoA synthetase (*SUCLA2*) in encephalomyopathic MDS, and deoxyguanosine kinase (*DGUOK*), the catalytic subunit of mtDNA polymerase (*POLG*) and *MPV17* in hepatocerebral MDS.

Four genes have so far been described in disorders with multiple deletions or depletion. Mutations in the polymerase portion of *POLG* are implicated in a heterogeneous group of syndromes (Horvath et al. 2006). They are the most common cause of dominant and recessive PEO. They are also associated with a large

variety of clinical features, among which is Alpers syndrome, a disorder of childhood characterized by liver insufficiency and grey matter disorder (Gordon 2006), SANDO (sensory ataxic neuropathy, dysarthria, ophthalmoplegia), deafness, hypogonadism, seizures, myoclonus, gastrointestinal dysmobility resembling MNGIE (mitochondrial neurogastrointestinal encephalomyopathy), and importantly, parkinsonism. The gene responsible for MNGIE encodes the enzyme thymidine phosphorylase (*TP*) (Hirano et al. 2005) and numerous mutations have already been described. Two others genes are responsible for autosomal dominant PEO and multiple DNA deletions in muscle, namely, *ANT1*, encoding an isoform of the adenine nucleotide transporter (Sharer 2005), and *twinkle*, encoding a mitochondrial helicase.

Mutations in additional nuclear genes are responsible for defective mitochondrial protein synthesis. *EFG1*, encoding an elongation factor, and *MRPS16*, encoding a mitochondrial ribosomal subunit, are linked to early hepatocerebral syndrome. *PUS1*, which encodes the mitochondrial enzyme pseudouridine synthetase is associated with myopathy, lactic acidosis and sideroblastic anaemia (MLASA) (Bykhovskaya et al. 2004).

At least some proteins are necessary for what we could call the 'maintenance' of the mitochondrion. Among these incompletely known aspects of mitochondrial dysfunctions is the Barth syndrome (X-linked mitochondrial myopathy, cardiomyopathy, neutropenia, and 3-methyl glutaconic aciduria) with low cardio-lipin levels due to mutations in the *tafazzin* gene. Cardiolipin, a major phospholipid component of the mitochondrial inner membrane, modulates the activities of several RC complexes. Defects in proteins required for mitochondrial mobility have been described in autosomal dominant hereditary spastic paraplegia with mutations in one kinesin gene (*KIFA*). Defects in proteins (dynamin) required for mitochondrial fusion have been reported in autosomal dominant optic atrophy (*OPA-1*) and in an autosomal dominant variant of Charcot–Marie–Tooth type 2A with defect in mitofussin 2 (*MNF2*).

Despite this increasing list and knowledge, it must be underlined that molecular investigations still fail to identify the responsible genetic defects in 80–90% of paediatric patients who on the clinical, biological and morphological evidence are obviously affected by RC disorders.

BIOLOGICAL FEATURES AND DIAGNOSTIC TESTS

In paediatric patients, the majority (90%) of proven RC defects present with raised lactate in blood, urine or CSF, often accompanied by a raised lactate to pyruvate ratio signifying a change in cellular redox state. Cerebral MR spectroscopy is a noninvasive and useful means to evaluate lactate accumulation in brain. In addition, it allows an easy diagnosis of the rare complex II deficiency by the presence of an abnormal peak of succinate (Lin et al. 2003, Brockmann et al. 2005). Some patients do not display lactic acidosis at rest, depending on the severity of the energy defect, the organ involvement, and the consequence of the primary defect on the oxidation rate. In some cases, lactic acidosis can spontaneously be precipitated by infection or functionally provoked by a glucose loading test. Those patients mostly affected with exercise intolerance may develop a severe hyperlactacidaemia after non-strenuous exercise. However, lactic acidosis is not an absolute requisite for diagnosis, especially in late childhood or adolescence. Apart from the usual lactaturia, rare patients have abnormal urinary excretion of Krebs-cycle intermediates such as fumarate, malate, alpha-ketoglutarate, succinate or 3-methyl-glutaconic acid. Mild methylmalonic aciduria has been found associated with a *SUCLA2* gene mutation responsible for mtDNA depletion (Carrozzo et al. 2007, Ostergaard et al. 2007). Ethylmalonic aciduria is indicative of ethylmalonic encephalopathy, a condition harbouring marked complex IV deficiency in muscle. High levels of thymidine, deoxyuridine and uracil in blood and urine are indicative of MNGIE with thymidine phosphorylase deficiency. Carnitine deficiency in serum and muscle may reflect inefficient fatty acid oxidation. Serum creatine kinase values, usually moderately elevated, can be high in myopathic forms of mtDNA depletion syndrome (MDS).

MR spectroscopy may be useful in children over 8 years of age, adolescents and adults. Measurement of the phosphocreatine/inorganic phosphorus ratio indicates ATP-synthesis defect during muscle exercise.

In patients with a clearly defined clinical syndrome it may be possible to confirm the diagnosis with a simple molecular genetic test carried out on DNA extracted from blood. Good examples of this are MNGIE (*TP*), the infantile encephalohepatopathy (*DGUOK*) and infantile encephalotubulopathy (*BCS1L*). Investigation in the remaining patients is more difficult, especially because pathogenic mutations may not be detectable in blood. If mitochondrial disease is suspected, muscle biopsy should be performed (Chinnery and Schon 2003).

A histochemical examination using Gomori, cytochrome *c* oxidase and succinate dehydrogenase (SDH) stains that revealed mitochondrial proliferation and mosaicism would be suggestive of mtDNA mutations and complex II or IV deficiencies.

Biochemical investigations include two main, and non-exclusive, procedures using mitochondria-enriched fraction from fresh tissue for polarographic studies or using frozen tissue for analysis of individual RC enzyme activities by spectrophotometry. For this purpose, skeletal muscle biopsy specimens are most often used. However, specific studies can be performed on fibroblasts, blood cells, liver, kidney or brain. In principle, the relevant tissue is the one that is clinically affected, i.e. investigation on a liver sample is recommended in hepatoencephalopathy. In case of dubious biochemical results while clinical level of suspicion is high, investigations in several tissues should be performed.

A structured approach to molecular investigations would start with a southern blot of muscle mtDNA looking for mtDNA rearrangement and a series of allele-specific assays looking for common point mutations. Further molecular screening, guided by the clinical phenotype, family history and results of biochemistry would help to define an increasing number of pathologies allowing proper genetic counselling (Chinnery and Schon 2003, DiMauro et al. 2004b). The major challenge to the accurate diagnosis of mitochondrial disease is the absence of a definitive biomarker that characterizes the disorder in all patients. To aid the interpretation, diagnostic schemes for infants and children have been established to categorize the likelihood of mitochondrial disease in a given patient as definite, probable, possible or unlikely (Bernier et al. 2002, Wolf and Smeitink 2002).

CLINICAL FEATURES

Due to the complexity of mitochondrial genetics and biochemistry, the clinical manifestations of these disorders are extremely heterogeneous. They range from lesions in a single tissue or organ such as the optic nerve in Leber's hereditary optic neuropathy, to more widespread lesions including myopathies, encephalomyopathies, cardiomyopathies or complex multisystem syndromes with onset ranging from the neonatal period to adulthood. Certain associations have long been identified as distinct entities such as Kearns–Sayre syndrome, MELAS, MERFF, NARP, Leigh syndrome and Alpers disease. However, not all patients with RC disorders may be so easily categorized, and many overlaps between categories have been documented. Consequently, RC disorder must be considered in patients presenting with an unexplained and progressive association of neuromuscular and non-neuromuscular symptoms (DiMauro and Schon 2003, Zeviani and Di Donato 2004, Robinson 2006).

MYOPATHIC FORMS

Myopathic forms are characterized by progressive weakness of the limbs with variable exercise intolerance, muscle pain, breathlessness, tiredness and nausea. Symptoms may appear within the first 2 years of life, with hypotonia and delayed motor skills, or later in childhood, adolescence or adulthood. Patients can die from early cardiorespiratory failure or remain stable for years. Lactataemia at rest can be normal or mildly increased. Short aerobic exercises can provoke severe lactic acidosis. Except in very young children, morphological and histochemical abnormalities in biopsied muscle are often characteristic. These isolated myopathic forms are associated with mtDNA point mutations in genes encoding subunits of complexes I, III (cytochrome *b*) or IV. Defect due to mutations in the cytochrome *b* gene is probably the most characteristic example as it mainly presents with isolated and progressive myopathy and exercise intolerance. Rare infantile or juvenile cases present with a predominant involvement of muscle, eventually associated with other organ involvement due to mutations in tRNA genes or with mitochondrial depletion (Alberio et al. 2007).

Primary CoQ10 deficiency, an autosomal recessive condition with a large clinical spectrum, has a pure juvenile myopathic form with exercise intolerance and eventually myoglobinuria. Other presentations are: (1) encephalomyopathy with brain involvement and recurrent myoglobinuria; (2) severe infantile multisystemic disease; (3) cerebellar ataxia; (4) Leigh syndrome with ataxia and deafness. These patients with ragged red fibres and undetectable CoQ10 in tissues are amenable to treatment with high doses of exogenous CoQ10. Mutation on the *COQ2* gene has been demonstrated in the infantile multisystemic form. It encodes the first enzyme required for CoQ10 biosynthetis (Quinzii et al. 2007).

The myopathic presentations of cytochrome *c* oxidase (complex IV) deficiency include three main variants: a fatal infantile myopathy, a benign reversible infantile myopathy, and a late-onset (adult) myopathy. Both fatal and benign forms present in newborns with severe and generalized weakness, respiratory distress and lactic acidosis. Patients with the fatal form usually die of respiratory failure within months. However, we have seen examples of survivors who at 7 years of age are still disabled by exercise intolerance but have normal cognitive development and educational course. Conversely, patients with the benign form improve spontaneously despite initial severe weakness, and are usually normal by early childhood. Some severe forms mimicking spinal muscular atrophy have been described with mutations in the nuclear-encoded *SCO2* gene, with the mitochondrial-encoded *COX1* gene, and with mtDNA depletion due to mutations in the nuclear gene encoding thymidine kinase 2 (*TK2*).

MULTISYSTEM DISORDERS

These involve mainly the CNS and present in the neonatal period or later in childhood, adolescence or even in adulthood.

FATAL INFANTILE FORM

This features neonatal lactic acidosis with hypotonia, seizures and respiratory distress, and results in death within a few months. As in complex IV deficiency, renal, cardiac and hepatic involvement may be seen. Severe hyperlactataemia is present, while morphological studies of muscle can be normal or reveal a nonspecific lipid–glycogen storage. CT and MRI may show cortical and subcortical atrophy and dysmyelination. This syndrome is frequently, but not exclusively, associated with complex I and complex IV deficiencies.

PROGRESSIVE ENCEPHALOPATHY/ENCEPHALOMYOPATHY

Severe encephalopathy may start later in infancy or childhood after a period of apparently normal development. Such 'undefined' types can feature various proportions of the following manifestations: developmental delay, hypotonia, weakness, ataxia, pyramidal signs, seizures, myoclonia, retinopathy, ptosis, PEO, sensorineural deafness, mild dysmorphism and growth retardation. Plasma lactate levels are mildly elevated or normal. In such cases, high CSF lactate and lactaturia are of great diagnostic value. Some patients present with bouts of drowsiness following intercurrent infections during which high plasma lactate levels and redox ratios may be found. Ragged red fibres are frequently associated with lipid–glycogen storage. CT and MRI may be normal or reveal cerebral and/or cerebellar atrophy and bilateral hyperdensity in the basal ganglia or white matter. Altered EMG, nerve conduction velocities and visual or brainstem evoked potentials can be found. Cases have been described with defects in all RC complexes due to various point mutations in either the mt- or nDNA. Specific associated neurological signs such as polymicrogyria, or associated visceral signs such as cardiomyopathy, nephropathy or hepatopathy may be helpful to lead to the diagnosis.

SUBACUTE NECROTIZING ENCEPHALOPATHY: LEIGH SYNDROME (LS)

LS is an inherited, progressive, metabolic disease of infancy and childhood. It causes striking neuropathological features of focal, bilateral and symmetrical necrotic lesions associated with demyelination, vascular proliferation, and gliosis in the brainstem, diencephalons, basal ganglia, cerebellum, and occasionally in the white matter (Farina et al. 2002). No clear boundaries seem to exist between LS and some of the 'undefined' encephalomyopathies.

The *neuropathological changes* involve most consistently the brainstem in a bilateral, roughly symmetrical distribution. The lesions are sharply delineated and cut across grey and white matter with preponderance in the former. The pathological complex of LS consists of a marked spongiosis involving mainly the neuropil, while neurons are relatively preserved. White matter lesions include loss of myelin and, eventually, of axons. An intense capillary proliferation with endothelial swelling is an essential feature (Fig. 8.26). The lesions are typically ischaemic in type but do not correspond to any vascular territory (Cavanagh and Harding 1994). Lesions of this type characteristically affect the tegmentum of midbrain and pons, the periaqueductal grey matter, the substantia nigra and posterior colliculi, the floor of

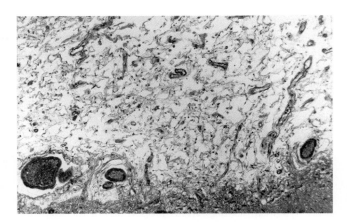

Fig. 8.26. Leigh syndrome. Typical histological appearance of tissues: note sharply demarcated area of marked spongiosis with intense capillary proliferation.

the fourth ventricle, and the dentate nuclei. Lesions of the basal ganglia, especially the putamen and caudate nucleus, are common. Cortical lesions are only uncommonly severe. Extensive leukoencephalopathy is found in rare cases (Bourgeois et al. 1992, Zafeiriou et al. 1995). The mamillary bodies are only rarely affected, which is important for distinguishing the condition from Wernicke disease in which similar lesions are present but regularly involve these structures.

The *clinical manifestations* are extremely variable, and the diagnosis is very difficult as no biochemical markers are available in a majority of cases. Some common features such as deterioration with slow recovery following infections, exercise intolerance, poor somatic growth and abrupt changes in respiratory or cardiac rate may suggest the diagnosis of mitochondrial disorder.

In the *infantile form*, signs usually appear within the first few years of life and consist of hypotonia, failure to thrive, psychomotor regression, pyramidal tract signs, and brainstem and basal ganglia dysfunction. This basal ganglia involvement results in ataxia, abnormal ocular movements such as ptosis or ophthalmoplegia, dystonia or rigidity, and swallowing difficulties. Movement disorders including choreoathetosis, dystonia and sometimes myoclonus are not infrequent. Episodes of stupor or of apnoea not related to the stupor state may supervene. Involvement of the peripheral nervous system is not rare (Jacobs et al. 1990). In a few cases, it may be the predominant manifestation and may simulate Guillain–Barré syndrome. Seizures occur in some patients and may present as infantile spasms. As a whole, the course is often rapidly progressive with alternating periods of remissions and exacerbations. These are often precipitated by infections or fasting. Acute fulminating cases, protracted forms with prolonged periods of stabilization, and cases with very slow progression have all been recorded.

Later forms are less commonly encountered but may occur throughout childhood and adolescence and well into adulthood. Predominant extrapyramidal manifestations such as dystonia or abnormal movements, hypokinesia and rigidity could be predominant signs. In some cases, mild psychomotor retardation

with slight neurological abnormalities may remain unchanged for years until rapid deterioration occurs, sometimes only in adulthood.

Although initial observations suggested an autosomal recessive inheritance, later reports of autosomal dominant, X-linked and maternally inherited cases have been reported indicating that causative genes exist in both the nuclear and the mitochondrial genome. This genetic heterogeneity has been confirmed with the identification of functional or molecular defects in several enzymes involved in the energy production, including pyruvate dehydrogenase, pyruvate carboxylase and RC complexes. As already described for unidentified encephalomyopathy, some specific clinical, biochemical or genetic features may be associated and lead to the final diagnosis.

In infancy, defects in each RC complex may present as LS. This presentation is the most common expression of isolated and profound COX deficiency. Associated with peripheral neuropathy, it is mainly due to mutations in the nuclear *SURF1* gene. LS is also a usual presentation of complex I deficiency secondary to mutations either in nuclear or in mitochondrial encoded subunits. Associated with hypertrophic cardiomyopathy it can indicate defect in the nuclear encoded subunits (*NDFS2*, *NDFS4*, *NDFS7* and *NDFS8*). Defect in complex II due to mutations in the *SDHA* gene is responsible for LS with a peculiar involvement of the white matter and a recognizable peak of succinate on brain MR spectroscopy (Brockmann et al. 2005). Mutation in *BCS1L*, an assembly gene for complex III, presents in early infancy with a specific combination of LS, liver insufficiency and tubulopathy, while deletion in subunit VII (*UQCRB*) caused lactic acidosis with hypoglycaemia. Mutations in mitochondrial *ATP6* gene producing complex V deficiency are responsible for either a maternally inherited LS when present at high heteroplasmy or neurogenic weakness, ataxia and retinitis pigmentosa (NARP syndrome) at low titres. In addition, early-onset LS can be associated with mitochondrial depletion syndromes such as *SUCLA2* and *POLG* where there is an associated hepatopathy.

Typical abnormalities visualized on CT and MRI are essential for the in vivo diagnosis of LS as they may be more characteristic than the combination of appropriate clinical features, lactic acidosis. Lesions are visible and hyperintense on proton density and T_2-weighted images, whereas they are hypointense, and usually less evident, on T_1-weighted images. Lesions are mainly found in the brainstem where they affect various structures of the medulla oblongata, the pons and the midbrain. Involvement of the cerebellum is frequent, mainly centred on the dentate nuclei with extension to the surrounding white matter. Basal ganglia, thalami and subthalamic nuclei are a third site (Fig. 8.27). Extensive lesions in the profound cerebral white matter and progressive cerebral atrophy or infarction may be additional features. There is no clear correlation between a specific enzymatic defect and the radiological patterns. This phenomenon is partly explained by the evolutivity of the CNS lesions and by the fact that a defect in a given complex may be due to different molecular alterations with varying consequences. However, a peculiar association of severe involvement of the brainstem and subthalamic lesions has

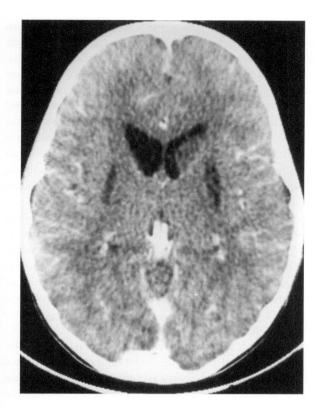

Fig. 8.27. Leigh necrotizing encephalomyelopathy. Cavitation of both lenticular nuclei. Head of left caudate nucleus is hypodense. There is marked atrophy of head of right caudate nucleus with widening of corresponding frontal horn.

been described in LS with COX deficiency due to *SURF1* mutations (Valanne et al. 1998, Arii and Tanabe 2000, Farina et al. 2002).

KEARNS–SAYRE SYNDROME (KSS)

KSS is usually a sporadic multisystemic disorder characterized by an invariant triad comprising onset before age 20 years, progressive external ophthalmoplegia (PEO) and pigmentary retinal degeneration, plus at least one of the following: heart block, elevated CSF protein content and cerebellar dysfunction (Zeviani and Di Donato 2004). Still other clinical abnormalities are present in many cases, and two constant pathological features have been described: ragged red fibres and spongy degeneration of the brain. The signs and symptoms may progress in various sequences.

Children with KSS usually have normal early development. In childhood, some patients may display episodes of aseptic meningitis. Ptosis and PEO are usually the first neurological manifestation of the disease, often associated with degenerative pigmentary retinopathy and sometimes with optic atrophy. The most common neurological feature is a cerebellar syndrome that may become severe. Mental retardation or regression may be present. Seizures do not occur, unless there is concomitant hypocalcaemia with hypoparathyroidism. Mild pyramidal signs, myopathy or peripheral neuropathy are not prominent. Heart block is a late sign that may be responsible for syncopal episodes

or sudden death despite pacemaker insertion. Rarely, congestive heart failure and supraventricular tachycardia are encountered. Associated endocrine disorders may include short stature with growth hormone defect, latent diabetes and hypoparathyroidism. Renal dysfunction often includes a proximal tubular defect, distal tubulopathy, glomerulopathy, and renal failure. Mild lactic acidosis and high CSF protein are typical laboratory findings.

Neuroimaging shows both grey and white matter lesions, most often localized in the brainstem tegmentum, cerebral and cerebellar white matter, and basal ganglia. Calcifications in the basal ganglia or deep white matter are commonly seen. Involvement of the subcortical U fibres with relative sparing of the periventricular white matter is typical of KSS. However, these classical lesions develop progressively with age, and MRI can be normal in early stages of the disease (Valanne et al. 1998). An extinguished ERG and abnormal visual evoked potentials may precede ophthalmoscopic evidence of retinopathy. EMG and nerve conduction velocity studies in some cases may indicate peripheral neuropathy or myopathic changes.

Histochemical and electron microscopic studies of skeletal muscle demonstrate ragged red fibres and altered mitochondria. Altered type I fibres lacking histochemical cytochrome *c* oxidase activity coexist with normal fibres. Eighty per cent of patients with KSS have a single deletion in mtDNA. However, KSS without deletion has been demonstrated, and not all patients with deleted mtDNA have KSS. Most often the KSS cases are sporadic, and only a few patients have a maternally inherited form of the disease.

Pearson syndrome, which can evolve into KSS with age, is characterized by connatal sideroblastic anaemia, and less frequently, severe exocrine pancreatic dysfunction. This syndrome represents an early and often fatal expression of KSS with similar large-scale single deletions/duplications of mtDNA.

PROGRESSIVE EXTERNAL OPHTHALMOPLEGIA (PEO)

PEO is a clinically and genetically heterogeneous condition associated with single or multiple mtDNA deletions and sporadic, autosomal dominant or autosomal recessive inheritance. Classically, the first signs arise in adulthood, with a few cases arising in adolescence or in early adulthood. Ophthalmoplegia, ptosis and muscle weakness with exercise intolerance are the main signs. Sensory motor neuropathy, sensorineural hearing loss, cataracts and cerebellar involvement are other progressive symptoms. Cognitive deterioration with psychiatric manifestations may develop. Similarly to KSS, single deletions/duplications in mtDNA are responsible for lactic acidosis, ragged red fibres and mosaic pattern of defective cytochrome *c* oxidase on muscle histochemical investigations. These KSS-related cases are most often sporadic.

Autosomal dominant forms of PEO (adPEO) are mainly caused by mutations in three nuclear genes: *POLG1*, *twinkle* and *ANT1*. They are associated with ragged red fibres in skeletal muscle and multiple deletions of mtDNA. The typical clinical features of adPEO are progressive muscle weakness, most severely affecting the external eye muscles. Ataxia, depression, hypogonadism, hearing loss, peripheral neuropathy and cataract are various other signs. Other sporadic or recessively transmitted PEO cases can be linked with *POLG* mutations (Zeviani and Di Donato 2004, Sharer 2005).

MYOCLONIC EPILEPSY WITH RAGGED RED FIBRES (MERRF)

MERRF is a maternally inherited encephalomyopathy, characterized by myoclonus, cerebellar ataxia and mitochondrial myopathy. Seizures, hearing loss, dementia, peripheral neuropathy and multiple symmetric lipomas are frequently associated (Zeviani and Di Donato 2004).

In most cases, symptoms begin between the ages of 5 and 13 years with a cerebellar ataxia, tremor and myoclonic jerks induced by action or intended movement. Many patients have generalized or massive myoclonic seizures and some become demented. Hearing loss, optic atrophy and proprioceptive sensory loss may occur. PEO, retinal degeneration or stroke-like episodes are not present. The severity of symptoms along a maternal lineage varies greatly from severe to mild manifestations, sometimes with only abnormal visual evoked response and EEG pattern. CSF and serum lactate levels may be slightly increased. Endocrine disorders may occur.

The EEG records abnormal background activity, variously associated with spike–wave patterns and a photoparoxysmal response. Visual, auditory and somatosensory evoked response studies may show abnormal latencies, while EMG shows myopathic changes. CT and MRI may indicate cerebral and cerebellar atrophy. At post-mortem examination, degeneration of the cerebral hemispheres, cerebellar dentate nuclei, posterior spinal column and spinocerebellar tracts has been found.

COX-depleted ragged red fibres and ultrastructurally abnormal mitochondria in biopsied muscle are constant and may be the only sign in asymptomatic individuals within a family. The typical mitochondrial DNA mutation is A8344G in the *tRNA^{lys}* gene. Other mutations in the same gene have been reported in association with MERRF, MERRF/MELAS overlap syndrome and other complex phenotypes.

MITOCHONDRIAL MYOPATHY, ENCEPHALOPATHY, LACTIC ACIDOSIS AND STROKE-LIKE EPISODES (MELAS)

MELAS generally presents in children or young adults after normal early development. Symptoms include recurrent vomiting, migraine-like headache, and recurrent stroke-like episodes causing cortical blindness, hemiparesis or hemianopsia. Seizures are often preceded by strokes or episodes of migraine with aura and are invariably partial motor in type. Intellectual regression and behavioural problems are prominent. The myopathy is usually asymptomatic or expressed as muscular weakness and mild amyotrophy. Additional features include short stature, diabetes mellitus, sensorineural hearing loss, mild retinal degeneration and cardiac involvement. Lactate levels in plasma and CSF are usually high, and creatine kinase is inconsistently increased. The CSF protein content is normal.

The EEG is usually abnormal, with occasional spike and wave or focal spike discharges. Neuroimaging shows focal lucencies or increased T_2 signal, generally not in a vascular distribution, affecting various sites of the white matter, cortex or brainstem, and areas of calcification or high T_2 signal in the basal ganglia. Cerebral and cerebellar atrophy may be associated. Focal necrosis and laminar cortical necrotic changes are the histopathological signs of the disease, together with neuronal degeneration and mineral deposits within the basal ganglia. The pathogenesis of the infarct-like lesions is presumably due to a mitochondrial microangiopathy with deficient energy metabolism in the endothelium of small pial arterioles and capillaries (Valanne et al. 1998). Ragged red fibres, lipid droplets and abnormal mitochondria are present in muscles.

The most common mtDNA mutation is A3243G in the *tRNA^{leu(UUR)}* gene. However, many other mutations are associated with MELAS. Conversely, this A3243G mutation has been detected in patients with maternally inherited PEO or diabetes mellitus and deafness, and isolated myopathy or cardiomyopathy.

ALPERS DISEASE

Alpers–Huttenlocher syndrome (AHS), an autosomal recessive hepatocerebral syndrome of early onset, is a degenerative disease that primarily affects the cerebral grey matter. The typical course of AHS includes severe developmental delay, intractable seizures, cortical blindness, progressive liver dysfunction and acute liver failure after exposure to valproic acid, and death in childhood. Biochemically, it has been associated with deficiencies of pyruvate carboxylase, pyruvate dehydrogenase and respiratory chain compounds. Most importantly, AHS is one clinical phenotype associated with mitochondrial depletion syndrome due to *POLG1* mutations resulting in mtDNA depletion and multiple RC defects in all affected tissues (Gordon 2006, Horvath et al. 2006). The clinical manifestations are considered in Chapter 9. Seizures and EEG abnormalities are much more prominent than in Leigh syndrome, which is a reflection of the extensive involvement of cortical grey matter. Variable visceral involvement may be associated.

MITOCHONDRIAL NEUROGASTROINTESTINAL ENCEPHALOMYOPATHY (MNGIE)

MNGIE is an autosomal recessive disease clinically defined by gastrointestinal dysmotility, cachexia, ptosis, ophthalmoparesis, peripheral neuropathy and white matter changes in brain MRI.

This devastating disorder is linked to nuclear mutations in the thymidine phosphrylase gene. They induce pathological accumulation of thymidine and deoxyuridine, and imbalance of the mitochondrial pool impairing mtDNA replication and/or maintenance, with depletion, multiple deletions and point mutations (Nishino et al. 2001).

MNGIE usually manifests in late adolescence with gastrointestinal dysmotility characterized by dysphagia, gastroparesis and recurrent vomiting that lead to cachexia. These signs could be due to a visceral myopathy especially affecting the external layer of muscularis propria (Giordano et al. 2006). Neurological impairments comprise ptosis and ophthalmoparesis, with late onset and progressive axonal and demyelinating sensorimotor poly-neuropathy. Cognitive impairment is typically absent. Lactic acidosis is usually mild, and protein level in CSF is increased in most patients. T_2-weighted and FLAIR MRI brain sequences show large confluent hyperintense signal changes indicating leukoencephalopathy. They are mainly localized in the periventricular areas, and may affect the cerebral peduncles, brainstem and pons.

TREATMENT
No satisfactory therapy is presently available for RC deficiency. Treatment remains largely supportive and does not alter the course of the disease.

Among the symptomatic therapies, seizures should not be treated with valproate, which inhibits the respiratory chain.

Primary deficiency of CoQ10 can be treated with large doses of ubidecarenone with notable improvement of the clinical course. However, it may not be sufficient to prevent neurological deterioration (Auré et al. 2004).

In MNGIE, several attempts to restore normal levels of thymidine are being pursued by dialysis, platelet transfusions and even bone marrow transplantation.

Beside these few specific aspects, various 'cocktails' of vitamins and cofactors are used including CoQ10, phylloquinone or menadione in conjunction with ascorbate, succinate, thiamine and riboflavin. Pharmaceutical therapy with dichloroacetate to treat lactic acidosis does not improve clinical outcome (Stacpoole et al. 2006). Creatine supplementation to allow storage of phosphocreatine (an energy compound) has variable effects (DiMauro et al. 2004a).

PYRUVATE DEHYDROGENASE DEFICIENCY

Pyruvate dehydrogenase complex (PDHc) deficiency is an important cause of encephalopathy associated with lactic acidosis. The clinical symptoms vary considerably ranging from early lactic acidosis to intermittent ataxia, Leigh syndrome and progressive neurodegenerative disease with mental retardation (Berendzen et al. 2006, Debray et al. 2006, De Meirleir et al. 2006).

BIOCHEMICAL AND GENETIC BACKGROUND
PDHc controls the entry of pyruvate, the glycolytic end-product, into mitochondria for oxidative metabolism and thus plays an important regulatory role in cellular energy metabolism in glycolytic-dependent organs such as the CNS. In the brain, PDHc is required for the formation of acetylcholine from acetyl-CoA. Thus PDHc defects are expected to involve the nervous system.

PDHc is a mitochondrial multienzyme complex comprising three catalytic enzymes (E1, E2, E3), two regulatory enzymes (PDH kinase and phosphatase), and three coenzymes (thiamine, lipoic acid, FADH2). Additionally, an E3 binding protein (E3BP) probably has a structural function. The E1 component is a hetero-tetramer of two alpha- and beta-subunits that share a thiamine pyrophosphate binding site. All components are encoded by nuclear genes located on autosome with the exception of the E1 alpha-subunit, which is located on chromosome Xp22.3.

The vast majority of patients have a defect in the E1 alpha-subunit with an X-linked transmission. Over 80 disease-causing mutations in the *PDHA1* gene have been identified. Most of the mutations originate de novo, and in 25% of cases the mother is a carrier. Males and females are equally affected with severely affected females not as common, depending on the X-inactivation pattern in different tissues, notably in the brain (Tulinius et al. 2005, Willemsen et al. 2006). There are more than 20 reported cases of E3 defect with a common mutation found particularly in Ashkenazi Jewish patients. About the same number of E3BP deficiency cases have been reported without prevalent mutations (Brown et al. 2006, Miné et al. 2006). Mutations in the genes for the defects in E1 beta-subunit, PDH-phosphatase and E2 component have been identified in a few patients (Head et al. 2005).

Genetic counselling is complex, and reliable antenatal diagnosis relies on molecular analyses in families whose molecular defect has been previously determined.

CLINICAL FEATURES
Male patients with PDHE1α deficiency present with an over-whelming lactic acidosis in the neonatal period or in infancy. Hypotonia and apnoeic spells are the most frequent features. Most patients die within the first few months of life after a clinical course marked by failure to thrive, developmental delay, hypotonia, respiratory difficulties and seizures. In some patients congenital brain malformations are present. Partial hypoplastic or thin corpus callosum, asymmetrical dilatation of ventricles and migrational defects are associated with null mutations. Rare females may have a similar early-onset form (Otero et al. 1995).

A second type of presentation includes *Leigh syndrome* or a progressive neurodegenerative disorder that affects both male and female patients. Symptoms occur after an apparently uneventful period of a few months. Seizures or episodes of weakness, respiratory failure, ataxia or dystonic posturing are the first manifestations. Later, these episodes may recur, and variable degrees of progressive neurological impairment and developmental delay are seen. Optic atrophy, ptosis, ophthalmoplegia and retinal degeneration have been mentioned. Atypical hypsarrhythmia or severe myoclonic seizures have been described in girls. Facial dysmorphism suggesting fetal alcohol syndrome has been described in patients with E1 deficiency. Many patients die within a few years but some survive with severe disability.

Finally, a small subset consists of patients who are clinically normal or have mild developmental delay and who experience intermittent neurological episodes of recurrent ataxia, acute dystonia, extrapyramidal movement disorders or muscle weakness with myopathy and/or peripheral neuropathy (Tulinius et al. 2005, Debray et al. 2006, Willemsen et al. 2006).

PDHE1α defects are the most frequent abnormality within these last two groups. However, the rare reported cases of PDHE2, PDHE3 and PDH phosphatase deficiencies can be associated with these clinical forms. E3BP deficiency may present in the neonatal period with lactic acidosis. However, most have survived well into childhood or even adulthood with variable impairment resembling the PDHE1α late-onset forms (Head et al. 2005, Brown et al. 2006, Schiff et al. 2006b).

In neonatal-onset forms, MRI studies have shown severe abnormalities including agenesis or dysgenesis of the corpus callosum, heterotopias and pachygyria, asymmetrical ventriculomegaly, periventricular and subependymal cysts, and hypomyelination (Otero et al. 1995). In late-onset forms, progressive lesions in basal ganglia and brainstem are common. High peak of lactate on brain MR spectroscopy is an indicative sign. Neuropathological findings confirm brain dysgenesis. Dysplasia and ectopia of the inferior olivary nuclei, dysplasia of dentate nuclei, absence or hypoplasia of the medullary pyramids, periventricular neuronal heterotopias and deficient myelination are other findings (Brismar and Ozand 1994a, Shevell et al. 1994, van der Knaap et al. 1996, Head et al. 2005).

BIOLOGICAL AND BIOCHEMICAL FEATURES

The most important laboratory tests for diagnosis are the measurement of lactate and pyruvate in blood and CSF. Both are usually elevated with a low to normal lactate to pyruvate ratio. These can be severe during the neonatal period or during episodes of deterioration, while in mildly affected patients abnormal lactate accumulation should be provoked by a glucose loading test (Benoist et al. 2003, Debray et al. 2007). A few patients are reported without lactate accumulation. In those PDHE2 cases, abnormal brain MRI with basal ganglia lesions has led to enzymatic evaluation (Head et al. 2005). Definite diagnosis is made by assay of PDHc activity and molecular investigations.

TREATMENT

Thiamine has been beneficial in a few patients (Pastoris et al. 1996). Dichloroacetate inhibits PDH kinase and is thereby effective to lower plasma lactate levels, although clinical improvement is not obvious (Berendzen et al. 2006, Stacpoole et al. 2006). A ketogenic diet by providing alternative energy fuel is probably the most effective therapeutic approach.

PYRUVATE CARBOXYLASE DEFICIENCY

This is a rare autosomal recessive disorder presenting with lactic acidosis and neurological involvement.

BIOCHEMICAL BACKGROUND

Pyruvate carboxylase (PC) is a biotin-containing enzyme that catalyses the first step of gluconeogenesis by converting pyruvate to oxaloacetate. PC also plays an anaplerotic role mainly in the brain and muscle by replenishing the tricarboxylic cycle. PC is an astrocytic-specific enzyme that allows neurotransmitter synthesis by supplying glutamine, and is a key factor for myelin synthesis by providing citrate (Brun et al. 1999). Pyruvate carboxylase activity is expressed in fibroblasts with various residual enzymatic activities without frank correlation with clinical phenotypes. The most severe form (French or B phenotype) is associated with

the absence of apoprotein on Western blot analysis, while in the milder form (North American or A phenotype) a detectable apoprotein is present. Various mutations in the *PC* gene have been found in both A and B phenotypes. Prenatal diagnosis is possible by measurement of PC activity in cultured amniocytes or in fresh chorionic villus samples, or by DNA analyses (De Meirleir et al. 2006).

CLINICAL FEATURES

Three different clinical presentations are described according to the severity of clinical and biochemical manifestations (De Meirleir et al. 2006, Garcia-Cazorla et al. 2006). The French phenotype is a neonatal-onset form with an overwhelming lactic acidosis. Patients present within the first hours of life with acute and relentless neurological deterioration and metabolic ketoacidosis. They have hypokinetic lethargy, axial hypotonia, large-amplitude tremors, seizures, and abnormal ocular movements such as nystagmus. Some patients have hepatic failure with persistent cytolysis and/or cholestasis. In addition, they may suffer a severe renal tubular acidosis with massive bicarbonaturia. Death in the first few months of age is the rule. Some rare patients may stabilize with symptomatic treatment and then develop moderate to severe developmental delay and spastic tetraparesis (Schiff et al. 2006a). Patients with the North American phenotype have a later onset with a progressive developmental delay, pyramidal signs, ataxia and nystagmus. In addition they suffer intermittent metabolic ketoacidosis exacerbated by intercurrent infections. They have longer survival. A third benign form has been described in rare patients with nearly normal development and who display intercurrent ketoacidosis that improve with symptomatic treatment.

The biochemical pattern in neonatal forms is notable for the presence of a secondary hyperammonaemia with citrullinaemia, and a very high lactate/pyruvate ratio contrasting with low beta-hydroxybutyrate/acetoacetate ratio. In CSF, lactate, lactate/pyruvate ratio, and alanine are increased and glutamine is decreased.

On neuroimaging reports, the most specific changes are ischaemic-like lesions with a diffuse white matter abnormality and periventricular cysts that are almost invariably haemorrhagic. Subdural, intraventricular and intracerebellar haemorrhages have also been reported. A similar description reported in two cases during the last trimester of pregnancy (Brun et al. 1999) underlines the prenatal severity and the irreversibility of brain involvement. In milder form leukodystrophy is the main sign. No basal ganglia lesions have been reported (Schiff et al. 2006a). CNS pathology has shown poor myelination involving cerebral and cerebellar white matter and sometimes the base of the pons, loss of neurons in the cerebral cortex, ventricular enlargement, thinning of the corpus callosum and proliferation of astrocytes (van der Knaap et al. 1996, Brun et al. 1999).

TREATMENT

Therapeutic trials have attempted to replenish the Krebs cycle using glutamate, aspartate, citrate and odd-numbered fatty acid (triheptanoine) supplementation, but all have failed to prevent neurological degradation (Ahmad et al. 1999, Mochel et al. 2005, Garcia-Cazorla et al. 2006).

DEFECTS OF THE KREBS CYCLE

These include fumarase, alpha-ketoglutarate dehydrogenase and lipoamide dehydrogenase deficiencies.

DIHYDROLIPOAMIDE DEHYDROGENASE (DLD) DEFICIENCY

DLD is a component of a number of mitochondrial multienzymes, including pyruvate dehydrogenase, alpha-ketoglutarate dehydrogenase and branched-chain alpha-ketoacid dehydrogenase (Cameron et al. 2006). The clinical phenotype of DLD deficiency may range from a severe neonatal disorder to less severe presentation in childhood. In infancy, patients present with intermittent ketoacidosis, neurological signs, microcephaly and Leigh syndrome resulting in mental retardation, ataxia, and hypotonia. A less severe form in childhood is characterized by episodic vomiting, ketoacidosis, liver dysfunction, hypotonia, and exercise intolerance between episodes in a few patients. Biologically, periods of decompensations are marked by hyperlactacidaemia accompanied by increased urinary excretion of alpha-ketoglutaric acid and, less constantly, by increased levels of branched-chain amino acids in plasma. Brain imaging investigations reveal various patterns from unspecific periventricular white matter lesions to signs of Leigh syndrome with involvement of basal ganglia. Mutations in the *DLD* gene have been reported, with a common mutation (229G>C in exon 9) in patients from Ashkenazi Jewish ancestry.

FUMARASE DEFICIENCY

Fumarase deficiency has been reported in a few children with severe neurological impairment (Kerrigan et al. 2000). The clinical phenotype is characterized in infancy by severe developmental delay with hypotonia, seizures, facial dysmorphism, growth failure, relative macrocephaly, and death in the first years of life. Hyperlactacidaemia can be mild, but urinary excretion of fumaric acid is diagnostic. On brain MRI, lesions can be severe with ventriculomegaly, polymicrogyria, agenesis of the corpus callosum, decreased white matter volume and relative hypoplasia of the brainstem. Autopsy in a case has revealed hypomyelination and heterotopia located in cerebellum, occipital and parietal areas (Gellera et al. 1990). The defect involves both cytosol and mitochondrial isoforms and appears to be autosomal recessive (Deschauer et al. 2006).

ALPHA-KETOGLUTARATE DEFICIENCY

Alpha-ketoglutarate deficiency has been described in a few neonates and infants (Bonnefont et al. 1992, Surrendran et al. 2002). The clinical presentation resembles that of early-onset PDH deficiency or the mitochondrial encephalomyopathies. Mild hyperlactataemia is associated with abnormal alpha-ketoglutaric acid in urine with or without increased excretion of other Krebs cycle intermediates. All patients had cortical atrophy and striatal necrosis in some cases.

MITOCHONDRIAL FATTY ACID BETA-OXIDATION DEFECTS

Inborn errors in mitochondrial fatty acid oxidation represent a group of disorders that affect energy metabolism during fasting and metabolic stress. As a consequence, common features include acute metabolic decompensations associated with fasting, recurrent hypoglycaemia, Reye-like syndrome and unexplained sudden infant death. Chronic involvement of fatty-acid-dependent tissues may result in myopathy and cardiomyopathy. About 20 different defects are known (Wanders et al. 1999, Tein 2002, Vockley 2002, Longo et al. 2006).

BIOCHEMICAL BACKGROUND

The general pathways of mitochondrial fatty acid oxidation and the sites of the different known enzymatic defects are shown in Figure 8.28. Long-chain fatty acids converted to their CoA-esters are transported into the mitochondria by a specific carnitine acyl-carnitine shuttle that comprises carnitine palmitoyltransferase I and II (CPT-I, CPT-II) and carnitine acyl-carnitine translocase (CAT). Medium- and short-chain acyl-CoAs readily diffuse into the mitochondria. Primary carnitine deficiency, CPT-I, CPT-II and translocase deficiencies impair mitochondrial transport of long-chain fatty acids and consequently beta-oxidation and ketogenesis. Further beta-oxidation involves four sequential steps with chain-length-specific enzymes. The first step requires four distinct acyl-CoA dehydrogenases, the very-long-, long-, medium- and short-chain acyl-CoA dehydrogenases (VLCAD, LCAD, MCAD, SCAD), which transform fatty acyl-CoA to enoyl-CoA. All four acyl-CoA dehydrogenases release electrons that pass to the respiratory chain via the electron-transfer flavoprotein system. The latter specific electron transfer sytem is shared with other flavoprotein dehydrogenases: glutaryl CoA- and isovaleryl CoA-dehydrogenases. The three remaining steps of long-chain beta-oxidation can be performed by either a single trifunctional protein (TFP) for longer chain substrates, or unifunctional enzymes for short- and medium-chain substrates. Each four-step beta-oxidation cycle releases acetyl-CoA, which enters the Krebs cycle in tissues such as heart and muscle. In liver, during the fasting state, acetyl-CoA is converted to ketones (ketogenesis), which are exported to peripheral organs, such as the brain, for final oxidation (ketolysis) and energy delivery. Known defects in mitochondrial beta-oxidation are summarized in Table 8.10. Multiple acyl-CoA dehydrogenase (MAD) deficiency, also called glutaric aciduria type II, is caused by a defect in the electron transfer system. Several alternative pathways become important when mitochondrial beta-oxidation is impaired. Omega-oxidation in microsomes results in the production of characteristic dicarboxylic acids, and intramitochondrial conjugation of acyl-CoA to glycine and carnitine is an important mechanism of detoxification.

The biochemical diagnosis is based on the identification of abnormal dicarboxylic acids and their by-products (glycine, carnitine) in urine. Glutaric and branched-chain organic acidurias are associated in MAD deficiency. It should be emphasized that

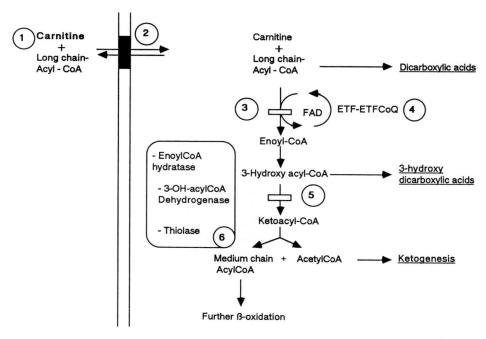

Fig. 8.28. Simplified schema of long-chain fatty acid beta-oxidation indicating sites of major inborn defects. Key: 1 = primary carnitine deficiency; 2 = carnitine acylcarnitine shuttle (carnitine palmityl transferase I and II, carnitine translocase); 3 = long- and very-long-chain acyl-CoA dehydrogenase (LCAD/VLCAD); 4 = electron transfer system (MAD, glutaric aciduria type II); 5 = long-chain 3-hydroxy-acyl-CoA dehydrogenase (LCHAD); 6 = trifunctional protein.

these specific patterns are best detected during an acute crisis, while in the basic state the most reliable tests are the determination of total and esterified plasma carnitine levels and the identification of an abnormal acyl-carnitine profile in plasma or dried blood spots. Measurement of fatty acid oxidation rate in fresh lymphocytes or cultured fibroblasts is a useful tool to narrow the search for the specific defect involved. Direct enzymatic assay may then be performed for definitive diagnosis. Most defects are expressed in cultured fibroblasts; however, certain of these defects, such as muscle CPT-I and SCHAD deficiencies, may be tissue-specific (Sim et al. 2002).

GENETIC BACKGROUND
Overall, these disorders are frequent, but MCAD and CPT-II deficiencies are the most common. All the disorders that have been identified are inherited as autosomal recessive traits. Heterozygotes are usually normal. However, heterozygote LCHAD mothers carrying an affected fetus may develop an acute fatty liver deficiency by the end of the pregnancy. All the implicated genes have been cloned, and various disease-causing mutations have been described. Prevalent mutations are associated with MCAD, adolescent–adult form of CPT-II deficiency, and alpha-subunit of TFP. Antenatal diagnosis is available by measuring the enzymatic activity in cultured amniocytes or in chorionic villus samples, and more reliably, by molecular analysis. The high frequency of these disorders associated with availability of effective treatments and/or preventive measures make them good candidates for an expanding neonatal screening. It has already been implemented

in many countries, especially for MCAD deficiency (Wilcken et al. 2003).

CLINICAL FINDINGS
Patients affected with fatty acid oxidation defects have in common some clinical presentations that are related to acute energy deprivation that can occur at any age from the neonatal period to adulthood (Table 8.10). However, neonates, infants and young children are the most susceptible to decompensate during metabolic stress due to their limited glucose reserves. At birth, the affected neonates are unable to cope with the energy demand. In infants and young children, prolonged fasting and intercurrent infections are the most frequent precipitating factors. In older children, infections, fever and prolonged exercise may induce decompensations.

Clinically, these acutely ill patients may manifest life-threatening episodes of hypoketotic hypoglycaemia, cardiomyopathy and arrhythmia, coma and multiorgan failure. Hepatic encephalopathy with lactic acidosis and hyperammonaemia has frequently been misdiagnosed as Reye syndrome. Various degrees of myolysis and/or cardiomyopathy are frequently associated. In some cases, rapid unexpected death may suggest sudden infant death syndrome. In most situations, this abrupt deterioration is associated with hypoketotic hypoglycaemia, lactic acidosis, hyperammonaemia, signs of liver failure, and muscular involvement with increased creatine kinase. Despite correction of blood glucose levels, some patients may display persistent lethargy, seizures, dystonic movements or opisthotonos due to concomitant cerebral oedema,

of penicillamine. Treatment should be started progressively and the dosage should be slowly increased. Side effects are frequent and may be severe in up to a quarter of cases. They include lupus erythematosus, nephrotic syndrome, fever, rashes, pyridoxine deficiency, thrombocytopenia and, rarely, myasthenic symptoms. Marked neurological deterioration on initiation of treament occurs in 40% of cases, so many authorities do not advise its use in neurological cases (Brewer 2005, Fink and Schilsky 2007).

Triethylene tetramine (trientine) at a dose of 40–50 mg/kg/day seems to be very efficacious; it is well tolerated and is regarded as the first-choice drug by some authorities (Brewer et al. 2006, Fink and Schilsky 2007). Its association with zinc seems particularly effective. It is clearly indicated when penicillamine is poorly tolerated or as initial treatment in moderate or severe forms of the disorder. However, it may also produce transient aggravation (Walshe and Munro 1995).

Tetrathiomolybdate is a promising agent that acts by forming a complex with copper and protein that can block the absorption of copper or render blood copper non-toxic (Brewer 2005), and very good results have been reported when followed by maintenance zinc therapy (Brewer et al. 1996, Brewer 2005).

Treatment with chelators must be closely monitored clinically and by watching copper excretion, which often increases dramatically upon starting treatment then returns to normal over a few months. When effective, the Kayser–Fleischer rings begin to fade in a few weeks and should disappear completely in about a year. A significant decrease of CT/MRI abnormalities should also be obtained as both indicate effective 'de-copperization'.

Oral zinc sulfate treatment, at a dosage of 300–600 mg/day (Hoogenraad 1996, 2006), is meant to decrease toxic free copper by binding it to metallothioneine, decreasing gut absorption of copper and rendering it non-toxic. It is often used as a complement to chelators and is also effective alone as shown by normalization or decrease of free blood copper and disappearance of Kayser–Fleischer ring. Some investigators consider it is the first-choice treatment (Hoogenraad 1996, 2006). Others prefer to use it together with trientine for moderate or severe forms and advise zinc for mild neurological cases or non-neurological presentations (Brewer et al. 2006). Zinc has been used successfully for presymptomatic children with subclinical liver involvement as indicated by high levels of transaminases (Marcellini et al. 2005). Gastrointestinal intolerance may occur. It does not produce iatrogenic paroxysmal intoxication. A low-copper diet is recommended in all cases.

Most children who have isolated hepatic disease usually do well on treatment. Approximately 40–50% of those with neurological manifestations become asymptomatic. Patients with advanced liver disease or acute liver failure can benefit from liver transplantation, which is often practiced in refractory disease (Dhawan et al. 2005).

VARIANTS AND RELATED DISORDERS
A few cases with features reminiscent of Wilson disease but with a different disturbance in copper metabolism have been reported.

Siblings with neurological signs, splenomegaly, absent Kayser–Fleischer ring, associated palsy of vertical gaze and an accumulation of copper in the mucosa of the lower intestine, clearly had a different condition to Wilson disease (Godwin-Austen et al. 1978). A few patients with prepubertal onset of neurological symptoms and some atypical features had marginally low ceruloplasmin, no Kayser–Fleischer rings and only mild accumulation of copper in their liver without hepatotoxic effect (Pall et al. 1987, Ono and Kurisaki 1988). The mechanism of such cases is not understood. Some patients may respond to penicillamine.

MENKES DISEASE (KINKY HAIR DISEASE, STEELY HAIR DISEASE, TRICHOPOLIODYSTROPHY)
Menkes disease is an uncommon X-linked disease (incidence 1 in 50,000 births) characterized pathologically by multiple focal involvement of the grey matter and chemically by low serum copper and ceruloplasmin. The gene (*MNK*) is located at Xq13.3 and codes for a copper-transporting ATPase (ATPase7 A). Deficiency of this protein results in lack of transport of copper to cellular organelles. There is secondary deficit of several copper-dependent enzymes including cytochrome *c* oxidase and lysine oxidase, accounting for bone and connective tissue abnormalities. The expression of the disease can be extremely diverse even with the same mutation (Borm et al. 2004). Many mutations have been identified, in particular splicing mutations resulting in an incomplete gene with partial activity responsible for allelic variants, especially the *occipital horn syndrome* (Qi and Byers 1998).

PATHOLOGY AND PATHOPHYSIOLOGY
Copper levels are low in the liver and brain but are elevated in intestinal mucosa and kidneys. Orally administered copper is poorly absorbed but intravenous copper produces a brisk rise of serum copper. The copper content of fibroblasts is markedly elevated. This suggests maldistribution of copper that becomes unavailable for the synthesis of copper-containing enzymes. Excessive uptake of copper by fibroblasts is the basis for prenatal diagnosis of this disease, which can also be done by measurement of copper in chorionic villus samples. DNA analysis may permit first-trimester diagnosis if the mutation in the family has been identified (Tümer et al. 1994).

Defective activity of metalloenzymes produces diffuse disturbances that particularly affect arteries in the brain and elsewhere, and extensive focal degeneration of the grey matter with neuronal loss and gliosis. There is profound involvement of the cerebellar cortex (Robain et al. 1988) with loss of Purkinje cells. Remaining cells show abnormal dendritic and axonal swellings (Menkes 1999).

CLINICAL MANIFESTATIONS
Clinical manifestations may be present from the neonatal period or after 2–3 months. Failure to thrive is the most striking feature. Seizures soon occur that can include infantile spasms (Bahi-Buisson et al. 2006, Bindu et al. 2007), and a profound deterioration with hypotonia becomes apparent. Hypothermia is an important

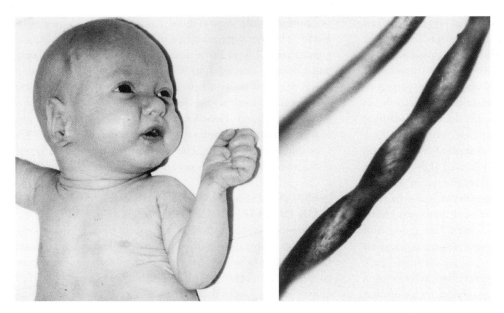

Fig. 8.31. Menkes kinky hair disease. Note chubby appearance of face. Head has a paucity of short, steely, twisted hair.

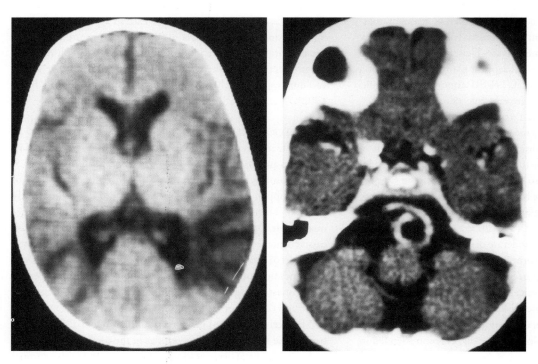

Fig. 8.32. Menkes kinky hair disease. *(Left)* CT shows extensive destructive lesions of vascular origin in both parietal regions. *(Right)* Enhanced CT shows dilatation, tortuosity and irregular calibre of basilar artery.

cue although commonly unrecognized. The hair is sparse, brittle, and grey or silvery. Microscopic examination easily confirms the diagnosis by showing pili torti (Fig. 8.31) and occasionally trichorrhexis nodosa. The cherubic appearance of affected infants is striking. In the first few weeks of life the primary hair may be normal; however, even neonatal hair may have a special appearance (Gu et al. 2005).

Hydroureters and hydronephrosis are common. Generalized osteoporosis, metaphyseal spurring, diaphyseal periosteal reaction, scalloping of the posterior aspect of the vertebral bodies and multiple wormian bones are often present. Angiography shows elongated and tortuous arteries but is not routinely indicated. However, tortuosity of intracranial arteries is well demonstrated by imaging (Fig. 8.32) and aneurysms may develop. Neuroimaging techniques show diffuse brain atrophy, defective myelination and often subdural haematoma. In some cases, more focal abnormalities with areas of cortical atrophy and associated hypodensity are seen (Takahashi et al. 1993).

The course is rapidly downhill and the mean age at death is 19 months. The diagnosis is easy, although bony lesions can suggest scurvy or the battered baby syndrome, the more so as subdural effusions are not unusual.

Early diagnosis may be difficult to make firmly as low copper levels may occur normally in the neonatal period and this may delay the diagnosis, which is highly regrettable as copper-histidine therapy should be started early and definitive laboratory diagnosis is complex and may take time. A low urine HVA/VMA (homovanillic/vanillylmandelic acid) ratio due to the decreased activity of the copper-dependent enzyme dopamine beta-hydroxylase may be suggestive (Matsuo et al. 2005). Prenatal diagnosis can be made by copper measurement in placenta or by genetic analysis when possible (Gu et al. 2002). Other early cues are a low birthweight and preterm birth, which are present in a third of cases, and the unusual coloration of the hair. Increased uptake by culture of fibroblasts is present from birth thus allowing diagnosis. Heterozygotes may be suspected by the presence of pili torti on low-power microscopy and confirmed by biological tests.

VARIANTS OF KINKY HAIR DISEASE
Mild cases of the condition are known and may present with ataxia and mild mental retardation (Kodama et al. 1999) and run a less malignant course. Other atypical cases have presented with hypotonia and hair anomalies but without seizures or hypothermia (Inagaki et al. 1988). The *occipital horn syndrome* features hyperelastic and bruisable skin, hyperextensible joints and calcification at the junction of neck muscles and occipital bones (Qi and Byers 1998). Abnormalities in copper metabolism are similar to those of Menkes disease, but less marked (Proud et al. 1996). There may be mental retardation.

TREATMENT
Treatment with parenterally administered copper restores blood levels but does not correct the neurological disease. Administration of copper-histidine not only corrects copper levels but results in clinical improvement, particularly if commenced early at 35 weeks gestational age (Tümer et al. 1996). Munakata et al. (2005) have shown that the treatment improves some of the biochemical disturbances (increased lactate and decreased N-acetyl aspartic acid as shown by MR proton spectroscopy). However, evaluation of results is still difficult.

MISCELLANEOUS METABOLIC DISORDERS

DISORDERS OF PURINE METABOLISM
LESCH–NYHAN DISEASE
Pathophysiology
Lesch–Nyhan disease is an X-linked disorder due to deficiency of the purine salvage enzyme hypoxanthine-guanine phosphoribosyltransferase (HGPRT). As a consequence of this defect,

hypoxanthine and guanine cannot be reutilized for the synthesis of the corresponding nucleotides guanosine monophosphate and inosine monophosphate. Hypoxanthine formed is catabolized to xanthine and uric acid or excreted. Depletion of hypoxanthine, which acts as a feedback regulator of uric acid synthesis, leads to markedly increased production of uric acid, resulting in hyperuricaemia and its consequences. The mechanism of neurological disturbances is still obscure and is unrelated to uric acid. They may result, at least in part, from a mixture of abnormal neurodevelopment and neurotransmitter abnormalities (Hyland et al. 2004, Deutsch et al. 2005). Failure of development of dopaminergic synaptic terminals has been demonstrated (Messina et al. 2005). The concentration of dopamine and the activity of enzymes involved in its synthesis are lessened, and this and other alterations in neurotransmitter balance within the basal ganglia are probably important.

There is a striking degree of genetic heterogeneity of HGPRT defects. Over 300 mutations of the *HGPRT* gene are currently known (Jinnah et al. 2004), and the spectrum of severity is extremely wide (Puig et al. 2001) from asymptomatic cases to the most severe classical syndrome, depending on the degree of residual enzyme activity and probably also on unknown factors. Many variants have been recognized variably due to small deletions or point mutations in the gene located at Xq26–q27, some of them with distinctive clinical concomitants.

Pathologically, no gross lesions have been recognized.

Clinical manifestations
The clinical manifestations are striking. They become apparent during the first year of life in the form of psychomotor retardation and generalized muscular hypotonia. Abnormal movements usually appear between 6 months to 1 year of age. Dystonia is constant; choreoathetosis or ballismus are subsequently superimposed in 44–90% of patients (Jinnah et al. 2006) but are not progressive after the first few years. Some degree of spasticity develops progressively. Ocular saccades are sometimes initiated by head movements or eye blinking, reflecting involvement of the basal ganglia (Jinnah et al. 2001). Seizures are uncommon but bouts of dystonic opisthotonus can occur and may wrongly suggest seizures. *Self-mutilation* is the most striking feature and one that raises major problems. The most common behaviours are biting of the fingers, lips and tongue that appear usually between 2 and 4 years of age but sometimes later. They often result in severe lesions of the mouth or hands that are difficult to prevent. Head banging, extension of the arms while being wheeled through doorways or putting fingers in the wheel spokes, and eye poking come next in frequency (Robey et al. 2003). Affected children are variably intellectually retarded, usually mildly or moderately, but most suffer from attention deficit and difficulties of comprehension of complex or lengthy speech and in multistep reasoning. They are severely disturbed by their compulsion to self-mutilate and appear happier when maintained in restraints.

In late childhood or adolescence haematuria, renal calculi and ultimately renal failure develop. Gouty arthritis and urate tophi can also be observed.

Diagnosis

The diagnosis is suggested by a high level of serum uric acid. However, urinary uric acid content is a better indicator, as serum uric acid may occasionally be normal. Enzymatic analysis of erythrocytes or fibroblasts confirms the diagnosis. Antenatal diagnosis is possible by enzymatic analysis of blood, skin fibroblasts or amniotic cells (Nyhan et al. 2003); identification of mutation is possible but the large number of mutations makes it difficult. It can also be used to detect female carriers in families in which the molecular defect has been established. Preimplantation diagnosis has been performed (Ray et al. 1999). Differential diagnosis is relatively easy even though hyperuricaemia is frequent and may be found in association with mental retardation and neurological deficits by mere coincidence. A different disorder with gout due to overproduction of uric acid as a result of overactivity of the enzyme phophoribosylpyrophosphate synthetase may be associated, in a few cases, with neurodevelopmental anomalies (Nyhan 2005) or sensorineural deafness (Becker et al. 1988).

Treatment

Treatment with allopurinol is effective in relieving symptoms due to high uric acid but has no action on neurological manifestations. Attempts at gene therapy are being pursued. Treatment of the neurological problem is mainly with behaviour modifiers and neurotransmitter therapy (reviewed in Olson and Houlihan 2000). Gabapentin has been reported to be efficacious in one patient (McManaman and Tam 1999).

Partial deficits in HGPRT and variants of Lesch–Nyhan syndrome

Deficits in HGPRT less complete than those in the classical Lesch–Nyhan syndrome (<1.3% of normal) can produce various clinical pictures. Patients with a level >8.5% of normal have no neurological symptoms but may have uric acid-related problems. At intermediate range, a neurological picture similar to Lesch–Nyhan syndrome but without mental retardation and self-mutilation may be observed (Puig et al. 2001). Other variants with mild mental retardation, spasticity and skeletal malformations, choreoathetosis, developmental delay and deafness have been described. Although intelligence is normal in most cases, comparison of patients with partial HGPRT deficiency with normal subjects has shown intermediate levels between those of controls and those with the classical syndrome (Schretlen et al. 2001). Rare cases of typical Lesch–Nyhan syndrome in girls are on record (Ogasawara et al. 1989).

ADENOSYLSUCCINATE LYASE DEFICIENCY

Jaeken and van den Berghe (1984) have reported on an autism syndrome with severe mental retardation in association with the presence of large amounts of succinyladenosine and succinylaminoimidazole carboxamide riboside in body fluids. CSF protein was described in affected children. Hypoplasia of the cerebellar vermis may be present (Chapter 2). Clinical features are variable. Developmental delay, hypotonia and seizures, often neonatal, are often associated with autistic symptoms (Nassogne

et al. 2000, Ciardo et al. 2001). In some infants, there may be only mild to moderate delay. Reduced myelination can be striking (Köhler et al. 1999). The diagnosis is confirmed by the presence of succinyl purines in the CSF. Many mutations are known. This disorder should be thought of in infants with early seizures and in investigation of autism spectrum disorders. Prenatal molecular diagnosis is possible (Marie et al. 2000). No treatment is known.

PURINE NUCLEOSIDE PHOSPHORYLASE DEFICIENCY

This rare disease is characterized by severe immunodeficiency. A neurological syndrome consisting of an association of diplegia and mental retardation seems to be an integral part of the disease (Tabarki et al. 2003, Ozkinay et al. 2007) Developmental delay has also been reported (Myers et al. 2004) (see also Chapter 10).

DISORDERS OF PYRIMIDINE DEGRADATION

Defects of *pyrimidine dehydrogenase* (van Gennip et al. 1994a) and of *dihydropyrimidinidine dehydrogenase* (Putman et al. 1997) have been reported in association with convulsions, mental retardation or choreoathetosis, sometimes associated with dysmorphism. In most cases, dihydropyrimidine dehydrogenase deficiency is expressed only by uraciluria in homozygotes. The neuropsychiatric manifestations described that are poorly correlated with the biochemical defect may be coincidental (van Kuilenburg et al. 1999). The metabolic defect is associated with a high frequency of severe toxicity of fluorouracil and is therefore important in many cancer patients (van Kuilenburg et al. 2003).

A second defect in this pathway is dihydropyriminidase deficiency (Assmann et al. 1997), which may also present with neurological signs. A third defect, beta-ureidopropionase deficiency, can result in severe dystonia, mental retardation and severe defect in myelination (Assmann et al. 2006a,b).

This group of conditions may represent a novel category of neurodevelopmental disorders and should be thought of in the investigation of obscure neurological conditions.

DISORDERS OF CREATINE SYNTHESIS AND TRANSPORT

Creatine (Cr) and phosphocreatine (PCr) are major components in energy storage and transmission. Creatine is mainly synthesized in the liver and the pancreas in a two-step mechanism from glycine, arginine and methionine and finally converted by non-enzymatic cyclization to creatinine (Fig. 8.33). Humans maintain their creatine pool by biosynthesis and nutritional uptake of 1–2g/day. Creatine is transported via blood and at the cellular level by the Cr-transporter system (CrT).

During the past few years inborn errors of metabolism of all three protein components have been identified in humans.

GUANIDINOACETATE-METHYLTRANSFERASE DEFICIENCY (GAMT-D)

The first patient with this disorder was reported by Stöckler et al. (1994). The child was normal at birth but became hypotonic, and developed extrapyramidal dystonic symptoms and

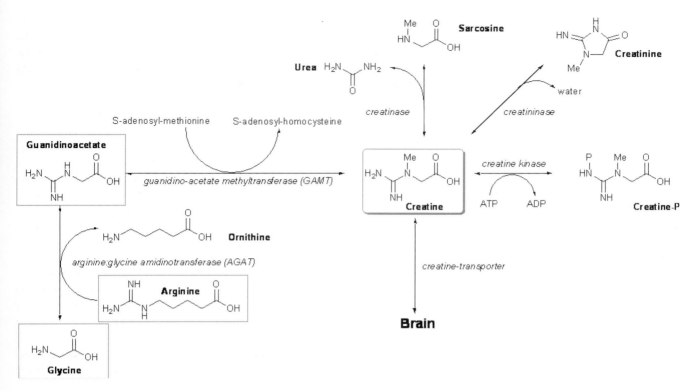

Fig. 8.33. Pathways of creatine synthesis and transport.

severe psychomotor retardation. The MRI at 12 months of age showed abnormal signals in the globus pallidus. Proton MR spectroscopy (MRS) revealed the absence of brain creatine and creatine phosphate signals, suggesting an inborn error of creatine synthesis. Deficient GAMT activity was confirmed in liver tissue. A number of patients with GAMT-D could be identified by the missing Cr/PCr signal in the brain detected by proton MRS (von Figura et al. 2000). Supplementation with creatine-mono-hydrate (4 g/day) produced considerable improvement and the MRS abnormalities in the putamen normalized. However, the Cr/PCr concentrations in the brain as measured by MRS remained below normal levels. At the age of 15 years the patient was able to walk but was severely mentally retarded with autistic self-injurious behaviour.

GAMT-D is an inherited autosomal disease; the gene maps to chromosome 19p13.3. Several GAMT-D mutant alleles have been characterized. The clinical manifestations of GAMT are variable: muscular hypotonia, dystonia, severe epilepsy and mental retardation have been observed.

The diagnosis of a creatine deficiency disorder should be suspected in patients with hypotonic–dystonic disorders with or without MRI abnormalities. Pathognomonic laboratory findings in GAMT-D consist of decreased concentration of creatine and creatinine in blood, CSF and urine, whilst guadinine acetate, the precursor of Cr, is elevated in blood, urine and CSF. The absence of a Cr/PCr signal in brain MRS is almost diagnostic. Further biochemical and genetic studies allow the identification of the underlying defect.

ARGININE:GLYCIN AMIDINOTRANSFERASE DEFICIENCY (AGAT-D)
In AGAT-D, first described in 2000, brain MRI is normal, but MRS reveals total absence of Cr/PCr. The diagnosis of AGAT-D was established in fibroblasts and lymphoblasts.

The patients had no epilepsy or other neuromuscular symptoms. Cr in serum was normal, GAA slightly decreased, the excretion of GAA in urine extremely low. Both patients responded favourably to supplementation of creatine (Schulze 2003).

X-LINKED CREATINE TRANSPORTER DEFICIENCY (CRT1-D)
This disorder features mild mental retardation and severe delay in the expression of speech and language function in boys. Apart from mild hypotonia, motor functions are normal. MRI and MRS reveal an almost complete absence of the Cr signal.

This inherited error of metabolism is caused by a genetic defect in the X-linked creatine transporter *SLC6A8* gene mapping to Xq28 (Salomons et al. 2003). More unrelated families with male patients and female carriers have been identified. The clinical characteristics of CrT1-D are mild muscular hypotonia, mental retardation, expressive speech and language delay, and epilepsy. Cr concentrations in plasma and urine are elevated, while GAA is normal. MRS is the most helpful non-invasive investigation. In a patient reported by Schulze (2003), treatment with oral Cr was ineffective in restoring normal Cr concentration in the brain as shown by MRS and did not improve symptoms.

315

PORPHYRIAS

This group of disorders is uncommon in childhood. The main clinical features of acute intermittent porphyria and of hereditary coproporphyria are described in Chapter 20.

DISORDERS OF DNA REPAIR

Defects in DNA repair mechanisms, especially excision of defective DNA and its replacement, play an important role in several neurological diseases. These include ataxia–telangiectasia (Chapter 3), trichothiodystrophy (Chapter 3), Cockayne syndrome (Chapter 9) and xeroderma pigmentosum.

Xeroderma pigmentosum is an autosomal recessive disease characterized by variably severe defects in DNA excision–repair mechanisms and extreme sensitivity of the skin to ultraviolet light. Development of cutaneous malignancies is extremely common and there is also an increased frequency of some brain tumours. At least nine genetic forms of the disease exist, eight of them with defective DNA nucleotide excision–repair (Robbins et al. 1991, Cleaver et al. 1999).

In its classical form (80% of cases), the disease affects mainly the skin. Even in this form, variable degrees of mental retardation are frequent and may remain stable. In about 20% of cases, especially in groups A and D, there is a progressive neurodegeneration due to selective neuronal death (Robbins et al. 1991, Rapin et al. 2000). These patients develop progressive neurological deficits that may start in infancy or before adolescence with intellectual impairment or dementia, microcephaly, abnormal movements and cerebellar signs. Retinopathy, cataracts and deafness occur, and peripheral mixed neuropathy is frequent. In the most severe cases there may be neonatal microcephaly, retarded growth and abnormal genitalia (*De Sanctis–Cacchione syndrome*). Milder forms also occur. Intermediate and late-onset forms tend to be less severe.

A rare association of xeroderma pigmentosum with Cockayne syndrome has been reported that combines the cutaneous features of xeroderma with the neurological manifestations of Cockayne syndrome such as intracranial calcification. This form is seen with some exceptional mutations (Lindenbaum et al. 2001).

CEREBROTENDINOUS XANTHOMATOSIS

Cerebrotendinous xanthomatosis is a rare inherited disorder of bile acid metabolism leading to accumulation of cholestanol and cholesterol in most tissues including the CNS. It is responsible for xanthomas, early cararact, severe neurological deterioration and premature atherosclerosis. In spite of its rarity, diagnosis is important because early treatment can halt and in some cases reverse the neurological impairment (Federico and Dotti 2003).

Cerebrotendinous xanthomatosis is an autosomal recessive disorder resulting from mutation of the 27-hydroxylase mitochondrial enzyme activity *CYP27A1* gene (Gallus et al. 2006). The defect impairs the mitochondrial part of bile acid synthesis from cholesterol and results in accumulation of cholestanol and cholesterol. In serum, cholesterol levels are normal but increased cholestanol levels result in an abnormal cholestanol/cholesterol ratio. The defect is responsible for a low synthesis of chenodeoxy-cholic acid, the end-product of bile acid synthesis. This, in turn, results in upregulation of the cholesterol 7-alpha-hydroxylase, the rate-limiting enzyme in bile acid synthesis, and further accumulation of bile acid intermediates. The enzymatic activity is expressed in cultured fibroblasts and liver.

NEUROPATHOLOGY

The cerebellar white matter, the optic pathways and the long tracts of the brainstem, spinal cord and spinal roots are most involved. Lesions are due to axonal degeneration with loss of myelinated fibres and accumulation of lipids. Cystic spaces and crystalline clefts surrounded by foamy cells, gliosis, axonal spheroids and multinucleated foreign giant cells are found in many parts of the CNS but especially in the cerebellum (Soffer et al. 1995). The sterol fraction from affected parts of the CNS and peripheral nerves is essentially made up of cholestanol.

CLINICAL FEATURES

The major clinical signs include xanthomas in the tendons and tuberous xanthomas, juvenile cataracts, progressive neurological dysfunction and dementia, and premature coronary heart disease or atherosclerosis. Onset is usually in adulthood but childhood cases are seen (Federico and Dotti 2003). Neurological signs include peripheral neuropathy, pyramidal and cerebellar signs with spasticity and ataxia, and convulsions in some cases (Kuriyama et al. 1991). Some patients may present with prominent psychiatric disorders (Berginer et al. 1988). Xanthomas may be absent in early stages of the disorder or even never develop, and a few patients have had normal intelligence in spite of neurological impairment such as ataxia, paresis or peripheral neuropathy (Björkhem et al. 1987). In the late and final stage, neurological deterioration is severe, speech becomes difficult, and swallowing difficulties and sphincter incontinence develop. MRI studies of the brain and spinal cord have demonstrated cerebral, cerebellar and spinal cord atrophy (Bencze et al. 1990) and demyelination in the cerebrum, cerebellum and brainstem (Federico and Dotti 2003). A spinal form has been described (Verrips et al. 1999). Results of neurophysiological studies are consistent with axonal and peripheral neuropathy (Arpa et al. 1995).

DIAGNOSIS

Biochemical diagnosis is made by the determination of excessive urinary excretion of bile alcohols and by the cholestanol/cholesterol ratio in serum (Björkhem et al. 1987, Arpa et al. 1995). The definitive diagnosis relies on measurement of 7-alpha-hydroxylase in cultured fibroblasts.

TREATMENT

By supplying the end-product of bile acid synthesis, supplementation with chenodeoxycholic acid decreases cholestanol accumulation and results in clear clinical, radiological and neurophysiological improvement (Björkhem et al. 1987). Addition of simvastatin, an inhibitor of 3-hydroxy-3-methyl-glutaryl-CoA reductase, may further improve the therapeutic effects.

REFERENCES

Abbott MH, Folstein SE, Abbey H, Pyeritz RE (1987) Psychiatric manifestations of homocystinuria due to cystathionine beta-synthase deficiency: prevalence, natural history, and relationship to neurologic impairment and vitamin B6-responsiveness. *Am J Med Genet* **26**: 959–69.

Abdenur JE, Abeling N, Specola N, et al. (2006) Aromatic L-amino acid decarboxylase: unusual neonatal presentation and additional findings in organic acid analysis. *Mol Genet Metab* **87**: 48–53.

Abeling NG, van Gennip AH, Overmars H, et al. (1994) Biogenic amine metabolite patterns in the urine of monoamine oxidase A-deficient patients. A possible tool for diagnosis. *J Inherit Metab Dis* **17**: 339–41.

Accardo AP, Pensiero S, Perisutti P (2005) Saccadic analysis for early identification of neurologic involvement in Gaucher Disease. *Ann NY Acad Sci* **1039**: 503–7.

Aerts JM, Hollak CE, Bock RG, et al. (2006) Substrate reduction therapy of glycosphingolipid storage disorders. *J Inherit Metab Dis* **29**: 449–56.

Ahmad A, Kahler SG, Kishnani P, et al. (1999) Treatment of pyruvate carboxylase deficiency with high doses of citrate and aspartate. *Am J Med Genet* **87**: 331–8.

Alberio S, Mineri R, Tiranti V, Zeviani M (2007) Depletion of mtDNA: syndromes and genes. *Mitochondrion* **7**: 6–12.

Amir N, Zlotogora J, Bach G (1987) Mucolipidosis type IV: clinical spectrum and natural history. *Pediatrics* **79**: 953–9.

Andersson U, Smith D, Jeyakumar M, et al. (2004) Improved outcome of N-butyldeoxygalactonojirimycin-mediated substrate reduction therapy in a mouse model of Sandhoff disease. *Neurobiol Dis* **16**: 506–15.

Andréasson S, Blennow G, Ehinger B, Strömland K (1991) Full-field electro-retinograms in patients with the carbohydrate-deficient glycoprotein syndrome. *Am J Ophthalmol* **112**: 83–6.

Andria G, Fowler B, Sebastio G (2006) Disorders of sulfur amino acid metabolism. In: Fernandes J, Saudubray JM, van den Berghe G, Walter JH, eds. *Inborn Metabolic Diseases. Diagnosis and Treatment, 4th edn.* Berlin: Springer-Verlag, pp. 273–82.

Aoki Y, Suzuki Y, Sakamoto O, et al. (1995) Molecular analysis of holocarboxylase synthetase deficiency: a missense mutation and a single base deletion are predominant in Japanese patients. *Biochim Biophys Acta* **1272**: 168–74.

Applegarth DA, Toone JR (2001) Nonketotic hyperglycinemia (glycine encephalopathy): laboratory diagnosis. *Mol Genet Metab* **74**: 139–46.

Applegarth DA, Toone JR (2004) Glycine encephalopathy (nonketotic hyperglycinemia): review and update. *J Inherit Metab Dis* **27**: 417–22.

Arbour L, Rosenblatt B, Clow C, Wilson GN (1988) Postoperative dystonia in a female patient with homocystinuria. *J Pediatr* **113**: 863–4.

Arii J, Tanabe Y (2000) Leigh syndrome: serial MR imaging and clinical follow-up. *AJNR* **21**: 1502–9.

Arpa J, Sánchez C, Vega A, et al. (1995) Cerebrotendinous xanthomatosis diagnosed after traumatic subdural haematoma. *Rev Neurol* **23**: 675–8.

Arvio M, Autio S, Louhiala P (1993) Early clinical symptoms and incidence of aspartylglucosaminuria in Finland. *Acta Paediatr* **82**: 587–9.

Ashorn M, Pitkänen S, Salo MK, Heikinheimo M (2006) Current strategies for the treatment of hereditary tyrosinemia type 1. *Pediatr Drugs* **8**: 47–54.

Assmann G, Seedorf U (1995) Acid lipase deficiency: Wolman disease and cholesterol ester storage disease. In: Scriver CR, Beaudet AL, Sly WS, Valle D, eds. *The Metabolic and Molecular Bases of Inherited Disease, 7th edn.* New York: McGraw-Hill, pp. 2563–8.

Assmann B, Hoffmann GF, Wagner I, et al. (1997) Dihydropyrimidinase deficiency and congenital microvillous atrophy: coincidence or genetic relation? *J Inherit Metab Dis* **20**: 681–8.

Assmann B, Göhlich G, Baethmann M, et al. (2006a) Clinical findings and a therapeutic trial in the first patient with beta-ureidopropionate deficiency. *Neuropediatrics* **37**: 20–5.

Assmann BE, van Kuilenburg AB, Distelmaier F, et al. (2006b) Beta-ureidopropionase deficiency presenting as febrile status epilepticus. *Epilepsia* **47**: 215–7.

Aubourg P (2007) [X-linked adrenoleukodystrophy.] *Ann Endocrinol* **68**: 403–11 (French).

Aubourg P, Blanche S, Jambaqué I, et al. (1990) Reversal of early neurologic and neuroradiologic manifestations of X-linked adrenoleukodystrophy by bone marrow transplantation. *N Engl J Med* **322**: 1860–6.

Aubourg P, Adamsbaum C, Lavallard-Rousseau MC, et al. (1992) Brain MRI and electrophysiologic abnormalities in preclinical and clinical adreno-myeloneuropathy. *Neurology* **42**: 85–91.

Aubourg P, Adamsbaum C, Lavallard-Rousseau M-C, et al. (1993) A two-year trial of oleic and erucic acids ("Lorenzo's oil") as treatment for adreno-myeloneuropathy. *N Engl J Med* **329**: 745–52.

Aula N, Aula P (2006) Prenatal diagnosis of free sialic acid storage disorders (SASD). *Prenat Diagn* **26**: 655–8.

Auré K, Benoist JF, Ogier de Baulny H, et al. (2004) Progression despite replacement of a myopathic form of coenzyme Q10 defect. *Neurology* **63**: 727–9.

Aydin K, Ozmen M, Tatli B, Sencer S (2003) Single voxel MR spectroscopy and diffusion-weighted MRI in two patients with L-2-hydroxyglutaric aciduria. *Pediatr Radiol* **33**: 872–6.

Bach G (2001) Mucolipidosis type IV. *Mol Genet Metab* **73**: 197–203.

Bachmann C (2003) Outcome and survival of 88 patients with urea cycle disorders: a retrospective evaluation. *Eur J Pediatr* **162**: 410–6.

Baethmann M, Wendel U, Hoffmann GF, et al. (2000) Hydrocephalus internus in two patients with 5,10-methylenetetrahydrofolate reductase deficiency. *Neuropediatrics* **31**: 314–7.

Bahi-Buisson N, Kaminska A, Nabbout R, et al. (2006) Epilepsy in Menkes disease: anlysis of clinical stages. *Epilepsia* **43**: 380–6.

Bamiou DE, Campbell P, Liasis A, et al. (2001) Audiometric abnormalities in children with Gaucher disease type 3. *Neuropediatrics* **33**: 146–51.

Bams-Mengerink AM, Majoie CB, Duran M, et al. (2006) MRI of the brain and cervical spinal cord in rhizomelic chondrodysplasia punctata. *Neurology* **66**: 798–803.

Barbot C, Martins E, Vilarinho L, et al. (1995) A mild form of infantile isolated sulphite oxidase deficiency. *Neuropediatrics* **26**: 322–4.

Bargal R, Goebel HH, Latta E, Bach G (2002) Mucolipidosis IV: novel mutation and diverse ultrastructural spectrum in the skin. *Neuropediatrics* **33**: 199–202.

Barth ML, Fensom A, Harris A (1994) The arylsulphatase A gene and molecular genetics of metachromatic leucodystrophy. *J Med Genet* **31**: 663–6.

Baulac S, Huberfeld G, Gourfinkel-An I, et al. (2001) First genetic evidence of GABA$_A$ receptor dysfunction in epilepsy: a mutation in the γ2-subunit gene. *Nat Genet* **28**: 46–8.

Baumgartner MR, Suormala T (2006) Biotin-responsive disorders. In: Fernandes J, Saudubray JM, van den Berghe G, Walter JH, eds. *Inborn Metabolic Diseases. Diagnosis and Treatment, 4th edn.* Berlin: Springer-Verlag, pp. 331–9.

Baxter P, Griffiths P, Kelly T, Gardner-Medwin D (1996) Pyridoxine-dependent seizures: demographic, clinical, MRI and psychometric features, and effect of dose on intelligence quotient. *Dev Med Child Neurol* **38**: 998–1006.

Beccari T, Bibi L, Ricci R, et al. (2003) Two novel mutations in the gene for human alpha-mannosidase that cause alpha-mannosidosis. *J Inherit Metab Dis* **26**: 819–20.

Becker MA, Puig JG, Mateos FA, et al. (1988) Inherited superactivity of phosphoribosylpyrophosphate synthetase: association of uric acid overproduction and sensorineural deafness. *Am J Med* **85**: 383–90.

Beckman DR, Hoganson G, Berlow S., Gilbert EF (1987) Pathological findings in 5,10-methylenetetrahydrofolate reductase deficiency. *Birth Defects Orig Artic Ser* **23**: 47–64.

Bencze KS, Vande Polder DR, Prockop LD (1990) Magnetic resonance imaging of the brain and spinal cord in cerebrotendinous xanthomatosis. *J Neurol Neurosurg Psychiatry* **53**: 166–7.

Bennet JK, Dembure PP, Elsas LJ (1995) Clinical and biochemical analysis of two families with type 1 and type II mannosidosis. *Am J Med Genet* **55**: 21–6.

Benoist JF, Alberti C, Leclercq S, et al. (2003) Cerebrospinal fluid lactate and pyruvate concentrations and their ratio in children: age-related reference intervals. *Clin Chem* **49**: 487–94.

Ben-Yoseph Y, Potier M, Mitchell DA, et al. (1987) Altered molecular size of N-acetylglucosamine 1-phosphotransferase in I-cell disease and pseudo-Hurler polydystrophy. *Biochem J* **248**: 697–701.

Berendzen K, Theriaque DW, Shuster J, Stacpoole PW (2006) Therapeutic potential of dichloroacetate for pyruvate dehydrogenase complex deficiency. *Mitochondrion* **6**: 126–35.

Berginer VM, Foster NL, Sadowsky M, et al. (1988) Psychiatric disorders in patients with cerebrotendinous xanthomatosis. *Am J Psychiatry* **145**: 354–7.

Bernier FP, Boneh A, Dennett X, et al. (2002) Diagnostic criteria for respiratory chain disorders in adults and children. *Neurology* **59**: 1406–11.

Bernsen PL, Wevers RA, Gabreëls FJ, et al. (1987) Phenotypic expression in mucopolysaccharidosis VII. *J Neurol Neurosurg Psychiatry* **50**: 699–703.

Berthier M, Oriot D, Bonneau D, Jaeken J (1995) Does a mutation of the glycine receptor modify GABA metabolism in startle disease? *Acta Paediatr* **84**: 5 (letter).

Bhala A, Willi SM, Rinaldo P, et al. (1995) Clinical and biochemical characterization of short-chain acyl-coenzyme A dehydrogenase deficiency. *J Pediatr* **126**: 910–5.

Bindu PS, Sinha S, Taly MB, et al. (2007) Menkes syndrome presenting as myoclonic szeizures: neuroimaging and EEG observations. *J Child Neurol* **22**: 42–5.

Björkhem I, Skrede S, Buchmann MS, et al. (1987) Accumulation of 7-alpha-hydroxy-4-cholesten-3-one and cholesta-4,6-dien-3-one in patients with cerebrotendinous xanthomatosis: effect of treatment with chenoxycholic acid. *Hepatology* **7**: 266–71.

Blom HJ (2000) Genetic determinants of hyperhomocysteinaemia: the roles of cystathionine β-synthase and 5,10-methylenetetrahydrofolate reductase. *Eur J Pediatr* **159**: S208–12.

Blom TS, Linder MD, Snow K, et al. (2003) Defective endocytic trafficking of NPC1 and NPC2 underlying infantile Niemann–Pick type C disease. *Hum Mol Genet* **12**: 257–72.

Bohu PA, Hannequin D, Hemet C, et al. (1995) [Late neurological complications of galactosaemia: study of three cases.] *Rev Neurol* **151**: 136–8 (French).

Bok LA, Struys E, Willemsen MA, Been JV, Jakobs C (2007) Pyridoxine-dependent seizures in Dutch patients: diagnosis by elevated urinary alpha-aminoadipic semialdehyde levels. *Arch Dis Child* **92**: 687–9.

Bonnefont J-P, Chretien D, Rustin P, et al. (1992) Alpha-ketoglutarate dehydrogenase deficiency presenting as congenital lactic acidosis. *J Pediatr* **121**: 255–8.

Borm BE, Muller LB, Hausser I, et al. (2004) Variable clinical expression of an identical mutation in the ATP7A gene for Menkes disease/occipital horn syndrome in three affected males in a single family. *J Pediatr* **145**: 119–21.

Boulat O, Benador N, Girardin E, Bachmann C (1995) 3-Hydroxyisobutyric aciduria with a mild clinical course. *J Inherit Metab Dis* **18**: 204–6.

Bourgeois M, Goutières F, Chrétien D, et al. (1992) Deficiency in complex II of the respiratory chain, presenting as a leukodystrophy in two sisters with Leigh syndrome. *Brain Dev* **14**: 404–8.

Bresolin N, Comi GP, Fortunato F, et al. (1993) Clinical and biochemical evidence of skeletal muscle involvement in galactose-1-phosphate uridyl transferase deficiency. *J Neurol* **240**: 272–7.

Brewer GJ (2005) Neurologically presenting Wilson's disease: epidemiology, pathophysiology and treatment. *CNS Drugs* **19**: 185–92.

Brewer GJ, Johnson V, Dick RD, et al. (1996) Treatment of Wilson disease with ammonium tetrathiomolybdate. II. Initial therapy in 33 neurologically affected patients and follow-up with zinc therapy. *Arch Neurol* **53**: 1017–25.

Brewer GJ, Askari F, Lorincz MT, et al. (2006) Treatment of Wilson disease with ammonium tetrahydromolybdate. IV. Comparison of tetrahydromolybdate and trientine in a double-blind study of treatment of neurologic presentation of Wilson disease. *Arch Neurol* **63**: 521–7.

Brismar J, Ozand PT (1994a) CT and MR of the brain in the diagnosis of organic acidemias: experiences from 107 patients. *Brain Dev* **16** (Suppl): 104–24.

Brismar J, Ozand PT (1994b) CT and MR of the brain in disorders of the propionate and methylmalonate metabolism. *AJNR* **15**: 1459–73.

Brockmann K, Bjornstad A, Dechent P, et al. (2005) Succinate in dystrophic white matter: a proton magnetic resonance spectrosopy finding characteristic for complex II deficiency. *Ann Neurol* **52**: 38–46.

Brown RM, Head RA, Morris AA, et al. (2006) Pyruvate dehydrogenase E3 binding protein (protein X) deficiency. *Dev Med Child Neurol* **48**: 756–60.

Broyer M, Tete MJ, Guest G (1996) Clinical molymorphism of cystinosis encephalopathy. Results of treatment with cysteamine. *J Inherit Metab Dis* **19**: 65–75.

Brun N, Robitaille Y, Grignon A, et al. (1999) Pyruvate carboxylase deficiency: prenatal onset of ischemia-like brain lesions in two sibs with the acute neonatal form. *Am J Med Genet* **84**: 94–101.

Burgard P, Link R, Schweitzer-Krantz S (2000) Phenylketonuria: evidence-based clinical practice. *Eur J Pediatr* **159** Suppl 2.

Buzzi A, Wu Y, Frantseva MV, et al. (2006) Succinic semialdehyde dehydrogenase deficiency: GABAB receptor-mediated function. *Brain Res* **1090**: 15–22.

Bykhovskaya Y, Casas K, Mengesha E, et al. (2004) Missense mutation in pseudouridine synthase 1 (PUS1) causes mitochondrial myopathy and siderobalstic anemia (MLASA). *Am J Hum Genet* **74**: 1303–8.

Cameron JM, Levandovskiy V, MacKay N, et al. (2006) Novel mutations in dihydrolipoamide dehydrogenase deficiency in two cousins with borderline-normal PDH complex activity. *Am J Med Genet A* **140**: 1542–52.

Cannizzaro LA, Chen YQ, Rafi MA, Wenger DA (1994) Regional mapping of the human galactocerebrosidase gene (GALC) to 14q31 by in situ hybridization. *Cytogenet Cell Genet* **66**: 244–5.

Cao Z, Natowicz MR, Kaback MM, et al. (1993) A second mutation associated with apparent beta-hexosaminidase A pseudodeficiency: identification and frequency estimation. *Am J Hum Genet* **53**: 1198–205.

Carrozzo R, Dionisi-Vici C, Steuerwald U, et al. (2007) SUCLA2 mutations cause mild methylmalonic aciduria, Leigh-like encephalomyopathy, dystonia and deafness. *Brain* **130**: 862–74.

Casteels I, Taylor DS, Lake BD, et al. (1992) Mucolipidosis type IV. Presentation of a mild variant. *Ophthal Paediatr Genet* **13**: 205–10.

Cavanagh JB, Harding BN (1994) Pathogenic factors underlying the lesions in Leigh's disease. Tissue responses to cellular energy deprivation and their clinico-pathological consequences. *Brain* **117**: 1357–76.

Chakrapani A, Sivakumar P, McKiernan PJ, Leonard JV (2002) Metabolic stroke in methylmalonic acidemia five years after liver transplantation. *J Pediatr* **140**: 261–3.

Charrow J, Hvizd MG (1986) Cardiomyopathy and skeletal myopathy in an unusual variant of GM1 gangliosidosis. *J Pediatr* **108**: 729–32.

Chemelli AP, Schocke M, Sperl W, et al. (2000) Magnetic resonance spectroscopy (MRS) in five patients with treated propionic acidemia. *J Magn Reson Imaging* **11**: 596–600.

Chen E, Nyhan WL, Jakobs C, et al. (1996) L-2-hydroxyglutaric aciduria: neuropathological correlations and first report of severe neurodegenerative disease and neonatal death. *J Inherit Metab Dis* **19**: 335–43.

Chinnery PF, Schon EA (2003) Mitochondria. *J Neurol Neurosurg Psychiatry* **74**: 1188–99.

Ciardo F, Salerno C, Guratolo P (2001) Neurologic aspects of adenosyl-lyase deficiency. *J Child Neurol* **16**: 301–8.

Clarke JT, Iwanochka RM (2005) Enzyme replacement therapy of Fabry disease. *Mol Neurobiol* **32**: 43–50

Clayton PT, Surtees RA, DeVile C, et al. (2003) Neonatal epileptic encephalopathy. *Lancet* **361**: 1614.

Cleaver JE, Alzal V, Feeney L, et al. (1999) Increased ultraviolet sensitivity and chromosomal instability related to P53 function in xeroderma pigmentosum variant. *Cancer Res* **59**: 1102–8.

Coman D, Klingberg S, Morris D, et al. (2005) Congenital disorder of glycosylation type Ia in a 6-year-old girl with a mild intelectual phenotype: two novel PMM2 mutations. *J Inherit Metab Dis* **28**: 1189–90.

Cordeiro P, Hectman P, Kaplan F (2000) The GM2 gangliosidosis databases: allelic variations in the HEXA, HEXB and GM2A gene loci. *Genet Med* **2**: 319–27.

Cormier-Daire V, Amiel J, Vuillaumier-Barrot S, et al. (2000) Congenital disorders of glycosylation IIa cause growth retardation, mental retardation, and facial dysmorphism. *J Med Genet* **37**: 875–7.

Cosma MP, Pepe L, Parenti G, et al. (2004) Molecular and functional analysis of SUMF1 mutations in multiple sulfatase deficiency. *Hum Mutat* **23**: 576–81.

Cox TM (2005) Substrate reduction therapy for lysosomal storage disorders. *Acta Paediatr Suppl* **94**: 69–75.

Debray FG, Lambert M, Vanasse M, et al. (2006) Intermittent peripheral weakness as the presenting feature of pyruvate dehydrogenase deficiency. *Eur J Pediatr* **165**: 462–6.

Debray FG, Mitchell GA, Allard P, et al. (2007) Diagnostic accuracy of blood lactate-to-pyruvate molar ratio in the differential diagnosis of congenital lactic acidosis. *Clin Chem* **53**: 916–21.

de Koning TJ (2006) Treatment with amino acids in serine deficiency disorders. *J Inherit Metab Dis* **29**: 347–51.

de Koning TJ, Klomp LW (2004) Serine-deficiency syndromes. *Curr Opin Neurol* **17**: 197–204.

de Koning TJ, Jaeken J, Pineda M, et al. (2000) Hypomyelination and reversible white matter attenuation in 3-phosphoglyrate dehydrogenase deficiency. *Neuropediatrics* **31**: 287–92.

Del Giudice E, Striano S, Andria G (1983) Electroencephalographic abnormalities in homocystinuria due to cystathionine synthase deficiency. *Clin Neurol Neurosurg* **85**: 165–8.

De Meirleir LJ, Van Coster R, Lissens W (2006) Disorders of pyruvate metabolism and the tricarboxylic acid cycle. In: Fernandes J, Saudubray JM, van den Berghe G, Walter JH, eds. *Inborn Metabolic Diseases: Diagnosis and Treatment, 4th edn.* Berlin: Springer-Verlag, pp. 161–74.

Demirkiran M, Jankovic J, Lewis RA, Cox DW (1996) Neurologic presentation of Wilson disease without Kayser–Fleischer rings. *Neurology* **46**: 1040–3.

den Boer ME, Dionisi-Vici C, Chakrapani A, et al. (2003) Mitochondrial trifunctional protein deficiency: a severe fatty acid oxidation disorder with cardiac and neurologic involvement. *J Pediatr* **142**: 684–9.

Deodato F, Boenzi S, Santorelli FM, Dionisi-Vici C (2006) Methylmalonic and propionic aciduria. *Am J Med Genet C Semin Med Genet* **142**: 104–12.

Deschauer M, Gizatullina Z, Schulze A, et al. (2006) Molecular and biological investigations in fumarase deficiency. *Mol Genet Metab* **88**: 146–52.

Deutsch SI, Long KD, Rosse R, et al. (2005) Hypothesized deficiency of guanine purines may contribute to abnormalities of neurodevelopment, neuromodulation, and neurotransmission in Lesch–Nyhan syndrome. *Clin Neuropharmacol* **28**: 28–37.

Dhawan A, Taylor RM, Cheeseman O, et al. (2005) Wilson's disease in children: 37-year experience and revised King's scores for liver transplantation. *Liver Transpl* **11**: 441–8.

DiMauro S, Hirano M (2005) Mitochondrial encephalomyopathies: an update. *Neuromusc Disord* **15**: 276–86.

DiMauro S, Schon EA (2003) Mitochondrial respiratory-chain diseases. *N Engl J Med* **348**: 2656–68.

DiMauro S, Mancuso M, Naini A (2004a) Mitochondrial encephalomyopathies: therapeutic approach. *Ann NY Acad Sci* **1011**: 232–45.

DiMauro S, Tay S, Mancuso M (2004b) Mitochondrial encephalomyopathies: diagnostic approach. *Ann NY Acad Sci* **1011**: 217–31.

Dinopoulos A, Matsubara Y, Kure S (2005) Atypical variants of nonketotic hyperglycinemia. *Mol Genet Metab* **86**: 61–9.

Divry P, Vianey-Liaud C, Gay C, et al. (1988) N-acetylaspartic aciduria: report of three new cases in children with a neurological syndrome associating macrocephaly and leukodystrophy. *J Inherit Metab Dis* **11**: 307–8.

Dobson CM, Gradinger A, Longo N, et al. (2006) Homozygous nonsense mutation in the MCEE gene and siRNA suppression of methylmalonyl-CoA epimerase expression: a novel cause of mild methymalonic aciduria. *Mol Genet Metab* **88**: 327–33.

Dobyns WB (1989) Agenesis of the corpus callosum and gyral malformations are frequent manifestations of non-ketotic hyperglycinemia. *Neurology* **39**: 817–20.

Drory VE, Birnbaum M, Peley L, et al. (2003) Hexosaminidase A deficiency is an uncommon cause of a syndrome mimicking amyotrophic lateral sclerosis. *Muscle Nerve* **28**: 109–12.

Dublin AB, Hald JK, Wootton-Gorges SL (2002) Isolated sulfite oxidase deficiency: MR imaging features. *AJNR* **23**: 484–5.

Elstein D, Guedalia J, Doniger GM, et al. (2005) Computerized cognitive testing in patients with type 1 Gaucher disease: effects of enzyme replacement and substrate reduction. *Genet Med* **7**: 125–30.

Eyskens F, Ceuterick C, Martin JJ, et al. (1994) Carbohydrate-deficient glycoprotein syndrome with previously unreported features. *Acta Paediatr* **83**: 892–6.

Fang J, Peters V, Körner C, Hoffmann GF (2004) Improvement of CDG diagnosis by combined examination of several glycoproteins. *J Inherit Metab Dis* **27**: 581–90.

Farina L, Chiapparini L, Uziel G, et al. (2002) MR findings in Leigh syndrome with COX deficiency and SURF-1 mutations. *AJNR* **23**: 1095–100.

Federico A, Dotti MT (2003) Cerebrotendinous xanthomatosis: clinical manifestations, diagnostic criteria, pathogenesis and therapy. *J Child Neurol* **18**: 633–6.

Feliz B, Witt DR, Harris BT (2003) Propionic acidemia: a neuropathology case report and review of prior cases. *Arch Pathol Lab Med* **127**: e325–8.

Ferdinandusse S, Denis S, Mooyer PA, et al. (2006) Clinical and biological spectrum of D-bifunctional protein deficiency. *Ann Neurol* **59**: 92–104.

Filocamo M, Mazzotti R, Strioppiano M, et al. (2004) Early visual seizures and progressive myoclonic epilepsy in neuronopathic Gaucher disease due to rare compound heterozygosity. *Epilepsia* **45**: 1154–7.

Fink JK, Brouwers P, Barton N, et al. (1989) Neurologic complications in long-standing nephropathic cystinosis. *Arch Neurol* **46**: 543–8.

Fink S, Shilsky ML (2007) Inherited metabolic disease of the liver. *Curr Opin Gastroenterol* **23**: 237–43.

Fiori L, Fiege B, Riva E, Giovannini M (2005) Incidence of BH4-responsiveness in phenylalanine-hydroxylase-deficient Italian patients. *Mol Genet Metab* **86** Suppl 1: S67–74.

Frei KP, Schiffmann R (2002) Myoclonus in Gaucher disease. *Adv Neurol* **89**: 41–8.

Froissart R, Moreira da Silva I, Guffon N, et al. (2002) Mucopolysaccharidosis type II—genotype/phenotype aspects. *Acta Paediatr Suppl* **91**: 82–7.

Froissart R, Cheillan D, Bouvier A, et al. (2005) Clinical, morphological, and molecular aspects of sialic aspects of sialic acid storage disease manifested in utero. *J Med Genet* **42**: 829–36.

Fyfe JC, Madsen M, Hojrup P, et al. (2004) The functional cobalamin(vitamin B12)-intrinsic factor receptor is a novel complex of cubilin and amnionless. *Blood* **103**: 1573–9.

Galjaard H, d'Azzo A, Hoogeveen A, Verheiven FW (1984) Combined beta-galactosidase-sialidase deficiency in man: genetic defect of a protective protein. In: Barranger JA, Brady RB, eds. *The Molecular Basis of Lysosomal Storage Disorders.* London: Academic Press, pp. 113–32.

Gallus GN, Dotti MT, Federico A (2006) Clinical and molecular diagnosis of cerebrotendinous xanthomatosis with a review of the mutations in the CYP27A1 gene. *Neurol Sci* **27**: 143–9.

Garcia-Cazorla A, Rabier D, Touati G, et al. (2006) Pyruvate carboxylase deficiency: metabolic characteristics and new neurological aspects. *Ann Neurol* **59**: 121–7.

Gärtner J (2000) Organelle disease: peroxisomal disorders. *Eur J Pediatr* **159** Suppl 3: S236–9.

Geller J, Kronn D, Jayabose S, Sandoval C (2002) Hereditary folate malabsorption: family report and review of the literature. *Medicine* **81**: 51–68.

Gellera C, Uziel G, Rimoldi M, et al. (1990) Fumarase deficiency is an autosomal recessive encephalopathy affecting both the mitochondrial and the cytosolic enzymes. *Neurology* **40**: 495–9.

Germain DP (2005) [Enzyme replacement therapies for lysosomal storage disorders.] *Med Sci* **21** (Suppl): 77–83 (French).

Gibbs TC, Payan J, Brett EM, et al. (1993) Peripheral neuropathy as the presenting feature of tyrosinemia type I and effectively treated with an inhibitor of 4-hydroxyphenylpyruvate dioxygenase. *J Neur Neurosurg Psychiatry* **56**: 1129–32.

Gieselmann V (2003) Metachromatic leukodystrophy: recent research developments. *J Child Neurol* **18**: 591–4.

Gillingham MB, Scott B, Elliott D, Harding CO (2006) Metabolic control during exercise with and without medium-chain triglycerides (MCT) in children with long-chain 3-hydroxy acyl-CoA dehydrogenase (LCHAD) or trifunctional protein (TFP) deficiency. *Mol Genet Metab* **89**: 58–63.

Giordano C, Sebastiani M, Plazzi G, et al. (2006) Mitochondrial neurogastrointestinal encephalomyopathy: evidence of mitochondrial DNA depletion in the small intestine. *Gastroenterology* **130**: 893–901.

Godwin-Austen RB, Robinson A, Evans K, Lascelles PT (1978) An unusual neurological disorder of copper metabolism clinically resembling Wilson's disease but biochemically a distinct entity. *J Neurol Sci* **39**: 85–98.

Goker-Alpan O, Hruska KS, Orvisky E, et al. (2005) Divergent phenotypes in Gaucher disease implicate the role of modifiers. *J Med Genet* **42**: e37.

Gordon BA, Gordon KE, Seo HC, et al. (1995) Fucosidosis with dystonia. *Neuropediatrics* **26**: 325–7.

Gordon N (2004) Succinic semialdehyde dehydrogenase deficiency (SSADH) (4-hydroxybutyric aciduria, γ-hydroxybutyric aciduria). *Eur J Paediatr Neurol* **8**: 261–5.

Gordon N (2006) Alpers syndrome: progressive neuronal degeneration of children with liver disease. *Dev Med Child Neurol* **48**: 1001–3.

Grabowski GA (2005) Recent clinical progress in Gaucher disease. *Curr Opin Pediatr* **17**: 519–24.

Grewal SS, Wynn R, Abdenur LG, et al. (2005) Safety and efficacy of enzyme replacement therapy in combination with hematopoietic stem cell transplantation in Hurler syndrome. *Genet Med* **7**: 143–6.

Gropman AL, Batshaw ML (2004) Cognitive outcome in urea cycle disorders. *Mol Genet Metab* **81**: S58–62.

Grosso S, Farnetani MA, Berardi R, et al. (2003) GM2 gangliosidosis variant B1: neuroradiological findings. *J Neurol* **250**: 17–21.

Grunewald S, Champion MP, Leonard JV, et al. (2004) Biotinidase deficiency: a treatable leukoencephalopathy. *Neuropediatrics* **35**: 211–6.

Gu YH, Kodama H, Sato E, et al. (2002) Prenatal diagnosis of Menkes disease by genetic analysis and copper measurement. *Brain Dev* **24**: 715–8.

Gu YH, Kodama H, Shiga K, et al. (2005) A survey of Japanese patients with Menkes disease from 1990 to 2003: incidence and early signs before typical syndrome onset, pointing the way to earlier diagnosis. *J Inherit Metab Dis* **28**: 473–8.

Gutierrez-Aguilar G, Abenia-Uson P, Garcia-Cazorla A, et al. (2005) Encephalopathy with methylmalonic aciduria and homocystinuria secondary to a deficient exogenous supply of vitamin B12. *Rev Neurol* **16**: 605–8.

Haas D, Kelley RJ, Hoffmann GF (2001) Inherited disorders of cholesterol biosynthesis. *Neuropediatrics* 32: 113–22.

Häberle J, Görg B, Rutsch F, et al. (2005) Congenital glutamine deficiency with glutamine synthetase mutations. *N Engl J Med* 353: 1926–33.

Häberle J, Görg B, Toutain A, et al. (2006) Inborn error of amino acid synthesis: human glutamine synthetase deficiency. *J Inherit Metab Dis* 29: 352–8.

Hagberg B (1984) Krabbe's disease: clinical presentation of neurological variants. *Neuropediatrics* 15 (Suppl): 11–5.

Hagberg BA, Blennow G, Kristiansson B, Stibler H (1993) Carbohydrate-deficient glycoprotein syndromes: peculiar group of new disorders. *Pediatr Neurol* 9: 255–62.

Hall CA (1990) Function of vitamin B12 in the central nervous system as revealed by congenital defects. *Am J Hematol* 34: 121–7.

Hanley WB (2004) Adult phenylketonuria. *Am J Med* 117: 590–5.

Hansen TW, Henrichsen B, Rasmussen RK, et al. (1996) Neuropsychological and linguistic follow-up studies of children with galactosaemia from an unscreened population. *Acta Paediatr* 87: 1197–202.

Haworth JC, Dilling LA, Surtees RA, et al. (1993) Symptomatic and asymptomatic methylenetetrahydrofolate reductase deficiency in two adult brothers. *Am J Med Genet* 45: 572–6.

Hayasaka K, Tada K, Fueki N, et al. (1987) Nonketotic hyperglycinemia: analyses of glycine cleavage system in typical and atypical cases. *J Pediatr* 110: 873–7.

Head RA, Brown RM, Zolkipli Z, et al. (2005) Clinical and genetic spectrum of pyruvate dehydrogenase deficiency: dihydrolipoamide acetyltransferase (E2) deficiency. *Ann Neurol* 58: 234–41.

Hedlund GL, Longo N, Pasquali M (2006) Glutaric aciduria type 1. *Am J Med Genet C Semin Med Genet* 142: 86–94.

Hendriksz CJ, Corry PC, Wraith JE, et al. (2004) Juvenile Sandhoff disease—nine new cases and a review of the literature. *J Inherit Metab Dis* 27: 241–9.

Hirano M, Lagier-Tourenne C, Valentino ML, et al. (2005) Thymidine phosphorylase mutations cause instability of mitochondrial DNA. *Gene* 354: 152–6.

Hobson EE, Thomas S, Crofton PM, et al. (2005) Isolated sulphite oxidase deficiency mimics the features of hypoxic ischaemic encephalopathy. *Eur J Pediatr* 164: 655–9.

Hoffman TL, Simon EM, Ficicioglu C (2005) Biotinidase deficiency: the importance of adequate follow-up for inconclusive newborn screening result. *Eur J Pediatr* 164: 298–301.

Hoffmann B, Mayatepek E (2005) Neurological manifestations of lysosomal storage disorders – from pathology to first therapeutic possibilities. *Neuropediatrics* 36: 285–9.

Hoffmann GF, Charpentier C, Mayatepek E, et al. (1993) Clinical and biochemical phenotype in 11 patients with mevalonic aciduria. *Pediatrics* 91: 915–21.

Hoffmann GF, Jakobs C, Holmes B, et al. (1995) Organic acids in cerebrospinal fluid and plasma of patients with L-2-hydroxyglutaric aciduria. *J Inherit Metab Dis* 18: 189–93.

Hoffmann GF, Assmann B, Bräutigam C, et al. (2003) Tyrosine hydroxylase deficiency causes progressive encephalopathy and dopa-nonresponsive dystonia. *Ann Neurol* 54 Suppl 6: S56–65.

Hoffmann GF, Schmitt B, Windfuhr M, et al. (2007) Pyridoxal 5′-phosphate may be curative in early-onset epileptic encephalopathy. *J Inherit Metab Dis* 30: 96–9.

Honavar M, Janota I, Neville BG, Chalmers RA (1992) Neuropathology of biotinidase deficiency. *Acta Neuropathol* 84: 461–4.

Hoogenraad TU (1996) *Wilson's Disease. Major Problems in Neurology, vol 30*. London: WB Saunders.

Hoogenraad TU (2006) Paradigm shift in treatment of Wilson's disease: zinc therapy now treatment of choice. *Brain Dev* 28: 141–6.

Hoover-Fong JE, Shah S, Van Hove JL, et al. (2004) Natural history of nonketotic hyperglycinemia in 65 patients. *Neurology* 63: 1847–53.

Horvath R, Hudson G, Ferrari G, et al. (2006) Phenotypic spectrum associated with mutations of the mitochondrial polymerase γ gene. *Brain* 129: 1674–84.

Houwen RH, Juyn J, Hoogenraad TU, et al. (1995) H714Q mutation in Wilson disease is associated with late, neurological presentation. *J Med Genet* 32: 480–2.

Huisman TA, Thiel T, Steinmann B, et al. (2002) Proton magnetic resonance spectroscopy of the brain of a neonate with nonketotic hyperglycinemia: in vivo-in vitro (ex vivo) correlation. *Eur Radiol* 12: 858–61.

Huttenlocher PR, Hillman RE, Hsia YE (1970) Pseudotumor cerebri in galactosemia. *J Pediatr* 76: 902–5.

Hyland K, Kasim S, Egami K, et al. (2004) Tetrahydrobiopterin deficiency and dopamine loss in a genetic model of Lesch–Nyhan disease. *J Inherit Metab Dis* 27: 165–78.

Ichinose H, Ohye T, Takahashi E, et al. (1994) Hereditary progressive dystonia with marked diurnal fluctuation caused by mutations in the GTP cyclohydrolase I gene. *Nat Genet* 8: 236–42.

Imrie J, Dasgupta S, Besley GT, et al. (2007) The natural history of Niemann–Pick type C in the UK. *J Inherit Metab Dis* 30: 51–9.

Inagaki M, Hashimoto K, Yoshino K, et al. (1988) Atypical form of Menkes kinky hair disease with mitochondrial NADH-CoQ reductase deficiency. *Neuropediatrics* 19: 52–5.

Ince Z, Çoban A, Peker Ö, et al. (1995) Gaucher disease associated with congenital ichthyosis in the neonate. *Eur J Pediatr* 154: 418 (letter).

Iturriaga C, Pineda M, Fernandez-Valero EM, et al. (2006) Nieman–Pick C disease in Spain: clinical spectrum and development of a disability scale. *J Neurol Sci* 249: 1–6.

Jackson GH, Meyer A, Lippmann S (1994) Wilson's disease. Psychiatric manifestations may be the clinical presentation. *Postgrad Med* 95: 135–8.

Jacobs JM, Harding BN, Lake BD, et al. (1990) Peripheral neuropathy in Leigh's disease. *Brain* 113: 447–62.

Jaeken J, van den Berghe G (1984) An infantile autistic syndrome characterised by the presence of succinylpurines in body fluids. *Lancet* 2: 1058–61.

Jaeken J, Casaer P, DeCock P, et al. (1984) Gamma-hydrobutyric acid-transaminase deficiency: a newly recognized inborn error of neurotransmitter metabolism. *Neuropediatrics* 15: 165–9.

Jaffe EK, Stith L (2007) ALAD porphyria is a conformational disease. *Am J Hum Genet* 80: 329–37.

Jain A, Buist NR, Kennaway NG, et al. (1994) Effect of ascorbate or N-acetylcysteine treatment in a patient with hereditary glutathione synthetase deficiency. *J Pediatr* 124: 229–33.

Jakobs C, Jaeken J, Gibson KM (1993) Inherited disorders of GABA metabolism. *J Inherit Metab Dis* 16: 704–15.

Jeyakumar M, Thomas K, Ellit-Smith E, et al. (2003) Central nervous system inflammation is a hallmark of pathogenesis in mouse models of GM1 and GM2 gangliosidosis. *Brain* 126: 974–87.

Jinnah HA, Lewis RF, Visser JE, et al. (2001) Ocular motor dysfunction in Lesch–Nyhan disease. *Pediatr Neurol* 24: 200–4.

Jinnah HA, Harris JC, Nyhan WL, O'Neill JP (2004) The spectrum of mutations causing HPRT deficiency: an update. *Nucleosides Nucleotides Nucleic Acids* 23: 1153–60.

Jinnah HA, Visser JE, Harris JC, et al. (2006) Delineation of the motor disorder of Lesch–Nyhan disease. *Brain* 129: 1201–17.

Johnson JL, Rajagopalan KV, Renier WO, et al. (2002) Isolated sulfite oxidase deficiency: mutation analysis and DNA-based prenatal diagnosis. *Prenat Diagn* 22: 422–36.

Kaback M, Lim-Steele J, Dabholkar D, et al. (1993) Tay–Sachs disease—carrier screeening, prenatal diagnosis, and the molecular era. An international perspective, 1970 to 1993. The International TSD Data Collection Network. *JAMA* 270: 2307–15.

Kanwar YS, Manaligod JR, Wong PW (1976) Morphologic studies in a patient with homocystinuria due to 5,10-methylenetetrahydrofolate reductase deficiency. *Pediatr Res* 10: 598–609.

Kappler J, Sommerlade HJ, von Figura K, Gieselmann V (1994) Complex arylsulfatase A alleles causing metachromatic leukodystrophy. *Hum Mutat* 4: 119–25.

Kato T, Kato Z, Kuratsubo I, et al. (2005) Mutational and structural analysis of Japanese patients with mucopolysaccharidosis type II. *J Hum Genet* 50: 395–402.

Kattner E, Schäfer A, Harzer K (1997) Hydrops fetalis: manifestation in lysosomal diseases including Farber disease. *Eur J Pediatr* 156: 292–5.

Kaye EM, Ullman MD, Wilson ER, Barranger JA (1986) Type 2 and type 3 Gaucher disease: a morphological and biochemical study. *Arch Neurol* 20: 223–30.

Kenworthy L, Park T, Charnas LR (1993) Cognitive and behavioral profile of the oculocerebrorenal syndrome of Lowe. *Am J Med Genet* 46: 297–303.

Kerrigan JF, Aleck KA, Tarby TJ, et al. (2000) Fumaric aciduria: clinical and imaging features. *Ann Neurol* 47: 583–8.

Kim W, Pyeritz RE, Bernhardt BA, et al. (2007) Pulmonary manifestations of Fabry disease and positive response to enzyme replacement therapy. *Am J Med Genet A* 143: 377–81.

Klarner B, Klünemann HH, Lürding R, et al. (2007) Neuropsychological profile of adult patients with Niemann–Pick C1 (NPC1) mutations. *J Inherit Metab Dis* 30: 60–7.

Knappskog PM, Flatmark T, Mallet J, et al. (1995) Recessively inherited L-dopa-responsive dystonia caused by a point mutation (Q381K) in the tyrosine hydroxylase gene. *Hum Molec Genet* 4: 1209–12.

Kodama H, Murata Y, Kobayashi M (1999) Clinical manifestations of Menkes disease and its variants. *Pediatr Int* 41: 423–9.

Koelink CJ, van Hasselt P, van der Ploeg A, et al. (2006) Tyrosinemia type 1 treated by NTBC: how does AFP predict liver cancer? *Mol Genet Metab* 89: 310–5.

Koenig M (2003) Rare forms of autosomal recessive neurodegenerative ataxia. *Semin Pediatr Neurol* 10: 183–92.

Köhler M, Assmann B, Bräutigam C, et al. (1999) Adenylosuccinase deficiency: possibly underdiagnosed encephalopathy with variable clinical features. *Eur J Paediatr Neurol* 3: 3–6.

Kölker S, ed (2004) Proceedings in glutaryl-CoA dehydrogenase deficiency: Report of the 3rd International Workshop on Glutaryl-CoA Dehydrogenase Deficiency and the 1st Guidelines Meeting for Glutaryl-CoA Dehydrogenase Deficiency. *J Inherit Metab Dis* 27: 797–926.

Kölker S, Koeller DM, Okun JG, Hoffmann GF (2004) Pathomechanisms of neurodegeneration in glutaryl-CoA dehydrogenase deficiency. *Ann Neurol* 55: 7–12.

Kölker S, Christensen E, Leonard JV, et al. (2007) Guidelines for the diagnosis and management of glutaryl-CoA dehydrogenase deficiency (glutaric aciduria type I). *J Inherit Metab Dis* 30: 5–22.

Korenke GC, Hunneman DH, Kohler J, et al. (1995) Glyceroltrioleate/glyceroltrierucate therapy in 16 patients with X-chromosomal adrenoleukodystrophy/adrenomyeloneuropathy: effect on clinical, biochemical and neurophysiological parameters. *Eur J Pediatr* 154: 64–70.

Korenke G, Christen HJ, Hyland K, et al. (1997) Aromatic L-aminoacid decarboxylase deficiency: an extrapyramidal movement disorder with oculogyric crises. *Eur J Paediatr Neurol* 1: 67–71.

Korman SH, Boneh A, Ichinohe A, et al. (2004) Persistent NKH with transient or absent symptoms and a homozygous GLDC mutation. *Ann Neurol* 56: 139–43.

Korman SH, Wexler ID, Gutman A, et al. (2006) Treatment from birth of non-ketotic hyperglycinemia due to a novel GLDC mutation. *Ann Neurol* 59: 411–5.

Kranz C, Ng BG, Sun L, et al. (2007) COG8 deficiency causes new congenital disorder of glycosylation type IIh. *Hum Mol Genet* 16: 731–41.

Kraut JA, Sachs G (2005) Hartnup disorder: unraveling the mystery. *Trends Pharmacol Sci* 26: 53–5.

Kudo M, Brem MS, Canfield WM (2006) Mucolipidosis II (I-cell disease) and mucolipidosis IIIA (classical pseudo-hurler polydystrophy) are caused by mutations in the GlcNAc-phosphotransferase alpha / beta -subunits precursor gene. *Am J Hum Genet* 78: 451–63.

Kudo Y, Boyd CA (1996) Placental tyrosine transport and maternal phenylketonuria. *Acta Paediatr* 85: 109–10.

Kuhn J, Miyajima H, Takahashi Y, et al. (2005) Extrapyramidal and cerebellar movement disorder in association with heterozygous ceruloplasmin gene mutation. *J Neurol* 252: 111–3.

Kuriyama M, Fujiyama J, Yoshidome H, et al. (1991) Cerebrotendinous xanthomatosis: clinical and biochemical evaluation of eight patients and review of the literature. *J Neurol Sci* 102: 225–32.

Lancet (1990) Hereditary tyrosinaemia. *Lancet* 335: 1500–1.

Land JM, Mistry S, Squier M, et al. (1995) Neonatal carnitine palmitoyl-transferase-2 deficiency: a case presenting with myopathy. *Neuromuscul Disord* 5: 129–37.

Largillière C, Van Schaftingen E, Fontaine M, Farriaux JP (1991) D-glyceric acidaemia: clinical report and biochemical studies in a patient. *J Inherit Metab Dis* 14: 263–4.

Lee PJ, Ridout D, Walter JH, Cockburn F (2005) Maternal phenylketonuria: report from the United Kingdom registry 1978–97. *Arch Dis Child* 90: 143–6.

Leib JR, Gollust SE, Hull SC, Wilford BS (2005) Carrier screening panels for Ashkenazi Jews. Is more better? *Genet Med* 7: 185–90.

Lenke RR, Levy HL (1980) Maternal phenylketonuria and hyperphenylalaninemia: an international survey of the outcome of untreated and treated pregnancies. *N Engl J Med* 303: 1202–8.

Leonard JV, McKiernan PJ (2004) The role of liver transplantation in urea cycle disorders. *Mol Genet Metab* 81 Suppl 1: S74–8.

Leonard JV, Morris AA (2002) Urea cycle disorders. *Semin Neonatol* 7: 27–35.

Leonard JV, Walter JH, McKiernan PJ (2001) The management of organic acidaemias: the role of transplantation. *J Inherit Metab Dis* 24: 309–11.

Leone L, Ippoliti PF, Antonicelli R, et al. (1995) Treatment and liver transplantation for cholesterol ester storage disease. *J Pediatr* 127: 509–10.

Leroy JG (2006) Congenital disorders of N-glycosylation including diseases associated with O- as well as N-glycosylation defects. *Pediatr Res* 60: 643–6.

Levy HL, Lobbregt D, Barnes PD, et al. (1996) Maternal phenylketonuria: magnetic resonance imaging of the brain in offspring. *J Pediatr* 128: 770–5.

Lin DD, Crawford TO, Barker PB (2003) Proton MR spectroscopy in the diagnostic evaluation of suspected mitochondrial disease. *AJNR* 24: 33–41.

Lin SP, Chang JH, de la Cadena MP, et al. (2007) Mutation identification and characterization of a Taiwanese patient with fucosidosis. *J Hum Genet* 52: 553–6.

Lindenbaum Y, Dickson D, Rosenbaum P, et al. (2001) Xeroderma pigmentosum/Cockayne syndrome complex: first neuropathological study and review of eight other cases. *Eur J Paediatr Neurol* 5: 225–42.

Linthorst GE, Hollak CE, Donker-Koopman WE, et al. (2004) Enzyme therapy for Fabry disease: neutralizing antibodies toward agalsidase alpha and beta. *Kidney Int* 66: 1589–95.

Longo N, Amat Di San Filippo C, Pasquali M (2006) Disorders of carnitine transport and the carnitine cycle. *Am J Med Genet C* 142: 77–85.

Lopez LC, Schuelke M, Quinzii CM, et al. (2006) Leigh syndrome with nephropathy and CoQ10 deficiency due to decaprenyl diphosphate, synthase subunit 2 (PDSS2) mutations. *Am J Hum Genet* 79: 1125–9.

Lücke T, Das AM, Hartmann H, et al. (2007) Developmental outcome in five children with Hurler syndrome after stem cell transplantation: a pilot study. *Dev Med Child Neurol* 49: 693–6.

Lüdecke B, Dworniczak B, Bartholomé K (1995) A point mutation in the tyrosine hydroxylase gene associated with Segawa's syndrome. *Hum Genet* 95: 123–5.

Lukong KE, Elsliger MA, Chang Y, et al. (2000) Characterization of the sialidase molecular defects in sialidosis patients suggests the structural organization of the lysosomal multienzyme complex. *Hum Mol Genet* 9: 1075–85.

Ly TB, Peters V, Gibson KM, et al. (2003) Mutations in the AUH gene cause 3-methylglutaconic aciduria type I. *Hum Mutat* 21: 401–7.

Lyon G, Kolodny EH, Pastores GM (2006) *Neurology of Hereditary Metabolic Diseases of Children, 3rd edn.* New York: McGraw-Hill.

Magera MJ, Gunawardena ND, Hahn SH, et al. (2006) Quantitative determination of succinylacetone in dried blood spots for newborn screening of tyrosinemia type 1. *Mol Genet Metab* 88: 16–21.

Mahmood A, Dubey P, Moser HW, Moser A (2005) X-linked adrenoleukodystrophy: therapeutic approaches to distinct phenotypes. *Pediatr Transplant* 9 Suppl 7: 55–62.

Man in't Veld AJ, Boomsma F, Moleman P, Schalekamp MA (1987) Congenital dopamine-beta-hydroxylase deficiency. A novel orthostatic syndrome. *Lancet* 1: 183–8.

Marcellini M, Di Commo V, Callea F, et al. (2005) Treatment of Wilson's disease with zinc in pediatric patients: a single hospital primary follow-up study. *J Lab Clin Med* 145: 139–43.

Marescau B, De Deyn PP, Lowenthal A, et al. (1990) Guanidino compound, analysis as a complementary diagnostic parameter for hyperargininemia: follow-up of guanidino compound levels during therapy. *Pediatr Res* 27: 297–303.

Marie S, Flipsen JW, Duran M, et al. (2000) Prenatal diagnosis in adenosyl succinic lyase deficiency. *Prenat Diagn* 20: 33–6.

Maroteaux P (1973) [A new type of mucopolysaccharidosis with athetosis and urinary excretion of keratan sulphate.] *Nouv Presse Med* 2: 975–9 (French).

Marquet J, Chadefaux B, Bonnefont JP, et al. (1994) Methylene-tetrahydrofolate reductase defiency: prenatal diagnosis and family studies. *Prenat Diagn* 14: 29–33.

Martin PT (2005) The dystroglycanopathies: the new disorders of O-linked glycosylation. *Semin Paediatr Neurol* 152: 152–8.

Martinez M (1996) Docosahexaenoic acid therapy in docosahexaenoic acid-deficent patients with disorders of peroxisomal biogenesis. *Lipids* 31 Suppl: S145–52.

Martinez M, Vazquez E (1998) MRI evidence that docosahexaenoic acid ethyl ester improves myelination in generalized peroxisomal disorders. *Neurology* 51: 26–32.

Martinez-Lage JF, Casas C, Fernández MA, et al. (1994) Macrocephaly, dystonia, and bilateral temporal arachnoid cysts: glutaric aciduria type I. *Childs Nerv Syst* 10: 198–203.

Matalon R, Michals K, Sebesta D, et al. (1988) Aspartoacylase deficiency and N-acetylaspartic aciduria in patients with Canavan disease. *Am J Med Genet* **29**: 463–71.

Matalon R, Michals K, Gao GP, et al. (1995) Prenatal diagnosis for Canavan disease: the use of DNA markers. *J Inherit Metab Dis* **18**: 215–7.

Matern D, He M, Berry SA, et al. (2003) Prospective diagnosis of 2-methyl-butyryl-CoA dehydrogenase deficiency in the Hmong population by newborn screening using tandem mass spectrometry. *Pediatrics* **112**: 74–8.

Matheus MG, Castillo M, Smith JK, et al. (2004) Brain MRI findings in patients with mucopolysaccharidosis types I and II with mild clinical presentation. *Neuroradiology* **46**: 666–72.

Matsuo M, Tasaki R, Kodama H, Hamasaki Y (2005) Screening for Menkes disease using the urine HVA/VMA ratio. *J Inherit Metab Dis* **28**: 89–93.

Mattson LR, Lindor NR, Goldman (1995) Central pontine myelinolysis as a complication of partial ornithine carbamoyl transferase deficiency. *Am J Med Genet* **60**: 210–3.

Matsuzawa F, Aikawa S, Sakuraba H, et al. (2003) Structural basis of the GM2 gangliosidosis B variant. *J Hum Genet* **48**: 582–9.

McKiernan PJ (2006) Nitisinone in the treatment of hereditary tyrosinemia type 1. *Drugs* **66**: 743–50.

McManaman J, Tam DA (1999) Gabapentin for self-injurious behavior in Lesch–Nyhan syndrome. *Pediatr Neurol* **20**: 381–2.

Medalia A, Isaacs-Glaberman K, Scheinberg H (1988) Neuropsychological impairment in Wilson's disease. *Arch Neurol* **45**: 502–4.

Menkes JH (1999) Menkes disease and Wilson disease: two sides of the same copper coin. Part I: Menkes disease. *Eur J Paediatr Neurol* **3**: 147–58.

Messina E, Micheli V, Giacomello A (2005) Guanine nucleotide depletion induces differentiation and aberrant neurite outgrowth in human dopaminergic neuroblastoma lines: a model for basal ganglia dysfunction in Lesch–Nyhan disease. *Neurosci Lett* **375**: 97–100.

Mills PB, Struys E, Jakobs C, et al. (2006) Mutations in antiquitin in individuals with pyridoxine-dependent seizures. *Nat Med* **12**: 307–9.

Miné M, Brivet M, Schiff M, et al. (2006) A novel gross deletion caused by non-homologous recombination of the PDHX gene in a patient with pyruvate dehydrogenase deficiency. *Mol Genet Metab* **89**: 106–10.

Mistry PK (1995) Genotype/phenotype correlations in Gaucher's disease. *Lancet* **346**: 982–3.

Mitchell G, Larochelle J, Lambert M, et al. (1990) Neurologic crises in hereditary tyrosinemia. *N Engl J Med* **322**: 432–7.

Mize C, Johnson JL, Rajagopalan KV (1995) Defective molybdopterin biosynthesis: clinical heterogeneity associated with molybdenum cofactor deficiency. *J Inherit Metab Dis* **18**: 283–90.

Mochel F, de Lonlay P, Touati G, et al. (2005) Pyruvate carboxylase deficiency: clinical and biochemical response to anaplerotic diet therapy. *Mol Genet Metab* **84**: 305–12.

Molinari F, Raas-Rothschild A, Rio M, et al. (2005) Impaired mitochondrial glutamate transport in autosomal recessive neonatal myoclonic epilepsy. *Am J Hum Genet* **76**: 334–9.

Monagle PT, Tauro GP (1995) Long term follow up of patients with transcobalamin II deficiency. *Arch Dis Child* **72**: 237–8.

Montano AM, Kaitila L, Sukagawa K, et al. (2003) Mucopolysaccharidosis IVA: characteristics of a common mutation found in Finnish patients with attenuated phenotype. *Hum Genet* **113**: 162–9.

Morel CF, Watkins D, Scott P, et al. (2005) Prenatal diagnosis for methylmalonic acidemia and inborn errors of vitamin B12 metabolism and transport. *Mol Genet Metab* **86**: 160–71.

Morton DH, Strauss KA, Robinson DL, et al. (2002) Diagnosis and treatment of maple syrup disease: a study of 36 patients. *Pediatrics* **109**: 999–1008.

Moser AB, Kreiter N, Bezman L, et al. (1999) Plasma very long chain fatty acids in 3,000 peroxisome disease patients and 29,000 controls. *Ann Neurol* **45**: 100–10.

Moser HW (1989) Peroxisomal diseases. *Adv Pediatr* **36**: 1–38.

Moser HW, Smith KD, Moser AB (1995) X-linked adrenoleukodystrophy. In: Scriver C, Beaudet AI, Sly WS, Valle D, eds. *The Metabolic and Molecular Bases of Inherited Disease, 7th edn.* New York: McGraw-Hill, pp. 2325–49.

Möslinger D, Mühl A, Suormala T, et al. (2003) Molecular characterisation and neuropsychological outcome of 21 patients with profound biotinidase deficiency detected by newborn screening and family studies. *Eur J Pediatr* **162**: S46–9.

Mudd SH, Skovby F, Levy HL, et al. (1985) The natural history of homocystinuria due to cystathionine beta-synthase deficiency. *Am J Hum Genet* **37**: 1–31.

Mudd SH, Levy HL, Skovby F (1995) The disorders of transulfuration. In: Scriver CR, Beaudet AL, Sly WS, Valle D, eds. *The Metabolic and Molecular Bases of Inherited Disease, 7th edn.* New York: McGraw-Hill, pp. 1279–327.

Munakata M, Sakamoto O, Kitamura T, et al. (2005) The effects of histidine therapy on brain metabolism in a patient with Menkes disease: a proton magnetic resonance spectroscopic study. *Brain Dev* **27**: 237–300.

Muntau AC, Röschinger W, Habich M, et al. (2002) Tetrahydrobiopterin as an alternative treatment for mild phenylketonuria. *N Engl J Med* **347**: 2122–32.

Muntoni F, Brockington M, Torelli S, Brown SC (2004) Defective glycosylation in congenital muscular dystrophies. *Curr Opin Neurol* **17**: 205–9.

Muntoni S, Wiebusch H, Funke H, et al. (1995) Homozygosity for a splice junction mutation in exon 8 of the gene encoding lysosomal acid lipase in a Spanish kindred with cholesterol ester storage disease (CESD). *Hum Genet* **95**: 491–4.

Muthane U, Chickabasaviah Y, Kaneski C, et al. (2004) Clinical features of adult GM1 gangliosidosis: report of three Indian cases. *Mov Disord* **19**: 1334–41.

Myall NJ, Wreden CC, Wlizla M, Reimer RJ (2007) G328E and G409E sialin missense mutations similarly impair transport activity, but differentially affect trafficking. *Mol Genet Metab* **92**: 371–4.

Myers LA, Hershfield MS, Neale WT, et al. (2004) Purine nucleoside phosphorylase deficiency (PPP-def) presenting with lymphopenia and developmental delay: successful correction with umbilical cord blood transplantation. *J Pediatr* **145**: 710–12.

Naidu S, Hofmann KJ, Moser HW, et al. (1988) Galactosylceramide-beta-galactosidase deficiency in association with cherry red spot. *Neuropediatrics* **19**: 46–8.

Nardocci N, Bertagnolio B, Rumi V, Angelini L (1992) Progressive dystonia symptomatic of juvenile GM2 gangliosidosis. *Mov Disord* **7**: 64–7.

Nardocci N, Bertagnolio B, Rumi V, et al. (1993) Chronic GM1 gangliosidosis presenting as dystonia: clinical and biochemical studies in a new case. *Neuropediatrics* **24**: 164–6.

Nassogne M, Henrot B, Aubert G, et al. (2000) Adenylosuccinase deficiency: an unusual cause of early-onset epilepsy associated with acquired microcephaly. *Brain Dev* **22**: 383–6.

Nassogne MC, Commare MC, Lellouch-Tubiana A, et al. (2003) Unusual presentation of GM2 gangliosidosis mimicking a brain stem tumor in a 3-year-old girl. *AJNR* **24**: 840–2.

Navon R, Khosravi R, Korczyn T, et al. (1995) A new mutation in the HEXA gene associated with a spinal muscular atrophy phenotype. *Neurology* **45**: 539–43.

Neudorfer O, Pastores GM, Zeng BJ, et al. (2005) Late-onset Tay–Sachs disease: phenotypic characterization and genotypic correlations in 21 affected patients. *Genet Med* **7**: 119–23.

Neumann LM, von Moers A, Kunze J, et al. (2003) Congenital disorder of glycosylation type 1a in a macrosomic 16-month-old boy with an atypical phenotype and homozygosity of the N2161 mutation. *Eur J Pediatr* **162**: 710–3.

Nguyen TV, Andresen BS, Corydon TJ, et al. (2002) Identification of isobutyryl-CoA dehydrogenase and its deficiency in humans. *Mol Genet Metab* **77**: 68–79.

Nishino I, Pinazzola A, Hirano M (2001) MNGIE: from nuclear DNA to mitochondrial DNA. *Neuromuscul Disord* **11**: 7–10.

Noelle V, Knuepfer M, Pulzer F, et al. (2005) Unusual presentation of congenital disorder of glycosylation 1a: congenital persistent thrombocytopenia, hypertrophic cardiomyopathy and hydrops-like aspect due to marked peripheral oedema. *Eur J Pediatr* **164**: 223–6.

Noll RB, Netzloff ML, Kulkarni R (1989) Long-term follow-up of biochemical and cognitive functioning in patients with mannosidosis. *Arch Neurol* **46**: 507–509.

Nordborg C, Hagberg B, Kristiansson B. (1991) Sural nerve pathology in the carbohydrate-deficient glycoprotein sybdrome. *Acta Paediatr Scand Suppl* **375**: 39–49.

North KN, Hoppel CL, De Girolami U, et al. (1995) Lethal neonatal deficiency of carnitine palmitoyltransferase II associated with dysgenesis of the brain and kidneys. *J Pediatr* **127**: 414–20.

Novotny EJ, Fulbright RK, Pearl PL, et al. (2003) Magnetic resonance spectroscopy of neurotransmitters in human brain. *Ann Neurol* **54** Suppl 6: S25–31.

Nyhan WL (2005) Disorders of purine and pyrimidine metabolism. *Mol Genet Metab* **86**: 25–33.

Nyhan WL, Vuong LU, Broock R (2003) Prenatal diagnosis of Lesch–Nyhan disease. *Prenat Diagn* 23: 807–9.

Oder W, Grimm G, Kollegger H, et al. (1991) Neurological and neuropsychiatric spectrum of Wilson's disease: a prospective study of 45 cases. *J Neurol* 238: 281–7.

Ogasawara N, Stout JT, Goto H, et al. (1989) Molecular analysis of a female Lesch–Nyhan patient. *J Clin Invest* 24: 1024–7.

Ogier de Baulny H, Superti-Furga A (2006) Disorders of mitochondrial fatty acid oxidation and ketone body metabolism. In: Blau N, Hoffmann GF, Leonard J, Clarke JT, eds. *Physician's Guide to the Treatment and Follow-up of Metabolic Diseases*. Berlin: Springer, pp. 147–60.

Ogier de Baulny H, Gérard M, Saudubray JM, Zittoun J (1998) Remethylation defects: guidelines for clinical diagnosis and treatment. *Eur J Pediatr* 157: S77–83.

Ogier de Baulny H, Benoist JF, Rigal O, et al. (2005) Methylmalonic and propionic acidemias: management and outcome. *J Inherit Metab Dis* 28: 415–23.

Olivos-Glander IM, Jänne PA, Nussbaum RL (1995) The oculocerebrorenal syndrome gene product is a 105-kD protein localized to the Golgi complex. *Am J Hum Genet* 57: 817–23.

Olson L, Houlihan D (2000) A review of behavioral treatments used for Lesch–Nyhan syndrome. *Behav Modif* 24: 202–22.

Ono S, Kurisaki H (1988) An unusual neurological disorder with abnormal copper metabolism. *J Neurol* 235: 397–9.

Ostergaard E, Hansen FJ, Sorensen N, et al. (2007) Mitochondrial encephalomyopathy with elevated methylmalonic acid is caused by SUCLA2 mutations. *Brain* 130: 853–61.

Otero LJ, Brown GK, Silver K, et al. (1995) Association of cerebral dysgenesis and lactic acidemia with X-linked PDH E1α subunit mutations in females. *Pediatr Neurol* 13: 327–32.

Ozand PT, Gascon G, Al Essa M, et al. (1998) Biotin-responsive basal ganglia disease: a novel entity. *Brain* 121: 1267–79.

Ozkinay F, Pehlivan S, Onay H, et al. (2007) Purine nucleoside phosphorylase deficiency in a patient with spastic paraplegia and recurrent infections. *J Child Neurol* 22: 741–3.

Pall HS, Williams AC, Blake DR, et al. (1987) Movement disorder associated with abnormal copper metabolism and decreased blood antioxidants. *J Neurol Neurosurg Psychiatry* 50: 1234–5.

Palomaki GE, Williams J, Haddow JE, Natowicz MR (1995) Tay–Sachs disease in persons of French-Canadian heritage in northern New England. *Am J Med Genet* 56: 409–12.

Pastores GT, Barnett NL, Kolodny EH (2005) An open-label, noncomparative study of miglustat in type I Gaucher disease: efficacy and tolerability over 24 months of treatment. *Clin Ther* 27: 1215–27.

Pastoris O, Savasta S, Foppa P, et al. (1996) Pyruvate dehydrogenase deficiency in a child responsive to thiamine treatment. *Acta Paediatr* 85: 625–8.

Pavlu-Pereira H, Asfaw B, Poupctová H, et al. (2005) Acid sphingomyelinase deficiency. Phenotype variability with prevalence of intermediate phenotype in a series of twenty-five Czech and Slovak patients. A multi-approach study. *J Inherit Metab Dis* 28: 203–27.

Pearl PL, Gibson KM (2004) Clinical aspects of the disorders of GABA metabolism in children. *Curr Opin Neurol* 17: 107–13.

Pearl PL, Novotny EJ, Acosta MT, et al. (2003) Succinic semialdehyde dehydrogenase deficiency in children and adults. *Ann Neurol* 54 Suppl 6: S73–80.

Pearl PL, Capp PK, Novotny EJ, Gibson KM (2005) Inherited disorders of neurotransmitters in children and adults. *Clin Biochem* 38: 1051–8.

Pedersen CB, Bischoff C, Christensen E, et al. (2006) Variations in IBD (ACAD8) in children with elevated C4-carnitine detected by tandem mass spectrometry newborn screening. *Pediatr Res* 60: 315–20.

Plecko B, Stockler-Ipsiroglu S, Paschka E, et al. (2000) Pipecolic acid elevation in plasma and cerebrospinal fluid of two patients with pyridoxine dependency. *Ann Neurol* 48: 121–5.

Poll-Thé BT, Gootjes J, Duran M, et al. (2004a) Peroxisome biogenesis disorders with prolonged survival: phenotypic expression in a cohort of 31 patients. *Am J Med Genet A* 126: 333–8.

Poll-Thé BT, Wanders RJ, Ruiter JP, et al. (2004b) Spastic diplegia and white matter abnormalities in 2-methyl-3-hydroxyisobutyryl-CoA dehydrogenase deficiency, a defect of isoleucine metabolism: differential diagnosis with hypoxic–ischemic brain diseases. *Mol Genet Metab* 81: 295–9.

Poll-Thé BT, Aubourg P, Wanders RJ (2006) Peroxisomal disorders. In: Fernandes J, Saudubray JM, van den Berghe G, Walter JH, eds. *Inborn Metabolic Diseases. Diagnosis and Treatment, 4th edn*. Berlin: Springer-Verlag, pp. 509–22.

Pons R, Ford B, Chiriboga CA, et al. (2004) Aromatic L-amino acid decarboxylase deficiency. *Neurology* 62: 1058–65.

Ponzone A, Spada M, Ferraris S, et al. (2004) Dihydropteridine reductase deficiency in man: from biology to treatment. *Med Res Rev* 24: 127-50.

Prella M, Baccala R, Hoesberger JD, et al. (2001) Haemolytic onset of Wilson disease in a patient with homologous truncation of ATP7B at Arg 1319. *Br J Haematol* 114: 230–32.

Prietsch V, Mayatepek E, Krastel H, et al. (2003) Mevalonate kinase deficiency: enlarging the clinical and biochemical spectrum. *Pediatrics* 111: 258–61.

Proud VK, Mussell HG, Kaler SG, et al. (1996) Distinctive Menkes disease variant with occipital horns: delineation and natural history and clinical phenotype. *Am J Med Genet* 65: 44–51.

Puig JG, Torres RJ, Mateos FA, et al. (2001) The spectruim of hypoxanthine-guanine-phosphoribosyl transferase (HPRT) deficiency. Clinical experience based on 22 patients from 18 Spanish families. *Medicine* 80: 102–12.

Putman CW, Rotteveel JJ, Wevers RA, et al. (1997) Dihydropyrimidinase deficiency, a progressive neurological disorder. *Neuropediatrics* 28: 106–10.

Qi M, Byers PH (1998) Constitutive skipping of alternatively spliced exon 10 in the ATP7A gene abolishes Golgi localization of the menkes protein and produces occipital horn syndrome. *Hum Molec Genet* 7: 465–9.

Qiu A, Jansen M, Sakaris A, et al. (2006) Identification of an intestinal folate transporter and the molecular basis for hereditary folate malabsorption. *Cell* 127: 917–28.

Quinzii C, DiMauro S, Hirano M (2007) Human coenzyme Q10 deficiency. *Neurochem Res* 32: 723–7.

Ramaekers VT, Blau N (2004) Cerebral folate deficiency. *Dev Med Child Neurol* 46: 843–51.

Ramaekers VT, Rotheberg SP, Sequeira JM, et al. (2005) Autoantibodies to folate receptors in the cerebral folate deficiency syndrome. *N Engl J Med* 352: 1985–91.

Rapin I, Goldfisher S, Katzman R, et al. (1978) The cherry-red spot myoclonus syndrome. *Ann Neurol* 3: 234–42.

Rapin I, Lindenbaum Y, Dickson DW, et al. (2000) Cockayne syndrome and xeroderma pigmentosum. *Neurology* 55: 1442–9.

Ray PF, Harper JC, Ao A, et al. (1999) Successful preimplantation genetic diagnosis for sex linked Lesch–Nyhan syndrome using specific diagnosis. *Prenat Diagn* 19: 1237–41.

Rees MI, Lewis TM, Kwook JB, et al. (2002) Hyperekplexia associated with compound heterozygote mutations of the human inhibitory glycine recptor (GLRB). *Hum Mol Genet* 11: 853–60.

Reiss J, Johnson JL (2003) Mutations in the molybdenum cofactor biosynthesis genes MOCS1, MOCS2, and GEPH. *Hum Mutat* 21: 569–76.

Renlund M, Kovanen PT, Raivio KO, et al. (1986) Studies on the defect underlying the lysosomal storage of sialic acid in Salla disease. *J Clin Invest* 77: 568–74.

Ries M, Gupta S, Moore DF, et al. (2005) Pediatric Fabry disease. *Pediatrics* 115: e344–55.

Rizzo WB, Dammann AL, Craft DA, et al. (1989) Sjögren–Larsson syndrome: inherited defect in the fatty alcohol cycle. *J Pediatr* 115: 228–34.

Robain O, Aubourg P, Routon MC, et al. (1988) Menkes disease: a Golgi and electron microscopic study of the cerebellar cortex. *Clin Neuropathol* 7: 47–52.

Robbins JH, Brumback RA, Mendiones M, et al. (1991) Neurological disease in xeroderma pigmentosum. Documentation of a late onset type of the juvenile onset form. *Brain* 114: 1335–61.

Robertson A, Singh RH, Guerrero NV, et al. (2000) Outcomes analysis of verbal dyspraxia in classic galactosemia. *Genet Med* 2: 142–8.

Robey KL, Beck JF, Giacomini KD, et al. (2003) Modes and patterns of self-mutilation in persons with Lesch–Nyhan disease. *Dev Med Child Neurol* 45: 167–71.

Robinson BH (2006) Lactic acidemia and mitochondrial disease. *Mol Genet Metab* 89: 3–13.

Robinson RO, Fensom AH, Lake BD (1997) Salla disease—rare or under-diagnosed? *Dev Med Child Neurol* 39: 153–7.

Roels F, Pauwels M, Poll-Thé BT, et al. (1988) Hepatic peroxisomes in adrenoleukodystrophy and related syndromes: cytochemical and morphometric data. *Virchows Arch A Pathol Anat Histopathol* 413: 275–85.

Roh JK, Lee TG, Wie BA, et al. (1994) Initial and follow-up brain MRI findings and correlation with the clinical course in Wilson's disease. *Neurology* 44: 1064–8.

Ron I, Horowitz M (2005) ER retention and degradation as the molecular basis underlying Gaucher disease heterogeneity. *Hum Molec Genet* 14: 2387–98.

Rosenblatt DS, Whitehead VM (1999) Cobalamin and folate deficiency: acquired and hereditary disorders in children. *Semin Hematol* 36: 19–34.

Rossi A, Cerone R, Biancheri R, et al. (2001) Early-onset combined methylmalonic aciduria and homocystinuria: neuroradiologic findings. *AJNR* 22: 554–63.

Roth A, Nogues C, Monnet JP, et al. (1985) Anatomo-pathological findings in a case of combined deficiency of sulphite oxidase and xanthine oxidase with a defect of molybdenum cofactor. *Virchows Arch A Pathol Anat Histopathol* 405: 379–86.

Roze E, Gervais D, Demeret S, et al. (2003) Neuropsychiatric disturbances in presumed late-onset cobalamin C disease. *Arch Neurol* 60: 1457–62.

Roze E, Paschke E, Lopez N, et al. (2005) Dystonia and parkinsonism in GM1 type 3 gangliosidosis. *Mov Disord* 20: 1366–9.

Rucker JC, Shapiro BE, Han YH, et al. (2004) Neuro-ophthamology of late-onset Tay–Sachs diseaase (LOTS). *Neurology* 63: 1918–26.

Sakuraba H, Itoh K, Shimmoto M, et al. (1999) GM2 gangliosidosis AB variant: clinical and biochemical studies of a Japanese patient. *Neurology* 52: 372–7.

Salomons GS, van Dooren SJ, Verhoeven NM, et al. (2003) X-linked creatine transporter defect: an overview. *J Inherit Metab Dis* 26: 309–18.

Salomons GS, Jakobs C, Landegge Pope L, et al. (2007) Clinical, enzymatic and molecular characterization of nine new patients with malonyl-coenzyme A decarboxylase deficiency. *J Inherit Metab Dis* 30: 23–8.

Saxonhouse MA, Behnke M, Williams JL, et al. (2003) Mucopolysaccharidosis type VII presenting with isolated ascites. *J Perinatol* 23: 73–5.

Scaglia F, Lee B (2006) Clinical, biochemical, and molecular spectrum of hyperargininemia due to arginase 1 deficiency. *Am J Med Genet C Semin Med Genet* 142C: 113–20.

Schaefer E, Mehta A, Gal A (2005) Genotype and phenotype in Fabry disease: analysis of the Fabry Outcome Survey. *Acta Paediatr Suppl* 94: 87–92; discussion 79.

Schiff M, Levrat V, Acquaviva C, et al. (2006a) A case of pyruvate carboxylase deficiency with atypical clinical and radiological presentation. *Mol Genet Metab* 87: 175–7.

Schiff M, Miné M, Brivet M, et al. (2006b) Leigh's disease due to a new mutation in the PDHX gene. *Ann Neurol* 59: 709–14.

Schmidt H, Ullrich K, von Lengerke HJ, et al. (1987) Radiological findings in patients with mucopolysaccharidosis I H/S (Hurler–Scheie syndrome). *Pediatr Radiol* 17: 409–14.

Schneider JF, Boltshauser E, Neuhaus TJ, et al. (2001) MRI and proton spectroscopy in Lowe syndrome. *Neuropediatrics* 32: 45–8.

Schretlen DJ, Harris JC, Park KS, et al. (2001) Neurocognitive functioning in Lesch–Nyhan disease and partial hypoxanthine-guanine-phosporibosyl transferase deficiency. *J Int Neuropsychol Soc* 7: 805–12.

Schuchman EH (1995) Two new mutations in the acid sphingomyelinase gene causing type A Niemann–Pick disease: N389T and R441X. *Hum Mutat* 6: 352–7.

Schuchman EH, Desnick RJ (1995) Niemann–Pick diseases types A and B: acid sphingomyelinase deficiency. In: Scriver CR, Beaudet AL, Sly WS, Valle D, eds. *The Metabolic and Molecular Bases of Inherited Disease, 7th Edn.* New York: McGraw-Hill, pp. 2601–24.

Schulze A (2003) Creatine deficiency syndromes. *Mol Cell Biochem* 244: 143–50.

Schwab MA, Sauer SW, Okun JG, et al. (2006) Secondary mitochondrial dysfunction in propionic aciduria: a pathogenic role for endogenous mitochondrial toxins. *Biochem J* 398: 107–12.

Segal S (1993) The challenge of galactosemia. *Int Pediatr* 8: 125–32.

Seijo-Martinez M, Navarro C, Castro del Rio M, et al. (2005) L-2-hydroxyglutaric aciduria: clinical, neuroimaging, and neuropathological findings. *Arch Neurol* 62: 666–70.

Selhub J, Miller JW (1992) The pathogenesis of homocysteinemia: interruption of the coordinate regulation by S-adenosylmethionine of the remethylation and transsulfuration of homocysteine. *Am J Clin Nutr* 55: 131–8.

Sener RN (2004) Lowe syndrome: proton MR spectroscopy, and diffusion MR imaging. *J Neuroradiol* 31: 238–40.

Sener RN (2005a) Brain magnetic resonance imaging in tyrosinemia. *Acta Radiol* 46: 618–20.

Sener RN (2005b) Tyrosinemia: computed tomography, magnetic resonance imaging, diffusion magnetic resonance imaging, and proton spectroscopy findings in the brain. *J Comput Assist Tomogr* 29: 323–5.

Sévin M, Lesca G, Baumann N, et al. (2007) The adult form of Niemann–Pick disease type C. *Brain* 130: 120–33.

Sharer JD (2005) The adenine nucleotide translocase type I (ANT1): a new factor in mitochondrial disease. *Life* 57: 607–14.

Shevell MI, Matthews PM, Scriver CR, et al. (1994) Cerebral dysgenesis and lactic acidemia: An MRI/MRS phenotype associated with pyruvate dehydrogenase deficiency. *Pediatr Neurol* 11: 224–9.

Shimizu N, Yamaguchi Y, Aoki T (1999) Treatment and management of Wison's disease. *Pediatr Int* 41: 418–32.

Sim KG, Hammond J, Wilcken B (2002) Strategies for the diagnosis of mitochondrial fatty acid ,-oxidation disorders. *Clin Chim Acta* 323: 37–58.

Simon A, Kremer HP, Wevers RA, et al. (2004) Mevalonate kinase deficiency: evidence for a phenotypic continuum. *Neurology* 62: 994–7.

Slaugenhaupt SA (2002) The molecular basis of mucolipidosis type IV. *Curr Mol Med* 2: 445–50.

Sleat DE, Wiseman JA, El-Banna M, et al. (2004) Genetic evidence for non-redundant functional cooperativity between NPC1 and NPC2 in lipid transport. *Proc Natl Acad Sci USA* 101: 5886–91.

Smith I, Brenton DP (1995) Hyperphenylalaninaemias. In: Fernandes J, Saudubray JM, van den Berghe G, eds. *Inborn Metabolic Diseases. Diagnosis and Treatment. 2nd edn.* Berlin: Springer-Verlag, pp. 147–60.

Smith W, Kishnani PS, Lee B, et al. (2005) Urea cycle disorders: clinical presentation outside the newborn period. *Crit Care Clin* 21 (Suppl): S9–17.

Soffer D, Benharroch D, Berginer V (1995) The neuropathology of cerebrotendinous xanthomatosis revisited: a case report and review of the literature. *Acta Neuropathol* 90: 213–20.

Sparks SE (2006) Inherited disorders of glycosylation. *Mol Genet Metab* 87: 1–7.

Spiegel R, Bach G, Sury V, et al. (2005) A mutation in the saponin A coding region of the prosaponine gene in an infant presenting as Krabbe disease: first report of saponin A deficiency in humans. *Mol Genet Metab* 84: 160–6.

Spiekerkoetter U, Bennett MJ, Ben-Zeev B, et al. (2004) Peripheral neuropathy, episodic myoglobinuria, and respiratory failure in deficiency of the mitochondrial trifunctional protein. *Muscle Nerve* 29: 66–72.

Stacpoole PW, Kerr DS, Barnes C, et al. (2006) Controlled clinical trial of dichloroacetate for treatment of congenital lactic acidosis in children. *Pediatrics* 117: 1519–31.

Steiner RD, Sweetser DA, Rohrbaugh JR, et al. (1996) Nonketotic hyperglycinemia: atypical clinical and biochemical manifestations. *J Pediatr* 128: 243–6.

Stibler H, Blennow G, Kristiansson B, et al. (1994) Carbohydrate-deficient glycoprotein syndrome: clinical expression in adults with a new metabolic disease. *J Neurol Neurosurg Psychiatry* 57: 552–6.

Stöckler S, Holzbach U, Hanefeld F, et al. (1994) Creatine deficiency in the brain: a new, treatable inborn error of metabolism. *Pediatr Res* 36: 409–13.

Straussberg R, Shorer Z, Weitz R, et al. (2002) Familial infantile bilateral striatal necrosis: clinical features and response to biotin treatment. *Neurology* 59: 983–9.

Stromme P, Maehlen J, Strom EH, Torvik A (1991) Postmortem findings in two patients with carbohydrate-deficient glycoprotein syndrome. *Acta Paediatr Scand Suppl* 375: 55–62.

Struys EA (2006) D-2-hydroxyglutaric aciduria: unravelling the biochemical pathway and the genetic defect. *J Inherit Metab Dis* 29: 21–9.

Subramanian I, Vanek ZF, Bronstein JM (2002) Diagnosis and treatment of Wilson's disease. *Curr Neurol Neurosci Rep* 2: 317–23.

Surrendran S, Michals-Matalon K, Krywawych S, et al. (2002) DOOR syndrome : Deficiency of E1 component of the 2-oxoglutarate dehydrogenase deficiency complex. *Am J Med Genet* 113: 371–4.

Surtees R (1998) Demyelination and inborn errors of the single carbon transfer pathway. *Eur J Pediatr* 157 Suppl 2: S118–21.

Surtees R (2001) Cobalamin and folate responsive disorders. In: Baxter P, ed. *Vitamin Responsive Conditions in Paediatric Neurology. International Review of Child Neurology Series.* London: Mac Keith Press for the International Child Neurology Association, pp. 96–108.

Suzuki Y, Shimozawa N, Orii T, et al. (1988) Molecular analysis of peroxisomal beta-oxidation enzymes in infants with Zellweger syndrome and Zellweger-like syndrome: further heterogenicity of the peroxisomal disorder. *Clin Chim Acta* 172: 65–76.

Suzuki Y, Sakuraba H, Oshima A, et al. (1991) Clinical and molecular heterogeneity in hereditary beta-galactosidase deficiency. *Dev Neurosci* 13: 299–303.

Swoboda KJ, Saul JP, McKenna CE, et al. (2003) Aromatic L-amino acid decarboxylase deficiency: overview of clinical features and outcomes. *Ann Neurol* 54 Suppl 6: S49–55.

324

Tabarki B, Yacoub M, Tlili K, et al. (2003) Familial spastic paraplegia as the presenting manifestation in patients with purine nucleoside phosphorylase deficiency. *J Child Neurol* **18**: 140–1.

Takahashi S, Ishii K, Matsumoto K, et al. (1993) Cranial MRI and MR angiography in Menkes' syndrome. *Neuroradiology* **35**: 556–8.

Takanashi J, Barkovich J, Cheng SF, et al. (2003) Brain MR imaging in neonatal hyperammonemic encephalopathy resulting from proximal urea cycle disorders. *AJNR* **24**: 1184–7.

Tan ES, Wiley V, Carpenter K, Wilcken B (2007) Non-ketotic hyperglycinemia is usually not detectable by tandem mass spectrometry newborn screening. *Mol Genet Metab* **90**: 446–8.

Tanaka R, Momoi T, Yoshida A, et al. (1995) Type 3 GM1-gangliosidosis: clinical and neuroradiological findings in an 11-year-old girl. *J Neurol* **242**: 299–303.

Tanzi RE, Petrukhin K, Chernov I, et al. (1993) The Wilson disease gene is a copper transport ATPase with homology to the Menkes disease gene. *Nat Genet* **5**: 344–50.

Tarini BA (2007) The current revolution in newborn screening: new technology, old controversies. *Arch Pediatr Adolesc Med* **161**: 767–72.

Tasso MJ, Martinez-Guttierez A, Carrascosa C, et al. (1996) GM1 gangliosidosis presenting as nonimmune hydrops fetalis: a case report. *J Perinat Med* **24**: 445–9.

Tatsumi N, Inui K, Sakai N, et al. (1995) Molecular defects in Krabbe disease. *Hum Mol Genet* **4**: 1865–8.

Tein I (2002) Role of carnitine and fatty acid oxidation and its defects in infantile epilepsy. *J Child Neurol* **17** Suppl 3: 3S57–82; discussion 3S82–3.

Thomas GR, Forbes JR, Roberts EA (1995) The Wilson disease gene: spectrum of mutations and their consequences. *Nat Genet* **9**: 210–7.

Tiranti V, Briem E, Lamantea E, et al. (2006) ETHE1 mutations are specific to ethylmalonic encephalopathy. *J Med Genet* **43**: 340–6.

Touati G, Rusthoven E, Depondt E, et al. (2000) Dietary therapy in two patients with a mild form of sulphite oxidase deficiency: evidence for clinical and biological improvement. *J Inherit Metab Dis* **23**: 45–53.

Tulinius M, Darin N, Wiklund LM, et al. (2005) A family with a pyruvate dehydrogenase complex deficiency due to a novel C>T substitution at nucleotide position 407 in exon 4 of the X-linked ε1α gene. *Eur J Pediatr* **164**: 99–103.

Tümer Z, Tønnesen T, Böhmann J, et al. (1994) First trimester prenatal diagnosis of Menkes disease by DNA analysis. *J Med Genet* **31**: 615–7.

Tümer Z, Horn N, Tønnesen T, et al. (1996) Early copper-histidine treatment for Menkes disease. *Nat Genet* **12**: 11–3.

Twomey EL, Naughten ER, Donoghue VB, Ryan S (2003) Neuroimaging findings in glutaric aciduria type 1. *Pediatr Radiol* **33**: 823–30.

Tyni T, Paetau A, Strauss AW, et al. (2004) Mitochondrial fatty acid β-oxidation in the human eye and brain: implications for the retinopathy of long-chain 3-hydroxyacyl-CoA dehydrogenase deficiency. *Pediatr Res* **56**: 744–50.

Uvebrant P, Lanneskog K, Hagberg B (1992) The epidemiology of progressive encephalopathies in childhood. I. Live birth prevalence in West Sweden. *Neuropediatrics* **23**: 209–11.

Valanne L, Ketonen L, Majander A, et al. (1998) Neuroradiologic findings in children with mitochondrial disorders. *AJNR* **19**: 369–77.

van den Brink DM, Brites P, Haasjes J, et al. (2003) Identification of PEX7 as the second gene involved in Refsum disease. *Am J Hum Genet* **72**: 471–7.

van der Knaap MS, Jakobs C, Valk J (1996) Magnetic resonance imaging in lactic acidosis. *J Inherit Metab Dis* **19**: 535–47.

van der Voorn JP, Kamphorst W, van der Knaap MS, Powers JM (2004) The leukoencephalopathy of infantile GM1 gangliosidosis: oligodendrocytic loss and axonal dysfunction. *Acta Neuropathol* **107**: 539–45.

van Geel BM, Assies J, Wanders RJ, Barth PG (1997) X linked adrenoleukodystrophy: clinical presentation, diagnosis, and therapy. *J Neurol Neurosurg Psychiatry* **63**: 4–14.

van Gennip AH, Abeling NG, Stroomer AE, et al. (1994a) Clinical and biochemical findings in six patients with pyrimidine degradation defects. *J Inherit Metab Dis* **17**: 130–2.

Vanier MT, Millat G (2003) Niemann–Pick disease type C. *Clin Genet* **64**: 269–81.

Vanier MT, Rodriguez-Lafrasse C, Rousson R, et al. (1991) Type C Niemann–Pick disease: spectrum of phenotypic variation in disruption of intracellular LDL-derived cholesterol processing. *Biochim Biophys Acta* **1096**: 328–37.

van Kuilenburg AB, Vreken P, Abeling NG, et al. (1999) Genotype and phenotype in patients with dihydropyrimidine dehydrogenase deficiency. *Hum Genet* **104**: 1–9.

van Kuilenburg AB, De Abreu RA, van Gennip AH (2003) Pharmacogenetic and clinical aspects of dihydropyrimidine dehydrogenase deficiency. *Ann Clin Biochem* **40**: 41–5.

Varho T, Jääskeläinen S, Tolonen U, et al. (2000) Central and peripheral nervous system dysfunction in the clinical variation of Salla disease. *Neurology* **55**: 99–104.

Verghese J, Goldberg RF, Desnick RJ, et al. (2000) Myoclonus from selective dentate nucleus degeneration in type 3 Gaucher disaease. *Arch Neurol* **57**: 389–95.

Verot L, Chikh K, Freydière E, et al. (2007) Niemann–Pick C disease: functional characterization of three NPC2 mutations and clinical and molecular update on patients with NPC2. *Clin Chim Acta* **71**: 320–30.

Verrips A, Nijeholt GJ, Barkhof F, et al. (1999) Spinal xanthomatosis: a variant of cerebrotendinous xanthomatosis. *Brain* **122**: 1589–95.

Vester V, Schubert M, Offner G, Brodehl J (2000) Distal myopathy in nephropathic cystinosis. *Pediatr Nephrol* **14**: 36–8.

Vockley J (2002) Defects of mitochondrial ,-oxidation: a growing group of disorders. *Neuromuscul Disord* **12**: 235–46.

Vockley J, Ensenauer R (2006) Isovaleric acidemia: New aspects of genetic and phenotypic heterogeneity. *Am J Med Genet C Semin Med Genet* **142**: 95–103.

von Figura K, Hanefeld F, Isbrandt D, Stockler-Ipsiroglu S (2000) Guanidinoacetate methyltransferase deficiency. In: Scriver C, Beaudet AL, Sly WS, Valle D, eds. *The Metabolic and Molecular Bases of Inherited Disease, 8th edn. Vol. 2.* New York: McGraw-Hill, pp. 1897–908.

Waggoner DD, Buist NR (1993) Long-term complications in treated galactosemia—175 U.S. cases. *Int Pediatr* **8**: 97–100.

Walshe JM (1996) Treatment of Wilson's disease: the historical background. *Q J Med* **89**: 553–5.

Walshe JM, Munro NA (1995) Zinc-induced deterioration in Wilson's disease aborted by treatment with penicillamine, dimercaprol, and a novel zero copper diet. *Arch Neurol* **52**: 10–1 (letter).

Walter U, Krolikowski K, Tarnaka B, et al. (2005) Sonographic detection of basal ganglia lesions in asymptomatic and symptomatic Wilson disease. *Neurology* **64**: 726–32.

Wanders RJ (2004) Metabolic and molecular basis of peroxisomal disorders: a review. *Am J Med Genet A* **126**: 355–75.

Wanders RJ, Vreken P, den Boer ME, et al. (1999) Disorders of mitochondrial fatty acyl-CoA beta-oxidation. *J Inherit Metab Dis* **22**: 442–87.

Waterham HR, Clayton PT (2006) Disorders of cholesterol synthesis. In: Fernandes J, Saudubray JM, van den Berg G, Walter JH, eds. *Inborn Metabolic Diseases. Diagnosis and Treatment, 4th edn.* Berlin: Springer-Verlag, pp. 411–9.

Watts RW, Gibbs DA (1986) Sphingolipidoses. In: Watts RW, Gibbs DA, eds. *Lysosomal Diseases: Biocemical and Clinical Aspects.* London: Taylor & Francis, pp. 43–117.

Weber P, Scholl S, Baumgartner ER (2004) Outcome in patients with profound biotinidase deficiency: relevance to newborn screening. *Dev Med Child Neurol* **46**: 481–4.

Weir DG, Scott JM (1995) The biochemical basis of the neuropathy in cobalamin deficiency. *Baillieres Clin Haematol* **8**: 479–97.

Wendel U, Claussen U, Dieckmann E (1983) Prenatal diagnosis of methylene tetrahydrofolate reductase deficiency. *J Pediatr* **102**: 938–40.

Whitehead VM (2006) Acquired and inherited disorders of cobalamin and folate in children. *Br J Haematol* **134**: 125–36.

Wilcken B, Don N, Greenaway R, et al. (1987) Sialuria: a second case. *J Inherit Metab Dis* **10**: 97–102.

Wilcken B, Wiley V, Hammond J, Carpenter K (2003) Screening newborns for inborn errors of metabolism by tandem mass spectrometry. *N Engl J Med* **348**: 2304–12.

Willems PJ, Gatti R, Dabry JK, et al. (1991) Fucosidosis revisited: a review of 77 patients. *Am J Med Genet* **38**: 111–31.

Willemsen M, Rodenburg RJ, Teszas A, et al. (2006) Females with PDHA1 gene mutations: a diagnostic challenge. *Mitochondrion* **6**: 155–9.

Williams JC, Butler IJ, Rosenberg HS, et al. (1984) Progressive neurologic deterioration and renal failure due to storage of glutamyl ribose-5-phosphate. *N Engl J Med* **311**: 152–5.

Wills AJ, Manning NJ, Reilly MM (2001) Refsum disease. *QJ Med* **94**: 403–6.

Wolf B (1995) Disorders of biotin metabolism. In: Scriver CR, Beaudet AL, Sly WS, Valle D, eds. *The Metabolic and Molecular Bases of Inherited Disease, 7th edn.* New York: McGraw-Hill, pp. 3151–77.

Wolf NL, Smeitink JA (2002) Mitochondrial disorders: a proposal for consensus diagnostic criteria in infants and children. *Neurology* **59**: 1402–5.

Wopereis S, Grünewald S, Huijben KM, et al. (2007) Transferrin and apolipoprotein C-III isofocusing are complementary in the diagnosis of N- and O-glycan biosynthesis defects. *Clin Chem* **53**: 180–7.

Wraith JE (2005) The first 5 years of clinical experience with laronidase enzyme replacement therapy for mucopolysaccharidosis I. *Expert Opin Pharmacother* 6: 489–506.

Xu X, Pin S, Gathinji M, et al. (2004) Aceruloplasminemia: an inherited neurological disease with impairment of iron homeostasis. *Ann NY Acad Sci* **1012**: 299–305.

Young ID, Young EP, Mossman J, et al. (1987) Neuraminidase deficiency: case report and review of the phenotype. *J Med Genet* **24**: 283–90.

Zafeiriou DI, Koletzko B, Mueller-Felber W, et al. (1995) Deficiency in complex IV (cytochrome c oxidase) of the respiratory chain, presenting as a leukodystrophy in two siblings with Leigh syndrome. *Brain Dev* 17: 117–21.

Zafeiriou DI, Augoustides-Savvopoulou P, Haas D, et al. (2007) Ethylmalonic encephalopathy: clinical and biochemical observations. *Neuropediatrics* **38**: 78–82.

Zarifi MK, Tzika AA, Astrakas LG, et al. (2001) Magnetic resonance spectroscopy and MRI findings in Krabbe disease. *J Child Neurol* **16**: 522–6.

Zeng WQ, Al-Yamani E, Acierno JS, et al. (2005) Biotin-responsive basal ganglia disease maps to 2q36.3 and is due to mutations in SLC19A3. *Am J Hum Genet* 77: 16–26.

Zeviani M, Di Donato S (2004) Mitochondrial disorders. *Brain* **127**: 2153–72.

9
HEREDODEGENERATIVE DISORDERS

Jean Aicardi and Folker Hanefeld

A significant proportion of genetically transmitted neurological diseases have not yet been linked with demonstrated metabolic errors, especially known enzymatic deficits. Many are characterized by early degeneration of one or more specific CNS areas or systems, perhaps related to defective maintenance of vital elements of certain neurons. Some demonstrate morphological evidence of storage at the microscopic or ultramicroscopic level. A majority show only 'degenerative' lesions of the brain and in some cases of the peripheral nervous system. There is little doubt, however, that many of these disorders are caused by as yet unknown genetic abnormalities of structural or enzyme proteins, and that many of these will be identified in the near future. These disorders are termed *heredodegenerative CNS disorders*. They share most of the clinical features of recognized metabolic diseases; in particular, they are progressive illnesses. A free interval and a loss of previously acquired skills are frequent but not constant features, so that the progressive nature of some may be difficult to determine. This group is highly heterogeneous, including many disorders with no real link between them. The various conditions studied in this chapter will be grouped mainly according to gross pathological criteria, e.g. on the system or part of the CNS that bears the brunt of the disease, although topographic delimitation is far from being always precise. Pathological location is relatively well correlated with the clinical features.

Heredodegenerative disorders can have their onset at any age, and age of onset is an important diagnostic clue (Lyon et al. 2006). Barth (1993) has drawn attention to the prenatal origin of a group of degenerative diseases that manifest clinically at birth.

Because no specific biological disturbance is known for several of these conditions, their diagnosis rests on clinical grounds, especially careful history taking, family investigation and neurological examination, and on certain laboratory tests – radiological, neurophysiological, ophthalmological or biochemical.

Brain biopsy that was used for the diagnosis of some heredodegenerative CNS disorders has been largely replaced, over the past two decades, by peripheral biopsies of muscle, gingiva, appendix and rectal plexuses. This has the advantage of allowing direct study of neuronal cells and may be the only way of confirming the diagnosis of disorders such as intraneuronal inclusion disease (Goutières et al. 1990) and some of the ceroid–lipofuscinoses (Barthez-Carpentier et al. 1991). Skin or conjunctival biopsy may be more efficient for the diagnosis of neuroaxonal dystrophy and related conditions.

Study of this group of disorders has been revolutionized by the progress of molecular genetics and the use of linkage techniques. These permit identification of mutations within or close to the relevant gene or in the proteins they code for making reliable diagnosis possible. When the gene has been mapped and cloned, appropriate methods can be applied to help determine the abnormal gene product and, hopefully, understand the mechanisms of the disease and eventually prepare possible therapies. DNA studies may permit prenatal diagnosis, and in some cases preimplantation diagnosis. With direct study of the gene sequence, mutations or deletions can be detected, enabling precise determination of the genotype and consequently of the subtype and genetic origin of the disorder.

Diagnosis by molecular genetic techniques has medical and ethical implications, in particular for prenatal and preimplantation diagnosis, which have to be carefully considered. There is no doubt though that they have opened exciting new perspectives in the field of heredodegenerative diseases.

For convenience, a few diseases that are not progressive but have similar clinical presentations and are also of genetic origin will be included in this discussion.

LEUKODYSTROPHIES

The leukodystrophies comprise a group of genetic diseases that affect the white matter of the brain and in a few disorders also peripheral myelin. There is no classification available that covers all aspects of clinical presentation, morphological alterations, or metabolic and genetic characteristics. In a broad sense leukodystrophies are defined as genetic white matter brain disorders. They belong to a larger group of conditions that also affect predominantly the white matter, termed leukoencephalopathies, which include many disorders involving the white matter but are acquired rather than genetically determined. The leukoencephalopathies produce imaging features that can closely resemble those of the leukodystrophies proper and constitute a major differential diagnosis (Table 9.1).

Originally the classification was based on morphological characteristics; examples are globoid cell leukodystrophy (Krabbe disease), metachromatic leukodystrophy, and sudanophilic leuko-

TABLE 9.1
Disorders involving the white matter of the cerebral hemispheres and which may cause abnormal density or signal on imaging

Disorders of genetic origin
- Leukodystrophies (see Table 9.2)
- Mitochondrial encephalomyopathies
- Leigh syndrome
- Refsum disease
- L-hydroxy-glutaric aciduria
- Phenylketonuria
- Maple syrup urine disease
- Mucopolysaccharidoses
- Giant axonal neuropathy
- Congenital muscular dystrophies
    - Fukuyama-type dystrophy
    - Laminin alpha 2 deficiency
- Cerebrotendinous xanthomatosis
- Trichothiodystrophies

Acquired disorders
- Diffuse post-anoxic encephalopathy
- Periventricular leukomalacia (extensive forms)
- Toxic leukoencephalopathy (e.g. methotrexate, X-ray therapy, immunosuppressive agents)
- Viral infections, e.g. acute encephalomyelitis, rare cases of subacute panencephalitis, congenital infections (TORCH)
- Diffuse vascular disorders (CADASIL*)
- Transependymal resorption of CSF in some cases of hydrocephalus
- Other diffuse white matter oedema

*Adults only.

TABLE 9.2
Classification of hereditary white matter disorders according to the organelles affected

Lysosomal disorders
- Metachromatic leukodystrophy (MLD)
- Globoid cell leukodystrophy (Krabbe, GLD)

Peroxisomal disorders
- Zellweger cerebro-hepato-renal syndrome
- X-linked adrenoleukodystrophy (X-ALD)
- Neonatal ALD
- Refsum disease (classic/infantile)

Mitochondrial encephalomyopathies/OXPHOS
- Succinate dehydrogenase deficiency
- Leigh syndrome
- Others

Disorders of amino and organic acid metabolism
- L-OH-glutaricaciduria
- Canavan disease
- Phenylketonuria
- Maple syrup urine disease
- Others

Mucopolysaccharidoses
- Hurler disease
- Hunter disease

Disorders of DNA repair
- Cockayne disease

Disorders of neurofilaments
- Alexander disease
- Leukoencephalopathy in giant axonal neuropathy

Disorders of extracellular matrix
- Congenital muscular dystrophy and leukoencephalopathy due to laminin α_2 deficiency
- Pelizaeus–Merzbacher-like disease

Leukoencephalopathy with hypomyelination
- Pelizaeus–Merzbacher disease
- Salla disease
- 18q– syndrome

Miscellaneous
- Megalencephalic leukoencephalopathy with subcortical cysts (MLC)
- Myelinopathia centralis diffusa (MCD)/vanishing white matter disease (VWM)
- Trichothiodystrophy
- Cerebrotendinous xanthomatosis
- Aicardi–Goutières syndrome

dystrophy. This last term has more or less disappeared as a result of advances in understanding of the genetic aetiology of most leukodystrophies. The terms demyelination, dysmyelination and hypomyelination describe the possible pathophysiological aspects. *Demyelination* refers to the breakdown of structurally and biochemically normal myelin (e.g. in multiple sclerosis), *dysmyelination* denotes a structurally and biochemically abnormal or unstable myelin (e.g. adrenoleukodystrophy), while *hypomyelination* indicates disturbance and delay in the formation of myelin (e.g. Pelizaeus–Merzbacher disease). Demyelination may occur in all three conditions, usually involving oligodendrocytes and macrophages as the major cellular components. Studies in recent years gave evidence for the involvement of the extracellular matrix proteins in the stabilization of the myelin membrane (e.g. alpha-sarcoglycanopathies). Axonopathies and disorders of neurofilaments may also play an important role in the maintenance of myelin. The role of astrocyte dysfunction has been recently discussed as a factor in demyelination (Seifert et al. 2006). Despite all diagnostic efforts and progress in modern neurological, radiological, biochemical and genetic techniques, a substantial proportion of leukodystrophies in childhood remains unclassified and the pathogenesis of many disorders of cerebral white matter remains unsolved. While onset of leukodystrophies is usually in early childhood, the age spectrum ranges from prenatal/congenital to adult-onset types in most entities. Leukodystrophies represent the classical type of white matter disorders. However, dysfunction of grey matter is increasingly recognized as a feature in many early onset types.

The classification of leukodystrophies as defined (Table 9.2) is primarily based on disturbances of cell organelles (lysosomes, peroxisomes, mitochondria), structural elements (neurofilaments, alpha-sarcoglycan), and metabolic processes. Table 9.3 classifies the leukodystrophies according to the presence or absence of known responsible metabolic or genetic defects. The large group of newly identified white matter diseases is described separately under the heading of 'miscellaneous' (Table 9.2). Future classifications will probably rely on the individual genetic defects. From the clinical point of view, the leukodystrophies are characterized clinically by the predominance of motor disturbances, especially pyramidal and cerebellar symptoms and signs, with slow mental deterioration and low incidence of seizures, myoclonus and paroxysmal EEG abnormalities. From the imaging point of view,

TABLE 9.3
Classification of the leukodystrophies according to genetic or metabolic defects

Leukodystrophies with known genetic or metabolic defect
   Lysosomal leukodystrophies
      Metachromatic leukodystrophy
      Globoid cell leukodystrophy
      Multiple sulfatase deficiency
   Peroxisomal leukodystrophies
      Adrenoleukodystrophy, juvenile
      Zellweger syndrome and infantile adrenoleukodystrophy
   Leukodystrophies with known genetic defect
      Alexander disease
      Canavan disease (aspartoacyclase deficiency)
      Megalencephalic leukodystrophy with subcortical cysts
      Vanishing white matter/myelinopathia centralis diffusa
      Pelizaeus and Pelizaeus-like leukodystrophy
      Salla disease
      18q– syndrome

Leukodystrophies without known genetic or metabolic defect
   Orthochromatic leukodystrophies[1]
   Unclassified leukodystrophies[2]
   Trichothiodystrophy
   Aicardi–Goutières syndrome

[1]See text.
[2]This group includes recently described leukodystrophies for which no sufficient genetic/metabolic data are yet available.

all share involvement of white matter, best demonstrated by MRI, which may be more or less obvious or may require the most recent techniques of imaging. The MRI features of white matter disease have been reviewed by van der Knaap and Valk (2005), and MR spectroscopic anomalies by Hanefeld et al. (2004).

LYSOSOMAL DISORDERS
METACHROMATIC LEUKODYSTROPHY
Metachromatic leukodystrophy (MLD) was first described by Scholz and Greenfield. Scholz realized the genetic origin of the disease and separated it from disorders described under the term of diffuse sclerosis. The typical staining properties, showing metachromasia after staining with kresyl violet or toluidine blue in an acid solution, separate the disease from the so-called orthochromatic or sudanophilic leukodystrophies. The staining appears to be specific for sulfatides, present not only in brain tissue but also in nerves and many somatic tissues like kidneys, liver and ovaries and also in urine. In addition to metachromasia, peripheral nerves may also show segmented demyelination. The detection of metachromatic material in urinary epithelial cells is still a useful diagnostic test.

MLD is an autosomal recessive disorder with an estimated prevalence of 1 in 40,000. It is caused by a deficiency of arylsulfatase A (ARSA). The deficiency of ARSA results in a storage of cerebroside sulfate (sulfatide). The genetic defect is localized on chromosome 22 (Polten et al. 1991). The accumulation of sulfatides leads to breakdown of central and peripheral myelin. Sulfatide concentration in affected tissue is increased and cerebroside concentration is decreased.

Besides the ARSA-alleles (frequency 0.5%) causing MLD, another ARSA allele (frequency 7–15%) exists, which has been called ARSA pseudodeficieny (*ARSA-PD*) gene (Gieselmann et al. 1991). Ten to 20 per cent of individuals homozygous for this allele have a low ARSA activity but show no clinical symptoms and no sulfatiduria. Homozygosity for ARSA-PD is frequent in the general population; patients with neurological symptoms of other causes and ARSA-PD may therefore be misdiagnosed as having MLD. The pseudodeficiency allele can be determined directly by DNA techniques. In addition, rare cases of MLD are caused by a different mutation involving an activator protein (saponin B) that is coded by a gene at 10q21–22. The activator protein activates not only the hydrolysis of sulfatides by ARSA but also the hydrolysis of GM1-gangliosides. Deficiency of saponin B may result in juvenile or rarely in late infantile phenotype of MLD but histologically also shows storage of gangliosides. The diagnosis can be confirmed in fibroblast cultures: pathological sulfatide metabolism can be corrected by the activator protein (Gieselmann 2003).

Three clinical types of MLD can be distinguished according to age of onset: late infantile type (40%), juvenile type (40%) and adult type (20%). The late infantile form is the most homogeneous group, which presents between the ages of 6 months and 2 years. Children show delayed development or deterioration of walking, some being never able to walk alone. The gait is characterized by spasticity and ataxia. Ankle reflexes may be absent, contrasting with the presence of a bilateral Babinski sign. Later in the course of the illness, optic atrophy and more generalized spasticity dominate the clinical picture (MacFaul et al. 1982). The prognosis is poor, with death occurring before the age of 10.

The juvenile type varies in onset and may show symptoms as early as 4–6 years. Gait disorders combined with educational and behavioural problems can be observed. Motor signs include cerebellar and pyramidal dysfunction as well as signs of a peripheral neuropathy. Seizures and dementia are late manifestations. In adult cases gait disorders, extrapyramidal symptoms and a psychiatric symptomatology dominate the clinical picture.

MLD should be suspected in all children with a progressive spastic–ataxic disorder and the paradoxical finding of a negative Achilles tendon reflex in the presence of exaggerated patellar tendon reflexes and Babinski sign. Fundi may show optic atrophy. The EEG is usually normal or may show some slow activity and epileptiform discharges late in the disease. The electroretinogram is preserved. Sensory and particularly motor nerve conduction velocities are decreased. In almost all cases there is an increased protein level in CSF. In all three types, CT and MRI show changes in the periventricular white matter with a frontal predominance (Fig. 9.1). U-fibres are spared, the corpus callosum is affected early during the disease, and pyramidal tracts may show signs of demyelination in juvenile and adult cases. The diagnosis is confirmed by measurement of ARSA and the demonstration of metachromatic material in urine.

No effective treatment is yet available. Bone marrow or haematopoietic stem cell transplantation has been tried with

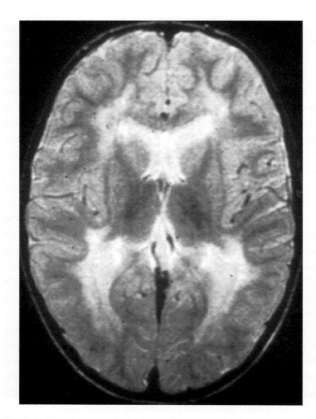

Fig. 9.1. Metachromatic leukodystrophy. T₂-weighted MRI shows high signal from the periventricular white matter.

conflicting results. Most recently the supplementation of aryl-sulfatase A has been discussed (Matzner and Gieselmann 2005).

MULTIPLE SULFATASE DEFICIENCY (MUCOSULFATIDOSIS, AUSTIN DISEASE)

Multiple sulfatase deficiency is a rare autosomal recessive disorder, combining features of both MLD and mucopolysaccharidosis, caused by the absence of arylsulfatase A, B and C and mucopoly-saccharide sulfatidase activity. Recently mutations in the gene encoding the human C-alpha-formylglycine generating enzyme have been descibed (Diercks et al. 2003). As a result of the deficit patients accumulate sulfatides and mucopolysaccharides in viscera and brain and there is an increased excretion of heparan sulfate in urine. Clinical manifestation includes coarse features, short stature, hepatosplenomegaly combined with skeletal changes, progressive neurodevelopmental deterioration and peripheral neuropathy. There is no corneal clouding. Three subtypes (neonatal, early childhood and juvenile) can be distinguished. Children with the most frequently occurring early childhood form learn to walk but develop a progressive encephalopathy combined with a peripheral neuropathy and the described somatic features around the age of 2 years. Progressive deterioration leads to early death. The diagnosis can be suspected in patients with neurological symptoms combined with skeletal dysplasia on X-ray and finally confirmed by the demonstration of arylsulfatase A, B and C deficiency. X-ray of lumbar spine may show anterior beaking

or ovoid vertebrae as in classical MPS disorders. The cranial MRI shows white matter changes similar to those in MLD.

GLOBOID CELL LEUKODYSTROPHY (KRABBE DISEASE)

Globoid cell leukodystrophy (GLD) is an autosomal recessive disorder caused by a deficiency of galactocerebroside-beta-galactosidase (galactocerebrosidase) (Suzuki et al. 1971). The gene maps to chromosome 14q24–32.1. Galactocerebrosides are the most specific myelin lipids in the brain; their concentration reflects maturation. Three subtypes of GLD have been delineated: the most common infantile form, and rare juvenile and adult subtypes. The neuropathology of Krabbe disease is characterized by a paucity of oligodendrocytes, lack of myelin, and proliferation of glial cells in affected areas with mononuclear epitheloid cells and clusters of large multinucleated *globoid cells*. Involvement of the peripheral nervous system is common but may be less pronounced than in MLD. The deficiency of galactocerebroside-beta-galactosidase results in accumulation of cerebrosides and psychosine (galactosyl sphingosine). Many symptoms observed in GLD are related to the increase of psychosine, which acts as a toxic substance (Suzuki 2003).

The most common infantile form presents initially with hypotonia before 6 months of age. In addition extreme irritability, especially marked sound-induced startle, and progressive stiffness are characteristic early symptoms. Increased muscle tone and pyramidal tract signs are found on examination, and opisthotonic spasms with head retraction are often precipitated by external stimuli. Convulsions are frequent and may present as infantile spasms with atypical hypsarrhythmic EEG pattern. Absence of deep tendon reflexes frequently contrasts with the spasticity. Optic atrophy and blindness develop. The disease is rapidly progressive and death usually occurs before the age of 2 years. The clinical stages of Krabbe disease have been delineated by Hagberg et al. (1969).

In all infantile cases high CSF protein (above 70 mg/dL) is found and nerve conduction velocities are decreased. In late-onset forms of GLD, CSF protein may be normal. MRI detects T₁ hypointensity and T₂ hyperintensity in cerebral and cerebellar white matter (Fig. 9.2). MR spectroscopy revealed pronounced elevation of myo-inositol and choline containing compounds in affected white matter, reflecting demyelination and glial proliferation, accompanied by a decrease of N-aspartyl acetate as a sign of neuroaxonal loss (Brockmann et al. 2003a).

The diagnosis of GLD is based on the characteristic clinical symptoms, raised CSF protein and MRI findings. In late-onset cases symptoms are less characteristic and include walking difficulties, fading vision, and learning problems. In any leukodystrophy combined with a mild peripheral neuropathy GLD must be suspected. The diagnosis is confirmed by measuring galactocerebroside-beta-galactosidase in white blood cells or fibroblasts. Molecular analysis may demonstrate one of the more than 60 mutations that have been described in association with Krabbe disease (Kleiyer et al. 1997, Wenger et al. 1997).

Treatment is symptomatic. High doses of benzodiazepines were useful in relieving the extreme irritability and opisthotonus

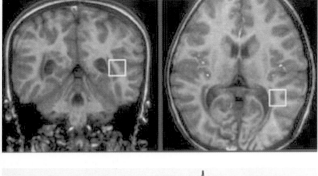

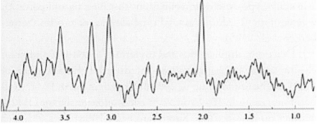

Fig. 9.2. Juvenile Krabbe disease. *(Top)* MRI shows only mild signal abnormalities of white matter. Note low signal from the thalami. *(Bottom)* MR spectroscopy shows high peaks of choline and myoinositol and reduced peak of N-acetylaspartic acid.

in some of our patients. Haematopoietic stem cell transplantation has been tried with doubtful results (Krivit et al. 1998). Most recently the restoration of normal blood levels of galacto-cerebrosidase was achieved in 11 asymptomatic newborn and 14 symptomatic infants with Krabbe disease by the transplantation of umbilical cord blood from unrelated donors (Escolar et al. 2005). Infants who underwent transplantation before the onset of symptoms showed progressive central myelination and gained developmental skills and age-appropriate cognitive function at a mean follow-up of three years. Transplantation after onset of symptoms did not result in substantive neurological improvement.

X-Linked Adrenoleukodystrophy (X-ALD)

X-ALD is the most frequently occurring leukodystrophy in males, with an estimated incidence of 1:20,000. The disorder was initially described as "encephalitis periaxialis diffusa" by Schilder in 1913 and in a case report of "diffuse sclerosis" combined with adrenal atrophy by Siemerling and Creutzfeldt in 1923. Almost half a century later the defect in peroxisomal beta-oxidation leading to characteristic excess of very long chain fatty acids in plasma, blood cells and altered fibroblasts was discovered. The gene for X-ALD has been mapped to Xq28 and found to encode a peroxisomal membrane protein of the ATP-binding cassette (ABC) transporter family. More than 200 mutations have been identified.

The transporter is necessary for transferring very long chain fatty acids (VLCFAs) or VLCFA-CoA into the peroxisomes, where they are metabolized. This process depends on a number of peroxisome-biogenesis genes or peroxines (PEX). No correlation has been found between the nature of a mutation and the

clinical phenotype (Powers and Moser 1998, Dubois-Dalcq et al. 1999).

A selective susceptibility of adrenal glands and neuronal tissue, with lesions especially involving the spinal cord and brain, is the morphological hallmark of X-ALD. In contrast to the adult adrenomyeloneuropathy (AMN), the childhood form of X-ALD is associated with an inflammatory reaction in the cerebral white matter. There is a confluent loss of myelin, usually symmetrical and most prominent in the parieto-occipital regions. U-fibres are relatively spared, but corpus callosum, the posterior part of the internal capsule, the corticospinal tract, the pons and the medulla are also involved.

Histological study reveals a loss of myelinated axons and oligodendrocytes, reactive astrocytosis and later cavitations and astrogliosis. The active edge of demyelination shows intensive perivascular inflammation and accumulation of lipophages. Perivascular cell collections contain macrophages and particularly lymphocytes. Hypertrophic GFAP-positive astrocytes and macrophages express cytokines like tumour necrosis factor alpha (TNF-alpha) and interleukin 1 (IL-1).

Three main phenotypes of X-ALD occur in males and three further subtypes are known. AMN can be observed in women carriers of the mutated gene.

1. The cerebral childhood form (frequency 30–40%): onset by 3–10 years of age, rapidly progressive
2. Adolescent ALD (4–7%): onset by age 11–21 years, slower progression
3. Adult AMN (40%): onset by mean age 28 years (SD 9 years), spinal cord involvement
4. Adult ALD (2–5%): marked by psychiatric symptoms and dementia
5. Addison only: onset before 7–8 years; most patients eventually develop AMN, the frequency of which varies with age
6. Asymptomatic cases: biochemical and genetic defect only.

Of 84 cases of X-ALD seen at the Department of Child Neurology in Göttingen (Germany), 51 were classified as symptomatic cerebral ALD and 10 as asymptomatic ALD, while 23 showed only symptoms of Addison's disease (FH, unpublished personal observations).

The cerebral childhood form of ALD has an initial slowly progressing phase followed by rapid deterioration. Initial symptoms are difficulties at school, combined with behavioural disturbances. Impaired hearing or hearing loss may be an early symptom. Impaired vision, dementia, seizures, and difficulties in walking, speech and handwriting develop fast following the onset of first neurological symptoms. Once neurological symptoms become manifest, progression is rapid and an apparent vegetative state develops in a few years. Mean age of death was 9.4 years (SD 2.7 years, range 5.1–19 years) in a series of patients reported from the Kennedy Krieger Institute in Baltimore (Powers and Moser 1998).

Hyperpigmentation typical for Addison disease may be present before neuropsychological disturbances occur.

X-linked ALD must be excluded in every boy with adrenal insufficiency. The diagnosis is based on the demonstration of

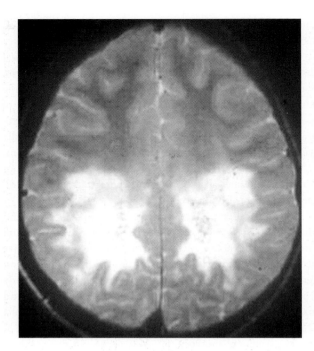

Fig. 9.3. X-linked adrenoleukodystrophy. T$_2$-weighted MRI shows high signal from the posterior part of both hemispheres. Note preservation of the arcuate fibres.

increased concentrations of VLCFA (c22:0, c24:0, c26:0) in plasma. Prenatal diagnosis is possible by measurements of VLCFA in cultured amniocytes and mutation analysis. The demonstration of cerebral demyelination by MRI is of great value and in many cases almost diagnostic. Cerebral demyelinating lesions usually start in the splenium of the corpus callosum and slowly progress symmetrically into the parieto-occipital white matter. Arcuate fibres are spared (Fig. 9.3). Using contrast agents the most severely affected area of the brain shows a rim of enhancement. The posterior limb of the internal capsule, pyramidal tract, pons and brainstem may also be involved. In about 10% of cases demyelination may also start frontally with involvement of the anterior limb of the internal capsule. Symmetrical involvement of the cerebellar white matter is also possible.

The *differential diagnosis* of X-ALD includes amongst others brain tumour, other leukodystrophies, encephalitis, subacute sclerosing panencephalitis, multiple sclerosis and acute demyelinating encephalitis.

Adrenal insufficiency can be effectively corrected by hormone replacement, but substitution does not prevent or alter the neurological manifestations. A diet with unsaturated fatty acids (Lorenzo's oil) lowers the levels of VLCFA but does not improve neurological symptoms already present and does not prevent progression of the disease. A follow-up study of 49 asymptomatic patients with ALD treated with Lorenzo's oil was able to show a reduced risk of developing MRI abnormalities (Moser et al. 2005). The most effective treatment so far has been the haematopoietic stem cell transplantation in the early stage of the disease (Shapiro et al. 2000).

PELIZAEUS–MERZBACHER DISEASE (PMD)

The classical X-linked type of PMD was first described by Pelizaeus in 1885. Merzbacher in 1910 described the neuropathology of the original family examined by Pelizaeus and conceived the disorder to be the result of a congenital aplasia of myelin sheaths. Much later biochemical analysis of cerebral white matter revealed a pattern consistent with that found in fetal myelin including a reduction of the proteolipid protein (PLP). Seitelberger added a congenital variant (type II). According to severity a transitional type III has also been defined.

The neuropathology of classical PMD (type I) is described as patchy hypo- and dysmyelination (so-called tigroid pattern), whereas type II exhibits almost total absence of myelin (Seitelberger et al. 1995).

Deletions, duplications and mutations of the *PLP1* gene on chromosome Xq22 give rise to the disorder. Duplications of *PLP1* can be found in up to 20% of all patients with PMD, and point mutations in 10–25%. *PLP1* codes additionally for DM20, another protein in CNS (Sistermans et al. 1998).

In a recent study five boys with a severe congenital form of PMD have been described with three and more copies of the proteolipid protein PLP1 (Wolf et al. 2005). There is also a clinical continuum between mild forms of PMD and X-linked spastic paraplegic type 2 (SPG2), which also results from mutations in the *PLP1* gene.

Clinical and radiological criteria for the diagnosis of PMD have been published (Boulloche and Aicardi 1986). They include the occurrence in a male patient of delayed motor development before 3 years of age and most often from a few months of age, and ophthalmological and neurological signs. Nystagmus is often the first detected manifestation. Hypotonia, choreoathetosis, and later on ataxia and spasticity develop progressively. Most patients show slow improvement until the age of 10–12 years. The majority of patients learn to sit; some are able to walk with aid but rarely independently. A minority develop active language. Most patients reach a plateau in development followed by a slow regression with dystonia, increasing ataxia, spasticity, and the development of optic atrophy.

The congenital type II (Haenggeli et al. 1989) shows a more severe course with limited development before deterioration, even though its onset may not be much earlier than in the classical type. The five patients described by Wolf et al. (2005) developed severe symptoms before the age of 3 months with hypotonia, nystagmus, stridor and seizures. Two died at 7 and 9 months respectively; three suffered from severe epilepsy.

An array of clinical, electrophysiological and neuroradiological signs leads to the diagnosis. Early developmental impairment, nystagmus, muscular hypotonia and choreiform movements are characteristic clinical symptoms. Nystagmus may disappear before the age of 2 years. Disturbance of cerebral conduction of auditory and/or visual evoked potentials and a diffuse hyperintensity of the white matter on T$_2$-weighted MRI are almost diagnostic for PMD.

High signal intensity is seen in all unmyelinated white matter structures on T$_2$-weighted images (Fig. 9.4), and low signal

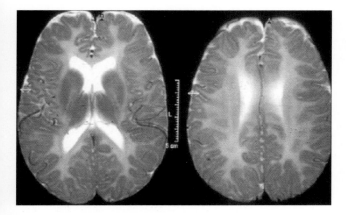

Fig. 9.4. Pelizaeus–Merzbacher disease. T$_2$-weighted MRI shows moderately increased signal from the periventricular white matter.

intensity on T$_1$-weighted images. However, CT may be deceptively normal or show only some atrophy. MR spectroscopy (MRS) reveals a metabolic pattern of white matter similar to grey matter with increased concentrations of N-acetylaspartate (NAA), glutamine, myo-inositole, creatine and phosphocreatine, while the concentration of choline-containing component is reduced. The proton MRS profile of PMD therefore differs from the pattern commonly observed in other leukodystrophies (Hanefeld et al. 2005).

The PMD phenotype has frequently been observed in patients without mutations or duplications of the *PLP1* gene and this is now classified as *PMD-like disease*. Recently, mutations in the gene encoding gap junction protein alpha 12 (connexin 46.6) have been implicated as the cause of PMD-like disease (Uhlenberg et al. 2004). In addition to the PMD-like clinical picture the patients also showed signs of a peripheral neuropathy and sporadic seizures. This variant follows an autosomal recessive trait. Other atypical forms with a similar clinical presentation probably belong to other disorders. Only symptomatic treatment is available for PMD and PMD-like disease.

ALEXANDER DISEASE (AXD)
AXD is the first described disorder caused primarily by a dysfunction of astrocytes (Hanefeld 2004, Mignot et al. 2004). It was first described by Alexander in 1949 in an 18-month-old boy with macrocephaly. The neuropathological hallmark on examination was the presence of 'rod-shaped fuscinophil bodies' in the white matter of his brain, which were later identified as Rosenthal fibres. Glial fibrilary acid protein (GFAP) is present in high concentration in Rosenthal fibres and is therefore used as a histological marker. Mutations of the *GFAP* gene (on chromosome 17q21) in patients with AXD have subsequently been discovered to be the cause of this autosomal recessive disease (Brenner et al. 2001).

According to the clinical presentation three different types of AXD can be distinguished: infantile, juvenile and adult cases. The most common infantile type belongs to the group of macrocephalic white matter diseases. Affected children are normo-

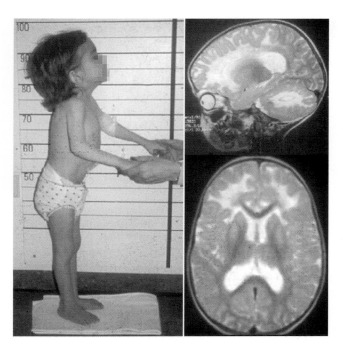

Fig. 9.5. Alexander disease. *(Left)* Macrocephaly in a 4-year-old girl. *(Right)* MRI sagittal T$_2$-weighted sequence shows high signal from the anterior white matter; note cerebellar involvement.

cephalic at birth and develop a slowly progressive megalencephaly combined with symptoms of spasticity, irritability and epileptic seizures (Pridmore et al. 1993). Acute episodes of intracranial hypertension are frequently observed following mild head trauma. Death may occur before the age of 10 years. Apart from this infantile progressive type, AXD has also been diagnosed in juvenile and adult patients. One peculiarity in the cases of older patients is the increasing involvement of brainstem and bulbar structures. Older patients are usually normocephalic. The symptoms are sometimes misdiagnosed as brainstem neoplasms. Single families with several affected members have been described, as well as monozygotic twins (Meins et al. 2002). The disease has been reviewed by Mignot et al. (2004).

The diagnosis in classical cases of AXD is based on the clinical presentation with macrocephaly, regression, seizures and the presence of bulbar symptoms in older patients. The EEG may show generalized slow activity and some focal discharges. The most important information is provided by cranial CT and MRI. Van der Knaap et al. (2001) described neuroradiological characteristics that are almost diagnostic for AXD. These include extensive signal enhancement of cerebral white matter with frontal predominance, a periventricular rim with high signal on T$_1$-weighted and a low signal on T$_2$-weighted images, abnormalities in basal ganglia, thalami and brainstem, and contrast enhancement of particular grey and white matter structures. MR spectroscopy reveals a strong elevation of myo-inositol and a decline of NAA accompanied by accumulation of lactate in affected cerebral and cerebellar white matter. Myo-inositol was elevated in white matter as well as in grey matter and in basal ganglia (Fig. 9.5).

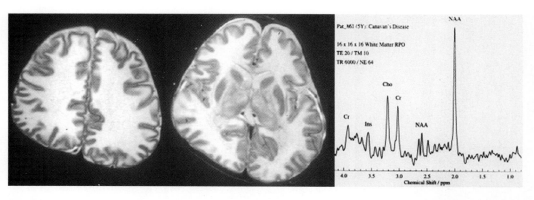

Fig. 9.6. Canavan disease. *(Left)* T$_2$-weighted MRI shows extensive high signal from both central and peripheral white matter. *(Right)* MR spectroscopy shows very high peak of acetylaspartic acid.

The pattern reflects glial (astrocytic) proliferation as well as active demyelination and neuroaxonal degeneration. Most recently, increased levels of GFAP in CSF in all three subtypes of AXD were described by Kyllerman et al. (2005). The diagnosis is confirmed by molecular genetic analysis of the *GFAP* gene.

Only symptomatic treatment is available for AXD.

CANAVAN DISEASE (ASPARTOACYLASE DEFICIENCY)

Canavan disease was first described in 1931 under the designation "Schilders Enzephalitis periaxialis diffusa" and in 1949 was recognized by van Bogaert and Bertrand as a rare autosomal recessive disease entity including leukoencephalopathy and macrocephaly. In 1988 a deficiency of aspartoacylase (Matalon et al. 1989) leading to an increased concentration of NAA in urine and plasma was correlated with Canavan disease. The genetic defect is caused by mutations in the gene for aspartoacylase (*ASPA*) located on chromosome 17pter–p13 (Kaul et al. 1993). Canavan disease is also characterized by macrocephaly combined with hypotonia, irritability and feeding difficulties. Patients suffering from the most frequent infantile type develop spasticity and blindness, and death occurs before 3 years of age. A severe congenital form resembles a metabolic encephalopathy, while the very rare juvenile form has a normal head circumference and shows a more protracted course. Neuropathology is characterized by degeneration and rarefaction of neural tissue (status spongiosus).

The cranial CT shows diffuse symmetrical hypodensity of white matter; MRI reveals a centripetal pattern of demyelination starting in the U-fibres and progressing to the periventricular regions (Fig. 9.6). NAA as one of the major metabolites detected by MRS shows an increased signal in the brain of patients with Canavan disease (Grodd et al. 1990). The increased concentration of NAA in proton MR spectra of the brain is almost diagnostic for the disease. The diagnosis is confirmed by the demonstration of increased concentrations of NAA in plasma and urine and a mutation in the gene of aspartoacylase. Prenatal diagnosis is possible in cultured amniocytes. The course is progressive, although the rate of progression may be variable (Traeger and Rapin 1998). There is no known treatment.

NEWLY IDENTIFIED GENETIC DISORDERS AFFECTING THE WHITE MATTER

As a result of systematic analysis of progressive white matter diseases and the introduction of modern radiological and genetic techniques, a number of 'new' disease entities have been identified amongst the inherited white matter diseases. Many had been described in single case reports previously.

Myelinopathia centralis diffusa (MCD); vanishing white matter disease; childhood ataxia with CNS hypomyelination (CACH)

This disorder, now called vanishing white matter disease (VWMD), represents one of the most prevalent inherited childhood white matter disorders (van der Knaap et al. 2006). Following the description in earlier case reports, the disease was described in 1993 by Hanefeld et al. as diffuse white matter disease with unique features on MRI and proton MRS. These authors described three children, including male and female siblings, who developed ataxia, following a mild head trauma and an unspecific infection respectively. The third patient, a boy, became atactic following mild head trauma. Ataxia persisted over three days. A CT taken at the time showed diffuse white matter changes. The boy made an initial recovery but became ataxic again following mild head traumas or unspecific febrile illness. At the age of 4 years he was referred with a spastic–atactic gait, brisk reflexes, clonus and bilateral Babinski sign. During the following months and years he developed optic atrophy, swallowing difficulties and major seizures. Later he died from bronchopneumonia. His sister followed almost the same clinical course. MRI in both siblings showed almost identical diffuse white matter abnormalities. The MRS done at the same time revealed a complete loss of all metabolites in affected white matter, whilst brain spectra of grey matter revealed only mild but definite decrease of NAA. The MRS appearance of white matter resembled CSF with a marked elevation of lactate (Fig. 9.7). Similar cases were described in large numbers during the following years (Schiffmann et al. 1994, van der Knaap et al. 1997). Leegwater et al. (2001) and van der Knaap et al. (2002a) were able to demonstrate mutations in all subunits of the eukaryotic translation initiation factor *eIF2B*. Most cases seem to be recessively inherited. A dominant inheritance was

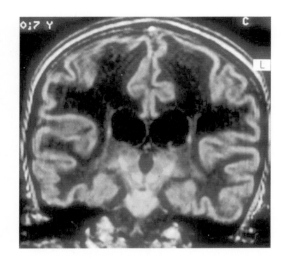

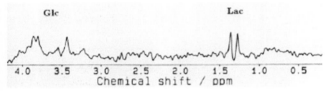

Fig. 9.7. Vanishing white matter disease. *(Top)* MRI shows virtually complete disappearance of the white matter of both hemispheres with CSF-like signal. *(Bottom)* MR spectroscopy shows almost complete absence of all normal peaks.

suggested in an adult family reported by Labauge et al. (2005). Further studies showed that early-onset variants including the Cree-leukoencephalopathy (Black et al. 1988) are caused by a mutation in *eIF2B5* (Fogli et al. 2002a,b). This mutation has also been described in other cases with a severe, lethal ante- and perinatal onset of the leukoencephalopathy. In addition other abnormalities are often present such as oligohydramnios, intrauterine growth retardation, cataract, pancreatitis, hepatosplenomegaly, hypoplasia of kidneys and ovarian dysgenesis (van der Knaap et al. 2003a). The combination of white matter disease with ovarian dysgenesis had already been described by Schiffmann et al. (1997). It has now become obvious that VWMD shows a wide spectrum of clinical manifestations, from the rare acute early onset types, the classical VWMD/MCD syndrome, to milder late-onset and adult cases (Fogli and Boespflug-Tanguy 2006, van der Knaap et al. 2006). Despite the large number of patients and mutations described so far, the genotype–phenotype relationship in eIF2B disorders, as they are now called, is still weak and poorly understood.

Neuropathological investigations have demonstrated age-dependent abnormalities. Cystic cavitations are described in advanced cases. Microscopically there is a loss of myelin but no inflammatory reaction. Grey matter is generally spared but axonal loss in areas of cavitation is complete. Oligodentrocytes are severely affected, showing apoptosis in early-onset cases (Brück et al. 2001) and increased density of oligodendrocytes in long-standing cases (Rodriguez et al. 1999, van Haren et al. 2004). A recent study of cell cultures from the brain of a boy who died

at the age of 12 years showed in vitro a rapid generation of oligodendrocytes but a severely compromised reduction of GFAP-positive astrocytes. A deficiency of normal astrocyte function may therefore be involved in the pathogenesis of VWMD.

The diagnosis in the classical type of VWMD/MCD is based on the clinical presentation and course: normal early development during the first 2–3 years, followed by ataxia and spasticity, usually in the context of mild trauma, or unspecific febrile illness, rapid progression with loss of motor function, seizures and late mental deterioration. There are no signs of peripheral neuropathy. Alternatively, recovery, often only partial, may occur with later recurrences leading to progressive decline.

MRI shows diffuse white matter disease with a characteristic early involvement of the central tegmental tract. MRS confirms a loss of myelin, revealing a metabolic pattern, different from CSF only by the presence of lactate. The disease progresses to severe disability, and most children with the classical phenotype die before the age of 20 years.

An elevation of glycine and a decreased concentration of asialotransferrin has been described as a possible marker of the disease (van der Knaap et al. 1999). However, MRI criteria, as formulated by van der Knaap, are primarily used for diagnosis. In view of the wide phenotypic variability in *eIF2B* disorders the diagnosis has to be confirmed by genetic analysis.

Prenatal diagnosis of eIB2B disorders is available. No treatment is known.

Megaloencephalic leukoencephalopathy with subcortical cysts (MLC)

In 1995 van der Knaap et al. described the clinical and pathological findings of a "leukoencephalopathy with swelling and a discrepantly mild clinical course" in 8 children. Family studies suggested an autosomal recessive mode of inheritance; the gene was mapped to chromosome 22qter by Topçu et al. (2000) and identified by Leegwater et al. (2001, 2002). The disease was characterized by megalencephaly and leukoencephalopathy, with onset during the first year of life and a slowly progressive neurological deterioration. Brain biopsy in one of the patients revealed a spongiform leukoencephalopathy with vacuolization and splitting of the outer lamellae of the myelin sheaths (van der Knaap et al. 1995). Singhal et al. (1996) described 30 patients from an ethnic group in India with similar clinical presentation.

The clinical symptomatology consists of macrocephaly, ataxia, spasticity, seizures and mild intellectual deterioration. Remarkably, cognitive functions are well preserved in many patients up to adolescence. The EEG may show epileptiform activity, a photoconvulsive response and generalized slowing (Topçu et al. 1998). The MRI reveals extensive signal changes of hemispherical white matter early in the disease and the development of subcortical cysts predominantly in the temporal and parietal regions.

Mejaski-Bosnjak et al. (1997) reported the MRS features of an 8-year-old girl with a severe clinical course of MLC that had led to wheelchair dependency at age 5 years. Localized MRS of the affected white matter showed a loss of all metabolites, pointing to a complete disintegration of neuroaxonal and glial tissue

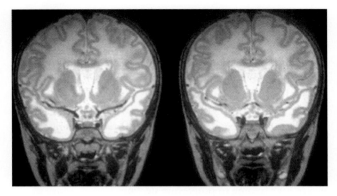

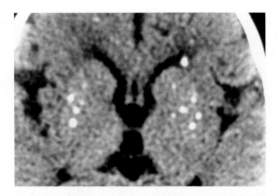

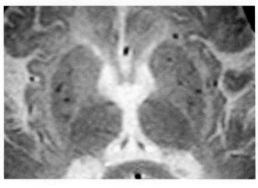

Fig. 9.8. Megalencephalic leukodystrophy with cysts. MRI shows extensive white matter involvement and cysts in the anterior part of the temporal lobe.

Fig. 9.9. Leukodystrophy with calcification of the basal ganglia (Aicardi–Goutières syndrome). *(Top)* Axial MRI shows punctate calcification in the basal ganglia, low signal from the frontal lobes, and diffuse moderate atrophy of the brain. Note the presence of calcification in the white matter. *(Bottom)* MRI of the basal ganglia: punctate calcifications are well shown as low-intensity signals.

(Fig. 9.8). A 37-year-old cognitively normal woman was studied for increasing gait disturbance caused by spasticity and ataxia in our institution (Brockmann et al. 2003b). MRI showed enlargement of ventricles and subarachnoid spaces. Cerebral white matter was characterized by diffuse T_2-hyperintensity with numerous subcortical cysts present.

Diagnosis is based on clinical findings, in particular megalencephaly, well-preserved cognitive function and characteristic MRI findings. No treatment for the disease is available.

Unclassified leukoencephalopathies
Amongst the unclassified leukoencephalopathies a new syndrome characterized by *hypomyelination with atrophy of the basal ganglia and cerebellum (H-ABC)* was described by van der Knaap et al. (2002b) with a distinct MRI pattern consisting of hypomyelination and atrophy of the cerebellum and basal ganglia that develop over time. The patient presented with absent motor development, already evident during the first months of life. Later spasticity, extrapyramidal symptoms with rigidity, dystonia and choreoathetosis developed in the most severe cases. Two patients were able to walk at the age of 2.5 years and 14 months respectively. All patients showed learning difficulties but no obvious decline of their cognitive functions. Seizures occurred in two patients. MRS and MRI were consistent with hypomyelination.

Another clinical entity described by the same group featured *brainstem and spinal cord involvement and high lactate* (van der Knaap et al. 2003b). The patients studied presented with slowly progressive pyramidal and cerebellar dysfunction. Early motor development was normal or mildly delayed. Loss of unsupported walking occurred in two patients at the age of 14 years. All patients showed ataxia and spastic paraparesis. In 4 cases posterior column dysfunction was registered. The MRI pattern is described as distinct with inhomogeneous white matter abnormalities and selective tract involvement. The pyramidal tract was affected over its entire length. Involvement of dorsal columns and cerebellar peduncles as well as of the intraparenchymal trajectories of the trigeminal nerve was a remakably consistent finding. MRS revealed a decrease of NAA, an increase of myo-inositol and

choline, and an elevated lactate concentration in white matter of all patients.

LEUKODYSTROPHY WITH CALCIFICATION OF THE BASAL GANGLIA AND LYMPHOCYTOSIS OF CSF (AICARDI–GOUTIÈRES SYNDROME)
This is an autosomal recessive condition, and its pathology is poorly known but indicates a microvasculitis. In similar cases, an inflammatory meningeal reaction was found in addition to patchy leukodystrophy with preserved islands of myelin. The clinical features include a very early onset in the first weeks or months of life so that deterioration, if any, is far from obvious. The general condition of the patient is poor, there is marked hypotonia interrupted by opisthotonic episodes, failure to develop, febrile episodes, and death in a state of decerebration within a few years, although some children survive for several years (Aicardi and Goutières 1984, Goutières et al. 1998). However, cases of later onset after the age of 6–12 months may run a less severe course (Rice et al. 2007), The two major diagnostic features are: (1) the presence of calcification of the basal nuclei, sometimes also of the periventricular white matter and the dentate nuclei, associated with hypodensities of the white matter and brain atrophy (Fig. 9.9); and (2) a persistent mild CSF lymphocytosis (10–80 cells/mm³) that is not constant and tends to decrease with time.

Cutaneous lesions (chilblain-like) are present in about half the cases. Moderately elevated levels of interferon alpha are present in CSF in most cases, at least in the first years of the disease (Lebon et al. 1988) and to a lesser extent in the blood. Similar cases have been reported as 'Cree encephalitis' from highly inbred Indian communities of Northern Quebec (Black et al. 1988). Aicardi–Goutières syndrome is genetically heterogeneous and four different loci have been shown to be linked with the disease. Recently, mutations in the subunits of four genes encoding the ribonuclease TREX1 (on chromosome 3p21) and the genes encoding three subunits of the ribonuclease H2 protein complex have been demonstrated (Crow et al. 2006, Rice et al. 2007). The disease should be distinguished from congenital viral infections especially with cytomegalovirus and HIV and from cases of calcification of the basal ganglia without evidence of white matter disease, sometimes with brain atrophy and without pleocytosis, which may not be present or will eventually disappear. Such cases are not rare (Billard et al. 1989) and probably represent a sequela to several nonprogressive, nongenetic disorders, although they may also occur with metabolic diseases (see Table 9.1). HIV infection should be systematically looked for in such cases.

NUCLEOTIDE EXCISION–DNA REPAIR SYNDROMES

Xeroderma pigmentosum (XP), Cockayne syndrome (CS) and trichothiodystrophy (TTD) are rare DNA-repair syndromes with photosensitivity of the skin, hair and skin abnormalities, short stature, microcephaly, mental retardation and various neurological abnormalities. An overlap between XP and TTD, as well as between XP and CS, may be observed clinically and has also been demonstrated by complementation analysis of cell fusions. Hereditary mutations in the repair and transcription factor DFIIH are associated with all three syndromes. White matter abnormalities are restricted mainly to CS and TTD.

Cockayne syndrome

CS is a rare but clinically characteristic disorder first described in 1936 as "dwarfism with retinal atrophy and deafness". It follows an autosomal recessive inheritance. Most CS cases are due to mutations of the CS-A gene on chromosome 5 and the *CS-B* gene on chromosome 10q (Cleaver et al. 1999). Nance and Berry (1992) reviewed 140 cases and distinguished three clinically different types of the disease: (1) classical CS (the majority); (2) early-onset severe, rapidly progressive type CS II; and (3) mild, late-onset, slowly progressive form.

Affected children show characteristic cachectic dwarfism, and a progeroid facial appearance with prominent chin and nose and large ears. The enophthalmia (sunken eyes) is due to the lack of subcutaneous orbital fat. Decreased height and weight, microcephalus, hearing loss, pigmentary retinopathy and cataracts develop. Patients walk with a characteristic stoop, and develop pyramidal and cerebellar symptoms (Rapin et al. 2000).

A peripheral neuropathy with reduced nerve conduction velocity and segmental demyelination in teased sural nerve preparation has been reported (Moosa and Dubowitz 1970). A recent analysis of 13 cases by Pasquier et al. (2006) described a

wide clinical variability of symptoms including conjunctival teleangiectasia and skeletal dysplasia with flat vertebral bodies. Neuropathology described thickened leptomeninges, features of a calcifying vasopathy, cerebral and cerebellar atrophy, and lack of myelin with a tigroid pattern due to preserved islands of myelin. Calcium deposits may be found in basal ganglia and dentate nuclei as well as in white matter and cortex of the brain.

CT and MRI show calcifications of basal ganglia, white matter abnormalities (hypomyelination) and cerebellar atrophy (Adachi et al. 2006). CSF may show high lactate levels. Abnormal excretion of organic acids has also been observed. The diagnosis is based on the hypersensitivity to UV light of cultured cells (Lehmann et al. 1993). Prenatal diagnosis of CS is possible (Kleijer et al. 2006). No treatment is available, the management is symptomatic.

18q– SYNDROME AND SALLA DISEASE

These are not usually described with the leukodystrophies, although involvement of the white matter is a prominent feature of both.

18q– syndrome is an autosomal recessive disorder caused by a deletion that includes the locus for the myelin basic protein gene (18q22–23). The clinical presentation is variable including generalized dysmorphic signs like microcephaly, high or cleft palate, narrow ear canals, clinodactyly, congenital heart disease and short stature. Mental retardation may be combined with hypotonia, choreoathetosis, poor coordination, nystagmus and seizures. Behavioural problems can be prominent. In a case of a 5-year-old girl with known 18q– syndrome studied in Göttingen, a general developmental retardation, clumsiness, a peculiar broad-based gait and marked impairment of active speech were the most prominent findings (FH, unpublished personal observations). MRI shows delay in myelination, most pronounced in older patients. In infants a poor differentiation between white and grey matter is present. T_2-weighted images may show widespread patches of hypomyelination.

Salla disease was first described in Finland by Aula et al. (1979). The name refers to the birth-place of the first patients, three brothers and their female cousin. It belongs to the group of sialic acid storage diseases. The efflux of sialic acid from lysosomes is disturbed by a transporter defect. The related gene *SLC17A5* (also called *AST*: anion sugar transport gene) is located on chromosome 6q14–15 (Haataja et al. 1994).

Symptoms appear at 6–9 months of age in the form of hypotonia, ataxia, athetosis and transient nystagmus. Later, spastic symptoms, growth retardation and dysmorphic, gargoyle-like features develop. Cognitive development and speech are affected. Most patients use only single words or short sentences, severely mentally retarded adult patients have been described by Haataja et al. (1994). Milder variants and single patients living outside Finland have also been diagnosed (Varho et al. 2002). Growth retardation becomes obvious, with varying endocrine abnormalities. Coarse facial features resemble storage disease involving the skeletal system. Plain X-ray of the lumbar spine may demonstrate ovoid-shaped vertebrae on lateral views. MRI in Salla disease shows generalized deficiency of myelin with a thin corpus callosum. Later, atrophy becomes evident that may also affect the cerebellum.

As in other mucolipidoses the EEG shows low voltage traces. Motor and sensory nerve conduction velocities are reduced. The increased excretion of sialic acid in urine is used for diagnostic purposes.

No causal treatment is available for patients with Salla disease.

RARE TYPES OF LEUKODYSTROPHY
A form of *leukodystrophy with pigmented glial cells and macrophages (van Bogaert–Nyssen disease)* has been only exceptionally observed in children (Seiser et al. 1990). Leukodystrophy with palmoplantar keratosis has been described in adults (Lossos et al. 1995). Skin abnormalities were also present in the cases of 'dermatoleukodystrophy' described by Matsuyama et al. (1978) in which spheroids were prominent in the white matter. Rare cases known as non-calcifying meningeal angiomatosis of Divry and van Bogaert appear to be the consequence of cortical microangiomatosis rather than true leukodystrophies. Such cases may be associated with cutaneous livedo reticularis. Labrune et al. (1996) reported three sporadic cases of diffuse white matter disease, extensive calcification and cyst formation with resulting hydrocephalus, and suggested that a diffuse vasculopathy was responsible. A rare type of prenatal leukodystrophy, probably autosomal recessive, known as Wiedeman–Rautenstrauch syndrome features progeroid features in association with demyelination of early onset (Martin et al. 1984). Leukodystrophy with congenital cataracts is due to mutation in the gene of hyalin (Biancheri et al. 2007).

DISORDERS INVOLVING PREDOMINANTLY THE GREY MATTER

These include the neuronal ceroid–lipofuscinoses, which also feature more diffuse involvement of the CNS, and a group of imperfectly defined conditions known as the poliodystrophies.

POLIODYSTROPHIES
Poliodystrophies form a heterogeneous group of disorders known collectively as Alpers or Alpers-like disease. The poliodystrophies are characterized pathologically by predominant involvement of the grey matter, which is reduced in volume and of abnormally firm consistency. At a late stage, the brain is usually grossly atrophic, the so-called 'walnut brain'. Neurons are greatly reduced or lacking altogether, or in a focal or laminar topography. There is marked glial proliferation, often associated with a spongy appearance of the neuropil, hence the term *glioneuronal spongy degeneration* used by some authors. At an early stage, the focal distribution of lesions is remarkable and they may be minimal. Such grey matter degeneration is difficult to differentiate from other conditions such as hypoxic sequelae, hypoglycaemia or postepileptic encephalopathy, and undoubtedly some such cases have been included among reports of poliodystrophy. Therefore,

the diagnosis should be based not only on pathological findings but also on the notion of a progressive illness. Most authentic cases of poliodystrophy have an established or probable genetic origin with an autosomal recessive inheritance.

The best-defined group among the poliodystrophies is the *progressive neuronal degeneration of childhood (PNDC) with hepatic involvement*, also known as *Alpers–Huttenlocher syndrome*. The onset of this disorder is usually wihin the first two years of life, and in most cases before 6 years, but same late cases even in adulthood are possible. Seizures and developmental regression appear insidiously, often in a child whose initial development had been somewhat slow. Generalized or multifocal myoclonus is a frequent feature, and epilepsia partialis continua is suggestive of the diagnosis. Bilateral spasticity, opisthotonus and decerebration eventually set in, often after several episodes of partial status epilepticus. Blindness is common and may be due either to occipital cortical involvement, which is often prominent, or to optic atrophy. The EEG is always severely abnormal with multifocal paroxysmal activity. Boyd et al. (1986) emphasized the occurrence of large slow waves with superimposed small-amplitude polyspikes often asymmetrically located over the occipital regions. Visual evoked potentials are grossly abnormal, with a normal ERG. CSF protein may be increased. Neuroimaging indicates progressive brain atrophy without signal change. PNDC runs a fatal course. Signs of hepatic disease that may end in terminal liver failure often become obvious only late in the course (Harding et al. 1995). Similar cases occur without hepatic failure (Bourgeois et al. 1992). The age of onset is variable, and late cases with atypical features may suggest spinocerebellar degeneration (Harding et al. 1995).

Although PNDC is probably heterogeneous, its features are suggestive of a mitochondrial disorder. Mutations in the *POLG1* (polymerase gamma) gene, involved in the replication and repair of the mitochondrial genome, with mtDNA depletion, have been demonstrated in several cases (Davidzon et al. 2005). Mutations in this gene can also be associated with other mitochondrial disorders involving muscle and/or CNS. A point mutation in the mtDNA gene-encoding subunit II of cytochrome *c* oxidase has been documented (Uusimaa et al. 2003).

Such cases may be easily mistaken for valproate hepatotoxicity (Delarue et al. 2000) and may account for some of the reported cases in which an early age of onset and the presence of seizures and severe neurological signs are often prominent (Bicknese et al. 1992; personal cases).

THE CEROID–LIPOFUSCINOSES (NEURONAL CEROID–LIPOFUSCINOSES, BATTEN DISEASE)
The neuronal ceroid–lipofuscinoses (CLNs) are a heterogeneous group of disorders characterized by the storage of certain lipopigments that present morphological and tinctorial similarities with lipofuscin, an autofluorescent pigment found in many animal tissues. Although the term lipofuscin, which designates the pigment that accumulates in neurons with age, is often used, the lipopigments that constitute the storage substance, termed ceroid, differ (Seehafer and Pearce 2006). Their ultrastructural appearance is also distinct. The chemical nature of these pigments is not fully

characterized. Lipofuscin normally accumulates in neural cells with ageing, although in variable amounts, and is regarded as a normal wear and tear substance. A major component of the pigment stored in infantile and juvenile ceroid–lipofuscinosis comprises subunit c of the respiratory chain enzyme ATP-synthase. Ceroid accumulates mainly in lysosome-like structures that give a positive acid phoshatase reaction.

CLNs are one of the most common degenerative conditions in childhood. Eight major types and a number of incompletely characterized forms have been described. At least six different genes are currently isolated and characterized, located on different chromosomes (Mole et al. 2004, 2005) (Table 9.4). The ceroid–lipofuscinoses are genetically determined progressive degenerative disorders affecting the CNS and retinae. The childhood forms are autosomal recessive diseases. The major neurological manifestations, epilepsy, myoclonus and cognitive deterioration express the predominant involvement of the grey matter (Santavuori et al. 2001).

The CLNs are a panethnic group of diseases; however, local variations are marked. The infantile form, which is rare in most countries, is frequent in Finland, with an incidence of 7.7 per 100,000 live births, while the juvenile form in common in the UK and Germany, and other types (CLN8) are also found preferentially in some populations (Goebel and Wisniewski 2004, Mole 2004). The ceroid–lipofuscinoses may be regarded as lysosomal diseases. In fact, deficiency of lysosomal enzymes has been demonstrated in some forms (see below) but abnormalities and dysfunction of structural proteins is also involved in the pathogenesis (Goebel and Winiewski 2004).

The term neuronal ceroid–lipofuscinosis is not entirely accurate as the lipopigment is also found in many extraneural tissues, which is still the basis for diagnosis of some CLNs. However, identification of several gene mutations now allows molecular diagnosis in several forms. Classification of the CLNs recognizes four major forms: CLN1 or classic infantile type, CLN2 or classic late infantile type, CLN3 or juvenile type, and CLN4 or adult form. Several variants of the late infantile form are known (Goebel et al. 1995). Goebel and Wisniewski (2004) could not classify 20% of the 520 cases they reviewed.

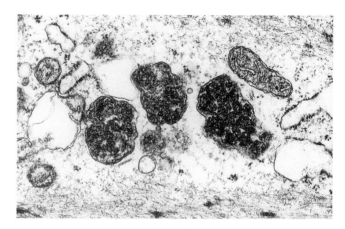

Fig. 9.10. Infantile neuronal ceroid–lipofuscinosis. Three electron-dense granular inclusions within a sweat gland cell. (Courtesy Dr M-L Arsenio-Nunes, Hôpital de la Salpétrière, Paris.)

electric tracing ('vanishing EEG') during the third year of life (Santavuori 1988). From 3 to 4 years of age, the disease appears to be 'burnt out', and the children remain without contact with their surroundings until death.

The disease produces an extraordinary degree of brain atrophy. This is well demonstrated by MRI that shows, in addition, hypodensity of the thalami, a peripheral ring of increased T_2 signal around the ventricles and a reversal of the normal white–grey contrast in late stages (Vanhanen et al. 1995). Surviving neurons, as well as a number of extraneural cells contain large amounts of ceroid with a homogeneous, finely granular internal structure (Fig. 9.10). Molecular diagnosis by demonstration of low activity of the enzyme PPT1 or by analysis of the mutation is possible. Death occurs following variable periods of vegetative state. In a few cases, a picture reminiscent of the Lennox–Gastaut syndrome is seen at onset of the disease.

Distinct mutations of the same gene can express in adolescents and adults (see below). In such cases, the course is much slower, and storage of granular osmiophilic deposits (GRODs) identical to those in the infantile form can be demonstrated by biopsy (Mitchison et al. 1998).

INFANTILE CLN (SANTAVUORI–HALTIA–HAGBERG DISEASE, CLN1)

This form is due to a mutant gene on chromosome 1 (1p33–p35) that codes for the enzyme *palmitoyl protein thioesterase (PPT1)*, a lysosomal enzyme whose function is still unknown. The early development of affected infants is normal. From 6 to 12 months of age, intellectual deterioration and ataxia are the main features. Anxiety and autistic-like features may be prominent, together with the abnormal stereotypic hand movements ('knitting movements') that may wrongly suggest the diagnosis of Rett syndrome. Myoclonic jerks appear during the second year of life and there is progressive microcephaly. Macular and retinal degeneration and optic atrophy are frequent, and the ERG is always extinguished, except perhaps in the first few months of the illness. The EEG shows progressive slowing and loss of amplitude leading to an iso-

LATE INFANTILE CLN (JANSKY–BIELCHOWSKY DISEASE, CLN2)

The responsible gene maps to chromosome 11p15 and codes for the lysosomal enzyme *tripeptyl peptidase 1*, which allows diagnosis by demonstration of low activity or molecular analysis. The onset is between 18 months and 4 years of age. The first symptom is arrest and rapid regession of development. Epilepsy is the prominent feature but usually begins after 30 months of age, soon followed by dementia and ataxia. Seizures are often myoclonic in type and are associated with erratic and intention myoclonus. Loss of motor skills and spasticity develop rapidly and the children become bedridden by 3.5–6 years of age. Visual failure is usually late after age 6 years. There is macular and retinal degeneration and optic atrophy but these usually appear by 3–4 years of age, and at onset even the ERG may be normal.

TABLE 10.4
Main types of neuronal ceroid–lipofuscinosis (CLN)

	Infantile (Santavuori–Hagberg) CLN1	Infantile CLN1 (GRODs variant)	Late infantile (Jansky–Bielschowski) CLN2	CLN2 variants CLN5 (late)	CLN6	Juvenile (Spielmeyer–Vogt) CLN3	Adult (Kufs) CLN4
Age at onset	6–18 months	Late childhood	18 months – 4 years	4–7 years	2–10 years	4–8 years	Occasionally in children
Early features	Deterioration, autism	Deterioration	Deterioration, seizures	Deterioration, ataxia	Deterioration	Visual failure	Behaviour, cognitive
Late manifestations Deterioration	Rapid	Often slow	Rapid	Variable	Marked	Psychiatric disturbances prominent	Slow
Epilepsy	Inconstant	Inconstant	Prominent[1]	Present, late	Present	Present	Present in some
Myoclonus	Early			Late or absent		Present	Possible
Acquired microcephaly	Marked	Usually absent	Absent	Absent		Absent	Absent
Ataxia	Present	Present	Marked	Marked			Some cases
Extrapyramidal signs	Inconstant	Often present	Present	Marked (dysarthria)		Marked (dysarthria)	Marked (not all)
Visual deficit	Inconspicuous	Present	Present, late	Early, marked	Present	Early blindness	Absent
Neurophysiology EEG	Vanishing EEG	Nonspecific	SW, IPS	SW		SW, runs of slow waves	SW, IPS in some cases
ERG	Extinguished	Decreased or absent	Extinguished, at times late	Extinguished, late		Extinguished	Normal
VEP	Abolished		Giant	Extinghished, late			
Vacuolated lymphocytes	Absent	Absent	Absent	Absent		Present	Absent
Major cytosome type	Granular	Granular (GRODs)	Curvilinear	Fingerprints and curvilinear		Fingerprints	Mostly granular
Course duration	Death or burnt-out state <5 years	May be long	Death 5–15 years	Death <15 years		Slow	Slow
Biopsy diagnosis	Lymphocytes, skin, conjunctiva		Lymphocytes, Ur	Lymphocytes, Ur		Lymphocytes	Idem; rectal biopsy may be required
Molecular biology diagnosis	Absent/decreased PTT1	Absent/decreased PTT1					
Prenatal diagnosis	Absent/decreased PTT1	Absent/decreased PTT1	AFC, Ur			Biopsy but molecular	Biopsy
Gene (chromosome)	PTT1 (1p33–p35)	PTT1 (1p33–35)	(11p15)	(13q31–32)	(15q21–23)	(16p2)	

[1]May simulate Lennox–Gastaut syndrome or other myoclonic epilepsies.

Abbreviations: AFC = amniotic fluid cells; ChV = chorionic villus biopsy; GRODs = granular osmiophilic deposits; IPS = response to slow photic stimulation; PTT1 = palmitoyl protein thioesterase; SW = spike–wave complexes; Ur = urinary sediment biopsy.

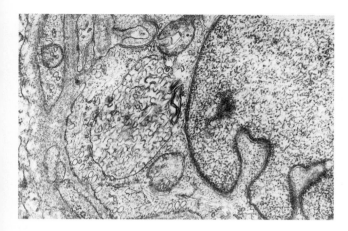

Fig. 9.11. Late infantile neuronal ceroid–lipofuscinosis. Skin biopsy: inclusion containing curvilinear profiles. (Courtesy Dr M-L Arsenio-Nunes, Hôpital de la Salpétrière, Paris.)

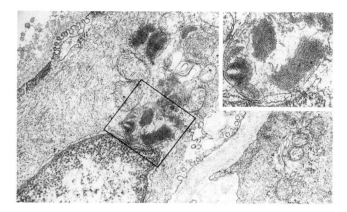

Fig. 9.12. Juvenile neuronal ceroid–lipofuscinosis. 'Fingerprint' inclusions within an endothelial cell of a skin capillary. Insert shows detail of inclusion with closely packed membranes. (Courtesy Dr M-L Arsenio-Nunes, Hôpital de la Salpétrière, Paris.)

The neurophysiological picture is characteristic. The EEG shows, in addition to multifocal spikes and slow background rhythm, a peculiar response to photic stimulation at a low rate, each flash producing a spike in the posterior scalp regions (Harden and Pampiglione 1982). The ERG is extinguished. Visual evoked potentials (VEPs) and somatosensory evoked responses are also very large, although VEPs may become abolished at a late stage.

Neuroimaging demonstrates brain atrophy less marked than in the infantile type. No vacuolated lymphocytes are found. Skin or conjunctival biopsy may show cytosomes containing predominantly curvilinear profiles (Fig. 9.11). Death occurs between 6 and 15 years of age.

Several variants of the late infantile type have been described. They are genetically heterogeneous and the resulting dieases are mostly seen in specific populations. A *Finnish variant (CLN5)* (Wisniewski et al. 1993) is due to mutations of a gene that maps to chromosome 13q31–q32 and codes for a membrane protein with 407 amino acids (Savukosky et al. 1998). The onset is around 5 years of age with mental deterioration or ataxia. Visual symptoms, epileptic manifestations and neurophysiological abnormalities are observed after 7–8 years of age, and the course is slower than in the late infantile type. Most cytosomes are of the 'fingerprint' type (containing linear, curved patterns reminiscent of fingerprints), but the neurophysiological features are similar to those of the late infantile type. CLN6 is due to several mutations of a gene mapping to chromosome 15q21.23 that codes for a membrane protein with 311 amino acids whose function is not determined (Sharp et al. 2003). CLN7 has been described in Turkish patients (Ranta et al. 2004, Topçu et al. 2004). The clinical picture was similar to that of the Finnish variant but with a greater severity. No mutant gene has been identified. The disorder seems to be genetically heterogeneous and the same clinical picture has been observed with mutations in the *CLN6* and especially of the *CLN8* genes (Siintola et al. 2005). Mutations in the *CLN8* gene with a similar clinical presentation are also encountered in other Mediterranean countries (Striano et al. 2007) with a clinical picture different from that of Northern epilepsy (see below).

Other variants including a Gypsy Indian form exist and the distribution of individual mutations may vary with the ethnic origin.

JUVENILE CLN (SPIELMEYER–VOGT–SJÖGREN DISEASE, CLN3)

The gene for this form maps to chromosome 16p2 and codes for a novel membrane protein of 438 amino acids. The onset is between 4 and 7 years. It is marked by failing vision that begins with hemeralopia and leads to very low acuity in about two years. Seizures appear in most cases after two or three years. Deterioration is initially absent or mild but behavioural disturbances may be prominent, often leading to a misdiagnosis of a psychiatric condition. A special type of dysarthria with precipitate and indistinct emission becomes obvious by 10–15 years of age. Neurological signs develop slowly and include extrapyramidal manifestations (tremor and rigidity) and slight cerebellar and pyramidal signs. Myoclonic seizures are common but generalized, and partial seizures may also supervene.

Ophthalmological examination reveals macular degeneration with pigment aggregates, present from 10 years onward.

The EEG may show pseudoperiodic bursts of high-amplitude slow waves or a low-amplitude, rather featureless tracing (Harden and Pampiglione 1982). The ERG and VEPs are decreased or abolished early in the course. Neuroimaging shows mild to moderate atrophy. Extensive calcification is present pathologically and may be apparent on CT.

Vacuolated lymphocytes are usually present, and ultrastructural examination of the skin and conjunctiva, lymphocytes and tonsillar tissue shows a predominance of fingerprint profiles (Fig. 9.12). The diagnosis can now be effectively made by studying the gene mutations (International Batten Disease Consortium 1995). The course is relentlessly progressive leading to death between 15 and 30 years of age.

An *early juvenile variant* has its onset between 3 and 5 years of age (Lake and Cavanagh 1978). The inclusions are both fingerprint and curvilinear profiles.

Juvenile-onset ceroid–lipofuscinosis with granular osmiophilic deposits (GRODs)

A clinical picture clinically indistinguishable from CLN3 has been encountered in some adolescent and adult patients (Mitchison et al. 1998). However, homogeneously granular cytosomes (GRODs) constitute the storage substance (Lake et al. 1996). This variant does not map to the CLN3 locus and is due to mutation of the *PPT1* gene, but the mutations are different to those of the early infantile type (Kalviainen et al. 2007). It is therefore considered a *late form of CLN1*.

Other cases, including a protracted form, have been reported (Wisniewski et al. 1998).

PROGRESSIVE EPILEPSY WITH MENTAL RETARDATION (NORTHERN EPILEPSY, CLN8)

CLN8 has been decribed so far only in Finland. The clinical onset is at about 8–10 years followed by a slowly progressive cognitive and neurological deterioration and progressive cerebral atrophy.

Northern epilepsy is allelic to another disorder, the Turkish variant of the late infantile form that was reported as CLN7. However, further reported cases whose clinical manifestations are more similar to those of the other forms of ceroid–lipofuscinosis (Ranta et al. 2004) proved to be usually due to mutations in the CLN8 gene (Siintola et al. 2005, Striano et al. 2007).

ADULT NEURONAL CEROID–LIPOFUSCINOSIS (KUFS DISEASE, CLN4)

Despite its denomination, adult CLN may have its onset in childhood or adolescence and the first symptoms may appear as early as 3 years of age (Berkovic et al. 1988). They develop insidiously and consist mainly of cognitive and behavioural disturbances. Mild dementia is evident eventually. Late in the course extrapyramidal signs may appear, especially facial dyskinesia. There are no ophthalmological abnormalities or visual failure. Some patients may develop myoclonic seizures. Berkovic et al. (1988) separate two types: one of progressive myoclonic epilepsy and neuropsychiatric changes, also observed by Sadzot et al. (2000), and one of dementia and motor, cerebellar and extrapyramidal manifestations. The EEG may show a remarkable response to photic stimulation, with high-amplitude spikes synchronous to flashes at low rhythm of repetition. Most reported cases have been sporadic, probably autosomal recessive in inheritance. In rare families, a dominant inheritance is likely.

Cytosomes containing granular osmiophilic inclusions can be found but they may be difficult to find in non-neural tissues.

OTHER ATYPICAL TYPES

Such types may account for 10–20% of cases in some series (Dyken and Wisniewski 1995, Goebel and Wisniewski 2004). Several classifications have been proposed, some containing as many as 15 different types (Dyken and Wisniewski 1995), but none has been generally adopted. Whether some of the minor forms are actually different entities or only 'variants' of more classic forms remains to be established.

Several cases of *congenital CLN (Norman–Wood type)* have been reported by Dyken and Wisniewski (1995). This presents as a devastating disease with rapidly fatal respiratory insufficiency and status epilepticus, and has recently been suggested to result from lysosomal cathepsin D deficiency (Siintola et al. 2006). The onset is marked by visual difficulties, and the slow development of seizures and dementia. The predominance of curvilinear profiles and visual failure separate these cases from the adult form. A *pigment variant* (Goebel et al. 1995) begins in childhood and also has a protracted course, but differs by the appearance of the storage product. *Chronic infantile* (Dyken and Wisniewski 1995) and childhood cases, and isolated cases with chorea, spinocerebellar signs, neuropathy and a slow progression have been described. A few *cases associated with osteopetrosis* are on record (Takahashi et al. 1990) and may have a prenatal onset.

DIAGNOSIS

The diagnosis of CLN may be difficult in the less usual types. Neurophysiological features, especially an abnormal ERG and a peculiar response of the EEG to slow light stimulation (1–3 Hz), are of value in late infantile and some 'adult' forms. Brain atrophy on neuroimaging is usually present early but may not be found in the first year of illness. A decreased T_2 signal in the thalami found in CLNs 1, 2, 3, 5, 6 and the Turkish variant of late infantile CLN is suggestive but not specific (Autti et al. 2007).

Molecular genetic testing for the classical types (CLNs 1, 2 and 3) by assay of palmitoyl-protein thioesterase in CLN1 and of tripeptyl-peptidase 1 activity in CLN2 (Young et al. 2001) is the most effective method. Mutation analysis is possible for those types in which the gene has been cloned (Zhong 2001). For rare forms, it is still a reseach investigation. For several forms, demonstration of the characteristic inclusions in lymphocytes, skin, conjunctiva or other extraneural tissues is still the only available test. No type of inclusion is completely specific for one form, although there is usually one predominant type. Biopsy of extraneural tissue is occasionally negative. In such cases, rectal biopsy may show inclusion-containing neurons.

Prenatal diagnosis can be established by the same molecular techniques in the forms in which a gene is known. It can also be made on the morphological appearance of inclusions in amniotic fluid cells or chorionic villus biopsies (Chow et al. 1993), or on the presence of subunit C of mitochondrial ATPase in CLNs 2 and 3, combined with DNA linkage in CLNs 1 and 3 (Goebel et al. 1995). Detection of carriers is possible in selected cases of CLN1.

TREATMENT

Antioxidant treatment with vitamins E and C and selenium has been proposed (Santavuori et al. 1985) but the results are unfortunately limited. Anticonvulsant treatment is essential in most types. Sodium valproate and/or clonazepam are often effective, but antiepileptic treatment should be individualized and seizures may be totally refractory.

Supportive care to the patients and families is essential and helps lessen the impact of these devastating diseases.

STEREOTYPIES AND MANNERISMS

Such phenomena are frequent in children with autism and other behaviour disturbances (Jankovic 2005). They are a major manifestation of Rett syndrome. They are also common in normal children (Mahone et al. 2004) and may take extraordinary forms in some cases. When isolated, they are a benign phenomenon but they may raise difficult differential diagnostic problems with movement disorders or epilepsy. Distinction from epileptic phenomena may be all the more difficult as epileptic stereotypies have been recognized (Deonna et al. 2002). Although most stereotypies in normal children do not require therapy, some cases such as self-injuring stereotypies can raise difficult therapeutic problems. A special type of head and eye movement reminiscent of those in the bobble head phenomenon (Chapter 6) and interpreted as a stereotypy, associated with hypotonia, axial ataxia, motor and language delay has been observed in 8 children (Hottinger-Blanc et al. 2002). In 2 of these, imaging demonstrated abnormalities of the cerebellum, suggesting a developmental cerebellar disorder.

OTHER ABNORMAL MOVEMENTS

TARDIVE DYSKINESIA

This is a common type of secondary dystonia observed only in persons receiving or having received neuroleptic drugs, especially phenothiazines, butyrophenones or diphenylbutylpiperidine, although it is rare in children (Jankovic 2005). The incidence is poorly known. Several types can occur. Tardive dyskinesia proper usually appears in children who have been receiving high doses of these medications for months or years, or with an increase in dosage. However, even low doses for short periods have uncommonly been responsible. The most usual type of movement is orofacial dyskinesia with stereotypic protrusion of the tongue, lip smacking or chewing motions. The intensity is variable.

Other types of dyskinesia may be observed such as dystonic or choreic movements. The abnormal movements can improve following discontinuation of the responsible drug over a period of several months but are permanent in about one third of patients.

Various types of dyskinesia may supervene on withdrawal of neuroleptics. These do not usually include orofacial movements, and they tend to disappear in a few weeks or months.

The mechanisms of tardive dyskinesia are imperfectly understood. Supersensitivity of dopamine receptors induced by the medication plays a major role. However, why only some patients are affected is unexplained.

Treatment of tardive dyskinesia is unsatisfactory. Drugs used in the treatment of movement disorders such as tetrabenazine or clonidine are rarely effective. Limitation of the use of neuroleptics in children is strongly advised.

OTHER TOXIN-INDUCED ABNORMAL MOVEMENTS

Many chemicals, including in particular a wide range of pharmaceuticals, can be responsible for abnormal movements (see also Chapter 16). These include, among others, dopaminergic, antiemetic, anticonvulsant and antidepressant drugs, and may produce variable dyskinesias (Elzinga-Huttenga et al. 2006).

MIRROR MOVEMENTS

Mirror movements are involuntary, symmetrical, identical movements associated with a voluntary movement carried out by the contralateral limb, in particular finger motions. They may be congenital and familial, following a dominant mendelian pattern (Rasmussen 1993), and are not associated with any brain pathology. In some cases, cervical abnormalities such as Klippel–Feil syndrome may be associated. They may occur with cervical spina bifida, so an X-ray of the spinal cord should be obtained. They may be associated with Kallmann syndrome (Farmer et al. 2004; see Chapter 20). Mirror movements may also occur in patients with childhood hemiparesis (Cohen et al. 1991). The mechanism of mirror movement is variable. In some cases, bilateral activation of the motor cortex or defective crossing of pyramidal tracts has been demonstrated (Farmer et al. 2004). The abnormal movements tend to decrease with age but they often persist into adulthood.

THE PROGRESSIVE MYOCLONIC EPILEPSIES (MYOCLONUS–EPILEPSIES)

The progressive myoclonic epilepsies are a group of symptomatic generalized epilepies caused by rare diseases, most of them of genetic origin (Shahwan et al. 2005). Mitochondrial disorders, especially the syndrome of myoclonic encephalopathy with ragged red fibres (MERRF), however, can produce a similar clinical picture (see Chapters 8, 21). Myoclonic epilepsies with known metabolic defects have been considered in Chapter 8. This paragraph deals with the so-called 'degenerative' types (Marseille Consensus Group 1990; Berkovic et al. 1991, 1993) and Lafora disease. Both disorders combine generalized tonic–clonic seizures or massive myoclonic jerks, localized myoclonus that may be spontaneous but is often induced by external stimuli such as touch, action or intention, and various degrees of neurological and mental deterioration. The main disorders featuring myoclonus and myoclonic epilepsy are shown in Table 9.13. Before accepting the diagnosis of idiopathic progressive myoclonic epilepsy one should always first exclude the diagnosis MERRF, if necessary by muscle biopsy and by searching for the mitochondrial DNA mutation.

UNVERRICHT–LUNDBORG DISEASE (BALTIC MYOCLONUS, RAMSAY HUNT SYNDROME, EPM1)

This disorder is the best example and the most common of the degenerative myoclonic epilepsies. It is transmitted as an autosomal recessive condition and is due to an unstable dodecamer repeat located in the promotor region of the *cystatin B* gene, a cysteine protease inhibitor, on chromosome 21. This mutation is associated with a deficiency of cystatin B messenger RNA in some cell types. In some cases, other mutations such as splicing error or other point mutations resulting in loss of function of cystatin B have been reported (Lehesjoki 2003). The pathology is limited to the cerebellum with loss of Purkinje cells and sometimes of neurons in deep cerebellar nuclei and inferior olive (Friede 1989, Koskiniemi et al. 1994). Onset of the clinical

TABLE 9.13
Diseases featuring progressive myoclonic epilepsy (PME)

Diseases in which PME is pure or in forefront of clinical picture
Lafora disease (PME1, PME2A, PME2B)
Unverricht–Lundborg disease[1]
Myoclonic epilepsy with ragged-red fibres (MERRF) (Chapter 8)
Juvenile Gaucher disease (type III) (Chapter 8)
Hereditary dentatorubral–pallidoluysian degeneration
PME with lipomas (Ekbom syndrome) (Berkovic et al. 1993)[2]
PME with deafness (May–White syndrome)[2]
PME with renal failure (Badhwar et al. 2004)

Diseases in which PME is atypical or associated with other manifestations
Neuronal ceroid–lipofuscinosis (several types)
Alpers poliodystrophy and related mitochondrial disorders[2]
Mitochondrial encephalomyopathy with lactic acidosis and stroke-like episodes (MELAS)
Huntington chorea (myoclonic form) (Gambardella et al. 2001)
Hallervorden–Spatz disease
Biopterin deficiency (Chapter 8)

Diseases in which PME is overshadowed by other manifestations
Nonketotic hyperglycinaemia
D-glyceric aciduria
Biopterin deficiency
Menkes disease
Krabbe disease
Tay–Sachs disease
Sandhoff disease
Niemann–Pick disease
Spinal muscular atrophy and progressive myoclonic epilepsy (Striano et al. 2004)
Myoclonic epilepsy and acute intermittent porphyria (Varsik et al. 2005)

Unless indicated, see text for references.
[1]The same (or a very similar) disorder is referred to as Ramsay Hunt syndrome in some publications (Genton et al. 2005).
[2]These syndromes are probably related to mitochondrial disorders.

manifestations occurs between 6 and 16 years with tonic–clonic seizures in 50% of cases and myoclonic seizures in the other half (Koskiniemi et al. 1974a). The myoclonus disappears during sleep or rest and is induced by external stimuli but mainly by maintenance of posture or intended movement. Its intensity increases progressively and it may become totally incapacitating in adulthood. Epileptic seizures are seldom severe and include generalized tonic–clonic seizures, often occurring on awakening, and massive myoclonic jerks very similar to those in juvenile myoclonic epilepsy (Chapter 15). Absences or drop-attacks are observed in a minority of patients. Intelligence is relatively preserved but in most cases there is a slow and mild deterioration that has been attributed most often to phenytoin treatment. Kyllerman et al. (1991) reported the occurrence of 'cascades' of seizures and myoclonic jerks. Neurological signs such as intention tremor tend to appear after a few years, but pyramidal tract signs are seen in only one third of cases (Berkovic et al. 1993). Cerebellar signs are very difficult to assess because of the intention myoclonus. The EEG seems to show variable slowing of background activity with superimposed paroxysmal activity (Koskiniemi et al. 1974b). In some cases the background rhythm remains normal for many years aside from paroxysmal abnormalities identical to

those in the primary generalized epilepsies. Runs of spikes appear at the vertex during REM sleep. Such differences are considered to be of nosological significance by some investigators who preferred to separate a subgroup of Mediterranean myoclonus from the Baltic form that corresponds to the original description of Unverricht. It is apparent that cases reported as Baltic myoclonus by some groups and as Mediterranean myoclonus or Ramsay Hunt syndrome by others (Tassinari et al. 1989) in fact represent the same disease; both types are linked to the same locus on chromosome 21 (Cochius et al. 1993), and the same mutation has been found in both Finnish and Italian cases (Parmeggiani et al. 1997). Giant somaesthetic evoked potentials are present in all cases, indicating a cortical-type myoclonus (Shibasaki et al. 1986). The treatment is that of intention myoclonus, and the use of polytherapy with sodium valproate, primidone, clonazepam and 5-hydroxytryptophan may be effective (Obeso et al. 1989). Piracetam in very large doses has been shown to be efficacious on the myoclonus, and levetiracetam may also be of benefit (Crest et al. 2004). Phenytoin may aggravate incapacity and is contraindicated. The prognosis is poor from a functional standpoint, but with modern treatment the disease is rarely life threatening. The term Ramsay Hunt syndrome is better abandoned. For some investigators it designates a disorder identical with or similar to Unverricht–Lundborg disease. For other authors (Marseille Consensus Group 1990) it applies to a progressive ataxia associated with intention myoclonus, with or without epilepsy but accompanied by cerebellar signs.

A second type of recessive progressive myoclonic epilepsy with similar clinical features but without mutations in the *cystatin B* gene has recently been described in an inbred Arab family, mapping to the pericentric region of chromosome 12 (Berkovic et al. 2005).

LAFORA DISEASE (EPM2)

Lafora disease is the best defined type of myoclonus epilepsy with a detectable storage. Lafora (amyloid) bodies are found within neurons throughout the neuraxis, especially in the substantia nigra, dentate nucleus, reticular substance and hippocampus. They are also present in muscle and liver, and in sweat gland ducts in the skin, thus permitting diagnosis by skin biopsy. Biochemically, Lafora bodies consist of a glucose polymer chemically related to glycogen in association with protein. These neurotoxic poyglucosans accumulate in the endoplasmic reticulum where they are normally cleared by the protein laforin, a dual-action phosphatase. The disease is inherited as an autosomal recessive trait, and two different loci and genes have been found: *EPM2A* has been mapped to chromosome 6q24 and codes for laforin; *EPM2B* on chromosome 6p22 codes for a different protein (Chan et al. 2003). There is evidence for a third locus (Chan et al. 2004). The *EPM2A* and *EPM2B* mutations were responsible respectively for 70% and 27% of the 54 cases studied by Gomez-Abad et al. (2005), but the proportions vary with the populations studied (Franceschetti et al. 2006). The phenotypes of both types are similar, although the 2B genotype is possibly milder.

of cerebellar and hippocampal cortex. *J Child Neurol* **2**: 279–86.

Chow CW, Borg J, Billson VR, Lake BD (1993) Fetal tissue involvement in the late infantile type of neuronal ceroid lipofuscinosis. *Prenat Diagn* **13**: 833–41.

Christodoulou K, Deymeer F Serdaroglu P, et al. (2001) Mapping of the second Friedreich's ataxia gene (FRDA2) locus to chromosome 9p23–p11: evidence for further locus heterogeneity. *Neurogenetics* **3**: 127–32.

Chuang S (1989) Vascular diseases of the brain in children. In: Edwards MSB, Hoffman HJ, eds. *Cerebral Vascular Disease in Children and Adolescents.* Baltimore: Williams & Wilkins, pp. 69–93.

Church AJ, Dale RC, Lees AJ, et al. (2003) Tourette's syndrome: a cross sectional study to examine the PANDAS hypothesis. *J Neurol Neurosurg Psychiatry* **74**: 602–7.

Chutorian AM, Nygaard TG, Waran S (1994) Dopa-responsive dystonia. *Int Pediatr* **9** Suppl: 49–54.

Cif L, Valente EM, Hemm S, et al. (2004) Deep brain stimulation in myoclonus–dystonia syndrome. *Mov Disord* **19**: 724–7.

Cleaver JF, Thompson LH, Richardson AS, States JC (1999) A summary of mutations in the UV-sensitive disorders: xeroderma pigmentosusm, Cockayne syndrome, and trichothiodystrophy. *Hum Mutat* **14**: 9–22.

Cochius JL, Figlewicz DA, Kälviäinen R, et al. (1993) Unverricht–Lundborg disease: absence of nonallelic genetic heterogeneity. *Ann Neurol* **34**: 739–41.

Cohen LG, Meer J, Tarkka I, et al. (1991) Congenital mirror movements. Abnormal organization of motor pathways in two patients. *Brain* **114**: 381–403.

Coleman RJ, Robb SA, Lake B, et al. (1988) The diverse neurological features of Niemann–Pick disease type C. *Mov Disord* **3**: 275–9.

Comella CL, Thompson PD (2006) Treatment of cervical dystonia with botulinum toxins. *Eur J Neurol* **13** Suppl 1: 16–20.

Comings DE (1990) *Tourette Syndrome and Human Behavior.* Duarte, CA: Hope Press.

Connelly KP, De Witt LD (1994) Neurologic complications of infectious mononucleosis. *Pediatr Neurol* **10**: 180–4.

Costeff H, Gadoth N, Apter N, et al. (1989) A familial syndrome of infantile optic atrophy, movement disorder and spastic paraplegia. *Neurology* **39**: 595–7.

Cotter M, Connell T, Colhoun E, et al. (2005) Carbonic anhydrase II deficiency: a rare autosomal recessive disorder of osteopetrosis, renal tubular acidosis, and cerebral calcification. *J Pediatr Hematol Oncol* **27**: 115–7.

Coubes P, Cif L, El Fertit H, et al. (2004) Elecrical stimulation of the globus pallidus internus in patients with primary generalized dystonia: long-term results. *J Neurosurg* **101**: 189–94.

Crest C, Dupont S, Leguern E, et al. (2004) Levetiracetam in progressive myoclonic epilepsy: an exploratory study in 9 patients. *Neurology* **62**: 640–3.

Crow YJ, Leitch A, Hayward BE, et al. (2006) Mutations in genes encoding ribonuclease H2 subunits cause Aicardi–Goutières syndrome and mimic congenital viral brain infection. *Nat Genet* **38**: 910–6.

Danek A, Robio JP, Rapoldi L, et al. (2001) The chorea of McLeod syndrome. *Ann Neurol* **50**: 755–64.

Danek A, Jung HH, Melone MA, et al. (2005) Neuroacanthocytosis: new developments in a neglected group of dementing disorders. *J Neurol Sci* **299–300**: 171–86.

Davidzon G, Mancuso M, Ferraris S, et al. (2005) POLG mutations and Alpers syndrome. *Ann Neurol* **57**: 921–3.

De Carvalho Aguiar PM, Ozelius LJ (2002) Classification and genetics of dystonia. *Lancet Neurol* **1**: 316–25.

De Carvalho Aguiar P, Sweadner KJ, Penniston JT, et al. (2004) Mutations of the Na+/K+ –ATPase alpha3 gene ATP1A3 are associated with rapid-onset dystonia parkinsonism. *Neuron* **43**: 169–75.

De Koning TJ, de Vries LS, Groenendal F, et al. (1999) Pontocerebellar hypoplasia associated with respiratory chain defects. *Neuropediatrics* **30**: 93–5.

Delarue A, Paut O, Guys JM, et al. (2000) Inappropriate liver transplantattion in a child with Alpers–Huttenlocher syndrome misdiagnosed as valproate-induced acute liver failure. *Pediatr Transplant* **4**: 170–2.

De León GA, Crawford SE, Stack C, et al. (1996) Amylaceous (polyglucosan) bodies in familial cerebral atrophy of early onset. *J Child Neurol* **11**: 58–62.

DeMichele G, Filla A, D'Armiento FP, et al. (1990) Cerebellar ataxia and hypogonadism. A clinicopathological report. *Clin Neurol Neurosurg* **92**: 67–70.

DeMichele G, Filla A, Cavalcanti F, et al. (1994) Late onset Friedreich's disease: clinical features and mapping of mutation to the FRDA locus. *J Neurol Neurosurg Psychiatry* **57**: 977–9.

DeMichele G, Di Maio L, Filla A, et al. (1996) Childhood onset of Friedreich

ataxia: a clinical and genetic study of 36 cases. *Neuropediatrics* **27**: 3–7.

Deonna T, Roulet E, Ghika J, Zesiger P (1997) Dopa-responsive childhood dystonia: a forme fruste with writer's cramp, triggered by exercise. *Dev Med Child Neurol* **39**: 49–53.

Deonna T, Fohlen M, Jalin C, et al. (2002) Epileptic stereotypies in children. In: Guerrini R, Aicardi J, Andermann F, Hallett M, eds. *Epilepsy and Movement Disorders.* Cambridge: Cambridge University Press, pp. 318–32.

de Rijk-Van Andel JF, Gabreels FJ, Geurtz B, et al. (2000) L-dopa-responsive infantile hypokinetic rigid parkinsonism due to hydroxylase oxidase deficiency. *Neurology* **55**: 1926–8.

Deuschl G, Toro C, Valls-Solé J, et al. (1994) Symptomatic and essential palatal tremor. 1. Clinical, physiological and MRI analysis. *Brain* **117**: 775–88.

Di Donato S, Gellera C, Mariotti C (2001) The complex clinical and genetic classification of inherited ataxias. II: Autosomal recessive ataxias. *Neurol Sci* **22**: 219–28.

Dierks T, Schmidt B, Borissenko LV, et al. (2003) Multiple sulfatase deficiency is caused by mutations in the gene encoding the human C(alpha)-formylglycine generating enzyme. *Cell* **113**: 435–44.

Di Mario FJ, Clancy R (1989) Symmetrical thalamic degeneration with calcification of infancy. *Am J Dis Child* **143**: 1056–60.

Dobson-Stone C, Velayos-Baeza A, Fillipone LA, et al. (2004) Chorein detection for the diagnosis of choreo-acanthocytosis. *Ann Neurol* **56**: 299–302.

Dooling EC, Schoene WC, Richardson EP (1974) Hallervorden–Spatz syndrome. *Arch Neurol* **30**: 70–83.

Dorfman LJ, Pedley TA, Tharp BR, Scheithauer BW (1978) Juvenile neuroaxonal dystrophy: clinical, electrophysiological and neuropathological features. *Ann Neurol* **3**: 419–28.

Dubois-Dalcq M, Feigenbaum V, Aubourg P (1999) The neurobiology of X-linked adrenoleukodystrophy, a demyelinating peroxisomal disorder. *Trends Neurosci* **22**: 4–12.

Dueñas AM, Goold R, Giunti P (2006) Molecular pathogenesis of spinocerebellar ataxias. *Brain* **129**: 1357–70.

Dürr A, Cossee M, Agid Y, et al. (1996a) Clinical and genetic abnormalities in patients with Friedreich's ataxia. *N Engl J Med* **335**: 1169–75.

Dürr A, Stevanin G, Cancel G, et al. (1996b) Spinocerebellar ataxia 3 and Machado–Joseph disease: clinical, molecular, and neuropathological features. *Ann Neurol* **39**: 490–9.

Dürr A, Camuzat A, Colin E, et al. (2004) Atlastin1 mutations are frequent in young-onset autosomal dominant spastic paraplegia. *Arch Neurol* **61**: 1867–72.

Dwork AJ, Balmaceda C, Fazzini EA, et al. (1993) Dominantly inherited early-onset parkinsonism: neuropathology of a new form. *Neurology* **43**: 69–74.

Dyken P, Wisniewski K (1995) Classification of the neuronal ceroid lipofuscinoses: expansion of the atypical forms. *Am J Med Genet* **57**: 150–4.

Eda I, Takashima S, Takeshita K (1983) Acute hemiplegia with lacunar infarct after varicella infection in childhood. *Brain Dev* **5**: 494–9.

Edwards M, Wood N, Bhatia K (2003) Unusual phenotypes in DYT1 dystonia: a report of five cases and a review of the literature. *Mov Disord* **18**: 706–11.

El-Khamisy SF, Saifi GM, Weinfeld M, et al. (2005) Defective DNA single-strand break repair in spinocerebellar ataxia with axonal neuropathy-1. *Nature* **434**: 108–13.

Elzinga-Huttenga J, Hekster Y, Bijl A, Rotteveel J (2006) Movement disorders induced by gastrointestinal drugs: two paediatric cases. *Neuropediatrics* **37**: 102–6.

Enevoldson TP, Sanders MD, Harding AE (1994) Autosomal dominant cerebellar ataxia with pigmentary macular dystrophy. A clinical and genetic study of eight families. *Brain* **117**: 445–60.

Engert JC, Berube P, Mercier J, et al. (2000) ARSACS, a spastic ataxia common in northeastern Quebec, is caused by mutations in a new gene encoding an 11.5-kb ORF. *Nat Genet* **24**: 120–5.

Escolar ML, Poe MD, Provenzale JM, et al. (2005) Transplantation of umbilical-cord blood in babies with infantile Krabbe's disease. *N Engl J Med* **352**: 2069–81.

Esscher E, Flodmark O, Hagberg G, Hagberg B (1996) Non-progressive ataxias: origins, brain pathology and impairments in 78 Swedish children. *Dev Med Child Neurol* **38**: 285–96.

Everett CM, Wood NW (2004) Trinucleotide repeats and neurodegenerative disease. *Brain* **127**: 2385–405.

Evidente VG, Advincula J, Esteban R, et al. (2002) Phenomenology of "Lubag" or X-linked dystonia–parkinsonism. *Mov Disord* **17**: 1271–7.

Evidente VG, Nolte D, Niemann S, et al. (2004) Phenotypic and molecular analyses of X-linked dystonia–parkinsonism ("lubag") in women. *Arch Neurol* **61**: 1956–9.

Fahn S, Bressman SB, Marsden CD (1998) Classification of dystonia. *Adv Neurol* **78**: 1–10.

Farmer SF, Harrison LM, Mayston MJ, et al. (2004) Abnormal cortex–muscle interactions in subjects with X-linked Kallman's syndrome and mirror movements. *Brain* **127**: 385–97.

Fasano A, Nardocci N, Elia AE, et al. (2006) Non-DYT1 early-onset primary torsion dystonia: comparison with DYT1 phenotype and review of the literature. *Mov Disord* **21**: 1411–8.

Fenichel GM, Phillips JA (1989) Familial aplasia of the cerebellar vermis. Possible X-linked dominant inheritance. *Arch Neurol* **46**: 582–3.

Fernandez-Alvarez E, Aicardi J (2001) *Movement Disorders in Children. International Review of Child Neurology Series*. London: Mac Keith Press for the International Child Neurology Association.

Ferrer I, Campistol J, Tobeña L, et al. (1987) Dégénérescence systématisée optico-cochléo-dentelée. *J Neurol* **234**: 416–20.

Fink JK (2002) Hereditary spastic paraplegia. *Neurol Clin* **20**: 711–26.

Fink JK, Hereda P (1999) Hereditary spastic paraplegia: genetic heterogeneity and genotype–phenotype correlations. *Semin Neurol* **19**: 301–9.

Fisher M, Sargent J, Drachman D (1979) Familial inverted choreoathetosis. *Neurology* **29**: 1627–31.

Fletcher NA, Harding AE, Marsden CD (1990) A genetic study of idiopathic torsion dystonia in the United Kingdom. *Brain* **113**: 379–95.

Fogli A, Bespflug-Tanguy O (2006) The large spectrum of eIF2B-related diseases. *Biochem Soc Trans* **34**: 22–9.

Fogli A, Dionisi-Vici C, Deodato F, Bartuli A, et al. (2002a) A severe variant of childhood ataxia with central hypomyelination/vanishing white matter leukoencephalopathy related to EIF21B5 mutation. *Neurology* **59**: 1966–8.

Fogli A, Wong K, Eymard-Pierre E, et al. (2002b) Cree leukoencephalopathy and CACH/VWM disease are allelic at the EIF2B5 locus. *Ann Neurol* **52**: 506–10.

Fortini D, Cricchi F, Di Fabio R, et al. (2003) Current insights into familial spastic paraparesis: new advances in an old disease. *Funct Neurol* **18**: 43–9.

Fowler WE, Kriel RL, Krach LE (1992) Movement disorders after status epilepticus and other brain injuries. *Pediatr Neurol* **8**: 281–4.

Franceschetti S, Gambardella A, Canafoglia L, et al. (2006) Clinical and genetic findings in 26 Italian patients with Lafora disease. *Epilepsia* **47**: 640–3.

Friede RL (1989) *Developmental Pathology, 2nd edn*. Berlin: Springer Verlag.

Funata N, Maeda Y, Koike M, et al. (1990) Neuronal intranuclear hyaline inclusion disease: report of a case and review of the literature. *Clin Neuropathol* **9**: 89–96.

Gadisseux JF, Rodriguez J, Lyon G (1984) Pontoneocerebellar hypoplasia—a probable consequence of prenatal destruction of the pontine nuclei and a possible role of phenytoin intoxication. *Clin Neuropathol* **3**: 160–7.

Gambardella A, Muglia M, Labate A, et al. (2001) Juvenile Huntington's disease presenting as progressive myoclonic epilepsy. *Neurology* **57**: 708–11.

Ganesh S, Delgado-Escueta AV, Suzuki T, et al. (2002) Genotype–phenotype correlations for EPM2A mutations in Lafora's progressive myoclonus epilepsy: exon 1 mutations associate with an early-onset cognitive deficit subphenotype. *Hum Mol Genet* **11**: 1263–71.

Gascon GG, Ozand PT, Brismar J (1994) Movement disorders in chilldhood organic acidurias. Clinical, neuroimaging, and biochemical correlations. *Brain Dev* **16** Suppl: 94–103.

Genton P, Malafosse A, Moulard B, et al. (2005) Progressive myoclonus epilepsies. In: Roger J, Bureau M, Dravet C, et al., eds. *Epileptic Syndromes in Infancy, Childhood and Adolescence, 4th edn*. Eastleigh, Hants: John Libbey, pp. 441–65.

Gieron MA, Gilbert-Barness E, Vonsattel JP, Korthals JR (1995) Infantile progressive striato–thalamic degeneration in two siblings: a new syndrome. *Pediatr Neurol* **12**: 260–3.

Gieselmann V (2003) Metachromatic leukodystrophy: recent research developments. *J Child Neurol* **18**: 591–4.

Gieselmann V, Fluharty AL, Tonnesen T, von Figura K (1991) Mutations in the arylsulfatase A pseudodeficiency allele causing metachromatic leukodystrophy. *Am J Hum Genet* **49**: 407–13.

Giunti P, Sweeney MG, Spadaro M, et al. (1994) The trinucleotide repeat expansion on chromosome 6p (SCA1) in autosomal dominant cerebellar ataxias. *Brain* **117**: 645–9.

Giunti P, Sweeney MG, Harding AE (1995) Detection of the Machado–Joseph disease/spinocerebellar ataxia three trinucleotide repeat expansion in families

with autosomal dominant motor disorders, including the Drew family of Walworth. *Brain* **118**: 1077–85.

Glass H, Boycott KM, Adams C, et al. (2005) Autosomal recessive cerebellar hypoplasia in the Hutterite population. *Dev Med Child Neurol* **47**: 691–5.

Goebel HH, Wisniewski KE (2004) Current state of clinical and morphological features in human NCL. *Brain Pathol* **14**: 61–9.

Goebel HH, Bode G, Caesar R, Kohlschütter A (1981) Bulbar palsy with Rosenthal fiber formation in the medulla of a 15-year-old girl. Localized form of Alexander's disease? *Neuropediatrics* **12**: 382–91.

Goebel HH, Vesa J, Reitter B, et al. (1995) Prenatal diagnosis of infantile neuronal ceroid–lipofuscinosis: a combined electron microscopic and molecular genetic approach. *Brain Dev* **17**: 83–8.

Gomez-Abad C, Gomez-Garre P, Gutierrez-Delicado E, et al. (2005) Lafora disease due to EPM2B mutations. *Neurology* **64**: 982–6.

Gordon N (2000) Cerebellar ataxia and gluten sensitivity: a rare but possible cause of ataxia, even in childhood. *Dev Med Child Neurol* **42**: 283–6.

Goutières F, Mikol J, Aicardi J (1990) Neuronal intranuclear inclusion disease in a child: diagnosis by rectal biopsy. *Ann Neurol* **27**: 103–6.

Goutières F, Aicardi J, Barth PG, Lebon P (1998) Aicardi–Goutières syndrome: an update and results of interferon-alpha studies. *Ann Neurol* **44**: 900–7.

Goutières F, Dollfus H, Becquet F, Dufier JL (1999) Extensive brain calcification in two children with bilateral Coats' disease. *Neuropediatrics* **30**: 19–21.

Gouw LG, Digre KB, Harris CP, et al. (1994) Autosomal dominant cerebellar ataxia with retinal degeneration: clinical, neuropathologic, and genetic analysis of a large kindred. *Neurology* **44**: 1441–7.

Gradstein G, Danek A, Grafman J, Fitzgibbon EJ (2005) Eye movements in chorea–acanthocytosis. *Invest Ophthalmol Vis Sci* **46**: 1979–87.

Greene P (1995) Medical and surgical therapy of idiopathic torsion dystonia. In: Kurlan R, ed. *Treatment of Movement Disorders*. Philadelphia: Lippincott, pp. 153–81.

Grodd W, Krageloh-Mann I, Petersen D, et al. (1990) In vivo assessment of N-acetylaspartate in brain in spongy degeneration (Canavan's disease) by proton spectroscopy. *Lancet* **336**: 437–8.

Grosso S, Mostardini R, Cioni M, et al. (2002) Pontocerebellar hypoplasia type 2: further clinical characterization and evidence of positive response of dyskinesia to levodopa. *J Neurol* **249**: 596–600.

Gunawardena S, Goldstein LS (2005) Polyglutamine diseases and transport problems: deadly traffic jams on neuronal highways. *Arch Neurol* **62**: 46–51.

Guzzetta F, Mercuri E, Bonanno S, et al. (1993) Autosomal recessive congenital cerebellar atrophy. A clinical and neuropsychological study. *Brain Dev* **15**: 439–45.

Haataja L, Schleutker J, Laine AP, et al. (1994) The genetic locus for free sialic acid storage disease maps to the long arm of chromosome 6. *Am J Hum Genet* **54**: 1042–9.

Hadders-Algra M, Bos AF, Martijn A, Prechtl HFR (1994) Infantile chorea in an infant with severe bronchopulmonary dysplasia: an EMG study. *Dev Med Child Neurol* **36**: 177–82.

Haenggeli CA, Engel E, Pizzolato GP (1989) Connatal Pelizaeus–Merzbacher disease. *Dev Med Child Neurol* **31**: 803–7.

Hagberg B, Sanner G Steen M (1972) The dysequilibrium syndrome in cerebral palsy. Clinical aspects and treatment. *Acta Paediatr Scand Suppl* **226**: 1–63.

Hagberg B, Kollberg H, Sourander P, Akesson HO (1969) Infantile globoid cell leucodystrophy (Krabbe's disease). A clinical and genetic study of 32 Swedish cases 1953–1967. *Neuropadiatrie* **1**: 74–88.

Hageneh J, Saunders-Pullman R, Hedrich K, et al. (2004) High mutation rate in dopa-responsive dystonia: detection with comprehensive GCH1 screening. *Neurology* **64**: 908–11.

Haltia M, Somer M (1993) Infantile cerebello-optic atrophy. Neuropathology of the progressive encephalopathy syndrome with edema, hypsarrhythmia and optic atrophy (the PEHO syndrome). *Acta Neuropathol* **85**: 241–7.

Hanefeld FA (2004) Alexander disease: past and present. *Cell Mol Life Sci* **61**: 2750–2.

Hanefeld F, Holzbach U, Kruse B, et al. (1993) Diffuse white matter disease in three children: an encephalopathy with unique features on magnetic resonance imaging and proton magnetic resonance spectroscopy. *Neuropediatrics* **24**: 244–8.

Hanefeld F, Brockmann K, Dechent P (2004) MR spectroscopy in pediatric white matter disease. In: Gillard JH, Waldman AD, Barker PB, eds. *Clinical*

MR Neuroimaging. Cambridge: Cambridge University Press, pp. 755–79.

Hanefeld FA, Brockmann K, Pouwels PJ, et al. (2005) Quantitative proton MRS of Pelizaeus–Merzbacher disease: evidence of dys- and hypomyelination. *Neurology* 65: 701–6.

Hanna MG, Davis MB, Sweeney MG, et al. (1998) Generalized chorea in two patients harboring the Friedreich's ataxia gene trinucleotide repeat expansion. *Mov Disord* 13: 339–40.

Hannan AJ (2004) Huntington's disease: which drugs might help patients? *Drugs* 7: 351–8.

Happle R, Traupe H, Gröbe H, Bonsmann G (1984) The Tay syndrome (congenital ichthyosis with trichothiodystrophy). *Eur J Pediatr* 141: 147–52.

Harden AE, Pampiglione G (1982) Neurophysiological studies (EEG/EG/VEP/SEP) in 88 children with so-called ceroid lipofuscinosis. In: Armstrong D, Koppang N, Ridder JH, eds. *Ceroid–Lipofuscinosis (Batten's Disease).* Amsterdam: Elsevier, pp. 61–70.

Harding AE (1981a) Early onset cerebellar ataxia with retained tendon reflexes: a clinical and genetic study of a disorder distinct from Friedreich's ataxia.' *J Neurol Neurosurg Psychiatry* 44: 503–8.

Harding AE (1981b) Friedreich's ataxia: a clinical and genetic study of 90 families with an analysis of early diagnostic criteria and intrafamilial clustering of clinical features. *Brain* 104: 589–620.

Harding AE (1981c) Hereditary "pure" spastic paraplegia: a clinical and genetic study of 22 families. *J Neurol Neurosurg Psychiatry* 44: 871–83.

Harding AE (1993) Clinical features and classification of inherited ataxias. In: Harding AE, Deufel T, eds. *Advances in Neurology, vol. 61. Inherited Ataxias.* New York: Raven Press, pp. 1–14.

Harding BN, Boyd SG (1991) Intractable seizures from infancy can be associated with dentato-olivary dysplasia. *J Neurol Sci* 104: 157–65.

Harding BN, Brett EM (1995) Familial cerebellar degeneration of early onset. *J Neurol Neurosurg Psychiatry* 54: 469 (letter).

Harding BN, Alsanjari N, Smith SJM, et al. (1995) Progressive neuronal degeneration of childhood with liver disease (Alpers' disease) presenting in young adults. *J Neurol Neurosurg Psychiatry* 58: 320–5.

Hart PE, Lodi R, Rajagopalan B, et al. (2005) Antioxidant treatment of patients with Friedreich ataxia: four-year follow-up. *Arch Neurol* 62: 621–6.

Hartig MB, Hörtnagel K, Garavaglia B, et al. (2006) Genotypic and phenotypic spectrum of PANK2 mutations in patients with neurodegeneration with brain iron accumulation. *Ann Neurol* 59: 248–56.

Harwood G, Hierons R, Fletcher NA, Marsden CD (1994) Lessons from a remarkable family with dopa-responsive dystonia. *J Neurol Neurosurg Psychiatry* 57: 460–3.

Hedrich K, Eskelson C, Wilmot B, et al. (2004) Distribution, type, and origin of Parkin mutations: review and case studies. *Mov Disord* 19: 1146–57.

Higgins JJ, Patterson MC, Papadopoulos NM, et al. (1992) Hypoprebetalipoproteinemia, acanthocytosis, retinitis pigmentosa, and pallidal degeneration (HARP syndrome). *Neurology* 42: 194–8.

Higgins JJ, Lombardi RQ, Tan EK, et al. (2004) Haplotype analysis of the ETM2 locus in a Singaporean sample with familial essential tremor. *Clin Genet* 66: 353–7.

Ho LN, Carmichael J, Swartz J, et al. (2001) The molecular biology of Huntington's disease. *Psychol Med* 31: 3–14.

Hoffmann GF, Assmann B, Bräutigam C, et al. (2003) Tyrosine hydroxylase deficiency causes progressive encephalopathy and dopa-nonresponsive dystonia. *Ann Neurol* 54 Suppl 6: S56–65.

Hortnagel K, Nardocci N, Zorzi G, et al. (2004) Infantile neuroaxonal dystrophy and pantothenate-kinase-associated neurodegeneration: locus heterogeneity. *Neurology* 63: 922–4.

Hottinger-Blanc PM, Ziegler AL, Deonna T (2002) A special type of head stereotypies in children with developmental (?cerebellar) disorder: description of 8 cases and literature review. *Eur J Paediatr Neurol* 6: 143–52.

Howard RS, Greenwood R, Gawler J, et al. (1993) A familial disorder associated with palatal myoclonus, other brainstem signs, tetraparesis, ataxia and Rosenthal fibre formation. *J Neurol Neurosurg Psychiatry* 56: 977–81.

Ichinose H, Ohye T, Takahashi E, et al. (1994) Hereditary progressive dystonia with marked diurnal fluctuation caused by mutations in the GTP cyclohydrolase I gene. *Nat Genet* 8: 236–42.

Illaroshkin SN, Tanaka, H., Markova, E.D., et al. (1996) X-linked nonprogressive congenital cerebellar hypoplasia: clinical description and mapping to chromosome Xq. *Ann Neurol* 40: 75–83.

Illune N, Reske-Nielsen E, Skovby F, et al. (1988) Lethal autosomal recessive arthrogryposis multiplex congenita with whistling face and calcifications of the nervous system. *Neuropediatrics* 19: 186–92.

International Batten Disease Consortium (1995) Isolation of a novel gene underlying Batten disease, CLN3. *Cell* 82: 949–57.

Iriarte LM, Mateu J, Cruz G, Escudero J (1988) Chorea: a new manifestation of mastocytosis. *J Neurol Neurosurg Psychiatry* 51: 1457–8 (letter).

Jan MM (2004) Misdiagnoses in children with dopa-responsive dystonia. *Pediatr Neurol* 31: 298–303.

Jankovic J (1994) Post-traumatic movement disorders: central peripheral mechanisms. *Neurology* 44: 2006–14.

Jankovic J (2005) Stereotypies in autistic and other childhood disorders. In: Fernandez-Alvarez E, Arzimanoglou A, Tolosa E, eds. *Paediatric Movement Disorders: Progress in Understanding.* London: John Libbey Eurotext, pp. 247–60.

Jankovic J, Fahn S (1986) The phenomenology of tics. *Mov Disord* 1: 17–26.

Jankovic J, Orman J (1988) Tetrabenazine therapy of dystonia, chorea, tics, and other dyskinesias. *Neurology* 38: 391–4.

Jankovic J, Madisetty J, Vuong KD (2004) Essential tremor among children. *Pediatrics* 114: 1203–5.

Jarman PR, Wood NW, Davis MT, et al. (1997) Hereditary geniospasm: linkage to chromosome 9q13–q21 and evidence for genetic heterogeneity. *Am J Hum Genet* 61: 928–33.

Kabakci K, Isbruch K, Schilling K, et al. (2005) Genetic heterogeneity in rapid onset dystonia–parkinsonism: description of a new family. *J Neurol Neurosurg Psychiatry* 76: 860–2.

Kalviainen R, Eriksson K, Losekoot M, et al. (2007) Juvenile-onset neuronal ceroid lipofuscinosis with infantile CLN1 mutation and palmitoyl-protein thioesterase deficiency. *Eur J Neurol* 14: 369–72.

Kaul R, Gao GP, Balamurugan K, Matalon R (1993) Cloning of the human aspartoacylase cDNA and a common missense mutation in Canavan disease. *Nat Genet* 5: 118–23.

Keen-Kim D, Freimer NB (2006) Genetics and epidemiology of Tourette syndrome. *J Child Neurol* 21: 665–71.

Kendall B, Cavanagh N (1986) Intracranial calcification in paediatric computed tomography. *Neuroradiology* 28: 324–30.

Khan NL, Wood NW, Bhatia KP (2003) Autosomal recessive, DYT2-like primary torsion dystonia: a new family. *Neurology* 61: 1801–3.

Khateeb S, Flusser H, Ofir R, et al. (2006) PLA2G6 mutation underlies infantile neuroaxonal dystrophy. *Am J Hum Genet* 79: 942–8.

Kiechl-Kohlendorfer U, Ellemunter H, Kiechl S (1999) Chorea as the presenting clinical feature of primary antiphospholipid syndrome in childhood. *Neuropediatrics* 30: 96–8

Kleber S, Azzedine H, Dürr A, et al. (2006) Autosomal recessive spastic paraplegia (SPG30) with mild ataxia and sensory neuropathy maps to chromosome 2q37.3. *Brain* 129: 1456–62.

Kleijer WJ, van der Sterre ML, Garritsen VH, et al. (2006) Prenatal diagnosis of the Cockayne syndrome: survey of 15 years experience. *Prenat Diagn* 26: 980–4.

Klein C, Liu L, Doheny D, et al. (2002) Epsilon-sarcoglycan mutations found in combination with other dystonia gene mutations. *Ann Neurol* 52: 675–9.

Kleiner-Fisman G, Rogaeva E, Halliday W, et al. (2003) Benign hereditary chorea: clinical, genetic, and pathologic findings. *Ann Neurol* 54: 244–7.

Klein-Schwartz W, McGrath J (2003) Poison centers' experience with methylphenidate abuse in pre-teens and adolescents. *J Am Acad Child Adolesc Psychiatry* 42: 288–94.

Klockgether T, Petersen D, Grodd W, Dichgans J (1991) Early onset cerebellar ataxia with retained tendon reflexes. Clinical, electrophysiological and MRI observations in comparison with Friedreich's ataxia. *Brain* 114: 1559–73.

Kobari M, Nogawa S, Sugimoto Y, Fukuuchi Y (1997) Familial idiopathic brain calcification with autosomal dominant inheritance. *Neurology* 48: 645–9.

Kobayashi H, Garcia CA, Alfonso G, et al. (1996a) Molecular genetics of familial spastic paraplegia: a multitude of responsible genes. *J Neurol Sci* 137: 131–8.

Kobayashi H, Garcia CA, Tay PN, Hoffman EP (1996b) Extensive heterogeneity in the "pure" form of autosomal dominant familial spastic paraplegia (Strümpell's disease). *Muscle Nerve* 19: 1435–8.

Kobor J, Javaid A, Omojola MF (2005) Cerebellar hypoperfusion in neuroaxonal dystrophy. *Pediatr Neurol* 32: 132–9.

Koenig M (2003) Rare forms of autosomal recessive ataxia. *Semin Pediatr Neurol* 10: 183–92.

Koeppen AH (2005) The pathogenesis of spinocerebellar ataxias. *Cerebellum* 4: 62–73.

Koletzko S, Koletzko B, Lamprecht A, Lenard HG (1987) Ataxia–deafness–

retardation syndrome in three sisters. *Neuropediatrics* **18**: 18–21.

Kong CK, Ko CH, Tong SF, Lam CW (2001) Atypical presentation of dopa-responsive dystonia: generalized hypotonia and proximal weakness. *Neurology* **57**: 1121–4.

Korf B, Wallman JK, Levy HL (1986) Bilateral lucency of the globus pallidus complicating methylmalonic acidemia. *Ann Neurol* **20**: 364–6.

Koskiniemi M, Donner M, Majuri H, et al. (1974a) Progressive myoclonus epilepsy. A clinical and histopathological study. *Acta Neurol Scand* **50**: 307–32.

Koskiniemi M, Toivakka E, Donner M (1974b) Progressive myoclonus epilepsy. Electroencephalographical findings. *Acta Neurol Scand* **50**: 333–59.

Koskiniemi M, Donner M, Majuri H, et al. (1994) Progressive myoclonus epilepsy. A clinical and histopathological study. *Acta Neurol Scand* **50**: 307–32.

Kovach MJ, Ruiz J, Mueed S, et al. (2001) Genetic heterogeneity of autosomal dominant essential tremor. *Genet Med* **3**: 197–9.

Kramer PL, Mineta M, Klein C, et al. (1999) Rapid-onset dystonia–parkinsonism: linkage to chromosome 19q13. *Ann Neurol* **46**: 176–82.

Krauss JK, Nobbe F, Wakhloo AK, et al. (1992) Movement disorders in astrocytomas of the basal ganglia and the thalamus. *J Neurol Neurosurg Psychiatry* **55**: 1162–7.

Krauss JK, Loher TJ, Weigel R, et al. (2003) Chronic stimulation of the globus pallidus internus for treatment of DYT1 generalized dystonia and choreoathetosis: 2-year follow up. *J Neurosurg* **98**: 785–92.

Kremer B, Goldberg P, Andrew SE, et al. (1994) A worldwide study of the Huntington's disease mutation. The sensitivity and specificity of measuring CAG repeats. *N Engl J Med* **330**: 1401–6.

Krivit W, Shapiro EG, Peters C, et al. (1998) Hematopoietic stem-cell transplantation in globoid-cell leukodystrophy. *N Engl J Med* **338**: 1119–26.

Kulikova-Schupak R, Knupp KG, Pascual JM, et al. (2004) Rectal biopsy in the diagnosis of neuronal intranuclear hyaline inclusion disease. *J Child Neurol* **19**: 59–62.

Kupke KG, Lee LV, Viterbo GH, et al. (1990) X-linked recessive torsion dystonia in the Philippines. *Am J Med Genet* **36**: 237–42.

Kyllerman M, Forsgren L, Sanner G, et al. (1990) Alcohol-responsive myoclonic dystonia in a large family: dominant inheritance and phenotypic variation. *Mov Disord* **5**: 270–9.

Kyllerman M, Sommerfelt K, Hedström A, et al. (1991) Clinical and neurophysiological development of Unverricht–Lundborg disease in four Swedish siblings. *Epilepsia* **32**: 900–9.

Kyllerman M, Sanner G, Forsgren L, et al. (1993) Early onset dystonia decreasing with development. Case report of two children with familial myoclonic dystonia. *Brain Dev* **15**: 295–8.

Kyllerman M, Mansson JE, Lichtenstein M, et al. (2001) Distal neuroaxonal dystrophy—a new familial variant with perineuronal argyrophilic bodies. *Acta Neuropathol* **102**: 83–8.

Kyllerman M, Rosengren L, Wiklund LM, Holmberg E (2005) Increased levels of GFAP in the cerebrospinal fluid in three subtypes of genetically confirmed Alexander disease. *Neuropediatrics* **36**: 319–23.

Labauge P, Fogli A, Castelnovo G, et al. (2005) Dominant form of vanishing white matter-like leukoencephalopathy. *Ann Neurol* **58**: 634–9.

Labrune P, Lacroix C, Goutières F, et al. (1996) Extensive brain calcifications, leukodystrophy, and formation of parenchymal cysts: a new progressive disorder due to diffuse cerebral microangiopathy. *Neurology* **46**: 1297–301.

Lake BD, Cavanagh NP (1978) Early-juvenile Batten's disease—a recognizable sub-group distinct from other forms of Batten's disease. Analysis of 5 patients. *J Neurol Sci* **36**: 265–71.

Lake BD, Brett EM, Boyd SG (1996) A form of juvenile Batten disease with granular osmiophilic deposits. *Neuropediatrics* **27**: 265–9.

Larsen TA, Dunn HG, Jan JE, Calne DB (1985) Dystonia and calcification of the basal ganglia. *Neurology* **35**: 533–7.

Larson PS (2008) Deep brain stimulation for psychiatric diseases. *Neurotherapeutics* **5**: 50–8.

Le Ber I, Moreira MC, Rivaud-Péchoux S, et al. (2003) Cerebellar ataxia with oculomotor apraxia type 1: clinical and genetic studies. *Brain* **126**: 2761–72.

Le Ber I, Bouslam N, Rivaud-Péchoux S, et al. (2004) Frequency and phenotypic spectrum of ataxia with oculomotor apraxia 2: a clinical and genetic study of 18 patients. *Brain* **127**: 759–67.

Le Ber I, Brice A, Dürr A (2005) New autosomal recessive cerebellar ataxias with oculomotor apraxia. *Curr Neurol Neurosci Rep* **5**: 411–7.

Lebon P, Badoual J, Ponsot G, et al. (1988) Intrathecal synthesis of interferon-

alpha in infants with progressive familial encephalopathy. *J Neurol Sci* **84**: 201–8.

Lee MS, Rinne JO, Ceballos-Baumann A, et al. (1994) Dystonia after head trauma. *Neurology* **44**: 1374–8.

Lee S, Park YD, Yen SH, et al. (1989) A study of infantile motor neuron disease with neurofilament and ubiquitin immunocytochemistry. *Neuropediatrics* **20**: 107–11.

Leegwater PA, Vermeulen G, Konst AA, et al. (2001) Subunits of the translation initiation factor eIF2B are mutated in leukoencephalopathy with vanishing white matter. *Nat Genet* **29**: 383–8.

Leegwater PA, Boor PK, Yuan BQ, et al. (2002) Identification of novel mutations in MLC1 responsible for megalencephalic leukoencephalopathy with subcortical cysts. *Hum Genet* **110**: 279–83; erratum **111**: 114.

Lehesjoki AE (2003) Molecular background of progressive myoclonus epilepsy. *EMBO J* **22**: 3473–8.

Leone M, Rocca WA, Rosso MG, et al. (1988) Friedreich's disease: survival analysis in an Italian population. *Neurology* **38**: 1433–8.

Leube B, Hendgen T, Kessler KR, et al. (1997) Sporadic focal dystonia in northwest Germany: molecular basis on chromosome 18p. *Ann Neurol* **42**: 111–4.

Ley CO, Gali FG (1983) Parkinsonian syndrome after methanol intoxication. *Eur Neurol* **22**: 405–9.

Leys A, Gilbert HD, Van de Sompel W, et al. (2000) Familial spastic paraplegia and maculopathy with juxtafoveolar retinal telangiectasis and subretinal neovascularization. *Retina* **20**: 184–9.

Licht DJ, Lynch DR (2002) Juvenile dentatorubral–pallidoluysian atrophy: new clinical features. *Pediatr Neurol* **26**: 51–4.

Logigian EL, Kolodny EH, Griffith JF, et al. (1986) Myoclonus epilepsy in two brothers: clinical features and neuropathology of a unique syndrome. *Brain* **109**: 411–29.

Longman C, Sewry CA, Muntoni F (2004) Muscle involvement in the cerebro-oculolo-facio-skeletal syndrome. *Pediatr Neurol* **30**: 125–8.

Lonnqvist T, Paetau A, Nikali K, et al. (1998) Infantile onset spinocerebellar ataxia (IOSCA): neuropathological features. *J Neurol Sci* **161**: 57–65.

Lossos A, Cooperman H, Soffer D, et al. (1995) Hereditary leukoencephalopathy and palmoplantar keratoderma: a new disorder with increased skin collagen content. *Neurology* **45**: 331–7.

Lossos A, Dobson-Stone C, Monaco AP, et al. (2005) Early clinical heterogeneity in choreo-acanthocytosis. *Arch Neurol* **62**: 611–4.

Lott IT, Williams RS, Schnur JA, Hier DB (1979) Familial amentia, unusual ventricular calcifications, and increased cerebrospinal fluid protein. *Neurology* **29**: 1571–7.

Lou JS, Jankovic J (1991) Essential tremor: clinical correlates in 350 patients. *Neurology* **41**: 234–8.

Louis ED (2005) Essential tremor. *Lancet Neurol* **4**: 100–10.

Louis ED, Fernandez-Alvarez E, Dure LS, et al. (2005) Association between male gender and pediatric essential tremor. *Mov Disord* **20**: 904–6.

Lucking CB, Durr A, Bonifati V, et al. (2000) Association between early-onset Parkinson's disease and mutations in the parkin gene. *N Engl J Med* **342**: 1560–7.

Lüdecke B, Knappskog PM, Clayton PT, et al. (1996) Recessively inherited L-DOPA-responsive parkinsonism in infancy caused by a point mutation (L205P) in the tyrosine hydroxylase gene. *Hum Mol Genet* **5**: 1023–8.

Lynch BJ, Becich MJ, Torack RM, Rust RS (1992) Arrested maturation of cerebral neurons, axons and myelin: a new familial syndrome of newborns. *Neuropediatrics* **23**: 180–7.

Lynch T, Sano M, Marder KS, et al. (1994) Clinical characteristics of a family with chromosome 17-linked disinhibition–dementia–parkinsonism–amyotrophy complex. *Neurology* **44**: 1878–84.

Lyon G, Arita F, Le Galloudec E, et al. (1990) A disorder of axonal development, necrotizing myopathy, cardiomyopathy, and cataracts: a new familial disease. *Ann Neurol* **27**: 193–9.

Lyon G, Kolodny EH, Pastores GM (2006) *Neurology of Hereditary Metabolic Diseases of Children, 3rd edn.* New York: McGraw Hill.

MacFaul R, Cavanagh N, Lake BD, et al. (1982) Metachromatic leucodystrophy: review of 38 cases. *Arch Dis Child* **57**: 168–75.

Mahmoud F, King MD, Smyth OP, Farrell MA (1998) Familial cerebellar hypoplasia and pancytopenia without chromosomal breakage. *Neuropediatrics* **29**: 302–6.

Mahone EM, Bridges D, Prahme C, Singer HS (2004) Repetitive hand movements (complex stereotypies) in children. *J Pediatr* **145**: 391–5.

Malandrini A, Scarpini C, Palmeri S, et al. (1996) Palatal myoclonus and unusual MRI findings in a patient with membranous lipodystrophy. *Brain Dev* 18: 59–63.

Manji H, Howard RS, Miller DH, et al. (1998) Status dystonicus: the syndrome and its management. *Brain* 121: 243–52.

Manto MU (2005) The wide spectrum of spinocerebellar ataxias (SCAs). *Cerebellum* 4: 2–6.

Manyam BV, Bhatt MH, Moore WD, et al. (1992) Bilateral striopallidodentate calcinosis: cerebrospinal fluid, imaging, and electrophysiological studies. *Ann Neurol* 31: 379–84.

Margolis RL, Holmes SE, Rosenblatt A, et al. (2004) Huntington's disease-like 2 (HDL2) in North America and Japan. *Ann Neurol* 56: 670–4; erratum 911.

Mariotti C, Gellera C, Rimoldi M, et al. (2004) Ataxia with isolated vitamin E deficiency: neurological phenotype, clinical follow-up and novel mutations in TTPA gene in Italian families. *Neurol Sci* 25: 130–7.

Marsden CD, Marion MH, Quinn N (1984) The treatment of severe dystonia in children and adults. *J Neurol Neurosurg Psychiatry* 47: 1166–73.

Marsden CD, Lang AE, Quinn NP, et al. (1986) Familial dystonia and visual failure with striatal CT lucencies. *J Neurol Neurosurg Psychiatry* 49: 500–9.

Marseille Consensus Group (1990) Classification of progressive myoclonus epilepsies and related disorders. *Ann Neurol* 28: 113–6.

Martin JJ, Martin L, Ceuterick C (1977) Encephalopathy associated with lamellar residual bodies in astrocytes (Towfighi, Grover and Gonatas 1975): a new observation. *Neuropädiatrie* 8: 181–9.

Martin JJ, Ceuterick CM, Leroy JG, et al. (1984) The Wiedemann–Rautenstrauch or neonatal progeroid syndrome. Neuropathological study of a case. *Neuropediatrics* 15: 43–8.

Marzan KAB, Barron TF (1994) MRI abnormalities in Behr syndrome. *Pediatr Neurol* 10: 247–8.

Matalon R, Michals-Matalon K (1998) Molecular basis of Canavan disease. *Eur J Paediatr Neurol* 2: 69–76.

Matalon R, Kaul R, Casanova J, et al. (1989) SSEIM Award. Aspartoacylase deficiency: the enzyme defect in Canavan disease. *J Inherit Metab Dis* 12 Suppl 2: 329–33.

Matarin MM, Singleton AB, Houlden H (2006) PANK2 gene analysis confirms genetic heterogeneity in neourodegeneration with brain iron accumulation (NBIA) but mutations are rare in other types of adult neurodegenerative disease. *Neurosci Lett* 407: 162–5.

Matsuyama H, Watanabe I, Mihm MC, Richarsdson EP (1978) Dermatoleukodystrophy with neuroaxonal spheroids. *Arch Neurol* 35: 329–36.

Matzner U, Gieselmann V (2005) Gene therapy of metachromatic leukodystrophy. *Expert Opin Biol Ther* 5: 55–65.

Mejaski-Bosnjak V, Besenski N, Brockmann K, et al. (1997) Cystic leukoencephalopathy in a megalencephalic child: clinical and magnetic resonance imaging/magnetic resonance spectroscopy findings. *Pediatr Neurol* 16: 347–50.

Melone MA, Jori FP, Peluso G (2005) Huntington's disease: new frontiers for molecular and cell therapy. *Curr Drugs Targets* 6: 43–56.

Meltzer E, Steinhauf S (2002) The clinical manifestations of lithium intoxication. *Isr Med J* 4: 265–7.

Mignot C, Boespflug-Tanguy O, Gelot A, et al. (2004) Alexander disease: putative mechanisms of an astrocytic encephalopathy. *Cell Mol Life Sci* 61: 369–85.

Minami T, Otsuka M, Ichiya Y, et al. (1994) Different patterns of [18F]dopa uptake in siblings with hereditary dentato-rubro-pallido-luysian atrophy. *Brain Dev* 16: 335–8.

Mirowitz SA, Westrich TJ, Hirsch JD (1991) Hyperintense basal ganglia on T1-weighted MR images in patients receiving parenteral nutrition. *Radiology* 181: 117–20.

Mitchison HM, Hoffmann SL, Becerra CH, et al. (1998) Mutations in the palmitoyl-protein thioesterase gene (PTT; CLN1) causing juvenile neuronal ceroid lipofuscinosis with granular osmiophilic deposits. *Hum Molec Genet* 7: 291–7; erratum 765.

Miyoshi K, Matsuoka T, Mizushima S (1969) Familial holotopistic striatal necrosis. *Acta Neuropathol* 13: 240–9.

Mole SE (2004) The genetic spectrum of human ceroid lipofuscinoses. *Brain Pathol* 14: 70–6.

Mole SE, Williams RE, Goebel HH (2005) Correlation between genotype, ultrasound morphology, and clinical phenotype in the neuronal ceroid lipofuscinoses. *Neurogenetics* 6: 107–26.

Molinuevo JL, Marti MS, Blesa R, Tolosa E (2003) Pure akinesia: an unusual phenotype of Hallervorden–Spatz disease. *Mov Disord* 18: 1351–3.

Montermini L, Richter A, Morgan K, et al. (1997) Phenotypic variability in Friedreich ataxia: role of the associated GAA triplet repeat expansion. *Ann Neurol* 41: 675–82.

Moosa A, Dubowitz V (1970) Peripheral neuropathy in Cockayne's syndrome. *Arch Dis Child* 45: 674–7.

Morita M, Tsuge I, Matsuoka H, et al. (1998) Calcification of the basal ganglia with chronic active Epstein–Barr virus infection. *Neurology* 50: 1485–8.

Moser HW, Raymond GV, Lu SE, et al. (2005) Follow-up of 89 asymptomatic patients with adrenoleukodystrophy treated with Lorenzo's oil. *Arch Neurol* 62: 1073–80.

Mostofsky SH, Blasco PA, Butler IJ, Dobyns WB (1996) Autosomal dominant torsion dystonia with onset in infancy. *Pediatr Neurol* 15: 245–8.

Mussell HG, Dure LS, Percy AK, et al. (1997) Bobble-head doll syndrome: report of a case and review of the literature. *Mov Disord* 12: 810–4.

Nagashima K, Suzuki S, Ichikawa E, et al. (1985) Infantile neuroaxonal dystrophy: perinatal onset with symptoms of diencephalic syndrome. *Neurology* 35: 735–8.

Nance MA, Berry SA (1992) Cockayne syndrome: review of 140 cases. *Am J Med Genet* 42: 68–84.

Nardocci N, Zorzi G, Grisoli M, et al. (1996) Acquired hemidystonia in childhood: a clinical and neuroradiological study of thirteen patients. *Pediatr Neurol* 15: 108–13.

Nardocci N, Farina L, Bruzzone MG, et al. (1999a) Infantile neuroaxonal dystrophy: neuroradiological studies in 11 patients. *Neuroradiology* 41: 378–80.

Nardocci N, Zorzi G, Farina L, et al. (1999b) Infantile neuroaxonal dystrophy: clinical spectrum and diagnostic criteria. *Neurology* 52: 1472–9.

Nardocci N, Zorzi G, Blau N, et al. (2003) Neonatal dopa-responsive extrapyramidal syndrome in twins with recessive GTPCH deficiency. *Neurology* 60: 335–7.

Nardocci N, Temudo T, Echenne B, et al. (2005) Status dystonicus in children. In: Fernández-Alvarez E, Arzimanoglou A, Tolosa E, eds. *Paediatric Movement Disorders: Progress in Understanding*. London: John Libbey Eurotext, pp. 71–6.

Neville BG, Parascandalo R, Farrugia R, Felice A (2005) Sepiapterin reductase deficiency: a congenital dopa-responsive motor and cognitive disorder. *Brain* 128: 2291–6.

Nicolaides P, Baraitser M, Brett EM (1993) Two siblings with mental retardation and progressive spasticity. *Clin Genet* 43: 312–4.

Nishimura N, MitoT, Takashima S, et al. (1987) Multisystem atrophy with retinal degeneration in a young child. *Neuropediatrics* 18: 91–5.

Nordstrom DM, West SG, Andersen PA (1985) Basal ganglia calcifications in central nervous system lupus erythematosus. *Arthritis Rheum* 28: 1412–6.

Novotny EJ, Singh G, Wallace DC, et al. (1986) Leber's disease and dystonia: a mitochondrial disease. *Neurology* 36: 1053–60.

Nygaard TG (1995) Dopa-responsive dystonia. *Curr Opin Neurol* 8: 310–3.

Obeso JA, Artieda J, Rothwell JC, et al. (1989) The treatment of severe action myoclonus. *Brain* 112: 765–7.

Ohlsson A, Cummings WA, Paul A, Sly WS (1986) Carbonic anhydrase II deficiency syndrome: recessive osteopetrosis with renal tubular acidosis and cerebral calcification. *Pediatrics* 77: 371–81.

Osborne JP, Munson P, Burman D (1982) Huntington's chorea. Report of 3 cases and review of the literature. *Arch Dis Child* 57: 99–103.

Østergaard JR, Christensen T, Hansen KN (1995) In vivo diagnosis of Hallervorden–Spatz disease. *Dev Med Child Neurol* 37: 827–33.

O'Sullivan JD, Hanagasi HA, Daniel SE, et al. (2000) Neuronal intranuclear inclusion disease and juvenile parkinsonism. *Mov Disord* 15: 990–5.

Ozand PT, Gascon GG, Al Essa S, et al. (1998) Biotin-responsive basal ganglia disease: a novel entity. *Brain* 121: 1267–80.

Palau F, De Michele G, Vilchez JJ, et al. (1995) Early-onset ataxia with cardiomyopathy and retained tendon reflexes maps to the Friedeich's ataxia locus on chromosome 9q. *Ann Neurol* 37: 359–62.

Pandolfo M (2003) Friedreich ataxia. *Semin Pediatr Neurol* 10: 163–72.

Parmeggiani A, Lehesjoki AE, Carelli V, et al. (1997) Familial Unverricht–Lundberg disease: a clinical, neurophysiologic, and genetic study. *Epilepsia* 38: 637–41.

Pascher P, Feng Y, Pakstis AJ, et al. (2004) Indication of linkage ansd association of Gilles de la Tourette syndrome in two independent family samples: 17q25 is a putative susceptibility region. *Am J Hum Genet* 75: 545–60.

Pascual-Castroviejo I, Guttierez M, Morales C, et al. (1994) Primary degeneration of the granular layer of the cerebellum. A study of 14 patients and review of the literature. *Neuropediatrics* 25: 183–90.

Pasquier L, Laugel V, Lazaro L, et al. (2006) Wide clinical variability among 13 new Cockayne syndrome cases confirmed by biochemical assays. *Arch Dis Child* 91: 178–82.

Patel H, Droukakis C, Cross H (2004) Troyer syndrome revisited. A clinical and radiological study of a complex hereditary spastic paraplegia. *J Neurol* 251: 1105–10.

Pavone L, Fiumara A, Barone R, et al. (1996) Olivopontocerebellar atrophy leading to recognition of carbohydrate-deficient glycoprotein syndrome type 1A. *J Neurol* 243: 700–5.

Pellecchia MT, Valente EM, Cif L, et al. (2005) The diverse phenotype and genotype of pantothenate kinase-associated neurodegeneration. *Neurology* 64: 1810–2.

Pinto F, Amantini A, de Scisciolo G, et al. (1988) Visual involvement in Friedreich's ataxia: PERG and VEP study. *Eur Neurol* 28: 246–51.

Pizzato MR, Castroviejo I (2001) [Behr syndrome: account of seven cases.] *Rev Neurol* 32: 142–6 (Spanish).

Polo JM, Calleja J, Combarros O, Berciano J (1993) Hereditary "pure" spastic paraplegia: a study of nine families. *J Neurol Neurosurg Psychiatry* 56: 175–81.

Polten A, Fluharty AL, Fluharty CB, et al. (1991) Molecular basis of different forms of metachromatic leukodystrophy. *N Engl J Med* 324: 18–22.

Powers JM, Moser HW (1998) Peroxisomal disorders: genotype, phenotype, major neuropathologic lesions, and pathogenesis. *Brain Pathol* 8: 101–20.

Pozzan GB, Battistella PA, Rigon F, et al. (1992) Hyperthyroid-induced chorea in an adolescent girl. *Brain Dev* 14: 126–7.

Pranzatelli MR (1996) Antidyskinetic drug therapy for pediatric movement disorders. *J Child Neurol* 11: 355–69.

Pranzatelli MR, Mott SH, Pavlakis SG, et al. (1994) Clinical spectrum of secondary parkinsonism in childhood: a reversible disorder. *Pediatr Neurol* 10: 131–40.

Pridmore CL, Baraitser M, Harding B, et al. (1993) Alexander's disease: clues to diagnosis. *J Child Neurol* 8: 134–44.

Puig JG, Torres RJ, Mateos FA, et al. (2001) The spectrum of hypoxanthine–guanine–phosphoribosyl transferase (HPRT) deficiency. Clinical experience based on 22 patients from 18 Spanish families. *Medicine* 80: 102–12.

Quinn NP (1996) Essential myoclonus and myoclonic dystonia. *Mov Disord* 11: 119–24.

Rajab A, Mochida GH, Hill A, et al. (2003) A novel form of pontocerebellar hypoplasia maps to chromosome 7q11–21. *Neurology* 60: 1664–7.

Rajput AH, Gibb WRG, Zhong XH, et al. (1994) Dopa-responsive dystonia: pathological and biochemical observations in a case. *Ann Neurol* 35: 396–402.

Ramaekers VT, Lake BD, Harding B, et al. (1987) Diagnostic difficulties in infantile neuroaxonal dystrophy. A clinicopathological study of eight cases. *Neuropediatrics* 18: 170–5.

Ramaekers VT, Heiman G, Revel J, et al. (1997) Genetic disorders and cerebellar abnormalities in childhood. *Brain* 120: 1739–51.

Rampoldi L, Danek A, Monaco AP (2002) Clinical features and molecular bases of neuroacanthocytosis. *J Mol Med* 80: 475–91.

Ranta S, Topçu M, Tegelberg S, et al. (2004) Variant late infantile neuronal ceroid lipofuscinosis in a subset of Turkish patients is allelic to Northen epilepsy. *Hum Mutat* 23: 300–5.

Rapin I, Lindenbaum Y, Dickson DW, et al. (2000) Cockayne syndrome and xeroderma pigmentosum. *Neurology* 55: 1442–9.

Rasmussen P (1993) Persistent mirror movements: a clinical study of 17 children, adolescents and young adults. *Dev Med Child Neurol* 35: 699–707.

Raspall-Chauré M, Solano A, Vazquez E, et al. (2004) [A patient with bilateral lesion in the striatum and slowly progressive dystonia secondary to T14487C mutation in the ND6 gene of complex I of the mitochondrial respiratory chain.] *Rev Neurol* 39: 1129–32 (Spanish).

Reuter I, Hu MT, Andrews TC, et al. (2000) Late onset levodopa responsive Huntington's disease with minimal chorea masquerading as Parkinson plus syndrome. *J Neurol Neurosurg Psychiatry* 68: 238–41.

Rice G, Newman WG, Dean J, et al. (2007) Heterozygous mutations in TREX1 cause familial chilblain lupus and dominant Aicardi–Goutières syndrome. *Am J Hum Genet* 80: 811–5.

Rivier F, Echenne B (1992) Dominantly inherited hypoplasia of the vermis. *Neuropediatrics* 23: 206–8.

Robinson RO, Samuels M, Pohl KRE (1988) Choreic syndrome after cardiac surgery. *Arch Dis Child* 63: 1466–9.

Rodriguez D, Gelot A, della Gaspera B., et al. (1999) Increased density of oligodendrocytes in childhood ataxia with diffuse central hypomyelination

(CACH) syndrome: neuropathological and biochemical study of two cases. *Acta Neuropathol* 97: 469–80.

Ronen G, Donat JR, Hill A (1986) Hemifacial spasm in children. *Can J Neurol Sci* 13: 342–3.

Rosenberg RN (1995) Autosomal dominant cerebellar phenotypes: the genotype has settled the issue. *Neurology* 45: 1–5.

Roubertie A, Bioli B, Rivier F, et al. (2003) Ataxia with vitamin E deficiency and severe dystonia: report of a case. **Brain Dev** 25: 442–5.

Rudnik-Schoneborn S, Sztriha L, Aithala GR, et al. (2003) Extended phenotype of pontocerebellar hypoplasia with infantile spinal muscular atrophy. *Am J Med Genet A* 117: 10–7.

Rump P, Hamel BC, Pinckers AJ, van Dop PA (1997) Two sibs with chorioretinal dystrophy, hypogonadotrophic hypogonadism, and cerebellar ataxia: Boucher–Neuhauser syndrome. *J Med Genet* 34: 767–71.

Rustin P, Bonnet D, Rotig A, et al. (2004) Idebenone treatment in Friedreich patients: one-year-long randomized placebo-controlled trial. *Neurology* 62: 524–5.

Ryan MM, Cooke-Yarborough CM, Procopis PG, Ouvrier RA (2000) Anterior horn cell disease and olivopontocerebellar hypoplasia. *Pediatr Neurol* 23: 180–4.

Sadzot B, Reznik M, Arrese-Estrada JF, Franck G (2000) Familial Kufs disease presenting as a progressive myoclonic epilepsy. *J Neurol* 247: 447–54.

Saïd G, Marion MH, Selva J, Jamet C (1986) Hypotrophic and dying-back nerve fibers in Friedreich's ataxia. *Neurology* 36: 1292–9.

Saint-Hilaire MH, Saint-Hilaire JM, Granger L (1986) Jumping Frenchmen of Maine. *Neurology* 36: 1269–71.

Saint-Hilaire MH, Burke RE, Bressman SB, et al. (1991) Delayed-onset dystonia due to perinatal or early childhood asphyxia. *Neurology* 41: 216–22.

Saito Y, Oguni H, Hawaya Y, et al. (2001) Phenytoin-induced choreoathetosis in patients with severe myoclonic epilepsy in infancy. *Neuropediatrics* 32: 231–5.

Sakuraba H, Matsuzawa F, Aikawa S, et al. (2004) Structural and immuno-cytochemical studies on alpha-N-acetylgalactosaminidase deficiciency (Schindler Kanzaki disease). *J Hum Genet* 49: 1–8.

Salazar-Grueso EF, Holzer TJ, Gutierrez RA, et al. (1990) Familial spastic paraparesis syndrome associated with HTLV-I infection. *N Engl J Med* 323: 732–7.

Salman MS, Blaser S, Bunkic JR, et al. (2003) Pontocerebellar hypoplasia type 1: new leads for an earlier diagnosis. *J Child Neurol* 18: 220–5.

Salonen R, Somer M, Haltia M, et al. (1991) Progressive encephalopathy with edema, hypsarrhythmia, and optic atrophy (PEHO syndrome). *Clin Genet* 39: 287–93.

Samuel M, Kleiner-Fisman G, Lang AE (2004a) Voluntary control and a wider clinical spectrum of essential palatal tremor. *Mov Disord* 19: 717–9.

Samuel M, Torun N, Tuite PJ, et al. (2004b) Progressive ataxia and palatal tremor (PAPT). Clinical and MRI assessment with review of palatal tremors. *Brain* 127: 1252–68.

Santavuori P (1988) Neuronal ceroid–lipofuscinoses in childhood. *Brain Dev* 10: 80–3.

Santavuori P, Westermarck T, Rapola J, et al. (1985) Antioxidant treatment in Spielmeyer–Sjögren's disease. *Acta Neurol Scand* 71: 136–45.

Santavuori P, Vanhanen SL, Autti T (2001) Clinical and neuroradiological diagnostic aspects of neuronal ceroid lipofuscinosis disorders. *Eur J Paediatr Neurol* 5 Suppl A: 157–61.

Savoiardo M, Halliday WC, Nardocci N, et al. (1993) Hallervorden–Spatz disease: MR and pathologic findings. *AJNR* 14: 155–62.

Savukoski M, Klockars T, Holmberg V, et al. (1998) CLN5, a novel gene encoding a putative transmembrane protein mutated in Finnish variant late infantile ceroid lipofuscinosis. *Nat Genet* 19: 286–8.

Sawada Y, Takahashi M, Ohashi N, et al. (1980) Computerised tomography as an indication of long-term outcome after acute carbon monoxide poisoning. *Lancet* 1: 783–4.

Schiffmann R, Moller JR, Trapp BD, et al. (1994) Childhood ataxia with diffuse central nervous system hypomyelination. *Ann Neurol* 35: 331–40.

Schiffmann R, Tedeschi G, Kinkel RP, et al. (1997) Leukodystrophy in patients with ovarian dysgenesis. *Ann Neurol* 41: 654–61.

Schneider SA, Mohire MD, Trender-Gerhard I, et al. (2006) Familial dopa-responsive cervical dystonia. *Neurology* 66: 599–601.

Schols L, Amoiridis G, Buttner T, et al. (1997) Autosomal dominant cerebellar ataxia: phenotypic differences in genetically defined subtypes? *Ann Neurol* 42: 924–32.

10
INFECTIOUS DISEASES

Cheryl Hemingway, Hermione Lyall

Infections of the CNS remain common life-threatening conditions. Despite recent advances in health care, and the development of new antibacterial and antiviral agents, they still are associated with an unacceptably high mortality and morbidity. Over the past few decades, many different therapeutic agents have been trialled, but few have resulted in any significant improvements in outcome. Early diagnosis and institution of treatment, careful monitoring of its efficacy and rapid detection of emerging complications give the best chances of an optimal outcome; but until we gain a greater understanding of the pathogenesis and pathophysiology of acute CNS infections, outcome will not improve significantly.

ACUTE BACTERIAL MENINGITIS IN INFANTS AND CHILDREN

Every year, over 1.2 million people develop acute bacterial meningitis, resulting in more than 170,000 deaths, the majority of which are in children (WHO 1998, 2008). Despite new antibiotics and treatments, mortality has remained essentially unchanged over the past 20 years. In those who survive, nearly half have neurological or other sequelae of disease. Several factors contribute toward this disappointing situation: delayed diagnosis because of the nonspecific character of the symptoms, the emergence of resistant strains of common pathogens, the weakness of the immunological defenses of the newborn infant, and our inability as yet to prevent the damage caused by the host inflammatory response through adjunctive neuroprotective or anti-inflammatory mechanisms.

EPIDEMIOLOGY

The relative incidence of acute bacterial meningitis varies according to age, socio-economic conditions, geographic location and immunization policies. In the developed world over the past decade the epidemiology of acute bacterial meningitis has undergone a dramatic change and the incidence has fallen to around 4–5/100,000, whereas in many developing countries it remains high at around 40–50/100,000.

Vaccination has brought about a radical change in the relative frequency of the three main pathogens – *Haemophilus influenzae*, *Neisseria meningitidis* and *Streptococcus pneumoniae*. *H. influenzae* type B (HiB) used to be the most common form of childhood

bacterial meningitis in the UK, with incidence rates ranging from 21 to 44 per 100,000 in those under 5 years of age, a peak age of 6–7 months, and case fatality rates of 2.4–4.3% (Booy and Moxon 1993, Booy et al. 1993, Anderson et al. 1995, Heath and McVernon 2002). Following the introduction in the early 1990s in many countries of the HiB protein–polysaccharide conjugate vaccine, the number of cases of *H. influenzae* meningitis dropped by more than 90% (Schuchat et al. 1997), leaving *S. pneumoniae* and *N. meningitides* as the commonest pathogens.

In Europe, pneumococcal meningitis currently has an incidence of around 0.5/100,000; associated mortality is 25% but can reach 45% in the very young. Over 30% of survivors are left with permanent neurological sequelae (Lexau et al. 2005). These figures are substantially worse in the developing world. There is a seasonal variation, with a peak in the winter months. Younger children are most affected, with 60% of cases occurring under 2 years of age. A 7-valent pneumococcal protein–polysaccharide conjugate vaccine became available in 2000 and was included on the UK national immunization schedule in 2006.

Those countries where it is included in their immunization programme have been seeing dramatic reductions in invasive pneumococcal disease, leaving *N. meningitidis* as the commonest pathogen. The incidence of *N. meningitidis* is around 1–3/100,000 in Europe, with the commonest serotypes being Groups B and C. Vaccination is available, but as yet only for groups A, C, Y and W135, with a polysaccharide–protein conjugate vaccine only against group C. This has now been included on many developed countries' immunization protocols, with introduction into the UK in 1999. A tetravalent conjugate vaccine for the other groups (A, C, Y and W135) has recently being launched in North America (Pace and Pollard 2007). Development of group B conjugate vaccines has been delayed by concerns of cross-reactivity with host antigens; however, phase 3 trials are currently being undertaken with new vaccine candidates that have emerged following the sequencing of the group B meningococcus. The highest burden of meningococcal disease occurs in sub-Saharan Africa, in an area known as the 'meningitis belt', an area that stretches from Senegal in the west to Ethiopia in the east. In the dry season (December–June) large epidemics with incidence rates up to 1000 per 100,000 can occur, mainly due to serogroups A, C and W135. Current global immunization campaigns (e.g. the GAVI Alliance) are promoting vaccination in these at-risk regions.

Another worrying epidemiological trend is the emergence of drug-resistant pathogens, the most serious of which cuurently is the penicillin-resistant pneumococcus (PRP), which occurs following mutations in one or more of the penicillin binding proteins. PRP appears to be directly linked to frequency of anti-microbial use, and certain countries have a far greater problem than others. Currently less than 3% of pneumococci in the UK are PRP, with higher incidences in Spain, USA and South Africa. Pneumococcus resistance is tested for in the laboratory using minimum inhibitory concentration (MIC) assay and can also be rapidly determined in specialized laboratory tests using polymerase chain reaction (PCR) assay for the penicillin binding protein 2b (PBP2B) gene. Penicillin and chloramphenicol resistance in meningococci is also increasing but fortunately is still rare.

PATHOPHYSIOLOGY AND IMMUNOLOGY

Effective invasion of the CNS involves four stages: first, adherence and colonization of the pathogen frequently from commensals in the nasopharynx; second, mucosal invasion and subsequent multiplication and bacteraemia; third, traversing the blood–brain barrier (BBB) to enter into the subarachnoid space – the exact mechanism of how this occurs is still unclear; and finally multiplication within the subarachnoid space, generating a host inflammatory response.

- *Adherence and colonization.* The exact mechansims by which bacteria attach to and penetrate the mucosal surface are still unclear. Multiple surface proteins on the organism are involved (e.g. choline binding proteins, sialic acid, and neuraminidase on *S. pneumoniae* and K1 polysaccharide on *E. coli*) (Koedel et al. 2002) as well as specific host receptors (e.g. pIgR). In the case of meningococcus the pili adhere to CD46 and 66 receptors of mucosal cells.
- *Invasion and multiplication.* To overcome host defences and survive within the bloodstream, surface proteins (e.g. Psp A and C) and the capsule help resist against complement destruction and phagocytosis respectively in the pneumococcus.
- *CNS penetration.* For pathogens to penetrate the CNS, the BBB and blood–CSF barrier have to be breached. Here various glycoconjugates and receptors (e.g. PAF-platelet activating factor) are involved. The size of the inoculum of bacteria in the blood has been shown to be important in producing meningitis in experimental animals, and this may also be the case in humans (Moxon et al. 1974).
- *Multiplication.* Once inside the CSF, an area of impaired host defence, the pathogens are likely initially to survive and multiply. However, their presence stimulates leukocyte migration into the CSF through a multistep process incorporating different adhesion molecules and ligands (e.g. selectins and integrins) with emigration along a chemotactic gradient. These then destroy the pathogens, and it is this destruction that precipitates the inflammatory cascade that causes the secondary tissue damage. The stimulation occurs though cell wall components (e.g. LPS from the gram-negative organisms such as *N. meningitidis* and *H. influenzae*, and peptidoglycans from gram-positive organisms such as *S. pneumoniae*) (Tuomanen et al. 1985),

directly from pneumolysins (Friedland et al. 1995), and through the bacterial DNA itself (Deng et al. 2001). After a time-lag of a few hours, proinflammatory cytokines including TNFα (Bazzoni and Beutler 1996) and interleukins 1β, 6 and 8 are induced. These precipitate a cascade of other cytokines, chemokines, proteolytic enzymes and reactive oxygen species and nitrogen intermediates from macrophages, neutrophils and platelets. In experiments in rats, administration of dexamethasone and antioxidants has been shown to partially diminish this untoward effect (Auer et al. 2000). Vascular congestion and increased vessel permeability result with cytotoxic and vasogenic brain oedema and increased intracranial pressure (ICP), further decreasing cerebral perfusion pressure (CPP), increasing the risk of herniation and irreversible brain damage. The CSF volume increases during the first two or three days of disease (Ashwal et al. 1992), and the levels of endotoxin (Mertsola 1991) and of other cytokines (Arditi et al. 1989) are correlated to the severity of the disorder (Dulkerian et al. 1995). Vasculitis is a frequent complication and can lead to infarction in 2–19% of cases. Cerebral blood flow is decreased by 30–70% in 30% of patients (Ashwal et al. 1992), but autoregulation of blood flow is generally maintained (Ashwal et al. 1990).

PATHOLOGY

The fundamental pathological change is inflammation of the two meningeal coverings of the brain and spine (arachnoid and pia mater) with initial hyperaemia, followed by migration of neutrophils into the subarachnoid space and the production of a purulent exudate. This exudate rapidly increases and extends into the Virchow–Robin spaces and along the penetrating vessels. Within 48–72 hours, inflammatory involvement of vessels is seen, initially of the subarachnoid arteries and then of the meningeal veins. Such changes can produce thrombosis of involved vessels with haemorrhagic cortical infarction and secondary necrosis. The necrosis may be limited to one vascular territory or diffusely involve a large portion or the whole of the cerebral cortex (Dodge and Swartz 1965). Oedema (cytotoxic, vasogenic and interstitial) is often present and, in isolation or in association with acute obstructive hydrocephalus due to purulent cisternal exudate, can be responsible for intracranial hypertension and secondary herniation of brain tissue. This in turn can further impede cerebral perfusion (Minns et al. 1989), setting the stage for a vicious circle. Apoptotic neuronal damage also occurs, particularly in the dentate gyrus of the hippocampus. This is of particular importance, as there is evidence that this damage is the cause of meningitis-related learning difficulties (Loeffler et al. 2001). The damage appears to be executed through amongst others caspase-3, an effector caspase, and in animal experiments blocking caspase-3 activation or administering specific caspase-3 inhibitors significantly reduced hippocampal damage (Braun et al. 1999). Organization of the meningeal exudate may lead to chronic hydrocephalus, especially in young infants. Hydrocephalus can also result from aqueductal stenosis that may supervene as a consequence of ventriculitis. The latter is extremely common in neonates, being found in as many as 92% of autopsy cases

(Berman and Banker 1966), but exists also in a lower proportion of older children (around 10%).

CLINICAL MANIFESTATIONS AND DIAGNOSIS

The importance of an early diagnosis is self-evident. Late diagnosis remains frequent, however, because meningitis is relatively rarely seen in general practice, compared with the frequency of common, mostly viral, febrile diseases. Meningitis is often preceded for a few days by fever so that it may be impossible to determine its actual onset; as a result, 33–40% of patients have received antibiotics prior to diagnosis (Kaplan et al. 1986). The mode of onset is an important prognostic feature: a progressive onset merging with previous disease often predicts a favourable outcome, while a fulminating onset is of ominous significance (Radetsky 1992, Kilpi et al. 1993). Fever, nausea and vomiting headache and lethargy and some disturbance of consciousness (more commonly mild stupor than coma) should suggest the diagnosis (Gururaj et al. 1973). Stiffness of the neck, and sometimes also of the back, and Kernig's sign make lumbar puncture imperative. In very early cases, mild irritability and change in mood together with fever may be the only signs. Generalized seizures occur in 30–40% of children with acute bacterial meningitis, especially children under 4 years of age. In one series of 328 children reviewed with first febrile seizures and no meningeal signs, meningitis was diagnosed in only 4 children by lumbar puncture (1.2%). All 4 were less than 18 months of age (Rutter and Smales 1977). So, although lumbar puncture should not routinely be performed in febrile seizures, for children under 18 months of age, in whom meningeal signs may be absent, a lumbar puncture should be performed if the child does not revert to a completely normal state soon after the seizure. Likewise, a lumbar puncture should also be performed in infants below 1 year of age if the slightest doubt persists. Neonates with meningitis may be febrile or hypothermic, and display feeding or respiratory difficulties. Nuchal rigidity and fontanelle changes are not typical. Lumbar puncture should be routinely performed in any septic screen of an unwell neonate.

The presence of a maculopapular rash can be an early sign of meningococcal sepsis, or represent a viral illness. Petechiae or a purpuric rash is suggestive of meningococcal disease, although can also occasionally be found in association with sepsis secondary to HiB, pneumococcus or some viral illnesses (e.g. echo 9). Focal neurologic signs such as cranial nerve palsies or hemiparesis usually develop late in the course of bacterial meningitis, or can occur earlier as a complication of raised ICP (particularly VIth nerve palsies). Papilloedema is rarely evident early on; in fact the presence of papilloedema should raise suspicion of a focal intracranial process such as brain abscess or a mass lesion, and is an indication for neuroimaging prior to lumbar puncture.

Although concern has arisen regarding the potential risks of lumbar puncture in the case of meningitis with raised ICP (Klein et al. 1986), failure to perform an early lumbar puncture can seriously compromise patient care. A CSF diagnosis has been shown to have changed management in 72% of cases, and delaying the lumbar puncture until after administration of antibiotics increases the rate of a sterile CSF from 3% to 44%. The concern is the risk of herniation, with the estimated risk of death from herniation thought to be between 4.3% (Rennick et al. 1993) and 6% (Wright et al. 1993, Lambert 1994). Lumbar puncture is felt to precipitate coning, although insufficient data exist to prove this as cause and effect, and herniation may have occurred in those cases spontaneously. The use of CT in detecting oedema or increased ICP is extremely limited (Pike et al. 1990, Heyderman et al. 1992), and it cannot predict the risk of coning. CT has been shown to change management in less than 5% of cases, and it delays lumbar puncture on average by 2.5 hours (Gopal et al. 1999). In addition, a normal CT does not mean it is safe to perform a lumbar puncture, and in 36% of those that showed coning, the CT had been normal. By using stringent patient selection, the use of CT can be dramatically reduced (Hasbun et al. 2001). Mellor (1992) advised deferring lumbar puncture for at least 30 minutes following seizures as these are known to produce a transient increase in ICP, and administration of mannitol before lumbar puncture is indicated in doubtful cases as it has been shown to effectively reduce ICP and increase CPP and blood flow velocity (Goh and Minns 1993). Another contraindication to lumbar puncture is the need for urgent treatment of shock (Lambert 1994). This applies especially to meningococcal disease, whose diagnosis can be made by blood culture. In summary, it therefore seems reasonable to defer lumbar puncture when the level of consciousness is severely depressed, when the child is shocked, and when there are dilated pupils, ophthalmoparesis or papilloedema.

LABORATORY DIAGNOSIS
CSF

Examination of the CSF is the essential step. Characteristically, the CSF is under increased pressure (>18 cmH$_2$0) and cloudy. In some children, however, the fluid may initially be clear and contain only a few cells or be altogether normal with a negative culture but subsequently demonstrate a positive culture when re-examined 48–72 hours later (Teele et al. 1981). Cultures may be positive for pathogenic bacteria in the presence of normal cytological and chemistry findings, if the lumbar puncture is done after bacterial invasion but before the inflammatory response (Onorato et al. 1980). If clinical suspicion persists, repeat lumbar puncture is indicated within 6–12 hours.

The cells present in CSF in bacterial meningitis usually number between 1000 and 10,000/mm^3, and initially a polymorphonuclear leukocyte response predominates, but anything over 5 mononuclear cells is abnormal, and in 10% of cases an early lymphocyte predominance is seen. Normal CSF does not contain neutrophils, but in cytocentrifuged samples, the occasional neutrophil can be normal. In a traumatic tap, a ratio of 1 neutrophil to 700 red blood cells (RBCs) would be expected if the peripheral RBC and white blood cell (WBC) counts are normal.

Organisms may be seen intracellularly and extracellularly in smears. Gram stains are positive in 25% of cases, depending on the concentration of pathogens in the CSF (Onorato et al. 1980). Staining with acridine orange, a fluorochrome that stains nucleic

TABLE 10.1
Causes of the 'aseptic meningitis syndrome'

Infectious causes

Bacteria: *Actinomyces* spp., *Borrelia burgdorferi* (Lyme disease), *Brucella melitensis, Leptospira* spp., *Mycoplasma pneumoniae* and *M. hominis, Mycobacterium tuberculosis*, atypical mycobacteria, *Nocardia* spp., *Rickettsia rickettsii* (Rocky Mountain spotted fever), *Treponema pallidum*. Bacterial endocarditis, brain abscess and parameningeal suppuration, partially treated meningitis, sinus thrombophlebitis, children with systemic infection[1]

Viruses: Arboviruses, arenaviruses (lymphocytic choriomeningitis), enteroviruses (e.g. polio, coxsackie, echo), adenoviruses, herpes viruses (e.g. HSV-1 /2, HHV-6/7, varicella, cytomegalovirus and Epstein–Barr virus), retroviruses (e.g. human immunodeficiency virus), paramyxoviruses (e.g. mumps, measles), orthomyxoviruses (e.g. influenza), parvovirus, live viral vaccines[2]

Fungi: *Blastomyces dermatidis, Candida* spp., *Coccidioides immitis, Cryptococcus neoformans, Histoplasma capsulatum, Sporotrichum schenkii*

Protozoa: Amoebae (*Naegleria* spp.), *Plasmodium falciparum, Toxoplasma gondii*, visceral larva migrans

Cestodes: Cysticercosis

Noninfectious causes

Malignancies: Leukaemia, lymphoma, metastatic brain tumours

Granulomatous disease: Sarcoidosis, Langerhans histiocytosis

Collagen and vascular diseases: Lupus erythematosus, panarteritis, other vasculitides

Trauma following lumbar puncture, subarachnoid haemorrhage, postoperative meningitis

Toxic causes: Intrathecal contrast media, anaesthetics, systemic toxicity (lead, mercury), catheters[3]

Drug-induced meningitis (azathioprine, cytosine-arabinoside, isoniazid, nonsteroidal anti-inflammatory drugs, penicillin, cephalosporins[4])

Immunological causes: High-dose immunoglobulins

Status epilepticus

Unknown mechanisms

Multiple sclerosis; Schilder disease; uveomeningitis syndromes (Behçet, Harada–Vogt–Koyanagy); Kawasaki disease; Mollaret meningitis; meningitis following heart transplant

[1]Carraccio et al. (1995).
[2]Rare complication, mainly with poliomyelitis vaccine, measles vaccine.
[3]A similar syndrome may occur with dermoid tumours as a result of chemical meningitis due to rupture of cyst (Erdem et al. 1994).
[4]Mainly in patients with collagen vascular disorders but also in healthy persons (Gordon et al. 1990, River et al. 1994, Creel and Hurtt 1995).

acid of some bacteria, may be positive in some patients with a negative gram stain (Kleiman et al. 1984), especially if partially treated. Cultures on blood agar or chocolate agar plate and in broth should always be obtained, even when the fluid is clear. Counting the number of colony-forming units (CFUs) gives an idea of the concentration of organisms in the CSF and is important for therapeutic purposes. It is possible to isolate an organism and determine its sensitivity to antibiotics in 90% of untreated cases of bacterial meningitis (Bohr et al. 1983). In partially treated meningitis, oral antibiotics appear to affect total WBC count, protein concentration, and gram stain and culture results, although when duration of illness is taken into account the effects are less dramatic (Kaplan et al. 1986). Intravenous antibiotics are likely to sterilize the CSF within 24 hours (Blazer et al. 1983).

A raised protein level (>0.4g/L) is usual, both as a result of disruption of the BBB and from local production of immuno-globulins (Maida and Horvatits 1986). The CSF–blood glucose ratio is usually reduced below the normal value of 0.66. Blood and CSF glucose levels should therefore be determined simultaneously (Donald et al. 1983). A normal glucose level is found in up to 20% of cases (Lambert 1994) and does not exclude the diagnosis. CSF lactate is nonspecific and, although frequently positive in bacterial meningitis, provides little additional information. Abnormal C-reactive protein level in the CSF can be a useful test to distinguish bacterial from viral meningitis (Gray et al. 1986).

PCR assay using specific primers to amplify bacterial genome can add useful information in culture-negative cases, as can the nonspecific 16S ribosomal PCR, which is useful in revealing the presence of bacterial components. Latex particle agglutination can be used for the detection of the three common pathogens and group B streptococci. The test is highly sensitive, but nonspecific agglutination may occur (Feigin et al. 1992). Cytokine analysis for the presence of IL-6 and TNFα in CSF reliably identifies purulent meningitis (Dulkerian et al. 1995).

In patients with meningitis but no bacteria grown from the CSF or other body fluids, the physician must consider other causes of the aseptic meningitis syndrome. Many aseptic meningitides are due to viral infections, but other causes are possible (Table 10.1). Such children should have a skin test for tuberculosis, and exclusion of other possibly treatable causes is a major consideration. Careful clinical, neuroradiological and laboratory examinations should be considered, as applicable to the individual child.

Other laboratory procedures

Blood cultures are positive in 80–90% of untreated cases of meningitis. Occasionally blood cultures are positive at the same time as CSF cultures are negative and thus give useful guidelines for therapy. Nose and throat cultures are neither sensitive nor specific. Urine cultures and gram-stained smears of skin lesions may provide clues to the identity of pathogens, the latter immediately. Bacteriological study of the middle ear fluid obtained by aspiration in the case of associated otitis media may show the same organism as is present in the CSF but this is inconstant, and even when the same bacterium is found in both sites, it is not uncommonly of a different strain. Blood cell counts and tests of inflammatory response should be performed. There is usually a high WBC and elevated C-reactive protein (Hansson et al. 1993).

NEUROIMAGING

Imaging early on may be normal, or may show meningeal enhancement with contrast, but its main use is in the exclusion of other CNS pathologies and for the diagnosis of complications (Klein et al. 1986) (see below). Riordan et al. (1993) list the following indications for CT: prolonged depressed consciousness, prolonged partial or late seizures, focal neurological abnormalities, enlarging head circumference, evidence of continuing infection, and recurrence of symptoms and signs. MRI has the added

TABLE 10.2

Preferred first-line antibiotic therapy for acute bacterial meningitis (children >2 months)

Organism	Antibiotic
Haemophilus influenzae	Ceftriaxone
Neisseria meningitidis	Ceftriaxone
Streptococcus pneumoniae	Ceftriaxone
Group B streptococcus	Ceftriaxone
Listeria monocytogenes	Ampicillin and aminoglycoside[1]
Escherichia coli	Ceftriaxone
Pseudomonas aeruginosa	Meropenem + aminoglycoside
	Ceftazidime + aminoglycoside
Proteus mirabilis	Meropenem + aminoglycoside
Staphylococcus aureus	Flucloxacillin (high dose) + rifampicin (vancomycin + rifampicin for methicillin-resistant staphylococcus)
Pasteurella spp.	Ampicillin
	Penicillin + chloramphenicol
Citrobacter spp.	Meropenem + aminoglycoside (sensitivities required)
Klebsiella pneumoniae	Ceftriaxone
Yersinia pestis	Chloramphenicol + gentamicin
	Tetracyclines
Unknown	Ceftriaxone

Always attempt to obtain antibiotic sensitivities where cultures are positive, and confer with a microbiologist concerning the most appropriate therapy. Be aware of local antibiotic sensitivity patterns. Use high doses for CNS penetration.

[1]Ototoxicity and renal toxicity.

advantage of increased sensitivity and no radiation, but is not always readily available.

MANAGEMENT

ANTIBACTERIAL CHEMOTHERAPY (Table 10.2)

The aim of chemotherapy is to select an antimicrobial agent to which the organisms are susceptible, and which reaches the CSF in sufficient concentration to kill the pathogens. Inhibition of growth is not enough, and bacterial concentrations may need to be 10–30 times the minimum inhibitory concentration (Table 10.3) (Quagliarello and Scheld 1997). This can be achieved, in most cases, with adequate plasma concentration; direct instillation of the drug into the ventricles is only very rarely indicated (Feigin et al. 1992). The initial choice of antibiotic depends on the likely causative organism in that age group (Table 10.2). However, treatment must be started without delay and thus often without a complete bacteriological diagnosis. All antibiotics should be given intravenously. For neonates, as gram-negative bacilli, group B streptococci and listeria are the most common organisms, a third-generation cephalosporin plus ampicillin is recommended, with or without an aminoglycoside. For infants over 2 months and children, the third-generation cephalosporins tend to be preferred, and vancomycin should be added if the local incidence of PRP is high. Selection of a particular cephalosporin must be based on personal experience and dosing schedules (Marks et al. 1986, Rodriguez et al. 1986, Hart et al. 1993). Once

the results of cultures and sensitivities become available, treatment can be modified. Penicillin G and ampicillin are usually satisfactory for most strains of *N. meningitidis*, but as the incidence of penicillin-resistant meningococci is increasing, in most cases in developed countries cefotaxime or ceftriaxone would be the drug of choice. Ceftriaxone has the advantage of once-a-day administration; however, biliary pseudolithiasis has been demonstrated by ultrasound study to be present in more than half of patients having received ceftriaxone for several days. Clinical manifestations were present in some of these children but the outcome was generally favourable (Schaad et al. 1988). As discussed earlier, the incidence of penicillin-resistant *S. pneumoniae* is increasing, resulting in vancomycin being routinely added to treatment regimes; vancomycin-tolerant pneumococci have also now been isolated, and in these cases meropenem may be effective. *H. influenzae* strains resistant to both chloramphenicol and ampicillin, once the mainstay of treatment and still commonly used in developing countries, are becoming increasingly common, and obviously demand the use of the cephalosporins (Klass and Klein 1992). Cephalosporin resistance in haemophilus has not as yet been described. Ampicillin together with an aminoglycoside is the drug of choice for *L. monocytogenes* (Klein et al. 1986), and vancomycin together with rifampicin (Peters et al. 1994) is effective against methicillin- and cephalosporin-resistant staphylococci, and is indicated in such cases even though it is potentially ototoxic and nephrotoxic.

DURATION OF TREATMENT

The duration of antibiotic therapy is dependent on clinical response, age and causative organism. Seven days of treatment suffice for meningococcal meningitis. Children with meningitis due to *H. influenzae* or *S. pneumoniae* are traditionally treated for at least 10–14 days or until afebrile for five full days, although 7-day treatment has been found to be no less effective and to be attended by no more complications or sequelae than 10- to 14-day treatment (Lin et al. 1985, Jadavji et al. 1986). Organisms such as staphylococcus and listeria warrant 3–4 weeks' treatment.

MONITORING OF TREATMENT

Patients with meningococcal and pneumococcal meningitis whose disease runs a smooth, uncomplicated course do not need a control lumbar puncture, and the same applies to H. influenzae meningitis. 'End of treatment' lumbar puncture is useless in regular cases of childhood meningitis as the cell and chemical composition of the CSF is extremely variable (Schaad et al. 1981, Durack and Spanos 1982). However, any child who remains febrile and who does not appear to be responding to treatment, warrants a repeat lumbar puncture.

ADJUVANT AND SUPPORTIVE TREATMENT

Corticosteroids remain controversial in treatment of acute bacterial meningitis, although there is now clear evidence of benefit (McIntyre et al. 1997, de Gans and van de Beek 2002, van de Beek et al. 2004). A recent Cochrane review concluded that steroids were associated with a lower case fatality, and lower rates of hearing loss and long-term neurological sequelae, in meningitis caused by *H.*

TABLE 10.3
Minimum inhibitory concentrations (MIC) against common meningeal pathogens*

	H. influenzae	S. pneumoniae	N. meningitidis	E. coli
Penicillin	1	0.015[1]	0.03	64
Ampicillin	0.05	0.02–0.05	0.05	5
Chloramphenicol	0.2–3.5	0.06–12.5	0.78–6.25	3.0–50.0
Cefotaxime	0.008–0.064	<0.01–0.25	<0.025	<0.1–8.0
Cefuroxime	0.5	<0.125	0.5	2.9
Ceftazidime	0.25	2	N/A	0.25
Ceftriaxone	0.003	0.012–0.1	<0.0016	0.0125–25

*Kucers et al. (1997)

[1]In the case of Pen-intermediate/resistant Strep pneumo the MIC is significantly raised: Pen-sensitive pneumo – MIC <0.12 mg/L; Pen-intermediate pneumo – MIC 0.12–1.0 mg/L; Pen-resistant pneumos have MIC >1.0 mg/L.

influenzae as well as other bacteria (van de Beek et al. 2007). Ideally dexamethasone should be given empirically with or before the first dose of antibiotic at a dose of 0.15 mg/kg 6-hourly for the first 48–72 hours. The concern raised has been that steroids may delay sterilization of the CSF; however, in children with cephalosporin-resistant pneumococci, CSF penetration of vancomycin seemed unaffected by adjunctive use of corticosteroids (Morris 2004).

New potential targets for adjuvant therapy are urgently being sought. The cascade of cytokines, chemokines, proteases, antioxidants and apoptotic enzymes, amongst others, that are induced by the host inflammatory response provide many potential targets for neuroprotection. A few therapies have revealed encouraging results. Anti-TNFα (cytokine) medications have been trialled, with some effect, as have MMP-9 (a protease) inhibitors (Leib et al. 2000, Leib et al. 2001). Caspase (an apoptotic enzyme) inhibitors have been shown to limit hippocampal damage in experimental pneumococcal meningitis and inhibit leukocyte migration into the CSF (Braun et al. 1999). Anti-oxidants have also been shown to decrease apoptosis (Auer et al. 2000) and protect the dentate gyrus.

Careful management of fluid and electrolyte balance is essential in meningitis, as both over- and under-hydration are associated with adverse outcomes. Although a recent Cochrane review (Oates-Whitehead et al. 2005) found insufficient evidence to guide practice, fluid restriction is no longer routinely indicated for patients with meningitis, and sufficient amounts of fluids are essential for the prevention of shock. Hyponatraemia frequently represents dehydration, rather than the syndrome of inappropriate antidiuretic hormone (SIADH), and fluid restriction may further compromise cerebral circulation. Arginine–vasopressin concentrations in blood normalize when children with meningitis are given adequate maintenance and replacement fluid therapy, indicating that high levels are a response to dehydration (Powell et al. 1990).

Convulsions should be treated with intravenous midazolam or lorazepam. If unsuccessful, benzodiazepines should be replaced by phenytoin in doses adequate for treatment of status epilepticus (Chapter 15). Preventive treatment is used in some centres, although it is not routinely advocated.

COMPLICATIONS

Vasculitis is a component of the pathological complex of purulent meningitis (Fig. 10.1). It can cause thrombosis of veins or of small or occasionally larger arteries with secondary necrosis (Taft et al. 1986). The location of ischaemic foci is variable, from localized well-defined areas to diffuse necrotic lesions that may be responsible for multicystic encephalomalacia. Ischaemic lesions can be found in the absence of vascular thrombosis. The inflammatory disruption of small vascular walls within the CNS can permit organisms to invade the parenchyma, producing small foci of septic necrosis. It seems likely that such foci give rise to the cerebral abscesses that in rare cases complicate bacterial meningitis. Vasculitis of the bridging veins also plays a prominent role in the genesis of subdural effusions. Focal cerebral signs such as hemiplegia or monoplegia are also a consequence of vasculitis. Spinal cord infarction is an uncommon complication related to vascular involvement. Exceptionally it has been seen as a presenting feature (Boothman et al. 1988). The appearance of bilateral sensory or motor deficit in the course of bacterial meningitis should suggest spinal cord infarction (Glista et al. 1980). Other unusual neurological abnormalities include movement disorders (Burstein and Breningstall 1986), hypothalamic dysfunction and central diabetes insipidus (Greger et al. 1986). Neuroimaging procedures permit a good assessment of the type and location of the responsible lesions. They usually present as areas of hypodensity that can be located to an arterial territory or they may be more diffuse. Such lesions may be partly haemorrhagic.

Focal cerebral signs, such as paralysis of the IIIrd, VIth, or less commonly the VIIth cranial nerves, occur as they cross the inflamed leptomeningeal spaces. Such palsies usually remit following resolution of the meningitis. Opsoclonus has been reported (Rivner et al. 1982).

Seizures, which occur in 30–40% of children with acute bacterial meningitis, may be secondary to fever or cerebral irritation, when they are generalized and occur early in the course. Focal seizures are due to localized involvement of the hemispheres, usually as a result of vasculitis. In some cases status epilepticus occurs and requires emergency treatment to prevent further long-term damage (Chapter 15).

Subdural effusions have been increasingly recognized as a

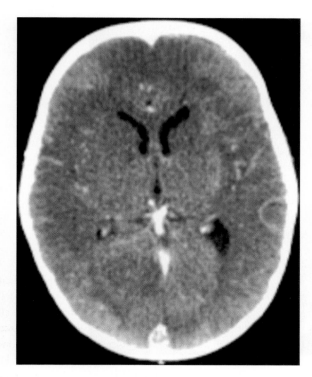

Fig. 10.1. Contrast-enhanced CT of 10-month-old boy with pneumococcal meningitis showing cerebral infarction secondary to vasculopathy, small left subdural empyaema, and a thrombus within the posterior saggital sinus. (Courtesy Dr A Jeanes, St Mary's Hospital, London.)

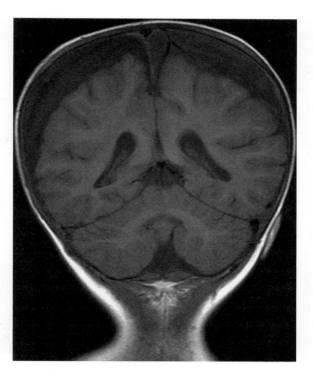

Fig. 10.2. T₁-weighted MRI showing bilateral sizeable extra-axial collections predominantly in the subdural space in a child with pneumococcal meningitis.

complication of acute bacterial meningitis and occur in 20–50% of children with meningitis but are usually of limited thickness and volume and clinically of little significance (Syrogiannopoulos et al. 1986, Cabral et al. 1987). Most effusions are located over the frontoparietal region bilaterally. The subdural fluid is rarely bloody but has a disproportionately high albumin to globulin ratio (Rabe et al. 1968). Persistent or recurring fever, focal neurological signs and persistently positive CSF cultures are probably more closely related to cortical damage than to the presence of an effusion (Syrogiannopoulos et al. 1986, Snedeker et al. 1990). Large effusions with enlargement of the head or signs of increased ICP are rare but necessitate drainage. Most subdural collections resolve spontaneously. Snedeker et al. (1990) found that patients with effusion were more likely to have neurological abnormalities and seizures during the acute illness, but that hearing loss, seizures and developmental delay were not more frequent at follow-up. *Subdural empyaema* is rare (Jacobson and Farmer 1981). It is often marked by the persistence of fever and infective symptoms and signs in association with focal signs such as convulsions and hemiplegia. The diagnosis is made by neuroimaging that shows an extra-axial collection with peripheral enhancement (Fig. 10.2). Diffuse weighted imaging (DWI) has been found helpful in distinguishing effusion and empyema (Hunter and Morriss 2003).

Raised intracranial pressure (ICP) of a severe degree is a serious complication of bacterial meningitis and can be due to different mechanisms: hydrocephalus from altered CSF absorption or obstructed flow, or cerebral oedema. *Acute hydrocephalus* is caused by increased resistance to the circulation and resorption of CSF, as a result of the presence of thick leptomeningeal exudate in the basal cisterns or over the cerebral convexity in the vicinity of the granulations of Pacchioni, or consequent to ventriculitis with obstruction of the aqueduct. It is usually transient but can lead to late hydrocephalus if extensive meningeal fibrosis develops. *Cerebral oedema* probably results from several mechanisms. These include cytotoxic oedema precipitated by cell damage from the infection, vasogenic oedema due to increased capillary permeability related to the inflammatory response to infection, and interstitial oedema from disturbance to CSF resorption by the normal route. SIADH can occur with acute bacterial meningitis (Kaplan and Feigin 1978) and lead to hyponatraemia and hypotonic extracellular fluid, which can exacerbate the cerebral oedema. The clinical manifestations of high ICP may not always be obvious. They include a decrease in the level of consciousness, headache and vomiting, tense fontanelle and split sutures, abnormal pupillary response and hypertension with bradycardia (Cushing reflex). Papilloedema is rare, particularly early on. CT may show loss of grey–white differentiation, compression of the ventricles and sulci, and small basal cisterns. MRI may show gyral swelling, and DWI can be useful in distinguishing cytotoxic oedema (restricted diffusion) from vasogenic oedema. Monitoring of ICP may be a necessary part of treatment in cases of marked or sustained intracranial hypertension (Goitein et al. 1983, Minns et al. 1989). Treatment consists of raising the head to approximately 30° and administering mannitol or other hyperosmolar agents (to reduce cytotoxic oedema). More aggressive measures

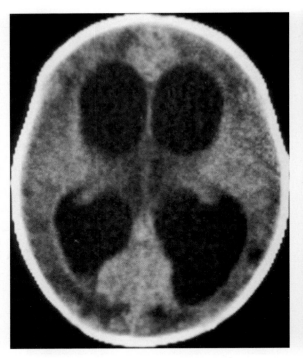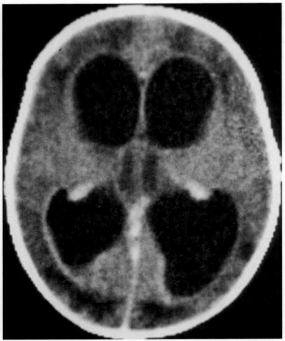

Fig. 10.3. *(Left)* Pre- and *(right)* post-contrast CT showing ventriculitis and secondary hydrocephalus as a complication of bacterial meningoencephalitis. (Courtesy Dr K Chong, Great Ormond Street Hospital for Sick Children, London.)

are described in Chapter 13. Intracranial hypertension is associated with reduced brain perfusion and reduced cerebral blood flow velocity (McMenamin and Volpe 1984), so even moderate episodes of systemic hypotension can have serious consequences and should be avoided (Kaplan and Fishman 1988).

Ventriculitis is almost constant in neonatal meningitis but is relatively uncommon in older children. When ventriculitis is associated with stenosis of the sylvian aqueduct, the infection becomes localized (pyocephalus) and may behave as a cerebral abscess. In most cases, ventriculitis is diagnosed because of persistence of positive CSF cultures with or without clinical signs. Neuroimaging may allow identification of ventriculitis (Fig. 10.3), with abnormal enhancement of the ventricular surface and oedema of adjacent periventricular white matter. Debris may be present in the ventricular cavities (Fukui et al. 2001). Ventriculitis may respond to massive doses of parenteral antibiotics, but local treatment and drainage may become necessary. If not rapidly treated, hydrocephalus is prone to develop in survivors.

Persistent fever and other septic complications are the result of concurrent bacteraemia. They include septic arthritis, pericarditis, pneumonia, endophthalmitis and hypopyon (Kaplan and Fishman 1988). Arthritis appearing after five to seven days of antibiotic therapy is probably mediated by an immune mechanism and frequently responds to anti-inflammatory agents (Rush et al. 1986). Gastrointestinal bleeding, anaemia and disseminated intravascular coagulation can be observed in severe cases, especially but not exclusively with meningococcal meningitis. Fever is prolonged for 10 days or longer in 13% of patients, particularly in pneumococcal disease, and recurs secondarily in 16% (Lin et al. 1984). Fever may be due to the persistence of foci of inflammation, superficial thrombophlebitis from intravenous infusions, nosocomial infections, or septic or aseptic abscesses. More commonly, no cause is found. In such cases, lumbar puncture is indicated. If the child appears well and CSF values are approaching normal, antimicrobial therapy can generally be discontinued at the usual time.

NEUROLOGICAL SEQUELAE
Neurological sequelae affect nearly half of all meningitis survivors, and even in those with normal cognition compared to before, quality of life assessment is significantly diminished. The commonest problems seen after meningitis are learning and neuromotor difficulties, hearing loss, seizure disorders, speech and language problems, scarring (especially after meningococcal disease), visual and ocular problems and behavioural problems. Considerable variation exists between different studies, and also depending on organism involved.

Severe *learning or neuromotor deficits* are found in 5–10% of children (Grimwood et al. 1995, 2000; Bedford et al. 2001) following bacterial meningitis, with a slightly worse outcome in neonates (11%) (Stevens et al. 2003) and in those in the developing world. The vast majority of these children receive special educational provision or have placements in special schools. Those children with higher rates of complications have a worse outcome. There is some discrepancy between the results of various studies. Feldman and Michaels (1988) reported that the academic achievements of children tested 10–12 years after recovering from *H. influenzae* meningitis did not differ markedly from those of their siblings, and there was no specific pattern of learning disabilities, attentional deficits or behaviour problems. Pomeroy et al. (1990) and Taylor et al. (1990) also both found a much lower incidence of persistent sequelae (around 14% in total), with only 1% and 4% respectively being severely disabled. Baraff et al. (1993) reviewed the outcome in 4920 children with meningitis in 45 published reports after 1955. Of these children, 1602 had been enrolled in 19 prospective studies from developed countries and were investigated for sequelae after discharge: 4.2% had learning difficulties or mental retardation; 3.5% had spasticity or paresis; 4.2% had seizures; and 16.4% had at least one major adverse outcome including intellectual sequelae, neurological deficits, seizures or deafness. Different pathogens were associated with different outcomes; those with pneumococcal meningitis had the worst outcome, 15.3% developing sequelae, compared with 7.5% of children with *N. meningitidis* and 3.8% with *H. influenzae*. Grimwood et al. (1995) studied 158 survivors of meningitis incurred between 1983 and 1986 (74% with HiB): 8.5% were found to have major deficits (IQ<70, seizures, hydrocephalus, spasticity, blindness or profound deafness), while 18.5% had minor deficits (school difficulties, behaviour problems or mild hearing loss) as compared to 10.8% of control children. However, an unusually high proportion of these patients had had a complicated course (coma in 18.2%, seizures in 32%, paresis or marked hypotonia in 10.7%).

Sensorineural hearing loss of a severe to profound degree occurs in about 10% of children with meningitis (Pomeroy et al. 1990, Taylor et al. 1990, Baraff et al. 1993) and is bilateral in 4–5%. Hearing loss is thought to result from labyrinthitis, presumably due to extension of inflammation from the subarachnoid space through the cochlear aqueduct (Kaplan et al. 1981, Eavey et al. 1985). The risk of deafness is increased if the CSF glucose concentration on admission is less than 1.1 mmol/L (Dodge et al. 1984), if seizures occur before admission and if sterilization of the CSF is delayed. Cefuroxime treatment is associated with delayed CSF sterilization compared to ceftriaxone and this may have influenced early dexamethasone trials (Schaad et al. 1990, van de Beek et al. 2007). Deafness appears to set in early in the course of meningitis. It is difficult to detect clinically, therefore systematic assessment of hearing should be performed before hospital discharge by evoked response audiometry (Vienny et al. 1984, Cohen et al. 1988). Repeat examination is recommended after discharge if the results of the initial examination are abnormal. Early evoked responses may be transiently abnormal in approximately 20% of cases, with recovery in one or two months (Vienny et al. 1984). The occurrence of deafness is not correlated to the age of the patient or the duration of illness before hospitalization, thus it is unlikely to be prevented by an early diagnosis. The use of dexamethasone treatment decreases the incidence of hearing loss. Deafness is frequently present in children with ataxia but occurs in its absence in most patients. Ataxia seems to be of vestibular origin, although cerebellar dysfunction may be operative in some cases (Kaplan et al. 1981). Virtually all patients are able to compensate for balance deficits in a few weeks or months.

Permanent seizure disorder is found in 2–5% of individuals (Pomeroy et al. 1990, Taylor et al. 1990, Baraff et al. 1993). This can be isolated but is often associated with learning difficulties and other neurological sequelae of variable severity. Such sequelae are the consequence of parenchymal changes resulting from the direct and toxic action of the organisms, vasculitis, and perhaps hypoxia and increased ICP.

Chronic hydrocephalus is uncommon following acute childhood bacterial meningitis. It is due to meningeal fibrosis of the basal cisterns or of the brain convexity or to stenosis of the aqueduct of Sylvius by granular ependymitis. Chronic hydrocephalus may follow early obstructive hydrocephalus. More commonly it develops insidiously and may not be recognized for weeks or months. Therefore systematic ultrasound examination of the CNS is indicated following neonatal meningitis, as ventricular dilatation may occur long before any increase in head circumference. Management is by an external drain in early cases, later by insertion of a shunt.

Other neurological sequelae include hemiplegia, quadriplegia and limb impairments, and occur in 1–4% of individuals. Blindness following purulent meningitis is rare. It may be due to intraocular pathology or optic neuritis, or be of cortical origin.

PECULIARITIES OF PARTICULAR FORMS OF ACUTE BACTERIAL MENINGITIS

NEISSERIA MENINGITIDIS (MENINGOCOCCUS)

N. meningitidis, a gram-negative diplococcus, is the commonest cause of bacterial meningitis in most western countries, occurring predominantly in the winter months, and with a primary peak incidence in the under-5s and a secondary peak in teenagers. Thirteen subtypes or serogroups have been identified, with four serogroups (A, B, C and Y) causing the majority of cases, and four having potential to cause epidemics (A, B, C and W135). Average incubation is 4 days, ranging between 2 and 10 days. Risk factors for younger children have been identified as a preceding upper respiratory tract infection, mannose binding lectin (MBL) deficiency, overcrowding, poverty and passive smoking. Risk factors for older children include dormitory living, kissing and preterm birth (Tully et al. 2006).

The organism is carried in the nasopharynx asymptomatically, and it is estimated that 10–25% of the population carry *N. meningitidis* at any given time, and more during epidemics. There are two different forms of meningococcal disease – a fulminant meningococcal septicaemia, and a more gradual form with development of meningitis alone. Meningococcaemia, which can develop in a few hours, starts with a rash in 50–75% of cases that may be petechial, maculopapular or morbilliform (Swartz and Dodge 1965). Bacteria can be found in petechial lesions. Rapid extension of the skin lesions may be of ominous significance as it often heralds intravascular coagulation leading to purpura fulminans. This is due to the endotoxin of the organism, which also induces shock, bilateral adrenal haemorrhage and other bacterial emboli which may result in metastatic infection to the lungs, pericardium, joints or eye. Eye lesions include hypopyon and panophthalmitis (Edwards and Baker 1981). Mortality, even with early diagnosis, is high at 5–15%, with significant sequelae in 10–20% of survivors. Outcome for meningitis alone is better. Chronic meningococcaemia is rare and is marked by fever, fleeting rashes, joint pain or effusion. Spontaneous remission is possible. Meningeal involvement is rare in such cases. Meningococcal meningitis may manifest as progressive hydrocephalus with mild fever and variable CSF pleocytosis. This form was formerly known as 'posterior basilar meningitis' and is now rare. Diagnosis can be made by isolating bacteria from the skin lesions, the blood or CSF. Antigen testing can be used for rapid detection in the blood, CSF and urine of infected patients, as can PCR.

Specific treatment is with penicillin G or a third-generation cephalosporin. Shock needs to be vigorously treated, and inotropic support is frequently required. Specific treatments with steroids, heparin, fresh frozen plasma or plasmapharesis have not revealed benefit. Activated protein C trials (PROWESS) showed some benefits (Vincent et al. 2003, Laterre et al. 2004).

Recurrent meningococcal meningitis is seen in patients with IgG2 subclass deficiency (Bass et al. 1983) and in patients with acquired or genetic deficiency of the complement system (Ross and Densen 1984), especially the C5–C9 terminal fraction (Davis et al. 1983, Ross and Densen 1984). Meningitis associated with such complement deficiency is often mild and due to uncommon serogroups (Fijen et al. 1989). The risk of developing the disease for household contacts is about 1000 times the endemic attack rate. Rifampicin prophylaxis is therefore recommended for household, day-care centre and nursery school contacts of a patient with meningococcal meningitis. Vaccination for certain serotypes is available (see Epidemiology, p. 383).

STREPTOCOCCUS PNEUMONIAE (PNEUMOCOCCUS)
S. pneumoniae, a gram-positive paired diplococcus, is the commonest cause for invasive disease worldwide, and accounts for 250,000-400,000 deaths, but epidemiology is currently changing with new vaccination schedules (Whitney et al. 2003). It is also a winter disease, and has a bimodal age distribution, being found mainly in the very young and the elderly. Sixty per cent of cases occur in the under-2 years age group, with 39% of cases in those less than 1 year old. There are currently over 90 serotypes known, but most disease is caused by only a few serotypes. The current 7-valent conjugate vaccine covers 75–80% of cases in the developed world, less in the developing world, and the 23-valent polysaccharide vaccine covers 95%. The incubation period is 1–3 days. Risk factors include splenic dysfunction, including those with sickle cell disease, abnormal humoral immunity, CSF shunts and previous head injury. Most cases are due to bacteraemia, but direct extension from a septic focus in the ears, or following a skull fracture with CSF leak, or following cochlear implants is possible. Recurrent attacks can occur, and the causal organisms often appear to be unusual strains. When associated with ear infection, organisms isolated from the middle ear are not always the same as those from the CSF.

The organism is again carried asymptomatically in the nasopharynx and is spread through respiratory droplets or direct oral contact. Pneumococcal meningitis has the highest mortality and complication rate of the three common bacterial meningitides of childhood, with convulsions occuring in up to 44% of patients and coma being frequent. Hearing loss is seen in more than 20% of cases, and ataxia was found in 17 of 93 patients by Bohr et al. (1984). Hydrocephalus is also more frequent than in the other acute bacterial meningitides, and this may be related to the greater thickness and abundance of purulent exudate. In overwhelming infection, the CSF may contain fewer than 75 cells/mm³ and more than 10 organisms per high-power field on first examination. Diagnosis is again made by either isolating the organism from blood or CSF, or from rapid antigen testing or PCR. The increasing incidence of PRP has modified recommendations for treatment, and in high-incidence areas vancomycin needs to be added to the cephalosporin of choice. All isolates should be sent for MIC or *PBP2B* testing to determine sensitivities (see epidemiology).

HAEMOPHILUS INFLUENZAE TYPE B
H. influenzae, a small gram-negative pleomorphic coccobacillus, is now a rare cause of meningitis and invasive disease in the developed world, thanks to the introduction of the type b conjugate vaccine. However, it is still common in those countries where vaccination is not available, and acounts for over 150,000 deaths/year (WHO 1998). HiB meningitis is primarily a disease of infants and preschool children, with more than 95% of cases occurring before 2 years of age, and with minimal seasonal variation. *H. influenzae* is either encapsulated or unencapsulated, with encapsulated strains being typable. Encapsulated strains are classified into six types (a–f), with over 90% of disease being caused by type b. Symptoms of upper respiratory tract infection, including otitis media, frequently precede the onset of meningitis, which is thus less abrupt than that of meningococcal or pneumococcal meningitides. This is a cause for both delayed treatment and the 'blind' administration of antibiotics with resulting sterile CSF. A sparse petechial rash may be present, and purpura fulminans is on record (Jacobs et al. 1983). Diagnosis again is confirmed through isolation of the organism or by PCR. The mortality rate is 3–4%, but much higher in the developing world. Sequelae occur in 9–20% of children, with a poorer outcome in more complicated cases. Subdural effusions complicate the disease in approximately 15% of patients but are of limited clinical significance. Hearing loss is a major problem, occurring in approximately 10% of cases. Treatment is with ceftriaxone or similar third generation cephalosporins, and as yet no resistance has been reported. Prevention in preschool unvaccinated contacts is recommended with rifampicin.

RARER CAUSES OF PURULENT MENINGITIS
Staphylococcal meningitis, caused by *S. aureus* or *S. epidermidis*, is often due to secondary invasion of the CNS as a result of wounds, surgery or nearby infections, and is a common pathogen in patients with ventriculoperitoneal or ventriculo-atrial shunts (25–40%). Other rare pathogens associated with shunt infections include enteric bacilli (10%) (Hirsch and Hoppe-Hirsch 1988) and diphtheroids (Everett et al. 1976) (see Chapter 6). Unhanand

TABLE 10.4
TABLE 10.4
Causes of recurrent bacterial meningitis

Cause	References
Surgical causes	
Post-traumatic fistulae following fractures of the cribriform plate, petrous pyramids, frontal, ethmoidal or sphenoidal sinuses	Wilson et al. (1990, 1991)
Nontraumatic fistulae	Ommaya (1976), Steele et al. (1985)
Congenital dehiscence of the cribriform plate	
Defects of the foot plate of the stapes	
Defects of the middle ear	
Congenital defects of the tegmen tympani	
Mondini syndrome	
Congenital dermal sinus with or without intraspinal or intracranial dermoid cyst (lumbosacral, cervico-occipital)	Chapter 2; Schwartz and Balentine (1978)
Craniopharyngioma and other intracranial dermoid or epidermoid cysts	Kitai *et al.* (1992)
Myelomeningoceles and meningoencephaloceles including occult forms such as sphenoidal or basioccipital meningoencephaloceles or neurenteric cysts	Chapter 2; Hemphill et al. (1982)
Shunt-treated hydrocephalus	Hirsch and Hoppe-Hirsch (1988)
Nonsurgical causes	
Congenital agammaglobulinaemia (or hypogammaglobulinaemia)	Bass et al. (1983)
Deficiency of the terminal components of complement (C5–C9)	Davis et al. (1983)
Splenectomy in infancy	
Mixed immunological deficiency	
Sickle cell anaemia	Nottidge (1983)
Unknown causes	
Pneumococci are the most common pathogens in post-traumatic cases, in children with congenital defects of nose and ear, and following splenectomy; gram-negative bacteria and staphylococci are common with dermal sinuses and neural tube defects; *S. epidermidis* in patients with shunt; and meningococci in children with complement deficiency	

et al. (1993) reviewed 98 cases of meningitis due to gram-negative bacilli both in neonates and in infants; a predisposing factor such as neural tube defect or urinary tract anomaly was present in 25% of cases. *E. coli* organisms accounted for 53% of cases, *Klebsiella/Enterobacter* for 16%, *Salmonellae* for 9%, and rare organisms for the rest. Other rare causes of acute purulent meningitis include *Bacillus* spp. (Feder et al. 1988), *Pasteurella multocida* (Kolyvas et al. 1978), *Yersinia pestis* (Mann et al. 1982), *Salmonella* spp. (Appelbaum and Scragg 1977), *Acinetobacter* spp. (Graber et al. 1965), *Serratia marcescens* (Campbell et al. 1992), nonanthrax *Bacillus* (Weisse et al. 1991) and *Burkholderia pseudomallei*, the agent of melioidosis, which is common in some tropical countries (Visudhiphan et al. 1990). This bacterium may also be the cause of brain abscess and empyaema. Meningitis caused by anaerobic bacteria is rare, except following rupture of a brain abscess. Other causes are secondary to chronic otitis media, mastoiditis, sinusitis, head trauma and prior neurosurgical procedures. Although all rare, bacteroides, peptostreptococci, fusobacterium, clostridium and actinomyctes species have all been isolated.

RECURRENT MENINGITIS
Recurrent meningitis usually occurs in children with an underlying dural fistula (congenital or acquired) facilitating infection of the nervous system (Table 10.4). *S. pneumoniae* is responsible in about three quarters of cases, with *S. aureus*, *S. epidermidis*, *Pseudomonas* spp., *Klebsiella* spp. and *H. influenzae* accounting

for the remainder. The clinical manifestations are often relatively mild, but severe cases can occur. Approximately 1% of cases of head injury requiring hospitalization develop CSF fistulae with a leak that become a source of infection in 10–24%. A low glucose and β-transferrin testing of the fluid identifies it as CSF. Infection is usually an early event but may be delayed for months or even years; it may occur even in the absence of CSF rhinorrhoea or otorrhoea. Nontraumatic fistulae, that represent congenital defects, are located along the craniospinal axis and often are difficult to detect and necessitate careful examination of the lumbosacral and the cervico-occipital area. Occipital sinuses may be especially difficult to detect, and shaving of the region is imperative as the external orifice may be pinpoint. Detailed otological examination, high-resolution neuroimaging and occasionally isotopic examination with radioiodinated albumin or technetium injected intrathecally may also be necessary. Imaging of the head may show a dermoid cyst of the posterior fossa. Sphenoidal and basioccipital meningoceles (Hemphill et al. 1982) may also be difficult to recognize, emphasizing the necessity for a careful neuroradiological examination. Treatment of recurrent meningitis is directed primarily against respiratory pathogens in the case of CSF fistulae and against enteric organisms in cases of dermal sinus. Pneumococcal vaccine may be useful for some patients. Prophylactic antibiotics are used by some clinicians but may favour the emergence of resistant bacteria. There is a consensus that surgical correction of fistulae lasting more than

4–6 weeks and surgical intervention for chronic otitis, sinusitis or mastoiditis should be performed. Dermoid tracts need total removal.

Mollaret meningitis (not bacterial) is a rare syndrome of recurrent attacks of aseptic meningitis, of undetermined but not necessarily single cause, which after a sudden onset subside within a few days. Preceding viral infections, including HSV2, are sometimes demonstrated (Graman 1987, Mirakhur and McKenna 2004). The patient usually presents with a high fever, headaches, myalgias and neck stiffness. Brudzinsky and Kernig's sign may be positive. CSF reveals initially a polymorphonuclear predominance with 'endothelial' or Mollaret's cells, followed later by a lymphocytic pleocytosis. Connective tissue diseases, epidermoid and intraspinal tumouts, and other infections (e.g. fungal) need to be excluded. The prognosis is excellent, with antiviral or antibiotic treatment having little effect.

BACTERIAL MENINGITIS IN NEWBORN INFANTS
Meningitis in the first 28 days of life differs in many ways from that in older children; not only are the organisms different, but the characteristics of the neonatal brain as well as the immature mechanisms of defence against infection result in a different picture and outcome. In the first week of life, vertical transmission accounts for the majority of cases, with group B streptococcus (GBS) predominating (42%), followed by *E. coli* (16%) (particularly K1 strains), enteroviruses (7%) and *L. monocytogenes* (3%). Meningitis of later onset may be nosocomial or community acquired, and can be caused by other gram-negative organisms, as well as *S. pneumoniae* and *Staphylococcus*. The incidence of neonatal meningitis in the UK is around 0.21/1000 births, increasing in preterm and low birthweight infants, and where there is a history of prolonged rupture of membranes or of maternal pyrexia. Boys are more commonly affected than girls, especially with gram-negative infections (Holt et al. 2001). In newborn infants diagnostic difficulties are often considerable, and meningitis should be thought of in any unwell infant who is drowsy or irritable. Apnoeic attacks, vomiting, low-grade fever and other systemic manifestations such as jaundice or respiratory distress are common but nonspecific. Convulsions, usually focal in type, are a clear indication to perform lumbar puncture. Meningeal signs are rare, and a full or bulging fontanelle is present in less than one third of patients. On account of the nonspecific features, a CSF study is thus mandatory in every case of suspected neonatal infection.

Interpretation of the results of lumbar puncture may be difficult in neonates because of the characteristics of the CSF at this age (Rodriguez et al. 1990). In one study, Bonadio et al. (1992) found that 31% of infants under 8 weeks old had more than 10 white blood cells/mm³ of CSF and that only 10% had no white blood cells. The majority of the white cells were polymorphs. The protein level was on average 0.44g/L in preterm infants, and figures as high as 1.5g/L are known to occur. Low glucose levels are frequent in neonates and especially in infants aged between 4 and 8 weeks. In addition, traumatic lumbar puncture is frequent in this age group, and up to 4% of newborn babies with meningitis,

especially preterm infants, may have a normal CSF at the first examination. This emphasizes the need for repeat lumbar puncture 6–12 hours after the first tap in case of doubt. Up to 30% of neonates with GBS meningitis may have fewer than 30 white blood cells/mm³, while the same is rare with *E. coli* meningitis. However, Klein et al. (1986) reported that less than 1% of patients had completely normal CSF (including cell count, protein and sugar). There are few contraindications to a lumbar puncture, even in sick neonates, in whom a modified left lateral position with flexure of the hips but without flexure of the neck can be used and is better tolerated.

Antibiotic use initially is empirical, with most neonatal units using a combination of a third generation cephalosporin, ampicillin (for listeria), and an aminoglycoside. If herpes encephalitis is suspected, aciclovir is added. Once the organism and sensitivities are known, antibiotic use can be rationalized. GBS meningitis is effectively treated with ceftriaxone. Listeria meningitis responds to ampicillin alone or in combination with aminoglycosides but not to cephalosporins (Kessler and Dajani 1990), and gram-negative enteric bacteria are best treated with a combination of cephalosporins and aminoglycosides. Intrathecal or intraventricular administration of antibiotics is no longer recommended. There have been no trials on duration of therapy, but current practice in the UK is between 2 and 3 weeks; usually 2 weeks for GBS and 3 weeks for *E. coli*. A lumbar puncture to confirm sterilization of the CSF is recommended at 24–48 hours (Heath et al. 2003) but not at the end of treatment (Schaad et al. 1981). Adjunctive therapy with dexamethasone has not been shown to have any benefits, and currently is not recommended. Trials with other adjuncts (GSCF, EPO, IgG) have not as yet shown definite benefit.

Imaging is used to detect complications of meningitis, such as hydrocephalus, empyaema and brain abscesses (associated particularly with *Enterobacter sakazaki*, *Morganella morganii* or *Citrobacter koseri*) (Fig. 10.4). Ultrasound, CT and MRI all have a role to play. Compartmentalization of the cerebral ventricles, especially at the level of the foramen of Monro, may lead to localized hydrocephalus (Kalsbeck et al. 1980), although diffuse hydrocephalus due to cisternal blockage is much more frequent. In newborn infants with brain abscesses, especially due to *Proteus* or *Citrobacter* spp., drug treatment is often sufficient. Drainage of the larger cavities is indicated when they are large and/or produce increased ICP.

The outcome of neonatal meningitis is far worse than that in older childen. Although mortality has decreased substantially over the past decade from around 24% to 6.6% (Holt et al. 2001), morbidity remains dismally high, with a 10-fold increase in the risk of moderate or severe disability following neonatal meningitis (Bedford et al. 2001). Over 50% of affected neonates have some disability, whether intellectual or motor, sensorineural hearing loss or seizures. The EEG may have predictive value as very slow tracings are of unfavourable prognostic significance (Chequer et al. 1992). The key to improvement in neonatal menigitis lies in prevention, with maternal vaccination for GBS and *E. coli* having the potential to prevent the majority of cases of neonatal meningitis.

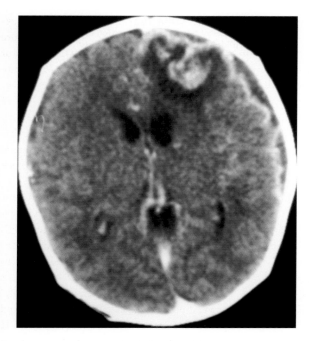

Fig. 10.4. Contrast-enhanced CT of 4-week-old infant with *Salmonella* meningitis showing left-sided meningeal enhancement and left fronto-parietal infarction. In addition there is a small left-sided subdural fluid collection and small amount of midline shift (courtesy Dr J Danin, St Mary's Hospital, London).

In infants 28 days to 3 months of age, there is overlap between the organisms responsible for neonatal and childhood meningitis (Baumgartner et al. 1983). However, the pathogens of childhood meningitis are occasionally the cause of neonatal disease.

SUBACUTE OR CHRONIC AND GRANULOMATOUS BACTERIAL MENINGITIS

TUBERCULOUS MENINGITIS

With over one third of the world's population infected with *Mycobacterium tuberculosis*, tuberculous meningitis (TBM) remains a major cause of childhood death and neurological disability in developing countries. Although strictly speaking it is an acute disorder with a mean duration without treatment of 20–30 days, it is usually seen as a chronic process as it is virtually always treated at some stage. With the recent resurgence of tuberculosis in the developed world, TBM in children is currently on the increase, and the diagnosis needs to be considered in every child with a possible history of exposure and clinical symptoms of meningitis, as delay in diagnosis directly affects mortality and morbidity, with the incidence of neurological sequelae being much higher when treatment is delayed.

PATHOLOGY AND PATHOGENESIS

Most cases of TBM are caused by *M. tuberculosis*; 5% are caused by *M. bovis*, mainly where unpasteurised milk is consumed, and

occasional cases are due to *atypical mycobacteria*. Exceptional cases have been observed following BCG immunization in immunodeficient and even occasionally in normal children (Tardieu et al. 1988). The majority of cases begin as a primary focus in the lung following inhalation of the acid-fast bacillus. The primary focus is frequently asymptomatic, and develops over weeks, until it invades the lymphatics, spreads to regional lymph nodes, and the lymph node then ruptures into the blood stream, resulting in haematogenous dissemination. These disseminated bacilli lodge in the brain and meninges, and provoke an inflammatory response, resulting in a granuloma. This can either be contained by the immune system, or the bacilli can continue to multiply until the focus ruptures into the subarachnoid space, with dissemination of the mycobacteria throughout the CSF, and TBM follows. Miliary tuberculosis is seen in approximately 30% of cases (Fig. 10.5) as bacilli have disseminated throughout the body. Meningitis may rarely be caused by dissemination from other visceral foci or by extension of spinal or cranial osteitis. The infection generates a cascade of inflammatory mediators, with secondary generation of a thick exudate that settles along the base of the brain. This in turn induces a vasculitis with secondary thrombosis of adjacent arteries and veins, resulting in embolization and infarction, particularly in the small lenticulostriate vessels supplying the basal ganglia, as well as in the cerebral cortex, pons and cerebellum (Poltera 1977). Over time, the exudate fills the basal cisterns, resulting in entrapment of cranial nerves and blockage of CSF drainage pathways resulting in secondary hydrocephalus (communicating or obstructive). Large tuberculomas are still relatively common in Asiatic and African countries and may be supratentorial or involve the brainstem. A tuberculous encephalopathy has been described in some cases of tuberculous meningitis (Dastur et al. 1970). The condition is characterized by oedema and, less frequently, perivascular myelin loss with vasculitis of capillary and small vessels. This might result from an allergic reaction to proteins liberated from lysed tubercle bacilli in partially immune children and can occur with little or no evidence of meningitis. In partially immune patients, localized forms are common and are apt to produce a wide variety of lesions, including localized meningitis of the posterior fossa with cerebellar signs and hydrocephalus, chiasmatic involvement with visual deficits (Silverman et al. 1995) or brainstem damage with alternative syndromes.

The efficacy of BCG is extremely variable (0–90%) (Fine 1995), with the greatest efficacy demonstrated in those countries with the lowest incidence of TB. This is thought to be due to the increased exposure of the children in a developing country at a young age to environmental mycobacteria. Even in these circumstances, BCG does seem to protect against the severest forms of TB, such as TBM and miliary TB.

CLINICAL MANIFESTATIONS

The clinical manifestations of TBM are extremely variable (Table 10.5) so that the diagnosis may be very difficult. Virtually any neurological picture can be seen. The majority of cases occur in children below 5 years of age, and progress over three successive

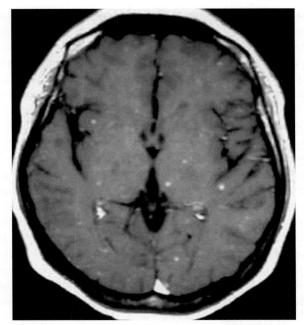

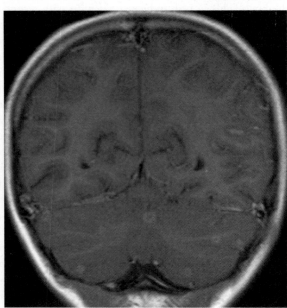

Fig. 10.5. Post-contrast T$_1$-weighted MRI showing enhancing miliary tubercles from disseminated *Mycobacterium tuberculosis* in two different patients.

TABLE 10.5
Clinical features at presentation of children with tuberculous meningitis*

Nuchal rigidity	77%
Apathy	72%
Fever	47%
Vomiting	30%
Drowsiness	23%
Headache	21%
Coma	14%
Papilloedema	9%
Convulsions	9%
Facial palsy	9%
VIth nerve palsy	9%
IIIrd nerve palsy	9%
Hemiparesis	5%
VIIIth nerve involvement	2%
Diabetes insipidus	2%

*Data from Idriss et al. (1976).

signs appear, and paralysis of cranial nerves III, IV, VI and VII is frequently present. Hemiplegia and movement disorders due to frequent involvement of the basal ganglia are often observed (Gelabert and Castro-Gago 1988). During the third stage, stupor and coma replace apathy. Symptoms and signs of increased ICP are obvious. The pupils are fixed, respiration is irregular, and signs of decerebration with tonic extensor spasms develop. Hydrocephalus is present in the majority of patients at this stage. Atypical manifestations are common. A febrile convulsion may occur at onset. Focal neurological deficits preceding the classical meningeal irritation have been reported in all large series and include field defects, aphasia, hemiparesis, monoparesis and abnormal movements. Isolated high fever, severe convulsions and features mimicking intracranial tumours may be observed (Udani and Bhat 1974). A spinal form of TBM may manifest as fever and meningeal signs rapidly followed by paraplegia, with secondary intracranial spread. Such cases are apt to be mistaken for acute viral meningomyelitis. Tuberculous encephalopathy (Udani and Dastur 1970) is characterized by convulsions and coma. The CSF is usually normal or shows only a mild increase of protein and cells. A diffuse encephalopathy may develop in a child already treated for TBM.

DIAGNOSIS

The diagnosis classically rests on a history of exposure to persons with pulmonary tuberculosis, often an asymptomatic older relative, a positive tuberculin skin test (TST) in association with a compatible clinical picture, chest X-ray changes, a CSF with lymphocytosis and elevated protein, and neuroimaging revealing the classic triad of infarction, hydrocephalus and basal enhancement. However, in practice diagnosis is often extremely difficult. Frequently there is no history of prior exposure, skin anergy is present in 10–40% of cases (Doerr et al. 1995) and a weakly positive TST may be difficult to interpret in patients immunized with BCG vaccine. The chest X-ray is abnormal in just over half the patients, revealing either a miliary picture or the primary complex.

stages, which if untreated results in death in 3–4 weeks. The prodromal stage is seen in 60% of cases and usually lasts 2–3 weeks. It is marked by apathy, irritability, disturbances of sleep, vomiting, abdominal pain and low-grade fever. At this stage, there are no neurological manifestations. Headache is uncommonly complained of by children under 3 years, but abdominal pain is present in 15% of cases. As the disease progresses to stage 2, mental changes are present in 80% of patients and focal neurological signs in approximately one third of cases (Waecker and Connor 1990, Curless and Mitchell 1991, Davis et al. 1993). Meningeal

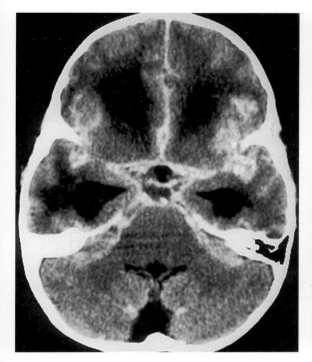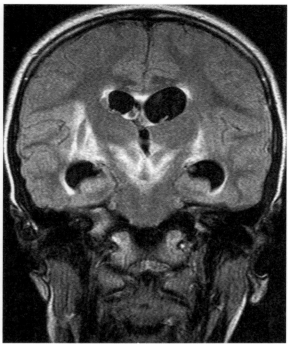

Fig 10.6. *(Left)* Contrast-enhanced CT showing the classic triad in tuberculous meningitis (TBM) of thickened enhancing basal leptomeninges, vascular infarction and obstructive hydrocephalus (courtesy Prof J Schoeman, Tygeberg Hospital, South Africa). *(Right)* Coronal fluid attenuated inversion recovery (FLAIR) image showing high-signal regions of oedema in the basal ganglia and subthalamic regions, as well as hydrocephalus. The oedema results from a combination of inflammation and vascular infarction.

The presence of retinal tubercules or hepatosplenomegaly with granuloma visualized on abdominal ultrasound may aid diagnosis. The CSF findings although fundamental are not always unequivocal. The fluid may be crystal-clear or have a ground-glass appearance. It contains normally between 10 and 400 cells/mm³, which in over 85% of cases are lymphocytes. It can be acellular, or polymorphonuclear leukocytes may outnumber lymphocytes in the early stages; and occasionally polymorphonuclear pleocytosis may occur during later stages (Teoh et al. 1986). Repeat lumbar puncture may be helpful in such cases for distinguishing partially treated acute bacterial meningitis from TBM (Feigin and Shackelford 1973). CSF protein is almost always raised, often to 2 g/L or more, and glucose is frequently lowered, in 80% of cases to below 1.5 mmol/L (Lambert 1994). Chloride is usually low. Direct visualization of acid-fast organisms is uncommon, particularly in children in whom CSF volumes are low. Definitive diagnosis by culture of CSF is positive in only approximately 30% of cases and results are available only after weeks, hence treatment should often be started on indirect evidence, and a significant proportion of the cases of TBM remain unproved (Traub et al. 1984). Rapid diagnosis using enzyme-linked immunosorbent assay (ELISA) (Sada et al. 1983), latex particle agglutination of mycobacterial antigens (Krambovitis et al. 1984), adenosine deaminase activity of CSF (Ribera et al. 1987) or radioactive bromide partition between CSF and serum (Coovadia et al. 1986) has been reported. None of these have gained widespread acceptance, on account of lack of sensitivity or specificity. Diagnosis

by PCR for IS 6110 (Shankar et al. 1991, Lin et al. 1995, Smith et al. 1996) can be obtained rapidly, and is the most promising, but again is positive in only approximately 30% of cases, and is often not available where TBM is most common. Recent studies using interferon-gamma release assays to mycobacterial proteins such as ESAT-6 and CFP-10 are still being evaluated (Pai 2005). CT findings vary with the stage at which examination is performed. Meningeal enhancement (Fig. 10.6) is present in two thirds of the patients (Kingsley et al. 1987, Teoh et al. 1989). Enhancement usually persists for months even when the course is favourable. Hydrocephalus may be present from stage I but increases in degree and frequency in later stages. Infarction is more common in children than in older patients. It involves especially the central grey matter (Teoh et al. 1989). Multiple hypodensities in the central grey matter or in the territory of the anterior or middle cerebral arteries on CT are characteristic. MRI gives similar results (Kumar et al. 1993) showing parenchymal enhancement with gadolinium and brainstem damage (Offenbacher et al. 1991). Imaging is also of diagnostic importance as it excludes other conditions such as cerebral abscess, which may mimic tuberculous meningitis. Pathological studies have emphasized the frequency of vasculitis (Poltera 1977), which may also be demonstrated by angiography. *Tuberculomas* may be seen initially. Brainstem tuberculomas are still frequently observed in developing countries (Talamas et al. 1989). A tuberculoma appears on CT or MRI as a round mass, sometimes with a necrotic, clear centre (ring lesion). They may be polycystic in contour and

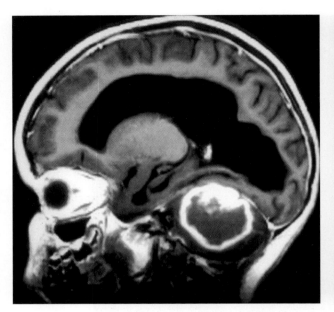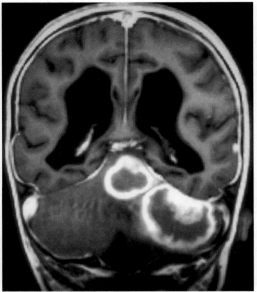

Fig. 10.7. *(Left)* Lateral and *(right)* frontal post-contrast T$_1$-weighted MRI showing two large ring-enhancing posterior fossa tuberculomas with secondary obstructive hydrocephalus.

behave as space-occupying lesions (Fig. 10.7). Occasionally they may be poorly limited and surrounded by extensive oedema. Calcification is common.

Oedema and signs of diffuse encephalopathy may also be detected (Trautmann et al. 1986). The finding of an entirely normal scan (with contrast) in a drowsy patient virtually excludes a diagnosis of TBM.

DIFFERENTIAL DIAGNOSIS

The differential diagnosis of TBM includes a large part of the neurological pathology of childhood, in particular other lymphocytic meningitides and aseptic meningitis. Neoplastic meningitis that occurs in cases of metastatic tumours, especially germinomas, ependymomas, choroid plexus tumours, medulloblastomas and sarcomas, may mimic TBM. The CSF in such cases contains lymphocytes or shows a mixed pleocytosis, protein is raised, and hypoglycorrhachia is frequent. The diagnosis is usually made by CT or MRI. Malignant cells may be demonstrated in the fluid following cytospin. The diagnosis of partially treated bacterial meningitis can usually be ruled out on history and CSF features. In case of doubt repeat CSF study settles the issue. The diagnoses of viral meningoencephalitis or myelitis should not be accepted without reservation. In cases where doubt exists, antituberculous drug treatment should be started and discontinued later. Tuberculomas can occur in the absence of meningeal involvement as a first CNS manifestation as well as during the course of meningitis (Dastur and Desai 1965).

TREATMENT

The optimal treatment for TBM is controversial with different centres using different drug regimes and very variable durations of treatment. We would recommend chemotherapy initially with

a four-drug regime, including pyrazinamide, isoniazid and rifampicin with either ethionamide or ethambutol. If the patient is extremely ill and cannot take oral medication, rifampicin, together with an aminoglycoside and ciprofloxacin/ofloxacin can be given intravenously. Pyrazinamide concentration in CSF is 75–110% of that in blood, and that of isoniazid is approximately equal, whereas rifampicin penetrates uninflamed meninges poorly. Ethionamide reaches high concentration in the CSF and, for that reason, is preferred to ethambutol. Ethionamide can produce optic neuritis, so visual acuity should be monitored. Isoniazid can induce a peripheral neuropathy, although this is mainly seen in adults, and is prevented by the administration of vitamin B$_6$. Resistance to any of these antibiotics can develop when they are given alone, and administration of several drugs simultaneously largely prevents the emergence of resistant strains (Iseman 1993). With the increasing emergence of multi-drug-resistant TB, determination of the sensitivity of the organism, if cultured, should be obtained where possible and treatment adjusted accordingly. The benefits of adjunctive use of corticosteroid treatment (usually prednisone) are becoming clearer (Schoeman et al. 1997), and we recommend their use for a period of 1–3 months in an effort to prevent meningeal fibrosis and vasculitis and to limit the degree of intracranial hypertension. Total duration of treatment is usually 9–12 months. However, some centres treat for 18 months, whilst others have shown that short-term supervised inpatient treatment (for 6 months) gives similar results (Alarcón et al. 1990, Donald et al. 1998). Indications for surgical treatment include high ICP, and especially hydrocephalus, which often requires the placement of a shunt (Bullock and Van Dellen 1982). Communicating hydrocephalus can often be successfully treated with a combination of acetazolamide and furosemide (Donald et al. 1991, Schoeman et al. 1991), avoiding the complications of

during the first two days of the major illness. The common spinal poliomyelitis is characterized by asymmetrical flaccid paralysis involving the legs, arms and/or trunk with absent tendon reflexes. Urinary retention is present at onset in 20–30% of cases. The bulbar form is rarely isolated as at least the cervical cord is involved in 90% of cases. All cranially innervated muscles may be affected. In addition, respiratory failure and hypertension may result from involvement of the brainstem reticular substance. Encephalitic signs may be associated but they may also be due to respiratory insufficiency consequent upon paralysis of diaphragmatic and intercostal muscles.

Examination of the CSF shows 30–200 cells/mm^3. Initially, these are predominantly polymorphonuclear cells, followed after 5–7 days by a lymphocytic pleocytosis. The protein content rises late, reaching a maximum about the 25th day of illness.

On MRI, swelling of the spinal cord with an abnormal signal from its central part has been reported (Kibe et al. 1996). Before clinical onset the virus can be isolated from the stools and oropharynx as early as 19 days and as late as 3 months after the first clinical features (mean 5 weeks). Typing of the virus shows one of the three types of poliovirus. Serological diagnosis is made by demonstration of an elevation of the titre of neutralizing or complement-fixing antibodies.

The prognosis of paralytic poliomyelitis depends on the extent of involvement. Recovery in some affected muscles is frequent for up to one year or more, but muscles still totally paralysed after one month usually remain so definitively. A progressive motor neuron disease (post-polio syndrome) resembling amyotrophic sclerosis is sometimes observed in adults 20 or more years after an acute attack (Dalakas et al. 1986).

Cases of paralytic poliomyelitis due to live vaccine may occur in immunocompromised patients receiving the vaccine or in contacts (Nkowane et al. 1987, Sen et al. 1989, Groom et al. 1994). Such cases may have an atypical presentation. As rare cases of poliomyelitis may also occur in nonimmunosuppressed children who receive live vaccine (Dussaix et al. 1987), with the waning incidence of disease worldwide most industrialized countries now use killed injected polio vaccine in their routine immunization schedules to avoid this complication.

The diagnosis is easy provided the disease is kept in mind. Guillain–Barré syndrome differs in its mode of onset, the symmetrical distribution of weakness and CSF characteristics. Rare cases of paralytic disease due to other viruses have been recorded (Kyllerman et al. 1993). West Nile virus has been responsible for epidemics of a disorder closely similar to paralytic poliomyelitis. Cases of intoxication by chemicals or insect bites may also clinically mimic the condition (Gear 1984).

Enteroviruses

The original classification of the enteroviruses, prior to genomic analysis, was according to cytopathic effects on different tissue culture cells and infected animals. Three types of poliovirus, 24 coxsackie A and 6 coxsackie B viruses, and 34 types of echoviruses were identified. Subsequent isolates were assigned an enterovirus number, carrying on from enterovirus 68 without further

subdivision. Subsequent, genomic sequence analysis partially supports the original culture based classification.

These viruses enter the host via the gastrointestinal tract, replicate there and induce a viraemia that may lead to infection of the CNS. Most cases will have a mild gastrointestinal viral prodrome, and there is often a contact history with other family members having gastrointestinal symptoms. Most patients have a benign course and make a rapid recovery. The organisms can be amplified by PCR or isolated from the CSF and also from blood, stool and oropharynx. Rapid diagnosis by PCR in the CSF may give a result within hours. Infection can occur at any age, including the first weeks of life (Kaplan et al. 1983).

Enteroviruses commonly associated with aseptic meningitis are coxsackie B1–5 and coxsackie A7, 9 and 25, echoviruses 4, 6, 9, 11, 14, 16, 18, 20 and 30, as well as polioviruses. Acute epidemic conjunctivitis due to enterovirus 70 can be complicated by meningitis, cranial nerve palsy or limb involvement, isolated or associated. Severe pain and fasciculations are common (Wadia et al. 1983, Chopra et al. 1986).

Group A coxsackie virus meningitis may be associated with or preceded by herpangina, respiratory infections and parotitis. In group B disease, pleurodynia (Bornholm disease or epidemic myalgia) or diarrhoea may occur. Myocarditis and encephalitis may complicate meningitis, especially in young infants (Kaplan et al. 1983). With echovirus infections, both sporadic and epidemic infections may occur. A maculopapular rash is common, especially in echovirus 4, 9 and 16 infections. Rashes sometimes occur also in coxsackie A9 and A23 disease. Rashes may also be petechial.

Sequelae of enteroviral meningitis have been reported (Kaplan et al. 1983). It is likely that sequelae are the result of encephalitic involvement, concomitant with meningitis. They are especially common in neonatal enteroviral meningitides, which also feature fever, poor feeding, diarrhoea, hepatomegaly and rashes (Huang et al. 2003).

Enteroviruses may also cause other CNS disease manifestations, including: lower motor neuron paralysis (coxsackie A4, 7, 9, B5, echovirus 70); Guillain–Barré syndrome and transverse myelitis (coxsackie A9, B1, 4, Echovirus 6, 70); cerebellar ataxia (coxsackie A9, 4, 7, B3, 4, echovirus 6, 9, 71); peripheral neuritis (echovirus 9). Enteroviruses usually cause self-limited disease, which, although associated with morbidity, is rarely fatal. However, in certain more vulnerable patient populations (e.g. infants or the immunocompromised), enteroviruses may cause life-threatening infections. Pleconaril is an antiviral compound that integrates into the capsid of picornaviruses, including enteroviruses, preventing the virus from attaching to cellular receptors and releasing viral RNA into the cell. Treatment studies of pleconaril have demonstrated some efficacy in patients with severe disease (Rotbart and Webster 2001); unfortunately the drug has not been commercially developed.

Mumps virus

In unimmunized populations, mumps is the most frequently identified cause of viral aseptic meningitis. The classic clinical picture of leptomeningitis is encountered in 0.5–2% of patients with mumps. However, pleocytosis has been observed in 56% of those with parotitis (Russell and Donald 1958). Parotitis may be absent in 30–40% of cases (Levitt et al. 1970), and in such cases the diagnosis can be made by PCR amplification of the viral genome in CSF, or serologically. Symptoms of meningitis have their onset from eight days before to 20 days after the appearance of parotitis. A high fever often occurs concomitantly.

The CSF shows lymphocytic pleocytosis often of marked intensity with several hundreds of cells/mm^3. The glucose content may be reduced (Wilfert 1969). Although the course is usually benign, pleocytosis may last for up to several months and there is protracted persistence of specific intrathecally produced oligoclonal IgG (Vandvik et al. 1978a).

Complications are uncommon, but hearing loss is the most common severe sequela (Hall and Richards 1987). Ataxia and opsoclonus (Ichiba et al. 1988) and vestibular neuritis (Thomke and Hopf 1992) are on record. Hydrocephalus (Yanofsky et al. 1981, Lahat et al. 1993) has been rarely reported. Vertigo and optic nerve atrophy have been occasionally reported (Wilfert 1969). Meningoencephalitis or myelitis may occur and occasionally become chronic (Ito et al. 1991). The occurrence of multifocal epileptic seizures has been recorded (Parain and Boulloche 1988).

Herpes viruses
Several members of the herpes virus group cause lymphocytic meningitis.

• *Herpes simplex virus.* HSV type 2 (Nahmias et al. 1982) is more often responsible than type 1, which mainly causes encephalitis. HSV-2 meningitis may be a manifestation of primary infection in the sexually active adolescent. Rarely, mild cases of HSV-1 infection can manifest only by meningeal irritation (Whitley et al. 1982a), and patients recover in 7–14 days.

• *Varicella-zoster virus.* VZV can cause an aseptic meningitis as well as more complex involvement of the CNS, described in a later section. Pre-eruptive neurological manifestations may occur (Tsolia et al. 1995). In that study, two children with encephalitis also had concomitant ataxia. Focal neurological deficits other than ataxia developed in 7 children: 3 with facial nerve palsy, 1 with concomitant hemiplegia, 2 with paresis of the arm, 1 with radiculitis resulting in paresis of the leg, and 1 with abducens nerve palsy. Two children had isolated meningitis. In this cohort, only 2 children experienced long-term sequelae, 1 with persistent paralysis of the arm, and 1 with abducens nerve palsy.

Other CNS syndromes associated with VZV infections include varicella myositis, zoster radiculopathy, zoster myelitis, and delayed hemiparesis following chickenpox (Kamholz and Tremblay 1985, Ichiyama et al. 1990, Rosenfeld et al. 1993, Herrold and Hahn 1994, Gilden 2004, Mariotti et al. 2006). Involvement of the basal ganglia (Silverstein and Brunberg 1995) and lateral medullary syndrome (Kovacs et al. 1993) have also been reported. Ischaemic vascular events, often involving large brain arteries, have been frequently reported after chicken-pox (Amlie-Lefond et al. 1995, Tsolia et al. 1995, Lanthier et al. 2005, Losurdo et al. 2006). Acute arteriopathies leading to ischaemic strokes may be aetiological in up to a quarter of cerebral arterial thrombosis cases in childhood; one study suggested that varicella was the likely aetiologic factor in up to 60% of cases (Guillot et al. 2005). There is probably more than one mechanism for these postinfectious events, and inflammatory changes in arterial tissue as well as increased secretion of procoagulants such as anticardiolipin may be important in some cases (Kurugol et al. 2000, 2001).

In addition, the host immune response to VZV includes antibodies that may cross-react with and inactivate the important host anticoagulant factor protein S. This may lead to a hypercoagulable state with development of purpura fulminans as well as post-VZV ischaemic stroke (Josephson et al. 2001).

• *Epstein–Barr virus (EBV).* The majority of EBV infections in early life are asymptomatic, and neurological complications are rare; they may include aseptic meningitis, encephalitic presentation and several other CNS complications (Hung et al. 2000). Meningitis may herald several other nervous complications such as infectious polyneuritis (the Guillain–Barré syndrome), encephalomyelitis or cranial nerve involvement (Hausler et al. 2002) or parkinsonism (Hsieh et al. 2002). About one third of patients with infectious mononucleosis have ≥5 cells/mm^3 on examination of CSF and these levels may persist for months, often after complete clinical recovery (Pejme 1964). Full recovery may be delayed for several weeks or months.

• *Cytomegalovirus (CMV).* Rare cases of CMV infection in non-immunodepressed children are on record. In one such case CMV infection presented as a transverse myelitis (Miles et al. 1993).

• *Human herpes virus (HHV) 6 and 7.* HHV-6 infection, the agent of exanthema subitum, can rarely cause meningoencephalitis in previously healthy children (Asano et al. 1992, Jones et al. 1994). Although most primary infections with HHV-6 and the closely related virus HHV-7 are asymptomatic, both of these viruses have been associated with up to 30% of febrile convulsions occurring in the first two years of life (Hall et al. 1994, Barone et al. 1995, Ward 2005).

Adenovirus infections
There are many types of adenoviruses; most cause mild gastrointestinal, respiratory or renal infections, and only rarely do they cause CNS syndromes. CNS presentations include aseptic meningitis, myelitis, subacute focal encephalitis, Reye-like syndrome, and transient encephalopathy (Linssen et al. 1991, Straussberg et al. 2001).

Parvovirus B19
Most infections with parvovirus B19 are asymptomatic, but symptomatic infections in children usually consist of fever and rash, and in adults there may also be associated arthropathy.

Rare cases of CNS infection have also been reported with a meningoencephalitic presentation and viral DNA detected in the CSF (Barah et al. 2001, 2003). The host immune response to parvo B19 in the CNS has been suggested as the cause of the inflammation with evidence of increased cytokines in the CSF as well as specific HLA genetics in the host (Kerr et al. 2002).

Lymphocytic choriomeningitic virus (LCMV)
LCMV infection is a human zoonosis caused by a rodent-borne arenavirus, which primarily infects wild mice. LCMV infection is transmitted to humans after contact with excreta of infected mice, guinea pigs or hampsters. In humans in-utero infection may lead to fetal damage (Barton and Mets 2001, Barton et al. 2002), whereas postnatal infection is usually either asymptomatic or an influenza-like illness, but a CNS syndrome can occur (Barton and Hyndman 2000).

Other and undetermined viruses
These are probably the cause of the many cases – indeed a majority – in which no pathogenic organism can be isolated. Understandably, as the number of possible viral agents is high, and because the disease is most often benign, complex investigations are not pursued.

ENCEPHALITIS AND MENINGOENCEPHALITIS

Encephalitis is an inflammatory process involving the brain. In most cases the meninges are also affected, and myelitis may be part of the process, hence the terms meningoencephalitis and encephalomyelitis that apply to the same spectrum of diseases. Encephalitides can be acute or chronic. The two types will be described separately as they pose completely different problems. Acute encephalitides are a major cause of acute neurological disease in childhood and have to be distinguished from a number of other infectious and metabolic processes that require immediate diagnosis. Subacute and chronic encephalitides raise the issue of degenerative or other slowly evolving disorders.

ACUTE ENCEPHALITIS
Acute encephalitides are the most common cause of acute non-suppurative neurological disease in children. Several other conditions produce an 'encephalitic-like illness' or 'acute encephalopathy', require different therapy and have different outcomes so that an accurate diagnosis is very important.

AETIOLOGY
The vast majority of cases of acute encephalitis are caused by viruses. However, some other organisms can be responsible. *M. pneumoniae* is of particular importance and was implicated in 13.1% of cases in Finland (Koskiniemi et al. 1991, Rantala et al. 1991). Other bacteria such as *Legionella, Campylobacter jejuni* (Nasralla et al. 1993) and *Bordetella pertussis* are rarely a cause, but in as many as a third of cases no responsible agent can be identified. The incidence of encephalitis varies greatly in different countries and during different seasons of the year, due to seasonal variation in incidence of common viral infections and to the geographical restriction of some agents such as the arboviruses.

The relationship between the occurrence of encephalitis and viral or bacterial infections is complex, and several mechanisms are at play in different cases. Two major mechanisms are recognized. The first mechanism is operative in the primary encephalitides in which the virus is present in the CNS and actually replicates within neurons, glial cells or macrophages leading to cell death and tissue destruction. The second mechanism involves a virally initiated, host-generated autoimmune response within the CNS, similar to that observed in experimental allergic encephalitis (Johnson 1982b) and applies to the *postinfectious meningoencephalitides*.

A distinction between the various mechanisms reponsible for encephalitis-like illnesses can be made on a pathological basis in at least some autopsied cases. The presence of viral genome, inflammatory infiltrates, round cells of glial nodules, neuronal necrosis, and sometimes intranuclear inclusions in the primary encephalitides or perivenous demyelination in postinfectious cases (ADEM) allows separation of *primary and postinfectious cases*, and the absence of inflammatory signs excludes the diagnosis of encephalitis. In clinical practice, however, a pathological distinction between primary and postinfectious encephalitis, or even between encephalitis and parainfectious encephalopathies, is rarely possible as very few cases proceed to diagnostic brain biopsy.

CLINICAL FEATURES, DIAGNOSIS AND MANAGEMENT OF ACUTE MENINGOENCEPHALITIS (REGARDLESS OF AETIOLOGY AND MECHANISMS)
Clinical features
The major clinical manifestations of encephalitis are deteriorating consciousness with confusion, drowsiness or coma, altered behaviour, convulsions and a variety of neurological signs. These usually appear acutely but there may be a prodromal phase with memory and behavioural disturbances. Neurological manifestations referable to any part of the CNS involve mostly the cerebral hemispheres (hemiplegia, aphasia) but may affect the brainstem or cerebellum, with ataxia present in 58% of cases in one series (Rantala et al. 1991), or the spinal cord with a picture of acute myelitis. Additional signs can include involvement of the cranial nerves, or of the hypothalamus with lethargy, or of the basal ganglia with rigidity or abnormal movements.

An abnormal EEG is virtually always present, the most common manifestation being generalized or predominantly unilateral slowing. The CSF opening pressure is usually raised, and the CSF is usually abnormal with a pleocytosis consisting of lymphocytes and mononuclear cells, an elevated protein level and a normal glucose level. The CSF cell count varies from a few to several hundred cells/mm^3, in most cases with a majority of mononuclear cells, although polymorphonuclear cells may predominate in very acute cases with necrotic lesions, and in such cases red blood cells may also be present. The CSF protein content may be increased; however, the CSF remains normal in a considerable proportion of cases (Rautonen et al. 1991).

TABLE 10.8
Differential diagnosis of the acute encephalitides

Intracranial infections
Bacterial or viral meningitis
Tuberculous meningitis
Brain abscess
Cerebral malaria

Para-infectious encephalopathies
Reye syndrome
Haemorrhagic shock and encephalopathy
Toxic shock syndrome

Metabolic disorders
Fluid, electrolyte and acid-base disorders
Inherited metabolic diseases
    Amino acid and organic acids
    Urea cycle disorders
    Lactic acidosis

Hypoxic–ischaemic injuries
Vascular collapse and shock of various causes
Cardiorespiratory arrest
Near-miss sudden infant death syndrome

Vascular diseases
Stroke of embolic or thrombotic origin
Haemorrhage from vascular malformations
Venous thrombosis

Toxic injuries
Endogenous (diabetes, uraemia, liver failure)
Exogenous (drugs or household agents)

Seizure disorders
Status epilepticus
Hemiconvulsions–hemiplegia syndrome

Increased intracranial pressure
Tumours
Haematomas
Acute hydrocephalus
Lead poisoning

Neuroimaging and some clinical features may help to distinguish some forms of encephalitis such as herpes simplex encephalitis. Early after presentation, CT and even MRI may be normal but often CT shows multiple areas of low density and contrast enhancement while MRI shows increased signal on T_2-weighted images (Kesselring et al. 1990). Diffusion imaging is more sensitive than conventional MRI in acute cases of encephalitis in children (Teixeira et al. 2001). Abnormalities involve mainly the white matter in postinfectious encephalitis but also the cortical grey matter in primary encephalitides. The time course of acute encephalitis may be fulminating. In many cases, however, new symptoms and signs appear over a few days to weeks. This is an important diagnostic feature, as in many other acute encephalopathies the full picture is abruptly completed.

Differential diagnosis
The differential diagnosis of meningoencephalitis includes a large number of encephalopathies and other disorders marked by disturbances of consciousness that may arise with pathology outside the CNS (Table 10.8). Because the clinical features are not specific, special attention should be given to disorders that require immediate effective therapy, especially bacterial meningitis, tuberculous meningitis and brain abscesses. Lumbar puncture is needed to exclude meningitis; however, it may be dangerous in the face of raised ICP, which is not excluded by the absence of papilloedema or a 'normal' CT scan. Neuroimaging may ultimately help to identify the underlying cause, but early in the encephalitic process abnormalities may be subtle and difficult to detect. In some patients, the diagnosis of tuberculosis or even of bacterial meningitis may remain a possibility even after CSF study. Exclusion of cerebral abscess may be difficult in the early stage of bacterial cerebritis. Contrast enhancement is important as it may demonstate the peripheral round-ring image suggestive of suppuration. The CT appearance of tuberculous meningitis is characteristic. Treatment with antibiotics and/or antituberculous agents may have to be started in dubious cases together with treatment for herpes simplex encephalitis, until the diagnosis is clarified. Cerebral thrombophlebitis usually produces characteristic CT images (Chapter 14). Occasionally, an acute arterial thrombosis mimics an encephalitic process. Cryptogenic status epilepticus may be accompanied by pleocytosis (Chapter 15). Acute metabolic diseases should also be excluded. Therefore, blood sugar, serum electrolytes, blood ammonia level and, in selected cases, amino acid and organic acid profiles should be obtained. These will help to rule out Reye syndrome or an intermittent and/or late manifesting form of aminoaciduria or organic aciduria. In some patients examination of urine for toxic substances may be useful, although the course of intoxication is generally much faster and there are no focal neurological signs or meningeal involvement. Lead intoxication can simulate encephalitis, but CSF shows high protein with only a few or no cells, and other features of lead toxicity are present.

Management
The general management of acute encephalitis is the same as that of other acute encephalopathies and is a paediatric emergency. Priority must be given to ensuring a patent airway and maintaining adequate circulation. A complete assessment of the child is then in order (Table 10.9). Neurological examination is essential in establishing the correct diagnosis, evaluating prognosis and planning therapy.

Critically ill children with a very depressed level of consciousness are best treated in intensive care units and this applies particularly to those with evidence of high ICP (Tasker et al. 1988a). Maintenance of an adequate cardiac output to support effective cerebral perfusion is essential, alongside close monitoring of respiration, blood pressure and body temperature to maintain homeostasis. Hyperthermia and seizures must be kept under control as far as possible. When available, EEG monitoring is extremely useful in detecting subclinical seizure activity and evaluating the degree of brain dysfunction (Tasker et al. 1988b). Monitoring of ICP is not generally required in acute encephalitis but may be essential in some related conditions such as Reye syndrome (see below). Treatment of high ICP is discussed in Chapter 13. Osmotic agents and, in some cases, corticosteroids may be needed.

410

TABLE 10.9
Assessment and emergency management of the child with acute encephalopathy

History
Details of acute events: time of year; current local epidemics; prodromal illness; recent history of: infectious disease, travel, human contacts, animal contacts, insect contacts, drugs/toxins, recent immunizations

Past medical history: early development; seizures; consanguinity; family history; metabolic history; immune status; immunization status

General physical examination
Vital signs (respiratory rate, blood pressure, temperature)

Skin and mucous membranes (exanthema, herpes)

Visceral examination

Lymphadenopathy

Status of peripheral circulation

Neurological examination
Level of consciousness using paediatric modifications of the Glasgow Coma Scale (Chapter 12)

Ocular responses (Chapter 12) including corneal reflex, pupillary responses, oculocephalic reflex (doll's eye manoeuvre), oculovestibular response

Motor asymmetry; response to noxious stimulation (appropriate withdrawal, decorticate or decerebrate posturing)

Signs of increased intracranial pressure (Chapter 13), especially examination of the fundi

Laboratory investigations
Blood gases, urea, electrolytes, creatinine, sugar

Full blood count

Labstix on urine (sugar, ketone bodies, organic acids)

Chest X-ray

CT/MRI

Blood biochemistry: liver enzymes, ammonia, calcium, clotting factors

More complete metabolic investigations (lactic acid, amino acids, organic acids) in selected cases (preserve blood and CSF)

EEG when available without delaying therapy; ideally polygraphic recording

CSF examination. Lumbar puncture should be deferred when patient deeply unconscious, evidence of high intracranial pressure or unstable vital conditions

Toxicology in urine

Microbiology
CSF sugar (paired with blood); protein; microscopy; gram stain; rapid antigen; culture; viral PCRs (select the most appropriate according to epidemiology)

If indicated:

Mycobacterial culture and staining (Zeil–Neelson/auramine)

Fungal culture and staining (India ink)

Cytology to exclude malignant cells

Blood, urine, stool, throat, nasopharyngeal aspirate, skin lesions: culture/antigen testing/PCR for appropriate infections

Serum paired base line and convalescent titres for evidence of seroconversion, ASOT (antistreptolysin O) for evidence of streptococcal infection

Immediate therapeutic measures
Ensure safe i.v. access (using large veins if necessary)

Ensure adequate airway

Maintain adequate blood pressure with i.v. fluids and pressor agents (e.g. dopamine) if necessary

Lowering of very high temperature

Control seizures

Administer appropriate antimicrobial therapy

Intensive care treatment usually required, especially when assisted ventilation is required

PRIMARY ENCEPHALITIDES

Primary encephalitides are characterized by the presence of viruses and their replication in target-cells within the CNS. Although a large number of viruses can induce a primary encephalitis, the single most common agent in Western Europe is the herpes simplex virus. Enteroviruses can also produce a primary encephalitis. In other parts of the world including North America, however, arboviruses are important causal agents.

HUMAN HERPESVIRUSES AND ENCEPHALITIDES
Herpes simplex encephalitis
At least 90% of cases are caused by HSV-1, although HSV-2 is the most common cause of disseminated infection and encephalitis in neonates (Kennedy and Chaudhuri 2002). Before treatment with aciclovir was available the mortality from HSV encephalitis was over 70% and fewer than 3% of individuals survived without severe sequelae. The frequency at all ages is between 1 in 200,000 and 1 in 400,000 persons per year in Western countries, which represents about 10% of all severe viral CNS infections. Thirty-one per cent of cases occur in patients below 20 years of age and 12% in those between 6 months and 10 years (Whitley et al. 1982b, Whitley and Kimberlin 2005).

Initially most cases were considered to be due to reactivation of latent virus but genomic analysis of viral strains from patients has demonstrated encephalitis cases caused by primary infection, reactivation of latent infection and reinfection with new strains (Whitley and Alford 1982). Primary infection is the norm in neonates and young infants. Latent HSV-1 can persist in the trigeminal ganglia (Johnson 1982b) and lead to recurrent cutaneous or mucosal infections by means of dendritic spread. The virus may occasionally spread along meningeal branches and this might give it access to the brain. Entry into the CNS may also be from the nasal mucosa through the cribriform plate to involve the parenchymal cells of the olfactory bulb (Johnson 1982a).

HSV encephalitis is highly cytopathic, pathologically characterized by necrotic lesions, which are often haemorrhagic with gross softening, and in severe cases, loss of all neural and glial elements. Damage predominates in the orbital, mesial temporal, cingulate and insular cortex, and in some cases may extend to the brainstem (Duarte et al. 1994). In perinatally infected neonates damage is usually much more diffuse throughout the brain. Intranuclear eosinophilic inclusions (Cowdry type A bodies) are recognized in neurons, oligoglial cells and astrocytes, and virus may be amplified from tissue and CSF.

The clinical symptoms of encephalitis are preceded in 60% of cases by prodromal symptoms that may be purely systemic such as fever and malaise, but are sometimes more suggestive when disturbances of memory or behaviour are prominent. The prodromal phase often lasts a few days, with increasing symptoms of reduced consciousness, abnormal behaviour and a high fever. The full-blown picture includes the symptoms common to all cases of encephalitis, i.e. lethargy, obtundation or coma and convulsive seizures. Seizures are particularly frequent and often repeated in cases of HSV infection, and they are almost always focal, especially facial and upper limb, reflecting the gross asymmetry

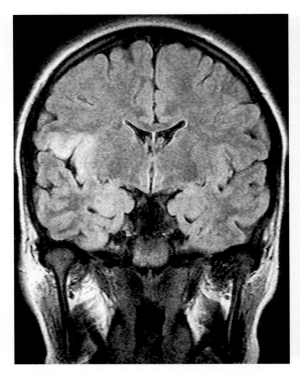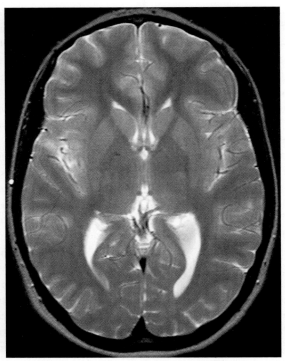

Fig. 10.9. FLAIR *(left)* and T₂-weighted *(right)* MRI showing hyperintensity in the right insular cortex and frontal operculum secondary to herpes encephalitis.

of lesions that is apparent pathologically. Unilateral status epilepticus may also occur. Increased ICP is frequent, and papilloedema is present in 15% of cases. Hemiplegia often develops, and aphasia may be a prominent and initial finding in older children and adolescents. Changes pointing to focal necrosis of the temporobasal structures such as anosmia, olfactory hallucinations and disordered behaviour may be prominent (Whitley et al. 1981). In many cases, however, clinical features are uncharacteristic, but HSV should always be considered because of its frequency, the potential severity of the outcome and because it is treatable (Rose et al. 1992). In infants and young children, febrile seizures, usually partial, are often the dominant symptom and may remain isolated for several days. Such cases may pose particularly difficult diagnostic problems. Puchhammer-Stöckl et al. (1993) reported five cases presenting as 'complicated febrile convulsions' among 151 cases of HSV encephalitis diagnosed by PCR. In three of these the CSF contained no cells, and in only one was the MR image suggestive of the diagnosis.

In some patients the disease appears more progressively. Aphasia or sensory abnormalities precede the more severe neurological signs by several days. A bilateral opercular syndrome, reminiscent of the Foix–Chavany–Marie syndrome caused by vascular lesions in adults, may occur as a result of the predominant basal involvement (Rantala et al. 1991). Atypical forms with only mild encephalitic involvement and spontaneously favourable outcome in the absence of therapy are rare (Marton et al. 1995), and where there is doubt treatment is always indicated. Focal forms with pseudotumoural features are on record (Counsell et

al. 1994). Since the advent of more sensitive PCR diagnosis of HSV encephalitis, the spectrum of CNS disease caused by this virus in adults and children has broadened to include milder and atypical presentations (Dennett et al. 1996). A more chronic presentation of disease has also been recognized in immunosuppressed patients (Kleinschmidt-DeMasters and Gilden 2001).

Contrary to the diffuse slow waves that are seen on EEG in other meningoencephalitides, the tracings in HSV cases are usually *very* asymmetrical and often exhibit clear foci of spikes on an abnormally slow background. Low amplitude in one or more regions, especially over the temporal lobe, is not unusual. Periodic complexes 1–3 seconds apart are frequent in the same area but are often only transient (Mizrahi and Tharp 1982). The periodic complexes occur most commonly between the second and fifteenth day of the disease and are rarely seen thereafter (Schauseil-Zipf et al. 1982). They are not specific, however, and may occur with encephalitis caused by *M. pneumoniae* (Hulihan et al. 1992) or Epstein–Barr virus.

Neuroimaging may appear normal within the first 24–48 hours after onset, and changes on MRI are seen before CT changes (Kapur et al. 1994). MRI may show focal oedema in the medial region of the temporal and orbital surface of the frontal lobes, insular cortex, and angular gyrus (Fig. 10.9). When CT is abnormal it usually shows reduced attenuation in one or both frontal or temporal lobes and sometimes areas of hyperintensity representing small haemorrhages, and there may be midline shift in up to 50% of cases (Greenberg et al. 1981, Dutt and Johnston 1982).

During the course of the illness, there may be an initial increase in the extent of abnormalities (Koskiniemi and Ketonen 1981). Later on, atrophy of the parenchyma with a marked peri-sylvian and temporal predominance progressively appears and will persist, and calcification may develop. Total disappearance of CT abnormalities is rare in infants but may be seen in older patients.

The CSF may be normal in 20–25% of patients. In most cases it is under increased pressure and contains an excess number of cells, usually lymphocytes, with fewer than 50 mononuclear cells/mm3 in about a quarter of cases (Whitley et al. 1982b). The CSF is frequently haemorrhagic or xanthochromic because of the necrotic and haemorrhagic character of the lesions.

Diagnosis of HSV encephalitis depends on PCR amplification of HSV DNA from CSF. This is highly sensitive (>95%) and specific (>95%), but false-negative PCR results may occur in samples taken early within the first 24–48 hours or late after 10–14 days, and indeed where the patient has been treated with aciclovir (Lakeman and Whitley 1995, Koskiniemi et al. 1996, Davis 2000). A quantitive relationship between HSV DNA copies per millilitre of CSF and CNS damage has not so far been established (Tyler 2004). Where PCR is negative a demonstration of a fourfold rise of antibody titre against HSV-1 infection in the CSF is significant but requires at least 10–14 days to appear (Koskiniemi et al. 1984). The antibodies initially belong to the IgM class and later switch to IgG type. They are associated with the presence of an oligoclonal protein pattern in the CSF (Mathiesen et al. 1988). The antibodies and the oligoclonal pattern may persist for years following an attack of herpes encephalitis (Tardieu and Lapresle 1980), reflecting the persistence of HSV within the CNS.

When the history, clinical and/or neuroimaging features are suggestive of HSV encephalitis, treatment (see below) should be started immediately. Brain biopsy is only very rarely indicated in children when, after neuroimaging, another diagnosis requiring different treatment is suspected, rather than for confirmation of the HSV diagnosis. Such diagnoses may include brain abscess, tumour or granulomatous meningitis (Whitley et al. 1989). Other conditions that may mimic HSV encephalitis such as paraneoplasic limbic encephalitis or mitochondrial encephalomyopathy with lactic acidosis and stroke-like episodes (MELAS) (Johns et al. 1993) are rare in children.

Treatment of HSV encephalitis is with the nucleoside analogue, aciclovir, which inhibits the HSV DNA polymerase and thus viral replication (Skoldenberg et al. 1984, Whitley et al. 1986). Aciclovir is phosphorylated to the active form by the viral thymidine kinase in HSV infected cells and is therefore non-toxic to uninfected host cells. In the original randomized controlled trial of Skoldenberg et al., adult mortality with aciclovir was 19%, significant sequelae occurred in 14%, and 56% of patients recovered fully, in contrast to a mortality of over 70% without treatment. In children, even with early administration of therapy after the onset of disease, nearly two thirds of survivors will have significant residual neurologic deficits, and infants below 12–18 months of age have the most unfavourable outlook

in terms of morbidity and mortality (Whitley and Kimberlin 2005). Sequelae include hemiplegia (Rautonen et al. 1991), bilateral opercular syndrome (van der Poel et al. 1995) and severe epilepsy which, in infants, may manifest as infantile spasms. Behavioural sequelae are frequent. Aphasia, which may be global or more specialized, is common because of the frequent temporal location of the lesions.

Resistant strains of HSV are rarely encountered in children; they are most common in immunocompromised patients who may have been frequently exposed to aciclovir, and such cases may require treatment with other antivirals such as foscarnet or cidofovir (Whitley 2002). Administration of corticosteroids together with antiviral drugs has been used to reduce oedema, but due to the concomitant risk of diminishing the host response they are not recommended (Wood et al. 1994).

As in adults, the treatment dose of aciclovir for children is 10 mg/kg (or 500 mg/m^2) intravenously 8 hourly (the mg/m^2 dose gives a slightly higher total daily dose than the mg/kg). Intravenous therapy is required to maintain adequate CNS penetration. In general, children tolerate aciclovir very well, although at high dose aciclovir may cause renal toxicity if the patient is not well hydrated. A course of 21 days of therapy is given in confirmed cases; shorter courses of treatment have been associated with an increased risk of relapse, and younger children and infants appear to be at more at risk or relapse (Davis 2000, Ito et al. 2000, Love et al. 2004, Valencia et al. 2004). Although in some cases relapse is due to recurrence of virus in the CNS, in others an immune-mediated mechanism may be the aetiology and this may be associated with secondary demyelinization (Barthez et al. 1987; Pike et al. 1991; Rautonen et al. 1991; De Tiège et al. 2003, 2005). Relapse in children may be associated with a choreoathetoid presentation, which has a poor prognosis (Barthez et al. 1987, Shanks et al. 1991, Wang et al. 1994, Valencia et al. 2004). Relapse may also be associated with lack of HSV antibody production in the CSF (De Tiège et al. 2006).

In neonates, a higher aciclovir dose of 20 mg/kg intravenously 8 hourly for 21 days has been demonstrated to have increased efficacy in terms of mortality and morbidity (Kimberlin et al. 2001). This increased dose was associated with a mild degree of neutropaenia in most patients, but if more severe could be supported by granulocyte colony stimulating factor. As a consequence of the more extensive and diffuse CNS infection and more immature immune response in neonates, repeat CSF PCR is advised at the end of intravenous treatment to confirm viral clearance (Kimberlin 2004). In addition, ongoing prophylaxis with high-dose oral aciclovir treatment for the first 1–2 years of life is advised to reduce the risk of reactivation and further CNS damage (Tiffany et al. 2005). Whether such prophylaxis should be considered in infants and children presenting beyond the perinatal period remains controversial.

A common clinical dilemma occurs when a patient presenting with a febrile encephalitis and treated initially with aciclovir is found to have a negative HSV PCR. Once started, can the aciclovir be stopped early, especially as three weeks of intravenous treatment is quite onerous in small children? If no other diagnosis is identified, our pragmatic approach, in such circumstances, is to stop aciclovir early only if: the clinical condition of the child is returned to normal; the EEG is normal; and cranial imaging after at least 5–7 days demonstrates no abnormality. However, if the imaging or EEG demonstrates a focal abnormality, then a full 21 days of treatment is completed.

Atypical forms of HSV encephalitis have been reported. Brainstem encephalitis with involvement of cranial nerves has been shown to result from herpes infection in some cases (Duarte et al. 1994). Acute myelitis due to HSV is also on record (Wiley et al. 1987). The latter is seen mainly with type 2 HSV, which also causes most neonatal HSV infections. These include encephalitis, associated with disseminated viral infection in two thirds of cases (Chapter 1). Encephalitis due to HSV-2 infection is more severe than type 1 disease (Corey et al. 1988) and may lead to diffuse encephalomalacia. In the neonate, the presence of a multifocal periodic pattern on the EEG, together with an inflammatory CSF, is highly suggestive of herpetic encephalitis and may occur before any abnormal image is visible on CT or MRI. In older patients, cases of severe temporal lobe epilepsy have been attributed to smouldering HSV-2 infection (Cornford and McCormick 1997).

Other herpesvirus encephalitides
These are much less common and may more often be due to mechanisms other than direct invasion.

• *Varicella-zoster virus.* Primary infection with VZV (chicken-pox) may cause both postinfectious encephalitis, usually a cerebellitis, and primary encephalitis, usually a more diffuse presentation occurring in the first few days along with cropping of new vesicular lesions. An early pre-eruptive onset of encephalitis has been reported in a few cases (Maguire and Meissner 1985). CNS manifestations of VZV also occur after recurrence of VZV with shingles or even without any cutaneous lesions, although this is more common in adults or the immunocompromised (Koskiniemi et al. 2002). Quantification of VZV DNA in the CSF has demonstrated higher levels in those with more severe disease (Aberle et al. 2005). Varicella may also induce Reye syndrome (see below).

Chicken-pox cerebellitis is usually mild, presenting as an acute ataxia in a child with a history of recent infection, and most cases show full recovery within a few weeks. In one small study a proportion of children with this postinfectious condition had evidence of high titre autoantibodies that reacted with cerebrum and cerebellar tissue (Adams et al. 2000). Treatment with aciclovir ($500\,mg/m^2$/dose 8 hourly) may be effective for the acute encephalitis, but is not necessary for the postinfectious cerebellitis.

• *Human herpesvirus 6 and 7.* Primary infection with HHV-6 is most often asymptomatic, but can be associated with the childhood infectious syndrome named 'exanthem subitum' or 'roseola infantum' (Asano et al. 1992, 1994). Primary infection has also been assoctaed with febrile convulsions, and in a large epidemiological study in the USA at least a third of febrile convulsions

were associated with seroconversion (Hall et al. 1994). The natural history of primary infection with HHV-7 is less well understood, but it may also be associated with exanthem subitum and CNS effects (Ward 2005). A prospective study of children under 3 years of age presenting with febrile encephalitis in the UK demonstrated 17% had primary infection with either HHV-6 or HHV-7, and two had primary infection with both viruses (Ward et al. 2005). Diagnosis of encephalitis with HHV-6/7 depends on amplification of the virus from CSF and/or seroconversion in the blood. These viruses have also been associated with encephalitis in immunosuppressed children (see below).

• *Epstein–Barr virus.* The majority of children are infected with EBV asymptomatically in early life; those infected later may present symptomatically with infectious mononucleosis. Neurological manifestions of infection with this B cell lymphotropic herpes virus are rare, but primary infection can be associated with an encephalitic presentation (Domachowske et al. 1996, Hung et al. 2000). Other neurological presentations of EBV infection include: acute parkinsonism with subsequent full recovery (Hsieh et al. 2002); brainstem encephalitis, which may mimic tumour (Angelini et al. 2000); and postinfectious encephalitic syndromes (Weinberg et al. 2002). Reactivation of latent EBV infection may also manifest as neurological disease, and in one study was associated with long-term sequelae including hippocampal sclerosis (Hausler et al. 2002). EBV DNA can be amplified from the CSF during acute encephalitis, although the highest levels of EBV DNA are found in immunocompromised patients with EBV-driven CNS lymphoma (Weinberg et al. 2002).

• *Cytomegalovirus.* Fetal infection with CMV may lead to severe damage within the CNS, whereas primary infection in childhood is usually asymptomatic, although rarely an infectious mononucleosis-type illness may occur. In common with all the other herpesviruses after primary infection latency is established and subsequent reactivation may occur. This is also usually asymptomatic, except in the immunocompromised host where symptomatic multisystem disease may occur (see below).

ARBOVIRUS (ARTHROPOD-BORNE) ENCEPHALITIDES
Worldwide, arboviruses are the most important causes of severe encephalitis. There are more than 400 types of arboviruses, most of which are RNA viruses from a number of different viral families, and they are transmitted between susceptible vertebrate hosts by bloodsucking arthropods (Rehle 1989). Infection with arboviruses is often asymptomatic or produces only a mild nonspecific disease; less commonly it results in serious neurological disease. Knowledge of local epidemiology and outbreaks is important, as with modern patterns of rapid global travel infections may rapidly establish in new sites. Details of some the more common and emergent arbovirus infections causing CNS disease are given below; Table 10.10 lists some of the main members of the group.

• *West Nile virus (WNV).* WNV is a mosquito-borne flavivirus,

TABLE 10.10
Main arbovirus encephalitides

Name	Genus	Distribution	Vector
Japanese encephalitis	Flavivirus	Asia	Mosquito
West Nile encephalitis	Flavivirus	Worldwide	Mosquito
Saint Louis encephalitis	Flavivirus	Americas	Mosquito
Murray Valley encephalitis	Flavivirus	Australia	Mosquito
Tick-borne encephalitides (incl. Russian spring–summer encephalitis)	Flavivirus	Russia, eastern and central Europe	Ticks
Powassan encephalitis	Flavivirus	North America	Ticks
California encephalitis	Bunyavirus	North America	Mosquito
Eastern equine encephalitis	Alphavirus	Americas	Mosquito
Western equine encephalitis	Alphavirus	Americas	Mosquito
Venezuelan equine encephalitis	Alphavirus	Americas	Mosquito

a human, equine and avian neuropathogen. It is indigenous to Africa, Asia, Europe and Australia, and has recently caused large epidemics in Romania, Russia and Israel. Birds are the natural reservoir (amplifying) hosts, and WNV is maintained in nature in a mosquito–bird–mosquito transmission cycle primarily involving *Culex* species mosquitoes. WNV was introduced to North America in 1999, causing an epidemic of meningoencephalitis in New York City (Campbell et al. 2002). Most human WNV infections are subclinical; symptomatic infections may range from mild fever to fatal meningoencephalitis. Severe manifestations are far more common in adults than in children, but 105 cases of neuroinvasive WNV disease were reported among children in the USA in 2002 (Hayes and O'Leary 2004). WNV infection can be diagnosed by detecting antibody in CSF or serum, or by detecting the virus or viral nucleic acid in CSF, blood or tissues. No WNV-specific treatment or vaccine is available, and prevention depends on vector mosquito control and public education.

• *Tick-borne encephalitis (TBE).* TBE is caused by a flavivirus, for which a number of types of tick may act as the insect vector. Although most infections are not or only mildly asymptomatic, manifestations may include meningitis, meningoencephalitis, meningoencephalomyelitis and meningoradiculoneuritis. TBE is a vaccine-preventable disease, which is a public health problem in central Europe (Kunze et al. 2004). The disease in children is generally milder than in adults, although severe illness may occur and even lead to long-term neuropsychological sequelae. Immunization should be offered to all children living in or travelling to endemic areas. In central Europe, although TBE is the most prevalent tick-transmitted disease it has to be distinguished from other tick-borne infections that may also present with neurological symptoms, such as ehrlichiosis and Lyme disease (*B. burgdorferi*) (Cizman et al. 2000). Childhood presentation with TBE is more common during the summer months, and up to a half of cases will have noticed a tick bite before admission. Two thirds of symptomatic children present with meningitis, and a third with meningoencephalitis. A biphasic course of illness may occur, but full recovery is the norm (Lesnicar et al. 2003). Diagosis may be by PCR of CSF or confirmation of seroconversion.

• *Japanese encephalitis virus (JEV).* JEV is a *Culex* mosquito-borne flavivirus, annually causing an estimated 35,000–50,000 encephalitis cases and 10,000–15,000 deaths in Asia. Infection transfers from birds to pigs, which are the most important source of viral amplification, and then to humans. There is no antiviral treatment for this infection, but immunization is effective. Again most infections are asymptomatic, but symptomatic infections follow a series of clinical stages. A febrile prodrome of 2–3 days with headache and vomiting is succeeded by an encephalitic phase (5–7 days) with seizures and coma; this is followed by a sub-acute phase (10–12 days) with increased tone and abnormal movements; finally gradual convalesence can take weeks to months. Disease is more severe in young children and the elderly, and long-term neuopsychiatric sequealae are common in survivors. The role played by the immune response in determining the outcome of human infection with JEV is poorly understood, although in animal models of flavivirus encephalitis, unregulated proinflammatory cytokine responses can be detrimental. During JEV infection, elevated levels of proinflammatory cytokines and chemokines in the CSF are associated with a poor outcome, but whether they are simply a correlate of severe disease or contribute to pathogenesis is yet to be understood (Winter et al. 2004).

• *Dengue.* The human arbovirus infection dengue is a flavirus infection transmitted by day-biting mosquitos that is highly prevalent is south-east Asia and South/Central America. Severe forms of dengue are associated with haemorrhagic disease and a generalized vascular leak syndrome, but encephalitic presentations may rarely occur in adults and children with or without other features of the disease (Solomon et al. 2000).

RABIES VIRUS (see also Chapter 20)
Rabies is rare in industrialized countries, but in the USA a third of cases occur in children. The virus is in the saliva of infected mammals (e.g. bats, dogs, foxes, cats, racoons, etc.) and is transmitted to man through a bite or skin abrasion and occasionally through intact skin or mucous membranes. A history of animal bite is absent in many cases (Fishbein and Robinson 1993). The virus replicates locally in the skin, then reaches the CNS by

retrograde axonal transportation via peripheral nerves. The incubation period lasts from 10 days to 8 months.

A brief premonitory period of fever and malaise precedes a second phase of excitement during which hyperacusis and hydrophobia with pharyngeal spasms are the most striking manifestations. A third, paralytic, phase may be seen if the patient survives the second phase or, on occasion, from onset. Although most cases of rabies still have a fatal outcome, with modern intensive care support paediatric survivors have been reported (Willoughby et al. 2005). Characteristic viral inclusions (Negri bodies) are found in the neurons, especially in the pyramidal cells of the hippocampus. PCR amplification and/or antigen detection can also be undertaken on brain biopsy, and should be considered cases of encephalopathy where exposure may have occurred (Hughes et al. 2004).

Where a suspected exposure has occurred, prevention of rabies may be achieved by rapid post-exposure prophylaxis, (a) passively with human rabies immunoglobulin, and (b) actively with a vaccine series of five rabies immunizations on days 0, 3, 7, 14 and 28 (Willoughby and Hammarin 2005).

OTHER AGENTS (WHOSE NEUROLOGICAL COMPLICATIONS MAY OR MAY NOT BE PRIMARY ENCEPHALITIS OR POSTENCEPHALITIC ILLNESS)
Mycoplasma
Although not a virus, mycoplasma also requires the host cell's mechanisms for replication. Encephalitis may be a rare acute manifestation of mycoplasma infection occurring simultaneously with respiratory symptoms, or more commonly a secondary phenomenon, related to an aberrant host immune response to the infection within the CNS (Abramovitz et al. 1987). In one study the long-term neurological outcome for patients with mycoplasma encephalitis was poor (Koskiniemi et al. 1991). Diagnosis of infection is by amplification of DNA in the CSF and/or serologically with production of mycoplasma IgM, IgG and IgA in blood and/or CSF (Bencina et al. 2000). Although macrolide antibiotics are effective antimycoplasmal agents and should be used in acute systemic infection, in individual cases it may be difficult to ascertain whether the encephalitis is primary or immune reactive. However, macrolide CNS penetration is poor, and efficacy in the brain beyond the blood–brain barrier is uncertain.

Respiratory virus infections
• *Influenza A and B.* Although the majority of infants and children infected with influenza have a mild respiratory illness, more severe manifestations of disease, including neurological symptoms, may occur (Wang et al. 2003, Maricich et al. 2004). Neurological involvement is often consistent with serious sequelae or death and includes acute encephalitis, Reye syndrome, acute necrotizing encephalopathy and myelitis, as well as autoimmune conditions such as Guillain–Barré syndrome. Virological diagnosis is based on virus isolation or antigen detection from nasopharyngeal secretions, as well as RNA detection by PCR in CSF, or seroconversion (Studahl 2003). An increasing incidence of influenza-associated encephalitis/encephalopathy was originally reported in Japanese children. In one study 89 children with a mean age of 3.8 years, none of whom had received aspirin, developed this disease during eight influenza seasons (1994–2002) (Togashi et al. 2004). After a short respiratory prodrome most patients rapidly became comatose with or without convulsions; 37% died and 19% had neurological sequelae. Interleukin-6 (IL-6) and tumour necrosis factor-alpha (TNF-α) were markedly elevated in serum and CSF samples from two patients who died after a rapidly fulminant course. Post-mortem examination of one fatal case revealed vasogenic brain oedema with generalized vasculopathy, suggesting impairment of vascular endothelial cells probably caused by highly activated cytokines. Other studies have demonstrated elevated levels of systemic and CSF cytokines in influenza encephalitis (IL-6 and TNF-α) as well as elevated cytochrome C suggestive of apoptotic cell death secondary to hypercytokinaemia (Hosoya et al. 2005, Nunoi et al. 2005). Highest levels were found in those with a fatal outcome.

• *Avian influenza.* To date, avian influenza A (H5N1) has passed to a small number of humans, usually where there has been contact with sick birds (de Jong et al. 2006). As well as severe respiratory disease there may also be multisystem involvement with coma, and the outcome for most patients has been fatal.

• *Adenovirus infections.* These are common in children, usually manifesting as mild respiratory or gastrointestinal disease. More severe manifestations include respiratory failure and encephalopathy, and chronic sequelae include bronchiolitis obliterans and long-term CNS damage (Chuang et al. 2003). Adenovirus may cause aseptic meningitis, although certain strains, such as adenovirus type 7, are often responsible for a meningoencephalitis with a rather severe course. Other neurological syndromes associated with adenovirus are myelitis, subacute focal adenovirus encephalitis, and Reye-like syndrome (Straussberg et al. 2001). In the immunocompromised patient, adenovirus may cause multisystem failure with encephalitis, hepatitis coagulopathy and death. Diagnosis of infection is by virus isolation or antigen detection from nasopharyngeal secretions or stool, as well as DNA detection by PCR in CSF.

Gastrointestinal viruses
Encephalitic disease may also follow a gastrointestinal prodrome. Enteroviruses (including the polio viruses, coxsackie viruses and echo viruses) may all cause a spectrum from a 'pure' encephalitic disease to 'pure' meningitis. These frequently happen in outbreaks where only a small proportion of individuals have the more severe encephalitic presentation (Huang et al. 2003). To make a diagnosis, virus may be amplified from CSF by PCR, isolated in stool or throat swabs, or seroconversion subsequently confirmed. Treatment with pleconaril may be considered (Rotbart and Webster 2001). Recent epidemics of enterovirus 71 infection have led to severe and fatal disease in some children. In one study, all of the fatal cases had evidence of rhombencephalitis, brainstem encephalitis and heart failure. It appeared that in most cases heart failure was not caused by myocarditis but possibly by neurogenic

cardiac damage secondary to brain inflammation/infection (Fu et al. 2004).

A rare encephalopathic presentation has been seen with rotavirus gastroenteritis, but this does not seem to be associated with viral penetration of the CNS (Nakagomi and Nakagomi 2005). Encephalitic presentations with seizures and disturbances of consciousness may be a complication of other nonviral diarrhoeal diseases, including *Shigella* (Mulligan et al. 1992) and *C. jejuni* enteritis infection (Nasralla et al. 1993).

POSTINFECTIOUS ENCEPHALITIDES

Postinfectious encephalitis is probably the most common type of acute encephalitis in European coutries. As no virus can be demonstrated in these cases, they are probably not the result of direct viral invasion of the CNS but rather due to a response of the immune system to the presence of virus in the host by mechanisms discussed under ADEM in Chapter 11.

Most cases of postinfectious encephalitis are complication of exanthematous diseases. However, many cases occur following undiagnosed infectious diseases (Table 10.11). The frequency of postinfectious encephalitis can only be estimated as in many cases no data are available on the pathology and mechanism of an acute encephalitic picture. Thus, in mumps, meningitis is very common but evidence of perivenous encephalitis is present in only a very few cases (Johnson 1982a). In a number of cases, the disease that precedes the onset of encephalitis is not diagnosed and, even in retrospect, no virus can be identified. The diagnosis of viral infection is then inferred from the clinical manifestations and course of the prodromal illness.

Measles is the most common cause post exanthem; thus, the incidence of encephalitis will depend upon the incidence of measles and the rate of immunization against measles in any population. Acute measles encephalitis has its onset 6–8 days after commencement of the rash and occurs in up to 1 per 1000 cases (Johnson et al. 1984). Although of variable intensity, the disease is often severe with a 10% mortality and frequent sequelae including seizures, motor imparement and mental retardation. Learning difficulties and behavioural disturbances are common in children who had an apparently complete recovery. Rare cases of postinfectious encephalitis following measles immunization have occurred but their frequency is considerably lower than that of encephalitis following wild measles (Landrigan and Witte 1973). Postinfectious encephalitis associated with 5th disease (parvovirus B19) and exanthem subitum (HHV-6 and 7) are very rare.

In countries with MMR vaccination, *rubella* (German measles) is now a rare disease and cases of acute rubella encephalomyelitis are consequently exceedingly rare. Postinfectious rubella encephalitis is a severe illness with a mortality of about 20%, occurring in 1 per 5000 acute cases of rubella. It may occur simultaneously with the rash or even up to a week or so later.

PATHOLOGY

The pathology of postinfectious encephalitis is distinctive. Numerous foci of perivenous demyelination are present. Axis

TABLE 10.11
Relative frequency of the occurrence of encephalitis in the course of various viral infections*

Virus disease	Frequency of encephalitis
Measles	1:1000
Mumps	1:2000
Chickenpox	1:10,000
Epstein–Barr virus	1:10,000
Rubella	1:20,000
Adenovirus	<1:1,000,000
Influenza A	<1:1,000,000
Parainfluenza	<1:1,000,000

*After Gibbons et al. (1956).

cylinders are usually better preserved than myelin. Cuffing of veins and venules by mononuclear cells is prominent, and microglial cells and macrophages are seen in the demyelinated areas.

CLINICAL FEATURES

The clinical manifestations are those already described for all types of encephalomyelitis. In a majority of cases, the onset is abrupt with disturbances of consciousness and seizures. These symptoms appear on average 6 days (up to 21 days) after the occurrence of an upper respiratory tract infection or an exanthematous disease, in most cases in a child over the age of 2 years. Various neurological signs may be seen, including hemiparesis, extrapyramidal signs, ataxia, facial palsy, nystagmus and cranial nerve involvement (Kennard and Swash 1981, Marks et al. 1988). Neuroimaging may be negative, but MRI usually shows areas of increased signal predominating in the hemispheral white matter and sometimes involving the cerebellum (Figs. 10.9, 10.10). Involvement of the thalamus and basal ganglia is common. The course is variable from case to case and depends on the causal agent. The death rate is low. In over three quarters of cases the duration is brief with recovery in less than 2 weeks.

Another variant of postinfectious encephalitis is *acute haemorrhagic leukoencephalitis*. This is a fulminating disease, which is characterized by the rapid evolution of focal neurological symptoms and signs, especially hemiplegia, accompanied by confusion, coma and fever. The CSF is xanthochromic in 20% of cases and shows a polymorphonuclear pleocytosis. A striking leukocytosis is often present in the peripheral blood. A biphasic course is possible. The demyelinating lesions are haemorrhagic, due to a necrotizing angiitis of venules and capillaries. CT and MRI may help to make the diagnosis by showing the presence of large areas of hypodensity sometimes with a haemorrhagic component (Watson et al. 1984, Huang et al. 1988). Herpesvirus DNA and RNA has been amplified from some cases of acute haemorrhagic leukoencephalitis, but whether this implicates these viruses in the process is still uncertain (An et al. 2002). The treatment of postinfectious encephalitis is mainly that of all acute encephalitic illnesses (see above). The value of steroid treatment remains uncertain, although its immediate effectiveness may be spectacular in some cases (Pasternak et al. 1980). Intravenous immuno-

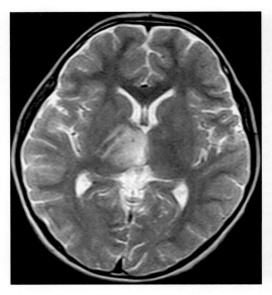 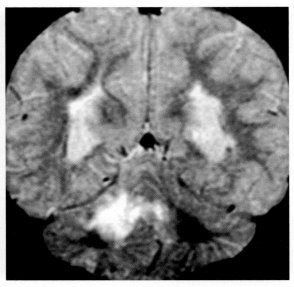

Fig. 10.10. *(Left)* T₂-weighted MRI showing signal abnormality of right thalamus and midbrain caused by parainfectious lymphocytic meningoencephalitis. *(Right)* MRI, T₂-weighted spin–echo sequence showing more extensive zone of intense signal from right cerebellar hemisphere and bilateral intense signal from supratentorial hemispheric white matter. (4-year-old girl with cerebellar ataxia of sudden onset lasting for several weeks associated with mild stupor that disappeared in a few days. All clinical and imaging abnormalities disappeared eventually.)

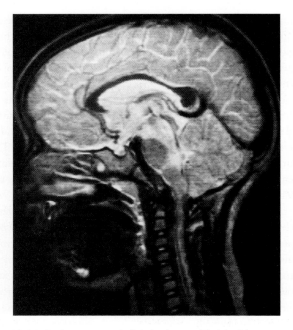

Fig. 10.11. Brainstem encephalitis in 4-year-old girl with stupor and multiple cranial nerve palsies. T₂-weighted MRI shows intense signal from cerebral peduncles and dorsal aspect of pons. Repeat MRI 2 months later was completely normal.

globulins have been used in a few cases (Kleiman and Brunquell 1995).

BRAINSTEM AND CEREBELLAR ENCEPHALITIS
The brainstem may be involved radiologically in cases of acute disseminated encephalitis. Localized brainstem involvement is

uncommon and may occur both with primary encephalitides (Kaplan and Koveleski 1978, North et al. 1993, Duarte et al. 1994) and, less rarely, with the postinfectious type.

The clinical presentation consists of fever, systemic symptoms and aseptic meningitis, in association with symptoms and signs of brainstem dysfunction. Involvement of ocular motor nerves and lower facial pairs is prominent and may be associated with obtundation and signs of involvement of the long tracts with resulting pyramidal and cerebellar manifestations. Cranial nerve involvement and ataxia may mimic the Miller Fisher syndrome (Chapter 20) that has been considered by some authors to be a form of brainstem encephalitis. MRI may demonstrate increased signal in the cerebral peduncles, pons, cerebellum and medulla (Ormerod et al. 1986, Hosoda et al. 1987) and is required to distinguish encephalitis from brainstem tumour, abscesses or other neurosurgical problems (Fig. 10.11). The possibility of *L. monocytogenes* rhombencephalitis should always be kept in mind as antibiotic treatment is effective (Frith et al. 1987).

Predominant involvement of the cerebellum is frequently observed with the varicella virus and occasionally with mumps (Cohen et al. 1992). Marked swelling of the cerebellum with consequent obstructive hydrocephalus has been reported in varicella virus infection (Hurst and Mehta 1988), in Epstein–Barr virus infection and with undetermined viral agents (Roulet Perez et al. 1993) and may run a fatal course. Severe cerebellar atrophy with persistent cerebellar signs may follow the acute attack (Hayakawa and Katoh 1995).

ACUTE FOCAL ENCEPHALITIS
Acute focal encephalitis affecting a limited territory during infection with coxsackie A9 (Roden et al. 1975) and echovirus 25

(Peters et al. 1979) can produce acute hemiplegia or hemichorea. Lacunar lesions in the central grey matter or internal capsule may result from vascular infarction or focal cerebritis.

CHRONIC ENCEPHALITIS

Most of the chronic encephalitides of children are primary encephalitides with presence of the responsible organism in the CNS; they form a heterogeneous group that includes well-defined types (e.g. subacute sclerosing panencephalitis, rubella panencephalitis, human immunodeficiency virus encephaolpathy, human T lymphocytic virus myelitis, and prion diseases) and poorly understood cases that are possibly not directly due to virus infection. The mechanisms of chronic viral encephalitis are complex and vary according to the interaction between the infecting agent and the host immune response. The well-defined types will be discussed below.

SUBACUTE SCLEROSING PANENCEPHALITIS (SSPE)

SSPE is a devastating long-term degenerative complication of continued aberrant measles virus replication in the CNS subsequent to primary infection (Connolly et al. 1967). Onset of SSPE occurs in up to 2 per 100,000 natural infections, with an incubation period of up to 7 years, and it is more common in children who had primary measles under 2 years of age. This compares with a rate of 1 per 1,000,000 in vaccinated children, with an incubation of 3–4 years. However, the majority of SSPE cases in vaccinacted individuals have been caused by wild type not vaccine strains of measles (Jin et al. 2002, Miller et al. 2004).

Early clinical diagnosis is difficult, with onset of subtle progressive symptoms during the first stage of the illness (Honarmand et al. 2004). In two thirds of cases there are personality changes and a subtle intellectual deterioration with an aphasic–apractic–agnosic predominance. Often, such children are regarded as suffering from psychological problems and referred to psychiatric clinics. In a quarter of patients neurological signs or seizures that may be atonic, myoclonic or even partial (Kornberg et al. 1991) are the first manifestations.

Involuntary movements usually appear within 2–3 months and are characteristic of the second stage. The movements may be myoclonic jerks. More often, they are more complex, involving in succession several segments in a repetitive pattern. Onset of each movement is abrupt, but the duration is longer than that of a common myoclonic jerk, often lasting several seconds. Abnormal movements recur periodically, although the intervals between two jerks are not equal and may vary from day to day in the same patient. The movements are usually bilateral, but strictly unilateral jerks may occur. They are absent during sleep and may disappear and reappear without apparent reason. In some patients, they may be replaced or preceded by periodic manifestations more typical of epilepsy, in particular by atonic seizures with head nods or complete falls, or rarely by typical myocolonias. Generalized epileptic seizures, absence-like fits or partial seizures are uncommon (Andermann 1967, Kornberg et al. 1991). In the third stage, extrapyramidal or pyramidal dysfunction or both become prominent. Extrapyramidal dyskinesias

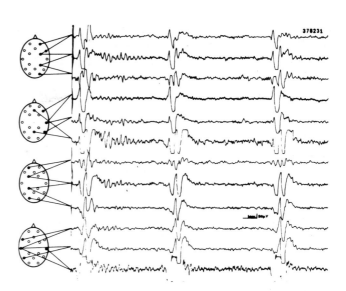

Fig. 10.12. Subacute sclerosing panencephalitis: pseudo-periodic EEG complexes. Note that the complexes are identical in any given lead.

may appear, and parkinsonian rigidity is frequent. Dementia is severe and the child is bedridden. In the terminal stage, progressive unresponsiveness, with increasing hypotonia and decerebrate rigidity, is associated with increasing swallowing and respiratory difficulties and with autonomic dysfunction.

The median duration of the disease is about 12 months and the course is usually regularly progressive. Subacute forms, lethal in as little as six weeks, are occasionally seen (Nihei et al. 1977). Contrariwise, long periods of arrested progression may occur. Periods of spontaneous remission may last up to several years (Risk and Haddad 1979).

Ophthalmic manifestations consist mainly of choroidoretinitis, which preferentially involves the macular area and may be associated with pallor of the disc. These may appear months or even years before the classical manifestations (Robb and Watters 1970). Cortical blindness is uncommon, but optic atrophy is frequent. Papilloedema can be observed with transient increases of ICP. The ERG is normal but visual evoked potentials are impaired.

Cases with lateralizing or other focal features may pose diagnostic problems. Spastic hemiplegia and unilateral spasms may occur. Some cases present with cortical blindness or hemianopia and may be confusing. Occasionally, signs of intracranial hypertension in association with focal features may wrongly suggest a tumour (Glowacki and Goscinski 1973).

Characteristic EEG abnormalities can be observed before any clinical manifestation (Wulff 1982). Paroxysmal EEG complexes typically are formed of high-voltage slow waves recurring periodically at the time of clinical jerks (Fig. 10.12). They are usually identical in shape in any given lead. They may occur in the absence of clinical manifestations and are seen at some stage in about 80% of patients. In some cases bursts of spike–wave activity may replace the typical complexes. Background tracings may be initially normal but become progressively slower while the

419

amplitude diminishes. Diagnosis of SSPE is confirmed by evidence of high titre measles antibody (IgG) in CSF and serum, with a very high CSF:serum antibody titre ratio. The CSF contains no cells, and the total protein is normal or slightly elevated. The virus cannot usually be amplified from the CSF, although viral genome may be amplified from brain tissue.

CT is usually normal in the weeks following onset. Diffuse swelling with ventricular compression may be seen. Focal hypodense areas are rare. Later, cerebral atrophy sets in and the white matter takes a hypodense appearance. In the early stages MRI may be normal or demonstrate lesions usually involving parieto-occipital corticosubcortical regions asymmetrically. In time, symmetric periventricular white-matter changes become more prominent but there is no good correlation between clinical stage and MRI findings (Ozturk et al. 2002).

Despite multiple attempts, no satisfactory treatment for SSPE has been developed. Isoprinosine seems to be able to induce remission in some cases (DuRant et al. 1982). A combination of intraventricular interferon and isoprinosine was reported to increase the rate of remissions from 5–10% to 45% (Yalaz et al. 1992, Gascon et al. 1993), but late recurrences may occur after several years of remission (Anlar et al. 1997). In a small randomized controlled trial, oral isoprinosine alone was compared with oral isoprinosine and intraventricular interferon-alpha2b. Neither Kaplan–Meier survival rates nor morbidity comparisons of clinical classification of outcomes showed statistically significant differences between groups. However, the observed rates of satisfactory outcome (stabilization or improvement) of around 35% were higher than the historical spontaneous remission rates of 5–10% reported in the literature, suggesting that treatment was superior to no treatment (Gascon 2003). Other combination treatments used have included ribavirin (both intraventricular and intravenous) with isoprinosine (Aydin et al. 2003, Hosoya et al. 2004).

PROGRESSIVE RUBELLA PANENCEPHALITIS
A few children with congenital rubella (Townsend et al. 1975) and an occasional patient with acquired rubella (Lebon and Lyon 1974) have developed this very rare, fatal panencephalitis with prominent cerebellar involvement about 10 years after initial infection. Insidiously progressive dementia is the first manifestation, followed by ataxia and myoclonic seizures. CSF examination shows mononuclear pleocytosis and increased protein with massively raised IgG globulins. Rubella virus has been isolated from the brain and leukocytes. Oligoclonal virus-specific antibodies are found in the CNS (Vandvik et al. 1978b). Pathologically, inflammatory infiltrates and astrocytosis are prominent (Townsend et al. 1982, Frey 1997). The course is fatal in several years. No treatment is known.

HUMAN IMMUNODEFICIENCY VIRUS (HIV) INFECTION
HIV-1 is a retrovirus that infects cells that carry the CD4 receptor and a chemokine co-receptor (e.g. CCR5, CXCR4), including helper T lymphocytes (CD4 cells) and monocytes. Infants may be infected with HIV in utero, at birth, or during breastfeeding,

but the majority are infected around the time of delivery. Maternal plasma HIV viral load is the most important predictor of infant infection with HIV, but preterm delivery, prolonged rupture of membranes, presence of other sexually transmitted infections, chorioamnionitis and interventional vaginal delivery all increase the risk of transmission (Abrams et al. 1995, Peckham and Gibb 1995). In non-breastfeeding populations, 15–20% of infants are infected compared to 30–40% in breastfeeding populations (European Collaborative Study 1991, 1994; Newell et al. 2004). Interventions including antiretroviral therapy in pregnancy, during delivery and post-partum; pre-labour caesarean section; and avoidance of breastfeeding can reduce mother to child transmission of HIV to less than 1% (Hawkins et al. 2005).

HIV is a neurotropic virus, although productive infection in the CNS is probably limited to macrophages and microglia. Brain involvement occurs very soon after infection, and infected microglia have been identified as early as seven days after transfusion of infected blood. In vitro, HIV infection leads to activation of brain endothelium, increasing the risk of entry of cells and viral particles into the CNS. HIV-induced expression of ICAM-1 on human brain microvascular endothelial cells increases the margination of inflammatory cells in the brain vasculature, leading to increased targets for HIV infection within the CNS (Stins et al. 2003). A small paediatric study demonstrated a relationship between T cell inflammatory mediators in CSF and CSF HIV viral load (McCoig et al. 2004). HIV in the CNS promotes an inflammatory process, which leads over time to cell death and neuronal loss, probably by the process of apoptosis (Epstein and Gendelman 1993). Pathological findings (Sharer et al. 1986) include diminished brain weight for age. Inflammatory cell infiltrates consisting of microglia, lymphocytes, plasma cells and, especially, multinucleated giant cells are distributed throughout the brain but are more prominent in the deep structures, including the basal ganglia and brainstem. Prominent inflammatory changes and calcification of small or medium-sized vessels are present, especially in the deep brain structures. These may explain the occurrence of ischaemic infarcts and strokes in children with HIV (Frank et al. 1989, Park et al. 1990). The spinal cord only rarely shows the vacuolar myelopathy, which is frequent in adults (Dickson et al. 1989).

The original Centre for Disease Control (CDC) classification of HIV disease in children included a number of different presentations of 'HIV encephalopathy': failure to attain or loss of developmental milestones and intellectual ability; impaired brain growth or an acquired microcephaly; and acquired symmetrical motor deficit (CDC 1994). These different clinical presentations have differing aetiologies relating not just to activity of HIV in the CNS but also to progression of immune deficiency and opportunisitic infections manifesting in the CNS (Mitchell 2001).

Around 20% of HIV-infected children become severely symptomatic or die in the first year of life. These 'rapid progressor' infants are more likely to be born to mothers with more advanced HIV disease, and they are at highest risk of early presentation with HIV encephalopathy (Blanche et al. 1994, Lobato et al. 1995, Tardieu et al. 2000). Overall, up to 10% of HIV-infected children

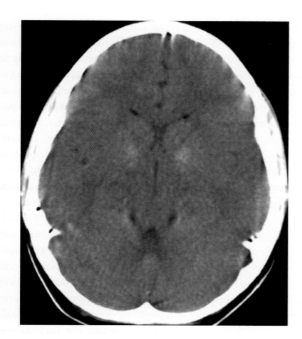

Fig. 10.13. CT of child with HIV encephalopathy showing basal ganglia calcification.

have signs of encephalopathy, usually presenting with motor impairment and developmental delay. More subtle cognitive abnormalities occur in at least 30% of children with HIV, and many have speech and language difficulties and problems with school performance (Tardieu et al. 1995, Pearson et al. 2000). Infants classically present with developmental delay, microcephaly and a diplegic motor imparement. This is often in association with other opportunistic infections including cytomegalovirus and *Pneumocystis carinii* pneumonia. In one detailed study from the USA, infants infected with both HIV and CMV had a significantly increased risk of CNS disease and a worse long-term neurological prognosis (Kovacs et al. 1999). These infants present like other children with cerebral palsy with a fixed neurological insult and developmental problems; they do not demonstrate a pattern of dementia as seen in adults or older children infected with HIV when the brain is more mature (Tardieu et al. 2000).

CT in symptomatic children has demonstrated brain atrophy in over three quarters of cases, and increased white matter attenuation and calcification of the basal ganglia in approximately a quarter (Belman et al. 1986, DeCarli et al. 1993, Pearson et al. 2000) (Fig. 10.13). MRI shows high signal from the white matter and cortical atrophy in most cases (Chamberlain et al. 1991, Pavlakis et al. 1995). In a small study of 39 children (aged from <1 year to 13 years), the level of HIV viral load in the CSF was related to severity of cortical atrophy, but not to intracerebral calcification (Brouwers et al. 2000). In addition, basal ganglia calcification was not related to the severity of the neurological symptoms. In HIV encephalopathy the CSF is most often normal but may contain a mild excess of lymphocytes associated with a modest, often transient, elevation of protein.

In younger children, due to persistance of transplacental maternal antibodies, direct methods of identification must be used, including either the HIV RNA PCR, HIV bDNA PCR, or proviral HIV DNA amplification. Advancement of HIV disease and requirement for antiretroviral treatment is defined by clinical assessment and measurement of the CD4 count and plasma HIV viral load.

In the era before successful treatment of HIV, only around 50% of affected children survived to 10 years of age, and those with neurological signs or symptoms had a very high risk for rapid disease progression at all ages (Pearson et al. 2000). With the advent of combination antiretroviral therapy (ART), the majority of HIV-infected children are likely to survive long-term (Gibb et al. 2003). Early identification of HIV-infected infants who may be at risk of encephalopathy is crucial, so that treatment may be started early enough to prevent permanent neurotoxic damage, if that is possible (Sanchez-Ramon et al. 2003). Within a French observational cohort, 40 infants who received ART before 6 months of age did not have early-onset severe HIV disease including encephalopathy during the first 24 months of life, whereas in the deferred therapy group (n=43), 3 developed encephalopathy (Faye et al. 2004). Although these numbers are small, treatment in infancy seems reasonable to attempt to prevent permanent neurological complications. However, where neurotoxic motor damage has already occurred in infancy, it is not surprising that it cannot be reversed by combination ARTs (Foster et al. 2006). However, it has been suggested that ART may prevent or improve more subtle neuropsychological problems (Sanchez-Ramon et al. 2003). Whether or not ART-treated survivors of vertical HIV infection will have an increased risk of early onset of HIV dementia or other neurological syndromes in adult life can only be speculated at this stage.

HUMAN T LYMPHOCYTE VIRUS (HTLV) INFECTION (see also Chapter 22)

As well as adult T cell leukaemia/lymphoma, HTLV-1 is also a causal agent of 'tropical spastic paraplegia' (HTLV-1-associated myelopathy HAM/TSP), which occurs most commonly in the Caribbean, West Africa and Southern Japan. HAM/TSP is usually manifest in only 1–5% of infected adults (Shibasaki et al. 1988). Most individuals are likely infected with HTLV-1 via breast milk, although other blood-borne routes of infection are possible. Mothers who breastfeed for longer, have higher breast milk viral load and have greatest HLA concordance with their children are more likely to transmit (Wiktor et al. 1997, Li et al. 2004, Biggar et al. 2006). Rare cases of HAM/TSP have been reported in children as young as 6 or 7 years of age (Roman 1988, Gessain and Gout 1992), and occasional familial cases are on record (Mori et al. 1988). HTLV-1 is also associated with a severe infective dermatitis in vertically infected children, which may occur along with early onset of HAM/TSP. Both conditions are probably related to the host anti-HTLV-I immune response as well as HTLV-1 viral load (de Oliveira Mde et al. 2004, Maloney et al. 2004). A rare smoldering retinal vasculitis with ultimate retinal degeneration has been reported in Japanese adolescents with HTLV-1 (Nakao and Ohba 2003).

Pathologically, there are chronic inflammatory signs in the spinal cord, and the virus has been shown to be present locally (Kuroda et al. 1994, Hollsberg and Hafler 1995, Lehky et al. 1995). Development of HAM/TSP is associated with higher viral load in the CNS (Taylor et al. 1999, Lezin et al. 2005), and the host HLA immune response type may also be important (Sabouri et al. 2005). In about half the cases, MRI of the brain may show disseminated lesions, but these are not specific and there is poor correlation between imaging and clinical findings (Gessain and Gout 1992, Bagnato et al. 2005). Optic atrophy and cerebellar signs are found in some patients and may occasionally be prominent (Kira et al. 1993). HTLV-2 virus infection in adult patients may produce the related clinical picture of tropical ataxic neuropathy (Harrington et al. 1993). Randomized controlled studies of antiretroviral and immune modulating therapies for HAM/TSP with the aim of halting neurological progression are currently being undertaken (Taylor and Matsuoka 2005).

PRION DISEASES

Human prion diseases can be classified as sporadic, hereditary or acquired. The cause of sporadic prion disease is unknown, hereditary cases are associated with mutations of the prion protein gene (*PRNP*), and acquired forms are caused by the transmission of infection from human to human or, as a zoonosis, from cattle to human (Prusiner and Hsiao 1994, Will 2003). Prion diseases include Kuru, Creutzfeld–Jakob disease, Gerstmann–Sträussler–Scheinker disease (Brown et al. 1994) and fatal familial insomnia (Medori et al. 1992) in humans, and scrapie and bovine spongiform encephalopathy (BSE) in domestic animals. Pathologically, prion diseases are characterized by a spongiform encephalopathy with the presence in some cases of amyloid plaques. Prions are 'infectious pathogens' composed of abnormal forms of a protein, which is encoded in the host genome (Collinge 2005). Prion disease is associated with the accumulation of the disease-related isoform of the normal cellular prion protein [PrP (Sc)]. Different strains of prions occur despite the absence of any agent-specific genetic material, and folding of the proteins themselves may encode strain diversity with subsequent different effects on the host.

Clinically affected individuals present with slowly progressive disturbances, mainly dementia, myoclonus and cerebellar signs. Neuropsychiatric symptoms such as depression or mood swings may be the earliest symptoms. Cases of Creutzfeld–Jakob disease have been reported in children who became infected through treatment of short stature with human growth hormone extracted from cadaveric brain tissue (Billette de Villemeur et al. 1996, Billette de Villemeur 2003). The disorder was marked initially by cerebellar signs followed by deterioration and myoclonus, leading to death in a few months (Brown et al. 1994). Cases have been observed in adolescents following accidental intracerebral inoculation of the agent through improperly sterilized EEG depth electrodes. Iatrogenic cases run a faster course than the classical types and show cerebellar involvement pathologically (Brown et al. 1994, Deslys et al. 1994).

Due to changes in animal feeding and abattoir procedures, the prion strain causing BSE in cattle infected humans in the UK in the 1990s leading to a novel human prion disease, variant Creutzfeldt–Jakob disease (vCJD) (Will et al. 1996, Epstein and Brown 1997). Variant CJD has occurred more frequently in young adults, where the sporadic and hereditary forms tend to occur at an older age. Since the number of people currently incubating this disease is unknown, there are concerns that prions might be transmitted iatrogenically via blood transfusion, tissue donation, and, since prions resist routine sterilization, contamination of surgical instruments. Such risks remain unquantified. Although vCJD can be diagnosed during life by tonsil biopsy, a prion-specific blood test is still under developement to assess and manage this potential threat to public health (Collinge 1999).

Epidemiological surveillance of human prion diseases across Europe, Australia and Canada, 1993–2002, identified 3720 cases of sporadic CJD, 455 genetic cases, 138 iatrogenic cases, and 128 vCJD cases. The overall annual mortality rate between 1999 and 2002 was 1.67 per million. There was heterogeneity in the distribution of cases by aetiologic subtype with an excess of genetic cases in Italy and Slovakia, of iatrogenic cases in France and the UK, and of vCJD in the UK (Ladogana et al. 2005). In 2002, 17 people died from vCJD in the UK, compared with 20 in 2001 and 28 in 2000 (Andrews et al. 2003). Encouragingly, in the UK, the death rate from vCJD peaked in 2000 suggesting that due to public health measures new infections were no longer occurring. However, uncertainties regarding the length of the incubation period in genetically different individuals may lead to an increased mortality again in the future. A paediatric surveillance was set up in the UK to identify childhood cases of vCJD and obtain information about the paediatric causes of progressive intellectual and neurological deterioration (PIND) (Devereux et al. 2004). After five years of surveillance, only six definite or probable vCJD cases were reported out of 798 PIND cases. Most of the other cases were diagnosed to have an underlying neurodegenerative condition, and consanguinity was a common finding.

Randomized controlled trials of anti-prion treatments as well as immunomodulatory therapies are in progress (Mallucci and Collinge 2004).

CNS VIRAL INFECTIONS IN THE IMMUNOCOMPROMISED

Opportunistic infections of the CNS may occur in immunocompromised children, and the spectrum of infection depends on the cellular nature of their immunodeficiency, whether congenital or iatrogenic (Cunha 2001). There are increasing numbers of children with iatrogenic immunosuppresion of varying degrees, from severe immune oblation for organ transplantation to chronic use of steroids for inflammatory conditions. Infections with opportunistic organisms, usually non-pathogenic to the human host, may occur as well as unusual disorders secondary to common viral pathogens. In general, those with T lymphocyte deficiency are most at risk, and a wide variety of viral, bacterial, fungal and protozoal infections may occur. Those with B lymphocyte deficiency are less at risk of CNS infections, but a well-recognized syndrome of chronic enterovirus infection may occur.

Delayed type of acute measles encephalitis in the immunocompromised

Acute delayed measles encephalitis is observed mainly in immunocompromised patients (Murphy and Yunis 1976), although it occasionally occurs in children with apparently normal immune mechanisms. Contrary to what occurs in the usual postinfectious encephalomyelitides, the measles virus is present in large quantities within the brain and nucleocapsids are seen by electron microscopy in the nuclei of glial cells and neurons. The inflammatory reaction is variable but often inconspicuous (Lacroix et al. 1995). The disease occurs 2–6 months following measles or contact with cases of measles. Epileptic seizures are often a prominent symptom, and epilepsia partialis continua is the first manifestation in many cases (Aicardi et al. 1977, Luna et al. 1990, Barthez Carpentier et al. 1992). Progressive deterioration with obtundation and coma rapidly appears, and focal signs, especially hemiplegia, are common. New neurological signs continue to appear for variable durations. In some patients, a retinopathy is present (Haltia et al. 1977). The diagnosis may be difficult as CSF may be normal or show only slight changes. In a majority of cases, there is intrathecal synthesis of specific anti-measles antibodies and a high titre of antibodies against measles virus in the serum and CSF. In the most severely immunosuppressed children, however, antibody production may be impaired.

CT usually gives normal images. Hypodense images in the central grey matter have been reported (Colamaria et al. 1989). MRI may show areas of intense signal in T_2-weighted sequences (Barthez Carpentier et al. 1992). The EEG may show slowing of the basal activity with repetitive slow-wave complexes at a rate of about 1 Hz (Aicardi et al. 1977, Colamaria et al. 1989). The course of the illness is usually fatal. Arrest of the disease may occur but the rare survivors are left with severe sequelae (Mustafa et al. 1993).

Human herpesvirus infections

All of the herpesviruses may cause serious disease in the immunocompromised child with impaired T lymphocyte function, including organ transplant recipients, HIV-infected children and those with congenital immune deficiency. Disease may occur as a result of primary infection in the non-immune host, or as a result of reactivation of latent infection during immunosuppresion. Disease may be limited to an organ or disseminate to involve multiple organs, and usually there is a high level of plasma viraemia. Although antiviral treatments are available, complete recovery often depends on improvement of immune function.

Vision-threatening viral retinitides are primarily caused by members of the herpesvirus family; clinical syndromes include acute retinal necrosis (ARN) (Bonfioli and Eller 2005), progressive outer retinal necrosis (PORN) (Purdy et al. 2003), multifocal choroiditis, serpiginous choroiditis and other viral retinopathies (CMV retinitis, see below). HSV retinitis is more common in immunocompetent persons, while VZV affects both immunocompetent and immunosuppressed patients equally. As penetration of the eye from systemic therapy is poor due to the restricted blood supply, treatment for severe disease may require both systemic and direct intra-ocular antiviral therapy (Scott et al. 2002).

• *Cytomegalovirus.* Disseminated CMV infections may occur in the severely immunocompromised. There is usually high-level CMV viraemia in the blood, and end organ disease may be found in brain, retinae, lungs, bone marrow, liver and gut. Prognosis is guarded without improved immune function. Treatment with gancyclovir, foscarnet or cidofovir may be effective; however, these are toxic agents and require close metabolic monitoring. Ganciclovir is the first-line compound used, followed by foscarnet and cidofovir; longer-term oral maintainance suppressive therapy can be considered with oral valganciclovir (Kimberlin 2002, Griffiths 2004). CMV retinitis is well recognized in advanced HIV infection; where this occurs in infants in contrast to adults or older children, the macula rather than the peripheral retina is first affected, causing immediate risk to central vision (Wren et al. 2004). Other CNS manifestations of CMV disease in the immunocompromised include focal and generalized encephalitis, cranial nerve palsies, transverse myelitis, radiculitis and Guillain–Barré syndrome. Success of therapy is monitored by end organ response as well as blood viraemia level. CMV disease in the CNS, including retinitis, may become acutely symptomatic in patients with HIV once they start antiretroviral therapy as a manifestation of immune reconstitution inflammatory syndrome (IRIS). IRIS is more common in patients who start treatment with advanced disease and very low CD4 counts, and it requires careful management with treatment of the CMV, HIV and immune modulation to reduce symptoms (Griffiths 2004).

• *Herpes simplex virus.* Severe HSV infections may occur in the immunocompromised. The mouth, skin, lungs and gut are most often affected, whilst the CNS is rarely specifically involved. High-dose intravenous aciclovir should be effective, although resistance may occur in patients with repeated exposure, especially to lower oral doses. CSF HSV PCR is important in diagnosis and monitoring of treatment in the immunocompromised (Cinque et al. 1998).

• *Varicella-zoster virus.* Disseminated encephalomyelitis due to VZV infection has been reported in adults and children with immunosuppression (Carmack et al. 1993, Herrold and Hahn 1994). This may occur with or without rash. Reactivation of latent VZV during immunosuppression is common, and dermatomal shingles may be severe and even progress to disseminated disease. Disseminated VZV infection may lead to multi-organ failure with disseminated intravascular coagulation.

• *Human herpesviruses 6 and 7.* HHV-6 reactivation occurs in nearly 50% of all bone marrow and in 20–30% of solid-organ transplant recipients, 2–3 weeks following the procedure. Clinical symptoms include fever, skin rash, pneumonia, bone marrow suppression, encephalitis and graft rejection (Yoshikawa 2003). Development of limbic encephalitis is associated with high blood

HHV-6 DNA viral load post-transplant (Ogata et al. 2006). HHV-7 viraemia after stem-cell transplant has also been associated with encephalitis (Chan et al. 2004). Treatment with ganciclovir may be effective.

• *Epstein–Barr virus.* EBV infection may be responsible for a severe and often fatal illness in certain families in which a potentially fatal sensitivity to EBV is transmitted as an X-linked character. This disease is known as the X-linked lymphoproliferative (XLP) syndrome (Grierson and Purtilo 1987) and variably features fatal infectious mononucleosis, malignant lymphoma, acquired hypo- or agammaglobulinaemia, and virus-associated haemophagocytic syndrome (Tiab et al. 2000, Gilmour and Gaspar 2003). The gene defective in XLP has been identified and designated *SH2D1A*; it encodes an adaptor protein SAP [signalling lymphocytic activation molecule-associated (SLAM-associated) protein]; measurement of this protein can be used to diagnose the condition (Gilmour et al. 2000). XLP is associated with a high morbidity, and overall outcome is poor. At present, allogeneic stem cell transplantation is the only curative treatment (Lankester et al. 2005).

A similar syndrome of mono- or polyclonal lymphocyte proliferation driven by EBV, known as post-transplant lymphoproliferative disease (PTLD), may occur in immunosuppressed patients, especially in transplant recipients (Randhawa et al. 1992). PTLD may present with multi-organ involvement, infrequently including the CNS. Brain involvement in transplant recipients with PTLD carries a poor prognosis; however, isolated CNS involvement has a better prognosis than CNS plus extracranial involvement (Buell et al. 2005). It has been demonstrated, in a study of paediatric liver transplant patients, that monitoring of EBV viral load with early intervention can reduce the incidence of PTLD (Lee et al. 2005). Combination treatment with immune modulation, the antivirals, and the anti-B-cell monoclonal antibody rituximab has some efficacy (Nozzoli et al. 2006).

In patients with more advanced HIV immunosuppression, EBV may drive the development of lymphoma. This may present solely as a CNS lymphoma or the CNS may be involved when there is more widespread disease (Nadal et al. 1994). More effective treatments for EBV-driven lymphoma in HIV patients involving antiretroviral therapy, chemotherapy and immune modulators such as rituximab are now being developed.

Human polyomavirus infection
JC virus is a human neurotropic polyomavirus that causes progressive multifocal leukoencephalopathy (PML), a fatal demyelinating disease, in immunocompromised patients. It has been reported in children with HIV, after treatment for malignancy, and in children with congenital immunodeficiency (Redfearn et al. 1993, Bezrodnik et al. 1998, Angelini et al. 2001, Nuttall et al. 2004, Demir et al. 2005). Presentation may be insidious with cognitive impairment or more rapidly progressive with seizures, hemiparesis, movement disorders or visual loss. White- and grey-matter lesions may be widespread on cranial MRI. Outcome without treatment and immune reconstitution

is usually fatal within a few months. Patients with advanced HIV may become actuely symptomatic with PML soon after starting antiretroviral treatment, and this is thought to be another manifestation of immune reconstitution inflammatory syndrome (Nuttall et al. 2004).

Poliovirus infection (wild type and post-vaccination)
Poliovirus in immunodepressed patients can induce a typical picture of paralytic poliomyelitis. This has been reported in X-linked hypogammaglobulinaemia (Wright et al. 1977) and in T-cell disorders. An exceptional patient may develop a more diffuse disease with encephalitic involvement and calcification of the thalami following immunization with live, attenuated virus (Davis et al. 1977).

Chronic enterovirus infection in children with X-linked hypogammaglobulinaemia
Children with X-linked hypogammaglobulinaemia (Bruton disease) often suffer viral CNS infections in addition to bacterial complications (purulent meningitis). The most common such infections are caused by enteroviruses (Cooper et al. 1983). The commonest clinical picture is of chronic lymphocytic meningitis with variable features of brain involvement such as disturbances of consciousness and focal seizures or neurological deficits. Other presentations include progressive myelopathy, myelopathy progressing to encephalopathy, pure encephalopathy, retinopathy, sensorineural hearing loss, and dermatomyositis (Rudge et al. 1996). The course is chronic and often fatal. Diagnosis is by PCR in the CSF or in some cases on biopsy tissue, and quantitative PCR may be used to monitor treatment efficacy (Quartier et al. 2000). Treatment by intrathecal and intraventricular injection of gammaglobulins may help to improve symptoms, but does not clear infection (Erlendsson et al. 1985, Johnson et al. 1985).

ENCEPHALOPATHIES OF OBSCURE ORIGIN THAT MAY BE RELATED TO VIRAL INFECTIONS
Several syndromes of CNS disease not associated with an abnormal CSF and not accompanied pathologically by inflammatory lesions of the brain have been reported. Such syndromes occur in close temporal relationship to a defined or an undetermined viral infection and are probably a consequence of such an infection. These include Reye syndrome (Crocker 1979) and the syndrome of haemorrhagic shock and encephalopathy (Levin et al. 1983) as well as nonsyndromic cases. Clearly, these acute parainfectious, noninflammatory encephalopathies form a heterogeneous group with diverse mechanisms. Some cases may be represented by episodes of status epilepticus or accidental complications of epileptic seizures as a result of choking on food or inhalation. Others may be the consequence of shock or circulatory failure in the course of a severe viral infection (Lyon et al. 1961). Still other cases are yet unexplained. In the majority of cases, acute encephalopathies appear as a secondary event in the course of a definite or probable viral disorder. Their onset is marked by a rapid change in consciousness often in association

with repeated vomiting. Convulsions are frequent. The CSF remains normal throughout the course of the illness, which is monophasic without the appearance of new signs and symptoms after the first few hours or days. Progressive recovery of neurological functions in nonfatal cases may be rapid or extend over weeks or months.

REYE SYNDROME

Reye syndrome is characterized pathologically by an acute encephalopathy with brain oedema, associated with microvesicular fatty degeneration of the liver and sometimes the kidneys (Devivo and Keating 1976). The aetiology of the condition is multiple but in most cases there is a clear association with a viral illness, especially varicella (Hurwitz et al. 1982) and influenza B (Norman 1968). Other viruses have also been implicated: the condition occurs most commonly following a respiratory disease (60–70% of cases), varicella (20–30% of cases) and gastrointestinal illnesses with diarrhoea (5–15% of cases) (Committee on Infectious Diseases 1982). The association of the syndrome with the use of salicylates for treatment of the fever accompanying the antecedent illnesses was first suggested by epidemiological studies. Subsequently a dramatic decrease in frequency of Reye syndrome was been observed, probably related to diminished use of aspirin (Hurwitz et al. 1987, Hall et al. 1988). In the USA, after a peak of 555 cases reported in 1980, there were no more than 36 cases per year after 1986 (Belay et al. 1999). As Reye syndrome is now very rare, any infant or child suspected of having this disorder should undergo extensive investigation to rule out treatable inborn metabolic disorders that may mimic the syndrome.

The clinical manifestations of Reye syndrome appear after the symptoms of the premonitory disease have subsided and in the absence of fever. Initial symptoms include repeated vomiting with progressive deterioration of consciousness to stupor and coma over a few hours. Convulsions may occur and changes in muscle tone in the form of opisthotonus or decorticate or decerebrate rigidity are frequent. Central neurogenic hyperventilation can be seen in late stages. The liver is enlarged in about half the cases. The clinical picture is conspicuous by the absence of focal signs and of icterus, and by the normal CSF. Clinical manifestations of high ICP are in the forefront and may include papilloedema and signs such as mydriasis and decerebrate attitude that indicate brainstem dysfunction. The CSF pressure is high, but it may be safer to measure it by an intracranial strain gauge rather than by lumbar puncture, which may be dangerous in such critically ill patients. Elevated transaminases (aspartate transaminase and alanine transaminase) are an early biological feature. Hyperammonaemia is almost constant but may be transient and is relatively late. Bilirubin is below 50 mmol/L (3 mg/dL). Hypoglycaemia is present in about half the cases, especially in infants (Glasgow 1984). A prolonged prothrombin time and an elevated creatine-kinase level are inconstant features.

The course of Reye syndrome is severe but the case fatality rate for children has regularly decreased over the years from 50–60% in the early 1970s to less than 30% in the early '80s (Glasgow 1984). In the USA the case fatality rate was highest in

TABLE 10.12
Inborn errors of metabolism that may produce a Reye-like picture

Systemic carnitine deficiency
Muscle carnitine deficiency
Late-onset glutaric aciduria type II
Medium-chain acyl-CoA dehydrogenase deficiency (MCAD)
Long-chain acyl-CoA dehydrogenase deficiency (LCAD)
ETF dehydrogenase deficiency ⎫ Glutaric aciduria type 2
Multiple dehydrogenase deficiency ⎭

children under 5 years of age and in those with a serum ammonia level above 45 µg/dL (26 µmol/L) (Belay et al. 1999).

The pathogenesis of Reye syndrome remains enigmatic (DeLong and Glick 1982). Most hypotheses are based on the presence of biochemical and pathological changes indicative of mitochondrial dysfunction (Table 10.12). Direct mitochondrial involvement by a virus is conceivable but no virus has ever been isolated from the liver or brain (Trauner et al. 1988). Another possibility would be the decompensation of a latent innate metabolic abnormality by the viral aggression. A third possibility would be the action of a cofactor to the viral infection, such as aspirin. The treatment of Reye syndrome is supportive. Careful attention to metabolic and physiological disturbances including hypoglycaemia, correction of electrolyte imbalance and bleeding diathesis may suffice in many early cases. In more severe cases, an aggressive therapeutic approach seems justified given the high mortality rate. Intensive care, mechanical ventilation, correction of metabolic abnormalities and treatment of intracranial hypertension are essential. A high ammonia level at presentation is associated with a poor prognosis (Fitzgerald et al. 1982).

HAEMORRHAGIC SHOCK AND ENCEPHALOPATHY

Haemorrhagic shock and encephalopathy is thought to be due to sepsis but the aetiology remains unknown (Whittington et al. 1985, Levin et al. 1989). A defect in the synthesis or reuptake of protease inhibitors (alpha-2-antitrypsin and alpha-2-macroglobulin) could be involved and these changes can be used to assist the diagnosis (Jardine and Bratton 1995). Most affected children are under 1 year of age. The onset is abrupt with unresponsiveness, fever and convulsions. Fever of 39.5°C to over 40.1°C is a constant feature. The skin is mottled, and oozing of blood occurs at all puncture sites as a result of intravascular coagulopathy. Profound hypotension is the rule (Chaves-Carballo et al. 1990, Bacon and Hall 1992).

Corrigan (1990) has emphasized the diagnostic importance of hyperpyrexia, which may also be of aetiological significance. The EEG may be of diagnostic importance by showing runs of paroxysmal discharges, rapidly changing in amplitude, rate and morphology often with shifting focal distribution, which have been termed 'electrical storms' (Harden et al. 1991). MRI may show haemorrhages and areas of ischaemia (Glauser et al. 1992).

The course is often fatal and neurological sequelae are present in survivors, although complete recovery has been documented

(Bonham et al. 1992). The CSF is normal. Treatment is symptomatic. Plasmapheresis has been proposed (Roth et al. 1987).

ACUTE NECROTIZING ENCEPHALOPATHY
Acute necrotizing encephalopathy is a rare, severe and often fatal condition, also termed symmetrical thalamic necrosis (Yagishita et al. 1995, Mizuguchi 1997). Affected infants develop a sudden quadriplegia and are usually left with severe sequelae. The condition can be caused by both influenza A and B (Voudris et al. 2001, Grose 2004, Huang SM et al. 2004) and by other viruses including herpes virus 6 (Oki et al. 1995). The acute necrotizing encephalopathy is not associated with any elevation of ammonia levels, and consists of multifocal and symmetric brain lesions affecting the bilateral thalami, brainstem tegmentum, cerebral periventricular white matter or cerebellar medulla. Symmetrical thalamic and brainstem lesions may be seen on MRI. The prognosis is poor, and less than 10% of patients recover completely. This condition has most often been described in Japanese children, suggesting there may be some genetic susceptibility. Treatment with the neuraminidase inhibitor oseltamivir may be helpful in some cases of influenza-associated encephalitis, but only if started very promptly (Straumanis et al. 2002). Vaccination of children against influenza is likely to be the best way to protect them against these severe manifestations of the infection (Sugaya 2002).

INFANTILE BILATERAL STRIATAL NECROSIS (IBSN)
IBSN is an acute neurological disorder marked by fever and often CSF pleocytosis, obtundation and sometimes seizures, followed within a few days by the appearance of extrapyramidal rigidity and dystonia, exacerbated intermittently by stereotyped attacks of paroxysmal tonic contractions, usually in flexion, with facial grimacing and protracted monotonous whining. CT and MRI show bilateral hypodensities involving predominantly the putamina in a symmetrical manner (Fig. 10.14). Considerable oedematous swelling initially extends into the neighbouring white matter but progressively disappears. The clinical abnormalities tend to decrease over weeks or months and may even disappear (Fujita et al. 1994), and no recurrences have been reported. Extrapyramidal sequelae persist in most cases (Goutières and Aicardi 1982, Rosemberg et al. 1992) but mild cases with full recovery occur (Kim et al. 1995). The nature of this syndrome is unclear. The acute onset, fever, and association, in some cases, with evidence of *M. pneumoniae* infection (Saitoh et al. 1993, Larsen and Crisp 1996) suggest an infectious process, and a relationship to encephalitis lethargica has been discussed (Al-Mateen et al. 1988). Alternatively, a metabolic abnormality such as mitochondrial disorder or organic aciduria, decompensated by an intercurrent disease, might be responsible. De Meirleir et al. (1995) have reported IBSN of a less acute form in a child with a mutation in the mitochondrial ATPase 6 gene. Acute bilateral infarction of the striatum may be seen following trauma (Brett 1991) or spontaneously (Bogousslavsky et al. 1988) but the clinical picture differs by the absence of inflammatory features. Cases with similar imaging features but with a chronic course and often a familial transmission are discussed in Chapter 9 (Roig

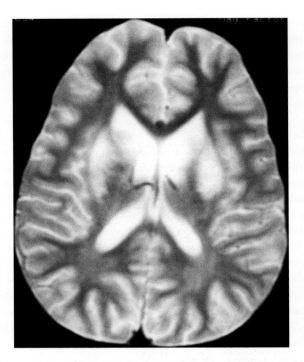

Fig. 10.14. Acute bilateral striatal necrosis. T$_2$-weighted MRI showing low signal from the basal ganglia extending into surrounding white matter. 4-year-old child with acute onset of fever, disturbances of consciousness and convulsions with subsequent development of rigidity and dystonia. Pleocytosis in CSF and negative metabolic studies. (Courtesy Dr A Arzimanoglou, Hôpital Robert Debré, Paris.)

et al. 1993, Vasel-Banagaite et al. 2006) and may represent mitochondrial disorders.

BEHÇET SYNDROME (see Chapter 11)
Behçet syndrome is rare in children but has been reported in infants as young as 2 months (Ammann et al. 1985). A transient form has been observed in babies born to affected mothers (Lewis and Priestley 1986). The disease features recurrent ulcerations of the mouth and genitalia, skin lesions often resembling erythema nodosum, anterior uveitis, keratitis, hypopyon and, less commonly, retinal involvement that in some cases may be isolated. CNS involvement is present in up to 25% of patients and may rarely precede the oculocutaneous manifestations. Neurological manifestations include involvement of the cerebral hemispheres, spinal cord, cerebellum or brainstem (Nakamura et al. 1994). Pseudotumour cerebri with or without sinus thrombosis may be observed (Shakir et al. 1990). MRI may show disseminated areas of intense signal in T$_2$ sequences (Wechsler et al. 1992, Saltik et al. 2004). The brainstem is consistently involved. Perivenous infiltrates with or without thrombosis are frequent (Wechsler et al. 1992). The disease may present as a cerebrovascular disease (Iragui and Maravi 1986) or as a chronic brainstem encephalitis (Ito et al. 1991). The diagnosis may be helped by the cutaneous sensitivity to mechanical trauma (pathergy).

Behçet syndrome has a complex genetic aetiology; it is most common in those of Mediterranean and Eastern origin, although

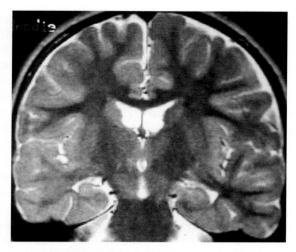

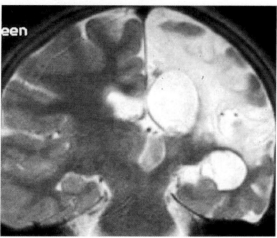

Fig. 10.15. T$_2$-weighted MRI showing early *(right hemisphere of top image)* and late *(left hemisphere of bottom image)* phases of Rasmussen encephalitis. The early disease manifests as T$_2$ signal change in the grey matter, which later evolves into extensive cortical and subcortical atrophy. (Courtesy Dr K Chong, Great Ormond Street Hospital for Sick Children, London.)

it also affects Caucasians. An enhanced inflammatory response and overexpression of proinflammatory cytokines are the prominent features of Behçet syndrome. This likely antigen-driven immune response in Behçet syndrome is possibly triggered by an infectious agent in a genetically susceptible host. Supporting this is the consistent association of disease susceptibility with polymorphisms in the human leukocyte antigen complex, particularly HLA-B*51. The diagnosis is a clinical one, and so far there is no single laboratory test specific for the diagnosis of Behçet syndrome (Uziel et al. 1998, Marshall 2004). The immune modulating agents cyclosporin and azathioprine have performed well in clinical trials, and evidence is accumulating for the efficacy of anti-tumour necrosis factor therapy for certain types of Behçet syndrome.

Rasmussen Encephalitis (see also Chapter 15)
Rasmussen encephalitis is a chronic epileptic disorder characterized clinically by progressive neurological deterioration, focal

seizures often progressing to intractable epilepsy, cognitive decline and hemispheric atrophy (Deb et al. 2005) (Fig. 10.15) The aetiology of this encephalitis remains unknown, and an autoimmune response triggered by a viral infection is a possibility. The multifocal distribution of pathological changes, as well as the heterogeneity in the stages of cortical damage in each patient, are consistent with an ongoing and progressive immune-mediated process of neuronal damage that involves neuroglial and lymphocytic responses, resembling other autoimmune CNS disorders such as multiple sclerosis (Pardo et al. 2004). A formal set of diagnostic criteria and a therapeutic pathway for the management have been proposed (Bien et al. 2005).

MYCOTIC INFECTIONS OF THE NERVOUS SYSTEM

Mycotic infections of the nervous system produce granulomatous meningitis or abscesses. In the majority of cases, mycotic infections occur as opportunistic infections in patients with immunodeficiency, indwelling devices or structural defects. The immunodeficent patients most at risk of CNS fungal infection include: those undergoing treatment for haematological malignancies; recipients of solid organ and bone marrow transplants; neonates; patients with advanced HIV disease; and patients with chronic granulomatous disease who have deficient phagocytic function.

As these infections are rare, advice regarding the most appropriate and up-to-date treatment should always be sought from microbiological specialists in the field.

ASPERGILLUS INFECTION
Invasive aspergillosis is an uncommon but often lethal complication in severely immunocompromised patients. *A. fumigatus* is the most common human pathogen in the genus *Aspergillus*. The most common primary infections are maxillary sinusitis of dental origin or lung infections. The eye and orbital structures may also become involved, leading to proptosis or ophthalmoplegia. Infection reaches the brain directly from the nasal sinuses or is blood borne from the lungs and gastrointestinal tract. Single or multiple abscess formation with blood vessel invasion leading to thrombosis is a characteristic feature on neuropathological examination (Kleinschmidt-DeMasters 2002). Aspergillosis should always be considered in immunocompromised patients with acute onset of focal neurological deficits. Diagnosis of an intracranial mass lesion should be confirmed with neuroimaging. Dual infections with other fungi may also occur, especially where the sinuses are the source. Direct examination and culture of tissue specimens is required to confirm the diagnosis, but treatment should be started on suspicion.

A combined approach with antifungal treatment and neurosurgical intervention with stereotactic removal of *Aspergillus* abscesses, granulomas and focally infected brain has demonstrated improved survival (Middelhof et al. 2005). Where possible, immunosuppressive treatment should be reversed and immune modulation to improve phagocytic function applied. The antifungal, voriconazole, which has excellent CNS penetration, appears to have the most promising treatment results (Schwartz et al. 2005, Theuretzbacher et al. 2006). Studies are currently underway to identify whether combination with other antifungals such as amphoteracin may improve efficacy.

CANDIDA INFECTIONS

Candida species may invade the meninges from the bloodstream in cases of disseminated candidiasis. Such cases occur most commonly in relatively immune-incompetent preterm infants with prolonged hospital stay and frequent antibiotic exposure. Infants with congenital anomalies, with central venous access, receiving total parenteral nutrition, or with shunted hydrocephalus are most at risk of candidal invasion of the CNS (Devlin 2006). Most neonatal fungal infections are due to *C. albicans*. The sources of candidiasis in neonatal intensive care units are often endogenous following superficial colonization. About 10% of babies are colonized in the first week of life and up to two thirds by 4 weeks of hospital stay. Disseminated candidiasis presents like bacterial sepsis and can involve multiple organs such as the kidneys, brain, eye, liver, spleen, bone, joints, meninges and heart.

Rarely, candidal invasion of the CNS may also occur in children receiving myelosuppressive chemotherapy, most often for haematological malignancies. A more protracted period of neutropaenia and receiving total parenteral nutrition increased the risk for CNS candida for these patients (McCullers et al. 2000). Confirming the diagnosis is difficult and requires culture of the organism from blood or other sterile bodily fluids: a high index of suspicion is required. Other candidal species, such as *C. tropicalis*, may also invade the CNS, and culture is important to ascertain sensitivity to antifungal treatment. Diagnosis is often made only shortly before death as there are few suggestive signs and the organism is difficult to culture. Yet, in infants and children with risk factors, even a single colony of yeast in the CSF should not be considered a contaminant and treatment should be commenced before positive identification (Faix 1984). Treatment with high-dose liposomal amphotericin B is effective if given relatively early (Juster-Reicher et al. 2003).

CRYPTOCOCCUS NEOFORMANS INFECTION

Cryptococcosis is a systemic fungal infection now most commonly seen in adults with advanced HIV disease; it is rarely seen in HIV-infected children. CNS involvement is the most serious complication, and spread is usually haematogenous from the lungs. The organism produces a granulomatous arachnoiditis that may cause hydrocephalus, cranial nerve palsies and vasculitis of large vessels. The disease may very rarely occur in previously well children (Tjia et al. 1985). Headache and back pain are the usual presenting symptoms. Fever is only inconstantly present. Disturbances of consciousness, cranial nerve involvement, especially of the VIth nerve, papilloedema and other signs of raised ICP are commonly seen. The diagnosis of cryptococcosis is difficult, especially in immunosuppressed patients. Blood cultures as well as CSF cultures should be undertaken. The CSF usually shows moderate lymphocytic pleocytosis, increased protein and low sugar. India ink staining demonstrates yeasts in only 60% of patients with positive culture. Cultures may take many days to yield growth and may be initially negative in up to 25% of cases. Demonstration of the presence of antigen in the blood and CSF may be helpful. The CSF may be normal in some cases, hence the need to repeat lumbar puncture and to culture large amounts of fluid. Neuroimaging may show cerebral oedema, hydrocephalus and occasionally mass lesions (Fujita et al. 1981). Repeated lumbar puncture may be required to reduce ICP during the acute phase; however, some patients will require shunting. Untreated CNS cryptococcocis is regularly fatal. Sequelae in late-treated cases may include blindness, deafness and chronic hydrocephalus. Antifungal combination treatment initially with amphoteracin-B and flucytosine has been demonstrated to be most effective (Brouwer et al. 2004); subsequent prophylaxis to prevent remission is advised with fluconazole where there is ongoing immunosuppression (Bicanic and Harrison 2004).

OTHER MYCOTIC INFECTIONS

Mucormycosis is a rare fungal infection that usually infects the sinuses and in the immunocompromised may penetrate locally into surrounding tissues including the eye and brain. Combined infections with aspergillis may also occur. Local surgical treatment as well as antifungal therapy may be required, Voriconazole and amphoteracin are the most effective treatments (Ladurner et al. 2003, Alfano et al. 2006).

CNS infections caused by *Coccidioides immitis*, *Histoplasma capsulatum* or *Blastomyces dermatitidis* are rare in Western Europe. These fungal infections are common in some regions of the Americas, Africa and Asia. CNS infection usually occurs as part of a disseminated infection in the immunocompromised and usually with pulmonary manifestations. Clinical features include headaches, low-grade fever, weight loss and minimal meningeal signs; hydrocephalus may occur. The diagnosis is suggested by the presence of pulmonary lesions, which may remain quiescent for many years. Liposomal amphoteracin is probably the most effective treatment (Wheat et al. 2005, Panicker et al. 2006).

Scedosporium apiospermum is a fungus found in the soil and contaminated water, and rarely CNS infection has been reported in paediatric cases of near drowning (Chakraborty et al. 2005). Many other rare forms of fungal infection may occur, and should be considered in the immunocompromised with poor phagocyctic function. Expert advice should be sought for treatment and management; often a combined surgical and drug treatment may be required, especially if there is abcess formation.

PROTOZOAN AND PARASITIC INFESTATION OF THE CNS

With the exception of toxoplasmosis and, to a certain extent, neurocysticercosis, protozoan or parasitic involvement of the CSF is rare in developed countries. Malaria is, however, of increasing importance because mass travel to infested countries has developed enormously and because preventive treatment is not always taken or effective. Table 10.13 lists the main clinical features and available treatments for some protozoan and parasitic diseases.

TABLE 10.13
Some protozoan and parasitic infestations of the CNS, and their treatment*

Disease (organism)	Main clinical features	Treatment
African trypanosomiasis (*T. gambiense* or *T. rhodesiense*)	Convulsions, disturbed consciousness, sometimes focal deficits (hemiplegia), spastic diplegia, choreoathetosis	Stage 1 – pentamidine (*T. gambiense*) suramin (*T. rhodesiense*) Stage 2 – melarsoprol, melarsoprol–nifurtimox combination
Amoebiasis (*Naegleria*)	Meningoencephalitis	Amphotericin B, miconazole and rifampicin
Amoebiasis (*Entamoeba histolytica*)	Brain abscess secondary to hepatic and pulmonary involvement	Metronidazole, tinidazole
Echinococcus	Raised intracranial pressure, focal deficits	Albendazole ± corticosteroids
Malaria	Encephalopathy, seizures, fever	Quinidine, quinine, artemether
Neurocysticercosis	Seizures, encephalopathy	Albendazole, praziquantel ± corticosteroids
Schistosomiasis (*S. japonicum, S. mansoni, S. haematobium*)	Transverse myelitis, granuloma of spinal cord, radiculitis, encephalopathy	Praziquantel, oxamniquine
Trichinosis (*T. spiralis*)	Fever, myalgia, encephalopathy, focal signs, papilloedema	Thiabendazole ± corticosteroids
Visceral larva migrans (*Toxocara canis* or *T. cati*)	Encephalopathy, seizures, optic neuritis, myelitis	Mebendazole, albendazole, thiobendazole ± corticosteroids

*Adapted from Abramowicz (2004).

MALARIA

At least 1 million children are estimated to die from malaria annually in Africa alone (Snow et al. 2005) and cerebral involvement is a major cause of death, with the peak incidence of cerebral malaria in children aged between 2 and 6 years. Malaria is caused by four species of the genus *Plasmodium*: *P. vivax*, *P. falciparum*, *P. malariae* and *P. ovale*, and cerebral malaria is a severe complication associated with *P. falciparum* infestation. Cerebral malaria in children is defined by three criteria: disturbances of consciousness with inability to localize pain (Blantyre coma score <3/5) more than 1 hour after a seizure; presence of *P. falciparum* parasitaemia; and absence of other causes of encephalopathy. The histopathological hallmark is engorgement of the cerebral capillaries and venules with parasitized and non-parasitized red blood cells (MacPherson et al. 1985). The earliest symptom is usually fever, followed by signs of respiratory distress (secondary to metabolic acidosis and/or anaemia), convulsions and decreased level of consciousness. Movement disorders and abnormal postures are common. Seizures, which may occur in any form of malaria, are common, and can be generalized or focal. Some may be subclinical. They are associated with a poorer outcome, particularly if prolonged. Status epilepticus is present in 10–20% of cases. Hypoglycaemia is present in 30% of patients and is of severe prognostic significance (Molyneux et al. 1989). Raised ICP is present in most children (Newton et al. 1991) with cerebral malaria, and is thought to be due to increased cerebral blood volume. Those children with a markedly elevated ICP have a higher mortality, and greater incidence of long-term sequelae.

Diagnosis is generally made on history, clinical examination, and examination of thick and thin blood smears. The CSF findings are usually unremarkable, and if pleocytosis is seen on CSF, meningitis or encephalitis becomes a more likely diagnosis. Treatment should be started without definite proof in case of doubt in any person who may have been exposed in the past three months, or 1 year if they have been on prophylaxis (Newton and Warrell 1998). Parenteral administration of cinchona alkaloids (quinine or quinidine in the USA) is the mainstay of treatment. Artemisinin derivatives (artesunate and artemether) are increasingly being used; although they appear to clear parasitaemia quicker, they have shown no benefit over the cinchona alkaloids on mortality rates. They have the advantage of being able to be administered rectally, although due to concerns about neurotoxicity raised by animal studies, they have limited use. Recommended supportive measures are: antipyretics for fever, fluids for hypovolaemia, anticonvulsants for the control of seizures, osmotic agents (e.g. mannitol) to reduce ICP, glucose for hypoglycaemia, and blood transfusion in certain settings for anaemia and possibly high peripheral parasitaemia (>10% of red blood cells affected). Corticosteroids were strongly recommended in the past but their use has no definite pathophysiological basis and they are now no longer recommended. Other ancillary measures such as desferrioxamine, malaria hyperimmune globulin, anti-TNFα and pentoxifylline have shown no clear benefit, and some have caused harm, so until further research is available they should not be used (Warrell 1999). The average mortality rate of cerebral malaria is between 15% and 20% (Marsh et al. 1995, Idro et al. 2005), with residual disability present in about 10–15% of survivors. Some sequelae are transient, e.g. ataxia, others may improve partially over months (motor disorders such as hemiparesis and cortical blindness), while others remain a problem (e.g. seizures). In addition, subtle cognitive defects are present in a high proportion of survivors (Kihara et al. 2006).

ACQUIRED TOXOPLASMOSIS

Infection with *T. gondii* is usually mild or asymptomatic, but the CNS can be infected and cause meningoencephalitis in an immunocompetent host, encephalitis and choroidoretinitis in neonates following transplacental infection, choroidoretinitis as

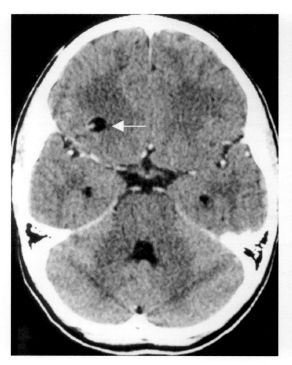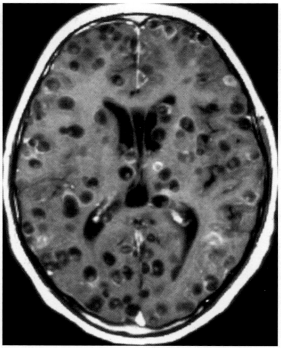

Fig. 10.16. T₁-weighted MRI showing intramural nodule of single neurocysticercosis *(left: arrow)* and multiple neurocysticercotic lesions *(right)*.

NEUROCYSTICERCOSIS

Neurocysticercosis (NCC) is the most common helminthic disease of the CNS, and is a major health problem in many developing countries. The disease results from poor sanitation, when humans become the intermediate host in the life cycle of *Taenia solium*, by ingesting the eggs of the tapeworm. Infestation by the encysted form of *T. solium* may then occur within brain parenchyma, the basilar cisterns or rarely the spinal cord, causing inflammation, oedema and residual calcification. NCC usually presents in children when cysts start dying, and provoke inflammation. They present with prolonged focal or generalized seizures, or occasionally with signs of raised ICP secondary to cysticercotic encephalitis or hydrocephalus, caused by a racemose cysticercus in the basal cistern or the ventricular system. Diagnosis is made by demonstrating either a single ring-enhancing lesion with surrounding oedema on neuroimaging (Fig. 10.16) or by seeing multiple lesions, some of which may be calcified. MRI may reveal a scolex. Differentiation of a single lesion from other single granulomata, such as a tuberculoma, without biopsy is difficult. Serum antibodies against cysticercus can help make the diagnosis, although in endemic areas exposure can lead to a high false positive rate. Del Brutto et al. (2001) have proposed a set of diagnostic criteria for NCC to aid in diagnosis. Treatment with albendazole (15 mg/kg/day for 8 days) has proved effective, with steroids added in cases of heavy infestation or when side effects develop with treatment. As most patients come to medical attention as a result of dying cysts, treatment was once not recommended; however, recent studies have shown that the use of albendazole appears to decrease the long-term risk of seizures (Garcia et al. 2004).

ECHINOCOCCOSIS

Human infestation by the dog tapeworm, *Echinococcus*, is known as hydatid disease and is common in sheep-raising countries. Humans are infected by ingesting the ova shed by dogs (the definitive hosts). *Echinococcus granulosus* causes cystic hydatid disease, and is mainly responsible for liver and lung hydatids, although in 5% cysts develop in the CNS. As the cysts are slow growing, they frequently remain asymptomatic until they reach considerable dimensions. Clinical features are mainly symptoms and signs of intracranial hypertension, while focal neurological deficits are rare. On CT or MRI, the cysts appear as round or oval masses with a smooth border and a content of CSF density (Fig. 10.17). Midline shift and ventricular distortion may occur (Tüzün et al. 2002). ELISA or IHA (indirect haemagglutination) for echinococcal antigens may be helpful. Treatment of choice is surgical removal, taking care to prevent rupture of the cyst. For large lesions, treatment with albendazole prior to surgery appears to improve outcome (Altinors et al. 2000).

EOSINOPHILIC MENINGITIS

Parasitic or protozoan diseases are the most common cause of eosinophilic meningitis; however, a high proportion of eosinophilic cells (>4%) may also be present in cases of infectious or postinfectious meningitis secondary to fungal, rickettsial, my-

Koskiniemi M, Ketonen L (1981) Herpes simplex virus encephalitis: progression of lesion shown by CT. *J Neurol* 225: 9–13.

Koskiniemi M, Vaheri A (1989) Effects of measles, mumps, rubella vaccination on pattern of encephalitis in children. *Lancet* 1: 31–4.

Koskiniemi M, Vaheri A, Taskinen E (1984) Cerebrospinal fluid alterations in herpes simplex virus encephalitis. *Rev Infect Dis* 6: 608–18.

Koskiniemi M, Rautonen J, Lehtokoski-Lehtiniemi E, Vaheri A (1991) Epidemiology of encephalitis in children: a 20-year survey. *Ann Neurol* 29: 492–7.

Koskiniemi M, Piiparinen H, Mannonen L, et al. (1996) Herpes encephalitis is a disease of middle aged and elderly people: polymerase chain reaction for detection of herpes simplex virus in the CSF of 516 patients with encephalitis. The Study Group. *J Neurol Neurosurg Psychiatry* 60: 174–8.

Koskiniemi M, Rantalaiho T, Piiparinen H, et al. (2001) Infections of the central nervous system of suspected viral origin: a collaborative study from Finland. *J Neurovirol* 7: 400–8.

Koskiniemi M, Piiparinen H, Rantalaiho T, et al. (2002) Acute central nervous system complications in varicella zoster virus infections. *J Clin Virol* 25: 293–301.

Kovacs A, Schluchter M, Easley K, et al. (1999) Cytomegalovirus infection and HIV-1 disease progression in infants born to HIV-1-infected women. Pediatric Pulmonary and Cardiovascular Complications of Vertically Transmitted HIV Infection Study Group. *N Engl J Med* 341: 77–84.

Kovacs SO, Kuban K, Strand R (1993) Lateral medullary syndrome following varicella infection. *Am J Dis Child* 147: 823–5.

Krambovitis E, McIllmurray MB, Lock PE, et al. (1984) Rapid diagnosis of tuberculous meningitis by latex particle agglutination. *Lancet* 2: 1229–31.

Kucers A, Crowe SM, Grayson ML, Hoy JF, eds (1997) *The Use of Antibiotics: a Clinical Review of Antibacterial, Antifungal, and Antiviral Drugs, 5th edn.* Oxford: Butterworth–Heinemann.

Kumar A, Montanera W, Willinsky R, et al. (1993) MR features of tuberculous arachnoiditis. *J Comput Assist Tomogr* 17: 127–30.

Kunze U, Asokliene L, Bektimirov T, et al. (2004) Tick-borne encephalitis in childhood—consensus 2004. *Wien Med Wochenschr* 154: 242–5.

Kuroda Y, Matsui M, Kikuchi M, et al. (1994) In situ demonstration of the HTLV-I genome in the spinal cord of a patient with HTLV-I-associated myelopathy. *Neurology* 44: 2295–9.

Kurugol Z, Vardar F, Ozkinay F, et al. (2000) Lupus anticoagulant and protein S deficiency in otherwise healthy children with acute varicella infection. *Acta Paediatr* 89: 1186–9.

Kurugol Z, Vardar F, Ozkinay F, et al. (2001) Lupus anticoagulant and protein S deficiency in a child who developed disseminated intravascular coagulation in association with varicella. *Turk J Pediatr* 43: 139–42.

Kyllerman MG, Herner S, Bergström TB, Ekholm SE (1993) PCR diagnosis of primary herpesvirus type I in poliomyelitis-like paralysis and respiratory tract disease. *Pediatr Neurol* 9: 227–9.

Lacroix C, Blanche S, Dussaix E, Tardieu M (1995) Acute necrotizing measles encephalitis in a child with AIDS. *J Neurol* 242: 249–51.

Ladogana A, Puopolo M, Croes EA, et al. (2005) Mortality from Creutzfeldt–Jakob disease and related disorders in Europe, Australia, and Canada. *Neurology* 64: 1586–91.

Ladurner R, Brandacher G, Steurer W, et al. (2003) Lessons to be learned from a complicated case of rhino-cerebral mucormycosis in a renal allograft recipient. *Transpl Int* 16: 885–9.

Lahat E, Aladjem M, Schiffer J, Starinsky R (1993) Hydrocephalus due to bilateral obstruction of the foramen of Monro: a 'possible' late complication of mumps encephalitis. *Clin Neurol Neurosurg* 95: 151–4.

Lakeman FD, Whitley RJ (1995) Diagnosis of herpes simplex encephalitis: application of polymerase chain reaction to cerebrospinal fluid from brain-biopsied patients and correlation with disease. National Institute of Allergy and Infectious Diseases Collaborative Antiviral Study Group. *J Infect Dis* 171: 857–63.

Lambert HP (1994) Meningitis. *J Neurol Neurosurg Psychiatry* 57: 405–15.

Landrigan PJ, Witte JJ (1973) Neurologic disorders following live measles-virus vaccination. *JAMA* 223: 1459–62.

Lankester AC, Visser LF, Hartwig NG, et al. (2005) Allogeneic stem cell transplantation in X-linked lymphoproliferative disease: two cases in one family and review of the literature. *Bone Marrow Transplant* 36: 99–105.

Lanthier S, Armstrong D, Domi T, deVeber G (2005) Post-varicella arteriopathy of childhood: natural history of vascular stenosis. *Neurology* 64: 660–3.

Larsen PD, Crisp D (1996) Acute bilateral striatal necrosis associated with Mycoplasma pneumoniae infection. *Pediatr Infect Dis J* 15: 1124–6.

Laterre PF, Levy H, Clermont G, et al. (2004) Hospital mortality and resource use in subgroups of the Recombinant Human Activated Protein C Worldwide Evaluation in Severe Sepsis (PROWESS) trial. *Crit Care Med* 32: 2207–18.

Lebech AM, Hansen K (1992) Detection of Borrelia burgdorferi DNA in urine samples and cerebrospinal fluid samples from patients with early and late Lyme neuroborreliosis by polymerase chain reaction. *J Clin Microbiol* 30: 1646–53.

Lebon P, Lyon G (1974) Letter: Non-congenital rubella encephalitis. *Lancet* 2: 468.

Lee TC, Tsai CP, Yuan CL, et al. (2003) Encephalitis in Taiwan: a prospective hospital-based study. *Jpn J Infect Dis* 56: 193–9.

Lee TC, Savoldo B, Rooney CM, et al. (2005) Quantitative EBV viral loads and immunosuppression alterations can decrease PTLD incidence in pediatric liver transplant recipients. *Am J Transplant* 5: 2222–8.

Legg NJ, Gupta PC, Scott DF (1973) Epilepsy following cerebral abscess. A clinical and EEG study of 70 patients. *Brain* 96: 259–68.

Lehky TJ, Fox CH, Koenig S, et al. (1995) Detection of human T-lymphotropic virus type I (HTLV-I) tax RNA in the central nervous system of HTLV-I-associated myelopathy/tropical spastic paraparesis patients by in situ hybridization. *Ann Neurol* 37: 167–75.

Leib SL, Leppert D, Clements J, Tauber MG (2000) Matrix metalloproteinases contribute to brain damage in experimental pneumococcal meningitis. *Infect Immun* 68: 615–20.

Leib SL, Clements JM, Lindberg RL, (2001) Inhibition of matrix metalloproteinases and tumour necrosis factor alpha converting enzyme as adjuvant therapy in pneumococcal meningitis. *Brain* 124: 1734–42.

Leonard HL, Swedo SE (2001) Paediatric autoimmune neuropsychiatric disorders associated with streptococcal infection (PANDAS). *Int J Neuropsychopharmacol* 4: 191–8.

Leotta N, Chaseling R, Duncan G, Isaacs D (2005) Intracranial suppuration. *J Paediatr Child Health* 41: 508–12.

Lesnicar G, Poljak M, Seme K, Lesnicar J (2003) Pediatric tick-borne encephalitis in 371 cases from an endemic region in Slovenia, 1959 to 2000. *Pediatr Infect Dis J* 22: 612–7.

Levin M, Hjelm M, Kay JD, et al. (1983) Haemorrhagic shock and encephalopathy: a new syndrome with a high mortality in young children. *Lancet* 2: 64–7.

Levin M, Pincott JR, Hjelm M, et al. (1989) Hemorrhagic shock and encephalopathy: clinical, pathologic, and biochemical features. *J Pediatr* 114: 194–203.

Levitt LP, Rich TA, Kinde SW, et al. (1970) Central nervous system mumps. A review of 64 cases. *Neurology* 20: 829–34.

Lewis DW, Tucker SH (1986) Central nervous system involvement in cat scratch disease. *Pediatrics* 77: 714–21.

Lewis MA, Priestley BL (1986) Transient neonatal Behçet's disease. *Arch Dis Child* 61: 805–6.

Lexau CA, Lynfield R, Danila R, et al. (2005) Changing epidemiology of invasive pneumococcal disease among older adults in the era of pediatric pneumococcal conjugate vaccine. *JAMA* 294: 2043–51.

Leys D, Destee A, Petit H, Warot P (1986) Management of subdural intracranial empyemas should not always require surgery. *J Neurol Neurosurg Psychiatry* 49: 635–9.

Lezin A, Olindo S, Oliere S, et al. (2005) Human T lymphotropic virus type I (HTLV-I) proviral load in cerebrospinal fluid: a new criterion for the diagnosis of HTLV-I-associated myelopathy/tropical spastic paraparesis? *J Infect Dis* 191: 1830–4.

L'Hommedieu C, Stough R, Brown L, et al. (1979) Potentiation of neuromuscular weakness in infant botulism by aminoglycosides. *J Pediatr* 95: 1065–70.

Li HC, Biggar RJ, Miley WJ, et al. (2004) Provirus load in breast milk and risk of mother-to-child transmission of human T lymphotropic virus type I. *J Infect Dis* 190: 1275–8.

Lin JJ, Harn HJ, Hsu YD, et al. (1995) Rapid diagnosis of tuberculous meningitis by polymerase chain reaction assay of cerebrospinal fluid. *J Neurol* 242: 147–52.

Lin TY, Nelson JD, McCracken GH (1984) Fever during treatment for bacterial meningitis. *Pediatr Infect Dis* 3: 319–22.

Lin TY, Chrane DF, Nelson JD, McCracken GH (1985) Seven days of ceftriaxone therapy is as effective as ten days' treatment for bacterial meningitis. *JAMA* 253: 3559–63.

Linssen WH, Gabreëls FJ, Wevers RA (1991) Infective acute transverse myelopathy. Report of two cases. *Neuropediatrics* 22: 107–9.

Lobato MN, Caldwell MB, Ng P, Oxtoby MJ (1995) Encephalopathy in children with perinatally acquired human immunodeficiency virus infection. Pediatric Spectrum of Disease Clinical Consortium. *J Pediatr* **126**: 710–5.

Loeffler JM, Ringer R, Hablützel M, et al. (2001) The free radical scavenger alpha-phenyl-tert-butyl nitrone aggravates hippocampal apoptosis and learning deficits in experimental pneumococcal meningitis. *J Infect Dis* **183**: 247–252.

Long SS, Gajewski JL, Brown LW, Gilligan PH (1985) Clinical, laboratory, and environmental features of infant botulism in Southeastern Pennsylvania. *Pediatrics* **75**: 935–41.

Losurdo G, Giacchino R, Castagnola E, et al. (2006) Cerebrovascular disease and varicella in children. *Brain Dev* **28**: 366–70.

Louis ED, Lynch T, Kaufmann P, et al. (1996) Diagnostic guidelines in central nervous system Whipple's disease. *Ann Neurol* **40**: 561–8.

Love S, Koch P, Urbach H, Dawson TP (2004) Chronic granulomatous herpes simplex encephalitis in children. *J Neuropathol Exp Neurol* **63**: 1173–81.

Luna D, Williams C, Dulac O, et al. (1990) [Delayed acute measles encephalitis.] *Arch Fr Pediatr* **47**: 339–44 (French).

Lyon G, Dodge PR, Adams RD (1961) The acute encephalopathies of obscure origin in infants and children. *Brain* **84**: 680–708.

MacPherson GG, Warrell MJ, White NJ, et al. (1985) Human cerebral malaria. A quantitative ultrastructural analysis of parasitized erythrocyte sequestration. *Am J Pathol* **119**: 385–401.

Maguire JF, Meissner HC (1985) Onset of encephalitis early in the course of varicella infection. *Pediatr Infect Dis* **4**: 699–701.

Maida E, Horvatits E (1986) Cerebrospinal fluid alterations in bacterial meningitis. *Eur Neurol* **25**: 110–6.

Mallucci G, Collinge J (2004) Update on Creutzfeldt–Jakob disease. *Curr Opin Neurol* **17**: 641–7.

Maloney EM, Nagai M, Hisada M, et al. (2004) Prediagnostic human T lymphotropic virus type I provirus loads were highest in Jamaican children who developed seborrheic dermatitis and severe anemia. *J Infect Dis* **189**: 41–5.

Mann JM, Shandler L, Cushing AH (1982) Pediatric plague. *Pediatrics* **69**: 762–7.

Marcus JC (1982) Congenital neurosyphilis: a re-appraisal. *Neuropediatrics* **13**: 195–9.

Maricich SM, Neul JL, Lotze TE, et al. (2004) Neurologic complications associated with influenza A in children during the 2003–2004 influenza season in Houston, Texas. *Pediatrics* **114**: e626–33.

Mariotti P, Colosimo C, Frisullo G, et al. (2006) Relapsing demyelinating disease after chicken pox in a child. *Neurology* **66**: 1953–4.

Marks WA, Stutman HR, Marks MI, et al. (1986) Cefuroxime versus ampicillin plus chloramphenicol in childhood bacterial meningitis: a multicenter randomized controlled trial. *J Pediatr* **109**: 123–30.

Marks WA, Bodensteiner JB, Bobele GB, et al. (1988) Parainflammatory leukoencephalomyelitis: clinical and magnetic resonance imaging findings. *J Child Neurol* **3**: 205–13.

Marsh K, Forster D, Waruiru C, et al. (1995) Indicators of life-threatening malaria in African children. *N Engl J Med* **332**: 1399–404.

Marshall SE (2004) Behçet's disease. *Best Pract Res Clin Rheumatol* **18**: 291–311.

Marshall WC (1983) Infections of the nervous system. In: Brett EM, ed. *Paediatric Neurology*. Edinburgh: Churchill Livingstone, pp. 508–567.

Marton R, Gotlieb-Stematsky T, Klein C, et al. (1995) Mild form of acute herpes simplex encephalitis in childhood. *Brain Dev* **17**: 360–1.

Mathiesen T, Linde A, Olding-Stenkvist E, Wahren B (1988) Specific IgG subclass reactivity in herpes simplex encephalitis. *J Neurol* **235**: 400–6.

Mauser HW, Van Houwelingen HC, Tulleken CA (1987) Factors affecting the outcome in subdural empyema. *J Neurol Neurosurg Psychiatry* **50**: 1136–41.

McCoig C, Castrejón MM, Saavedra-Lozano J, et al. (2004) Cerebrospinal fluid and plasma concentrations of proinflammatory mediators in human immunodeficiency virus-infected children. *Pediatr Infect Dis J* **23**: 114–8.

McCullers JA, Vargas SL, Flynn PM, et al. (2000) Candidal meningitis in children with cancer. *Clin Infect Dis* **31**: 451–7.

McIntyre PB, Berkey CS, King SM, et al. (1997) Dexamethasone as adjunctive therapy in bacterial meningitis. A meta-analysis of randomized clinical trials since 1988. *JAMA* **278**: 925–31.

McMenamin JB, Volpe JJ (1984) Bacterial meningitis in infancy: effects on intracranial pressure and cerebral blood flow velocity. *Neurology* **34**: 500–4.

Medori R, Montagna P, Tritschler HJ, et al. (1992) Fatal familial insomnia, a prion disease with a mutation at codon 178 of the prion protein gene. *N Engl J Med* **326**: 444–9.

Mell LK, Davis RL, Owens D (2005) Association between streptococcal infection and obsessive–compulsive disorder, Tourette's syndrome, and tic disorder. *Pediatrics* **116**: 56–60.

Mellor DH (1992) The place of computed tomography and lumbar puncture in suspected bacterial meningitis. *Arch Dis Child* **67**: 1417–9.

Mertsola J (1991) Cytokines in the pathogenesis of bacterial meningitis. *Trans R Soc Trop Med Hyg* **85** Suppl 1: 17–8.

Middelhof CA, Loudon WG, Muhonen MD, et al. (2005) Improved survival in central nervous system aspergillosis: a series of immunocompromised children with leukemia undergoing stereotactic resection of aspergillomas. Report of four cases. *J Neurosurg* **103** (4 Suppl): 374–8.

Miles C, Hoffman W, Lai CW, Freeman JW (1993) Cytomegalovirus-associated transverse myelitis. *Neurology* **43**: 2143–5.

Miller C, Andrews N, Rush M, et al. (2004) The epidemiology of subacute sclerosing panencephalitis in England and Wales 1990–2002. *Arch Dis Child* **89**: 1145–8.

Miller ES, Dias PS, Uttley D (1987) Management of subdural empyema: a series of 24 cases. *J Neurol Neurosurg Psychiatry* **50**: 1415–8.

Mills RW, Schoolfield L (1992) Acute transverse myelitis associated with Mycoplasma pneumoniae infection: a case report and review of the literature. *Pediatr Infect Dis J* **11**: 228–31.

Minns RA, Engleman HM, Stirling H (1989) Cerebrospinal fluid pressure in pyogenic meningitis. *Arch Dis Child* **64**: 814–20.

Mirakhur B, McKenna M (2004) Recurrent herpes simplex type 2 virus (Mollaret) meningitis. *J Am Board Fam Pract* **17**: 303–5.

Mitchell W (2001) Neurological and developmental effects of HIV and AIDS in children and adolescents. *Ment Retard Dev Disabil Res Rev* **7**: 211–6.

Mizrahi EM, Tharp BR (1982) A characteristic EEG pattern in neonatal herpes simplex encephalitis. *Neurology* **32**: 1215–20.

Mizuguchi M (1997) Acute necrotizing encephalopathy of childhood: a novel form of acute encephalopathy prevalent in Japan and Taiwan. *Brain Dev* **19**: 81–92.

Molyneux ME, Taylor TE, Wirima JJ, Borgstein A (1989) Clinical features and prognostic indicators in paediatric cerebral malaria: a study of 131 comatose Malawian children. *Q J Med* **71**: 441–59.

Morandi X, Mercier P, Fournier HD, Brassier G (1999) Dermal sinus and intramedullary spinal cord abscess. Report of two cases and review of the literature. *Childs Nerv Syst* **15**: 202–6; discussion 207–8.

Mori M, Ban N, Kinoshita K (1988) Familial occurrence of HTLV-I-associated myelopathy. *Ann Neurol* **23**: 100.

Morris AM (2004) Review: adjuvant corticosteroid therapy reduces death, hearing loss, and neurologic sequelae in bacterial meningitis. *ACP J Club* **140**: 34.

Moxon ER, Smith AL, Averill DR, Smith DH (1974) Haemophilus influenzae meningitis in infant rats after intranasal inoculation. *J Infect Dis* **129**: 154–62.

Mulligan K, Nelson S, Friedman HS, Andrews PI (1992) Shigellosis-associated encephalopathy. *Pediatr Infect Dis J* **11**: 889–90.

Murphy JV, Yunis EJ (1976) Encephalopathy following measles infection in children with chronic illness. *J Pediatr* **88**: 937–42.

Mustafa MM, Weitman SD, Winick NJ, et al. (1993) Subacute measles encephalitis in the young immunocompromised host: report of two cases diagnosed by polymerase chain reaction and treated with ribavirin and review of the literature. *Clin Infect Dis* **16**: 654–60.

Nadal D, Caduff R, Frey E, et al. (1994) Non-Hodgkin's lymphoma in four children infected with the human immunodeficiency virus. Association with Epstein–Barr virus and treatment. *Cancer* **73**: 224–30.

Nahmias AJ, Whitley RJ, Visintine AN, et al. (1982) Herpes simplex virus encephalitis: laboratory evaluations and their diagnostic significance. *J Infect Dis* **145**: 829–36.

Nakagomi T, Nakagomi O (2005) Rotavirus antigenemia in children with encephalopathy accompanied by rotavirus gastroenteritis. *Arch Virol* **150**: 1927–31.

Nakamura Y, Takahashi M, Ueyama K, et al. (1994) Magnetic resonance imaging and brain-stem auditory evoked potentials in neuro-Behçet's disease. *J Neurol* **241**: 481–6.

Nakao K, Ohba N (2003) Human T-cell lymphotropic virus type 1-associated retinal vasculitis in children. *Retina* **23**: 197–201.

Nasralla CA, Pay N, Goodpasture HC, et al. (1993) Postinfectious encephalopathy in a child following Campylobacter jejuni enteritis. *AJNR* **14**: 444–8.

Newell ML, Coovadia H, Cortina-Borja M, et al. (2004) Mortality of infected and uninfected infants born to HIV-infected mothers in Africa: a pooled analysis. *Lancet* **364**: 1236–43.

Newton CR, Kirkham FJ, Winstanley PA, et al. (1991) Intracranial pressure in African children with cerebral malaria. *Lancet* **337**: 573–6.

Nihei K, Kamoshita S, Mizutani H, et al. (1977) Atypical subacute sclerosing panencephalitis. *Acta Neuropathol* **38**: 163–6.

Nkowane BM, Wassilak SG, Orenstein WA, et al. (1987) Vaccine-associated paralytic poliomyelitis. United States: 1973 through 1984. *JAMA* **257**: 1335–40.

Norman MG (1968) Encephalopathy and fatty degeneration of the viscera in childhood: I. Review of cases at the Hospital for Sick Children, Toronto (1954–1966). *Can Med Assoc J* **99**: 522–6.

North K, de Silva L, Procopis P (1993) Brain-stem encephalitis caused by Epstein–Barr virus. *J Child Neurol* **8**: 40–2.

Nottidge VA (1983) Pneumococcal meningitis in sickle cell disease in childhood. *Am J Dis Child* **137**: 29–31.

Nozzoli C, Bartolozzi B, Guidi S, et al. (2006) Epstein–Barr virus-associated post-transplant lymphoproliferative disease with central nervous system involvement after unrelated allogeneic hematopoietic stem cell transplantation. *Leuk Lymphoma* **47**: 167–9.

Nunoi H, Mercado MR, Mizukami T, et al. (2005) Apoptosis under hypercytokinemia is a possible pathogenesis in influenza-associated encephalopathy. *Pediatr Int* **47**: 175–9.

Nuttall JJ, Wilmshurst JM, Ndondo AP, et al. (2004) Progressive multifocal leukoencephalopathy after initiation of highly active antiretroviral therapy in a child with advanced human immunodeficiency virus infection: a case of immune reconstitution inflammatory syndrome. *Pediatr Infect Dis J* **23**: 683–5.

Oates-Whitehead RM, Maconochie I, Baumer H, Stewart ME (2005) Fluid therapy for acute bacterial meningitis. *Cochrane Database Syst Rev* (3): CD004786.

Offenbacher H, Fazekas F, Schmidt R, et al. (1991) MRI in tuberculous meningoencephalitis: report of four cases and review of the neuroimaging literature. *J Neurol* **238**: 340–4.

Ogata M, Kikuchi H, Satou T, et al. (2006) Human herpesvirus 6 DNA in plasma after allogeneic stem cell transplantation: incidence and clinical significance. *J Infect Dis* **193**: 68–79.

Oki J, Yoshida H, Tokumitsu A, et al. (1995) Serial neuroimages of acute necrotizing encephalopathy associated with human herpesvirus 6 infection. *Brain Dev* **17**: 356–9.

Olinsky A (1970) Precocious sexual development following tuberculous meningitis: a case report. *S Afr Med J* **44**: 1189–90.

Ommaya AK (1976) Spinal fluid fistulae. *Clin Neurosurg* **23**: 363–92.

Onorato IM, Wormser GP, Nicholas P (1980) 'Normal' CSF in bacterial meningitis. *JAMA* **244**: 1469–71.

Ormerod IE, Bronstein A, Rudge P, et al. (1986) Magnetic resonance imaging in clinically isolated lesions of the brain stem. *J Neurol Neurosurg Psychiatry* **49**: 737–43.

Ozturk A, Gurses C, Baykan B, et al. (2002) Subacute sclerosing panencephalitis: clinical and magnetic resonance imaging evaluation of 36 patients. *J Child Neurol* **17**: 25–9.

Pace D, Pollard AJ (2007) Meningococcal A, C, Y and W-135 polysaccharide-protein conjugate vaccines. *Arch Dis Child* **92**: 909–15.

Pachner AR (1989) Neurologic manifestations of Lyme disease, the new great imitator. *Rev Infect Dis* **11** Suppl 6: S1482–6.

Pachner AR, Delaney E (1993) The polymerase chain reaction in the diagnosis of Lyme neuroborreliosis. *Ann Neurol* **34**: 544–50.

Pachner AR, Steere AC (1985) The triad of neurologic manifestations of Lyme disease: meningitis, cranial neuritis, and radiculoneuritis. *Neurology* **35**: 47–53.

Pai M (2005) Alternatives to the tuberculin skin test: interferon-gamma assays in the diagnosis of mycobacterium tuberculosis infection. *Indian J Med Microbiol* **23**: 151–8.

Panicker J, Walsh T, Kamani N (2006) Recurrent central nervous system blastomycosis in an immunocompetent child treated successfully with sequential liposomal amphotericin B and voriconazole. *Pediatr Infect Dis J* **25**: 377–9.

Parain D, Boulloche J (1988) [Multifocal epileptic crises following mumps.] Neurophysiol Clin 18: 187–91 (French).

Pardo CA, Vining EP, Guo L, et al. (2004) The pathology of Rasmussen syndrome: stages of cortical involvement and neuropathological studies in 45 hemispherectomies. *Epilepsia* **45**: 516–26.

Park YD, Belman AL, Kim TS, et al. (1990) Stroke in pediatric acquired immunodeficiency syndrome. *Ann Neurol* **28**: 303–11.

Pascual J, Combarros O, Polo JM, Berciano J (1988) Localized CNS brucellosis: report of 7 cases. *Acta Neurol Scand* **78**: 282–9.

Pasternak JF, De Vivo DC, Prensky AL (1980) Steroid-responsive encephalomyelitis in childhood. *Neurology* **30**: 481–6.

Pavlakis SG, Lu D, Frank Y, et al. (1995) Magnetic resonance spectroscopy in childhood AIDS encephalopathy. *Pediatr Neurol* **12**: 277–82.

Peacock JE, McGinnis MR, Cohen MS (1984) Persistent neutrophilic meningitis. Report of four cases and review of the literature. *Medicine* **63**: 379–95.

Pearson DA, McGrath NM, Nozyce M, et al. (2000) Predicting HIV disease progression in children using measures of neuropsychological and neurological functioning. Pediatric AIDS clinical trials 152 study team. *Pediatrics* **106**: E76.

Peckham C, Gibb D (1995) Mother-to-child transmission of the human immunodeficiency virus. *N Engl J Med* **333**: 298–302.

Pejme J (1964) Infectious mononucleosis. A clinical and haematological study of patients and contacts, and a comparison with healthy subjects. *Acta Med Scand Suppl* **413**: 1–83.

Pelekanos JT, Appleton DB (1989) Melioidosis with multiple cerebral abscesses. *Pediatr Neurol* **5**: 48–52.

Peters AC, Vielvoye GJ, Versteeg J, et al. (1979) ECHO 25 focal encephalitis and subacute hemichorea. *Neurology* **29**: 676–81.

Peters MJ, Pizer BL, Millar M (1994) Rifampicin in pneumococcal meningoencephalitis. *Arch Dis Child* **71**: 77–9.

Pike MG, Wong PK, Bencivenga R, et al. (1990) Electrophysiologic studies, computed tomography, and neurologic outcome in acute bacterial meningitis. *J Pediatr* **116**: 702–6.

Pike MG, Kennedy CR, Neville BG, Levin M (1991) Herpes simplex encephalitis with relapse. *Arch Dis Child* **66**: 1242–4.

Poltera AA (1977) Thrombogenic intracranial vasculitis in tuberculous meningitis. A 20 year post mortem survey. *Acta Neurol Belg* **77**: 12–24.

Pomeroy SL, Holmes SJ, Dodge PR, Feigin RD (1990) Seizures and other neurologic sequelae of bacterial meningitis in children. *N Engl J Med* **323**: 1651–7.

Powell KR, Sugarman LI, Eskenazi AE, et al. (1990) Normalization of plasma arginine vasopressin concentrations when children with meningitis are given maintenance plus replacement fluid therapy. *J Pediatr* **117**: 515–22.

Prusiner SB, Hsiao KK (1994) Human prion diseases. *Ann Neurol* **35**: 385–95.

Puchhammer-Stöckl E, Heinz FX, Kundi M, et al. (1993) Evaluation of the polymerase chain reaction for diagnosis of herpes simplex virus encephalitis. *J Clin Microbiol* **31**: 146–8.

Purdy KW, Heckenlively JR, Church JA, Keller MA (2003) Progressive outer retinal necrosis caused by varicella-zoster virus in children with acquired immunodeficiency syndrome. *Pediatr Infect Dis J* **22**: 384–6.

Quagliarello VJ, Scheld WM (1997) Treatment of bacterial meningitis. *N Engl J Med* **336**: 708–16.

Quartier P, Foray S, Casanova JL, et al. (2000) Enteroviral meningoencephalitis in X-linked agammaglobulinemia: intensive immunoglobulin therapy and sequential viral detection in cerebrospinal fluid by polymerase chain reaction. *Pediatr Infect Dis J* **19**: 1106–8.

Rabe EF, Flynn RE, Dodge PR (1968) Subdural collections of fluid in infants and children. A study of 62 patients with special reference to factors influencing prognosis and the efficacy of various forms of therapy. *Neurology* **18**: 559–70.

Radetsky M (1992) Duration of symptoms and outcome in bacterial meningitis: an analysis of causation and the implications of a delay in diagnosis. *Pediatr Infect Dis J* **11**: 694–8; discussion 698–701.

Randhawa PS, Jaffe R, Demetris AJ, et al. (1992) Expression of Epstein–Barr virus-encoded small RNA (by the EBER-1 gene) in liver specimens from transplant recipients with post-transplantation lymphoproliferative disease. *N Engl J Med* **327**: 1710–4.

Rantala H, Uhari M, Uhari M, et al. (1991) Outcome after childhood encephalitis. *Dev Med Child Neurol* **33**: 858–67.

Rautonen J, Koskiniemi M, Vaheri A (1991) Prognostic factors in childhood acute encephalitis. *Pediatr Infect Dis J* **10**: 441–6.

Redfearn A, Pennie RA, Mahony JB, Dent PB (1993) Progressive multifocal leukoencephalopathy in a child with immunodeficiency and hyperimmunoglobulinemia M. *Pediatr Infect Dis J* **12**: 399–401.

Rehle TM (1989) Classification, distribution and importance of arboviruses. *Trop Med Parasitol* **40**: 391–5.

Renier D, Flandin C, Hirsch E, Hirsch JF (1988) Brain abscesses in neonates. A study of 30 cases. *J Neurosurg* **69**: 877–82.

Rennick G, Shann F, de Campo J (1993) Cerebral herniation during bacterial meningitis in children. *BMJ* **306**: 953–5.

Ribera E, Martinez-Vazquez JM, Ocana I (1987) [Adenosine deaminase in the quick diagnosis of tuberculous meningitis.] *Neurologia* **2**: 19–22 (Spanish).

Riordan FA, Thomson AP, Sills JA, Hart CA (1993) Does computed tomography have a role in the evaluation of complicated acute bacterial meningitis in childhood? *Dev Med Child Neurol* **35**: 275–6.

Risk WS, Haddad FS (1979) The variable natural history of subacute sclerosing panencephalitis: a study of 118 cases from the Middle East. *Arch Neurol* **36**: 610–4.

River Y, Averbuch-Heller L, Weinberger M, et al. (1994) Antibiotic induced meningitis. *J Neurol Neurosurg Psychiatry* **57**: 705–8.

Rivner MH, Jay WM, Green JB, Dyken PR (1982) Opsoclonus in Hemophilus influenzae meningitis. *Neurology* **32**: 661–3.

Robb RM, Watters GV (1970) Ophthalmic manifestations of subacute sclerosing panencephalitis. *Arch Ophthalmol* **83**: 426–35.

Roden VJ, Cantor HE, O'Connor DM, et al. (1975) Acute hemiplegia of childhood associated with Coxsackie A9 viral infection. *J Pediatr* **86**: 56–8.

Rodriguez AF, Kaplan SL, Mason EO (1990) Cerebrospinal fluid values in the very low birth weight infant. *J Pediatr* **116**: 971–4.

Rodriguez WJ, Puig JR, Khan WN, et al. (1986) Ceftazidime vs. standard therapy for pediatric meningitis: therapeutic, pharmacologic and epidemiologic observations. *Pediatr Infect Dis* **5**: 408–15.

Roig M, Calopa M, Rovira A, et al. (1993) Bilateral striatal lesions in childhood. *Pediatr Neurol* **9**: 349–58.

Roman GC (1988) The neuroepidemiology of tropical spastic paraparesis. *Ann Neurol* **23** Suppl: S113–20.

Rose JW, Stroop WG, Matsuo F, Henkel J (1992) Atypical herpes simplex encephalitis: clinical, virologic, and neuropathologic evaluation. *Neurology* **42**: 1809–12.

Rosemberg S, Amaral LC, Kliemann SE, Arita FN (1992) Acute encephalopathy with bilateral striatal necrosis. A distinctive clinicopathological condition. *Neuropediatrics* **23**: 310–5.

Rosenfeld J, Taylor CL, Atlas SW (1993) Myelitis following chickenpox: a case report. *Neurology* **43**: 1834–6.

Ross SC, Densen P (1984) Complement deficiency states and infection: epidemiology, pathogenesis and consequences of neisserial and other infections in an immune deficiency. *Medicine* **63**: 243–73.

Rotbart HA, Webster AD; Pleconaril Treatment Registry Group (2001) Treatment of potentially life-threatening enterovirus infections with pleconaril. *Clin Infect Dis* **32**: 228–35.

Roth B, Younossi-Hartenstein A, Schroder R, et al. (1987) Haemorrhagic shock–encephalopathy syndrome: plasmapheresis as a therapeutic approach. *Eur J Pediatr* **146**: 83–5.

Roulet Perez E, Maeder P, Cotting J, et al. (1993) Acute fatal parainfectious cerebellar swelling in two children. A rare or an overlooked situation? *Neuropediatrics* **24**: 346–51.

Rudge P, Webster AD, Revesz T, et al. (1996) Encephalomyelitis in primary hypogammaglobulinaemia. *Brain* **119**: 1–15.

Rush PJ, Shore A, Inman R, et al. (1986) Arthritis associated with Haemophilus influenzae meningitis: septic or reactive? *J Pediatr* **109**: 412–5.

Russell RR, Donald JC (1958) The neurological complications of mumps. *BMJ* **2**: 27–30.

Rutter N, Smales OR (1977) Lumbar puncture in children with convulsions. *Lancet* **2**: 190–1.

Sabouri AH, Saito M, Usuku K, et al. (2005) Differences in viral and host genetic risk factors for development of human T-cell lymphotropic virus type 1 (HTLV-1)-associated myelopathy/tropical spastic paraparesis between Iranian and Japanese HTLV-1-infected individuals. *J Gen Virol* **86**: 773–81.

Sada E, Ruiz-Palacios GM, Lopez-Vidal Y, Ponce de Leon S (1983) Detection of mycobacterial antigens in cerebrospinal fluid of patients with tuberculous meningitis by enzyme-linked immunosorbent assay. *Lancet* **2**: 651–2.

Saitoh S, Wada T, Narita M, et al. (1993) Mycoplasma pneumoniae infection may cause striatal lesions leading to acute neurologic dysfunction. *Neurology* **43**: 2150–1.

Saltik S, Saip S, Kocer N, et al. (2004) MRI findings in pediatric neuro-Behçet's disease. *Neuropediatrics* **35**: 190–3.

Sanchez-Ramon S, Resino S, Bellon Cano JM, et al. (2003) Neuroprotective effects of early antiretrovirals in vertical HIV infection. *Pediatr Neurol* **29**: 218–21.

Sauerbrei A, Wutzler P (2002) Laboratory diagnosis of central nervous system infections caused by herpesviruses. *J Clin Virol* **25** Suppl 1: S45–51.

Schaad UB, Nelson JD, McCracken GH (1981) Recrudescence and relapse in bacterial meningitis of childhood. *Pediatrics* **67**: 188–95.

Schaad UB, Wedgwood-Krucko J, Tschaeppeler H (1988) Reversible ceftriaxone-associated biliary pseudolithiasis in children. *Lancet* **2**: 1411–3.

Schaad UB, Suter S, Gianella-Borradori A, et al. (1990) A comparison of ceftriaxone and cefuroxime for the treatment of bacterial meningitis in children. *N Engl J Med* **322**: 141–7.

Schauseil-Zipf U, Harden A, Hoare RD, et al. (1982) Early diagnosis of herpes simplex encephalitis in childhood. Clinical, neurophysiological and neuroradiological studies. *Eur J Pediatr* **138**: 154–61.

Schoeman J, Donald P, van Zyl L, et al. (1991) Tuberculous hydrocephalus: comparison of different treatments with regard to ICP, ventricular size and clinical outcome. *Dev Med Child Neurol* **33**: 396–405.

Schoeman JF, Van Zyl LE, Laubscher JA, Donald PR (1997) Effect of corticosteroids on intracranial pressure, computed tomographic findings, and clinical outcome in young children with tuberculous meningitis. *Pediatrics* **99**: 226–31.

Schreiner MS, Field E, Ruddy R (1991) Infant botulism: a review of 12 years' experience at the Children's Hospital of Philadelphia. *Pediatrics* **87**: 159–65.

Schuchat A, Robinson K, Wenger JD, et al. (1997) Bacterial meningitis in the United States in 1995. Active Surveillance Team. *N Engl J Med* **337**: 970–6.

Schwartz JF, Balentine JD (1978) Recurrent meningitis due to an intracranial epidermoid. *Neurology* **28**: 124–9.

Schwartz S, Ruhnke M, Ribaud P, et al. (2005) Improved outcome in central nervous system aspergillosis, using voriconazole treatment. *Blood* **106**: 2641–5.

Scott IU, Luu KM, Davis JL (2002) Intravitreal antivirals in the management of patients with acquired immunodeficiency syndrome with progressive outer retinal necrosis. *Arch Ophthalmol* **120**: 1219–22.

Selby G, Walker GL (1979) Cerebral arteritis in cat-scratch disease. *Neurology* **29**: 1413–8.

Sen S, Sharma D, Singh S, et al. (1989) Poliomyelitis in vaccinated children. *Indian Pediatr* **26**: 423–9.

Shah SS, Zaoutis TE, Turnquist J, et al. (2005) Early differentiation of Lyme from enteroviral meningitis. *Pediatr Infect Dis J* **24**: 542–5.

Shakir RA (1986) Neurobrucellosis. *Postgrad Med J* **62**: 1077–9.

Shakir RA, Sulaiman K, Kahn RA, Rudwan M (1990) Neurological presentation of neuro-Behçet's syndrome: clinical categories. *Eur Neurol* **30**: 249–53.

Shankar P, Manjunath N, Mohan KK, et al. (1991) Rapid diagnosis of tuberculous meningitis by polymerase chain reaction. *Lancet* **337**: 5–7.

Shanks DE, Blasco PA, Chason DP (1991) Movement disorder following herpes simplex encephalitis. *Dev Med Child Neurol* **33**: 348–52.

Sharer LR, Epstein LG, Cho ES, et al. (1986) Pathologic features of AIDS encephalopathy in children: evidence for LAV/HTLV-III infection of brain. *Hum Pathol* **17**: 271–84.

Shibasaki H, Endo C, Kuroda Y, et al. (1988) Clinical picture of HTLV-I associated myelopathy. *J Neurol Sci* **87**: 15–24.

Shope TR, Garrett AL, Waecker NJ (1994) Mycobacterium bovis spinal epidural abscess in a 6-year-old boy with leukemia. *Pediatrics* **93**: 835–7.

Silverman IE, Liu GT, Bilaniuk LT, et al. (1995) Tuberculous meningitis with blindness and perichiasmal involvement on MRI. *Pediatr Neurol* **12**: 65–7.

Silverstein FS, Brunberg JA (1995) Postvaricella basal ganglia infarction in children. *AJNR* **16**: 449–52.

Simon JK, Lazareff JA, Diament MJ, Kennedy WA (2003) Intramedullary abscess of the spinal cord in children: a case report and review of the literature. *Pediatr Infect Dis J* **22**: 186–92.

Sköldenberg B, Forsgren M, Alestig K, et al. (1984) Acyclovir versus vidarabine in herpes simplex encephalitis. Randomised multicentre study in consecutive Swedish patients. *Lancet* **2**: 707–11.

Smith HP, Hendrick EB (1983) Subdural empyema and epidural abscess in children. *J Neurosurg* **58**: 392–7.

Smith KC, Starke JR, Eisenach K, et al. (1996) Detection of Mycobacterium tuberculosis in clinical specimens from children using a polymerase chain reaction. *Pediatrics* **97**: 155–60.

Snedeker JD, Kaplan SL, Dodge PR, et al. (1990) Subdural effusion and its relationship with neurologic sequelae of bacterial meningitis in infancy: a prospective study. *Pediatrics* **86**: 163–70.

Snow RW, Guerra CA, Noor AM, et al. (2005) The global distribution of clinical episodes of Plasmodium falciparum malaria. *Nature* **434**: 214–7.

Solders G, Nennesmo I, Persson A (1989) Diphtheritic neuropathy, an analysis based on muscle and nerve biopsy and repeated neurophysiological and autonomic function tests. *J Neurol Neurosurg Psychiatry* **52**: 876–80.

Solomon T, Dung NM, Vaughn DW, et al. (2000) Neurological manifestations of dengue infection. *Lancet* **355**: 1053–9.

Sonnabend OA, Sonnabend WF, Krech U, et al. (1985) Continuous microbiological and pathological study of 70 sudden and unexpected infant deaths: toxigenic intestinal clostridium botulinum infection in 9 cases of sudden infant death syndrome. *Lancet* **1**: 237–41.

Stanek G, Strle F (2003) Lyme borreliosis. *Lancet* **362**: 1639–47.

Steele RW, McConnell JR, Jacobs RF, Mawk JR (1985) Recurrent bacterial meningitis: coronal thin-section cranial computed tomography to delineate anatomic defects. *Pediatrics* **76**: 950–3.

fStevens JP, Eames M, Kent A, et al. (2003) Long term outcome of neonatal meningitis. *Arch Dis Child Fetal Neonatal Ed* **88**: F179–84.

Stins MF, Pearce D, Di Cello F, et al. (2003) Induction of intercellular adhesion molecule-1 on human brain endothelial cells by HIV-1 gp120: role of CD4 and chemokine coreceptors. *Lab Invest* **83**: 1787–98.

Straumanis JP, Tapia MD, King JC (2002) Influenza B infection associated with encephalitis: treatment with oseltamivir. *Pediatr Infect Dis J* **21**: 173–5.

Straussberg R, Harel L, Levy Y, Amir J (2001) A syndrome of transient encephalopathy associated with adenovirus infection. *Pediatrics* **107**: E69.

Studahl M (2003) Influenza virus and CNS manifestations. *J Clin Virol* **28**: 225–32.

Sugaya N (2002) Influenza-associated encephalopathy in Japan. *Semin Pediatr Infect Dis* **13**: 79–84.

Swartz MN, and Dodge PR (1965) Bacterial meningitis—a review of selected aspects. I. General clinical features, special problems and unusual meningeal reactions mimicking bacterial meningitis. *N Engl J Med* **272**: 898–902.

Swedo SE, Grant PJ (2005) Annotation: PANDAS: a model for human autoimmune disease. *J Child Psychol Psychiatry* **46**: 227–34.

Swedo SE, Leonard HL, Garvey M, et al. (1998) Pediatric autoimmune neuropsychiatric disorders associated with streptococcal infections: clinical description of the first 50 cases. *Am J Psychiatry* **155**: 264–71; erratum 578.

Swedo SE, Garvey M, Snider L, et al. (2001) The PANDAS subgroup: recognition and treatment. *CNS Spectr* **6**: 419–22, 425–6.

Sweeney VP, Drance SM (1970) Optic neuritis and compressive neuropathy associated with cat scratch disease. *Can Med Assoc J* **103**: 1380–1.

Swift TR (1981) Disorders of neuromuscular transmission other than myasthenia gravis. *Muscle Nerve* **4**: 334–53.

Syrogiannopoulos GA, Nelson JD, McCracken GH (1986) Subdural collections of fluid in acute bacterial meningitis: a review of 136 cases. *Pediatr Infect Dis* **5**: 343–52.

Taft TA, Chusid MJ, Sty JR (1986) Cerebral infarction in Hemophilus influenzae type B meningitis. *Clin Pediatr* **25**: 177–80.

Talamas O, Del Brutto OH, Garcia-Ramos G (1989) Brain-stem tuberculoma. An analysis of 11 patients. *Arch Neurol* **46**: 529–35.

Tan TQ (2003) Chronic meningitis. *Semin Pediatr Infect Dis* **14**: 131–9.

Tardieu M, Lapresle J (1980) [Persistence of herpetic inflammation of the central nervous system four years after an episode of acute encephalitis.] *Rev Neurol* **136**: 67–9 (French).

Tardieu M, Truffot-Pernot C, Carriere JP, et al. (1988) Tuberculous meningitis due to BCG in two previously healthy children. *Lancet* **1**: 440–1.

Tardieu M, Mayaux MJ, Seibel N, et al. (1995) Cognitive assessment of school-age children infected with maternally transmitted human immunodeficiency virus type 1. *J Pediatr* **126**: 375–9.

Tardieu M, Le Chenadec J, Persoz A, et al. (2000) HIV-1-related encephalopathy in infants compared with children and adults. French Pediatric HIV Infection Study and the SEROCO Group. *Neurology* **54**: 1089–95.

Tasker RC, Boyd S, Harden A, Matthew DJ (1988a) Monitoring in non-traumatic coma. Part II: Electroencephalography. *Arch Dis Child* **63**: 895–9.

Tasker RC, Matthew DJ, Helms P, et al. (1988b) Monitoring in non-traumatic coma. Part I: Invasive intracranial measurements. *Arch Dis Child* **63**: 888–94.

Taylor GP, Matsuoka M (2005) Natural history of adult T-cell leukemia/lymphoma and approaches to therapy. *Oncogene* **24**: 6047–57.

Taylor GP, Tosswill JH, Matutes E, et al. (1999) Prospective study of HTLV-I infection in an initially asymptomatic cohort. *J Acquir Immune Defic Syndr* **22**: 92–100.

Taylor HG, Mills EL, Ciampi A, et al. (1990) The sequelae of Haemophilus influenzae meningitis in school-age children. *N Engl J Med* **323**: 1657–63.

Teele DW, Dashefsky B, Rakusan T, Klein JO (1981) Meningitis after lumbar puncture in children with bacteremia. *N Engl J Med* **305**: 1079–81.

Teixeira J, Zimmerman RA, Haselgrove JC, et al. (2001) Diffusion imaging in pediatric central nervous system infections. *Neuroradiology* **43**: 1031–9.

Tekkok IH, Erbengi A (1992) Management of brain abscess in children: review of 130 cases over a period of 21 years. *Childs Nerv Syst* **8**: 411–6.

Teman AJ (1992) Spinal epidural abscess. Early detection with gadolinium magnetic resonance imaging. *Arch Neurol* **49**: 743–6.

Teoh R, O'Mahony G, Yeung VT (1986) Polymorphonuclear pleocytosis in the cerebrospinal fluid during chemotherapy for tuberculous meningitis. *J Neurol* **233**: 237–41.

Teoh R, Humphries MJ, Hoare RD, O'Mahony G (1989) Clinical correlation of CT changes in 64 Chinese patients with tuberculous meningitis. *J Neurol* **236**: 48–51.

Theuretzbacher U, Ihle F, Derendorf H (2006) Pharmacokinetic/pharmacodynamic profile of voriconazole. *Clin Pharmacokinet* **45**: 649–63.

Thomke F, Hopf HC (1992) Unilateral vestibular paralysis as the sole manifestation of mumps. *J Neurol Neurosurg Psychiatry* **55**: 858–9.

Thompson JA, Glasgow LA, Warpinski JR, Olson C (1980) Infant botulism: clinical spectrum and epidemiology. *Pediatrics* **66**: 936–42.

Tiab M, Mechinaud F, Harousseau JL (2000) Haemophagocytic syndrome associated with infections. *Baillieres Best Pract Res Clin Haematol* **13**: 163–78.

Tiffany KF, Benjamin DK, Palasanthiran P, et al. (2005) Improved neurodevelopmental outcomes following long-term high-dose oral acyclovir therapy in infants with central nervous system and disseminated herpes simplex disease. *J Perinatol* **25**: 156–61.

Tjia TL, Yeow YK, Tan CB (1985) Cryptococcal meningitis. *J Neurol Neurosurg Psychiatry* **48**: 853–8.

Togashi T, Matsuzono Y, Narita M, Morishima T (2004) Influenza-associated acute encephalopathy in Japanese children in 1994–2002. *Virus Res* **103**: 75–8.

Townsend JJ, Baringer JR, Wolinsky JS, et al. (1975) Progressive rubella panencephalitis. Late onset after congenital rubella. *N Engl J Med* **292**: 990–3.

Townsend JJ, Stroop WG, Baringer JR, et al. (1982) Neuropathology of progressive rubella panencephalitis after childhood rubella. *Neurology* **32**: 185–90.

Traub M, Colchester AC, Kingsley DP, Swash M (1984) Tuberculosis of the central nervous system. *Q J Med* **53**: 81–100.

Trauner DA, Horvath E, Davis LE (1988) Inhibition of fatty acid beta oxidation by influenza B virus and salicylic acid in mice: implications for Reye's syndrome. *Neurology* **38**: 239–41.

Trautmann M, Kluge W, Otto HS, Loddenkemper R (1986) Computed tomography in CNS tuberculosis. *Eur Neurol* **25**: 91–7.

Tsolia M, Skardoutsou A, Tsolas G, et al. (1995) Pre-eruptive neurologic manifestations associated with multiple cerebral infarcts in varicella. *Pediatr Neurol* **12**: 165–8.

Tuerlinckx D, Bodart E, Garrino MG, de Bilderling G (2003) Clinical data and cerebrospinal fluid findings in Lyme meningitis versus aseptic meningitis. *Eur J Pediatr* **162**: 150–3.

Tully J, Viner RM, Coen PG, et al. (2006) Risk and protective factors for meningococcal disease in adolescents: matched cohort study. *BMJ* **332**: 445–50.

Tuomanen E, Liu H, Hengstler B, et al. (1985) The induction of meningeal inflammation by components of the pneumococcal cell wall. *J Infect Dis* **151**: 859–68.

Tüzün M, Altinörs N, Arda IS, Hekimolu B (2002) Cerebral hydatid disease CT and MR findings. *Clin Imaging* **26**: 353–7.

Tyler KL (2004) Update on herpes simplex encephalitis. *Rev Neurol Dis* **1**: 169–78.

Udani PM, Bhat US (1974) Tuberculosis of central nervous system. II. Clinical aspects. *Indian Pediatr* **11**: 7–17.

Udani PM, Dastur DK (1970) Tuberculous encephalopathy with and without meningitis. Clinical features and pathological correlations. *J Neurol Sci* **10**: 541–61.

Unhanand M, Mustafa MM, McCracken GH, Nelson JD (1993) Gram-negative enteric bacillary meningitis: a twenty-one-year experience. *J Pediatr* **122**: 15–21.

Uziel Y, Brik R, Padeh S, et al. (1998) Juvenile Behçet's disease in Israel. The Pediatric Rheumatology Study Group of Israel. *Clin Exp Rheumatol* **16**: 502–5.

Valencia I, Miles DK, Melvin J, et al. (2004) Relapse of herpes encephalitis after acyclovir therapy: report of two new cases and review of the literature. *Neuropediatrics* **35**: 371–6.

van de Beek D, de Gans J, McIntyre P, Prasad K (2004) Steroids in adults with acute bacterial meningitis: a systematic review. *Lancet Infect Dis* **4**: 139–43.

van de Beek D, de Gans J, McIntyre P, Prasad K (2007) Corticosteroids in acute bacterial meningitis. *Cochrane Database Syst Rev* (1): CD004405.

van der Poel JC, Haenggeli CA, Overweg-Plandsoen WC (1995) Operculum syndrome: unusual feature of herpes simplex encephalitis. *Pediatr Neurol* **12**: 246–9.

Vandvik B, Norrby E, Steen-Johnsen J, Stensvold K (1978a) Mumps meningitis: prolonged pleocytosis and occurrence of mumps virus-specific oligoclonal IgG in the cerebrospinal fluid. *Eur Neurol* 17: 13–22.

Vandvik B, Weil ML, Grandien M, Norrby E (1978b) Progressive rubella virus panencephalitis: synthesis of oligoclonal virus-specific IgG antibodies and homogeneous free light chains in the central nervous system. *Acta Neurol Scand* 57: 53–64.

van Toorn R, Weyers HH, Schoeman JF (2004) Distinguishing PANDAS from Sydenham's chorea: case report and review of the literature. *Eur J Paediatr Neurol* 8: 211–6.

Vienny H, Despland PA, Lütschg J, et al. (1984) Early diagnosis and evolution of deafness in childhood bacterial meningitis: a study using brainstem auditory evoked potentials. *Pediatrics* 73: 579–86.

Vincent JL, Angus DC, Artigas A, et al. (2003) Effects of drotrecogin alfa (activated) on organ dysfunction in the PROWESS trial. *Crit Care Med* 31: 834–40.

Visudhiphan P, Chiemchanya S, Dheandhanoo D (1990) Central nervous system melioidosis in children. *Pediatr Infect Dis J* 9: 658–61.

Voudris KA, Skaardoutsou A, Haronitis I, et al. (2001) Brain MRI findings in influenza A-associated acute necrotizing encephalopathy of childhood. *Eur J Paediatr Neurol* 5: 199–202.

Wadia NH, Wadia PN, Katrak SM, Misra VP (1983) A study of the neurological disorder associated with acute haemorrhagic conjunctivitis due to enterovirus 70. *J Neurol Neurosurg Psychiatry* 46: 599–610.

Waecker NJ, Connor JD (1990) Central nervous system tuberculosis in children: a review of 30 cases. *Pediatr Infect Dis J* 9: 539–43.

Walker KG, Lawrenson J, Wilmshurst JM (2005) Neuropsychiatric movement disorders following streptococcal infection. *Dev Med Child Neurol* 47: 771–5.

Wang HS, Kuo MF, Huang SC, Chou ML (1994) Choreoathetosis as an initial sign of relapsing of herpes simplex encephalitis. *Pediatr Neurol* 11: 341–5.

Wang YH, Huang YC, Chang LY, et al. (2003) Clinical characteristics of children with influenza A virus infection requiring hospitalization. *J Microbiol Immunol Infect* 36: 111–6.

Ward KN (2005) The natural history and laboratory diagnosis of human herpesviruses-6 and -7 infections in the immunocompetent. *J Clin Virol* 32: 183–93.

Ward KN, Andrews NJ, Verity CM, et al. (2005) Human herpesviruses-6 and -7 each cause significant neurological morbidity in Britain and Ireland. *Arch Dis Child* 90: 619–23.

Warrell DA (1999) Management of severe malaria. *Parassitologia* 41: 287–94.

Watson RT, Ballinger WE, Quisling RG (1984) Acute hemorrhagic leukoencephalitis: diagnosis by computed tomography. *Ann Neurol* 15: 611–2.

Wechsler B, Vidailhet M, Piette JC, et al. (1992) Cerebral venous thrombosis in Behçet's disease: clinical study and long-term follow-up of 25 cases. *Neurology* 42: 614–8.

Weinberg A, Li S, Palmer M, Tyler KL (2002) Quantitative CSF PCR in Epstein–Barr virus infections of the central nervous system. *Ann Neurol* 52: 543–8.

Weisberg L (1986) Subdural empyema. Clinical and computed tomographic correlations. *Arch Neurol* 43: 497–500.

Weisse ME, Bass JW, Jarrett RV, Vincent JM (1991) Nonanthrax Bacillus infections of the central nervous system. *Pediatr Infect Dis J* 10: 243–6.

Weller PF (1993) Eosinophilic meningitis. *Am J Med* 95: 250–3.

Wheat LJ, Musial CE, Jenny-Avital E (2005) Diagnosis and management of central nervous system histoplasmosis. *Clin Infect Dis* 40: 844–52.

Whitley RJ (2002) Herpes simplex virus infection. *Semin Pediatr Infect Dis* 13: 6–11.

Whitley RJ, Alford CA (1982) Herpesvirus infections in childhood: diagnostic dilemmas and therapy. *Pediatr Infect Dis* 1: 81–4.

Whitley RJ, Kimberlin DW (2005) Herpes simplex encephalitis: children and adolescents. *Semin Pediatr Infect Dis* 16: 17–23.

Whitley RJ, Soong SJ, Hirsch MS, et al. (1981) Herpes simplex encephalitis: vidarabine therapy and diagnostic problems. *N Engl J Med* 304: 313–8.

Whitley R, Lakeman AD, Nahmias A, Roizman B (1982a) Dna restriction-enzyme analysis of herpes simplex virus isolates obtained from patients with encephalitis. *N Engl J Med* 307: 1060–2.

Whitley RJ, Soong SJ, Linneman C, et al. (1982b) Herpes simplex encephalitis. Clinical Assessment. *JAMA* 247: 317–20.

Whitley RJ, Alford CA, Hirsch MS, et al. (1986) Vidarabine versus acyclovir therapy in herpes simplex encephalitis. *N Engl J Med* 314: 144–9.

Whitley RJ, Cobbs CG, Alford CA, et al. (1989) Diseases that mimic herpes simplex encephalitis. Diagnosis, presentation, and outcome. NIAD Collaborative Antiviral Study Group. *JAMA* 262: 234–9.

Whitney CG, Farley MM, Hadler J, et al. (2003) Decline in invasive pneumococcal disease after the introduction of protein–polysaccharide conjugate vaccine. *N Engl J Med* 348: 1737–46.

Whittington LK, Roscelli JD, Parry WH (1985) Hemorrhagic shock and encephalopathy: further description of a new syndrome. *J Pediatr* 106: 599–602.

WHO (1998) Epidemic meningococcal disease. WHO Fact Sheet 105. Geneva: World Health Organization.

WHO (2008) Bacterial infections. WHO Initiative for Vaccine Research. Geneva: World Health Organization (online at: http://www.who.int/vaccine_research/diseases/soa_bacterial/en/).

Wiktor SZ, Pate EJ, Rosenberg PS, et al. (1997) Mother-to-child transmission of human T-cell lymphotropic virus type I associated with prolonged breast-feeding. *J Hum Virol* 1: 37–44.

Wiley CA, VanPatten PD, Carpenter PM, et al. (1987) Acute ascending necrotizing myelopathy caused by herpes simplex virus type 2. *Neurology* 37: 1791–4.

Wilfert CM (1969) Mumps meningoencephalitis with low cerebrospinal-fluid glucose, prolonged pleocytosis and elevation of protein. *N Engl J Med* 280: 855–9.

Will RG (2003) Acquired prion disease: iatrogenic CJD, variant CJD, kuru. *Br Med Bull* 66: 255–65.

Will RG, Ironside JW, Zeidler M, et al. (1996) A new variant of Creutzfeldt–Jakob disease in the UK. *Lancet* 347: 921–5.

Williams CL, Strobino B, Lee A, et al. (1990) Lyme disease in childhood: clinical and epidemiologic features of ninety cases. *Pediatr Infect Dis J* 9: 10–4.

Williams DN, Schned ES (1990) Lyme disease. Recognizing its many manifestations. *Postgrad Med* 87: 139–40, 143–6.

Willoughby RE, Hammarin AL (2005) Prophylaxis against rabies in children exposed to bats. *Pediatr Infect Dis J* 24: 1109–10.

Willoughby RE, Tieves KS, Hoffman GM, et al. (2005) Survival after treatment of rabies with induction of coma. *N Engl J Med* 352: 2508–14.

Wilson NW, Copeland B, Bastian JF (1990) Posttraumatic meningitis in adolescents and children. *Pediatr Neurosurg* 16: 17–20; discussion 20.

Winter PM, Dung NM, Loan HT, et al. (2004) Proinflammatory cytokines and chemokines in humans with Japanese encephalitis. *J Infect Dis* 190: 1618–26.

Wokke JH, de Koning J, Stanek G, Jennekens FG (1987a) Chronic muscle weakness caused by Borrelia burgdorferi meningoradiculitis. *Ann Neurol* 22: 389–92.

Wokke JH, van Gijn J, Elderson A, Stanek G (1987b) Chronic forms of Borrelia burgdorferi infection of the nervous system. *Neurology* 37: 1031–4.

Wood MJ, Johnson RW, McKendrick MW, et al. (1994) A randomized trial of acyclovir for 7 days or 21 days with and without prednisolone for treatment of acute herpes zoster. *N Engl J Med* 330: 896–900.

Wormser GP, Ramanathan R, Nowakowski J, et al. (2003) Duration of antibiotic therapy for early Lyme disease. A randomized, double-blind, placebo-controlled trial. *Ann Intern Med* 138: 697–704.

Wren SM, Fielder AR, Bethell D, et al. (2004) Cytomegalovirus retinitis in infancy. *Eye* 18: 389–92.

Wright PF, Hatch MH, Kasselberg AG, et al. (1977) Vaccine-associated poliomyelitis in a child with sex-linked agammaglobulinemia. *J Pediatr* 91: 408–12.

Wright PW, Avery WG, Ardill WD, McLarty JW (1993) Initial clinical assessment of the comatose patient: cerebral malaria vs. meningitis. *Pediatr Infect Dis J* 12: 37–41.

Wulff CH (1982) Subacute sclerosing panencephalitis: serial electroencephalographic studies. *J Neurol Neurosurg Psychiatry* 45: 418–21.

Yagishita A, Nakano I, Ushioda T, et al. (1995) Acute encephalopathy with bilateral thalamotegmental involvement in infants and children: imaging and pathology findings. *AJNR* 16: 439–47.

Yalaz K, Anlar B, Oktem F, et al. (1992) Intraventricular interferon and oral inosiplex in the treatment of subacute sclerosing panencephalitis. *Neurology* 42: 488–91.

Yanofsky CS, Hanson PA, Lepow M (1981) Parainfectious acute obstructive hydrocephalus. *Ann Neurol* 10: 62–3.

Yogev R, Bar-Meir M (2004) Management of brain abscesses in children. *Pediatr Infect Dis J* 23: 157–9.

Yoshikawa T (2003) Human herpesvirus-6 and -7 infections in transplantation. *Pediatr Transplant* 7: 11–7.

11
PARAINFECTIOUS AND OTHER INFLAMMATORY DISORDERS OF IMMUNOLOGICAL ORIGIN

Folker Hanefeld and Jean Aicardi

This chapter is concerned with a heterogeneous collection of conditions often of an inflammatory type. In at least some of these diseases, the inflammatory reaction appears to result from an immunological response to various antigens, some of which may be of foreign – e.g. viral or bacterial – origin. However, the antigens, if any, responsible for the immune response often remain unknown and the factors that trigger the response remain obscure. In at least some cases, the immune response seems to be directed against components of the CNS of the host, an autoimmune process.

In all such cases, the result is that the immunological response itself, rather than the agent that originates it, is responsible for most of the harm produced, and therefore treatment may have to be directed against the response rather than against the initial cause, which is often unknown or beyond reach.

Several groups of disorders can be included among the inflammatory conditions of immunological origin. We will consider in succession: (1) demyelinating conditions, including multiple sclerosis; (2) rheumatic diseases; (3) cerebellar ataxias of unknown origin and the myoclonic encephalopathy of Kinsbourne; (4) virus-induced and familial haemophagocytic syndromes and related proliferative disorders; (5) neurological complications of immunization and serotherapy as well as other rare causes of CNS damage of allergic origin.

The postinfectious encephalitides belong to the group of disorders studied in this chapter. Their clinical aspects have been described in Chapter 10 because their clinical presentation and circumstances of occurrence make it difficult to dissociate them from the primary encephalitides and other neurological complications of viral infections. This chapter will more specifically discuss their situation with respect to the demyelinating disorders.

DEMYELINATING DISEASES

MULTIPLE SCLEROSIS AND RELATED DISORDERS
Multiple sclerosis (MS) was first recognized during the 19th century as the most common demyelinating disorder of the brain and spinal cord. Following its definition by Charcot in 1868/69, his pupil Pierre Marie had by 1883 already reported 13 cases of MS with onset in childhood. Since the late 1950s, paediatric MS has re-emerged as a disease entity, and studies in the 1950s established the occurrence of MS in childhood beyond doubt. With our current understanding of inherited leukodystrophies as well as MS, it is acknowledged that children can develop MS. The overlap in the clinical presentation of these disorders results in the difficulty of differential diagnosis of childhood MS. Paediatric MS has been reviewed in a recent report by Banwell (2004).

DEFINITION
MS is the most frequently occurring inflammatory autoimmune disorder of the CNS that is precipitated by undefined environmental factors (infections?) in a genetically predisposed host. MS is one of the major neurological problems in adult neurology. It is, however, rare in children under 10 years and uncommon in adolescents. In a recent study of 4632 cases of MS, only 125, or 2.7%, had their onset before 16 years of age. The mean age at onset in this group was 13 years, and in only 8 patients did the disorder manifest before age 11 years (Duquette et al. 1987). According to Hanefeld et al. (1991), 176 cases in patients under 18 years of age were published between 1980 and 1990, and cases may occur even in infants (Bye et al. 1985, Cole and Stuart 1995, Cole et al. 1995). Girls are more commonly affected than boys, especially among those older than 12 years (Hanefeld et al. 1991). Very early onset under 3 years of age has been reported (Bye et al. 1985, Hanefeld et al. 1991, Cole et al. 1995). The disease is characterized by the successive occurrence of foci of demyelination disseminated in various areas of the CNS white matter, including the periventricular region, spinal cord, brainstem, cerebellum and optic nerve.

From a diagnostic point of view, the essential feature of MS is the dissemination of lesions in both time and space.

MS typically affects young adults, with a frequency of 0.05–0.15% among Caucasians. About 5% of all MS patients experience their first clinical symptoms prior to 16 years of age.

A variety of terms are used to describe MS in children and adolescents, including early-onset MS, and childhood or paediatric (onset) MS. The term true childhood MS in contrast to juvenile MS was also proposed by us to differentiate between the very rare cases with onset before 10 years of age (puberty) and those with first symptoms occurring between 10 and 16 years. Most paediatric MS cases follow a remitting–relapsing course (95%), while primary progressive forms are extremely rare. A recent consensus conference agreed upon the terminology 'paediatric MS' for all cases with onset of the disease prior to the age of 18 years (Krupp et al. 2007).

PATHOLOGY

The classical pathological MS lesion is the plaque. Histopathological hallmarks are: (1) an inflammatory infiltration consisting of T-cells, macrophages and few B-cells; (2) demyelination of white and grey matter with loss of oligodendrocytes in chronic states; (3) damage to axons with significant axonal loss; and (4) gliosis with astrocytic proliferation.

Multiple lesions (plaques) are formed of round areas of greyish gelatinous appearance, scattered in the white matter. Within the plaques, which are generally located around small vessels, there is destruction of the myelin sheath with relative preservation of axons. In recent plaques, oedema and inflammatory cells can be seen and neutral lipids that represent myelin breakdown products are present. Old lesions are mostly gliotic with astrocytic proliferation (McDonald et al. 1992). Lesions have a predilection for the optic nerves, periventricular white matter, brainstem, cerebellum and spinal cord.

There is now agreement that the inflammatory reaction in MS is consistent with that of a T-cell-mediated immune reaction. Autoreactive T-cells cross the blood–brain barrier and activate microglia (macrophages). Binding of the putative MS antigen by the trimolecular complex – the T-cell receptor (TCR) and class II MHC molecules on antigen presenting cells – may trigger an enhanced immune response and via inflammatory CD4+ type 1 helper (TH1) cells ultimately immune-mediated injury of oligodendrocytes and myelin. Toxic inflammatory mediators (like the macrophage toxins, TNF-α, proteases) and nitric oxide (NO) are thought to damage myelin and axons, and at the same time these cytokines together with growth promoting factors released by astrocytes and microglia promote remyelination (Hemmer et al. 2002).

Since axonal loss is most prominent in secondary progressive MS, it is proposed that the chronic axonopathy is not due directly to inflammation, but results from loss of trophic support provided to axons.

Four subtypes of demyelination in MS based on immune-pathological findings have been defined (Lucchinetti et al. 2000, Lassmann et al. 2001). Subtypes 1 and 2 (autoimmune types) are characterized by macrophage/T-cell mediated demyelination and antibody-mediated demyelination respectively. In type 3, apoptosis of oligodendrocytes and loss of myelin-associated glycoprotein (MAG) are seen, while subtype 4 is considered a primary oligodendrocytopathy.

AETIOLOGY

The aetiology of MS remains unknown in spite of an enormous amount of investigation. Two main factors are usually considered as essential. Currently, the importance of dysfunction of the immunological system is accepted as a basic factor; however, the nature of the supposed precipitating factor remains elusive. Recent data suggest that the activity of the immune system in human beings is modulated by a network of regulatory controls mediated, in part, through inducer and suppressor T-cells. Abnormalities of circulating T-cell subsets have been demonstrated in both adults and children with multiple sclerosis (Hauser et al. 1983, Rose et al. 1988, Olsson 1992, Hohlfeld 1997). Loss of T-suppressor/cytotoxic cells with an increase in the ratio of inducer to suppressor cells (T4:T5) has been found during attacks. Other anomalies affect the production of immunoglobulins in the CSF, which in a majority of adults and children with MS are elevated and/or demonstrate oligoclonal banding.

The genetic predisposition to MS is verified by twin studies and the observation of recurrence of MS in families. Fifteen per cent of MS patients have affected relatives, and the recurrence risk is higher in siblings (3%), parents (2%) and children (2%), and lower for 2nd and 3rd degree relatives. Concordance in identical twins is at least 35%. Multiplex families indicate that genetic factors determine susceptibility and also the course of MS. Disability is highest in male offspring of affected fathers. So far, only the human leukocyte antigen (HLA) DR15 and DR6 alleles have been associated with the development of MS, and only in Caucasians. HLA DR15 alleles are associated with a lower age at onset of adult MS (reviewed by Compston and Svegard 2001).

An infectious origin of MS in childhood has long been suspected. However, in spite of extensive epidemiological studies, no single pathogen has been identified as a cause of the disease. During the last decade, interest has concentrated on *Chlamydia pneumoniae* and herpesviruses, in particular HHV-6 and Epstein–Barr virus (EBV). Sriram et al. (1999) suggested *C. pneumoniae* as a possible cause of MS; subsequent studies detected *C. pneumoniae* DNA in CSF of patients (including children) with definite MS (21%) as well as in CSF of patients with a variety of other neurological disorders (43%) (Gieffers et al. 2001). A high seroprevalence of EBV antibodies in MS patients has been found (Alotaibi et al. 2004). Vaccinations against hepatitis B, influenza, measles and rubella are not associated with an increased risk of MS or optic neuritis in adults (Confavreux et al. 2001, DeStefano et al. 2003) or in children (Mikaeloff et al. 2007).

CLINICAL FEATURES

MS can present in several different manners, from acute forms leading to death in only a few weeks to a completely asymptomatic disease incidentally discovered at autopsy. Reports on paediatric MS have been retrospective studies. The following description is therefore based on these reports and the personal experience from a prospective nationwide survey performed in Germany during a 3-year period between 1997 and 1999. The clinical features of MS result from an inflammatory reaction of white matter in the brain, optic nerves and spinal cord, separated

TABLE 11.1
The 2005 revisions to the McDonald diagnostic criteria for multiple sclerosis (MS)*

Clinical presentation	Additional data needed for MS diagnosis
Two or more attacks[1]; objective clinical evidence of two or of two or more lesions	None[2]
Two or more attacks[1]; objective clinical evidence evidence of one lesion	Dissemination in space, demonstrated by: • MRI or • Two or more MRI-detected lesions consistent with MS plus positive CSF[2] or • Await further clinical attack[1] implicating a different site
One attack[1]; objective clinical evidence of two or more lesions	Dissemination in time, demonstrated by: • MRI or • Second clinical attack[1]
One attack[1]; objective clinical evidence of one lesion (monosymptomatic presentation; clinically isolated syndrome)	Dissemination in space, demonstrated by: • MRI or • Two or more MRI-detected lesions consistent with MS plus positive CSF[2] and dissemination in time, demonstrated by: • MRI or • Second clinical attack[1]
Insidious neurological progression suggestive of MS	One year of dissemination in space demonstrated retrospectively or prospectively determined by two of the following: • Positive brain MRI (nine T_2 lesions or four or more T_2 lesions with positive VEP) • Positive spinal cord MRI (two focal T_2 lesions) • Positive CSF[2]

*Polman et al. (2005).

[1]An attack is defined as an episode of neurological disturbance for which causative lesions are likely to be inflammatory and demyelinating in nature. There should be subjective report (backed up by objective findings) or objective observation that the event lasts for at least 24 hours.

[2]Positive CSF determined by oligoclonal bands detected by established methods (isoelectric focusing) different from any such bands in serum, or by an increased IgG index.

TABLE 11.2
Initial symptoms in 100 cases of paediatric MS*

Monosymptomatic (n=54)	
Visual (optic neuritis)	19 (4)
Pyramidal	9
Cerebellar	3
Brainstem	9
Sensory	9
Bowel and bladder dysfunction	0
Cerebral/mental	1
Seizures	1
Acute encephalopathy	3
Polysymptomatic (n=46)	

*Unpublished data from the Göttingen study.

in space and time. Diagnostic criteria have been formulated by Poser et al. (1983) and McDonald et al. (2001). The McDonald criteria were revised by Polman et al. (2005) and are shown in Table 11.1.

These criteria can also be applied to paediatric MS, although elimination of conditions that may mimic the disease often demands further consideration. It can, however, be stated that MS in adults and children is basically the same disease (Hanefeld 1992). The Poser criteria have been used in most paediatric studies. It must be stressed, however, that Poser and McDonald criteria cannot be applied without careful examination of the patient in order to classify symptoms and signs as either uni- or multifocal.

The course of MS can be classified into three different types: primary progressive, relapsing–remitting, and secondary progressive MS. More than 95% of paediatric MS patients present with the relapsing–remitting type. Secondary progressive MS might evolve after a variable disease duration that seems to be longer than in adult MS patients. Over the 3 years from 1997 to 1999, the Göttingen Study recorded 132 patients with onset of MS before the age of 16 years; this yields an overall incidence in Germany of 0.3 cases of MS per 100,000 children per year. The diagnosis of MS was very rare for children younger than 10 years of age, while the number of cases increased particularly in the 13–15 years age group, especially in girls. Boys are equally represented in the very young group of MS patients. By 14–15 years of age, the female:male ratio has risen to 2.2, as it is in adult MS.

Primary symptoms of paediatric MS do not seem to differ substantially from those described for adult-onset MS. Frequent initial clinical features are deficits in visual, sensory, brainstem, cerebellar or motor functions. Vertigo is frequently reported as an early symptom. A polysymptomatic presentation is reported in about 50–60% of paediatric MS patients (Table 11.2).

Besides well-defined neurological symptoms, patients with early-onset multiple sclerosis (EOMS) may complain of fatigue and show emotional and learning problems at school. Several studies (Bye et al. 1985, Hanefeld et al. 1991, Sindern et al. 1992, Bauer and Hanefeld 1993) emphasized the relative frequency of systemic manifestations such as fever and vomiting, and of encephalopathic presentation, especially in cases of very early onset. Cognitive deficits have been demonstrated in EOMS patients by Banwell and Anderson (2005) and by Krupp and Macallister (2005). Remarkably, these deficits were already notable in children with no demonstrable physical disability. In one personal case, learning difficulties at school between the ages of 10 and 12 years were seen as the first symptom before a mild hemiparesis developed two years later. Child and mother went through an odyssey of diagnostic procedures before the correct diagnosis of MS was reached at the age of 14 years.

In the usual remittent–relapsing forms, the initial attack of paediatric MS is commonly followed by a near-complete to complete clinical recovery usually within 4–6 weeks. Sixty per cent of children relapse during the first year (Cole and Stuart 1995, Boiko et al. 2002, Ghezzi et al. 2002, Pohl et al. 2005). The mean rate of relapse in paediatric MS is 1.4 attacks per year, higher than in adult-onset MS (Weinshenker et al. 1989), but symptoms remit faster than in adult MS (Ruggieri et al. 2004).

A large series of acute inflammatory demyelination in childhood included 296 children under 16 years of age after an initial demyelinating episode (Mikaeloff et al. 2004b). The initial diagnosis was suggestive of MS in 96 (33%), of acute disseminating encephalomyelitis (ADEM) in 119 (40%), and of "a focal episode" in 81 of the affected children. At the end of follow-up (mean 2.9±3 years) 168 (57%) met the diagnosis of MS, while 85 (29%) were diagnosed with monophasic ADEM. One fifth of the patients with the final diagnosis of MS were considered to have ADEM at the clinical onset.

Optic neuritis (ON) was noticed amongst the symptoms at the first attack in 35%. ON, an age above 10 years, and an initial MRI with multiple well-defined periventricular or subcortical lesions were predictors for a second attack.

The same authors analysed prognostic MRI factors for relapse after acute CNS inflammatory demyelination in 116 children (Mikaeloff et al. 2004a). Patients with corpus callosum long axis perpendicular lesions and with the presence of well-defined other lesions showed a high rate of second attack.

Implications to be drawn from this and other studies are limited by the relatively short follow-up.

ON as primary symptom may present as sudden or progressive visual loss, loss of colour perception, or pain with ocular movements. Lucchinetti et al. (1997) reviewed the follow-up information of 94 cases with the initial diagnosis of idiopathic ON prior to the age of 16 years. By 10 years' follow-up, 13% had progressed to definite MS, a proportion that increased to 26% by 40 years. In a study of 21 children from Finland with ON, 9 developed clinically definite MS (Riikonen et al. 1988a).

NEUROIMAGING, NEUROPHYSIOLOGICAL AND OTHER LABORATORY FINDINGS
Neuroimaging
CT may show areas of low density and/or of contrast enhancement in 50–66% of patients. MRI abnormalities can be demonstrated in 70% to over 90% of patients with definite or possible MS (Ormerod et al. 1986, 1987; Paty et al. 1988; Millner et al. 1990). In most patients, several areas of increased signal appear on T_2-weighted sequences (Fig. 11.1). These areas are of variable size and may be located in the cerebellum, brainstem, spinal cord and hemispheric white matter. In this last case, their periventricular location is suggestive (Ormerod et al. 1984, Isaac et al. 1988, Miller et al. 1989, Willoughby et al. 1989), but the images are not specific as they have been reported in adults with vascular disorders (Ormerod et al. 1984), in patients with other

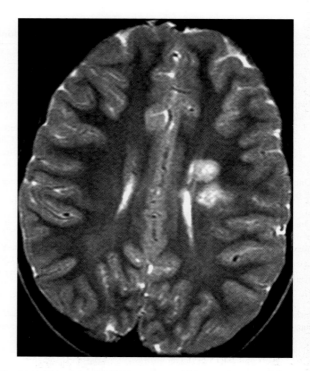

Fig. 11.1. T_2-weighted MRI in 10-year-old boy with MS showing two periventricular lesions.

inflammatory conditions, including HTLV-1 infection (Jacobson et al. 1990), in patients with Lyme disease (Chapter 10) and, occasionally, in subjects without evidence of neurological disease (Baker et al. 1985). In addition to its diagnostic value, MRI also indicates that new lesions frequently appear over a period of a few months in asymptomatic patients (Ormerod et al. 1987), thus posing the problem of definition of an attack (Millner et al. 1990). MRI following gadolinium enhancement enables recent lesions that take up the product, indicating impairment of the blood–brain barrier with consequent oedema, to be distinguished from old plaques that do not enhance and are probably mainly gliotic (Miller et al. 1988b). Lesions of the optic nerve can also be detected by MRI (Miller et al. 1988a, Koopmans et al. 1989). MRI in children seems to give similar results (Golden and Woody 1987, Haas et al. 1987, Millner et al. 1990).

MS in children under 10 years of age
In children below 10 years of age and especially in infants or children under 5 years, MS may have unusual features clinically and from the viewpoint of imaging. Seizures have been reported to occur more frequently than in adults, and acute encephalopathic states with diminished consciousness, seizures and pyramidal tract signs may occur (Bye et al. 1985, Shaw and Alvord 1987, Cole et al. 1995). Intellectual deterioration can be seen early in young patients (Bye et al. 1985).

In some cases diagnosed as MS, large lesions of the white matter (Maeda et al. 1989), atypical butterfly-like enhancement and ring enhancement have been reported (Ishihara et al. 1984, Morimoto et al. 1985). Some of these cases were also clinically

TABLE 11.3
**Frequency of CSF findings in early-onset MS (EOMS)
and adult-onset MS (AOMS)***

	EOMS	AOMS
Oligoclonal IgG	92%	98%
Normal blood–CSF barrier	87%	88%
Intrathecal IgG fraction >10%	69%	72%
Pleocytosis (>4/µL)	66%	58%

*Adapted from Pohl et al. (2004).

atypical, and the diagnosis of MS may not be demonstrated. However, a similar appearance has been described in adult patients (Vliegenthart et al. 1985). An association between certain mitochondrial mutations responsible for Leber hereditary optic neuropathy (especially the nt11778 mutation) and the development of an MS-like disease with prominent early optic nerve disease has been reported (Chalmers and Harding 1996, Funalot et al. 1996), especially in women. The significance of this association remains to be explored.

CSF studies (Table 11.3)
These are also largely identical to those in adults, especially regarding the presence of oligoclonal banding, which was present in 85% of the cases of Boutin et al. (1988). In children, however, pleocytosis is often more marked than in older patients, with 50–100 lymphocytes/mm^3 (Bye et al. 1985, Sindern et al. 1992).

The CSF analysis has to include the basic work-up (cell count, protein content) as well as lactate, cytology, and the determination of intrathecal IgG synthesis via detection of oligoclonal IgG bands not present in a parallel serum analysis. Pohl et al. (2004) studied the CSF in 136 patients with onset before 16 years. Cell counts at the first lumbar puncture were in the range of 0–61 cells/µL, and 66% of patients showed mild CSF pleocytosis. The total protein content, measured in 110 patients, was in the range of 100–700 mg/L (controls 130–450 mg/L). Intrathecal IgG synthesis was detectable in a total of 125 patients (92%) at the first analysis. Of 25 patients with onset of MS before the age of 10 years, 24 demonstrated oligoclonal IgG at the time of first spinal tap. In contrast, intrathecal IgA was detectable in only 6% of cases, and intrathecal IgM in 36%. The detection of intrathecal IgG is highly dependent on the method used. With respect to the wide range of differential diagnosis in EOMS, the analysis of oligoclonal IgG, if necessary by repeated spinal taps, is recommended as state of the art diagnostic in every child with suspected MS. In particular, the differentiation between MS and ADEM might become possible at an early stage of the disease.

Minimum blood testing in a child suspected of having MS should include complete blood count with differential, erythrocyte sedimentation rate, antinuclear antibody, *B. burgdorferi* and HIV serology.

Neurophysiological evaluations
These should comprise EEG and visual, somatosensory and auditory evoked potentials. Visual evoked potentials are fre-

quently abnormal (delayed or low amplitude) as a result of the predilection of the disease for the visual pathways.

DIAGNOSIS
The diagnosis of paediatric MS requires great accuracy, especially if established early in the disease course (e.g. before the second attack). The younger a child and the more atypical the presenting clinical, laboratory and neuroimaging features are, the more care is needed in establishing the diagnosis.

The diagnostic work-up should include MRI, neurophysiology, ophthalmology, CSF and blood analyses in every child. Depending on the clinical presentation, additional examinations like MR spectroscopy, angiography, CT, and skin or muscle biopsy might be indicated.

MRI should include cerebral and spinal cord imaging with and without gadolinium in order to determine disease burden and disease activity (Hahn et al. 2004, Mikaeloff et al. 2004a).

In spite of careful analysis of anamnestic, clinical and paraclinical findings, a substantial number of cases will remain unclassified following an initial demyelinating event (IDE). It is customary to separate cases of definite, probable and possible MS (Poser et al. 1983). Clinically, definite cases are characterized by the occurrence of two attacks and clinical evidence of two separate lesions, or two attacks and clinical evidence of one lesion plus paraclinical evidence of another separate lesion. The two attacks must involve different parts of the CNS, must be separated by a period of at least one month, and must last a minimum of 24 hours. Laboratory-supported definite MS consists of two attacks plus either clinical or paraclinical evidence of one lesion plus IgG oligoclonal banding in CSF, or one attack plus clinical evidence of two separate lesions, or one attack plus clinical evidence of one lesion and paraclinical evidence of another lesion.

The diagnostic criteria currently applied to children with suspected MS are based on observation in "classical MS seen in a typical adult population of western European ethnic origin" (Polman et al. 2005). The core concept of these criteria (Poser, McDonald) rests on determining dissemination of lesions in time and space. Although the revised McDonald criteria "cannot even be applied without careful clinical evaluation of the patient" (Polman et al. 2005), the diagnosis of MS relies heavily on different types of imaging criteria to demonstrate dissemination of lesions in time and space. In paediatric-onset MS cases, presenting features are more atypical and therefore less sensitive. The diagnosis of MS in children, in particular in those younger than 10–12 years of age, requires the elimination of alternative disorders causing demyelination and mimicking the disease.

The term 'clinically isolated syndrome' (CIS) has been introduced in adult neurology to designate suggestive acute or subacute episodes of neurological disturbance due to a white matter lesion, e.g. optic neuritis, isolated brainstem or partial spinal cord syndromes, that cannot be firmly diagnosed at the first episode. An IDE may be classified as either MS or ADEM if it presents with clear symptoms of encephalopathy, or as a CIS in a situation lacking these symptoms. It must, however, be stressed that in young children this might be especially difficult because

TABLE 11.4
Differential diagnosis of MS in childhood

Disease categories	Examples
Infectious (post-/parainfectious)	Neuroborreliosis (Lyme disease) HIV Subacute sclerosing panencephalitis (SSPE) Haemophagocytic syndromes
Genetic/metabolic leukodystrophies	Adrenoleukodystrophy (ALD) Metachromatic leukodystrophy (MCD)/vanishing white matter disease (VWMD)
Mitochondrial/OXPHOS	Mitochondrial encephalomyopathy with lactic acidosis and stroke-like episodes (MELAS) Leber hereditary optic neuropathy (LHON)
Macrophage activation syndromes	Familial hemphagocytic lymphohistiocytosis
Immunologic/rheumatic (incl. immune vasculitis)	Lupus erythematosus Behçet disease Antiphospholipid-antibody syndrome Neurosarcoidosis
Neoplastic/paraneoplastic	Lymphoma Histiocytosis (Langerhans)
Endocrine	Hashimoto leukencephalopthy
Toxic/nutritional	Methotrexate Vitamin B_{12} deficiency
Vascular	Moya moya CADASIL
Inflammatory demyelinating	Viral encephalitis

Isolated demyelinating syndromes	Acute disseminating encephalomyelitis (ADEM)
	Monophasic isolated demyelination:
	    Optic neuritis
	    Transverse myelitis
	Others

MS variants	Acute MS (Marburg) Neuromyelitis optica (Devic) Concentric sclerosis (Baló) Myelinoclastic diffuse sclerosis (Schilder)

of the presence of symptoms like headache, fever and clinical signs of raised intracranial pressure frequently occurring during an acute attack of MS. The differentiation between ADEM and an acute 'encephalitic' MS attack is sometimes impossible.

DIFFERENTIAL DIAGNOSIS
Differentiating ADEM from MS may be particularly difficult. Several so-called 'variants of MS' have been described, in addition to ADEM. They are described below. Their relation to classical MS remains unknown.

The differential diagnosis of MS includes a wide range of clinically fluctuating neurological diseases ranging from recurrent hemiplegia and moyamoya disease or lupus erythematosus to the metabolic crisis in adrenoleukodystrophy or mitochondrial disorders. The following table lists the main categories of differential diagnoses of MS in childhood. Clinical and diagnostic details of white matter disorders with prominent demyelination and a proven or probable genetic/metabolic defect are considered in Chapters 8, 10 and 13. The major conditions are listed in Table 11.4.

TREATMENT AND MANAGEMENT
No curative therapy for MS is yet available. Currently, the aim

of drugs that modify the cause of MS is to prevent or reduce the frequency of clinical relapses and the progression of disability.

Treatment of the acute attack and relapses
No therapeutic trial for relapses has yet been conducted in the paediatric MS population. Preventive therapy of relapses is therefore based on experience in the management of adult MS. Corticosteroids are the treatment of choice for the first attack and relapses associated with significant neurological impairment. The dose of 20–30 mg/kg/day methylprednisolone as a 1–2 hour infusion in the morning for 3–5 consecutive days is recommended. Steroid taper should be kept as short as possible. Most frequent side effects include facial flushing, sleeping difficulties and increased appetite. Intravenous immunoglobulins are an option in special situations. Plasma exchange has been proposed in children as an alternative treatment for recurrent relapses occurring in a short period.

Disease modifying therapy: immunomodulatory therapy
There is class I level evidence for the treatment with three preparations of interferon beta (IFNβ) and glatirameracetate. According to the American Academy of Neurology all four medications reduce the frequency of relapses by approximately

30% and reduce the disease activity seen on brain MRI. All have little or no effect on the progression of disability in adult patients. Two studies describe the tolerability and safety of IFNβ-1a (Rebif®) and IFNβ-1b (Betaseron®) in retrospectively analysed cohorts of 51 and 43 patients respectively.

IFNβ-1a (22 and 44μg) was found to be generally safe and well tolerated. Side effects included injection site reactions, flu-like symptoms, leukopenia, neutropenia and elevation in liver transaminases. The yearly relapse rate decreased from a mean pre-treatment value of 1.9 to 0.8. Twenty-one patients were relapse-free during treatment (mean treatment duration in this group was 1.5 years; range 6 months to 4.1 years). EDSS (Expanded Disability Status Scale) scores remained stable in 48 of the 51 treated patients (Pohl et al. 2005).

In a cohort of 43 children and adolescents treated for a mean of 29.2 months, safety and tolerability of IFNβ-1b (Betaseron®) were retrospectively reviewed by an international working group (Banwell et al. 2006). Mean age at start of treatment was 13 years, and 8 children were below the age of 10 years. Doses of 250μg (8 MIU) were given subcutaneously every other day. No serious adverse events were reported. Most common side effects included flu-like symptoms (15/43), abnormal liver function test (11/43) and injection site reactions (9/43).

IFNβ-1a (Avonex®) is administered intramuscularly in a dose of 30μg once a week. The spectrum of side effects is similar to that observed in the other interferons. No other data on large numbers of paediatric patients are available.

Glatiramer acetate (GA, Copaxone®) appeared to be safe and well tolerated in 7 children with MS at the daily adult dose of 20mg during a period of 24 months (Kornek et al. 2003).

Intravenous immunoglobulin therapy (IVIG, 0.4g/kg/day for 5 days) has been proposed for paediatric MS patients whose symptoms relapse within days or weeks of discontinuation of steroids (Banwell 2004).

Recommendations for disease-modifying therapies in paediatric MS:

- *Initiation:* Immunomodulatory treatment should be started in all children and adolescents with relapsing–recurring disease (defined clinically or by MRI) as soon as MS diagnosis has been secured. However, there is no consensus on the definition of active disease. The following definition seems reasonable: more than one exacerbation in a period of 1–2 years and/or new T_2 bright or gadolinium-enhancing lesions on repeat MRI over the same time frame.

- *Choice of drug:* First-line drugs approved for adult MS are IFNβ-1a and -1b, and GA. Azathioprine should remain a second-line drug. IVIG treatment may be considered for very young children.

Another FDA-approved immunosuppressive medication, mitoxanthrone (Novanthrone®) has been used for adult patients with worsening MS. Other immunosuppressive agents like metothrexate and cyclophosphamide should be considered as therapeutic options only in individual cases.

The management of MS in childhood has to consider medical problems (drugs, special diets, physiotherapy and occupational therapy) and issues of psychosocial support. The implications of the diagnosis of MS in childhood for the child and family include: (1) understanding the nature of the disease; (2) coping with disabilities, potential and real; (3) schooling and education; (4) choices for the professional life; and (5) partnership and family planning. These problems become particularly relevant in children with an affected mother or other relative with an advanced stage of the disease.

The treatment of pediatric MS has recently been reviewed by Krupp and Macallister (2005) and by Pohl et al. (2007).

OUTCOME
Within the first decade of the disease, most paediatric MS patients have a more favourable outcome as compared to adult MS patients. A transition to a progressive disease course, associated with a worse prognosis, is seen in only a relatively few paediatric MS patients during this time frame. The mean disease duration to acquire a moderate impairment as measured by the Expanded Disability Status Scale (EDSS) is about twice as long for paediatric as for adult MS patients (to reach EDSS 4, 11 years for adult MS patients as compared to 20 years for paediatric MS patients). On the other hand, due to the young age at onset, the same patients are significantly younger than their adult counterparts when a compromising level of disability has accumulated (32 years versus 41 years of age for EDSS 4) (Ghezzi et al. 2002). All these data originate from retrospective studies with obvious inherent difficulties in interpretation, and prospective longitudinal outcome studies for paediatric MS are needed to evaluate the prognosis of MS in childhood with greater accuracy.

MS VARIANTS
NEUROMYELITIS OPTICA (NMO) (DEVIC DISEASE)
Neuromyelitis optica is characterized clinically by the occurrence, simultaneously or in rapid succession, of optic neuritis and transverse myelitis and pathologically, by inflammatory and destructive lesions of the white matter with necrosis, cavitation and acute axonal damage. Perivascular immunoglobulin deposition and complement activation implicate their involvement in the pathogenesis of NMO and resemble the antibody/complement-mediated pattern of MS (type II). Diagnostic criteria have been formulated by Wingerchuk (2006). Necessary criteria are optic neuritis (ON), acute myelitis and no evidence of clinical disease outside the optic nerve or spinal cord. Supportive criteria include negative brain MRI at onset, spinal cord MRI with signal abnormality extending over more than three vertebral segments, and CSF pleocytosis of $>50 \times 10^6$/L white blood cells or $>5 \times 10^6$/L neutrophils. Minor supportive criteria include bilateral ON, severe ON with fixed visual acuity of less than 20/200 in at least one eye, and severe, fixed, attack-related weakness in one or more limbs.

An autoantibody (NMO-IgG) specifically associated with NMO has been recently identified (Lennon et al. 2004). NMO-IgG binds near or at the blood–brain barrier microvessels, pial, subpial and Virchow–Robin spaces at the site of aquaporin 4 expression (Pittock et al. 2006b). The autoantibody NMO-IgG distinguishes neuromyelitis optica from multiple sclerosis. However, the clinical diagnosis may be very difficult especially as a recurrent course may be observed (Wingerchuk and Weinschenker 2003, Pittock et al. 2006a). Successful treatment with plasmaexchange was reported in a steroid-unresponsive case (Cox et al. 2005). Single cases of possible NMO have been seen in children. The exact diagnosis has become feasible with the demonstration of NMO-IgG and should be considered in children presenting with suspicious clinical symptoms and paraclinical signs.

CONCENTRIC SCLEROSIS OF BALÓ

The classical lesion of Baló concentric sclerosis (BCS) consists of rings of myelin separated by rings of demyelination. BCS is an acute neurological illness with the profile of acute MS in young adults. There is still controversy whether BCS represents a variant of MS or a different clinical entity. BCS is recognizable on MRI and shows the alternating layers of myelinated and unmyelinated tissue. CSF may show intrathecal synthesis of IgG oligoclonal bands. Clinically, BCS presents as an acute, sometimes monophasic encephalopathy with a fulminant course that can be rapidly fatal. Imaging features are pathognomonic (Caracciolo et al. 2001, Kavanaagh et al. 2006). A BCS-like picture has been described in a 13-year-old girl with primary HHV-6 infection (Pohl et al. 2005). Treatment of BCS with steroids, other immunosuppressants and plasmapheresis has been tried with varying efficacy.

ACUTE MS OF MARBURG TYPE (ENCEPHALOMYELITIS PERIAXALIS SCLEROTICANS)

Acute sclerosis was first recognized as a variant of MS by Marburg in 1906. He reviewed 19 cases from the literature and added three of his own patients, describing clinical symptoms, course and pathological findings in great detail. The patients presented with a severe encephalopathy of acute onset with a progressive course leading to early death mainly due to brainstem involvement. Marburg's disease presents as severe demyelinating encephalomyelitis leading to death within one year of onset. About 5% of all MS patients can be categorized as having Marburg's variant (Mathews 1998). The prevalence in paediatric MS patients is unknown.

SCHILDER MYELINOCLASTIC DIFFUSE SCLEROSIS (ENCEPHALOMYELITIS PERIAXALIS DIFFUSA)

The term diffuse sclerosis was initially given to a demyelinating condition thought to represent a single disease (Poser et al. 1986). Based on the morphological descriptions in Schilder's first case report, Poser used the term Schilder's myelinoclastic diffuse sclerosis. It has since become clear that it includes several different disorders of inflammatory or metabolic origin. The recognition of inborn errors of metabolism as possible causes of demyelination in many white matter disorders might be an explanation for the confusion about what is currently known as Schilder disease, as some metabolic diseases, especially adrenoleukodystrophy, were not initially distinguished.

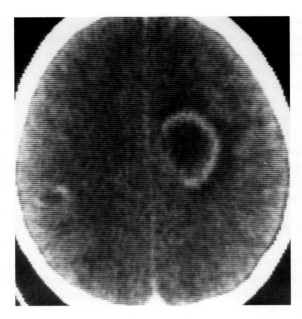

Fig. 11.2. Schilder disease. 11-year-old boy who presented with right hemiplegia of recent onset, headache and papilloedema. CT shows ring images in left central region and smaller lesion in opposite parietal area. Stereotaxic puncture yielded only yellow fluid with some necrotic debris. Clinical symptoms disappeared rapidly on steroid therapy. Repeat CT was normal but MRI showed persistence of small area of increased signal on T_2-weighted sequences.

This condition is currently defined as an acquired progressive subacute or chronic demyelinating disease of unknown origin. It causes large demyelinating lesions of the hemispheric cerebral white matter with relative sparing of the axons and sparing of subcortical U-fibres (Mehler and Rabinowich 1988). The histological characteristics of brain tissue are identical to those of MS (Kepes 1993, Afifi et al. 1994). At least one, and more commonly two or more roughly symmetrical bilateral plaques of large dimensions (>3.2 cm) are present in the centrum ovale and can be demonstrated by brain imaging. Imaging shows a low signal from the lesions, with peripheral enhancement after contrast. Cavitation may occur and can mimic a brain abscess. Smaller similar satellite lesions are often present. The histological characteristics of brain tissue are identical to those of MS. The clinical features include focal neurological signs (usually hemiplegia), which may be associated with cerebellar symptoms, progressive clumsiness, impaired vision, headaches, lethargy, behavioural deterioration and personality changes. Intracranial hypertension may occur and papilloedema may be found (Konkol et al. 1987).

Brain lesions in Schilder disease are extremely sensitive to steroids, which produce a rapid decrease in their size and disappearance of contrast enhancement. Hyperintense images on MRI appear to persist for prolonged periods (several years). T_1-weighted sequences show the persistence of focal loss of myelin.

The diagnosis remains one of exclusion and rests largely on neuroimaging techniques (Mehler and Rabinowich 1989). It should be consisered in children presenting with an 'ADEM-like' symptomatology with large asymmetrical, sharply outlined white matter lesions in one or both hemispheres on MRI. Exclusion of adrenoleukodystrophy by determination of very-long-chain fatty acid plasma level is an absolute requirement. Cerebral abscess is an essential consideration as ring images may be identical to those in Schilder disease (Fig. 11.2).

The relationship of Schilder disease to MS remains unclear (Poser et al. 1986). It is often regarded as a variant type. Whilst transitional forms with small satellite plaques in addition to the large ones have been described (Poser et al. 1986), the age of occurrence, clinical features and course, and the frequent absence of IgG oligoclonal CSF banding in cases of Schilder disease are clinically suggestive.

OPTIC NEURITIS (ON)

ON consists of involvement of the nerve by inflammation, degeneration or demyelination resulting in impaired function (Riikonen et al. 1988a, Balcer 2006). ON is often an early symptom of MS, and it has been suggested that both disorders have the same aetiology. This is in contrast with the experience of Riikonen et al. (1988a) who observed the development of MS in 12 of their 21 children. This discrepancy remains unexplained. The higher incidence in recent series may reflect the improvement of diagnostic methods for MS such as MRI.

A number of viral infections such as measles, varicella and mumps (Kline et al. 1982, Purvin et al. 1988, Lucchinetti et al. 1997) can also induce ON, either in isolation or associated with other manifestations of disseminated encephalomyelitis. ON may also follow immunization with live vaccines (Riikonen 1989) and has been reported in Miller Fisher syndrome (Toshniwal 1987). Interestingly, recurrent ON has been found in association with *C. pneumoniae* CNS infection (Pohl et al. 2006) and with varicella-zoster infection (Pless and Malik 2003).

Sudden monocular or binocular reduction of visual activity is the major manifestation. It may be preceded by headaches or painful eye movements (Riikonen et al. 1988a). Initially, there is blurred vision with progression within a few days to partial or complete blindness. Bilateral involvement is present in over half of cases and occurs either simultaneously or sequentially. It was observed in 58% in the recent US study of Wilejto et al. (2006). The neuritis may be retrobulbar, in which case fundoscopic examination is normal. In children, however, a swollen optic disc (neuropapillitis) is seen in three quarters of cases during the acute phase (Kriss et al. 1988). In some cases, vasculitic changes such as retinal exudates, local vessel tortuosity or sheathing of veins may be seen (Riikonen et al. 1988a). Visual field examination reveals central scotomas, and visual evoked responses are delayed, a finding that persists for several years even when recovery seems complete. Involvement of the optic chiasm can produce unusual visual field deficits (Newman et al. 1991).

Most patients recover normal or useful vision despite the frequent persistence of optic atrophy, but colour vision and stereoscopic vision may remain impaired. Persistent severe loss of vision is rare.

In diagnosing ON it is essential to exclude other causes of acute impairment of vision, in particular compression of the optic nerve, which may closely mimic unilateral ON (Chapter 17). Malingering and hysteria can be excluded, when necessary, by testing the visual evoked response. Papilloedema is not accompanied by early loss of vision and is therefore readily excluded when fundoscopic manifestations of neuropapillitis include severe disc swelling with haemorrhages. MRI may demonstrate demyelinating lesions in one or both optic nerves (Miller et al. 1988a, Jacobs et al. 1991).

The occurrence of ON raises the possibility of its being the first manifestation of MS. The risk was estimated to be lower in children than in adults, and was found to be 28% by Riikonen (1989). However, Wilejto et al. (2006) observed the development of MS in 13 of their 36 children after a 2-year follow-up. Contrary to most previous studies they found the risk to be greater in bilateral cases. Features predictive of MS include CSF pleocytosis and intrathecal IgG production of oligoclonal antibodies (Riikonen et al. 1988a,b). MRI is indicated in all cases. Wilejto et al. found that all of their 13 patients with brain lesions seen on MRI had developed MS after a 2-year follow-up whereas none of those with normal MR did. Areas of abnormal signal were found in 71% of cases in one series (Riikonen et al. 1988b). Their association with IgG oligoclonal bands in CSF and HLA Dr 2 group is indicative of a very high risk of developing disseminated disease (Jacobs et al. 1986). Recurrences of ON can rarely in patients who do not develop MS (Pless and Malik 2003). In such cases immunosuppressive treatment may allow discontinuation of corticoid treatment (Myers et al. 2006).

Treatment with corticosteroids is effective in shortening the duration of attacks but not on overall evolution or prevention of the development of MS. Corticosteroids, especially in the form of methylprednisolone (1 g/day for 3 days in adults, followed by prednisone 1 mg/kg/day for 2 weeks), have been advised (Beck et al. 1992, 1993). Withdrawal of steroids may be associated with rebounds and should be slow (Pless and Malik 2003).

ACUTE DISSEMINATED ENCEPHALOMYELITIS (ADEM)

ADEM has long been recognized after infectious childhood disease like measles, mumps, chickenpox, rubella and whooping cough, and with vaccination, but can occur with multiple infections (Chapter 10). Experimental allergic encephalomyelitis is considered as the animal model of ADEM. Perivenous demyelination was described as the pathological hallmark in early publications. Within these lesions axial cylinders are relatively unaffected. The relationship with immunization with Pasteur's rabies vaccine and smallpox vaccinations is undisputed, while a causal association with other immunizations is questioned. ADEM occurs predominantly, but not exclusively in children, frequently preceded by one or two weeks by a clearly identifiable infection.

Para-/postinfectious encephalomyelitis is often severe and constitutes with few exceptions a monophasic disease. This time course is the basis for considering ADEM as a disease entity. However, relapses of ADEM can be observed, making it difficult to distinguish it from MS (Tardieu and Mikaeloff 2004).

A recent review from the USA estimated an incidence of 0.4/100,000 amongst persons younger than 20 years of age. Only 5% of patients had received a vaccination within 4 weeks before the onset of ADEM, but 93% reported infections in the preceeding days (Leake et al. 2004).

The diagnosis of ADEM must be discussed in children with an acute onset of an encephalopathy with multiple variable symptoms such as headache, fever and a declining level of conciousness. Neurological symptoms include convulsions, paresis, frequently hemipareses, ataxia, cranial nerve palsies, visual loss due to optic neuritis (frequently bilateral) evolving over several days. Seizures occur more frequently below the age of 5 years.

The presence of severe disturbances of consciousness together with multifocal neurological symptoms and signs, especially in a child under 10 years of age, favours a diagnosis of ADEM rather than MS (Mikaeloff et al. 2004a,b).

Neuroimaging is an essential investigation for establishing the diagnosis of ADEM. T_2-weighted and FLAIR (fluid attenuated inversion recovery) sequences are best used. A variable number of large, bilateral, asymmetrical lesions in deep and subcortical white matter of the brain can be demonstrated. There is relative sparing of the periventricular white matter and the corpus callosum (20%). Basal ganglia and thalamus are more frequently involved than in classical MS (Mikaeloff et al. 2004a).

Lesions may also be demonstrated in the cerebellum, brainstem and optic nerves. Spinal cord involvement is often detectable on MRI even in the absence of clinical defects. It can lead to complete myelopathy (Kesselring et al. 1990).

In the CSF, a mild pleocytosis and elevated protein is usually present, but oligoclonal IgG bands are rare. The diagnosis of ADEM must be considered in every case presenting as acute encephalopathy and/or disseminated demyelination in childhood.

Investigations of suspected ADEM cases in childhood must therefore follow emergency guidelines that require excluding infectious and metabolic disorders in blood, urine and CSF. In oncological (immune suppressed) patients, toxic (e.g. methotrexate) or nutritional metabolic (e.g. thiamine deficiency, Wernicke encephalopathy) disorders may manifest as a sudden-onset encephalopathy with signs of demyelination on MRI that may mimic ADEM.

Dale et al. (2000) reported on 48 children with ADEM seen between 1985 and 1999 at the Great Ormond Street Hospital, London. Seven cases relapsed ("multiphasic ADEM" or MDEM). After a mean follow-up period of 5.6 years, 13 of the 48 children had developed MS. A history of "predemyelinating" infectious disease, polysymptomatic presentation, pyramidal signs, encephalopathy or bilateral optic neuritis was more commonly seen in ADEM/MDEM patients. Patients later diagnosed with MS showed more frequently intrathecal synthesis of oligoclonal bands on presentation, but this finding was not significant.

Tenembaum et al. (2002) reported on 84 consecutive children with ADEM observed in Buenos Aires between 1988 and 2000. The mean age at onset was 5.4±3.9 years. A preceding infection was described in 62%. Twenty-six per cent had no defined prodromes, and in 10 cases (12%) ADEM followed

TABLE 11.5
Differential diagnoses of ADEM (selected)

Bacterial and viral infections
Meningitis
Meningoencephalitis
Encephalitis
Brain abscess

Disorders of mitochondrial energy metabolism
Mitochondrial encephalomyopathy with lactic acidosis and stroke-like episodes (MELAS)
Myoclonic encephalopathy with ragged red fibres (MERRF)
Leigh syndrome

Syndromes with macrophage activation
Familial haemophagocytic lymphohistiocytosis
Chediak–Higashi disease
Griscelli syndrome

Autoimmune diseases
Behçet disease
Lupus erythematosus
Sjögren syndrome
Sarcoidosis

Malignancies
Lymphoma
Glioma

immunizations. The interval between the "febrile prodrome" and onset of ADEM symptomatology ranged from 2 to 30 days. Ataxia, acute hemiparesis with bilateral pyramidal tract signs, and impaired consciousness were the most frequent presenting features. A surprisingly high incidence of partial status epilepticus was observed in 35%. After a mean follow-up of 6.4±3.8 years, 90% showed a monophasic course and 10% a biphasic disease. The overall outcome was good. There was no significant association between findings on neuroimaging (large versus small lesions) and clinical outcome.

The studies by Dale and Tenembaum reflect the great regional differences in frequency and clinical presentation of ADEM, or of diagnostic criteria, as well as of outcome. Besides the classical monophasic form of ADEM, relapsing and recurrent forms have been observed. Three forms of ADEM have therefore been delineated: (1) classical monophasic ADEM; (2) recurrent ADEM (relapse with identical features); and (3) multiphasic ADEM (relapse with new features).

DIAGNOSIS

Multiple neurological disorders can have a presentation similar to ADEM (Table 11.5). Acute viral encephalitis cannot be clinically distinguished from ADEM (Chapter 10). It is important to recognize that metabolic or toxic disorders should be diagnosed as their treatment is different.

The most difficult differential diagnosis is that of MS. The possibility of subsequent episodes of CNS demyelination without encephalopathy and with evidence of dissemination in time demonstrated on MRI illlustates the close relationship of ADEM and MS. Mainly retrospective studies have reported that up to

20–30% of patients presenting with symptoms of ADEM ultimately fulfilled MS criteria (Hartung and Grossman 2001, Tardieu and Mikaeloff 2004). At present, there exists no biological marker for distinguishing between these two disorders. Careful and critical follow-up is therefore essential.

TREATMENT

High-dose steroid treatment is the most widely reported therapy in ADEM. It frequently results in a dramatic clinical improvement and clearing of lesions on MRI within weeks to months. Steroid treatment should therefore be started as soon as an infectious cause has been excluded. Intravenous methylprednisolone (max. 30 mg/kg/day up to 1 g/day) over 3–8 days, or i.v. dexamethasone, followed by oral steroid taper over 2–4 weeks are most frequently used. Full recovery has been reported in over 50% of patients. The recurrence of symptoms must be expected in some patients following discontinuation of treatment. Intravenous immunoglobulins or even plasma exchange may be considered in these cases. ADEM in childhood must be considered as a pediatric emergency and frequently needs intensive care during the acute phase.

ACUTE TRANSVERSE MYELITIS (ATM)

Transverse myelopathy or myelitis occurs often as one of the clinically isolated syndromes previously mentioned (see above), or as part of an encephalomyelitic illness. Several neuropathological processes may affect the spinal cord and give rise to this syndrome. These include postinfectious myelitis, MS, vascular insufficiency, diverse viral or bacterial infections, X-irradiation and vascular malformations. A long list of viruses have been associated with the syndrome including cytomegalovirus, herpes simplex virus, hepatitis A virus (Breningstall and Belani 1995) and adenoviruses (Linssen et al. 1991). Other infectious agents have been occasionally implicated, for example that causing Lyme disease (Rousseau et al. 1986, Linssen et al. 1991), *Mycoplasma pneumoniae* (Dewez et al. 1992, Logigian et al. 1994) and typhoid vaccine (Breningstall and Belani 1995). One third to one half of cases seem to be related to a viral infection, often an exanthematous disease. A cell-mediated immune response is a likely mechanism in many cases, as suggested by the observation that the lymphocytes of 7 of 10 patients with transverse myelitis responded to bovine myelin basic protein and to human peripheral nerve myelin P2 protein (Abramsky and Teitelbaum 1977).

Only idiopathic and postinfectious cases are considered here. In a series of 25 children reviewed by Paine and Byers (1953) and a further 21 cases reviewed by Dunne et al. (1986), the majority had a history of a recent infectious illness. There was a seasonal clustering with most patients presenting in late autumn, winter and early spring. Despite an extensive work-up some cases remain of unknown aetiology. Inclusion and exclusion criteria for the diagnosis of idiopathic ATM for were proposed in 2002 by the Transverse Myelitis Consortium Working Group (Table 11.6).

A multicentre study from neurological departments in France (de Sèze et al. 2005) reported 45 cases of idiopathic ATM,

TABLE 11.6
Diagnostic criteria for idiopathic acute transverse myelitis (ATM)*

Inclusion criteria
- Development of sensory, motor and autonomic dysfunction attributable to the spinal cord
- Bilateral signs or symptoms
- Clearly defined sensory level
- Exclusion of extra-axial compressive aetiology by neuroimaging
- Inflammation within the spinal cord demonstrated by CSF
- Progression to nadir between 4 hours and 21 days after the onset of symptoms

Diagnosis of idiopathic ATM is considered *definite* if all these criteria are met, and *possible* if the inflammation is not demonstrated by CSF cell count or gadolinium enhancement on spinal cord MRI

Exclusion criteria
- History of previous radiation of the spine within the past 10 years
- Clear arterial distribution of deficit consistent with thrombosis of the anterior spinal artery
- Abnormal flow voids on the surface of the spinal cord
- Serological or clinical evidence of connective tissue disease
- CNS manifestations of syphilis, Lyme disease, HIV, HTLV-I, mycoplasma or other viral infection
- Brain MRI abnormalities suggestive of MS
- History of clinically apparent optic neuritis

*Transverse Myelitis Consortium Working Group (2002).
HTLV-I = human T-cell lymphotrophic virus type I.

diagnosed out of a cohort of 288 cases with ATM. Spinal cord infarction, neuromyelits optica, MS, infectious or parainfectious and systemic diseases were diagnosed in the non-idiopathic group. Preceding illnesses/infections in children included measles, rubella, varicella, *M. pneumoniae*, *B. burgdorferi* and schistosomiasis.

CLINICAL FEATURES

Most cases occur in patients over 5 years of age; the youngest child reported was a 7-month-old boy who developed ATM after diphtheria–tetanus–pertussis vaccination (Riel-Romero 2006). The onset may be hyperacute and then marked by pain in the back and the abrupt development of paraplegia with sphincter paralysis and marked sensory disturbances. Another mode of onset is more progressive over days. In such cases, paraesthesiae and pain extend from the back in the groin and limbs, frequently asymmetrically. When asked, the patient complains of obstipation and urine retention. All patients develop weakness or flaccid paralysis usually of the lower extremities during the course of the illness, but weakness in the arms may also be present. Gross sensory disturbances are always present, but an upper sensory level is difficult to define. Involvement of respiratory muscles occurs in up to 20%. A fully developed Brown–Sequard syndrome is observed in rare cases. Pyramidal involvement gradually appears. In the study by Dunne et al. (1986), one group of patients with an acute onset of symptoms was unable to walk within hours, while the majority showed a slowly progressive evolution of symptoms. Most patients recovered within a period of 3 months. Eight out of 21 recovered without neurological sequelae. The outcome was fair or poor in 9 children, 2 became wheelchair dependent, and 3 had no sphincter control.

Pleocytosis and an increased level of protein are found in about a quarter of patients.

DIAGNOSIS

The diagnosis of ATM may be difficult. Exclusion of cord compression by a neoplasm or an abcess is an absolute requirement. MRI is now the gold standard of investigation. Typical presentations include swelling of the spinal cord and hyperintensity on T_2-weighted images as well as patchy enhancement with gadolinium; the extension of cord involvement does not correlate with the severity of presentation or outcome (Andronikou et al. 2003). Scanning of the head may be of interest as intracranial abnormalities are sometimes detected in patients with only clinical signs of cord involvement (Campi et al. 1995).

Other causes of the transverse myelitis syndrome such as lupus erythematosus, meningitis, schistosomiasis, and spontaneous or post-traumatic occlusive vascular disease (Linssen et al. 1990) should be excluded as far as possible. In cases with an apoplectic onset, the possibility of a vascular malformation of the spinal cord should always be kept in mind (Chapter 14). In all cases, epiduritis must be ruled out (Chapter 10). Polyradiculoneuritis in young patients may be difficult to distinguish from ATM because sensory disturbances and sphincter dysfunction are not always easy to appreciate in such instances.

ACUTE MYELOPATHIES OF OBSCURE ORIGIN

Myelopathies of noninflammatory cause are exceptional in children. The *vascular myelopathy* associated with AIDS is virtually limited to adults (Rosenblum et al. 1989), and HTLV-1-associated progressive myelopathy (Link et al. 1989) has only rarely been reported in children. HTLV-1 may be associated with the presence of disseminated areas of intense signal on T_2-weighted MRI, thus mimicking MS (Newton et al. 1987).

The association of central demyelination with peripheral demyelinating neuropathy is unusual.

COURSE AND PROGNOSIS

In large series of both adults and children (Ropper and Poskanzer 1978, Berman et al. 1981, Ponsot and Arthuis 1981, Dunne et al. 1986), approximately 60% of the patients made a good recovery that was rapid or extended over several months. Only 10–20% of patients fail to improve significantly. The development of MS following transverse myelitis is observed in less than 10% of adult patients and is exceptional in children. A normal MR scan is of considerable help in excluding MS. The most important prognostic factor is the mode of onset (Ropper and Poskanzer 1978). A large majority of patients with catastrophic onset of pain and paralysis are left with sequelae, whereas the reverse applies to those with a progressive onset (Dunne et al. 1986).

Treatment is purely symptomatic. Corticosteroids are not proven to be effective. However, high-dose pulses of methylprednisolone are often used in an attempt to reduce the frequent cord swelling (Sébire et al. 1997).

NEUROLOGICAL DISORDERS IN THE HAEMOPHAGOCYTIC SYNDROMES, SARCOIDOSIS AND RELATED PROLIFERATIVE DISORDERS

The exact nosological situation of the disorders considered in this section is still in doubt, and their aetiologies are multiple. Some of them, at least, represent an abnormal response of the histiocytic system or of blood cell precursors, or both, to various aggressions especially of viral nature. Others are clearly malignant in nature but are mentioned here for convenience as they share many features with the reactive types. A genetic predisposition is probably present in most cases (Risdall et al. 1979).

Bone marrow derived histiocytes play an important part in many disorders. The dentric cell types (including Langerhans cells of the skin) are mainly antigen presenting cells, while phagocytosis is the main function of macrophages. A monoclonal proliferation of the dentritic Langerhans cells causes Langerhans cell histiocytosis.

LANGERHANS CELL HISTIOCYTOSIS (LCH)

LCH includes eosinophilic granuloma (isolated bone histiocytosis), Hand–Schüler–Christian disease (triad of bone lesions, diabetes insipidus and hepatosplenomegaly) and Abt–Letterer–Siwe disease (disseminated involvement of skin and multiple organs). The three disorders were previously named histiocytosis X.

LCH usually occurs in childhood. Three major clinical groups can be distinguished (Grois 1998): (1) hypothalamic/pituitary type with diabetes insipidus as the main clinical feature; (2) extraparenchymal/space-occupying type originating from meninges and choroid plexus, which may cause symptoms of raised intracranial pressure; (3) neurodegenerative type mainly affecting cerebellum, pons and basal ganglia. Clinical symptoms include severe ataxia, tremor, dysarthria, behavioural and cognitive deficits. There is considerable overlap among these different types.

The pathogenesis of LCH in general and of the neurodegenerative type in particular is unknown. Under normal circumstances Langerhans cells do not divide any more while LCH cells proliferate in mesenchymal tissue. The triggering process or agent activating Langerhans cells is still unknown. The classical appearance in LCH is characterized by the presence of Langerhans cells but also of macrophages, eosinophiles and giant cells. Langerhans cells are identified by their morphological characteristics and a positive stain for CD1a antigen. Electron microscopy shows intracytoplasmatic organelles (Birbeck granules).

Neurological disease may be the presenting feature of LCH or appear only after an interval of many years following the initial diagnosis. The true incidence of CNS involvement is estimated to be around 3%.

MRI plays an important part in establishing the diagnosis and localization of the disease. Cerebellar lesions show high signal intensities symmetrically in the hilus of the dentate nucleus often with calcification and white matter of cerebellum and pons. Basal ganglia and supratentorial white matter may also be involved. Cerebellar atrophy has been observed in longstanding cases (Barthez et al. 2000). One peculiarity of the neurodegenera-tive type of LCH is the absence of Langerhans cells in the affected white matter. Massive neuronal and axonal destruction with sec-ondary demyelination different from that in MS was reported in a neuropathological study (Grois et al. 2005). A paraneoplastic aetiology has therefore been discussed.

Treatment depends on localization and stage of the disease. The aim is to correct dysfunction (e.g. diabetes insipidus) as well as to limit the spread of the disease. Surgery, chemotherapy, corticosteroids and local irradiation have been employed with varying results. The outcome of CNS LCH is poor. Long-term follow-up of 49 paediatric cases from one centre in Sweden found at least 90% of all LCH patients had CNS sequelae, 10% had died, and 51% were alive and well (Writing Group of the Histiocyte Society 1987, Bernstrand et al. 2005).

FAMILIAL AND ACQUIRED HAEMOPHAGOCYTIC LYMPHOHISTIOCYTOSIS (HLH)
HLH is a rare life-threatening disorder of childhood character-ized by massive infiltration of organs including the meninges and brain parenchyma by activated lymphocytes and macrophages. The present view is that the inability of natural killer cells or cytotoxic lymphocytes (CD8+ T-cells) to terminate an immune response leads to a proliferation of these cells. The result is widespread haemophagocytosis and overproduction of cytokines such as interferon gamma, TNF-alpha and interleukin 1 and 6. Two different forms are at presently recognized: primary HLH, an autosomal recessive disorder (familial HLH or FHL), in which HLH is the sole manifestation; and sporadic or secondary forms that can occur in association with immune deficiency in Chediak–Higashi syndrome, Griscelli syndrome, and X-linked lymphoproliferative syndrome. However, most patients with acquired HLH have no known underlying immune deficiency. Both forms are triggered by mainly viral infections. An associa-tion with Epstein–Barr virus has been frequently demonstrated. Familial forms are genetically heterogeneous and can be due to mutations in either the *perforin-1* gene or the *MUNC13-4* gene (Zur Stadt et al. 2006, Turtzo et al. 2007).

Biochemical markers of HLH include elevated triglycerids, elevated ferritin, and low fibrinogin in blood. Haemophagocytosis can be demonstrated in bone marrow, CSF or lymph nodes. Demonstration in bone marrow might be difficult during the ini-tial stage of the disease. Clincal features of HLH are recurrent fever, infections, cytopenia, and hepatosplenomegaly. Neurological symptoms can be extremely variable ranging from emotional changes and convulsions to focal symptoms like hemiparesis and cranial nerve palsy. They may occur as the first sign of the dis-ease in rare cases (Rostasy et al. 2004, Imashuku and Iwai 2006). CSF assay is inconclusive or normal in most cases. The MRI shows widespread involvement of white matter, cerebellum and brainstem. Cortical structures and basal ganglia may also be affected. A marked discrepancy between the extensive cerebral in-volvement and the severity of clinical symptoms can be observed.

The disease may follow a relapsing–remitting course mim-icking disorders of inflammatory origin like MS or ADEM. Next

to lethal multiorgan infection, CNS involvement is the second most frequent cause of death. Therapy aims at suppression of the increased inflammatory response by immunosuppressive/im-mune modulatory and cytotoxic drugs. Stem cell transplantation may be used in genetic cases (Janka and Zur Stadt 2005).

SARCOIDOSIS
Sarcoidosis is a chronic multisystemic granulomatous disorder that affects mainly young adults, rarely children. Sarcoidosis in-volves the CNS in 5–10% of cases. Pathologically it is charac-terized by the presence of non-necrotizing granulomas with giant cells and epitheloid cells. Clinical manifestations of paediatric neurosarcoidosis are cranial neuropathy (involving nerves II, VII and VIII), aseptic meningitis, hydrocephalus, hypothalamic dys-function, myelopathy, and involvement of the peripheral nervous system and muscles.

In children, the presentation is different from that in adults; seizures are a predominant feature in patients under 3 years old, while cranial nerve involvement increasingly occurs in older children and adolescents. Mass lesions may also be more common in young children (Baumann and Robertson 2003). The most common manifestation of sarcoidosis in children is *Heerfordt syn-drome* (McGovern and Merritt 1956). This consists of uveitis, optic neuritis associated with swelling of the parotic gland, and facial nerve palsy. Isolated CNS sarcoidosis is rare. Cranial neuro-pathy, which is the commonest feature of CNS sarcoidosis in adults, papilloedema and diabetes insipidus are rare in children. CSF examination may show mononuclear pleocytosis, blood–brain barrier damage and a decreased CSF–blood glucose ratio. Intrathecal injection of IgM and IgG has been reported. MRI may show lesions similar to those of MS in periventricular white matter, and diffuse enhancement of basal meninges and ten-torium and hydrocephalus may result. Granulomas can be demonstrated at the base of brain and scattered throughout the hemispheres.

The diagnosis rests on demonstration of associated lesions, especially hilar enlargement on chest X-ray, a positive Kveim test, hypercalcemia, and elevated levels of serum angiotensin-converting enzyme in 60% of patients. However, none of these tests is specific.

The course of the disorder is slow and partial, or complete remission may supervene.

GRISCELLI SYNDROME
Griscelli syndrome is a rare autosomal recessive disorder of partial albinism and immunodeficiency. During an accelerated phase of the disease a life-threatening haemophagocytic syndrome may develop due to uncontrolled lymphocyte and macrophage activa-tion, and proliferation may develop. Patients have characteristic silver-grey hair that under the light microscope shows big lumps of melanin. Late neurological manifestations include seizures, ataxia, hemiparesis and nystagmus. An early-onset neurological presentation with hypotonicity and delay in psychomotor de-velopment has also been described (Sanal et al. 2002). Recently a mutation in *LAB22A* in familial HLH related to Griscelli

syndrome has been identified. The diagnosis is based on the characteristic irregular large clumps of pigment distributed along the hair shafts viewed by light microscopy. Neurological presentation without abnormal haematology has been reported (Rajadhyax et al. 2007) The MRI may show white matter abnormalities, suggesting cellular infiltration.

Most of the CNS-involving inflammatory and autoimmune diseases are rare in childhood. However, due to the therapeutic implications, they present an important group of disorders to consider in the differential diagnosis of MS. The potentially great overlap with pediatric MS in regard to the clinical features and diagnostic tests may pose diagnostic difficulties, especially in the case of isolated CNS symptoms. CSF oligoclonal IgG may be present in most connective tissue diseases with a frequency of up to 50%, thereby causing further problems in the diagnostic process.

OPSOCLONUS–MYOCLONUS–ATAXIA SYNDROME (MYOCLONIC ENCEPHALOPATHY OF KINSBOURNE)

Opsoclonus–myoclonus syndrome (OMS) was first described in 1963 by Kinsbourne, who published under the title "myoclonic encephalopathy of infants" a series of cases identified by the late Paul Sandifer at the Hospital for Sick Children in Great Ormond Street, London.

OMS is an uncommon disorder characterized by three main symptoms: opsoclonus (rapid eye movement, asynchronous and oscillating), myoclonus, and cerebellar ataxia, along with neuropsychological signs (e.g. irritability, sleeplessness). These neurological signs may vary widely in their expression and are not necessarily present together (Kinsbourne 1963). OMS is less common in adults than in children. The vast majority of paediatric cases have their onset between 1 and 3 years of age (Plantaz et al. 2000). In both age groups the disease manifests either as a paraneoplastic syndrome or idiopathically without a clearly defined cause. Poliomyelitis or other enterovirus infections (Kuban et al. 1983, Sheth et al. 1995), mumps (Ichiba et al. 1988), and toxic and metabolic disorders have been reported as possible triggers of OMS. The paraneoplastic OMS in adults is mainly associated with small-cell lung or breast cancer, whereas children almost exclusively have neuroblastoma. OMS is present in about 3% of patients with neuroblastoma (Warrier et al. 1985). The incidence of neuroblastoma-associated and non-neuroblastoma-associated OMS is reported to be similar (Tate et al. 2005). However, the true frequency of neuroblastoma-associated OMS is assumed to be higher, since neuroblastomas are often occult and difficult to detect, and may regress spontaneously.

OMS is strongly suspected to be immune mediated, based on the observations of successful immunosuppressive treatments, the presence of hypergammaglobulinaemia, CSF pleocytosis with a predominant B-cell response (Pranzatelli et al. 2004) and intrathecal IgG synthesis. In addition, autoantibodies have been reported in different studies in adults and children with OMS, but a common cross-reactive autoantigen has not yet been found.

Anti-neurofilament antibodies have been described in some patients. Anti-neuronal antibodies were detected more frequently in neuroblastoma patients with OMS than in those without OMS (Antunes et al. 2000). In a recent report, autoantibodies binding to the surface of isolated rat cerebellar granular neurons were detected in 10 of 14 children with OMS (Blaes et al. 2005). Neuroblastoma associated with Kinsbourne syndrome has a better prognosis for survival than neuroblastoma in general, suggesting an autoimmune factor also confining the growth of the tumour (Altman and Baehner 1976). A recent case report of a neuroblastoma found only after rituximab treatment might be supportive of this hypothesis (Chang et al. 2006).

The clinical picture is distinctive and unlike that seen in any other condition. Onset is acute or subacute with gait or truncal ataxia, frequently followed by loss of the ability to walk or even sit within several days. The most remarkable feature is the presence of chaotic, rapid, multidirectional eye movements occurring in sudden bursts, frequently precipitated by changing fixation. Opsoclonus might appear only weeks after the onset of ataxia. It is almost always accompanied by violent myoclonus, exacerbated by attempted movements or emotional distress. The clinical myoclonus is unassociated with any paroxysmal EEG abnormality. It may involve all body parts including limbs, trunk and face. This remarkable association of eye and limb jerking has been termed 'dancing eyes, dancing feet syndrome'. The movement disorder is often accompanied by severe irritability, developmental regression, personality change and sleep disturbances. Occult neuroblastoma may present with some, but not all OMS symptoms. Therefore, neuroblastoma should be suspected in all patients with prolonged cerebellar ataxia of unknown aetiology.

The disease course is often prolonged, lasting months or even years, with recurrences precipitated by intercurrent respiratory infections or decreases in the dose of steroids (Pohl et al. 1996). Progressively, and especially with immunosuppressive therapy, the intensity of jerking diminishes and the opsoclonus often disappears, followed by the myoclonus of limbs.

Diagnostic work-up in patients with suspected OMS has to include in-depth search for neuroblastoma. Repeated complete investigations should be made, with rectal examination, careful palpation, ultrasound and MRI of the abdomen and pelvis, and multiple determinations of urinary vanillyl-mandelic and homovanillic acids (as the levels of these compounds may be only mildly and intermittently or not at all raised) (Mitchell and Snodgras 1990). Metaiodobenzylguanidine radionuclide scans may further increase the sensitivity of neuroblastoma detection.

There is no standard therapy regime, and no prospective trial addressing treatment in OMS has been published. Resection of a neuroblastoma may improve OMS in some patients, but most will require immunosuppressive treatment. Therapies with steroids, ACTH, plasmapheresis, immunoglobulins, cyclophosphamide and rituximab have been reported to be of varying efficacy (Pless and Ronthal 1996, Pohl et al. 1996, Plantaz et al. 2000, Hayward et al. 2001, Rudnick et al. 2001, Yiu et al. 2001, Mitchell et al. 2002, Armstrong et al. 2005, Pranzatelli et al. 2005, Chang et al. 2006, Burke and Cohn 2008). Long-term

TABLE 11.7
Major causes of acute ataxia*

Cause	Reference
Infectious and parainfectious cerebellar ataxia	
Viral infections (varicella, measles, mumps, herpes simplex, Epstein–Barr virus, coxsackie and echovirus, poliomyelitis)	This chapter
Bacterial infections	
Mycoplasma pneumoniae	Behan et al. (1986)
Legionella pneumophila	Nigro et al. (1983)
Toxic and metabolic causes	
Organic acid and mitochondrial disorders	Chapter 8
Benzodiazepines	Chapter 15
Phenytoin, barbiturates, carbamazepine[1]	Chapter 15
Antihistamine drugs	Chapter 12
Vitamin A	Chapter 22
Methotrexate	Chapter 13
Piperazine ('worm wobble')	Chapter 12
Acute ataxia revealing structural lesion of the posterior fossa	
Posterior fossa tumour	Chapter 13
Chiari I anomaly and other anomalies of the cervico-occipital region	Chapter 2
Vascular causes	
Basilar migraine[1]	Chapter 16
Basilar artery thrombosis or emboli	Echenne et al. (1983)
Cryptogenic ataxia	
Possibly related to unnoticed infections	This chapter
Ataxia due to peripheral nerve involvement	Chapter 20
Miller Fisher syndrome	
Other neuropathies	
Ataxia following an acute neurological disease	
Multiple sclerosis	This chapter
Head trauma	Chapter 12
Heat stroke	Chapter 12
Acute purulent meningitis	Chapter 10
Cerebellar abscess	Chapter 10
Pseudoataxia due to nonconvulsive epileptic activity[1]	Bennett et al. (1982)
Nonconvulsive status epilepticus	Chapter 15
Periods of uncontrolled activity in Lennox–Gastaut syndrome and myoclonic epilepsies	Guerrini et al. (1993)

*Excluding intermittent ataxias that are dealt with in Table 16.3 (p. 673).
In most cases of acute ataxia, it is difficult to distinguish between cerebellar, sensory or other (vestibular) causes, and additional signs of CNS involvement may be present.
[1]May be recurrent.

treatment over years is often required, and recurrences after dose-reduction or termination of therapy are common. No treatment to prevent the common neuropsychological sequelae has been established. Prompt and strong immunosuppression is recommended with the goal of minimizing residual disability, but has not yet been formally proven to be effective.

The outcome is unfavourable in many cases, and 70% to over 90% of childhood patients are reported to suffer from residual disabilities, mainly cognitive impairment, motor difficulties and speech disturbances (Pohl et al. 1996, Hayward et al. 2001, Rudnick et al. 2001, Mitchell et al. 2002). The question as to whether an early and aggressive treatment might improve the long-term prognosis has yet to be resolved. Neuroblastomas associated with Kinsbourne syndrome have a better prognosis for survival than neuroblastoma in general, suggesting that the neurological manifestations in these children may result from an unknown, perhaps autoimmune factor that is also effective in checking the growth of the tumour.

ACUTE AND SUBACUTE PARAINFECTIOUS CEREBELLAR ATAXIAS (Table 11.7)

These conditions are characterized by the sudden or rapid onset of ataxia, usually following a specific (e.g. varicella) or nonspecific infectious illness.

In some cases, a direct viral infection of the CNS is responsible for the clinical picture, even though there has been no direct demonstration of the presence of a virus in cerebellar cells. Several viruses have been isolated from the CSF or extraneural sites including polioviruses, echoviruses 9 and coxsackie B virus (Kuban et al. 1983), but these may have induced ataxia through an indirect mechanism similar to what occurs in postinfectious encephalomyelitis. Such is probably the causal mechanism for cases of acute ataxia following chicken-pox (Johnson and Milbourn 1970), mumps (Koskiniemi et al. 1983), varicella immunization (Sunaga et al. 1995) or other exanthematous diseases of childhood, and for the rare cases of ataxia that may be the initial feature of MS.

Acute cerebellar ataxia is a common CNS disorder in children. It may occur at any age, most commonly during the second year of life. In one series (Connolly et al. 1994), 26% of cases were associated with chicken-pox, 52% with other presumably viral illness, and 3% with immunizations. The clinical picture is marked by severe truncal ataxia and gait disturbance. Tremor of the extremities or head is less common. Nystagmus is present in 45% of patients. CSF pleocytosis is found in a quarter of the cases, and late increase in CSF protein has been observed.

Most patients recover spontaneously in a few weeks to six months. However, a residual cerebellar syndrome may persist in a quarter to a third of the patients, and persistence of an incapacitating ataxia may be seen. In such cases, CT may demonstrate residual cerebellar atrophy. Areas of altered signal in the cerebellum, sometimes with contrast enhancement, may be observed in the early stage of the illness and may persist for several months, although they are uncommon. Acute cerebellar swelling demonstrated by neuroimaging with symptoms and signs of high intracranial pressure may occur following varicella (Hurst and Mehta 1988) or undetermined, probably viral infections (Roulet Perez et al. 1993) and may be fatal in rare cases.

Acute cerebellar ataxia should not be confused with posterior fossa or other tumours. Acute labyrinthitis is difficult to separate from cerebellar ataxia. Nausea, intense vertigo and abnormal tests of labyrinthine function permit the diagnosis (Eviatar and Eviatar 1977). The course of acute vestibular ataxia is often briefer than that of cerebellar ataxia, and recovery is the rule. The most common differential diagnosis is from drug or other intoxications, which account for up to one third of cases of acute ataxia. Ataxia may also follow heat stroke (Freedman and Schenthal 1953), and a reversible although prolonged ataxic syndrome can be seen in severe epilepsies during periods of intense seizure activity (Bennett et al. 1982).

RHEUMATIC AND OTHER INFLAMMATORY DISORDERS

The rheumatic diseases include a series of disorders characterized by diffuse inflammatory changes in connective tissue. The exact nature of these disorders and their mutual relationships remain uncertain but CNS involvement is a feature of many of them.

SYDENHAM CHOREA
Sydenham chorea is the major neurological manifestation of rheumatic fever. Most cases of chorea are preceded by a streptococcal infection or by other manifestations of rheumatic fever. The disease is described in Chapter 10.

RHEUMATOID ARTHRITIS
Rheumatoid arthritis can be accompanied by a symmetrical sensorimotor neuropathy or by an encephalopathy with disturbances of consciousness, marked slowing of the EEG and, occasionally, neurological signs suggestive of intracranial hypertension such as decorticate rigidity (Jan et al. 1972). The possible role of salicylate toxicity has been considered. About 6% of patients with rheumatoid arthritis develop an acute encephalopathy that is usually spontaneously reversible. Myelopathy may result from cervical compression at the cervico-occipital junction, and focal neuropathies can also occur because of bone deformations.

CHRONIC INFANTILE, NEUROLOGICAL, CUTANEOUS AND ARTICULAR DISEASE (CINCA)
Also termed neonatal-onset multisystem inflammatory disease (NOMID), this disorder with neonatal or very early onset is marked by a skin rash, arthritis of the knees, ankles, elbows, wrists and hands, chronic aseptic meningitis that may lead to hydrocephalus, headaches, seizures and sometimes optic atrophy, deafness and hoarseness (Prieur and Griscelli 1981, Yarom et al. 1985, Prieur 2001). Mental retardation is common. Cerebral atrophy and sometimes areas of softening of probable vascular origin are present on CT. In about half the cases, mutations of the gene *CIAS1* are found (Feldmann et al. 2002, Hawkins et al. 2004). This gene codes for the protein cryopyrin that regulates inflammation (probably by acting as an inhibitor of interleukin-1 receptor).

Treatment is with anti-inflamatory drugs including thalidomide and immunosuppressors. Recently, anakinrin, an inhibitor of interleukin-1 receptor, has been found to be remarkably effective (Goldbach-Mansky et al. 2006).

SYSTEMIC LUPUS ERYTHEMATOSUS (SLE)
SLE is a multisystem disease affecting the joints, skin, kidneys, cardiovascular and respiratory systems, and the central and

TABLE 11.8
Neuropsychiatric manifestations of systemic lupus erythematosus

Central nervous system	Peripheral nervous system
Aseptic meningitis	Acute inflammatory demyelinating polyneuropathy (Guillain-Barré syndrome)
Cerebrovascular disease	
Demyelinating syndrome	
Headache (including migraine and benign intracranial hypertension)	Autonomic disorder
	Mononeuropathy, single or multiplex
Movement disorder (chorea)	
Myelopathy	Myasthenia gravis
Seizure disorders	Neuropathy, cranial
Acute confusional state	Plexopathy
Anxiety disorder	Polyneuropathy
Cognitive dysfunction	
Mood disorder	
Psychosis	

peripheral nervous systems. Children and adolescents represent about 20% of all patients with SLE (Stichweh et al. 2004), and neuropsychiatric symptoms may be the presenting features of SLE in childhood. The female to male ratio is reported to be about 5:1 (Carreno et al. 1999, Gutiérrez-Suárez et al. 2006).

Pathology of the brain reveals gross findings of large and small intracerebral haemorrhages and small areas of infarction. Microscopic abnormalities include diffuse perivascular infiltrations with inflammatory cells, increased peripapillary microglia, true vasculitis with inflammatory proliferative changes in the intima, and ischaemic lesions due to intimal proliferation of small cerebral arteries. Pathology appears most frequently in small blood vessels. Vascular changes and the resultant microinfarcts in the cerebral cortex and brainstem correlate well with the clinical abnormalities in most cases. The circulating antiphospholipid antibodies commonly present in SLE may play a role in the genesis of vascular thrombosis and thus contribute to brain damage.

The clinical manifestations of SLE can occur at any age, but there seems to be an incidence peak for girls around puberty, and in one large series reported by Lehman et al. (1989) 22% of cases occurred in the first decade. The characteristics of childhood- and juvenile-onset SLE are similar to those in adult-onset disease, but SLE that begins in childhood has been considered more severe than adult-onset SLE, with higher rates of organ involvement and a more aggressive clinical course (Tucker et al. 1995). It has been reported that paediatric patients with SLE may need high-dose corticosteroids and immunosuppressive agents for disease control more often than do their adult counterparts (Brunner et al. 1999).

Neuropsychiatric manifestations of SLE (Table 11.8) were defined in a consensus document and comprise CNS and peripheral nervous system involvement (ACR Ad Hoc Committee on Neuropsychiatric Lupus Nomenclature 1999). Children with SLE have an increased risk for neuropsychiatric involvement, present in 40% and 48% respectively in two large series (Parikh et al. 1995, Steinlin et al. 1995). An organic psychosis, probably due to toxic encephalopathy in which brain lesions, electrolyte disturbances and, in rare cases, steroid therapy may all play a role, may feature delirium, depression, delusions or hallucinations.

This syndrome may appear during acute exacerbations of the disease and subside with improvement of systemic manifestations. Neurological manifestations occur especially early in the disease course (i.e. in the first year after manifestation) (Gutiérrez-Suárez et al. 2006), although the reported frequencies of neurological symptoms in paediatric SLE are highly variable, ranging from 13% to 75% (reviewed by Schmutzler et al. 1997, Hussain and Isenberg 1999). The most frequent CNS manifestations of paediatric SLE are headache, seizures, movement disorders, disturbances of concentration or behaviour, and depression or frank psychosis. Headache is often migraine-like. Neurological symptoms and signs include focal or generalized seizures, and hemiplegia or diplegia, resulting from ischaemic cerebral events. Cranial nerve dysfunction, especially of the IIIrd and VIth pairs, and optic neuritis can occur (Yancey et al. 1981), as well as choreiform movement disorders. Chorea or hemichorea may occur in 1–28% of patients with SLE, especially in young patients (Parikh et al. 1995), and can precede systemic manifestations by several months or years.

Acute transverse myelitis may be associated with underlying SLE or be part of pediatric MS. Acute myelopathy (Provenzale and Bouldin 1992) can be the first manifestation of the disease (Linssen et al. 1988) and can simulate MS in juvenile patients.

Neurological complications have been exceptionally reported in infants with neonatal lupus erythematosus, a rare condition consisting of facial skin lesions, heart block and the passive transfer of maternal antibodies (Watson et al. 1984, Telang et al. 1993). Myelopathy is on record in one such case and has also been reported in infantile lupus associated with deficiency of complement components (Kaye et al. 1987).

CSF analysis may reveal a usually mild pleocytosis, raised protein content as a consequence of a blood–brain barrier dysfunction, and evidence for intrathecal IgG synthesis (raised IgG index or oligoclonal IgG). CT and MRI may show areas of infarction, haemorrhage or demyelination. MRI is more informative, but still may be normal even in the presence of acute neuropsychiatric symptoms.

Diagnosis of SLE is hampered by the fact that neuropsychiatric manifestations may be present long before serological confirmation is possible. Antinuclear antibodies are present in the vast majority of patients but are also found in patients with other autoimmune diseases like dermatomyositis, rheumatoid arthritis, chronic active hepatitis or MS. Antibodies against DNA are more specific and were found in 44 of 49 juvenile-onset SLE patients (Carreno et al. 1999). Antibodies against ribonucleoprotein and sm antigen may also contribute to confirm the diagnosis although they are less sensitive, with method-dependent seropositivity rates of 57% and 46%, respectively.

Treatment strategies for neuropsychiatric SLE are similar to those for other severe systemic manifestations of the disease and comprise various immunosuppressive drugs as well as immunoglobulins and plasmapheresis. Even for adult onset neuropsychiatric SLE, there is a shortage of randomized controlled treatment trials, and there is a lack of specific trials for paediatric-onset SLE. Methylprednisolone, cyclophosphamide, mycophenolate mofetil, chloroquine, methotrexate, cyclosporin and thalidomide all have been used with varying efficacy in SLE.

Prognosis of SLE depends on the timely implementation of effective treatment, and is best in countries with good medical care, with 10-year survival rates around 80% (reviewed by Ruiz-Irastorza et al. 2001). The outcome of neuropsychiatric SLE in children and adolescents has been reported to be favourable for the majority of patients, with mostly good functional recovery (Parikh et al. 1995, Steinlin et al. 1995).

HENOCH–SCHOENLEIN PURPURA
This disease is by far the most common vasculitis in childhood. It is characterized pathologically by a generalized small-vessel vasculitis of the hypersensitive type and can occur at any age, including infancy. Neurological manifestations occur in 2–7% of cases. Headache, changes in consciousness or behaviour and seizures are the usual manifestations and account for 25–50% of the neurological complications of Henoch–Schoenlein disease (Belman et al. 1985). Less frequent anomalies include focal deficits that may be hemiplegia, paraparesis, quadriplegia, cortical blindness or polyneuropathy (Ritter et al. 1983). Mononeuropathy and brachial plexopathy (Belman et al. 1985), and ataxia and peripheral neuropathy (Bulun et al. 2001) have been recorded. Some complications probably result from hypertension or renal involvement, but neurological symptoms may occur in the absence of any systemic disturbance and are probably caused by cerebral vasculitis.

KAWASAKI DISEASE
This disease, also known as mucocutaneous lymph node syndrome, is a disorder of obscure origin, although various pathogens including *Rickettsia*, *Propionibacterium acnes* and *Streptococcus sanguis* have been incriminated. An abnormal immune response to staphylococcal toxin (Leung et al. 1993) or parvovirus B19 (Sissons 1993, Nigro et al. 1994) has been proposed. Criteria for diagnosis of Kawasaki disease include a fever lasting five days or more, conjunctival injection, inflammation of respiratory mucous membranes, cutaneous abnormalities, in particular desquamation of the digital extremities, cervical adenitis, and the absence of a known cause to explain these features.

Kawasaki disease is complicated in 10–50% of cases by the occurrence of coronary artery aneurysms that may be responsible for death. The condition occurs in many parts of the world outside Japan and accounts for the cases of infantile periarteritis nodosa published before its description (see above). About 25% of the patients have aseptic meningitis with a mononuclear CSF pleocytosis of 25–100 cells/mm^3 (Bell et al. 1983). Hemiplegia, epilepsy and myositis have also been reported (Laxer et al. 1984). The incidence of neurological complications in one large series was 1.1% (Terasawa et al. 1983). CT changes may include diffuse or localized widening of sulci which appears to be reversible. Facial nerve paralysis of lower motor neuron type has occurred in several patients (Terasawa et al. 1983, Bushara et al. 1997). Sensorineural hearing loss has also been reported (Sundel et al. 1990).

Prevention of the development of coronary artery disease using high-dose intravenous globulin (400 mg/kg/day for 4 days) in combination with aspirin (3–10 mg/kg/day) is currently recommended for all cases (Bierman and Gersony 1987). However, uncertainties remain regarding the dose, schedule and indications for such treatment. Combination of intravenous globuli and corticosteroids may more effectively prevent coronary artery involvement (Inoue et al. 2006).

HAEMOLYTIC–URAEMIC SYNDROME

This condition has been associated with Shiga toxin-producing *Escherichia coli*, especially *E. coli* O157:H7 (Boyce et al. 1995), and with *Shigella dysenteriae* infection (Ashkenazi 1993). The presence of thrombocytopenia, haemolytic anaemia and azotaemia defines the syndrome. Two patterns of thrombi are encountered. In one, they form a loose fibrin meshwork. In the other, they appear as a coarse granular aggregation of eosinophilic material in the arterioles, capillaries and venules. Such abnormalities are not limited to the kidney and may be seen in the CNS. They may be responsible for small or large areas of infarction.

Neurological symptoms occur in 30–50% of cases (Sheth et al. 1986, Nadeau 2002). They consist of seizures, disturbances of consciousness such as stupor, hallucinations or coma, and focal deficits including extrapyramidal signs (Barnett et al. 1995, Bennett et al. 2003). They may occur in the absence of renal insufficiency and hypertension. Haemorrhagic infarction may occur and may be responsible for sequelae (Crisp et al. 1981). CSF protein is often raised in patients who have a poor outcome.

Imaging (Sherwood and Wagle 1991) often shows abnormal areas of ischaemic infarction and, sometimes, of haemorrhagic infarction. Involvement of the basal ganglia has been reported in patients who presented clinically with intractable seizures and intermittent decerebrate posturing. Even in such severe cases a satisfactory recovery remains possible, but sequelae persist in 10–20% of patients (Barnett et al. 1995).

BEHÇET DISEASE

Behçet disease is a chronic, relapsing–remitting, multisystem inflammatory disorder of unknown aetiology. The major pathologic feature of Behçet disease is a vasculitis with mucocutaneous, ocular, arthritic, vascular and other manifestations. Age at onset normally ranges from 20 to 35 years, but the disease can manifest in childhood, even as early as the first year of life (Kone-Paut et al. 2002). Oral ulcers are often the first manifestation of Behçet disease and are the sine qua non for the diagnosis. Genital ulcers, commonly leading to scar formation, may rarely occur at the onset of the disease. Other cutaneous manifestations include erythema nodosum-like lesions, folliculitis, acne-like lesions, superficial thrombophlebitis, cutaneous vasculitis and papulopustular lesions. Ocular involvement, most commonly recurrent anterior uveitis with hypopyon or posterior uveitis with retinal involvement, is usually episodic, but recurrent attacks may cause blindness. Non-deforming, non-erosive arthritis may occur. Vascular involvement includes both arterial and venous inflammation. Pulmonary, cardiac, gastrointestinal and urogenital symp-

TABLE 11.9
Clinical manifestations of neuro-Behçet disease

Hemispheral	Paresis, hypaesthesia, visual field defects, speech disorders, diabetes insipidus, seizures, psychological, psychiatric and cognitive disorders, parkinsonism, involuntary movements
Brainstem/cerebellar/spinal	Cranial nerve palsies, cerebellar and spinal symptoms, pseudobulbar palsy, emotional incontinence, palatal myoclonus, dysarthria, intranuclear ophthalmoplegia
Ophthalmic	Optic neuritis, ischaemic optic neuropathy
Otologic	Cochlear and neural hearing loss, vestibular complaints with similarities to Menière disease
Urologic	Bladder dysfunction with increased urinary frequency, sensation of urgency, incontinence, retention
Venous	Intracranial hyertension with headache, papilloedema, focal neurological deficits, seizures, VIth nerve palsy, altered consciousness due to dural sinus thrombosis
Arterial	Stenosis, aneurysm, dissection, followed by haemorrhage or infarct
Peripheral nervous system	Sensorimotor polyneuropathy, mononeuritis multiplex, autonomic neuropathy
Muscle	Necrotizing myositis

toms are rare. Erythrocyte sedimentation rate, C-reactive protein and immunoglobulins may be elevated, especially during active phases of the disease. The duration of attacks ranges from a few days to weeks. Attacks usually result in complete remission, but sequelae can also be found.

There is no diagnostic test for Behçet disease. Diagnostic criteria have been proposed (International Study Group for Behçet's Disease 1990).

Neurological manifestations of Behçet disease were first reported by Knapp in 1941. The frequency of neurological involvement shows a high degree of variation in different series, ranging from 2.5% to 49%. In an autopsy series, 20% of patients with Behçet disease presented neurological involvement (Lakhanpal et al. 1985). In the paediatric age group, neurological symptoms were reported in 20% of cases (Kone-Paut and Bernard 1993). Neurological involvement (Table 11.9) usually presents after systemic manifestations, but in a minority of patients, the disease manifests neurologically. Pathological findings include perivascular cuffing with lymphocytes or neutrophils or rarely eosinophils, demyelination with vasculitis, multifocal necrosis and glial proliferation. The most common sites involved are the brainstem and basal ganglia. Neurological involvement can present without orogenital ulcers, and true diagnosis of Behçet disease then can be made only at autopsy.

CNS manifestations of Behçet disease can be categorized into two main groups: the more common neurological CNS involvement (neuro-Behçet disease), and neurovasculo-Behçet including

Schonberger LB, Hurwitz ES, Katona P, et al. (1981) Guillain–Barré syndrome: its epidemiology and associations with influenza vaccination. *Ann Neurol* **9** Suppl: 31–8.

Sébire G, Hollenberg A, Meyer L, et al. (1997) High dose methylprednisolone in severe acute transverse myelitis. *Arch Dis Child* **76**: 67–8.

Shaw CM, Alvord EC (1987) Multiple sclerosis beginning in infancy. *J Child Neurol* **2**: 252–6.

Sherwood JW, Wagle WA (1991) Hemolytic uremic syndrome: MR findings of CNS complications. *AJNR* **12**: 703–4.

Sheth KJ, Swick HM, Haworth N (1986) Neurologic involvement in hemolytic–uremic syndrome. *Ann Neurol* **19**: 90–3.

Sheth RD, Horwitz SJ, Aronoff S, et al. (1995) Opsoclonus myoclonus syndrome secondary to Epstein–Barr virus infection. *J Child Neurol* **10**: 297–9.

Shields WD, Nielsen C, Buch D, et al. (1988) Relationship of pertussis immunization to the onset of neurologic disorders: a retrospective epidemiologic study. *J Pediatr* **113**: 801–5.

Sigal LH (1987) The neurologic presentation of vasculitic and rheumatologic syndromes. A review. *Medicine* **66**: 157–80.

Sindern E, Haas J, Stark E, Wurster U (1992) Early onset of MS under the age of 16: clinical and paraclinical features. *Acta Neurol Scand* **86**: 280–4.

Sissons JG (1993) Superantigens and infectious disease. *Lancet* **341**: 1627–9.

Sriram S, Stratton CW, Yao S, et al. (1999) Chlamydia pneumoniae infection of the central nervous system in multiple sclerosis. *Ann Neurol* **46**: 6–14.

Steinlin MI, Blaser SI, Gilday DL, et al. (1995) Neurologic manifestations of pediatric systemic lupus erythematosus. *Pediatr Neurol* **13**: 191–7.

Stichweh D, Arce E, Pascual V (2004) Update on pediatric systemic lupus erythematosus. *Curr Opin Rheumatol* **16**: 577–87.

Strebel PM, Sutter RW, Cochi SL, et al. (1992) Epidemiology of poliomyelitis in the United States one decade after the last reported case of indigenous wild virus-associated disease. *Clin Infect Dis* **14**: 568–79.

Sugiura A, Yamada A (1991) Aseptic meningitis as a complication of mumps vaccination. *Pediatr Infect Dis J* **10**: 209–13.

Sunaga Y, Hikima A, Otsuka T, Morikawa A (1995) Acute cerebellar ataxia with abnormal MRI lesions after varicella vaccination. *Paediatr Neurol* **13**: 340–2.

Sundel RP, Newburger JW, McGill T, et al. (1990) Sensorineural hearing loss associated with Kawasaki disease. *J Pediatr* **117**: 371–7.

Tardieu M, Mikaeloff Y (2004) What is acute disseminated encephalomyelitis? *Eur J Paediatr Neurol* **8**: 239–42.

Tate ED, Allison TJ, Pranzatelli MR, Verhulst SJ (2005) Neuroepidemiologic trends in 105 US cases of pediatric opsoclonus–myoclonus syndrome. *J Pediatr Oncol Nurs* **22**: 8–19.

Telang G, Leong KK, Koblenzer P, Tunnessen WW (1993) Picture of the month. Neonatal lupus erythematosus. *Am J Dis Child* **147**: 903–4.

Tenembaum S, Chamoles N, Fejerman N (2002) Acute disseminated encephalomyelitis: a long-term study of 84 pediatric patients. *Neurology* **59**: 1224–31.

Terasawa K, Ichinose E, Matsuishi T, Kato H (1983) Neurological complications in Kawasaki disease. *Brain Dev* **5**: 371–4.

Toshniwal P (1987) Demyelinating optic neuropathy with Miller Fisher syndrome. The case for overlap syndromes with central and peripheral demyelination. *J Neurol* **234**: 353–8.

Transverse Myelitis Consortium Working Group (2002) Proposed diagnostic criteria and nosology of acute transverse myelitis. *Neurology* **59**: 499–505.

Trump RC, White TR (1967) Cerebellar ataxia presumed due to live, attenuated measles virus vaccine. *JAMA* **199**: 129–30.

Tucker LB, Menon S, Schaller JG, Isenberg DA (1995) Adult- and childhood-onset systemic lupus erythematosus: a comparison of onset, clinical features, serology, and outcome. *Br J Rheumatol* **34**: 866–72.

Turtzo LC, Lin DD, Hartung H, et al. (2007) A neurologic presentation of familial hemophagocytic lymphohistiocytosis which mimicked septic emboli to the brain. *J Child Neurol* **22**: 863–8.

Vliegenthart WE, Sanders EA, Bruyn GW, Vielvoye GJ (1985) An unusual CT-scan appearance in multiple sclerosis. *J Neurol Sci* **71**: 129–34.

Warrier RP, Kini R, Besser A, et al. (1985) Opsomyoclonus and neuroblastoma. *Clin Pediatr* **24**: 32–4.

Watson RM, Lane AT, Barnett NK, et al. (1984) Neonatal lupus erythematosus: a clinical, serological and immunogenetic study with review of the literature. *Medicine* **63**: 362–78.

Wattigney WA, Mootrey GT, Braun MM, Chen RT (2001) Surveillance for poliovirus vaccine adverse events, 1991 to 1998: impact of a sequential vaccination schedule of inactivated poliovirus vaccine followed by oral poliovirus vaccine. *Pediatrics* **107**: E83.

Weinshenker BG, Bass B, Rice GP, et al. (1989) The natural history of multiple sclerosis: a geographically based study. I. Clinical course and disability. *Brain* **112**: 133–46.

Weintraub MI, Chia DTS (1977) Paralytic brachial neuritis after swine flu vaccination. *Arch Neurol* **34**: 518 (letter).

Wells CEC (1971) A neurological note on vaccination against influenza. *BMJ* **3**: 755–6.

Wilejto M, Schroff M, Buncic JR, et al. (2006) The clinical features, MRI findings, and outcome of optic neuritis in children. *Neurology* **67**: 258–62.

Willoughby EN, Grochowski E, Li DKB, et al. (1989) Serial magnetic resonance scanning in multiple sclerosis: a second prospective study in relapsing patients. *Ann Neurol* **25**: 43–9.

Wingerchuk DM (2006) Neuromyelitis optica. *Int MS J* **13**: 42–50.

Wingerchuk DM, Weinschenker BG (2003) Neuromyelitis optica: clinical predictors of a relapsing course and survival. *Neurology* **60**: 848–53.

Writing Group of the Histiocyte Society (1987) Histiocytosis syndromes in children. *Lancet* **1**: 208–9.

Yahr MD, Lobo-Antunes J (1972) Relapsing encephalomyelitis following the use of influenza vaccine. *Arch Neurol* **27**: 182–3.

Yancey CL, Doughty RA, Athreya BH (1981) Central nervous system involvement in childhood systemic lupus erythematosus. *Arthritis Rheum* **24**: 1389–95.

Yarom A, Rennebohm RM, Levinson JE (1985) Infantile multisystem inflammatory disease: a specific syndrome? *J Pediatr* **106**: 390–6.

Yiu VW, Kovithavongs T, McGonigle LF, Ferreira P (2001) Plasmapheresis as an effective treatment for opsoclonus–myoclonus syndrome. *Pediatr Neurol* **24**: 72–4.

Zur Stadt U, Beutel K, Kolberg S, et al. (2006) Mutation spectrum in children with primary hemophagocytic lymphohistiocytosis: molecular and functional analyses of PRF1, UNC13D, STX11, and RAB27A. *Hum Mutat* **27**: 62–8.

12
ACCIDENTAL AND NON-ACCIDENTAL INJURIES BY PHYSICAL AGENTS AND TOXIC AGENTS

J Keith Brown and Robert A Minns

Acute brain and spinal cord disease due to external agents can be divided into three main divisions: (a) traumatic encephalopathies (birth trauma, accidental trauma, non-accidental trauma); (b) exogenous toxic encephalopathies (e.g. lead poisoning, scalds, burns); and (c) asphyxiating or suffocating hypoxic–ischaemic encephalopathies (e.g. drowning, carbon monoxide poisoning).

TRAUMATIC ENCEPHALOPATHIES

ACCIDENTAL INJURIES
Accidents of all types are the most frequent cause of death and a leading cause of significant impairment and disability in children and adolescents between 5 and 19 years of age (Robertson 1992, WHO 1995). Adolescents have an overall higher frequency of accidents than younger patients and are especially exposed to traffic accidents and to sports-related accidents. More children attend accident and emergency (A&E) departments with injury (76%) than with illness (24%) (Hendry et al. 2005).

ACCIDENTAL HEAD INJURIES
About 10% of new attenders at A&E departments present with head injuries (Jennett 1998). The total annual incidence of all head trauma is around 200–300 per 100,000 population. Approximately 5% of these are severe with a Glasgow Coma Score (GCS) of 8 or less, 5–10% are moderate (GCS 9–12), and 85–90% are minor (GCS >12) (Miller 1992). Accidental head injuries are common in children and the majority will have a straightforward course with a good outcome. A small number of children will sustain brain injury with the potential for more serious lasting complications and long-term disability. The incidence of head injury in children is 290/100,000 child A&E attenders, and in 5–10% of these (14.5–29/100,000), the injury is severe (Brookes et al. 1990).

Head injuries account for approximately one-third of accidental deaths in children. Deaths have been falling for the last 40 years in the USA (National Center for Health Statistics 1987). In the UK, the number of children killed in accidents is now about one per day. The mean mortality for head injury in children aged 1–15 years calculated from 18 published studies is 5.1 (SD 2.39) per 100,000 children per year (Minns and Lo 2008).

Accidental head injury results mainly from falls from various heights and from road traffic related accidents (RTAs) (Table 12.1).

Preventative measures are now showing a gratifying reduction in the number of adults and children killed or seriously injured in RTAs in Britain (Fig. 12.1) and in several European countries. These include legislation and 'road safety campaigns' for compulsory wearing of seat belts, back-facing baby restrainer seats, speed control by cameras, traffic calming measures, spot speed checks, banning the use of hand-held mobile phones when driving, drink/driving laws, spot breathalyser tests and cycle helmets (Agran et al. 1985, Bull and Stroup 1985, Selbst et al. 1987). The largest cause of accidents is falls; many of these are from windows and balconies and so are also amenable to preventative measures such as safety rails, locks and better supervision, while playground injuries can be reduced by modifying play equipment and by providing a forgiving surface such as forest bark or rubber.

Mechanism of injury
The primary brain injury can be due to seven different external physical mechanisms: penetrating injuries, compression, impact acceleration, impact deceleration, rotation, whiplash, and vascular.

• *Penetrating injuries.* These are high-velocity, high-energy injuries acting over a small area and can penetrate bone. The most obvious is a gunshot wound. Knife and scissor blades or screwdrivers can penetrate the vault of the skull in malicious assault. Accidental penetrating injuries of the orbits with sticks, knitting needles, pencils and toy railway lines are seen. The stick may be broken off leaving a piece still in the frontal lobes as a source of infection. Penetrating injuries are non-rotational and so non-concussional and therefore consciousness is preserved unless raised intracranial pressure supervenes.

TABLE 12.1
Causes of traumatic brain injury (TBI) in children*

Cause	%
Falls	45.1
From bicycle	5.7
From horse	1.2
Dropped[1]	3.3
Other[2]	45.1
Road traffic accident (RTA)	21.1
Pedestrian	12.7
Passengers	3.5
Cyclist	3.4
Other	1.5
Hit by object	11.7
Assault[3]	3.5
Sport	2.7
Non-accidental head injury (NAHI)[4]	2.2
Other	0.8
Unknown	2.5

*Adapted from Hawley et al. (2003), data from 1553 cases admitted to hospital for ≥24 hours.

The frequency of causes of TBI changes with severity and age, i.e. more RTA patients are severely injured, NAHI patients are usually infants, and falls and bicycles occur mostly in the 5–10 years age group.

[1] Cases would have been included in the NAHI category only if there were sufficient grounds to disbelieve the story.

[2] Falls could be 'high' or 'low' and might include those from windows, balconies, stairs, furniture, baby walkers, play equipment, trees or walls.

[3] These were usually child-on-child and were witnessed.

[4] Predominantly unwitnessed. The distinction between 'dropped', other 'falls', 'hit by an object' or 'assault' vs NAHI were made according to review of what was recorded in the case notes.

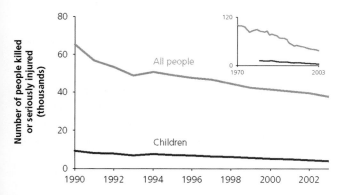

Fig. 12.1. Numbers of people and children killed or seriously injured in road traffic accidents (RTAs) in Great Britain, 1990–2003 (inset: 1970–2003). Adapted from Defra (2005).

In 1970 over 100,000 people were killed or seriously injured in RTAs. In 2003 the total was 37,500, a decrease of 63%.

The number of children killed or seriously injured in RTAs fell from 12,400 in 1979 to 4,100 in 2003, a decrease of 67%.

• *Compression injuries.* If the head is compressed between two surfaces, sat upon or stood on, a bursting fracture with suture diastases and a fractured base of the skull results. As there is no concussion, rotation or shearing, the child may be conscious even after severe injury.

Symptomatology varies with site of fracture. *Anterior cranial fossa fracture* may lead to anosmia, epistaxis, cerebrospinal fluid

(CSF) leakage from the nose (rhinorrhoea), subconjunctival haemorrhage, periorbital haemorrhage ('raccoon eyes'), optic nerve severance, squint, ptosis, and loss of sensation to forehead and cornea. *Middle cranial fossa fracture* may give rise to facial palsy, loss of sensation to lower face, haemotympanum, CSF leakage from the ear (otorrhoea), otalgia, deafness, tinnitus and dislocation of the stapes. *Posterior cranial fossa fracture* may be evidenced by ecchymosis behind the ear (Battle sign), impaired gag reflex, hypoventilation and ataxia.

• *Impact (contact) injuries.* The vast majority of accidental injuries in children are impact injuries. They may be accidental or non-accidental. They occur either when a moving force makes external contact with the head, causing it to accelerate (acceleration injury), or when the child's head is already moving and comes into contact with an unforgiving surface, causing it to suddenly decelarate (deceleration injury).

Acceleration injuries may be seen, for example, when the child is hit by a moving vehicle, fist, foot, hammer, golf club or milk bottle. If the child flies through the air some of the force is dissipated as the imparted motion.

Decceleration injuries occur in head-on car crashes; when children fall or are thrown from windows; and in falls from beds, incubators, changing mats, slides and ladders. Severity of injury depends on the forgiveness of the surface upon which the child lands, e.g. concrete, grass, sand or forest bark. Falls may be dissipated by a forgiving surface or by bounce, as on a trampoline or firefighter's safety net.

The force applied to the head depends on the size and weight of the child, the height of the fall, the speed of impact, and whether the child was stationary or moving at the time of the fall. If the impact force cannot be dissipated these deceleration impact injuries produce the most devastating type of head injury.

Head trauma generates physical forces that act upon the brain through acceleration–deceleration (linear or rotatory) and also by deformation. Brain damage that results from the action of these forces comes from percussion, compression, shearing or tearing of neural tissue occurring alone or successively, and may result in: (a) damage to the scalp with avulsion, skin bruising, subgaleal contusion and bleeding, and damage to the cranial skeleton in the form of fractures and extradural haematomas; (b) damage to the underlying dural sac with subsequent CSF rhinorrhoea or otorrhoea; (c) damage to the underlying brain tissue, including primary cerebral contusions (coup and contracoup), midbrain injury, subdural haematomas, intracerebral haematomas, cerebral lacerations or deep white matter shearing injuries (traumatic axonal injury).

• *Skull fractures.* Seventy to 80 per cent of skull fractures are linear fractures of the vault. Forty per cent of infants hospitalized with cranial trauma will have a skull fracture. Sequelae in the form of intracranial haematomas will develop in less than 20%. Leggate et al. (1989) showed that infants under 6 months of age operated on for evacuation of extradural haematoma, had either a skull fracture or suture separation seen on X-ray.

The poorly mineralized skull of the neonate bends and may indent causing the 'ping pong ball' or Pond fracture. Under these circumstances the skull offers little protection to the underlying brain, which is easily compressed. Severe local bruising and haemorrhage into the brain may then be seen associated with a minimal fracture.

Compound fractures secondary to penetration injuries may be obvious or subtle. Orbital trauma that penetrates the medial aspect of the orbit will pass into the ethmoid sinus and through the cribriform plate into the intracranial cavity. Another typical site for a penetrating injury is the squamous temporal region. In all such cases, extensive preoperative investigation is required, including CT and MR angiography prior to a thorough exploration of the penetrating tract, with debridement of damaged brain and formal closure of dura.

Fractures of the anterior fossa tear the roots of the olfactory nerve passing through the cribriform plate causing anosmia, and a dural tear causing CSF rhinorrhoea with a risk of meningitis. CSF rhinorrhoea is usually transient, disappearing in 70% of cases within 1 week and in a majority of the remaining cases within 6 months. Rhinorrhoea that persists more than 10 days is an indication for surgical repair. Prophylactic administration of antibiotics (ampicillin) does not reduce the incidence of meningitis and may change the flora to gram-negative organisms; it is preferable to watch the patients closely and to treat infection early. Periorbital echymosis ('racoon eyes') points to a possible anterior fossa fracture but can also be due to blood tracking down under the galea.

Fractures of the middle fossa involve the petrous temporal bone with haemotympanum, middle ear bleeding, dislocation of the ossicular chain and mastoid bruising (Battle sign). CSF otorrhoea may not be obvious if CSF passes down the eustachian tube and may be first heralded by pneumococcal meningitis. In the case of fracture of the petrous temporal bone there may be an ipsilateral facial nerve palsy or VIth nerve type squint which usually recovers spontaneously. Labyrinthine disturbances are due to haemorrhage or to a traumatic perilymphatic fistula. Vertigo, positional nystagmus, episodic vertigo, ataxia and hearing loss are uncommon.

Mechanism of primary brain injury in impact injury

There is very little that can be done to minimize the damage to the brain once the primary injury has occurred. Operation on the brain is mainly confined to removal of debris, bone and bullets as intracerebral haematomas are rarely evacuated. The major aim and thrust of modern head injury management is the prevention and treatment of the secondary injury.

• *Contusional or laceration injury.* Contusion or bruising of the brain occurs at the site of impact (coup) and then at the opposite side as the brain accelerates, forcibly hitting the other side of the skull, which suddenly stops moving before the brain (contracoup) and may then continue to rebound as the brain bounces inside the skull. The frontal and temporal lobes are accelerated and hit the bony buttress such as the sphenoid wing and ethmoidal

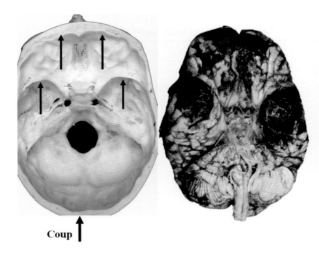

Fig. 12.2. Severe frontal and temporal contracoup contusion, caused by anterior bony buttresses, following occipital impact.

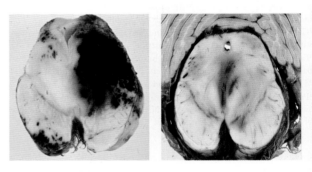

Fig. 12.3. Primary brainstem injury: *(left)* coup/contracoup from free edge of tentorium; *(right)* central midbrain injury from rotational trauma.

plate, so contusions are particularly likely on the under-surface of the frontal and temporal lobes and the anterior temporal pole (Fig. 12.2). The midbrain may be contused as it forcibly hits the free edge of the tentorium (Fig. 12.3). In a simple contusion, blood vessels rupture allowing red cells into the tissue spaces. Contusion of the brain presents as areas of gross or petechial haemorrhage with associated tearing of nerve fibres and cellular damage surrounded by oedema. Occipital pole lesions may occur with backward projection of the brain mass by frontal percussion. The brain architecture, however, is preserved, so that although there is temporary interference with function, good recovery is possible. If the brain is actually lacerated due to sphenoid impaction or tearing from impounded bone fragments then local atrophy and gliosis with less complete recovery is to be expected. Care must always be taken before prognosticating for recovery of function on the basis of an anatomical lesion on imaging. *Imaging studies* show that lesions are exclusively frontal or involve the frontal lobe in 80% of cases. In the remaining 20%, the lesions predominate in the temporal lobes. Cortical or cortico-subcortical contusions are very frequent with severe head trauma; MRI demonstrates such lesions in nearly all severe cases (Jenkins et al. 1986), twice as often as with CT.

improvement will continue to 18 months, but one cannot say that residual disability is permanent or will not improve further until 5 years post-injury. Care must be taken when prognosticating as there is now a suggestion of a late deterioration with loss of abilities in up to 7% of cases that may be due to seizures or hydrocephalus, but suspicion of a late cytokine-dependent regression following TBI is gaining support. The global outcome may be assessed at 6 and 12 months using such tools as the Glasgow Outcome Score (GOS) (Jennett and Bond 1975) or the KOSCHI score (Crouchman et al. 2001).

Cognitive and behavioural sequelae

Learning disorders, behavioural and motor deficits and epilepsy are the major sequelae of head injury. Post-traumatic epilepsy is considered below. Poor concentration and headache are the most frequent complaints on follow up. Cognitive difficulties, memory disturbance and behavioural problems are common after moderate to severe head trauma as might be expected with frontal and anteromedial temporal lobe damage. In children after severe TBI, the behavioural diagnosis of ADHD is associated with more difficulty in attention, executive functioning and memory than primary ADHD (Slomine et al. 2005).

Concentration is poor, memory deficiency may be severe enough to class as post-traumatic Korsakoff syndrome, personality changes and rage reactions may make the parents' life unbearable and yet little may be found on a superficial neurological examination or routine standardized psychometrics. However, the use of single photon emission computed tomography (SPECT) has shown that many children with pervasive learning or behaviour problems do have very definite residual pathology. The behaviour and learning problems are easily missed in a hurried follow-up examination.

Minor and mild injuries do not seem commonly to be associated with sequelae (Bijur et al. 1990), but a seemingly minor injury does not exclude secondary learning or behavioural sequelae and imaging with MRI and SPECT may show an unexpected pathological basis. Sequelae, however, are much more frequent following severe injury with coma, and there is a clear relationship between the duration of coma and the presence of sequelae (Mahoney et al. 1983, Filley et al. 1987). A period of coma exceeding 1 week in duration is associated with an increased incidence of cognitive deficits, while coma of less than a week is not (Jennett and Teasdale 1977, Chadwick 1985). A significant part of post-traumatic dysfunction in children appears to be reactive in origin and therefore preventable by correct psychological management during recovery. In children in whom behavioural problems were present before the accident, the brain injury may exacerbate these problems. Tentorial herniation with damage to the amygdala and hippocampus would be expected to cause severe memory defects, especially putting new memories into long-term stores (post-traumatic Korsakoff syndrome).

Some behaviour and personality changes may be secondary to stress from impaired perceptual and cognitive difficulties. Klonoff et al. (1993) found that the IQ in the post-acute phase was a reliable predictor of outcome. They reported that subjective sequelae, observed in 31% of 159 children followed for 23 years, were clearly related to the extent of head injury and a low IQ. The need for rehabilitation after severe head injury was assessed by Scott-Jupp et al. (1992) who found that 18 of 43 children had persistent neurological impairment and 15 needed special educational support.

Post-traumatic headaches and post-concussion subjective syndrome are much less frequent in children than in adults as sequelae to head injury (Barlow 1984). Post-traumatic migraine may be very troublesome in predisposed children after relatively minor trauma. Sleep disturbances are extremely common (Guilleminault et al. 1983). A 12-week course of a dopamine agonist, amantadine hydrochloride (AMH), used for neurobehavioural sequelae of paediatric TBI, was safe and, according to parent report, improved behaviour (Beers et al. 2005).

Visual deficits, especially optic atrophy, may occur, particularly as a result of hydrocephalus or haematoma (Gerber et al. 1992). Optic nerve trauma is seen in shaking injury, with bruising and haemorrhage in the optic nerve sheath. Complete severance of one optic nerve may occur by the sphenoid wing. This causes a fixed dilated pupil and a blind eye in a conscious patient with eye movements. Acute blindness lasting several days may occur after severe occipital contusional injuries, sometimes complicated by seizure discharges. Post-traumatic migraine with visual phenomena can also be severe in predisposed children. Cortical visual agnosia is seen from watershed zone infarction in the territory between middle and posterior cerebral arteries. Calcarine infarction with cortical blindness occurs from compression of the posterior cerebral arteries due to raised ICP with tentorial herniation.

Disorders of visual processing are more common than usually appreciated. The Winsconsin Card Sorting Test (Heaton 2005) will pick out problems following frontal lobe injury. Wrightson et al. (1995) compared 78 children with mild head trauma not requiring hospitalization and 86 control children who had incurred other forms of injury, and found that the former scored less than controls on reading and solving a visual puzzle.

Visual problems are particularly prevalent after non-accidental shearing head injuries due to primary retinal damage, white matter atrophy of the optic radiation or calcarine infarction secondary to severe cerebral oedema.

Deafness is uncommon and unilateral in most cases and easily missed. The potentially treatable traumatic dislocation of the stapes footplate should be borne in mind.

Post-traumatic epilepsy is discussed in Chapter 14.

NON-ACCIDENTAL HEAD INJURIES

Non-accidental head injuries are but one part of the wide domain of child abuse, which also includes emotional abuse, neglect and sexual abuse as well as other non-neurological physical injuries and less obvious forms of aggression such as the Munchausen syndrome by proxy.

We prefer the term non-accidental head injury (NAHI) to 'shaken baby syndrome' as this implies knowledge of a mechanism that one then has to try to prove (Minns and Brown 2005). The pathology is a traumatic brain injury. One has to establish the surety of diagnosis of non-accidental trauma, and then consider the mechanism. Who did it is not a medical consideration. NAHIs are the commonest type of head injury in children under 2 years of age. Billmire and Myers (1985) found that in children under 2 years, 64% of all head injuries (excluding uncomplicated skull fractures), and 95% of serious head injuries were of non-accidental origin. Physical abuse constitutes about one third of all child abuse (Minns and Brown 2005). In England there is a category of multiple abuse that includes physical abuse. Actual brain injury is rare and occurs in only 0.5% of all cases of abuse, and 1–3% of cases of physical abuse.

Hahn et al. (1988) considered that the head injuries in 4.4% of 318 children were the result of abuse, whereas Duhaime et al. (1992) found a much higher prevalence of 24% in 100 carefully studied children. The prevalence of NAHI in infants in the Lothian region of Scotland is 33 per 100,000 infants under 1 year of age (Minns et al. 2008).

MECHANISM OF INJURY

Any of the mechanisms described above under accidental head injury can occur as a non-accidental TBI. Penetrating injuries are uncommon from gunshot wounds or stabbings. Compression can occur from standing on the infant's head or even squeezing between an adult's knees. Impact injuries can be due to throwing the baby onto the ground, pushing down stairs, swinging by the legs and hitting the wall, or shaking and banging the head on the floor (hard impact) or on the crib (soft impact). Asphyxial injury is common due to primary cervico-medullary injury, the secondary injury with impaired cerebral perfusion, but also by suffocation, for example pressing a hand or pillow over the mouth to stop the noise from crying, or as a deliberate act, e.g. using a rolled towel. Because of the infant's size it is easily lifted so shaking is a mechanism of injury peculiar to the first year of life and will be considered in more detail. Shaking is thought to produce a rotational shearing injury but a mixed mechanism is probably at play in many cases (Zepp et al. 1992).

Shaking as a cause of head injury

Sufficient numbers of parents and carers have admitted to and described the manner of shaking to establish it as an unequivocal cause of NAHI (Minns 2005). Duhaime et al. (1987) and Kleinman et al. (1989) were doubtful that shaking alone was the mechanism because of the high incidence of associated findings indicating impact seen in the shaken human infant. If there is associated impact, for example by the head being banged against a hard surface repeatedly during the shaking, or the infant being thrown or dropped on the floor after the shaking (shake and throw away), the clinical features will confirm the impact injury. Soft impact, however, may be more devastating by causing acute deceleration and so more swirling of the brain within the skull, and yet leave no mark. The identical cerebral syndrome of encephalopathy, subdural haematoma and retinopathy is seen whether signs of impact, e.g. bruising, subgaleal bleeding,

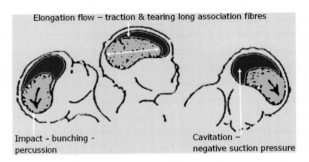

Fig. 12.15. Illustration of mechanism of axonal shearing due to flowing effect of jellyish brain causing bunch flow and cavitation 'bounce' within the skull.

fractures and extensive evidence elsewhere of trauma, are present or not.

Potential mechanisms of non-accidental shaking (brain trauma) include:

1. Shaking causes rotation of the brain, which bounces inside the skull causing rotational shearing injuries as well as repeated percussion/cavitation and flow, causing traction and tearing of white matter axons (Fig. 12.15).
2. Impact against a soft surface causing acute deceleration of the brain and vastly increasing the rotational torque forces inside the skull.
3. Hyperflexion and hyperextension injury from the whiplash causing repetitive subluxation (there is a physiological subluxation at extremes of movement in infants) of the cervical vertebrae resulting in injury to the cervical cord and medulla.
4. Shaking with hard impact causing skull fractures and contusional injuries in addition to the rotational injuries.
5. Primary hypoxic–ischaemic brain injury resulting from stem injury or suffocation with apnoea.

CLINICAL MANIFESTATIONS AND DIAGNOSIS OF NAHI

Most affected infants are generally unwell, refuse feeds, vomit, are irritable and resent handling. They may suddenly quieten (an ominous sign). Some may be pale, anaemic and shocked or have apnoea, cyanotic attacks or tachycardia (Brown and Minns 1993), and even with these nonspecific symptoms, brain injury should be suspected. The neurological presentation is thus of a nonspecific acute encephalopathy and so the true nature may not at first be obvious when meningitis, metabolic disease, poisoning, encephalitis and status epilepticus are suspected (Fig. 12.16). In a large Canadian Study (King et al. 2003) presenting complaints for the 364 children identified as having 'shaken baby syndrome' were seizure-like episodes (45%), decreased level of consciousness (43%) and respiratory difficulty (34%), though bruising was noted on examination in 46%. A temporal classification of neurological presentations has been suggested (Minns and Busuttil 2004) and is discussed in the following, numbered, sections.

1. Hyperacute cervico-medullary syndrome

This hyperacute presentation results from repetitive severe hyperflexion/hyperextension whiplash shaking forces and the infant's

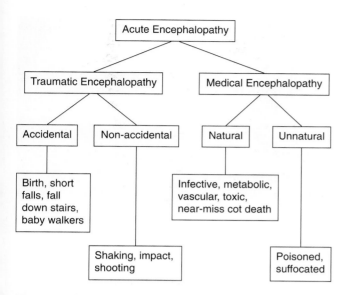

Fig. 12.16. Flow diagram of potential causes in a child presenting with an acute encephalopathy.

lower medulla and upper cervical cord receive a repeated percussion injury. Geddes et al. (2001) found localized axonal damage at the cranio-cervical junction, in the corticospinal tracts in the lower brainstem, and in the cervical cord roots. Additionally there is the possibility of traumatic thrombosis of the vertebral arteries as they wind through the foramina of the cervical vertebrae. These patients are infrequently seen by the clinician and are either dead on arrival at hospital or shortly thereafter (6%), and are the group most likely seen by the pathologists.

Combined sequential MRI and CT studies have given a much more dynamic picture of pathology than autopsy, which often occurs after a period of reanimation and secondary insult, or acutely before classical findings appear (Robert Minns and Karen Choo, unpublished observations). The cervical spine has not been routinely included with MRI of the head, but should be in all small infants with suspected trauma.

2. Acute encephalopathic presentation

This is characterized by seizures, decerebration, homeostatic derangements, bilateral large subdural haematomas and widespread haemorrhagic retinopathy. There may be additional skeletal fractures such as rib or metaphyseal 'corner' or 'chip' fractures or other evidence of non-accidental injuries such as bruising, cuts, cigarette burns, etc. This type of presentation is the commonest pattern seen by hospital paediatricians and has been the pattern frequently referred to as the classical "shaken baby syndrome" by clinicians. When there are additional signs of impact the syndrome may then be more accurately referred to as 'shaken impact syndrome'.

Failure of peripheral circulation causes cold extremities, decreased capillary return and low blood pressure, and these are serious signs of circulatory failure that could further interfere with CPP. Although the babies feel cold due to shock, hypothermia is rarely present. A depressed conscious state with floppiness and reduced movements is a common presentation (Minns and Brown 2005).

• *Respiratory symptomatology.* Respiratory distress appears as the ICP rises, but it may also represent direct medullary trauma or vertebral artery trauma due to the whiplashing. Abnormal breathing, such as apnoea and respiratory arrest, grunting respirations, shallow respirations or choking, features in approximately 40% of cases. Pallor or cyanosis is a presenting feature in approximately a third of cases. A history of previous respiratory symptoms, which may have required medical attention, or antibiotics in the weeks prior to presentation, may represent an earlier traumatic episode and old fractures of ribs should be carefully sought. Cardiorespiratory arrest occurred in 11 of 127 cases of 'suspected NAHI' (8.6%) in our Scottish database, and 34% (36/105) presented with apnoea and required subsequent ventilation for 1–22 days (personal data, unpublished).

• *Seizures.* Seizures present at the time of the acute encephalopathic presentation are described in approximately 20% of children. Decerebrate posturing due to the tonic phase of a seizure, postasphyxial rigidity or raised ICP was evident from the history in a third of cases. This highlights the need in neurointensive care units for continuous real-time EEG and ICP monitoring. Following admission to hospital two thirds of children have seizures, a much higher incidence than that occurring in accidental TBI. These epileptic seizures are often severe and drug resistant, reaching a climax at 24–48 hours but usually decreasing and ceasing by the fifth day. EEG recordings often show more discharges than those witnessed clinically. Seizures cause a further rise in ICP every time there is a clinical or electrical discharge. Barlow et al. (2000) have shown a significant relationship between the early post-traumatic seizures and outcome in NAHI.

• *Raised intracranial pressure.* Evidence of raised ICP is suggested by an increased head circumference, tense non-pulsatile anterior fontanelle, or distended scalp veins. Pupillary changes are not helpful. Cerebral oedema was evident on brain imaging in 25% of children at first imaging after admission (Kemp et al. 2003), and two thirds of children have documented raised ICP when objectively measured (Barlow and Minns 1999). The increased ICP together with shock and hypotension further reduces the CPP and increases the risk of secondary ischaemic brain damage. A low CPP is a good predictor of long-term disability (Barlow and Minns 1999).

• *Retinal haemorrhages.* Inflicted head injuries are associated with a high incidence of retinal haemorrhage (approximately 70% in the Scottish Database – Minns and Brown 2005). Retinal haemorrhages can be unilateral. They were reported to occur in 80% of cases of pure shaken baby syndrome (without evidence of impact) (Ludwig and Warman 1984).

In a typical angiopathic (traumatic) retinopathy the haemorrhages are not around the disc or flame shaped but tend to occur throughout the retina, usually bilaterally and extending to the periphery, but one eye may be much more seriously affected than the other. The retinal haemorrhages are multilayer, severe and extensive (too numerous to count) throughout the retina, and involve sub-retinal, intra-retinal (flame or dot/blot) and pre-retinal layers that may rupture into vitreous, and extend to the ora serrata. Traumatic retinoschisis is thought to be pathognomonic, being a shearing-type injury, and is seen only in NAHI in children under 5 years of age.

We have found retinal haemorrhages in almost 17% of accidental head injuries, and in 93% of NAHI cases (unpublished data). Plunket (2001) described an older group of children who sustained playground injuries that were witnessed. Retinal haemorrhages were noted in 4 of 6 children who had ophthalmological examinations. Retinal haemorrhages following accidental head injury are more likely to occur following high-velocity road traffic accidents involving side impact. They are exceptionally rare after cardiopulmonary resuscitation but are often florid if there has been chest compression in a traffic accident.

There may also be other ocular trauma including retinal folds, secondary retinal detachment and optic nerve percussion trauma. Papilloedema although not often recognized may also occur. Retinal scarring is highly suggestive of child abuse.

The infant retina is loosely attached at the macula and periphery and is easily damaged by vitreous traction resulting from a rotational injury to the head. This ties the lesions in the brain and those in the retina to a common shearing/rotational mechanism.

3. Non-encephalopathic subacute presentation
In this group the presentation is with subdural haemorrhage, retinal haemorrhages, bruising, and rib and other skeletal fractures, but an acute encephalopathy is not a prominent feature and the outcome is better than in the other groups. Timing of the injury, and hence identification of a perpetrator, may be more problematic.

4. Recurrent encephalopathy
This is the converse of number 3 above, when the child may present with a recurrent encephalopathy without fractures, subdural haemorrhage or retinopathy or any pointers to trauma, and when encephalitis or a metabolic cause is suspected, rather than repeated poisoning, suffocation or shaking (Rogers et al. 1976). The child may present with an isolated seizure from shaking or with status epilepticus. A proper examination of the fundi is indicated in infants presenting with unexplained seizures in the first year of life. Fabrication of symptoms especially seizures (fictitious epilepsy) is also a form of child abuse in Munchausen syndrome by proxy (Meadow 1984).

5. Chronic (non-encephalopathic) extracerebral presentation
This is the late-presenting subdural haematoma in a child with an expanding head circumference, vomiting, failure to thrive, hypotonicity and mild developmental delay. There are often no retinal haemorrhages, no encephalopathy, no accompanying fractures or bruising, and the acute subdural haemorrhage has

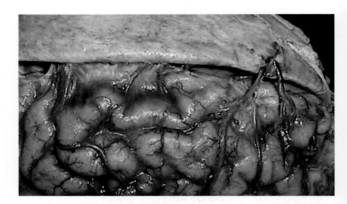

Fig. 12.17. Penetrating vessels anchoring the brain to the dura and inner skull, easily torn with brain rotation.

occurred weeks prior to presentation. These children are at risk of the effects of raised ICP and visual compromise, but the prognosis with recognition and appropriate treatment is good compared to the acute subdural haemorrhage with acute encephalopathy.

The differential diagnosis for chronic subdural space expansion encompasses a wide variety of conditions and these must be excluded by appropriate investigation. Although cases may be due to late presentation of NAHI, the possibility of some other cause including the nebulous idiopathic spontaneous subdural haemorrhage means that there is not sufficient evidence to start legal proceedings. One cannot give date or time, certainty of trauma or a possible mechanism. Suspicion may be strong in the mind of the paediatrician and social worker but proof is lacking unless skull, rib or old long-bone fractures are demonstrated.

SUBDURAL HAEMATOMA (SDH)
Bleeding from torn bridging veins running from the surface of the brain to the saggital sinus (Fig. 12.17) causes a surface and interhemispheric subdural and subarachnoid bleeding without any fracture being present. Such bleeding into the subdural space is the hallmark of non-accidental shaking injury in the first year of life, occurring in 90% of cases. It is bilateral in approximately 80% of cases. A unilateral SDH does not negate the diagnosis of NAHI. The subdural bleeding is usually most obvious over the surface convexity of the cerebral hemispheres but also occurs in the interhemispheric fissure, sub-temporally in the middle cranial fossa, and less often in the sub-occipital region tentorially or in the posterior fossa.

Subdural haematomas are usually classified as subdural haemorrhage, subdural haematoma and subdural effusion, or as acute, subacute and chronic, although there is no universally agreed definition as to the exact timing that differentiates one from the other. An acute SDH occurs within 3 days of the injury, a subacute SDH from 3 days to 3 weeks, and a chronic SDH more than 3 weeks from the time of the injury (Choux et al. 1986).

Chronic subdural haematoma
A chronic SDH is in most cases due to failure to resolve an acute

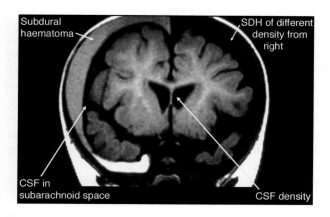

Fig. 12.18. MRI showing subdural collections of different densities, and external hydrocephalus with a deep subarachnoid space.

Labels on image:
- Subdural haematoma
- SDH of different density from right
- CSF in subarachnoid space
- CSF density

haematoma and has two components: a liquid low-haematocrit haematoma or effusion, and evidence of continued fresh bleeding, with fluid ingress causing dilution and expansion and eventually a membrane. Incorporation of the haematoma into the dura as a membrane is the basis of the healing process.

A chronic SDH is not a true haematoma but a subdural effusion in that it is mainly water not blood, with the haematocrit rarely exceeding 10%. After 3 weeks the colour turns from red to brown due to formation of methaemoglobin and the fluid is very xanthochromic on centrifugation. The density may be different between the two sides and this does not indicate a second injury. The SDH at the vertex compresses the subarachnoid space and sagittal sinus and impairs CSF absorption. Blood in the CSF also blocks the arachnoid granulations and so impairs CSF absorption, which results in expansion of the subarachnoid space as an 'external hydrocephalus' (Fig. 12.18). Although there are many causes of subdural haemorrhage and effusion, SDH of this age is more likely to be a traumatic lesion.

Treatment
SDH can be aspirated through the angle of the fontanelle in order to acutely relieve raised ICP. Some cases will rapidly come under control with a few needle aspirations (taps). Alternatively, burr hole drainage may be used. There is always the risk of infection, meningitis or a subdural empyema, so repeated tapping even under strict aseptic conditions with full skin preparation for more than 10 days is best avoided. In these circumstances a non-valved subdural/peritoneal shunt is preferred to continuous external drainage with tunnelling of the external catheter below the scalp. Small SDHs can be left alone and monitored by imaging if there is no rise in ICP. Overenthusiastic drainage after the head has expanded leaves 'craniocerebral disproportion' so there must be persistent extracerebral fluid to fill the increased volume.

DIAGNOSIS OF NAHI
A major reason for suspecting non-accidental trauma is the discrepancy between the severity of injury and the history of

trauma given by the parents or guardians. No spontaneous history of trauma is of less value than denial of trauma on direct questioning. A changing story or discrepancy between parents, both supposed witnesses of the same event, arouses suspicion.

Falls from heights of less than one meter are a common claim as a cause of the injury but are only exceptionally the cause of multiple injuries or brain injury (Plunkett 2001, Minns and Brown 2005). Kravitz et al. (1969) found only 3 skull fractures and 1 SDH in 330 children younger than 2 years old who fell from couches, dressing tables and cots, and less than 10% had evidence of minor concussion.

In infants less than 6 months of age, depressed or 'growing skull fractures' with brain injury, certain locations such as the occipital bone, scapula, multiple bilateral ribs, bucket handle fractures of long bones and multiple metacarpel bone fractures are virtually pathognomonic of abuse. The presence of multiple fractures of differing ages, especially metaphyseal injuries that give rise to characteristic X-ray images, is very suggestive (Kleinman 1987). Likewise, multiple cutaneous lesions such as bites, cigarette burns and ecchymoses are strong evidence of abuse. Cardiac massage in infants is only exceptionally associated with rib fractures, which are frequent in abused infants (Feldman and Brewer 1984), and is only rarely associated with retinal haemorrhage (Odom et al. 1997).

Although proof of the diagnosis may be difficult to provide, evidence of contact (impact) trauma is supported by the following: (i) history of trauma may be given even if not the true mechanism; (ii) bruising (cutaneous or subcuraneous), fractures, burns, knife cuts or obvious trauma; (iii) subgaleal haemorrhage; (iv) skull fracture; (v) extradural haemorrhage; (i) focal SDH; (vii) focal cerebral contusion; (viii) contracoup injury; (ix) metaphyseal or long bone fractures in a young infant who is incapable of independent movement.

Recurrent injuries may be sustained if the original diagnosis is missed. A high index of suspicion is therefore essential. One arrives at a decision as to the level of suspicion or probability of abuse with varying degrees of certainty. The diagnosis rests on a conjunction of features, i.e. a syndrome, rather than isolated symptoms, which can nearly always have alternative explanations and which rarely constitute adequate evidence of child abuse (Brown and Minns 1993). The shaken baby syndrome of encephalopathy, SDH, retinal haemorrhage with fractured ribs and metaphyseal injury, as originally described by Caffey (1972), is much more sound than an isolated subdural or retinal haemorrhage, although the latter features individually will raise suspicion in the paediatrician's mind. The circumstances of the abuse – e.g. in a preterm infant; accompanying failure to thrive; a single mother with cohabiting boyfriend who is not the biological father; previous court appearances for aggressive behaviour; social work involvement, or puerperal psychosis – may all be additionally suggestive but are not diagnostic. The paediatricians must ask a fundamental question about what is the 'relative probability' that these clinical findings are due to an accidental cause, a non-accidental cause, or other (medical) cause. Equally a diagnosis of non-accidental trauma should not be taken as automatically indicating a mechanism such as shaking. Factors such as the pattern of injuries or the presence or absence of contact will allow the paediatrician to offer an opinion as to the possible mechanism with which the injuries are consistent, e.g. impact, rotation, impact plus rotation, whiplash, compression, penetration or asphyxia.

The *differential diagnosis* includes unintentional trauma and benign subdural collections (Chapter 5). Osseous disorders associated with multiple metaphyseal lesions such as scurvy, rickets and copper deficiency may simulate the 'battered child syndrome'. Osteogenesis imperfecta, especially in its less severe forms (mild type I and type IV) may pose difficult diagnostic problems. The presence of many wormian bones, osteopenia, joint laxity and blue sclera are useful but not infallible clues. Biochemical analysis of type I collagen can be very helpful as 87% of patients have a demonstrable abnormality of procollagen (Gahagan and Rimsza 1991). A similar problem may arise with copper deficiency in preterm infants and in cases of Menkes disease (Chapter 8). Haematological diseases such as idiopathic thrombocytopenic purpura can also resemble the syndrome when associated with bone lesions.

Many children with non-accidental trauma have also been abused in other ways, and therefore accompanying short stature and low body weight may be an indication of possible neglect as well as abuse.

A special problem is posed by Munchausen syndrome by proxy (Meadow 1982, 1991; Rosenberg 1987) in which the child is abused in various manners by a parent – usually the mother. The parent submits the child to a form of abuse by fabricating or producing signs or symptoms of illness so that the child becomes involved in hospital investigations and procedures, often over a long period. Fabricated illness may also be initiated by poisoning, injecting insulin, putting blood in urine, feeding salt, or suffocation and strangulation to produce 'pseudoepileptic' attacks.

MANAGEMENT

The aim of intensive care management in inflicted TBI is to reduce the risk of death or secondary brain damage and hence resultant disability. It does not differ from the management of accidental head trauma described above. In our experience early CT and MRI are essential, as is follow-up imaging, at 2 weeks, 2 months, 6 months and 2 years, to determine the natural history of the injury – resolution of the acute injury and evolution of the long-term brain damage – which is useful from a medicolegal viewpoint. A skeletal survey and investigation of other confounding diseases, along with a thrombophilic profile, are indicated, which would not routinely be performed after accidental injury. The other big difference is the need to confront parents and record accurately their explanations. Most areas in the UK have a 'child protection team' who should be contacted on suspicion of a 'suspected NAHI' diagnosis or unexplained clinical features. They will involve social services and police as circumstantial evidence is vital to support clinical suspicion (Minns and Brown 2005).

PROGNOSIS

The proportion of children with serious morbidity is far worse with NAHI than with accidental head injury, not only because of the residual brain damage, but also because of the arrested skull and brain growth with progressive microcephaly and cerebral atrophy.

Thirty per cent of abused children have signs of severe disability (acquired cerebral palsy and severe mental retardation) due to permanent CNS damage, and 25% have moderate learning, perceptual, cognitive or memory deficits; 57% have an IQ ≤80. Bonnier et al. (1995) have emphasized the late effects of whiplash injury, after a 'sign free interval', that include arrest of brain and skull growth, long-tract signs, seizures, and increasingly obvious psychological and behavioural problems as the child grows older. Visual problems are also very much more common than after accidental injury as described above.

Emotional consequences are frequent in abused children (Friedman 1976) and, when adults, such individuals sometimes tend to reproduce the behaviour of their parents, towards their own children. There is evidence that even non-abused siblings of battered infants may have unsatisfactory mental and emotional development.

SPINAL CORD INJURY

Spinal injury as with head injury can be due to birth-related, accidental or non-accidental causes.

SPINAL DAMAGE IN THE INFANT

Trauma in utero can cause spinal injury, especially if the head is engaged and the maternal abdomen pendulous. Birth trauma to the cervical spine is well documented in breech delivery or forceps rotation, and was not a rare clinical diagnosis at the time when birth trauma was common, estimated to be present in 10–33% of neonatal deaths (Towbin 1970). Lifting the infant body over the mother's abdomen with the head still engaged may also cause fractures of the occipital bone and cerebellar haemorrhage or thoracolumbar injury. Spinal injury may be atlantoaxial, C5/T1, or less commonly thoracolumbar. Root pocket haemorrhage, spinal root avulsion, spinal epidural haemorrhage and intraparenchymatous cord haemorrhages were seen at autopsy (Yates 1959).

ACCIDENTAL INJURY

Accidental injuries to the spinal cord occur rarely in childhood. In one US study of 103 consecutively treated paediatric cervical spine injury patients (mean age approx. 10 years), motor vehicle accidents were the cause in 50% of cases and sports injuries in 25%, with falls the next most common (Brown et al. 2001). A recent series found motor vehicle accidents responsible for 40%, falls 35% and sports injuries 17.5% of cases (Leonard et al. 2007). Martin et al. (2004) in a large series of children on the UK Trauma Audit and Research Network Database 1989–2000, found 2.7% with spinal injury, 0.6% with spinal cord injury and 0.15% with spinal cord injury without radiological abnormality (SCIWORA).

NON-ACCIDENTAL INJURY

Concurrent injuries to the cervical spine with epidural spinal haemorrhage and bruising of the cervicomedullary junction are probably underestimated. They were found in 5 out of 6 fatal cases of whiplash shaking injury by Hadley et al. (1989). Geddes et al. (2001) have revisited the pathology of the spine and medulla in NAHI, and her cases showed spinal epidural bleeding, localized axonal damage to the cranio-cervical junction, and damage to the spinal nerve roots and brainstem in 11 out of 37 shaken infants. Patients presenting with apnoea or who die without significant SDH or cerebral oedema should be particularly suspect (see acute cervico-medullary syndrome above).

PATHOLOGY OF SPINAL CORD INJURY

The cervical spine is the most commonly injured area (C1–C2, C5–C6). T12–L1 and L2–L5 are other common sites of spinal injury. Dislocations are frequent in cervical cord injuries, and compression fractures in thoracolumbar insults. The thoracic spine is rigidly supported by the ribs, but when fractures occur, neurological damage is frequently seen. The spinal cord ends at the level of L1–L2 lumbar vertebrae and injury below this will damage only the cauda equina. These are lower motor neuron fibres and as such have the capacity to regenerate. Of 89 children with spinal fractures or fracture dislocations of the thoraco-lumbar region reviewed by Dogan et al. (2007), 85% had no serious irreversible cord damage. The odontoid peg on the axis has an epiphysis that does not fuse until 7 years of age and so odontoid epiphysiolysis with anterior dislocation is particularly an injury of very young children.

CLINICAL FEATURES

The clinical features of spinal cord injury vary with the location of the trauma, the structures affected, and with the severity of the insult.

Spinal injury in the newborn causes sudden death in labour or tetraparesis (which may resemble Werdnig–Hoffman spinal muscular atrophy), a flaccid paraparesis, bilateral Erb's palsy, or diaphragmatic and respiratory paralysis requiring continued ventilation. There may be very brisk spinal flexor withdrawal reflexes masking the true paraparesis.

Concussion of the spinal cord produces transient neurological deficits of unclear mechanism. Loss of function may be complete or partial but signs of recovery appear within hours or a few days. Recovery is often complete, but in more severe cases there may be only partial recovery with persisting physical signs or symptoms of cord dysfunction. Topographical syndromes of spinal cord involvement are indicated in Table 12.4.

In severe cord injury there occurs a period of *spinal shock* below the injured segment. It is characterized by complete loss of motor, sensory and sphincter functions with complete areflexia lasting 2–6 weeks. Gradually, a muscular response to stimuli in the involved territory appears, and spasticity with extensor plantar reflexes, mass flexion reflexes and increased deep tendon reflexes follows. Extensor reflexes (spasms) ultimately appear and become the dominant reflex activity.

TABLE 12.4
Neurological features of the commonest spinal cord injuries

Transverse lesions
C1–C2
    Complete quadriplegia
    Respiratory paralysis
C5–C6
    Quadriplegia
    Preservation of diaphragmatic movements
    Sensory level at upper thoracic level with preservation of sensation over lateral aspects of the arm
T1–L1
    Paraplegia
    Sensory level at inguinal folds
    Loss of sphincter control

Unilateral or predominantly unilateral lesions
Brown–Sequard syndrome
Unilateral paralysis ipsilateral to affected side
Unilateral disturbances of deep sensation
Disturbances of position and vibration sense ipsilateral to paralysis
Unilateral (contralateral to lesion) disturbances of superficial (pain and thermal) sensation
Incomplete forms frequent, e.g. spinal hemiplegias

Central cord lesions
Involvement of upper limbs greater than that of lower limbs (lesion affects the more medial segment of corticospinal tract)
Lower motor neuron involvement of upper limbs
Spasticity of the lower limbs
Bladder dysfunction
Disturbances in pain and thermal sensation below the level of the lesion

Anterior spinal syndrome
Paraplegia
Loss of pain and thermal sensation
Preservation of deep sensation
May be due to lesion of the anterior spinal artery

The eventual clinical picture of spinal cord injury may be one of purely reflex activity in the most severe cases, with variable degrees of preserved function in patients with less extensive damage. Three quarters of the patients of Hamilton and Myles (1992) with physiologically incomplete spinal cord deficit improved significantly and more than half made a complete recovery, whereas a similar improvement was seen in only 10% of those with physiologically complete section.

RADIOLOGY

Radiological investigations are imperative to diagnosis in cases of spinal cord trauma. Fracture or dislocation are often present, but special views with CT using 3-dimensional reconstructions may be necessary to demonstrate them. CT (especially helical CT) will show bony injury missed on plain radiographs. The patients however, should be manipulated with the utmost care to avoid provoking damage or exacerbating any prior insult.

MRI is nowadays mandatory to determine the presence or absence of compression and the extent to which nervous structures have been compromised. Multilevel injury may be seen in children, and the whole spine should be routinely imaged. This may show cord oedema, posterior swelling, ligamentous injury, bleeding into the cord, root pocket haemorrhages and nerve root tears. MRI provides considerable information about the cord itself: acute haemorrhage and syrinxes give a low signal on T_1-weighted sequences, whereas oedema and punctate haemorrhages are well demonstrated (Davis 1995). An haematomyelia on MRI carries a very poor prognosis. Late imaging studies may show cavitation of the spinal cord that may be progressive, whether originating from accidental or surgical trauma (Avrahami et al. 1989).

TREATMENT

Treatment of spinal cord injury in the acute stage includes positioning and prevention of movement, especially in cervical injuries (Sonntag and Hadley 1988). The relatively large head of children forces the neck into flexion if the child is simply laid flat on a hard surface. All serious accidents, especially head injuries, should be assumed to have a potential spinal injury and paramedics nowadays will routinely immobilise the cervical spine and move the patient as if a spinal injury is present until proved otherwise.

Conservative treatment is favoured if the spine is stable with no cord compression on imaging. The cervical spine can be immobilized by a Philadelphia collar or halo vest. Skeletal traction may be indicated in definite cases on a Stryker frame with or without cranial tongs. High-dose methylprednisolone (a 30 mg/kg bolus followed by 5.4 mg/kg/hour for 23 hours) is being evaluated. Although GM1 ganglioside has seemed encouraging, there is serious doubt about its efficacy and innocuity.

Surgical treatment is indicated (i) in the case of suspected spinal canal block, (ii) in wounds in which imaging shows bony fragments in the spinal canal, (iii) in cases in which the neurological deficit is shown to increase because of the possibility of a remediable spinal epidural haematoma (Tender and Awasthi 2004), and (iv) in cases of dislocation of the spine that cannot be reduced by traction. Cervical spine wiring and bone grafts may be required to restore stability.

Any surgical intervention should be monitored by somato-sensory evoked potentials; if these are absent or not improved by surgery, this carries a poor prognosis (Tsirikos et al. 2004).

INJURIES BY OTHER PHYSICAL AGENTS

EXOGENOUS TOXIC ENCEPHALOPATHY

The large group of exogenous toxic encephalopathies is due to externally administered agents which include all the poisonings from therapeutic drugs, recreational drugs, suicidal overdoses, deliberate poisonings, bites and stings, and environmental agents such as aflatoxins, heavy metals and insecticides, and also the toxins from bacteria.

The source of the exogenous toxic substance may not always be obvious, for example in bathing newborns with hexachlorophene antiseptics, unbalanced high glycine amino acid mixtures, hydrogen sulphide from burning coal bings (slag heaps), or aluminium in water used for dialysis of children with chronic renal failure (Moreno et al. 1991).

There may be selective damage to particular groups of cells in the central nervous system. The heavy metals such as copper, manganese, iron and thallium, along with hydrogen sulphide, affect the basal ganglia. Certain metabolic disorders (intermittent maple syrup urine disease, Hartnup disease, arginino-succinic aminoacidaemia, Leigh encephalopathy) have a predilection for the cerebellum. Cortical involvement may occur with pentazocine, hyoscine or nalidixic acid poisoning or porphyria. Lead poisoning and porphyria may also selectively affect the anterior horn cells of the spinal cord.

One of the problems in young children is that there may be no history of exposure, and Munchausen syndrome by proxy should be considered.

LEAD POISONING

Plumbism remains a significant problem in childhood. Measures to prevent exposure to lead have been implemented at different time periods in different countries. Putty and paint pigments are the main hazards, but other sources are soft water conveyed in lead pipes, lead-glazed ceramic vessels, the burning of storage battery cases (Dolcourt et al. 1981), and atmospheric pollution due to automobile emissions or in the neighbourhood of smelting works and factories making batteries (Rutter 1980). Eye shadow cosmetics containing lead sulfite applied to children in some third world countries were responsible for cases among immigrants to the United Kingdom.

Lead toxicity is mainly observed in toddlers with pica from low socio-economic circumstances, or with a perverted appetite, who ingest lead usually in the form of paint scrapings. Most absorbed lead is tightly bound to growing bone and some is deposited in the hair and nails. Only a small amount enters the brain, where it is present mostly in the cortical and central grey matter. Lead is thought to be toxic to glutamatergic synapses, and specifically the N-methyl-D-aspartate type of excitatory amino acid receptor is a direct target for Pb^{++} effects in the brain (Toscano and Guilarte 2005). Almost all the absorbed lead is eventually excreted in the urine, and the levels of lead in blood and urine are an index of exposure to the toxin. Acceptable levels remain controversial. In the 1960s and '70s a blood level of 30–60 μg/dL was accepted but by 1985 this had decreased to 25 μg/dL, and the present recommendation of the American Academy of Pediatrics Committee on Environmental Health (1993) is <10 μg/dL. Even low levels below 10–25 μg/dL partially inhibit haem synthesis and may be responsible for cognitive and behavioural problems (Rutter 1980). Levels in excess of 70 μg/dL are an indication for immediate chelation (American Academy of Pediatrics 1993).

Lead inhibits numerous sulfhydryl enzymes and interferes with haem synthesis with resultant inhibition of delta-aminolevulinic acid dehydratase in erythrocytes, a sensitive index of subclinical lead poisoning. Inhibition of coproporphyrin oxidase provokes an increased excretion of coproporphyrin III.

The *pathology* of lead toxicity is characterized by widespread capillary damage with consequent interstitial brain oedema. Axonal damage is prominent in peripheral nerves whose myelin is not affected.

The *early symptoms* of lead poisoning are often vague and

nonspecific. For several weeks, the child is irritable or apathic and pale, coordination may be poor, and recently acquired skills may be lost. There is constipation and poor appetite. Iron deficiency anaemia is almost always present.

Acute encephalopathy used to be most common between 12 and 36 months of age. Sudden onset of repeated generalized convulsions and altered consciousness interrupts the vague symptoms of the premonitory period. There is evidence of increased ICP with a bulging fontanelle and separation of sutures more commonly than papilloedema. Nuchal rigidity is common. Cerebellar ataxia is occasionally present, and optic neuritis is possible with sudden visual loss. A diagnosis of acute meningoencephalitis is frequently entertained. Lead toxicity may not be limited to acute encephalopathy and peripheral neuropathy. A low global IQ and impairment of fine motor coordination and visuomotor performance as well as behavioural disturbances have been noted in children with blood levels over 10–30 µg/dL, in those with increased lead content in hair or deciduous teeth, and in those with elevation of free erythrocyte protoporphyrin.

SCALDS ENCEPHALOPATHY
In scalds encephalopathy, the child may sustain a minor scald, but a few hours later, the hands will become shaky, s/he will begin to convulse (often misdiagnosed as a febrile convulsion), become unconscious, hyperpyrexial and hypertensive, and may die or survive only with severe disability. The fluid retention in children with minor scalds (not burns) appears to be enormous, and peptides in the blister fluid may be vasoactive in addition to the liberation of stress peptides and ADH resulting in cerebral oedema, which is potentially completely reversible. The scald swells at the same time as the encephalopathy appears and shrinks with the use of mannitol at the same time the child recovers. A likely cause is the use of osmotically free intravenous solutions in the presence of ADH. With modern fluid balance this is rare.

BURNS ENCEPHALOPATHY
Neurological manifestations occur in 5% (Mohnot et al. 1982) to 14% (Antoon et al. 1972) of burned children. This encephalopathy may begin 48 hours to several weeks after the burn. Only severe burns (30% or more of body surface) are associated with neurological symptoms. These include lethargy or coma, generalized or partial seizures, and sometimes hallucinations and personality change. In 3 of 13 children reported by Mohnot et al. (1982) a relapsing course was observed, and in 1 child temporary enlargement of the cerebral ventricles was seen on CT. The course is usually favourable and 11 of these children improved to normal. Although neurological disturbances may be seen in children with minor burns and do not have a recognizable cause (Warlow and Hinton 1969), in most cases the encephalopathy can be attributed to hypoxia, hypovolaemia, sepsis or hyponatraemia. Several factors are usually operative. Cortical venous thrombosis was the cause of focal seizures in one child (Antoon et al. 1972). Brain swelling has been found in lethal cases. Hypertension and hypercalcaemia are possible causes. Central pontine myelinolysis has been reported (Winkelman

and Galloway 1992). Polyneuropathy is a possible complication of extensive burns (Marquez et al. 1993).

NEAR-DROWNING
Near-drowning is one of the most common causes of hypoxic accidents, accounting for about 10% of accidental deaths in children (Orlowski 1987, Shaw and Briede 1989). In addition to acute asphyxia, drowning is associated with inhalation of water. In *freshwater drowning*, fluid enters the circulatory system and haemolysis, hyponatraemia and hypoproteinaemia develop. Ventricular fibrillation is a frequent terminal event. In *saltwater drowning*, a different sequence of events is observed. Saltwater is highly irritating for the alveolar membrane because of its hypertonic concentration and induces massive pulmonary oedema. Because of the large quantities of fluid that are drawn from the vascular sector, hypovolaemic shock and hypotension may be seen.

The prognosis is difficult to establish. The overall survival rate is 75–93%, and survival with intact CNS is 58–90% (Shaw and Briede 1989). All patients who are awake on arrival at the emergency room and 90% of those arousable have a normal neurological outcome, whereas this is the case for only 32–55% of those comatose on admission. Initial elevated blood glucose levels are highly predictive of death or persistent vegetative state (Ashwal et al. 1990). Noonan et al. (1996) proposed that the prognosis of freshwater near-drowning can be determined by 18 hours and that prolongation of hospitalization is unnecessary if the child is well after this period. Quan et al. (1990) reported that 32% of patients with cardiopulmonary arrest following submersion could be salvaged with prehospital care. Patients with submersion lasting more than 9 minutes and those who needed more than 25 minutes of cardiopulmonary resuscitation died or remained severely impaired.

CARBON MONOXIDE POISONING
Carbon monoxide poisoning causes hypoxia both by combining haemoglobin to form carboxyhaemoglobin that dissociates less than haemoglobin thus reducing delivery of oxygen to the tissues and by interfering with the function of cytochrome (Crocker and Walker 1985). Because of foams used in modern households, hydrogen cyanide may be combined with the carbon monoxide, making the tissue hypoxia worse. Hydrogen cyanide was present in 26 out of 64 post-mortem blood samples. Carboxyhaemoglobin (COHb) was found in 52 cases. The hydrogen cyanide levels ranged from 0.8 to 39.2 µg/L, and the COHb levels from 16% to 85% (Wardaszka et al. 2005).

Mild intoxication results in headaches, vomiting, sweating and dyspnoea. Severe intoxication results in coma, retinal haemorrhages, convulsions and cardiac irregularities. Poisoning is usually caused by malfunctioning household heating equipment or car exhausts. A delayed posthypoxic encephalopathy is observed in some severe cases (Zagami et al. 1993). The delayed encephalopathy occurs from 14 to 45 days after recovery from the acute stage. The clinical manifestations include cognitive impairment, akinetic mutism, sphincter incontinence, gait ataxia

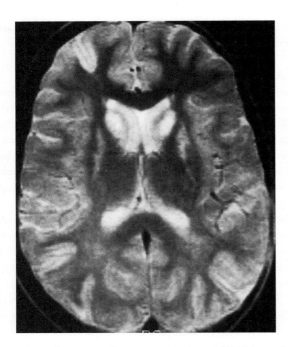

Fig. 12.19. Carbon monoxide poisoning in 11-year-old girl due to faulty heating apparatus. She demonstrated typical two-stage course with secondary deterioration but eventually regained consciousness. She was left with bilateral rigidity and significant loss of intellectual abilities. T_2-weighted MRI shows bilateral intense signal from heads of caudate nuclei. Note also two small areas of abnormal signal in right frontal and both parieto-occipital regions.

and extrapyramidal syndromes such as chorea, dystonia and parkinsonism (Hsiao et al. 2004).

Fleta Zaragozano et al. (2005) described 14 patients, with a mean age of 8.2 years, and a peak incidence was in the winter months. All poisonings took place in poorly ventilated rooms and were produced by gas inhalation due to incomplete combustion of organic fuels (charcoal, propane and butane). Clinical symptoms were gastrointestinal (nausea, vomiting, abdominal pain) and neurological (dizziness, headache and alterations in level of consciousness). COHb levels in blood were elevated (from 4.8% to 27.6% in the first determination). Outcome was favourable in all patients.

CT often shows a diffuse leukoencephalopathy with extensive demyelination and/or destructive lesions in the globus pallidus bilaterally in the form of hypodense areas that initially may enhance following injection of contrast (Vieregge et al. 1989). The most common finding on MRI is bilateral symmetric hyperintensity of the white matter, which is more obvious in the centrum semiovale, with relative sparing of the temporal lobes and anterior parts of the frontal lobes on T_2-weighted and FLAIR images in all patients. Cerebral cortical atrophy, mild atrophy of cerebellar hemispheres and vermian atrophy may develop. Basal ganglia lesions occur bilaterally, mostly in the globus pallidus, and to a lesser degree in the putamen and caudate, in some but not all patients (Fig. 12.19). The lesions are hypointense on T_1-weighted images and hyperintense on T_2-weighted and FLAIR images (Durak et al. 2005).

Residual deficits are frequent after acute CO poisoning and include extrapyramidal manifestations such as choreoathetosis, bradykinesia and tremor, cognitive manifestations such as dementia, dysphasia and dyspraxia, convulsions and peripheral neuropathy (Snyder 1970, Davous et al. 1986).

Treatment consists of removal of the patient from the CO atmosphere, supportive treatment and hyperbaric oxygen (Cregler and Mark 1986).

REFERENCES

Adams H, Mitchell DE, Graham DI, Doyle D (1977) Diffuse brain damage of immediate impact type. Its relationship to 'primary brain-stem damage' in head injury. *Brain* **100**: 489–502.

Agran PF, Dunkle DE, Winn DG (1985) Motor vehicle accident trauma and restraint usage patterns in children less than 4 years of age. *Pediatrics* **76**: 382–6.

Aicardi J, Goutieres F (1971) [Subdural effusions in infants.] *Arch Fr Pediatr* **28**: 233–47 (French).

Alexander MP (1995) Mild traumatic brain injury: pathophysiology, natural history, and clinical management. *Neurology* **45**: 1253–60.

American Academy of Pediatrics Committee on Environmental Health (1993) Lead poisoning: from screening to primary prevention. *Pediatrics* **92**: 176–83.

Anderson RC, Kan P, Klimo P, et al. (2004) Complications of intracranial pressure monitoring in children with head trauma. *J Neurosurg* **101** (Suppl): 53–8.

Antoon AY, Volpe JJ, Crawford JD (1972) Burn encephalopathy in children. *Pediatrics* **50**: 609–16.

Ashwal S, Schneider S, Tomasi L, Thompson J (1990) Prognostic implications of hyperglycemia and reduced cerebral blood flow in childhood near-drowning. *Neurology* **40**: 820–3.

Avrahami E, Tadmor R, Cohn DF (1989) Magnetic resonance imaging in patients with progressive myelopathy following spinal surgery. *J Neurol Neurosurg Psychiatry* **52**: 176–81.

Barlow CF (1984) Traumatic headache syndromes. In: *Headaches and Migraine in Childhood. Clinics in Developmental Medicine No. 91.* London: Spastics International Medical Publications, pp. 181–97.

Barlow KM, Minns RA (1999) The relationship between intracranial pressure and outcome in non-accidental head injury. *Dev Med Child Neurol* **20**: 220–5.

Barlow KM, Spowart JJ, Minns RA (2000) Early posttraumatic seizures in non-accidental head injury: relation to outcome. *Dev Med Child Neurol* **42**: 591–4.

Beers SR, Skold A, Dixon CE, Adelson PD (2005) Neurobehavioral effects of amantadine after pediatric traumatic brain injury: a preliminary report. *J Head Trauma Rehabil* **20**: 450–63.

Berger MS, Pitts LH, Lovely M, et al. (1985) Outcome from severe head injury in children and adolescents. *J Neurosurg* **62**: 194–9.

Bijur PE, Haslum M, Golding J (1990) Cognitive and behavioral sequelae of mild head injury in children. *Pediatrics* **86**: 337–44.

Billmire ME, Myers PA (1985) Serious head injury in infants: accident or abuse? *Pediatrics* **75**: 340–2.

Bonnier C, Nassogne M-C, Evrard P (1995) Outcome and prognosis of whiplash shaken infant syndrome; late consequences after a symptom-free interval. *Dev Med Child Neurol* **37**: 943–56.

BPNA (2001) Childs Glasgow Coma Scale. Online at: http://www.bpna.org.uk/audit/gcs.pdf.

Brookes M, MacMillan R, Cully S, et al. (1990) Head injuries in accident and emergency departments. How different are children from adults? *J Epidemiol Commun Health* **44**: 147–51.

Brown JK, Habel AH (1975) Toxic encephalopathy and acute brain-swelling in children. *Dev Med Child Neurol* **17**: 659–79.

Brown JK, Minns RA (1993) Non-accidental head injury, with particular reference to whiplash shaking injury and medico-legal aspects. *Dev Med Child Neurol* **35**: 849–69.

Brown RL, Brunn MA, Garcia VF (2001) Cervical spine injuries in children: a review of 103 patients treated consecutively at a level 1 pediatric trauma center. *J Pediatr Surg* **36**: 1107–14.

Bull MJ, Stroup KB (1985) Premature infants in car seats. *Pediatrics* 75: 336–9.

Caffey J (1972) On the theory and practice of shaking infants. *Am J Dis Child* 124: 161–9.

Chadwick O (1985) Psychological sequelae of head injury in children. *Dev Med Child Neurol* 27: 72–5.

Chambers IR, Stobbart L, Jones PA, et al. (2005) Age-related differences in intracranial pressure and cerebral perfusion pressure in the first 6 hours of monitoring after children's head injury: association with outcome. *Childs Nerv Syst* 21: 195–9.

Chambers IR, Jones PA, Lo TY, et al. (2006) Critical thresholds of intracranial pressure and cerebral perfusion pressure related to age in paediatric head injury. *J Neurol Neurosurg Psychiatry* 77: 234–40.

Choux M, Grisoli F, Peragut JC (1975) Extradural hematomas in children. 104 cases. *Childs Brain* 1: 337–47.

Choux M, Lena G, Genitori L (1986) Intracranial hematomas. In: Raimondi AJ, Choux M, Di Rocco C, eds. *Head Injuries in the Newborn and Infant.* Heidelberg: Springer-Verlag, pp. 203–16.

Cregler LL, Mark H (1986) Medical complications of cocaine abuse. *N Engl J Med* 315: 1495–500.

Crocker PJ, Walker JS (1985) Pediatric carbon monoxide toxicity. *J Emerg Med* 3: 443–8.

Crouchman M, Rossiter L, Colaco T, Forsyth R (2001) A practical outcome scale for paediatric head injury. *Arch Dis Child* 84: 120–4.

Davis PC (1995) Pediatric spinal disease. In: Faerber EN, ed. CNS *Magnetic Resonance Imaging in Infants and Children. Clinics in Developmental Medicine No. 134.* London: Mac Keith Press, pp. 236–78.

Davous P, Rondot P, Marion MH, Gueguen B (1986) Severe chorea after acute carbon monoxide poisoning. *J Neurol Neurosurg Psychiatry* 49: 206–8.

De Meirleir LJ, Taylor MJ (1987) Prognostic utility of SEPs in comatose children. *Pediatr Neurol* 3: 78–82.

Dearden NM (1985) Ischaemic brain. *Lancet* 2: 255–9.

Defra (2005) *Sustainable Development Indicators in Your Pocket.* London: Department for Environment, Food and Rural Affairs (available online at: www.sustainable-development.gov.uk).

Dias MS, Lillis KA, Calvo C, et al. (2004) Management of accidental minor head injuries in children: a prospective outcomes study. *J Neurosurg* 101 (Suppl): 38–43.

Dogan S, Safavi-Abbasi S, Theodore N, et al. (2007) Thoracolumbar and sacral spinal injuries in children and adolescents: a review of 89 cases. *J Neurosurg* 106 (Suppl): 426–33.

Dolcourt JL, Finch C, Coleman GD, et al. (1981) Hazard of lead exposure in the home from recycled automobile storage batteries. *Pediatrics* 68: 225–30.

Duhaime AC, Gennarelli TA, Thibault LE, et al. (1987) The shaken baby syndrome. A clinical, pathological, and biomechanical study. *J Neurosurg* 66: 409–15.

Duhaime AC, Alario AJ, Lewander WJ, et al. (1992) Head injury in very young children: mechanisms, injury types, and ophthalmologic findings in 100 hospitalized patients younger than 2 years of age. *Pediatrics* 90: 179–85.

Durak AC, Coskun A, Yikilmaz A, et al. (2005) Magnetic resonance imaging findings in chronic carbon monoxide intoxication. *Acta Radiol* 46: 322–7.

Feldman KW, Brewer DK (1984) Child abuse, cardiopulmonary resuscitation, and rib fractures. *Pediatrics* 73: 339–42.

Filley CM, Cranberg LD, Alexander MP, Hart EJ (1987) Neurobehavioral outcome after closed head injury in childhood and adolescence. *Arch Neurol* 44: 194–8.

Fleta Zaragozano J, Fons Estupiñá C, Arnauda Espatolero P, et al. (2005) [Carbon monoxide poisoning.] *An Pediatr* 62: 587–90 (Spanish).

Friedman R (1976) Child abuse: a review of the psychological research. In: *Four Perspectives on the Status of Child Abuse and Neglect Research.* Washington, DC: National Center on Child Abuse and Neglect, DHEW, pp. 19–23.

Gahagan S, Rimsza ME (1991) Child abuse or osteogenesis imperfecta: how can we tell? *Pediatrics* 88: 987–92.

Geddes JF, Hackshaw AK, Vowles GH, et al. (2001) Neuropathology of inflicted head injury in children. I. Patterns of brain damage. *Brain* 124: 1290–8.

Gentry LR, Godersky JC, Thompson B (1988) MR imaging of head trauma: review of the distribution and radiopathologic features of traumatic lesions. *Am J Radiol* 150: 663–72.

Gerber CJ, Neil-Dwyer G, Kennedy P (1992) Posterior ischaemic optic neuropathy after a spontaneous extradural haematoma. *J Neurol Neurosurg Psychiatry* 55: 630.

Gordon NS, Fois A, Jacobi G, et al. (1983) The management of the comatose child. *Neuropediatrics* 14: 3–5.

Graham DI, Ford I, Adams JH, et al. (1989) Ischaemic brain damage is still common in fatal non-missile head injury. *J Neurol Neurosurg Psychiatry* 52: 346–50.

Guilleminault C, Faull KF, Miles L, van den Hoed J (1983) Posttraumatic excessive daytime sleepiness: a review of 20 patients. *Neurology* 33: 1584–9.

Haas DC, Lourie H (1988) Trauma-triggered migraine: an explanation for common neurological attacks after mild head injury. Review of the literature. *J Neurosurg* 68: 181–8.

Hadley MN, Sonntag VK, Rekate HL, Murphy A (1989) The infant whiplash-shake injury syndrome: a clinical and pathological study. *Neurosurgery* 24: 536–40.

Hahn YS, Chyung C, Barthel MJ, et al. (1988) Head injuries in children under 36 months of age. *Childs Nerv Syst* 4: 34–40.

Hamilton MG, Myles ST (1992) Pediatric spinal injury: review of 174 hospital admissions. *J Neurosurg* 77: 700–4.

Hawley CA, Ward AB, Long J, et al. (2003) Prevalence of traumatic brain injury amongst children admitted to hospital in one health district: a population-based study. *Injury* 34: 256–60.

Heaton RK (2005) *Wisconsin Card Sorting Test Computer Version 4 Research Edition (WCST:CV4).* Lutz, FL: Psychological Assessment Resources.

Hendrick EB, Harwood-Hash DC, Hudson AR (1964) Head injuries in children: a survey of 4465 consecutive cases at the hospital for sick children, Toronto, Canada. *Clin Neurosurg* 11: 46–65.

Hendry SJ, Beattie TF, Heaney D (2005) Minor illness and injury: factors influencing attendance at a paediatric accident and emergency department. *Arch Dis Child* 90: 629–33.

Holsti M, Kadish HA, Sill BL, et al. (2005) Pediatric closed head injuries treated in an observation unit. *Pediatr Emerg Care* 21: 639–44.

Hsiao CL, Kuo HC, Huang CC (2004) Delayed encephalopathy after carbon monoxide intoxication—long-term prognosis and correlation of clinical manifestations and neuroimages. *Acta Neurol Taiwan* 13: 64–70.

Huttenlocher PR (1972) Reye's syndrome: relation of outcome to therapy. *J Pediatr* 80: 845–50.

Jenkins A, Teasdale G, Hadley MD, et al. (1986) Brain lesions detected by magnetic resonance imaging in mild and severe head injuries. *Lancet* 2: 445–6.

Jennett B (1998) Epidemiology of head injury. *Arch Dis Child* 78: 403–6.

Jennett B, Bond M (1975) Assessment of outcome after severe brain damage. A practical scale. *Lancet* 1: 480–4.

Jennett B, Teasdale G (1977) Aspects of coma after severe head injury. *Lancet* 1: 878–81.

Jennett B, Teasdale G (1981) *Management of Head Injuries.* Philadelphia: FA Davis.

Johnson MH, Lee SH (1992) Computed tomography of acute cerebral trauma. *Radiol Clin North Am* 30: 325–52.

Jones PA, Chambers IR, Minns RA, et al. (2008) Are head injury guidelines changing the outcome of head injured children? A regional investigation. *Acta Neurochir Suppl* (in press).

Kang JK, Park CK, Kim MC, et al. (1989) Traumatic isolated intracerebral hemorrhage in children. *Childs Nerv Syst* 5: 303–6.

Kaye EM, Herskowitz J (1986) Transient post-traumatic cortical blindness: brief v prolonged syndromes in childhood. *J Child Neurol* 1: 206–10.

Keenan HT, Nocera M, Bratton SL (2005) Frequency of intracranial pressure monitoring in infants and young toddlers with traumatic brain injury. *Pediatr Crit Care Med* 6: 537–41.

Kemp AM, Stoodley N, Cobley C, et al. (2003) Apnoea and brain swelling in non-accidental head injury. *Arch Dis Child* 88: 472–6.

King WJ, MacKay M, Sirnick A; Canadian Shaken Baby Study Group (2003) Shaken baby syndrome in Canada: clinical characteristics and outcomes of hospital cases. *CMAJ* 168: 155–9.

Kleinman PK (1987) *Diagnostic Imaging of Child Abuse.* Baltimore: Williams & Wilkins.

Kleinman PK, Blackbourne BD, Marks SC, et al. (1989) Radiologic contributions to the investigation and prosecution of cases of fatal infant abuse. *N Engl J Med* 320: 507–11.

Klonoff H, Clark C, Klonoff PS (1993) Long-term outcome of head injuries: a 23 year follow up study of children with head injuries. *J Neurol Neurosurg Psychiatry* 56: 410–5.

Kravitz H, Driessen G, Gomberg R, Korach A (1969) Accidental falls from elevated surfaces in infants from birth to one year of age. *Pediatrics* 44 (Suppl): 869–76.

Leggate JR, Lopez-Ramos N, Genitori L, et al. (1989) Extradural haematoma in infants. *Br J Neurosurg* 3: 533–9.

Leonard M, Sproule J, McCormack D (2007) Paediatric spinal trauma and associated injuries. *Injury* 38: 188–93.

Leonidas JC, Ting W, Binkiewicz A, et al. (1982) Mild head trauma in children: when is a roentgenogram necessary? *Pediatrics* 69: 139–43.

Ludwig S, Warman M (1984) Shaken baby syndrome: a review of 20 cases. *Ann Emerg Med* 13: 104–7.

Mahoney WJ, D'Souza BJ, Haller JA, et al. (1983) Long-term outcome of children with severe head trauma and prolonged coma. *Pediatrics* 71: 756–62.

Marquez S, Turley JJE, Peters WJ (1993) Neuropathy in burn patients. *Brain* 116: 471–83.

Martin BW, Dykes E, Lecky FE (2004) Patterns and risks in spinal trauma. *Arch Dis Child* 89: 860–5.

Mazza C, Pasqualin A, Feriotti G, Da Pian R (1982) Traumatic extradural haematomas in children: experience with 62 cases. *Acta Neurochir* 65: 67–80.

Meadow R (1982) Munchausen syndrome by proxy and pseudo-epilepsy. *Arch Dis Child* 57: 811–2.

Meadow R (1984) Fictitious epilepsy. *Lancet* 2: 25–8.

Meadow R (1991) Neurological and developmental variants of Munchausen syndrome by proxy. *Dev Med Child Neurol* 33: 270–2.

Miller JD (1992) Head injury. *J Neurol Neurosurg Psychiatry* 56: 440–7.

Minns RA (2005) Shaken baby syndrome: theoretical and evidential controversies. *J R Coll Physicians Edinb* 35: 5–15.

Minns RA, Busuttil A (2004) Patterns of presentation of the shaken baby syndrome: four types of inflicted brain injury predominate. *BMJ* 328: 766.

Minns RA, Brown JK (1978) Intracranial pressure changes associated with childhood seizures. *Dev Med Child Neurol* 20: 561–9.

Minns RA, Brown JK, eds. (2005) *Shaking and Other Non-Accidental Head Injuries in Children. Clinics in Developmental Medicine No. 162.* London: Mac Keith Press.

Minns RA, Lo TY (2008) Head and neck injury. In: Keeling J, Busuttil A, eds. *Paediatric Forensic Medicine and Pathology.* London: Hodder Arnold, pp. 277–311.

Minns RA, Jones PA, Mok JY (2008) Incidence and demography of non-accidental head injury in southeast Scotland from a national database. *Am J Prev Med* 31 (Suppl): S126–33.

Mizrahi EM, Kellaway P (1984) Cerebral concussion in children: assessment of injury by electroencephalography. *Pediatrics* 73: 419–25.

Mohnot D, Snead OC, Benton JW (1982) Burn encephalopathy in children. *Ann Neurol* 12: 42–7.

Moreno A, Dominguez P, Dominguez C, Ballabriga A (1991) High serum aluminium levels and acute reversible encephalopathy in a 4-year-old boy with acute renal failure. *Eur J Pediatr* 150: 513–4.

Morray JP, Tyler DC, Jones TK, et al. (1984) Coma scale for use in brain-injured children. *Crit Care Med* 12: 1018–20.

Natelson SE, Sayers MP (1973) The fate of children sustaining severe head trauma during birth. *Pediatrics* 51: 169–74.

National Center for Health Statistics (1987) *Advance Report of Final Mortality Statistics, 1985. NCHS Monthly Vital Statistics Report, vol. 36, no. 5. Suppl. DHHS pub. no. (PHS) 87-1120.* Hyattsville, MD: Public Health Service.

Noonan L, Howrey R, Ginsburg CM (1996) Freshwater submersion injuries in children: a retrospective review of seventy-five hospitalized patients. *Pediatrics* 98: 368–71.

Odom A, Christ E, Kerr N, et al. (1997) Prevalence of retinal hemorrhages in pediatric patients after in-hospital cardiopulmonary resuscitation: a prospective study. *Pediatrics* 99: E3.

Oi S, Matsumoto S (1987) Post-traumatic hydrocephalus in children. Pathophysiology and classification. *J Pediatr Neurosci* 3: 133–47.

Oka H, Kako M, Matsushima M, Ando K (1977) Traumatic spreading depression syndrome. Review of a particular type of head injury in 37 patients. *Brain* 100: 287–98.

Ommaya AK, Gennarelli TA (1974) Cerebral concussion and traumatic unconsciousness. Correlation of experimental and clinical observations of blunt head injuries. *Brain* 97: 633–54.

Orlowski JP (1987) Drowning, near-drowning, and ice-water submersions. *Pediatr Clin North Am* 34: 75–92.

Pang D, Horton JA, Herron JM, et al. (1983) Nonsurgical management of extradural hematomas in children. *J Neurosurg* 59: 958–71.

Plunkett J (2001) Fatal pediatric head injuries caused by short-distance falls. *Am J Forensic Med Pathol* 22: 1–12.

Povlishock JT, Becker DP, Cheng CL, Vaughan GW (1983) Axonal change in minor head injury. *J Neuropathol Exp Neurol* 42: 225–42.

Quan L, Wentz KR, Gore EJ, Copass MK (1990) Outcome and predictors of outcome in pediatric submersion victims receiving prehospital care in King County, Washington. *Pediatrics* 86: 586–93.

Raimondi AJ, Hirschauer J (1984) Head injury in the infant and toddler. Coma scoring and outcome scale. *Childs Brain* 11: 12–35.

Reed MJ, Browning JG, Wilkinson AG, Beattie T (2005) Can we abolish skull x rays for head injury? *Arch Dis Child* 90: 859–64.

Robertson LS (1992) *Injury Epidemiology.* New York: Oxford University Press.

Rogers D, Tripp J, Bentovim A, et al. (1976) Papers and originals. *BMJ* 1: 793–6.

Rosenberg DA (1987) Web of deceit: a literature review of Munchausen syndrome by proxy. *Child Abuse Negl* 11: 547–63.

Rosenthal BW, Bergman I (1989) Intracranial injury after moderate head trauma in children. *J Pediatr* 115: 346–50.

Ruijs MB, Gabreëls FJ, Keyser A (1993) The relation between neurological trauma parameters and long-term outcome in children with closed head injury. *Eur J Pediatr* 152: 844–7.

Ruijs MB, Gabreëls FJ, Thijssen HM (1994) The utility of electroencephalography and cerebral computed tomography in children with mild and moderately severe closed head injuries. *Neuropediatrics* 25: 73–7.

Rutter M (1980) Raised lead levels and impaired cognitive/behavioural functioning: a review of the evidence. *Dev Med Child Neurol Suppl* 42: 1–26.

Scott-Jupp R, Marlow N, Seddon N, Rosenbloom L (1992) Rehabilitation and outcome after severe head injury. *Arch Dis Child* 67: 222–6.

Selbst SM, Alexander D, Ruddy R (1987) Bicycle-related injuries. *Am J Dis Child* 141: 140–4.

Seshia SS, Seshia MM, Sachdeva RK (1977) Coma in childhood. *Dev Med Child Neurol* 19: 614–28.

Shaw KN, Briede CA (1989) Submersion injuries: drowning and near-drowning. *Emerg Med Clin North Am* 7: 355–70.

SIGN (2000) *Early Management of Patients with a Head Injury. SIGN Publication No. 46.* Edinburgh: Scottish Intercollegiate Guideline Network.

Simpson D, Reilly P (1982) Pediatric coma scale. *Lancet* 2: 450.

Sklar EM, Quencer RM, Bowen BC, et al. (1992) Magnetic resonance applications in cerebral injury. *Radiol Clin North Am* 30: 353–66.

Slomine BS, Salorio CF, Grados MA, et al. (2005) Differences in attention, executive functioning, and memory in children with and without ADHD after severe traumatic brain injury. *J Int Neuropsychol Soc* 11: 645–53.

Snyder RD (1970) Carbon monoxide intoxication with peripheral neuropathy. *Neurology* 20: 177–80.

Sonntag VK, Hadley MN (1988) Nonoperative management of cervical spine injuries. *Clin Neurosurg* 34: 630–49.

Taylor MJ, Farrell EJ (1989) Comparison of the prognostic utility of VEPs and SEPs in comatose children. *Pediatr Neurol* 5: 145–50.

Teasdale G, Jennett B (1974) Assessment of coma and impaired consciousness. A practical scale. *Lancet* 2: 81–4.

Tender G C, Awasthi D (2004) Spontaneous cervical spinal epidural hematoma in a 12-year-old girl: case report and review of the literature. *J Louisiana State Med Soc* 156: 196–8.

Toscano CD, Guilarte TR (2005) Lead neurotoxicity: from exposure to molecular effects. *Brain Res Brain Res Rev* 49: 529–54.

Towbin A (1970) Central nervous system damage in the human fetus and newborn infant. Mechanical and hypoxic injury incurred in the fetal–neonatal period. *Am J Dis Child* 119: 529–42.

Tsirikos AI, Aderinto J, Tucker SK, Noordeen HH (2004) Spinal cord monitoring using intraoperative somatosensory evoked potentials for spinal trauma. *J Spinal Disord Tech* 17: 385–94.

Vieregge P, Klostermann W, Blumm RG, Borgis KJ (1989) Carbon monoxide poisoning: clinical, neurophysiological, and brain imaging observations in acute disease and follow-up. *J Neurol* 236: 478–81.

Wardaszka Z, Niemcunowicz-Janica A, Janica J, Koc-Zorawska E (2005) [Levels of carbon monoxide and hydrogen cyanide in blood of fire victims in the autopsy material of the Department of Forensic Medicine, Medical University of Bialystok.] *Arch Med Sadowej Kryminol* 55: 130–3 (Polish).

Warlow CP, Hinton P (1969) Early neurological disturbances following relatively minor burns in children. *Lancet* 2: 978–82.

White RJ, Likavec MJ (1992) The diagnosis and initial management of head injury. *N Engl J Med* 327: 1507–11.

Winkelman MD, Galloway PG (1992) Central nervous system complications of thermal burns. A postmortem study of 139 patients. *Medicine* 71: 271–83.

Wrightson P, McGinn V, Gronwall D (1995) Mild head injury in preschool children: evidence that it can be associated with a persisting cognitive defect. *J Neurol Neurosurg Psychiatry* **59**: 375–80.

Yates PO (1959) Birth trauma to the vertebral arteries. *Arch Dis Child* **34**: 436–41.

Zagami AS, Lethlean AK, Mellick R (1993) Delayed neurological deterioration following carbon monoxide poisoning: MRI findings. *J Neurol* **240**: 113–6.

Zepp F, Bruhl K, Zimmer B, Schumacher R (1992) Battered child syndrome: cerebral ultrasound and CT findings after vigorous shaking. *Neuropediatrics* **23**: 188–91.

PART VI

TUMOURS AND VASCULAR DISORDERS

13

TUMOURS OF THE CENTRAL NERVOUS SYSTEM AND OTHER SPACE-OCCUPYING LESIONS

BRAIN TUMOURS

FREQUENCY AND AETIOLOGICAL FACTORS

Tumours of the CNS are the second most common malignancy of childhood, after leukaemia. The overall population incidence of intracranial neoplasms varies between 1 and 3 per 100,000 in different series (see Baldwin and Preston-Martin 2004). Approx-imately 10% of tumours occur in children under 2 years of age, 20% between 2 and 5 years, 25% between 3 and 10 years, and 45% over 10 years (Keene et al. 1999). However, the location varies with age. In infants, there is a predominance of supraten-torial tumours, especially astrocytomas, over infratentorial neo-plasms, mainly medulloblastomas and ependymomas. In children older than 4 years, infratentorial tumours, mostly cerebellar astrocytomas, medulloblastomas and ependymomas, are the most frequent, and this is enhanced in children over 8 years of age by an increase in cerebellar astrocytomas. Overall, supratentorial tumours account for about half the cases (Table 13.1).

The reasons for the changing age distribution of supraten-torial and infratentorial tumours, for the predominance of mid-line tumours, and for the predominance of neuroectodermal neoplasms in childhood are poorly understood (Bunin 2004).

Most tumours of the CNS occur in children without personal or familial predisposing conditions. However, predisposing con-ditions, e.g. neurofibromatosis, are known; several surveys of the incidence of neoplasms in relatives have demonstrated a higher incidence of CNS tumours and of leukaemia but not of other malignancies. Cases of familial tumours of various histological types are on record (Battersby et al. 1986, Vieregge et al. 1987) and may be part of genetic syndromes of predisposition to malig-nant tumours, e.g. Li–Fraumeni syndrome (Iwakuma et al. 2005); neurofibromatosis; some syndromes of multifocal cell prolifera-tion, e.g. the Turcot syndrome of colonic polyposis and brain tumours (Qualman et al. 2003); and some immunodeficiency syndromes, e.g. Wiskott–Aldrich syndrome and ataxia–telangiec-tasia, which are genetically transmitted and in which the incidence of tumours is high. The genetics of brain tumours have been the subject of intensive investigation over the past two decades, and

the development is so rapid that only a superficial overview can be attempted. In addition to evidence drawn from clinical obser-vation of familial cases, cytogenetics and molecular genetics have considerably increased our knowledge of some of the mechanisms of tumorogenesis in general, which can apply also to the common, apparently sporadic cases of neoplasms.

From the *cytogenetic* point of view, the development of cancer is a multistep process in which some cells acquire a series of genetic insults that disrupt their normal development and fate as a result of dysfunction of oncogenes, tumour supressor genes and stability genes (Vogelstein and Kinzler 2004, Gilbertson 2005). It has long been known that the cells of many tumours contain acquired chromosomal abnormalities (Biegel 1991) that result apparently from new mutations (e.g. deletions of certain chromosomes or part thereof) as they do not exist in the cells of other organs. Such chromosomal abnormalities (e.g. abnormal-ities of chromosome 22 in acoustic schwannomas) are frequently present in other tumour cells, for example deletions of 10q, 11 and 17p in medulloblastoma, and deletions of 1q and 19q in certain oligodendrogliomas (Bigner et al. 1997). Interestingly, these anomalies may differ among different cases of a same tumour type. In addition to the general interest of this finding in the understanding of mechanisms of non-genetic as well as of genetic neoplasms, it has come to have a practical value as their presence or absence can be of great prognostic value, e.g. the presence of the *p53* gene (Sung et al. 2000, Pollack et al. 2001) or the amplification of the *Myc* gene in neuroblastoma.

Molecular genetic studies (Gilbertson 2005) were developed as a consequence of the discovery of these chromosomal aberra-tions. They have led to breakthroughs in the understanding of the biology of tumours, with practical consequences. The role of certain genes has been found to be important for the develop-ment of neoplasms. Some genes have the property of opposing or slowing down their development (tumour-suppressor genes or anti-oncogenes), some stabilize signalling pathways, while others favour their growth (oncogenes) or predispose to certain types of cancer. The mechanisms are illustrated by the case of the retinoblastoma, a retinal neoplasm that usually develops in young

TABLE 13.1
Common brain tumours in childhood: location and histological nature*

Location	% of all brain tumours
Infratentorial	43–63
Medulloblastoma	20–25
Low-grade astrocytoma (cerebellar)	12–18
Ependymoma	4–8
Brainstem glioma	5–11
High grade	3–9
Low grade	3–6
Other	2–5
Supratentorial	22.5–58
Low-grade astrocytoma	8–20
Malignant astrocytoma	6–12
Ependymoma	2–5
Mixed glioma	1–5
Oligodendroglioma	1–2
Ganglioglioma	1–5
Other (choroid plexus, PNET, meningioma)	3.5–9
Supratentorial midline	7–13.5
Suprasellar	
Craniopharyngioma	6–9
Chiasmatic/hypothalamic glioma	4–8
Pituitary adenoma	0.5–2.5
Pineal region	
Germ-cell tumor**	1.5–4
Parenchymal tumours	0.5–2
Low-grade glioma	1–2

*Modified from Pollack (1994).
**Includes ectopic germ-cell tumours.

children below 4 years of age and often metastasizes to the CNS. Retinoblastoma may be familial (40% of patients), occurring in patients who have a heritable predisposition to the tumour as well as to a number of other cancers, especially osteosarcoma, or sporadic. The hereditary predisposition is determined by mutations at a locus within the q14 band of chromosome 13. Patients with non-hereditary retinoblastoma have somatic mutations at the same genetic locus. The gene for sensitivity to retinoblastoma normally functions as a dominant suppressor of tumour formation, and alterations or inactivation of both homologous alleles is necessary for the development of a retinoblastoma. In persons who have inherited a genetic mutation, a second, somatic mutation is sufficient to lead to clinical disease ('two-hit' hypothesis), wheras two somatic mutations are required for non-genetic cases, a much less likely event.

Such a model can apply to other familial (e.g. neurofibromatosis) or nonfamilial tumours. Its potential importance is considerable because: (1) detection of an abnormality at the specific locus can allow diagnosis of susceptibility to a tumour in the absence of clinical manifestations (Yandell et al. 1989); (2) it emphasizes the role of oncogenes in at least certain tumours (Slamon 1987) and establishes a link between chromosomal and gene abnormalities and carcinogenesis, and may have a prognostic significance: the presence of clones with specific deletions in human cerebral astrocytomas has been associated with an unfavourable outcome (Kimmel et al. 1992). There is evidence that such abnormalities may be associated with transformation of normal proto-oncogenes into oncogenes that are altered or overexpressed versions of their normal proto-oncogene counterparts (Druker et al. 1989, Krontiris 1995). Such a mechanism is at play in Burkitt lymphoma where the primary event is excessive expression of the *c-myc* proto-oncogene, itself resulting from translocation of the *c-myc* gene locus from band 8q24 on chromosome 14. In the process, the *c-myc* gene is deregulated, becoming an oncogene. Amplification of a nucleotide sequence that shares similarities with *c-myc* (*N-myc*) is associated with 20% of neuroblastomas and with rapid tumour progression and poor prognosis. Proto-oncogenes may normally code for growth factors or transcription factors (Druker et al. 1989). The role of oncogenes and of cell growth factors in the genesis of brain tumours, and the role they play in certain genetically determined cancers, are being studied (Krontiris 1995, Rubnitz and Crist 1997). The proto-oncogene *RET* is closely associated with the occurrence of multiple endocrine neoplasias (Eng 1996). Considerable attention has also been given to tumour-suppressor genes whose deletion or mutation can result in the occurrence of several types of malignancy (Stanbridge 1990), especially the *p53 tumour-suppressor gene* whose absence or abnormality in the germline is associated with half the cases of Li–Fraumeni syndrome and with many gliomas. The genes for types 1 and 2 neurofibromatosis also act as tumour suppressors. The gene for NF1 codes for a protein termed neurofibromin that seems to act as a negative regulator of the *p21ras* oncogene, thus preventing aberrant cellular transformation mediated by this oncogene. The gene for NF2 codes for a protein, termed merlin, that also has tumour-suppressive properties (MacCollin 1995). In both cases, the development of tumours may result from a somatic mutation occurring in persons already at severe disadvantage because they have a genetic defect involving an anti-oncogene. In addition to oncogenes and anti-oncogenes, genes of susceptibility to certain cancers (e.g. breast cancer) have been recognized and are important in the understanding of malignant processes and potentially in early detection of susceptible persons, which could lead to preventive measures.

Knowledge of genes associated wth carcinogenesis has made it possible to analyse the pathways they belong to and some possible modes of action (De Angelis 2001). In general, it appears that development of tumours or predispostion to their development (e.g. in persons with mutant *BCRA* genes) is due to either abnormalities either of signal transduction or of cell control cycle anomalies in developmental pathways that result in multiple phenotypic consequences at different points of these pathways that then go awry in very complex manners in multiple steps (Guha and Mukhergee 2004, Pietsch et al. 2004, Taillibert et al. 2004). Recent studies using DNA arrays have shown that multiple suppression or amplification of gene expression, resulting in complex interferences with the normal developmental metabolic pathways are common in tumour cells (Suarez-Merino et al. 2005) and account in part for the extreme complexity of the problem.

Acquired factors of carcinogenesis certainly exist but only very few of them are definitely established. The role of ionizing radiation is well demonstrated and it may be responsible for

5–10% of tumours. Certain chemicals such as those in tobacco smoke have a well-demonstrated effect on the incidence of some cancers, but associated factors are probably necessary to induce carcinogenesis. Other factors are certainly at play but their role is supposed mostly on indirect evidence drawn from international incidence comparisons and risk factor studies (Bunin 2004). A possible role of viruses as a causal factor of some brain tumours is suggested by the presence of viral DNA sequences in some choroid plexus papillomas and ependymomas (Bergsagel et al. 1992). Herpes and polyoma viruses may play an important role. Epstein–Barr and HIV infections may have a facilitating role, like other disorders of immunity, and the role of immunosurveillance in elimination of mutant cells is important. The possible roles of many other suspected agents or factors (e.g. waves from mobile telephones) have not been confirmed so far.

GENERAL PATHOLOGY

Tumours of the CNS may have variable grades of malignancy, from highly malignant tumours such as neuroblastomas and medulloblastomas to very indolent tumours, some of which may be considered as hamartomas (Russell and Rubinstein 1989). In such cases, the lesion grows at the same rate as the rest of the CNS (e.g. hamartomas of the tuber cinereum). The localization of the major types of brain tumours is shown in Table 13.1.

There is still much controversy regarding the classification of tumours according to their degree of evolutivity (Russell and Rubinstein 1989, Heffner 1994, Rorke-Adams and Biegel 2005). The World Heath Organization classification (Kleihues et al. 2002) is most used. The histological types of tumours in childhood series (Pollack 1994) are shown in Table 13.2.

It is important to note that even malignant CNS tumours rarely metastasize outside the CNS and those that do often metastasize only after operation. Most CNS tumours tend to metastasize along CSF pathways rather than by blood dissemination. It is also essential to realize that the clinical significance of pathological grading may be different from its biological value. A benign tumour that is strategically located so as to be impossible to remove while interfering with essential neural function is 'malignant' for the patient even if histologically benign. Pathological diagnosis may be difficult; in particular, some tumours may consist of histologically different areas. However, Revesz et al. (1993) found stereotactic biopsy reliable for diagnosis and grading of adult gliomas.

CLINICAL MANIFESTATIONS, DIAGNOSIS AND TREATMENT

The clinical symptomatology of intracranial tumours is often atypical, with only minor clinical symptoms that may not be different from those in common benign illnesses of children. Therefore, the possibility of a brain neoplasm should always be kept in mind even if it materializes only rarely. Symptoms and signs of brain tumours can result from increased intracranial pressure (ICP) and/or from focal effects of the tumour on neighbouring neural structures. The symptoms and signs differ with the location of the tumour and, to a certain extent, its histological nature (e.g. depending of the importance of the oedema produced), these two factors being related.

INTRACRANIAL HYPERTENSION
Headache due to intracranial hypertension may be intense and relieved by vomiting. More often it is mild and intermittent, but its persistence, especially if it occurs in the morning, must always

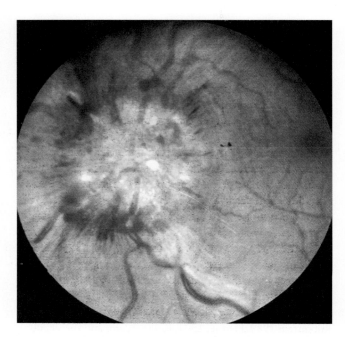

Fig. 13.1. Papilloedema in child with raised intracranial pressure. Optic nerve head protrudes above level of retina, and limits of disc are obscured by oedema and haemorrhage. (Courtesy Prof. J-L Dufier, Hôpital des Enfants Malades, Paris.)

attract the physician's attention. The headache of intracranial tumours, however, may be intermittent and may be relieved by usual analgesic agents. Headaches often awaken the patients at night or are present on arising, and these morning headaches characteristically tend to recur repeatedly. Moreover, the children are often less active and generally unwell.

Vomiting is the second most common symptom of intracranial hypertension. It is usually but not always associated with headaches, even in the case of posterior fossa tumours. Vomiting due to increased pressure is usually unremarkable except by its repetition and persistence and by its frequent morning occurrence. Changes in behaviour and personality are commonly an early manifestation of ICP (Cohen and Duffner 1994). Irritability or lethargy are especially of concern when associated with vomiting and headache.

Papilloedema (Fig. 13.1) although a major sign is absent in almost half the children with brain tumours, especially supratentorial tumours and those with a rapid course such as medulloblastoma. The presence of papilloedema makes an intracranial mass highly probable, but its absence in no way excludes such a diagnosis. Papilloedema should be distinguished from pseudo-papilloedema, a congenital anomaly consisting of excessive glial proliferation at the disk margins, and from drusen of the optic nerve head, which, in children, are usually buried within the disk and produce elevation of the nerve head (Chapter 17). In such cases there is no vascular congestion or vessel tortuosity. In difficult cases, fluorescein fundus angiography may be useful, as the increased capillary network and exudation of fluorescein out of the vessels with persistence of fluorescence at the disk margins

seen with papilloedema are absent in congenital disc anomalies. Papilloedema is, of course, not specific for brain tumours and can be present with increased ICP of other causes as well as in certain conditions unassociated with intracranial hypertension such as polyradiculoneuritis (Chapter 20) and optic neuritis. In the latter case it is associated with blindness or scotoma.

Less commonly, raised ICP may be associated with diplopia due to paralysis of the VIth cranial nerve, which may be unilateral or bilateral and may fluctuate.

Raised ICP from tumours or from other causes is dangerous because it leads to reduction of cerebral blood flow when the point is reached at which perfusion pressure (the difference between mean arterial pressure and ICP) falls to below 40 mmHg. Reduced blood flow can be responsible for lethargy, coma, and a number of autonomic manifestations generally attributed to brain herniation or 'coning'. Such manifestations may occur only transiently during the 'plateau waves' of ICP and disappear with decrease in pressure.

Mass movements of the brain as a result of asymmetrical or unequal expansion of one brain compartment due to the presence of a mass lesion can produce *herniation* of the cerebellar tonsils through the foramen magnum or of the uncus hippocampi through the tentorial opening. Both types of herniation may induce secondary brainstem dysfunction, by direct compression against the tentorium or by stretching brainstem vessels. Brainstem dysfunction can occur with global downward movement of the brain substance without lateral herniation. This central *syndrome of rostrocaudal deterioration* (Plum and Posner 1980) is common with bilateral supratentorial masses. It results in progressive functional impairment, involving in succession the diencephalon, the midbrain and upper pons, the lower pontine–upper medulla, and finally the medulla, with eventual death. Brain displacements can be demonstrated by MRI (Reich et al. 1993, Ropper 1993, Johnson et al. 2002), and correlations have been proposed between the magnitude of displacements and the patient's level of consciousness (Ropper 1989). Lateral displacement of the brainstem with uncus herniation is more frequent with unilateral masses. Fisher (1995) questioned the importance of downward displacements and suggested that herniation is a late phenomenon and that the clinical phenomena attributed to herniation may remain reversible for relatively long periods.

Herniations also produce localized signs, especially compression of the IIIrd cranial nerve by the uncus against the tentorial edge with unilateral pupillary dilatation. Rarely, there is compression of the posterior cerebral artery with occipital infarction. Paralysis of the last cranial pairs may occur with foramen magnum herniation, which can also be responsible for neck stiffness in children with posterior fossa tumours. Stiffness may be paroxysmal and associated with a rigid extension of the body, the so-called cerebellar fit of Jackson. A lesser degree of chronic herniation may account for the torticollis that is seen in children with posterior fossa tumours, a sign that mainly occurs with hemispheral cerebellar tumours.

Symptoms and signs or very high ICP threatening brain perfusion, and those of herniation (which are associated) are an indication of imminent danger and require emergency treatment (see below).

FOCAL FEATURES

Focal neurological features of brain tumours occur in less than 15% of cases and depend mainly on the location of the tumour. However, some focal signs are of no value in the presence of intracranial hypertension. This applies particularly to paralysis of the abducens nerve, as indicated above, and less commonly to paralysis of the IIIrd nerve. In general, compression of the ocular motor nerve by a herniated uncus produces only involvement of the pupillary fibres with unresponsive mydriasis. In rare cases there is complete paralysis of the IIIrd nerve with ptosis and extrinsic muscle deficit (Weiner and Porro 1965). Other false localizing signs include involvement of the IVth (Halpern and Gordon 1981), Vth and VIIth (Davie et al. 1992) nerves, which is probably due to compression of the nerve fibres stretched over angular bony structures (O'Connell 1978). Rarely, paradoxical mydriasis of the pupil contralateral to the side of the tumour is observed (Chen et al. 1994).

Ataxia, which is a major manifestation of cerebellar tumours, may also occur with frontal lesions. In this case, there is often no nystagmus, dysmetria or adiadochokinesia, and dysequilibrium is prominent.

DIAGNOSIS

The current diagnostic approach to a suspected brain tumour is primarily neuroimaging. Isotopic brain scan and ultrasonography have only limited indications.

Plain X-rays of the skull often show widening of sutures, abnormal digital markings, and rarefaction of the posterior clinoids and lamina dura in the pituitary fossa. Calcification may be seen in certain tumour types.

These signs are frequently absent, however, and CT used to be a major neuroradiological investigation. MRI is much more precise except for visualization of intracranial calcification (Renowden 2005). It provides better definition and is especially helpful in brainstem tumours and in small lesions located close to bony structures (Poussaint 2001). However, CT may be sufficient for the diagnosis and is less expensive and more readily available than MRI. The latter is currently clearly superior to CT for the diagnosis of all brain tumours, particularly for posterior fossa localization, because it is free from bony artefacts, and for certain midline tumours as images can be obtained in various planes, especially sagittal ones. Gadolinium-enhanced MRI is superior to CT for demonstrating some lesions that may be otherwise difficult to diagnose. MRI is also superior to CT for visualizing optic gliomas and CNS lymphomas (Zimmerman et al. 1992) and meningeal dissemination (River et al. 1996). MRI preferably with FLAIR sequence is now the essential tool for assessment of childhood brain tumours and of sequelae related to their treatment (Warren 2005). It can be completed by MRS (Tzika and Chang 2002, Curless et al. 2002a, Tzika et al. 2004), which can allow chemical characterization of paediatric brain tumours, and by the more recent techniques of diffusion-weighted and perfusion-weighted MRI (Chang et al. 2003) and tensor analysis for specific purposes. If only CT is available, it should be performed with and without injection of iodine contrast substance except in patients with allergy to iodine. Unenhanced scans may rarely fail to reveal existing tumours, and the presence and degree of enhancement provides information on the nature of the tumour. Functional imaging is less precise from a morphological point of view but may have specific indications, e.g. to localize essential functional areas that must be respected.

Examination of the CSF is usually not essential for the diagnosis. In specific cases study of the CSF may be indicated for cytology, especially for the detection of meningeal spread, and in cases of leukaemia, malignant meningeal tumours or melanomas. The presence of malignant cells in the CSF is not uncommon with malignant tumours such as medulloblastomas or ependymomas. Although false positives are rare, false negative results are fairly common (Glass et al. 1979). A search for markers (e.g. human chorionic gonadotropin or alphafetoprotein) for some types of embryonal tumours is sometimes useful (Edwards et al. 1985).

In most cases, the dangers of lumbar puncture probably outweigh the information that can be expected from its performance. How often a lumbar puncture produces or hastens the occurrence of transtentorial herniation is difficult to determine, and the literature presents conflicting opinions in this regard (for a review, see Plum and Posner 1980). It is thus safer to refrain from performing lumbar puncture except in cases in which essential information can be expected, e.g. when it is necessary to exclude meningitis. The advent of CT has considerably simplified this problem, and CT should be obtained before lumbar puncture when there is a suspicion of a mass lesion.

The *differential diagnosis* of brain tumours includes other intracranial mass lesions, hydrocephalus, intracranial haemorrhages and infections. Pseudotumour cerebri, lead encephalopathy and various types of brain oedema are described below.

TREATMENT: GENERAL CONSIDERATIONS

Surgery is generally the primary treatment for brain tumours. Total resection is always desirable as it is associated with the best results. It cannot be accomplished in many cases, but partial resection is useful to reduce the bulk of the tumour thus permitting destruction of the remaining malignant cells by irradiation and/or chemotherapy (Cohen and Duffner 1994, Estlin and Lowis 2005).

Radiation therapy aims at achieving selective death of tumour cells with as little damage as possible to the surrounding brain. The principles of radiation therapy are beyond the scope of this book: they have been recently reviewed (Estlin and Lowis 2005). Efforts are currently being made to increase the total dose of radiation delivered to neoplasms while minimizing damage to the surrounding CNS by more precise collimation and/or modifying the schedule of delivery of irradiation. Hyperfractionation, with division of the daily dose into more than one treatment, separated by a minimum of 6 hours (a time shown to permit most cellular repair), may improve the results of treatment of highly malignant inaccessible tumours and allows administration of a higher total dose. High-energy irradiation with photon (X-ray or ^{60}Co), electron or neutron beams is variably used. Currently, heavy charged particles (protons and helium ions) and sensitizers to X-rays are being tested. Stereotactic irradiation is used for tumours of limited volume difficult to remove surgically (Régis et al. 2004). Stereotactic neurosurgery has considerably developed, often in combination with minimally invasive endoscopic techniques.

Chemotherapy (Estlin 2005) is increasingly used in the treatment of tumours. A number of new drugs are available, and new treatment protocols are continuously being tested. The basic principles of chemotherapy have been reviewed (Cohen and Duffner 1994) but new developments are constantly taking place. Novel rescue techniques with autologous stem cells permit increased doses of radiation and/or chemotherapy to be given for highly malignant tumours resistant to conventional doses (Packer et al. 2003). Immunotherapy, using recombinant interferon and other lymphokine products including tumour necrosis factor and interleukin 2, as well as molecular genetic treatment of cancers and a large number of agents too numerous to be described in this book are under intensive investigation. The latter includes attempts at gene substitution to enhance resistance of patients and 'antisense therapy' blocking the expression of particular DNA sequences and others (Gilberson 2005).

CHARACTERISTICS OF INDIVIDUAL TUMOURS

POSTERIOR FOSSA TUMOURS

MEDULLOBLASTOMA

Medulloblastoma accounts for 14–20% of childhood intracranial tumours and is second only to cerebellar astrocytoma among posterior fossa tumours. Medulloblastoma is most frequent in the first decade of life and twice as common in boys as in girls. It has been reported in the neonatal period.

The medulloblastoma is a malignant and rapidly growing tumour arising from undifferentiated neural cells. Its precise histological classification is difficult because of its primitive nature. It has often been regarded as a primitive neuroectodermal tumour (PNET), although current thinking considers it distinct due to both histological and molecular differences (Rostomily et al. 1997, Nicholson et al. 1999). The latter include frequent anomalies of chromosome 17, in contrast with the mutations in the *HASH1* gene that are common in PNETs but are not found in medulloblastomas (Cohen and Duffner 1994, Ellison et al. 2003). Identification of *PTCH1* mutation in sporadic medulloblastoma has revealed the role of the 'sonic hedgehog' pathway mutations. Genetic disruption of this pathway in medulloblastoma results in inappropriate acivation of the signalling cascade and downstream tumourogenic effects (Taipale and Beachy 2001). A special prognostic importance is attached to staging of medulloblastoma, especially with regard to therapeutic strategies and prognosis (Packer et al. 1999). The tumour is poorly demarcated from normal tissue. It is very cellular and consists of small round cells without any definite pattern, with frequent mitotic figures. Medulloblastomas usually arise from the cerebellar vermis in the region of the roof of the fourth ventricle. They extend toward the

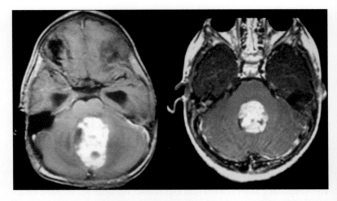
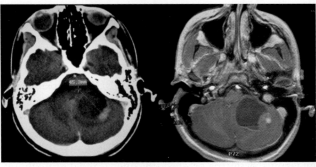

Fig. 13.2. Medulloblastoma: comparison with cerebellar astrocytoma. (In each pairing of images the left-hand scan is from a case of medulloblastoma and the right-hand scan from a case of cerebellar astrocytoma.)

(Top) Cerebellar medulloblastoma involving the vermis and compressing and invading the brainstem. MRI shows heterogeneous enhancement of the mass and hydrocephalus with dilatation of the temporal horns.

(Bottom) MRI of a different case illustrates the fact that some medulloblastomas can involve the cerebellar hemispheres and make differential diagnosis with cerebellar astrocytoma (a benign tumour) problematic.

dorsum of the cerebellar vermis and into the lumen of the fourth ventricle thus producing hydrocephalus. Metastases along the CSF pathways are frequent, and imaging of the spinal canal is useful to determine the extent of the tumour. Extraneural metastases may occur, especially following surgery, and involve preferentially bones and lymph nodes (Duffner and Cohen 1981).

The main clinical features are intracranial hypertension and ataxia. Ataxia is usually truncal or affects both lower limbs, with a tendency to fall backwards or forwards. Symptoms of raised ICP are prominent and may be isolated. The whole symptomatology develops rapidly in a few weeks and papilloedema is often lacking. Bilateral pyramidal tract signs may be present. Wasting is often marked. Occasionally, multiple cranial nerve involvement, spinal root pain or even paraplegia are seen early, indicating the presence of metastatic dissemination.

The imaging appearance of medulloblastoma on CT and MRI is highly suggestive. The tumour is median and rounded and has, on unenhanced scans, a slightly lower density than the surrounding parenchyma. The density increases homogeneously and markedly on contrast injection. In some cases, small cystic areas, haemorrhages or calcification are visible. Hydrocephalus is virtually constant (Fig. 13.2).

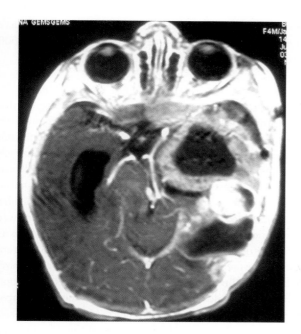

Fig. 13.9. Large pilocytic astrocytoma of the left temporal lobe. T_2-weighted MRI. The tumour is heterogeneous with a solid central part and cystic formation. The posterior cyst is thin-walled; the anterior cavity has a thick wall with irregular contrast enhancement and pushes the median vessels towards the right. In spite of its huge volume, the histological nature of the tumour was not malignant.

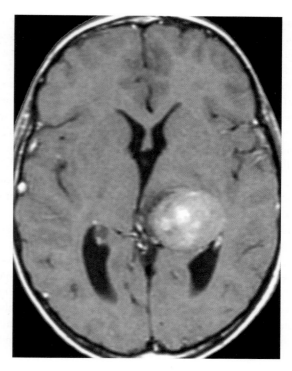

Fig. 13.10. Oligodendroglioma of the left cerebral hemisphere. T_2-weighted MRI showing heterogeneous areas of high signal and faintly visible areas of low signal. CT showed areas of high density indicating the presence of calcification at the periphery of the tumour.

et al. 1987). Seizures are the presenting feature in about one third of patients, but headache, hemiparesis and personality changes are more frequent. High-grade gliomas may evolve from a low-grade lesion, not infrequently following irradiation of the lesion, or be observed several years after treatment of acute lymphocytic leukaemia (Hoppe-Hirsch et al. 1993). Contrast enhancement in a ring-like formation is almost constant in glioblastoma but may be absent in anaplastic astrocytomas. Diffusion-weighted MRI and MR spectroscopy can help establish the nature of the tumour (Chang et al. 2003). However, large enhancing tumours are not necessarily malignant (Fig. 13.9). Metastases may occur (Duffner and Cohen 1994) but local invasion is the major problem. Surgical treatment is usually associated with radiation therapy. There is currently an increasing tendency to use chemotherapy, which has been found to be effective in improving the overall survival of children with these tumours, in contrast to what has been reported in adults (Dropcho et al. 1987; Pollack et al. 1999a,b). It is also increasingly used to delay or avoid radiotherapy for high-grade tumours. The prognosis is often more favourable than in adults with histologically similar tumours but remains poor with an actuarial probability of survival of 32%, three years after surgery. However, even with high-dose chemotherapy, the results are variable and mortality remains significant. An adverse outcome has been found to be significantly correlated with overexpression of the P53 protein in the tumours independently of histology, age and tumour location (Pollack et al. 2002). *Pleomorphic xanthoastrocytomas* have attracted some attention despite their rarity. They occur in young subjects, are almost always supratentorial and frequently in the temporal or frontal lobes, and present commonly as isolated seizures. They share many clinical features with the epileptogenic tumours such as ganglioglioma and developmental neuroepithelial tumours (see below), despite their specific histological features (Fouladi et al. 2001, Im et al. 2004).

Oligodendrogliomas are relatively rare tumours in childhood (about 20% of all supratentorial tumours). It has been observed recently that oligogliomas with partial deletion of chromosomes 1p or 19q in adults have a more benign evolution (Walker et al. 2005). However, these deletions seem to be rare in children (Kreiger et al. 2005). Oligogliomas are slow-growing tumours with a strong tendency to calcify. Tice et al. (1993) studied 39 cases, 32 of which were located in the frontal lobe. The most common presenting symptoms are convulsive seizures that occur in 50–70% of cases. The diagnosis is relatively easy by CT or MRI.

Oligogliomas are usually hypointense on T_1 sequences and give a high signal in T_2 images. About 40% are calcified and 60% have well-defined margins (Fig. 13.10). Less than half produce a mass effect and less than a quarter of the cases enhance with contrast. They may produce thinning of the inner skull table: this indicates a slowly enlarging lesion and can be seen with benign astrocytomas and with dysembryoplastic neuroepithelial tumours (Daumas-Duport et al. 1988). These are described in Chapter 15 as they usually present with isolated epilepsy.

The outcome following surgery is usually good, especially in young patients (Rizk et al. 1996), and the tumours tend to remain stable for long periods even following only partial resection, although a poor outcome is associated with coexisting neurological deficit at the time of diagnosis and the presence of nuclear polymorphism of the tumour (Wilkinson et al. 1987) on histological examination. This favourable outcome was recently confirmed by Peters et al. (2004) who reported post-surgery survival in 22 of 26 children with peripheral tumours. This was in marked contrast with the low survival rates for central oligodendrogliomas involving the basal nuclei. The prognosis of malignant oligogliomas is poor (Hoppe-Hirsch et al. 1993).

Ependymomas of the cerebral hemispheres represent 30–40% of intracranial ependymomas in children (Jayawickreme et al. 1995). Over 90% of ependymomas arise within the cranium, two thirds of them below the tentorium. Malignant ependymomas are more common in a supratentorial location (Pierre-Kahn et al. 1983, Hoppe-Hirsch et al. 1993). In Pierre-Kahn's series, 86% of supratentorial ependymomas were malignant. The biology of these tumours resembles that of other low-grade gliomas where local control is most important and only 5% of children present with metastatic disease. Metastases are mainly intracranial, in contrast with the spinal metastases of posterior fossa ependymomas (Allen et al. 1998). The main clinical manifestations are signs and symptoms of intracranial hypertension and focal deficits. Seizures are relatively uncommon. Neuroradiological appearance is nonspecific. Small multiple intratumoural calcification is frequent. Despite improvement in the past decade, the overall outcome is relatively poor with a 5-year survival rate of about 50% (Smyth et al. 2000, Agaoglu et al. 2005). A young age is the most important negative prognostic factor (Pierre-Kahn et al. 1983, Sala et al. 1998).

Treatment of low-grade brain gliomas in children
Surgery is clearly the initial approach and can give excellent results especially in astrocytomas and oligogliomas. Surgery can be a definitive treatment for astrocytomas. In one series of 43 children with benign astrocytomas and oligogliomas reported by Hirsch et al. (1989), 41 demonstrated progression-free survival at 5 years even though only 2 patients had had radiotherapy; similar results have been obtained by others (Pollack et al. 1995, Gajjar et al. 1997, Shaw and Wisoff 2003). However, complete excision may not be possible. Adjuvant treatment after partial excision is commonly with radiation, which has some effect on tumour volume, but chemotherapy currently has a major role as an adjuvant treatment as it is effective in children and avoids radiation damage (Packer 1999; Pollack et al. 1999b; Fouladi et al. 2003a,b; Duffner 2004) and combined treatment with surgery followed by chemotherapy is often employed. Cisplatin and etoposide seem especially effective (Massimino et al. 2002). However, Van Veelen-Vincent et al. (2002) found that for ependymomas chemotherapy was of no help but radiation was somewhat efficacious although the overall long-term results of treatment were disappointing. Irradiation is indicated for residual tumour or recurrences. It is probably desirable to differ it as much as possible as the growing CNS is particularly sensitive to radiation damage (Kortmann et al. 2003a,b). Favourable results of hyper-fractionated radiotherapy associated with chemotherapy have been obtained by some authors (Timmermann et al. 2000, Massimino et al. 2004).

OTHER TUMOURS OF THE CEREBRAL HEMISPHERES
Meningiomas are relatively rare in children, representing less than 2% of intracranial tumours. Most meningiomas are found in the convexity of the brain, but a higher incidence of location within the lateral ventricles than in adults, with absence of dural attachment, an origin in the posterior fossa and cyst formation characterize meningiomas found in childhood (Cohen and Duffner 1994). Ferrante et al. (1989) reviewed 178 cases from the literature and added 19 cases of their own. Sixteen per cent were intraventricular, 90% were supratentorial and 10% arose from the fourth ventricle. Perry and Dehner (2003) reported 13 cases and reviewed the literature extensively. Im et al. (2001) emphasized the large size of many of these tumours, their unusual location, the frequency of calcification and of cyst formation in the gingiva and characteristic radiological appearance. Most meningiomas in childhood are of the fibroblastic type, consisting of spindles of prominent fibroglia. The syncytial and angioplastic types are much less common. Sarcomatous meningiomas are more frequent in children than in adults (Cohen and Duffner 1994).

Increased ICP is responsible for most clinical manifestations but seizures are the presenting feature in 8–31% of cases. Intraventricular meningiomas are apt to present with signs of intermittent obstruction of CSF outflow tracts. Optic canal or orbital tumours produce central scotomas or variable field defects. They may be difficult to distinguish from gliomas of the optic pathway. Hyperostosis or bone destruction favour the diagnosis of meningioma. CT clearly demonstrates most meningiomas especially after contrast enhancement. The CT picture, however, may be less characteristic in children than in adults (Ferrante et al. 1989). Large cystic formations are frequent, especially in children under 2 years of age. MRI shows a decreased T_1 and increased T_2 signal, and usually demonstrates heterogeneity of the tumour due to tumour vascularity, cystic degeneration and calcification. It enables better delineation of the limits of the lesion and helps to indicate whether the tumour is intra- or extra-axial.

Therapy is basically surgical but radiation, especially stereotactic irradiation, may play a role for patients in whom total removal is impossible. However, 18 of 22 patients in the series of Davidson and Hope (1989) were doing well up to 18 years after operation, and the favourable outcome has been confirmed (Di Rocco and Di Rienzo 1999). Sarcomatous meningiomas show many mitotic figures and disorganized architecture. They have a strong tendency to local recurrence and can metastasize to the CNS or to remote tissues (Cohen and Duffner 1994).

Meningiomas are one type of post-irradiation secondary tumour. It is also a frequent tumour in patients with NF2 (Sadetzki et al. 2002, Ruggieri et al. 2005) (Chapter 3).

TUMOURS OF THE BASAL GANGLIA AND THALAMUS
These tumours represent 2–6% of intracranial tumours in children. Most are astrocytomas of various grades, from benign

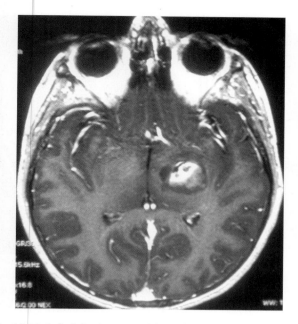

Fig. 13.11. Left thalamic tumour. T_2-weighted MRI after gadolinium shows high-signal tumour in the left thalamus with a cystic component. Note displacement and flattening of the third ventricle.

pilocytic lesions to anaplastic astrocytomas and glioblastoma multiforme (Bernstein et al. 1984).

The most common manifestation is progressive hemiparesis, which may be associated with unilateral dystonia or intention tremor. Krauss et al. (1992) in a review of 225 cases in adults and children found only 20 with a movement disorder, most commonly tremor or dystonia. Seventy per cent of the patients had signs of corticospinal tract involvement. Homonymous hemianopia, nystagmus and hearing loss may be observed. Sensory manifestations are exceptional. Martinez-Lage et al. (2002) studied 20 patients, 4 of whom presented with acute manifestations: intracranial hypertension was present in 13, motor deficit in 8, seizures in 7, behavioural or mental disturbance in 5, and abnormal movements in only 2 patients.

The diagnosis is readily suggested by CT or MRI, when the tumour is hypodense and when contrast enhancement is present (Lefton et al. 2000) (Fig. 13.11). The latter may occur in a ring-like manner. In some cases the tumour is infiltrating and its density does not differ, even after contrast injection, from that of the surrounding brain. In such cases recognition of the mass effect caused by the tumour is the only diagnostic criterion. Bilateral gliomas may raise a difficult diagnostic problem (Gudouris et al. 2002).

Complete surgical removal of tumours of the basal ganglia is not possible. Biopsy is advised by many authorities (see Bernstein et al. 1984), who reserve irradiation for malignant tumours (Souweidane and Hoffman 1996). Stereotactic biopsy is often used. Blind radiotherapy is probably best avoided.

GANGLIOGLIOMAS AND GANGLIOCYTOMAS
These are benign tumours of the cerebral hemispheres that are

characterized histologically by the presence of mature neuronal and glial cells and clinically by their isolated epileptic manifestations. Their outcome is benign. Luyken et al. (2004) recently reported 184 cases with a median follow-up at 8 years postsurgery. Removal of the lesion was associated with relief of seizures in 84% of patients. The survival rate at 7.5 years was 97% even in cases in which the tumour was not totally removed. These tumours may be intermediate between cortical dysplasias and more aggressive tumours (Duchowny et al. 1989, 1996). Gangliogliomas are particularly apt to present as cases of isolated, intractable epilepsy, usually of a focal type. In the series of Zentner et al. (1994), 84% of tumours were in the temporal lobe and 92% were revealed by epileptic seizures. They occur mainly in young children or even in neonates (Duchowny et al. 1989) without any sign of increased pressure. The diagnosis is often difficult. CT typically reveals hyperdense cortical lesions with gyriform or serpiginous outlines without marked mass effect. Most lesions are difficult to identify on T_1-weighted MRI sequences and may have low, intermediate or increased signal on T_2-weighted images. Gangliocytomas differ from gangliogliomas, which typically show cyst formation, calcification, contrast enhancement and mass effect. The recently described angiocentric neuroepithelial tumour (Lellouch-Tubiana et al. 2005) belongs to the same spectrum of neuroglial tumours.

Surgical removal often results in the cure of epilepsy. The long-term prognosis is favourable. The rare *desmoplastic infantile ganglioglioma* (Khaddage et al. 2004) is seen almost exclusively below 2 years of age. It presents as a large tumour with a large cystic component and a solid component that takes up contrast on T_1 sequences and appears hyperintense on T_2 sequences, often with meningeal enhancement (Tamburini et al. 2003, Trehan et al. 2004). Its main interest is that its diagnosis is difficult and it is often mistaken for a malignt tumour. Yet, resection leads to cure.

INTRAVENTRICULAR TUMOURS
Tumours of different histological types can be located within the lateral ventricles. These include intraventricular meningiomas, which are more frequent in children than in adults (Cohen and Duffner 1994), intraventricular neurocytomas, also known as intraventricular oligodendrogliomas (Nishio et al. 1988), intraventricular cysts, ependymomas and, especially, papillomas of the choroid plexus (Pascual-Castroviejo et al. 1983).

Papillomas arise from the epithelium of the plexus and are relatively common in infants, about 20% occurring below 1 year of age, but rare in older children. They are large, cauliflower-like tumours that present the structure of normal choroid plexus with a considerable degree of hyperplasia (Schijman et al. 1990, Sarkar et al. 1999).

The usual manifestation of choroid plexus papilloma in infants is hydrocephalus (Chapter 6), which is generally rapidly evolving and may be accompanied by papilloedema, an uncommon finding in nontumoural hydrocephalus. The diagnosis is easy because papillomas present as large intraventricular masses with massive enhancement after contrast injection (Fig. 13.12). The

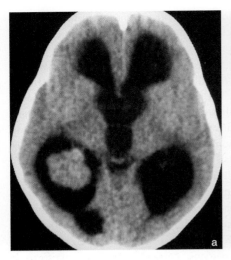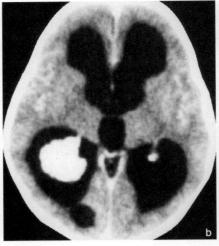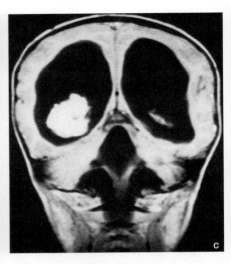

Fig. 13.12. Papilloma of right choroid plexus in 4-year-old boy with moderate psychomotor delay and large head. *(a,b)* CT before and after contrast injection. *(c)* MRI, coronal cut after gadolinium enhancement showing large papilloma in right ventricle and normal choroid plexus on left.

hydrocephalus is thought to result from hypersecretion of CSF by the tumour but it may also be due to meningeal fibrosis resulting from haemorrhage from the tumour. The CSF frequently contains an excess of protein.

In rare cases, choroid plexus papilloma may mimic a degenerative CNS disorder. In older children, papillomas are often located in the temporal lobe and produce seizures rather than hydrocephalus. Calcification is sometimes present.

Excision of the papilloma is the treatment of choice. Total excision was achieved in 20 of 24 children with choroid plexus tumours (16 papillomas and 8 carcinomas) reported by Lena et al. (1990). Overall, 6 opf the 24 patients died, while 5 of the 15 surviving papilloma patients had sequelae. Postoperative complications are unfortunately not rare (Nagib and O'Fallon 2000, Kumar and Singh 2005). In some cases, hydrocephalus persists following removal of the tumour and a shunt may be required. Radiation therapy is reserved for tumours having malignant histological patterns.

DYSEMBRYOPLASTIC NEUROEPITHELIAL TUMOURS (DNETS)

DNETs (Daumas-Duport et al. 1988) are probably related to gangliocytomas and gangliogliomas. Indeed, both terms may well be used for the same lesions by different investigators (see Chapter 15). They include a mixture of neuronal and glial elements, both oligocytes and astrocytes, and appear to be of developmental origin. It is likely that a significant proportion of the cases formerly diagnosed as low-grade oligoastrocytomas were in fact DNETs. These tumours are located cortically but may encroach on the underlying white matter. They are often found in the temporal or frontal lobes of children and adolescents with chronic focal seizures of early onset (Giulioni et al. 2005). They are of mixed density on CT, and only 18% enhance after contrast infusion. A quarter of them are calcified, and one third produce a focal cranial deformity as a result of erosion of the inner

skull table. They give a mixed signal on MRI, usually with low signal on T_1-weighted sequences and sometimes high signal on T_2-weighted sequences (Fig. 13.13). These lesions have little or no tendency to grow and usually remain stable on repeat examinations. They may be associated with some oedema of the white matter. However, a few mitoses can be seen (Raymond et al. 1994). Some of these tumours develop in areas of cortical dysplasia. They manifest clinically as isolated epilepsy (see Chapter 15). Surgical removal, even if subtotal, may give good results without recurrences (Murphy et al. 1995). Irradiation is clearly contraindicated.

OTHER CNS TUMOURS

PRIMARY CEREBRAL NEUROBLASTOMAS
Primary cerebral neuroblastomas occur in the first decade in 81% of cases and in 20% before the age of 2 years. Most are primary (Etus et al. 2002, Yaris et al. 2005). A few are cerebral relapses or metastases of peripheral neuroblastoma (Porto et al. 2005b). The clinical picture is that of hemispheric tumours in general. Survival following surgery and irradiation with or without chemotherapy reaches 3 years in 60% of patients and exceeds 5 years in 30% (Bennett and Rubinstein 1984).

PRIMITIVE NEUROECTODERMAL TUMOURS (PNETS)
PNETs are highly malignant neoplasms that occur mostly in children and young adults (Duffner et al. 1981). They consist of small, undifferentiated cells without observable cytoplasm, and dark oval or irregular nuclei. Numerous mitotic figures and necrosis are often present (Vogel and Fuller 2003). Occasional focal areas of differentiation toward neuronal or glial lines may often be recognized. By electron microscopy, the tumour cells have been reported to have similarities to the developing cortical plate of the fetus. PNETs are mainly hemispheric in location but may be found in the posterior fossa (Zagzag et al. 2000). They have similarities with medulloblastomas, from which thay are now

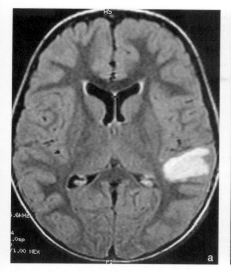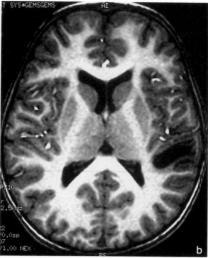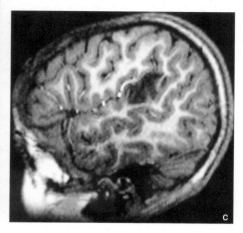

Fig. 13.13. Dysembroplastic neuroepithelial tumour (DNET). *(a)* Axial T₂-weighted image showing high cortical lesion. *(b)* Axial T₁-weighted image from the same area showing low signal. *(c)* Sagittal view. The tumour is entirely limited to the deep cortex. There is no oedema, and the shape of the involved convolution is not significantly modified.

separated, which are sometimes regarded as being posterior fossa PNETs (Ellison et al. 2003). Horten and Rubinstein (1976) have regarded PNETs as cerebral neuroblastomas. However, neuroblastomas are less malignant than PNETs, and histologically these neoplasms are not purely neuroblastic. Most PNETs have structural and/or numerical chromosomal abnormalities. Nerve growth factor receptors are demonstrated immunochemically in one third of cases.

The clinical features of PNETs are those of malignant supratentorial tumours, with hypertension and focal deficits being more common than seizures. The course is usually very brief. CT may show cystic formation and extensive calcification. Neoplastic meningitis may be the first manifestation.

Treatment is with as complete a resection as possible, followed by irradiation and chemotherapy. Stem cell rescue has permitted the use of increased doses of chemotherapy and/or radiation (Pérez-Martínez et al. 2004).

DIFFUSE GLIOMATOSIS (GLIOMATOSIS CEREBRI)
Gliomatosis cerebri is a rare neoplastic disorder involving large parts of the brain in a multicentric or diffuse overgrowth with cells of neuroglial, oligodendroglial or astroctytic lineage (Artigas et al. 1985, Caroli et al. 2005). The disorder has been described in a newborn infant and was originally mistakenly diagnosed as lissencephaly (Barth et al. 1988). Jennings et al. (1995) reviewed 160 cases from the literature plus three of their own, involving primarily the centrum semi-ovale, the mesencephalon, brainstem and basal ganglia. Clinical features included corticospinal tract deficits in 58%, dementia/mental retardation in 44%, headache in 39%, seizures in 38%, cranial neuropathy in 37%, raised ICP in 34% and spinocerebellar deficit in 33%. The diagnosis is often difficult as imaging is not characteristic, showing areas of nonspecific (diffusely increased) signal. Atypical clinical presenta-

tions have been reported, suggesting meningoencephalomyelitis (Jayawant et al. 2001) or even Rasmussen syndrome because of the presence of epilepsia partialis continua (Shahar et al. 2002). Chemotherapy (Sanson et al. 2004) appears to be the advised therapy for children.

METASTASES
Intracranial metastases of extracranial tumours are rare in childhood. Wilms tumours, osteosarcoma, rhabdomyosarcoma, melanoma and neuroblastoma are known occasionally to metastasize to the brain (Bouffet et al. 1997). Curless et al. (2002b) found that neuroblastomas, osteosarcomas, melanoblastomas, Ewing sarcomas and germ cell tumours were responsible for most haematogenous metastases in a review of 2040 tumour cases. Intracranial metastases have no distinctive features. They may be single or multiple and present as areas of hypodensity, which enhance following contrast injection, and surrounding oedema.

LIPOMAS (see also Chapter 2)
Lipomas are space-occupying lesions of malformative origin that do not behave as tumours. The most frequent location of lipomas is the region of the corpus callosum and the quadrigeminal cistern (Gomez-Gosalvez et al. 2003, Yilmaz et al. 2005). Lipomas are generally associated with total or partial agenesis of the callosal commissure. They may communicate through a narrow stalk with an extracranial lipoma in the region of the bregma. They should be distinguished from dermoid cysts of the anterior fontanelle (Saito et al. 1988, Aslan et al. 2004), encephaloceles, haemangiomas, lipomas, lymphangiomas and sinus pericranii (extracranial varicoceles) by using preoperative MRI.

Lipomas of the corpus callosum are often asymptomatic. Epilepsy is the most frequent manifestation of symptomatic lesions. The diagnosis is readily made by demonstrating the presence of a mass of fat density, usually surrounded by 'eggshell' calcification. Lipomas, usually of small size and asymptomatic, may be found in other locations, notably in the pineal region (Spallone and Pitskhelauri 2004).

SPECIFIC FEATURES AND OUTCOME OF BRAIN TUMOURS IN INFANTS AND CHILDREN

BRAIN TUMOURS IN INFANTS AND CHILDREN UNDER 2 YEARS OF AGE

These differ in location, pathology, clinical features and therapy from those of older children. The proportion of all childhood brain tumours occurring at this age may be at least 10% (Cohen and Duffner 1994). A significant number of these are definite 'congenital' tumours, i.e. they produce symptoms within the first two weeks of life, or 'probably congenital' tumours, i.e. they are present or recognized within the first year of life (Fort and Rushing 1997, Sarkar et al. 2005).

In infants under 6 months of age, supratentorial tumours account for 70–75% of all intracranial neoplasms. Cohen and Duffner (1994) found that 30% of children with brain tumours occurring under 2 years of age had ependymomas, 20% medulloblastomas, 15% astrocytomas, 8% glioblastomas and 22% an admixture of sarcomas, choroid plexus papillomas, pinealomas, PNETs, gangliogliomas and teratomas. Wakai et al. (1984) in a review of congenital brain tumours found that 46.1% were teratomas and 36.5% were of neuroepithelial origin, fewer than 10% being astrocytomas. The low incidence of dysontogenic tumours in the large series of Balestrini et al. (1994), in which 41% of tumours were astrocytomas and 20% medulloblastomas, is probably related to the fact that it included mostly children in the second year of life.

The *clinical features* of congenital and early-onset tumours are variable with the type and location of the tumour. Macrocrania, delayed milestones and behavioural disturbances are prominent. In the case of congenital tumours, fetal death and preterm birth are very frequent (Wakai et al. 1984). Intracranial haemorrhage can be the presenting manifestation. Vomiting, focal neurological signs, seizures and the diencephalic syndrome of emaciation (see p. 514) may also be early signs. Infantile spasms are an uncommon manifestation.

The *diagnosis* may be delayed if it is not suggested by relatively trivial symptoms such as delayed milestones or vomiting. Tumours manifested by hemiplegia may be difficult to separate from congenital static hemiplegia but brain imaging will resolve any doubt. CSF examination may be misleading as pleocytosis and increased protein are commonly found. CT and MRI will, in most cases, readily permit the diagnosis.

Historically, the *prognosis* of congenital tumours is poor (Sarkar et al. 2005). Radiation is highly dangerous for the very young developing brain and so has been almost completely abandoned. Surgery is difficult because of the large size of many tumours. Surgical mortality was 17.4% in 63 operated patients studied by Balestrini et al. (1994). Many tumours are malignant. The survival rate 5 years after diagnosis has varied between 23% and 54% in published series. In a recent report on 16 cases

(Young and Johnston 2004), 13 were alive at 5 years post-surgery including all cases of benign tumours and none of the malignant ones. The quality of life for survivors is often poor: 7 of the 13 patients suffered from epilepsy, 12 had serious cognitive difficulties and 8 had neurological deficit. Chemotherapy appears to be effective, and results are as good as or better than those achieved with standard radiation therapy. However, the possible late effects of chemotherapy are as yet poorly known.

OUTCOME OF BRAIN TUMOURS IN CHILDREN

The results of recent advances in therapy have been impressive, especially for certain types of tumours that were regularly fatal a few years ago, such as medulloblastomas. The survival of children with brain tumours (Duffner et al. 1986) varies with their nature and location. The worst prognosis is for children with diffuse brainstem tumours, whereas more than 90% of children with cerebellar astrocytoma, and 70–90% of those with low-grade hemispheric astrocytoma, have a 5-year survival. Children under 2 years of age with tumours have a lower survival rate (30–50%) than older children, and their quality of life is often poor. These figures apply to an unselected group of patients, and results in individual institutions with a special interest and experience in the treatment of neoplasms should be better.

The quality of survival is one of the major concerns with current therapeutic approaches. In a prospective study of a small group of children (Duffner 2004) most of the patients remained within the normal range of intelligence but their IQ scores declined over time. Learning disabilities were found in more than 90% of children after irradiation, and most required special educational services. Similar results, especially related to radiotherapy, have been reported by other investigators (Radcliffe et al. 1992, Garcia-Perez et al. 1993). In the series of Radcliffe et al., there was an average loss of 27 IQ points in children treated under 7 years of age, but no loss in children receiving therapy later, and Packer et al. (1989) reported that young age at the time of irradiation and adjuvant chemotherapy were risk factors associated with a decline in IQ. Radiotherapy for tumours is also associated with significant endocrinological complications (Cohen and Duffner 1994), mostly growth failure commonly caused by pituitary insufficiency but which may also result from irradiation of the spine. Thyroid and gonadal problems also occur. Finally, the risk of late development of secondary tumours, mostly meningiomas and gliomas, 2–40 years (average 20 years) after irradiation is small but real (Cohen and Duffner 1994). For these reasons, efforts are being made to explore forms of treatment avoiding some causes of complications, especially the replacement of radiation therapy with various chemotherapeutic regimens (Kalifa and Grill 2005).

The very long-term outcome for children with tumours is generally favourable in terms of mortality. However, multiple late complications may occur including late mortality, secondary tumours, small stature or low birthweight of offspring, and especially decreased level of education are significant problems, particularly frequent in high-risk groups (Anderson 2003, Packer 2005, Robison et al. 2005).

NEUROLOGICAL MANIFESTATIONS OF LEUKAEMIAS AND LYMPHOMAS AND OF THEIR TREATMENT

Neurological manifestations frequently occur as an initial feature or as a late complication of leukaemias and lymphomas and can be their presenting manifestation (Aysun et al. 1994). Complex neurological pictures are often observed at various stages of these diseases, and it has become extremely difficult to determine the cause of neurological manifestations as these may be due to the disease itself, to toxic complications of therapy, to viral or other opportunistic infections resulting from immuno-depression, or to haemorrhagic accidents. Appropriate therapy, however, depends on a correct diagnosis of the nature of the neurological abnormality.

Neurological Manifestations of Leukaemias

Complications of the leukaemic process may result from leukaemic infiltrations of the meninges, brain and cranial nerves, or may be due to haemorrhage or infections.

Meningeal leukaemia may occur at any stage of the disease. One third to one half of children are in complete remission when neurological complications appear. Leukaemic infiltration primarily affects the arachnoid, and infiltration of the brain tissue is found in less than 15% of the children who die in a relapse (Price 1983). Presenting features of CNS leukaemia include headache, vomiting and papilloedema. Seizures occur in about 10% of patients, and the risk of seizure is considerably greater in children receiving methotrexate therapy. Increased appetite and weight gain may occur consequent to hypothalamic infiltration. Cranial nerve palsies are frequently present. CT usually fails to demonstrate the leukaemic infiltrates (Chen et al. 1996), but MRI with gadolinium enhancement may show the meningeal involvement.

The CSF shows an increased cell count and blast cells are usually recognized. However, blast cells may be associated with a low CSF cell count (Mahmoud et al. 1993). The sugar content is low in about 50% of affected children. Eosinophilic or basophilic meningitis has been recorded (Budka et al. 1976).

Large intracranial or paraspinal masses (granulocytic sarcomas or chloromas) are uncommon (Brown et al. 1989). They occur with myeloblastic leukaemia. This often affects the spinal canal and produces spinal and radicular compression. Retinal lesions including haemorrhages and white exudates sometimes with swelling of the disc occur in about 20% of cases of leukaemia (Taylor 1990).

Prophylaxis of CNS involvement is part of the management of leukaemia and aims at preventing overt leukaemic infiltration of the nervous system.

A combination of radiotherapy in various doses and chemotherapy is used in most centres.

Intracranial haemorrhage is uncommon in acute lymphoblastic leukaemia but is a frequent cause of death in nonlymphoblastic types (Yamauchi and Umeda 1997). Subdural haematoma or subarachnoid haemorrhage usually indicates a poor prognosis.

Sinus thrombosis (Sébire et al. 2005) may present with seizures and symptoms of increased ICP. Cranial neuropathies resulting from leukaemic infiltration of the basilar meninges commonly involve the facial, abducens and auditory nerves. Epidural compression of the spinal cord may be an initial manifestation (Pui et al. 1985).

NEUROLOGICAL MANIFESTATIONS OF LYMPHOMAS

Non-Hodgkin Lymphomas

Although lymphomas are currently a common maligncy in adults (De Angelis 2001) they are still relatively rare in children and may be primary or occur as secondary tumours following leukaemia (Porto et al. 2005a). However, involvement of the CNS (Franssila et al. 1987) was observed in 25% of 63 children with lymphomas at the time of diagnosis by Bergeron et al. (1989). Of these 16 patients, 10 had clinical manifestations, with frequent involvement of cranial nerves, including hypoacusis and sudden amaurosis; 7 of these children had an abnormal CSF, and 6 had asymptomatic meningitis. The characteristics of the CSF are similar to those in leukaemia. Neuromeningeal relapses occurred in 19 children (30%). A peripheral neuropathy is sometimes seen in patients with lymphomas and is of ominous prognostic significance. Involvement of the venous sinuses may occur.

CNS involvement is much more frequent in lymphomas located in the cervical region than in those of abdominal or thoracic location. Various histological types are observed, including small-cell (Kai et al. 1998) and large-cell anaplastic lymphomas (Rowsell et al. 2004). Burkitt lymphomas seem to have a better prognosis than other types.

Primary lymphoma of the CNS is being recognized increasingly as a complication of the acquired immunodeficiency syndrome (AIDS), which accounts, together with the increased use of immunosuppressive thearpy, for its current incidence. Primary lymphoma has been reported in a few children with AIDS (Rodriguez et al. 1997). Lymphomas may be more common in children with AIDS than opportunistic CNS infections (Epstein et al. 1988). They present as focal mass lesions, hyperdense before contrast and with marked homogeneous enhancement, and give an intense signal on T_2-weighted MRI sequences. New lesions are apt to appear every few days. Two of the three children reported by Epstein et al. had large-cell neoplasms, one a Burkitt-type lymphoma. These lesions, which may be mistaken for inflammatory lesions, are highly sensitive to steroid treatment, although recurrence is ultimately inevitable. Lymphomas are very sensitive to irradiation, and the remission rate is high (80%).

The effects of lymphomas on the peripheral nervous system have been reviewed by Hughes et al. (1994).

Hodgkin Disease

Neurological complications of Hodgkin disease are uncommon in children (Sapozink and Kaplan 1983). They include intracerebral deposits that give rise to focal signs, basal meningeal involvement with cranial nerve palsies, and spinal extradural deposits that can produce paraplegia. These are usually associated with CSF abnormalities, occasionally in the form of an eosinophilic meningitis (Patchell and Perry 1981).

Another type of neural involvement results from direct extension into the nervous system of visceral disease, producing compression of the brainstem, the brachial plexus and the spinal roots (Mallouh 1989).

A polyneuropathy, due not to direct infiltration of the nerves but apparently to the remote effect of malignancy, has been reported in a child with Hodgkin disease. Such paraneoplastic disorders, which are common in adults, are exceptional in children. A paraneoplastic cerebellar syndrome manifesting as chronic ataxia has been reported in one child (Topçu et al. 1992, Hahn et al. 2000). Secondary tumours frequently occur several years after the cure of the disease (Lin and Teitell 2005).

All lymphomas may be associated with the same opportunistic infections as leukaemias.

COMPLICATIONS OF THE TREATMENT OF MALIGNANCIES IN CHILDREN

The effects of therapy of leukaemia on the nervous sytem, whether related to irradiation or to chemical toxicity, are a source of concern, and minimizing such effects is an important part of attempts to improve the treatment of leukaemia. It is often difficult to separate toxicity mainly due to irradiation from the toxic effects of drugs (Hanefeld and Riehm 1980), and indeed side effects are experienced in almost all cases. In a somewhat arbitrary manner I will describe in succession the complications attributed primarily to irradiation, those due to chemical toxicity, and those that result from opportunistic infections facilitated by or due to therapeutically induced immunosuppression. In fact, interaction of these multiple factors is probably at play in most cases.

COMPLICATIONS MAINLY DUE TO IRRADIATION

A *transient syndrome of somnolence and apathy* may develop in 58–63% of patients 1–2 months after completion of radiotherapy, with malaise, anorexia and vomiting (Hanefeld and Riehm 1980). The course is usually benign with resolution in 10–20 days. The EEG background frequencies decrease markedly during this syndrome, and learning disabilities and recurrent seizures seem to be more frequent in patients with the syndrome, suggesting that somnolence may be an indicator of long-term neurological sequelae after cranial irradiation. A similar syndrome may occur after irradiation of the spinal cord, appearing a few weeks to months after completion of treatment. The first symptom is often tingling in the back induced by neck flexion (Lhermitte sign). Paraesthesia may be a prominent feature but all symptoms abate after 2–8 weeks. An acute intermittent confusional state may occur several years after completion of radiotherapy and is probably due to ischaemia from irradiation vasculopathy.

Cerebrovascular accidents can be related to radiotherapy. Mitchell et al. (1991) reported 11 cases occurring 1–4 years after completion of treatment. Seven patients had also received chemotherapy, and 5 had repeated episodes. Santoro et al. (2005) studied retrospectively the incidence and type of 'ischaemic

stroke' in 2318 children treated for leukaemia. They found an incidence of 0.47%; all cases were of sinovenous origin. The response to anticoagulant treatment was satisfactory. Arterial lesions in the field of irradiation also exist; they may be more common in neurofibromatosis patients (see Chapter 3) but also occur in other patients (Kortmann et al. 2003a,b). Cerebrovascular accidents may also result from disseminated intravascular coagulation, especially at onset of treatment of promyelocytic leukaemia (Packer et al. 1985). In such cases, the symptoms and signs are recurrent and fluctuating, and the course is often lethal. Early anticoagulation may be effective in some cases. Packer et al. (1985) recognized four different syndromes in children treated for lymphoreticular malignancies and, less commonly, for solid tumours. These include, in addition to intravascular coagulation, acute neurological dysfunction in children treated for osteogenic sarcoma, acute hemiplegia in patients treated with L-asparaginase (see below), and a syndrome of impaired consciousness, seizures and focal neurological deficits produced by metastatic neuroblastoma compressing the torcular. The relationship of acute hemiplegia to irradiation is also suggested by reports of accelerated atherosclerosis following radiation therapy in adults and in children (Werner et al. 1988). Shuper et al. (1995) have reported "complicated migraine-like episodes" in four irradiated children. Severe headache was associated with transient hemiparesis and/or aphasia, as I have observed in one child in whom angiography demonstrated stenosis of the distal carotid artery following radiotherapy for a tumour of the hypothalamus.

Secondary tumours are well-recognized complications of irradiation (Vasquez et al. 2003, Broniscer et al. 2004, Kantar et al. 2004, Paulino and Fowler 2005). Meningiomas are frequent in adults (Mack and Wilson 1993) but rare in children.

CNS tumours are most frequent, but other tumours (lymphomas, neuroblastomas, retinoblastomas, leukaemia and thyroid cancer) are not rare. Glioblastoma multiforme is apt to develop in children with leukaemia treated with X-rays and methotrexate (Fig. 13.14). Multiple PNETs have been reported in the same circumstances. Therefore all children treated for malignancy should receive life-long surveillance. The development of tumours has also been observed following relatively low-dose irradiation for benign conditions such as tinea capitis. Other complications of irradiation, especially of brain tumours or of extracranial tumours, include radionecrosis and postradiotherapy thrombosis of the carotid artery with development of deep anastomotic vessels mimicking moyamoya syndrome.

Radionecrosis is a rare complication that usually becomes clinically manifest months to years after completion of the treatment, with a maximum frequency between 1 and 3 years. It occurs mainly following large doses of the order of 60 Gy or more. Pathologically, the lesions predominate in the white matter, with characteristic vascular changes (endothelial proliferation and fibrinoid necrosis) that may lead to complete occlusion. The clinical manifestations include insidious and progressive deterioration, with dementia, focal neurological signs and seizures, and frequently death. They are often interpreted as indicating tumour relapse, an impression that is also given by neuroradiological

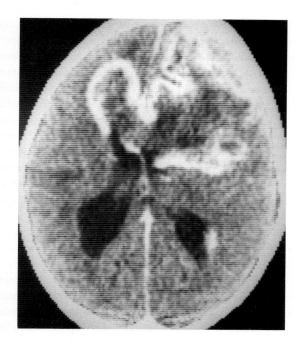

Fig. 13.14. Extensive glioblastoma multiforme in 9-year-old girl who had been treated for acute lymphocytic leukaemia at age 3 years and was subsequently retarded with a leukoencephalopathy due to methotrexate and X-irradiation. This is typical of a 'second tumour' probably induced by initial therapy.

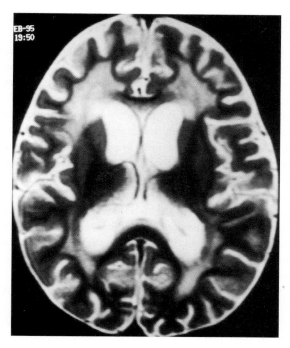

Fig. 13.15. Methotrexate encephalopathy. T$_2$-weighted MRI showing extensive leukoencephalopathy involving predominantly frontal and to a lesser extent occipital white matter. (Courtesy Dr Kling Chong, Great Ormond Street Hospital, London.)

findings, as neither CT nor MRI, even with gadolinium enhancement, can distinguish the mass effect of necrosis from that due to recurrence of a tumour. Excision of the lesion may be life-saving (Nelson et al. 1990) but is probably unnecessary in less severe cases (Woo et al. 1987). Radionecrosis has been reported following irradiation of extraneural tumours of the head or scalp (Vallée et al. 1984). For severe radiation-induced injury, treatment with heparin and warfarin (Glantz et al. 1994) may improve the outcome.

A more benign syndrome featuring hallucinations progressing to seizures, and areas of triangular hypodensity in watershed areas suggestive of infarcts, has been described by Pihko et al. (1993). This syndrome regresses without sequelae.

Radiation-induced lesions of the peripheral nerves are much rarer than CNS damage. A few cases are on record mainly in adults (Lamy et al. 1991).

COMPLICATIONS MAINLY DUE TO DRUG TOXICITY

All the drugs used in the treatment of cancer have significant toxicity.

High-dose administration of *methotrexate* by intravenous route has been associated with reversible dementia in a nonirradiated child with myelogenic leukaemia (Mittal et al. 2005). A variety of neurological manifestations, including cranial nerve palsies and focal and diffuse deficits, have been seen 1–2 weeks after i.v. administration for the treatment of osteogenic sarcoma (Fig. 13.15). Intrathecal methotrexate may be followed by a sudden

paraplegia that may be transient or persistent. A similar accident can be caused by intrathecal injection of vincristine (Bain et al. 1991) or of cytosine arabinoside (Özön et al. 1994). Both drugs given intrathecally more commonly induce arachnoiditis with signs of meningeal irritation, headache, vomiting and moderate pleocytosis (Hanefeld and Riehm 1980). *Necrotizing leukoencephalopathy* is usually attributed to methotrexate, although irradiation is also a significant factor in its genesis. Pathological lesions range from simple pallor of myelin to necrosis with cavitation. Numerous alterations of vessels with hyalinization and endothelial proliferation are present. Spinal involvement is usually absent, although it has occasionally been reported. The clinical features include a change of behaviour with apathy, slurred speech and depressed mood, followed by akinesia and muteness.

Spastic and ataxic gait later becomes evident. CSF protein levels are often raised. The syndrome appears 2–12 months after completion of treatment. Its mechanism is imperfectly understood. Both the dose of irradiation and that of methotrexate seem to play a role. However, similar CT findings have been found in patients receiving methotrexate who had not been irradiated and in patients who had received radiotherapy and cytosine arabinoside (Fusner et al. 1977). CT shows large, poorly limited areas of hypodensity of the white matter bilaterally. Enhancement of the white matter is sometimes observed. Multiple areas of calcification mainly located at the junction of the white and grey matter appear secondarily.

A variable degree of atrophy is associated with the white matter lesions. Transient atrophy has been recorded following prophylactic CNS treatment of lymphoblastic leukaemia (Lund and Hamborg-Pedersen 1984).

Calcification of the basal ganglia, especially the putamen, commonly appears approximately one year after irradiation in many children, the majority of whom remain asymptomatic. Calcification in other deep cortical regions may also be asymptomatic (Price 1983). Calcification appears to result from a microangiopathy with secondary calcium deposition. The angiopathy also plays an important role as a cause of the white matter hypodense areas reflecting demyelination, necrosis and glial damage so often shown by CT or MRI examination of irradiated children (Constine et al. 1988). There is no established relationship between the extent of MRI abnormalities and clinical features, although the most severe lesions tend to be frequently associated with dementia. Brainstem demyelination in the form of multifocal areas or as central pontine myelinolysis has been reported (LoMonaco et al. 1992).

Cerebellar degeneration may be induced by cytosine arabinoside.

Vincristine toxicity includes a neuropathy (Schiavetti et al. 2004; see also Chapter 20) and, rarely, an acute encephalopathic syndrome marked mainly by seizures that may be asociated with cortical blindness (Byrd et al. 1981) and other neurological deficits. Hyponatraemia is frequently present and plays a role in the origin of seizures, but direct cerebral involvement seems likely in some cases. Cerebral blindness has also been reported during treatment with cyclosporin A in association with other manifestations of toxic encephalopathy.

L-asparaginase can produce thrombosis of the cerebral veins or dural sinuses that may be associated with either haemorrhage or infarction (Feinberg and Swenson 1988). The thrombogenic effect of the drug seems to be mediated through transient deficiencies of plasma proteins important for coagulation and fibrinolysis.

Carmustine therapy in high doses has been responsible for an acute encephalopathic syndrome. Cytosine arabinoside, intraventricular methotrexate, cisplatin and virtually all drugs used in chemotherapy can also produce immediate or delayed toxicity. Rescue with bone marrow transplant or with stem cells is now used in order to allow more intensive therapies with larger doses and multiple drugs regimens.

Cisplatin can cause a peripheral neuropathy (Chapter 20) and involvement of the auditory nerve.

COMPLICATIONS RELATED TO OPPORTUNISTIC INFECTIONS

These include bacterial, viral, fungal and protozoan diseases that have been described in Chapter 10. In the series of Campbell et al. (1977), complicating infections were present in 21 of 438 children with leukaemia. Twelve were viral and 9 bacterial in origin. Mumps was the most common, occurring in 5 patients, 1 of whom died. The subacute measles encephalitis seen in children with treated lymphatic malignancies is described in Chapter 10. Immunological complications include in the first place the opsoclonus–myoclonus syndrome mainly observed with neuro-

blastoma but exceptionally with other tumours. Recently, rare cases of *paraneoplastic limbic encephalitis*, a complication well known in adults (Gultekin et al. 2000, Graus et al. 2001) have been reported in adolescents with ovarian and other tumours (Rosenbaum et al. 1998, Lee et al. 2003). They present clinically with subacute behavioural episodes that can be misdiagnosed as psychosis or drug abuse, seizures, and central hypoventilation that requires respiratory assistance (Vitaliani et al. 2006). The symptoms can respond to resection of the tumour or immunological therapy and recover completely. They are probably an immune response to tumour antigens. A few cases of transverse myelitis, possibly due to undetermined viral infection are on record (Ullrich et al. 2006).

LATE EFFECTS OF THE TREATMENT OF LEUKAEMIAS ON COGNITIVE DEVELOPMENT

Prophylactic treatment of the CNS of patients with various types of leukaemia may produce cognitive deficits, which are particularly frequent in children who developed the early somnolence syndrome. Although many children function within the normal range, children who received treatment at a young age tend to perform below their matched controls, especially on tasks measuring quantitative, memory and motor skills, but not on language tasks. Their academic results are even poorer than their IQ would suggest, and behavioural problems are common (Anderson et al. 1994, MacLean et al. 1995). Epilepsy, often of a resistant type, is frequently associated (Khan et al. 2003).

The mechanism of such deficits is probably multifactorial. Irradiation seems to play a prominent role but psychogenic factors are also probably operative to some extent. Persistent sequelae of the peripheral nervous system have been described (Lehtinen et al. 2002, Packer et al. 2003).

INTRACRANIAL CYSTS AND OTHER MASS LESIONS

The term cyst is loosely applied to a large number of intracranial cavities of multiple pathology and aetiologies such as anoxic necrosis, post-haemorrhagic lesions, vacular accidents, tumours, infections and infestations (Chapter 10), and neurodegenerative diseases. Cysts may be of any size from huge lesions to very small, often transient and usually insignificant formations such as subependymal or frontal horn cysts in neonates (Chang et al. 2006). Some rare cystic formations may raise diagnostic problems, e.g. rare cases of massive dilatation of the Virchow–Robin spaces whose significance is not fully understood (Rohlfs et al. 2005). This section considers only large primary cysts.

ARACHNOID CYSTS

Most large intracranial cysts are arachnoid cysts. The term designates fluid-filled cavities that develop either within a duplication of the arachnoid membrane or between the arachnoid and the pia mater (Gosalakkal 2002). Arachnoid cysts represent 1% of space-occupying lesions (Hanieh et al. 1988), and 60–90% of symptomatic lesions are recognized during childhood or

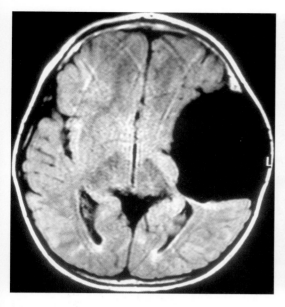 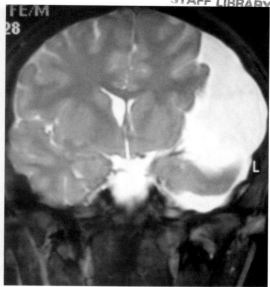

Fig. 13.16. Large sylvian arachnoid cyst. *(Left)* Axial cut showing large cavity filled with CSF-like fluid. *(Right)* Frontal cut showing displacement of median structures and small temporal lobe probably due to displacement and distortion rather than to atrophy.

adolescence. Cysts may be an incidental finding in up to 5% of cases in autopsy studies (Naidich et al. 1985–86). Arachnoid cysts are most usually malformations and only rarely follow arachnoiditis. Familial cases are rare and causes generally remain obscure (Arriola et al. 2005). Arachnoid cysts may or may not communicate with the subarachnoid space, whether located supratentorially or infratentorially.

SUPRATENTORIAL ARACHNOID CYSTS

These are the most common type of intracranial cysts. Middle fossa (sylvian) arachnoid cysts have the highest frequency in most series, followed by suprasellar cysts and cysts of the cerebral convexity (Hanieh et al. 1988). However, Pascual-Castroviejo et al. (1991) found, in a series of 67 arachnoid cysts, that interhemispheric cysts were almost as common as middle fossa cysts, and that posterior fossa cysts accounted for 42% of their cases. Middle fossa cysts are frequently asymptomatic and may be discovered incidentally on CT performed for various reasons (Robertson et al. 1989) (Fig. 13.16). They may be very large, pushing back the temporal lobe, which is compressed rather than atrophic. When of moderate size and found in later childhood or adolescence, these cysts may not require treatment. The most common clinical manifestations are a large head and temporal bossing. However, some recent reports challenge the benignity of these cysts. De Volder et al. (1994) described aphasia associated with a cyst that disappeared following drainage, and Millichap (1997) thought that attention deficit disorder that disappeared following drainage was a consequence of the lesion. According to Raeder et al. (2005), arachnoid cysts can cause cognitive deficits that disappear after treatment in adults. Until better confirmed, surgical indications are imperative only when symptoms of pressure (headache) are present and in large cysts.

Symptomatic sylvian cysts can give rise to signs of increased pressure, especially headache and papilloedema, or to seizures, usually focal (Van der Meché and Braakman 1983), or become manifest as a result of haemorrhagic complications. These include bleeding into the cyst, which may render the cavity invisible on CT, and subdural haematoma with or without associated intracystic haemorrhage. It seems likely that the 'juvenile relapsing subdural haematoma', characterized radiologically by bony changes similar to those of sylvian cysts, is a haematoma complicating a middle fossa cyst. Subdural haematoma may rarely be on the side opposite to the cyst. No treatment is ever indicated in such cases.

The diagnosis of temporal arachnoid cysts is generally easy. Large porencephalic lesions of the temporal pole may superficially mimic arachnoid cysts. Bilateral cysts of the temporal fossa have been reported in children with glutaric aciduria type I (Martinez-Lage et al. 1994). Such lesions are also reported as atrophy of the temporal lobe, a term that seems more appropriate than that of cyst, and are not an indication for surgery.

Treatment of sylvian cyst is best performed by cystoperitoneal shunting. However, drainage of huge cysts in children with closed fontanelles should be cautious as rapid decompression can produce mass brain displacement. It is not indicated for small asymptomatic cases, which are common.

Suprasellar cysts are manifested by hydrocephalus in 90% of cases. Visual abnormalities and ataxia are observed in a quarter of the cases. In some patients they are responsible for a slow anteroposterior to-and-fro movement of the head at a rhythm of 2–3 Hz known as the *'bobble-head doll syndrome'*. Partial hypopituitarism with especial involvement of corticotropin secretion is seen in 10% of patients (Brauner et al. 1987). The full spectrum of endocrinological disturbances may also include precocious puberty and growth hormone deficiency (Mohn et al. 1999).

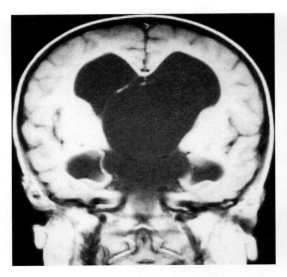 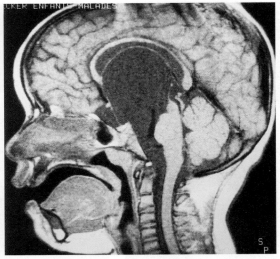

Fig. 13.17. Suprasellar arachnoid cyst. *(Left)* T₁-weighted MRI, frontal cut shows massive hydrocephalus of lateral ventricles. Third ventricle is entirely filled with a cyst, separated from lateral ventricle by a thin membrane, and with a fluid content slightly denser than CSF. *(Right)* Sagittal cut shows that the cyst extends upwards almost to the corpus callosum. (Courtesy Prof. F Brunelle, Hôpital des Enfants Malades, Paris.)

The CT appearance is typical with a large rounded suprasellar image of fluid density obstructing the foramina of Monro with resulting hydrocephalus (Fig. 13.17). MRI may show that the cyst and the third ventricle are distinct cavities separated by a thin membrane. Treatment may be with shunting of the cyst. Opening of the cyst membrane by an endoscopic or open approach is also possible (Decq et al. 1996).

Arachnoid cysts of the convexity can produce focal signs and raised ICP. Interhemispheric cysts may be difficult to separate from dorsal cysts associated with agenesis of the corpus callosum. Cysts in this location are apt to be dysembryoplastic with cuboid or columnar epithelium rather than arachnoidal cells.

Infratentorial Arachnoid Cysts

Infratentorial arachnoid cysts are the second most frequent form of intracranial cysts after middle fossa cysts. Their histological structure is diverse and only a few are true arachnoid cysts (Friede 1989). In fact, there is some confusion regarding what should be considered as a posterior fossa arachnoid cyst, because other fluid collections are common in the posterior fossa. These include Dandy–Walker syndrome, megacisterna magna, and even some cases of large but nonpathological cisterna magna (Chapter 2; see also Barkovich et al. 1989, Altman et al. 1992). Posterior fossa cysts are closed cavities that do not communicate with the fourth ventricle and are not associated with hypoplasia of the cerebellum. The most common clinical manifestations in infants and young children are macrocephaly and hydrocephalus, whereas typical posterior fossa syndrome is the presenting manifestation in older patients (Galassi et al. 1985, Harsh et al. 1986). The location of the cysts within the posterior fossa is variable. The majority are located behind the cerebellum, but some lesions may be supra-cerebellar, laterocerebellar or located to the cerebellopontine angle (Galassi et al. 1985, Pierre-Kahn and Sonigo 2003).

Cysts of the incisura are often both infratentorial and supra-tentorial and are located anteriorly to the cerebellar vermis, posterior to the pineal region and above the quadrigeminal plate, extending above the roof of the third ventricle below the corpus callosum (Fig. 13.18). In addition to hydrocephalus, they may be associated with Parinaud syndrome or ataxia. Some mesencephalic and third ventricle cysts may be secondary to arachnoiditis caused by thalamic haemorrhage, or to bacterial ventriculitis (Ramaeckers et al. 1994).

Treatment of posterior fossa cysts may be by direct operative approach (Hanieh et al. 1988). Derivation by cystoperitoneal shunting seems to be the method of choice and leads in many cases to complete disappearance of the lesion.

OTHER INTRACRANIAL CYSTS

Dermoid cysts are apt to be found in the sagittal plane of the skull. Caldarelli et al. (2004) studied 16 cases of dermoid and 3 of epidermoid cysts. These lesions can produce compression of intracranial structures. Some of the dermoids are connected by a tract to the skin and may give rise to infections. Imaging (Hakyemez et al. 2005) shows that epidermoids are well-demarcated lesions giving a high signal on T₂-weighted images and on water-diffusion MRI.

Colloid cysts of the third ventricle are rare in childhood. They are revealed by paroxysmal headaches, often of extreme intensity, that may be related to the movements or position of the patient. Sudden death may occur and has been ocasionally reported in childhood (Byard and Moore 1993). Nine familial cases are on record (Partington and Bookalil 2004).

Ependymal cysts are rare. Sundaram et al. (2001) found only 5 cases in their clinicopathological study of 145 cases of intracranial cysts. Their cavity is lined with an ependyma-like epithelium. They are supratentorial, intracerebral or convexity

signs of segmental spinal involvement, and signs resulting from interruption of long tracts within the spinal cord. The importance of back pain and, especially, of *spinal rigidity* as an early symptom of tumour of the cord has long been known. Pain may have a radicular distribution but is more often diffuse and is usually predominantly nocturnal. Rigidity is frequently associated with scoliosis. Segmental weakness, hyporeflexia, sensory disturbances and amyotrophy can result from involvement of the central grey matter or nerve roots. Segmental myoclonus is a rare presentation (Renault et al. 1995). Spasticity evolving into paraplegia, sphincter disturbances and sensory deficits results from long tract involvement. Disturbances of walking with claudication and stiffness may be present long before other symptoms. The presence of a definable sensory level, which may be difficult to demonstrate in young children, indicates the upper level of compression. Bilateral pyramidal tract signs are present with Babinski and Rossolimo* responses. Initial bladder symptoms are increased urgency followed by retention or incontinence. Sphincter disturbances, especially urinary retention, indicate urgent need for decompression.

The diagnosis of spinal cord tumour should be quickly confirmed because sudden aggravation with complete paraplegia due to compromised circulation in the anterior cerebral artery and its branches may occur at any time. One should be exceedingly suspicious of recurrent back pain and, in some patients, of recurrent abdominal pain. Atypical presentations with paroxysmal attacks of arm pain or isolated abdominal discomfort simulating an irritable bowel syndrome (Robertson 1992) may delay recognition of a tumour.

Plain X-rays of the spine may be diagnostic by showing bone destruction, erosion of the spinal pedicles or of the posterior vertebral bodies, and widening of both the anteroposterior and transverse diameters of the spinal canal. Currently MRI is the technique of choice. It clearly shows both intra- and extramedullary lesions and associated cystic formation, thus permitting separation of intramedullary tumours with associated cysts from syringomyelia. However, distinguishing a tumour from an area of increased signal due to oedema, haemorrhage or inflammation can be difficult. Gadolinium enhancement helps make such distinctions, and diffusion-weighted MRI may be useful in some cases (Pui et al. 2005). Transverse cuts should be obtained allowing detailed studies of the zones of interest discovered with sagittal cuts. MRI has supplanted myelography and avoids the reactions associated with the introduction of the contrast medium into the subarachnoid space. These are usually minor (headache, nausea and vomiting, radicular pain and hyperaesthesia) but may include in rare cases seizures, and minor status epilepticus has been observed following metrizamide myelography (Obeid et al. 1988).

CSF protein is usually increased below the level of the block. However, there is a serious risk of damage to the cord by lumbar

*The Rossolimo sign is obtained by flicking the toes upwards. A positive response is active flexion of the toes and is indicative of pyramidal tract involvement. It is more reliable than the Babinski sign in infants and young children.

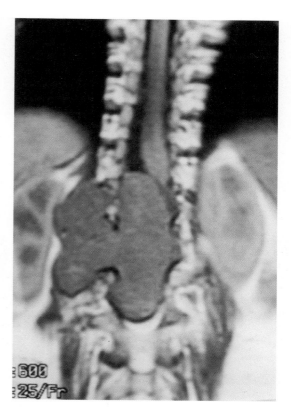

Fig. 13.19. Paraspinal neuroblastoma entering the spinal canal through intervertebral foramen and displacing and compressing the lower spinal cord and roots.

puncture at the site of compression possibly due to slight downward displacement of the cord.

EXTRAMEDULLARY TUMOURS

Approximately two thirds of the extramedullary tumours are extradural in origin (Albanese and Platania 2002), spreading from nearby bone or through intervertebral foramina. About a quarter are intradural. Neuroblastoma (Fig. 13.19) is the most frequent cause but other tumours of osseous or soft tissue origin such as rhabdomyosarcoma, Ewing sarcoma (Uesaka et al. 2003), aneurysmal cysts, metastases, lymphomas (Daley et al. 2003) or histiocytosis X can be the cause of spinal compression. Intradural tumours account for approximately 25% of cases, and meningiomas are the most common histological type followed by schwannomas (Fig. 13.20). Metastases from intracranial tumours, especially ependymomas and medulloblastomas, are usually multiple and may be especially difficult to evidence.

The diagnosis of extradural tumours is often facilitated by the demonstration on plain X-ray films of a mass lesion in the cervical region or posterior mediastinum or by the discovery of the adrenal calcification of a neuroblastoma.

Extramedullary tumours tend to manifest initially with unilateral pain in segmental distribution, often in association with paraesthesiae and weakness. Brown–Séquard syndrome is observed in a small proportion of children with extramedullary tumours. More commonly, there is only predominant weakness,

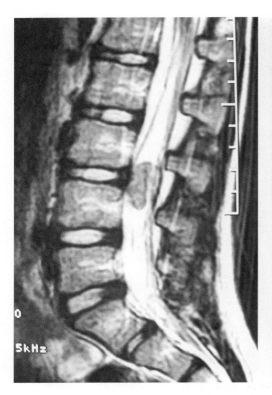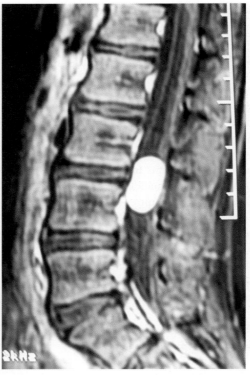

Fig. 13.20. Spinal schwannoma (neurinoma) of the cauda equina. *(Left)* T$_1$-weighted MRI shows well-limited rounded mass. *(Right)* T$_2$-weighted high-signal image.

spasticity and deep sensory loss on the side of the tumour, with more marked contralateral loss of pain and temperature sensation. *Schwannomas* (neurinomas) (Celli et al. 2005) are more common than meningiomas (Di Rocco et al. 1994).

The treatment of extramedullary tumours depends on their nature. For extraspinal tumours with intraspinal extension, surgical removal of the intraspinal tumours should be done on an emergency basis, and later completed by surgical excision and/or other treatment of the extraspinal mass according to its nature. Intraspinal tumours should be treated by surgery (neurinomas) or irradiation and chemotherapy. New neurosurgical techniques have considerably improved the quality of results (Albanese and Platania 2002) but sequelae are still frequent and early diagnosis is essential for good results.

INTRAMEDULLARY TUMOURS

Intramedullary tumours are mainly represented by astrocytomas and ependymomas. They are frequently associated with cystic cavitation of the central cord, which may be difficult to differentiate from purely cystic intramedullary lesions. They can produce symmetrical weakness of the limbs and are often unassociated with pain. Intramedullary tumours often do not produce a clear-cut sensory level and some of them may be surprisingly well tolerated for long periods despite a considerable extension (Pascual-Castroviejo 1990) (Fig. 13.21). *Astrocytomas* may extend over considerable lengths of cord. Yet, their removal has been made possible in some cases by modern neurosurgical techniques

(Epstein 1987, Allen et al. 1998). *Ependymomas* are uncommon. They may affect the conus medullaris (Nagib and O'Fallon 1997, Phan et al. 2000). *Gangliogliomas* (Jallo et al. 2004) are rare in children. *Haemangioblastomas* (Roig et al. 1988) are rare and may be a part of the von Hippel–Lindau complex. These tumours are often cystic and commonly extend over considerable lengths in the cervicodorsal part of the cord. Some of them also involve the lower brainstem.

Some spinal astrocytomas may present with the clinical manifestations of raised ICP without local signs (Gelabert et al. 1990, Rifkinson-Mann et al. 1990, Costello et al. 2002). Cinalli et al. (1995) reported 8 cases in which hydrocepahlus was the initial manifestation and reviewed 38 cases from the literature. Intracranial hypertension may result from metastatic disease, meningeal fibrosis due to haemorrhage from the tumour, or decreased resorption of CSF because of its high protein content 'clogging' the arachnoid granulations. There are cases, however, in which papilloedema and raised pressure are not associated with ventricular dilatation. In two personal cases a tumoural basal arachnoiditis appeared to be responsible for the hydrocephalus and continued to be present years after successful treatment of spinal astrocytoma. An unusual case presenting with the features of spinal muscular atrophy is on record (Aysun et al. 1993).

In one infant (personal case), an intramedullary tumour involving the whole length of the cord simulated Werdnig–Hoffmann disease, but a Rossolimo sign was present.

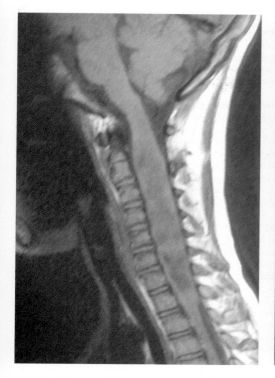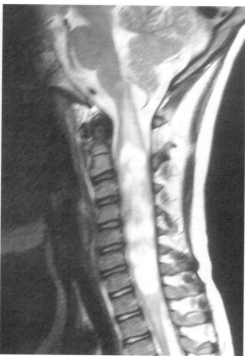

Fig. 13.21. Intramedullary astrocytoma of the spinal cord. *(Left)* T₁-weighted MRI showing enlarged cervical cord with multiple low-signal areas. *(Right)* High signal from the same areas on T₂-weighted sequence.

The special features of intraaxial tumours of the cervico-medullary junction have been described earlier (p. 510).

The diagnosis of intramedullary tumours has been facilitated by MRI, which allows separation of the cystic cavity from the solid part of the tumour (Williams et al. 1987).

Treatment of intramedullary tumours raises special problems (Houten and Weiner 2000). If removal proves impossible, decompression and irradiation may afford fairly long symptomatic relief in 30–50% of cases. Astrocytomas when removable may have a favourable outcome. They may, however, continue to be relatively well tolerated for long periods (Townsend et al. 2004). The overall long-term survival was only of the order of 50% in this study. Patients with malignant tumours such as glioblastomas mostly do poorly (Allen et al. 1998).

New forms of chemotherapy, especially cisplatin and vincristine, may improve the prognosis.

OTHER SPINAL COMPRESSIONS

Compression of the cord may occur with epidural infections and with traumatic or spontaneous haematomas (Pascual-Castraviejo 1990) (Chapters 10, 12).

Spinal arachnoid cysts can produce a slowly progressive myelopathy but, in some cases, symptoms can fluctuate with time and postural changes (Maiuri et al. 2006).

Spinal meningeal cysts (Richaud 1988) are a rare cause of cord compression, which is accessible to effective treatment. Extradural meningeal cysts are diverticuli of the arachnoid through a dural opening, extending on the back of the cord in the extradural space. Extradural cysts may be associated with acquired lymphoedema of the lower limbs and lower lid ectropion and distichiasis (double row of eyelashes) in a dominant syndrome.

Excessive growth of epidural fat has been reported in patients receiving corticosteroid therapy (Munoz et al. 2002) and, exceptionally, in patients with hypothyroidism (Toshniwal and Glick 1987). This is a dangerous condition for which treatment is difficult.

Bony compression of the cord is occasionally seen in patients with thalassaemia or, rarely, with other types of haemolytic anaemia or myelosclerosis as a result of overgrowth of the bone marrow encroaching on the spinal canal (Rutgers et al. 1979).

Other rare causes of spinal cord compression include chronic spinal arachnoiditis, which is a low-grade inflammatory reaction that may follow trauma, shunt procedures or infections, or be idiopathic, and congenital intraspinal lipomas or epidermoid tumours that can be a late consequence of lumbar puncture (MacDonald and Klump 1986).

REFERENCES

Aarsen FK, Van Dongen HR, Paquier PF, et al. (2004) Long-term sequelae in children after cerebellar astrocytoma surgery. *Neurology* 62: 1311–6.

Abel TW, Baker SJ, Fraser MM, et al. (2005) Lhermitte–Duclos disease: a report of 31 cases with immunohistochemical analysis of the PTEN/AKT/mTOR pathway. *J Neuropathol Exp Neurol* 64: 341–9.

Agaoglu FY, Ayan I, Dizdar Y, et al. (2005) Ependymal tumors in childhood. *Pediatr Blood Cancer* 45: 298–303.

Aicardi J (1994) Epilepsy as a presenting manifestation of brain tumors and other selected brain disorders. In: *Epilepsy in Children, 2nd edn.* New York: Raven Press, pp. 334–53.

Albanese V, Platania N (2002) Spinal intradural extramedullary tumors. Personal experience. *J Neorosurg Sci* **46**: 18–24.

Allen JC, Aviner S, Yates JA, et al. (1998) Treatment of high-grade spinal cord astrocytoma of childhood with "8-in-1" chemotherapy and radiotherapy: a pilot study of CCM-945. Children's Cancer Group. *J Neurosurg* **88**: 215–20.

Altman NR, Naidich TP, Braffman BH (1992) Posterior fossa malformations. *AJNR* **13**: 691–724.

Alvord EC, Lofton S (1988) Gliomas of the optic nerve or chiasm. *J Neurosurg* **68**: 85–98.

Anderson NE (2003) Late complications in childhood central nervous system tumour survivors. *Curr Opin Neurol* **16**: 677–83.

Anderson VA, Smibert E, Ekert H, Godber T (1994) Intellectual, educational and behavioural sequelae following cranial irradiation and chemotherapy. *Arch Dis Child* **70**: 476–83.

Appleton RE, Jan JE (1989) Delayed diagnosis of optic nerve glioma: a preventable cause of visual loss. *Pediatr Neurol* **5**: 226–8.

Aronica PA, Ahdab-Barmada M, Rozin L, Wecht CH (1998) Sudden death in an adolescent boy due to a colloid cyst of the third ventricle. *Am J Forensic Med* **19**: 119–22.

Arriola G, de Castro P, Verdu A (2005) Familial arachnoid cysts. *Pediatr Neurol* **33**: 146–8.

Artigas J, Cervos-Navarro J, Iglesias JR, Ebhardt G (1985) Gliomatosis cerebri: clinical and histological findings. *Clin Neuropathol* **4**: 135–48.

Arzimanoglou A, Hisch E, Aicardi J (2003) Hypothalamic hamartoma and epilepsy in children: illustrative cases and possible evolutions. *Epil Dis* **5**: 197–9.

Asamoto M, Ito H, Suzuki N, et al. (1994) Transient mutism after posterior fossa surgery. *Childs Nerv Syst* **10**: 275–8.

Aslan O, Ozveren F, Kotil K, et al. (2004) Congenital dermoid cysts of the anterior fontanelle in Turkish children—four case reports. *Neurol Med Chir* **44**: 150–2.

Aysun S, Cinbis M, Özcan O (1993) Intramedullary astrocytoma presenting as spinal muscular atrophy. *J Child Neurol* **8**: 354–6.

Aysun S, Topçu M, Günay M, Topaloglu H (1994) Neurologic features as initial presentations of childhood malignancies. *Pediatr Neurol* **10**: 40–3.

Babikian P, Corbett J, Bell W (1994) Idiopathic intracranial hypertension in children: the Iowa experience. *J Child Neurol* **9**: 144–9.

Bain PG, Lantos PL, Djurovic V, West I (1991) Intrathecal vincristine: a fatal chemotherapeutic error with devastating central nervous system effects. *J Neurol* **238**: 230–4.

Baker RS, Baumann RJ, Buncic JR (1989) Idiopathic intracranial hypertension (pseudotumor cerebri) in pediatric patients. *Pediatr Neurol* **5**: 5–11.

Balcer LJ, Liu GT, Heller G, et al. (2001) Visual loss in children with neurofibromatosis type 1 and optic pathway gliomas: relation to tumor location by magnetic resonance imaging. *Am J Ophthalmol* **131**: 442–5.

Baldwin RT, Preston-Martin S (2004) Epidemiology of brain tumors in childhood—a review. *Toxicol Appl Pharmacol* **199**: 118–31.

Balestrini MR, Micheli R, Giordano L, et al. (1994) Brain tumors with symptomatic onset in the first two years of life. *Childs Nerv Syst* **10**: 104–10.

Barkovich AJ, Kjos BO, Norman D, Edwards MS (1989) Revised classification of posterior fossa cysts and cystlike malformations based on the results of multiplanar MR imaging. *AJNR* **10**: 977–88.

Barnes D, McDonald WI, Johnson G, et al. (1987) Quantitative nuclear magnetic resonance imaging: characterisation of experimental cerebral oedema. *J Neurol Neurosurg Psychiatry* **50**: 125–33.

Barth PG, Uylings HBM, Stam FC (1984) Interhemispheral neuroepithelial (glio-ependymal) cysts, associated with agenesis of the corpus callosum and neocortical maldevelopment. A case study. *Childs Brain* **11**: 312–9.

Barth PG, Stam FC, Hack W, Delemarre-Van de Waal AH (1988) Gliomatosis cerebri in a newborn. *Neuropediatrics* **19**: 197–200.

Battersby RDE, Ironside JW, Maltby EL (1986) Inherited multiple meningiomas: a clinical, pathological and cytogenetic study of an affected family. *J Neurol Neurosurg Psychiatry* **49**: 362–8.

Bennett JP, Rubinstein LJ (1984) The biological behavior of primary cerebral neuroblastoma: a reappraisal of the clinical course in a series of 70 cases. *Ann Neurol* **16**: 21–7.

Berger MS, Wilson CB (1985) Epidermoid cysts of the posterior fossa. *J Neurosurg* **62**: 214–9.

Bergeron C, Patte C, Caillaud JM, et al. (1989) [Clinical, anatomo-pathological aspects and therapeutic results in 63 malignant ORL non-Hodgkin's lymphomas in children.] *Arch Fr Pediatr* **46**: 583–7 (French).

Bergsagel DJ, Finegold MJ, Butel JS, et al. (1992) DNA sequences similar to those of simian virus 40 in ependymomas and choroid plexus tumors of childhood. *N Engl J Med* **326**: 988–93.

Berkovic SF, Andermann F, Melanson D, et al. (1988) Hypothalamic hamartomas and ictal laughter: evolution of a characteristic epileptic syndrome and diagnostic value of magnetic resonance imaging. *Ann Neurol* **23**: 429–39.

Bernstein M, Hoffman HJ, Halliday WC, et al. (1984) Thalamic tumors in children. Long-term follow-up and treatment guidelines. *J Neurosurg* **61**: 649–56.

Biegel JA (1991) Cytogenetics and molecular genetics of child brain tumors. *Neurooncology* **1**: 139–151.

Bigner SH, McLendon RE, Frichs I, et al. (1997) Chromosomal characteristics of childhood brain tumors. *Cancer Genet Cytogenet* **77**: 127–35.

Binder DK, Horton JC, Lawton MT, McDermott MW (2004) Idiopathic intracranial hypertension. *Neurosurgery* **54**: 538–51; discussion 551–2.

Blumberg DL, Sklar CA, David R, et al. (1989) Acromegaly in an infant. *Pediatrics* **83**: 998–1002.

Boudreau EA, Liow K, Frattali CM, et al. (2005) Hypothalamic hamartomas and seizures: distinct natural history of isolated and Pallister–Hall syndrome cases. *Epilepsia* **46**: 42–7.

Bouffet E, Doumi N, Thiesse P, et al. (1997) Brain metastases in children with solid tumors. *Cancer* **79**: 405–10.

Bourgeois M, Sainte-Rose C, Lellouch-Tubiana A, et al. (1999) Surgery of epilepsy associated with focal lesions in childhood. *J Neurosurg* **90**: 833–42.

Brauner R, Pierre-Kahn A, Nemedy-Sandor E, et al. (1987) [Precocious puberty caused by a suprasellar arachnoid cyst. Analysis of 16 cases.] *Arch Fr Pediatr* **44**: 489–93.

Broniscer A, Gajjar A (2004) Supratentorial high-grade astrocytoma and diffuse brainstem glioma: two challenges for the pediatric oncologist. *Oncologist* **9**: 197–206.

Broniscer A, Ke W, Fuller CE, et al. (2004) Second neoplasms in pediatric patients with primary central nervous system tumors: the St. Jude Children's Research Hospital experience. *Cancer* **100**: 2246–52.

Brown LM, Daeschner C, Timms J, Crow W (1989) Granulocytic sarcoma in childhood acute myelogenous leukemia. *Pediatr Neurol* **5**: 173–8.

Budka H, Gusco A, Jellinger K (1976) Intermittent meningitic reaction with severe basophilia and eosinophilia in CSF leukemia. *J Neurol Sci* **28**: 459–68.

Bunin GR (2004) Nongenetic causes of childhood cancers: evidence from international variation, time trends, and risk factor studies. *Toxicol Appl Pharmacol* **199**: 91–103.

Byard RW, Moore L (1993) Sudden unexpected death in childhood due to a colloid cyst in the third ventricle. *J Forensic Sci* **38**: 210–3.

Byrd RL, Rohrbaugh TM, Raney RB, Norris DG (1981) Transient cortical blindness secondary to vincristine therapy in childhood malignancies. *Cancer* **47**: 37–40.

Calaminus G, Bamberg M, Baranzelli MC, et al. (1994) Intracranial germ cell tumors: a comprehensive update of the European data. *Neuropediatrics* **25**: 26–32.

Calaminus G, Bamberg M, Jürgens H, et al. (2004) Impact of surgery, chemotherapy and irradiation on long term outcome of intacranial malignant nongerminomatous germ cell tumors: results of the German cooperative trial MAKEI 89. *Klin Padiatr* **216**: 141–9.

Calaminus G, Bamberg M, Harms D, et al. (2005) AFP/β-HCG secreting CNS germ cell tumors: long-term outcome with respect to initial symptoms and primary tumor resection. Results of the cooperative trial MAKEI 89. *Neuropediatrics* **36**: 71–7.

Caldarelli M, Massimi L, Kondageski C, Di Rocco C (2004) Intracranial midline demoid and epidermoid cysts in children. *J Neurosurg* **100**: 473–80.

Campbell RHA, Marshall WC, Chessells JM (1977) Neurological complications of childhood leukaemia. *Arch Dis Child* **52**: 850–8.

Cannavo S, Venturino M, Curto L, et al. (2003) Clinical presentation and outcome of pituitary adenomas in teenagers. *Clin Endocrinol* **58**: 519–27.

Caroli E, Orlando ER, Ferrante L (2005) Gliomatosis cerebri in children. Case report and clinical considerations. *Childs Nerv Syst* **21**: 1000–3.

Cascino GD, Andermann F, Berkovic SF, et al. (1993) Gelastic seizures and hypothalamic hamartomas: evaluation of patients undergoing chronic intracranial EEG monitoring and outcome of surgical treatment. *Neurology* **43**: 747–50.

Celli P, Trillo G, Ferrante L (2005) Spinal extradural schwannoma. *J Neursurg Spine* **2**: 447–56.

Chamberlain MC, Silver P, Levin VA (1990) Poorly differentiated gliomas of the cerebellum. A study of 18 patients. *Cancer* **65**: 337–40.

Chan MY, Foong AP, Heisey DM, et al. (1998) Potential prognostic factors of relapse-free survival in childhood optic pathway glioma: a multivariate analysis. *Pediatr Neurosurg* **29**: 23–8.

Chang CL, Chiu NC, Ho CS, Li ST (2006) Frontal horn cysts in normal neonates. *Brain Dev* **28**: 426–30.

Chang YW, Yoon HK, Shan HJ (2003) MR imaging of glioblastoma in children: usefulness of diffusion/perfusion-weighted and MR spectroscopy. *Pediatr Radiol* **33**: 836–42.

Chen CY, Zimmerman RA, Faro S, et al. (1996) Childhood leukemia: central nervous system abnormalities during and after treatment. *AJNR* **17**: 295–310.

Chen R, Sahjpaul R, Del Maestro RF, et al. (1994) Initial enlargement of the opposite pupil as a false localising sign in intraparenchymal frontal haemorrhage. *J Neurol Neurosurg Psychiatry* **57**: 1126–8.

Chiechi MV, Smirnopoulos JC, Jones RV (1995) Intracranial subependymoma: CT and MR imaging features in 24 cases. *AJNR* **165**: 1245–50.

Chipkevitch E (1994) Brain tumors and anorexia nervosa syndrome. *Brain Dev* **16**: 175–9.

Cho BK, Wang KC, Nam DH, et al. (1998) Pineal tumors: experience with 48 cases over 10 years. *Childs Nerv Syst* **14**: 53–58.

Choi JU, Kim DS, Chang SS, Kim TS (1998) Efficacy of neuroendoscopic procedures in minimally invasive preferential management of pineal region tumors: a prospective study. *J Neurosurg* **93**: 245–53.

Cinalli G, Sainte-Rose C, Lellouch-Tubiana A, et al. (1995) Hydrocephalus associated with intramedullary low-grade glioma. Illustrative cases and review of the literature. *J Neurosurg* **83**: 480–5.

Coffin CM, Swanson PE, Wick MR, Dehner LP (1993) Chordoma in childhood and adolescence. A clinicopathologic analysis of 12 cases. *Arch Pathol Lab Med* **117**: 927–33.

Cognard C, Casasco A, Toevi M, et al. (1998) Dural arteriovenous fistulas as a cause of intracranial hypertension due to impairment of cranial venous outflow. *J Neurol Neurosurg Psychiatry* **65**: 308–16.

Cohen BH, Handler MS, De Vivo DC, et al. (1988) Central nervous system melanotic neuroectodermal tumor of infancy: value of chemotherapy in management. *Neurology* **38**: 163–4.

Cohen ME, Duffner PK (1994) *Brain Tumors in Children: Principles of Diagnosis and Treatment, 2nd edn.* New York: Raven Press.

Connolly MB, Farrell K, Hill A, Flodmark O (1992) Magnetic resonance imaging in pseudotumor cerebri. *Dev Med Child Neurol* **34**: 1091–4.

Constine LS, Konski A, Ekholm S, et al. (1988) Adverse effects of brain irradiation correlated with MR and CT imaging. *Int J Radiat Oncol Biol Phys* **15**: 319–30.

Conway PD, Oechler HW, Kun LE, Murray KJ (1991) Importance of histologic condition and treatment of pediatric cerebellar astrocytoma. *Cancer* **67**: 2772–5.

Costello F, Kardon RH, Weill M, et al. (2002) Papilledema as the presenting manifestation of spinal schwannoma. *J Neuroophthalmol* **22**: 199–203.

Couch R, Camfield PR, Tibbles JAR (1985) The changing picture of pseudotumor cerebri in children. *Can J Neurol Sci* **12**: 48–50.

Cruz J, Minoja G, Okuchi K, Facco E (2004) Successful use of the new high-dose mannitol treatment in patients with Glasgow Coma Scale scores of 3 and bilateral abnormal pupillary widening: a randomized trial. *J Neurosurg* **100**: 376–83.

Cuccia V, Rodríguez F, Palma F, Zuccaro G (2006) Pinealoblastomas in children. *Childs Nerv Syst* **22**: 577–85.

Curless RG, Bowen BC, Pattany PM, et al. (2002a) Magnetic resonance spectroscopy in childhood brainstem tumors. *Pediatr Neurol* **26**: 374–8.

Curless RG, Toledano SR, Ragheb J, et al. (2002b) Hematogenous brain metastases in children. *Pediatr Neurol* **26**: 219–21.

Daglioglu E, Cataltepe O, Akalan N (2003) Tectal gliomas in children: the implications for natural history and managemant strategy. *Pediatr Neurosurg* **38**: 223–31.

Daley MF, Partington MD, Kadan-Lottick N, Odom LF (2003) Primary epidural Burkitt lymphoma in a child: case presentation and literature review. *Pediatr Hematol Oncol* **20**: 333–8.

Daumas-Duport C, Scheithauer BW, Chodkiewicz JP, et al. (1988) Dysembryoplastic neuroepithelial tumor: a surgically curable tumor of young patients with intractable partial seizures. Report of thirty-nine cases. *Neurosurgery* **23**: 545–56.

Davidson GS, Hope JK (1989) Meningeal tumors of childhood. *Cancer* **63**: 1205–10.

Davie C, Kennedy P, Katifi HA (1992) Seventh nerve palsy as a false localising sign. *J Neurol Neurosurg Psychiatry* **55**: 510–1 (letter).

De Angelis LM (2001) Brain tumors. *N Engl J Med* **344**: 114–23.

De Angelis LM (2005) Chemotherapy for brain tumors—a new beginning. *N Engl J Med* **352**: 1036–8.

Decq P, Brugières P, Le Guerinel C, et al. (1996) Percutaneous endoscopic treatment of suprasellar arachnoid cysts: ventriculocystostomy or ventriculocystocisternostomy? Technical note. *J Neurosurg* **84**: 696–701.

Deliganis AV, Geyer JR, Berger MS (1996) Prognostic significance of type 1 neurofibromaosis (von Recklinghausen disease) in childhood optic glioma. *Neurosurgery* **38**: 1114–8; discussion 1118–9.

Delitala A, Brunori A, Chiappetta F, et al. (2004) Purely neuroendoscopic transventricular management of cystic craniopharyngiomas. *Childs Nerv Syst* **20**: 858–62.

De Vile CJ, Grant DB, Kendall BE, et al. (1996) Management of childhood craniopharyngioma: can the morbidity of radical surgery be predicted? *J Neurosurg* **85**: 73–81.

De Volder AG, Michel C, Thauvoy C, et al. (1994) Brain glucose utilisation in acquired childhood aphasia associated with sylvian arachnoid cyst: recovery after shunting as demonstrated by PET. *J Neurol Neurosurg Psychiatry* **57**: 296–300.

Dhiravibulya K, Ouvrier R, Johnston I, et al. (1991) Benign intracranial hypertension in childhood: a review of 23 patients. *J Paediatr Child Health* **27**: 304–7.

Di Rocco C, Di Rienzo A (1999) Meningiomas in childhood. *Crit Rev Neurosurg* **9**: 180–8.

Di Rocco C, Ianelli A, Colosimo C (1994) Spinal epidural meningiomas in childhood: a case report. *J Neurosurg Sci* **38**: 251–4.

Dogulu CF, Tsilou E, Rubin B, et al. (2004) Idiopathic intracranial hypertension in cystinosis. *J Pediatr* **145**: 673–8.

Dropcho EJ, Wisoff JH, Walker RW, Allen JC (1987) Supratentorial malignant gliomas in childhood: a review of fifty cases. *Ann Neurol* **22**: 355–64.

Druker BJ, Mamon AJ, Roberts TM (1989) Oncogenes, growth and signal transduction. *N Engl J Med* **321**: 1383–91.

Drummond BKJ, Rosenfeld JV (1999) Pineal region tumours in childhood. A 30-year experience. *Childs Nerv Syst* **15**: 119–26.

Duchowny MS, Resnick TJ, Alvarez L (1989) Dysplastic gangliocytoma and intractable partial seizures in childhood. *Neurology* **39**: 602–4.

Duchowny MS, Altman N, Bruce J (1996) Dysplastic gangliocytoma of the cerebral hemisphere. In: Guerrini R, Andermann F, Canapicchi R, et al., eds. *Dysplasia of Cerebral Cortex and Epilepsy.* Philadelphia: Lippincott-Raven, pp. 93–100.

Duffner PK (2004) Long-term effects of radiation therapy on cognitive and endocrine function in children with leukemia and brain tumors. *Neurologist* **10**: 293–310.

Duffner PK, Cohen ME (1981) Extraneural metastases in childhood brain tumors. *Ann Neurol* **10**: 261–5.

Duffner PK, Cohen ME (1994) Extraneural metastases in childhood brain tumors. In: Cohen ME, Duffner PK, eds. *Brain Tumors in Children: Principles of Diagnosis and Treatment, 2nd edn.* New York: Raven Press, pp. 423–36.

Duffner PK, Cohen ME, Heffner RR, Freeman AI (1981) Primitive neuroectodermal tumors of childhood. An approach to therapy. *J Neurosurg* **55**: 376–81.

Duffner PK, Cohen ME, Myers MH, Heise HW (1986) Survival of children with brain tumors: SEER Program, 1973–1980. *Neurology* **36**: 597–601.

Duntas LH (2001) Prolactinomas in children and adolescents—consequences in adult life. *J Pediatr Endocrinol Metab* **14** Suppl 5: 1227–1232; discussion 1261–2.

Edwards MSB, Davis RL, Laurent JP (1985) Tumor markers and cytologic features of cerebrospinal fluid. *Cancer* **56**: 1773–7.

Edwards MSB, Hudgins RJ, Wilson CB, et al. (1988) Pineal region tumors in children. *J Neurosurg* **68**: 689–97.

Eliash A, Roitman A, Karp M, et al. (1983) Diencephalic syndrome due to a suprasellar epidermoid cyst: case report. *Childs Brain* **10**: 414–8.

Ellison DW, Clifford SC, Gajjar A, Gilbertson RJ (2003) What's new in neuro-oncology? Recent advances in medulloblastoma. *Eur J Paediatr Neurol* **7**: 53–6.

Eng C (1996) The RET proto-oncogene in multiple endocrine neoplasia type 2 and Hirschsprung's disease. *N Engl J Med* **335**: 943–51.

Epstein F (1987) Intra-axial tumors of the cervico-medullary junction in children. *Concepts Pediatr Neurosurg* **7**: 117–33.

Epstein F, Wisoff JH (1988) Intrinsic brainstem tumors in childhood: surgical indications. *J Neurooncol* **6**: 309–17.

Epstein LG, Dicarlo FJ, Joshi VV, et al. (1988) Primary lymphoma of the central nervous system in children with acquired immunodeficiency syndrome. *Pediatrics* **82**: 355–63.

Ersahin Y, Yararbas U, Duman Y, Mutluer S (2002) Single photon emission tomography following posterior fossa surgery in patients with and without mutism. *Childs Nerv Syst* **18**: 318–25.

Estlin E (2005) General principles of chemotherapy. In: Estlin E, Lowis S, eds. *Central Nervous System Tumours in Childhood. Clinics in Developmental Medicine No. 166.* London: Mac Keith Press, pp. 179–89.

Estlin E, Lowis S, eds. (2005) *Central Nervous System Tumours of Childhood. Clinics in Developmental Medicine No. 166.* London: Mac Keith Press.

Etus V, Kurtkaya O, Sav A, et al. (2002) Primary central neuroblastoma: a case report and review. *Tohoku J Exp Med* **197**: 55–65.

Farah S, Al-Shubaili A, Montaser A, et al. (1998) Behçet's syndrome: a report of 41 patients with emphasis on neurological manifestations. *J Neurol Neurosurg Psychiatry* **64**: 382–4.

Farmer JP, Khan S, Khan A, et al. (2002) Neurofibromatosis type 1 and the pediatric neurosurgeon: a 20-year institutional study. *Pediatr Neurosurg* **37**: 122–36.

Favre J, Deruaz JP, Uske A, De Tribolet N (1994) Skull base chordomas: presentation of six cases and review of the literature. *J Clin Neurosci* **1**: 7–18.

Feinberg WG, Swenson MR (1988) Cerebrovascular complications of L-asparginase therapy. *Neurology* **38**: 127–33.

Fernandez C, Figarella-Branger D, Girard N, et al. (2003) Pilocytic astrocytomas in children: prognostic factors—a retrospective study of 80 cases. *Neurosurgery* **53**: 544–53; discussion 554–5.

Ferrante L, Acqui M, Mastronardi L, et al. (1989) Cerebral meningiomas in children. *Childs Nerv Syst* **5**: 83–6.

Fisher BJ, Bauman GS, Leighton CE, et al. (1998) Low-grade gliomas in children: tumor volume response to radiation. *J Neurosurg* **88**: 769–74.

Fisher CM (1995) Brain herniation: a revision of classical concepts. *Can J Neurol Sci* **22**: 83–91.

Fisher EG, Welch K, Shillito J, et al. (1990) Craniopharyngiomas in children. Long-term effects of conservative surgical procedures combined with radiation therapy. *J Neurosurg* **73**: 534–40.

Fisher PG, Jenab J, Goldthwaite, et al. (1998) Outcomes and failure patterns in childhood craniopharyngiomas. *Childs Nerv Syst* **14**: 558–63.

Fisher PG, Breiter SN, Carson BS, et al (2000) A clinicopathologic reappraisal of brainstem tumor classification. Identification of pilocytic astrocytoma and fibrillary astrocytoma as distinct entities. *Cancer* **89**: 1569–76.

Fohlen M, Lellouch A, Delalande O (2003) Hypothalamic hamartoma with refractory epilepsy: surgical procedures and results in 18 patients. *Epileptic Disord* **5**: 267–73.

Fort DW, Rushing EJ (1997) Congenital central nervous system tumors. *J Child Neurol* **12**: 157–64.

Fouladi M, Jenkins J, Burger P, et al. (2001) Pleomorphic xanthoastrocytoma: favorable outcome after complete surgical resection. *Neuro Oncol* **3**: 184–92.

Fouladi M, Hunt DL, Pollack IF, et al. (2003a) Outcome of children with centrally reviewed low-grade gliomas treated with chemotherapy with or without radiotherapy on Children's Cancer Group high-grade glioma study CCG-945. *Cancer* **98**: 1243–52.

Fouladi M, Wallace D, Langston JW, et al. (2003b) Survival and functional outcome of children with hypothalamic/chiasmatic tumors. *Cancer* **97**: 1084–92.

Franssila KO, Heiskala MK, Rapola J (1987) Non-Hodgkin's lymphomas in childhood. A clinicopathologic and epidemiologic study in Finland. *Cancer* **59**: 1837–46.

Freeman JH, Coleman LT, Wellard RM, et al. (2004) MR imaging and spectroscopic study of epileptogenic hypothalamic hamartoma: analysis of 72 cases. *AJNR* **25**: 450–62.

Friede R (1989) *Developmental Neuropathology, 2nd Edn.* Berlin: Springer.

Friedman DI, Jacobson DM (2002) Idiopathic intracranial hypertension. *J Neuroophthalmol* **24**: 138–45.

Fusner SE, Poplack DG, Pizzo PA, Di Chiro G (1977) Leukoencephalopathy following chemotherapy for rhabdomyosarcoma: reversibility of cerebral changes demonstrated by computer tomography. *J Pediatr* **91**: 77–9.

Gajjar A, Sanford RA, Heideman R, et al. (1997) Low-grade astrocytoma: a decade of experience at St. Jude Children's Research Hospital. *J Clin Oncol* **15**: 2792–9.

Galassi E, Tognetti F, Franck F, et al. (1985) Infratentorial arachnoid cysts. *J Neurosurg* **63**: 210–7.

Gangemi M, Maiuri F, Colella G, Buonamassa S (2001) Endoscopic surgery for pineal region tumors. *Minim Invasive Neurosurg* **44**: 70–3.

Garcia-Perez A, Narbona-Garcia J, Sierrasesumaga L, et al. (1993) Neuropsychological outcome of children after radiotherapy for intracranial tumours. *Dev Med Child Neurol* **35**: 139–48.

Gardner K, Cox T, Digre KB (1995) Idiopathic intracranial hypertension associated with tetracycline use in fraternal twins: case reports and review. *Neurology* **45**: 6–10.

Gelabert M, Bollar A, Paseiro MJ, Allut AG (1990) Hydrocephalus and intraspinal tumor in childhood. *Childs Nerv Syst* **6**: 110–2.

Gilbertson RJ (2005) Molecular approaches to the understanding and treatment of childhod CNS tumours. In: Estlin E, Lowis S, eds. *Central Nervous System Tumours of Childhood. Clinics in Developmental Medicine No. 166.* London: Mac Keith Press, pp. 129–50.

Giulioni M, Galassi E, Zucchelli M, Volpi L (2005) Seizure outcome of lesionectomy in glioneural tumors associated with epilepsy in children. *J Neurosurg* **102** (3 Suppl): 288–93.

Giunta F, Grasso G, Marini G, Zorzi F (1989) Brain stem expanding lesions: stereotactic diagnosis and therapeutical approach. *Acta Neurochirurg Suppl* **46**: 86–9.

Glantz MJ, Burger PC, Friedman AH, et al. (1994) Treatment of radiation-induced nervous system injury with heparin and warfarin. *Neurology* **44**: 2020–7.

Glass JP, Melamed M, Chernik NL, Posner JB (1979) Malignant cells in cerebrospinal fluid (CSF): the meaning of a positive CSF cytology. *Neurology* **29**: 1369–75.

Gnekow AK, Kortmann RD, Pietsch T, Emser A (2004) Low grade chiasmatic–hypothalamic glioma – carboplatin and vincristin therapy effectively defers radiotherapy within a comprehensive treatment stategy – report from the multicenter treatment study for children and adolescents with a low grade glioma – HIT-LGG 1996 – of the Society of Pediatric Oncology and Hematology (GPOH). *Klin Padiatr* **216**: 331–42.

Göbel U, Calaminus G, Engert J, et al. (1998) Teratomas in infancy and childhood. *Med Pediatr Oncol* **31**: 8–15.

Gomez-Gosalvez FA, Menor-Serrano F, Tellez de Meneses-Lorenzo M, et al. (2003) [Intracranial lipomas in paediatrics: a retrospective study of 20 patients.] *Rev Neurol* **37**: 515–21 (Spanish).

Gosalakkal JA (2002) Intracranial arachnoid cysts in children: a review of pathogenesis, clinical features, and management. *Pediatr Neurol* **18**: 93–8.

Graus F, Keime-Guibert F, Rene R, et al. (2001) Anti-Hu-associated paraneoplastic encephalomyelitis: analysis of 200 patients. *Brain* **124**: 1138–48.

Grill J, Pascal C, Kalifa C (2003) Childhood ependymoma: a systematic review of treatment options and strategies. *Pediatr Drugs* **58**: 533–43.

Gropman AL, Packer RJ, Nicholson HS, et al. (1998) Treatment of diencephalic syndrome with chemotherapy: growth tumor response and long-term control. *Cancer* **83**: 166–72.

Gudourius S, Engelbrecht V, Messing-Junger M, et al. (2002) Diagnostic difficulties in childhood bilateral thalamic astrocytoma. *Neuropediatrics* **33**: 331–5.

Guha A, Mukherjee J (2004) Advances in the biology of astrocytomas. *Curr Opin Neurol* **17**: 655–62.

Gultekin SH, Rosenfeld MR, Voltz R, et al. (2000) Paraneoplastic limbic encephalitis: neurological symptoms, immunological findings and tumour association in 50 patients. *Brain* **123**: 1481–94.

Hahn A, Claviez A, Brinkmann G, et al. (2000) Paraneoplastic degeneration in pediatric Hodgkin disease. *Neuropediatrics* **31**: 42–4.

Hakyemez B, Aksoy U, Yildiz H, Ergin N (2005) Intracranial epidermoid cysts: diffusion-weighted, FLAIR and conventional MR findings. *Eur J Radiol* **54**: 214–20.

Halpern JR, Gordon WH (1981) Trochlear nerve palsy as a false localizing sign. *Ann Ophthalmol* **13**: 53–6.

Han YN, Sun NZ (2002) An evidence based review on the use of corticosteroids in preoperative and critical care. *Acta Anaesthesiol Sin* **40**: 71–9.

Hanefeld F, Riehm H (1980) Therapy of acute lymphoblastic leukaemia in childhood: effects on the nervous system. *Neuropadiatrie* **11**: 3–16.

Hanieh A, Simpson DA, Worth JB (1988) Arachnoid cysts: a critical survey of 41 cases. *Childs Nerv Syst* **4**: 92–6.

Harsh GR, Edwards MSB, Wilson CB (1986) Intracranial arachnoid cysts in children. *J Neurosurg* **64**: 835–42.

Hart RG, Carter JE (1982) Pseudotumor cerebri and facial pain. *Arch Neurol* **39**: 440–2.

Härtel C, Schilling S, Neppert B, et al. (2002) Intracerebral hypertension in neuroborreliosis. *Dev Med Child Neurol* 44: 641–2.

Hasegawa T, Kondziolka D, Hadjipanayis CG, et al. (2003) Stereotactic surgery for CNS nongerminomatous germ cell tumors. Report of four cases. *Pediatr Neurosurg* 38: 329–33.

Heffner RR (1994) Principles of neuropathology. In: Cohen ME, Duffner PK, eds. *Brain Tumors in Children, 2nd edn.* New York: Raven Press, pp. 51–78.

Henry M, Driscoll MC, Millet M, et al. (2004) Pseudotumor cerebri in children with sickle cell disease: a case series. *Pediatrics* 113: 265–9.

Hexom B, Barthel RP (2004) Lithium and pseudotumor cerebri. *J Am Acad Child Adolesc Psychiatry* 43: 247–8.

Hirsch JF, Sainte-Rose C, Pierre-Kahn A, et al. (1989) Benign astrocytic and oligodendrocytic tumors of the cerebral hemispheres in children. *J Neurosurg* 70: 568–72.

Hoppe-Hirsch E, Hirsch JF, Lellouch-Tubiana A, et al. (1993) Malignant hemispheric tumors in childhood. *Childs Nerv Syst* 9: 131–5.

Horten BC, Rubinstein LJ (1976) Primary cerebral neuroblastoma. A clinicopathological study of 35 cases. *Brain* 99: 735–56.

Houten JK, Weiner HL (2000) Pediatric intramedullary spinal cord tumors: special considerations. *J Neurooncol* 47: 225–30.

Hughes RA, Britton T, Richards M (1994) Effects of lymphoma on the peripheral nervous system. *J R Soc Med* 87: 526–30.

Im SH, Wang KC, Kim SK, et al. (2001) Childhood meningioma: unusual location, atypical radiological findings, and favorable treatment outcome. *Childs Nerv Syst* 17: 656–62.

Im SH, Chung CK, Kim S, et al. (2004) Pleomorphic xanthoastrocytoma: a developmental glioneural tumor with prominent glioproliferative changes. *J Neurooncol* 66: 17–27.

Iwakuma T, Lozano G, Flores ER (2005) Li–Fraumeni syndrome: a p53 family affair. *Cell Cycle* 4: 865–7.

Jallo GL, Freed D, Epstein FJ, et al. (2004) Spinal cord ganglioglioma: a review of 56 patients. *J Neurooncol* 68: 71–7.

Janmohamed S, Grossman AB, Metcalfe K, et al. (2002) Suprasellar germ cell tumours: specific problems and the evolution of optimal management with a combined chemoradiotherapy regimen. *Clin Endocrinol* 57: 487–500.

Jayawant S, Neale J, Stoodley N, Wallace S (2001) Gliomatosis cerebri in a 10-year-old girl masquerading as diffuse encephalomyelitis and spinal cord tumour. *Dev Med Child Neurol* 43: 124–6.

Jayawickreme DP, Hayward RD, Harkness WF (1995) Intracranial ependymomas in childhood: a report of 24 cases followed for 5 years. *Childs Nerv Syst* 11: 409–13.

Jennings MT, Frenchman M, Shehab T, et al. (1995) Gliomatosis cerebri presenting as intractable epilepsy during early childhood. *J Child Neurol* 10: 37–45.

Johnson PL, Eckard DA, Chason DP, et al. (2002) Imaging of acquired cerebral herniations. *Neuroimaging Clin N Am* 12: 217–28.

Kai Y, Kuratsu J, Ushio Y (1998) Primary malignant lymphoma of the brain in childhood. *Neurol Med Chir* 38: 232–7.

Kalfas IH, Hahn JF (1986) Symptomatic subependymoma in a 14-year-old girl, diagnosed by NMR scan. *Childs Nerv Syst* 2: 44–6.

Kalifa C, Grill J (2005) The therapy of infantile malignant brain tumors: current status? *J Neurooncol* 75: 279–85.

Kantar M, Cetingul N, Kansoy S, et al. (2004) Radiation induced secondary cranial neoplasm in children. *Childs Nerv Syst* 20: 46–7.

Karahalios DG, Rekate HL, Khayata MH, Apostolides PJ (1996) Elevated intracranial venous pressure as a universal mechanism in pseudotumor cerebri of varying etiologies. *Neurology* 46: 198–202.

Karavitaki N, Brufani C, Warner JT, et al. (2005) Craniopharyngiomas in children and adults: systematic analysis of 121 cases with long-term follow-up. *Clin Endocrinol* 62: 397–409.

Kaufmann AM, Cardoso ER (1992) Aggravation of vasogenic cerebral edema by multiple-dose mannitol. *J Neurosurg* 77: 584–9.

Kava MP, Tullu MS, Deshmukh CT, Shenoy A (2003) Colloid cyst of the third ventricle: a cause of sudden death in a child. *Indian J Cancer* 40: 31–3.

Keene DL, Hsu HE, Ventureyra E (1999) Brain tumors in childhood and adolescence. *Pediatr Neurol* 20: 198–203.

Kermode AG, Plant GT, MacManus DG, et al. (1989) Behçet's disease with slowly enlarging midbrain mass on MRI: resolution following steroid therapy. *Neurology* 39: 1251–2.

Kesler A, Goldhammer Y, Hadayer A, Pianka P (2004) The outcome of pseudotumor cerebri induced by tetracycline therapy. *Acta Neurol Scand* 110: 408–11.

Khaddage A, Chambonniere ML, Morrison AL, et al. (2004) Desmoplastic infantile ganglioglioma: a rare tumor with an unusual presentation. *Ann Diagn Pathol* 8: 280–3.

Khan RB, Marshman KC, Mulhern RK (2003) Atonic seizures in survivors of childhood cancer. *J Child Neurol* 18: 397–400.

Kim RJ, Janss A, Shanis D, et al. (2004) Adult heights attained by children with hypothalamic/chiasmatic glioma treated with growth hormone. *J Clin Endocrinol Metab* 89: 4999–5002.

Kimmel DW, O'Fallon JR, Scheithauer BW, et al. (1992) Prognostic value of cytogenetic analysis in human cerebral astrocytomas. *Ann Neurol* 31: 534–42.

Kirkham FJ (1991) Intracranial pressure and cerebral blood flow in non-traumatic coma in childhood. In: Minns R, ed. *Problems of Intracranial Pressure in Childhood. Clinics in Developmental Medicine No. 113/114.* London: Mac Keith Press, pp. 283–348.

Kleihues P, Louis DN, Scheithauer BW, et al. (2002) The WHO classification of tumors of the nervous system. *J Neuropathol Exp Neurol* 61: 15–25.

Klein P, Rubinstein LJ (1989) Benign symptomatic glial cysts of the pineal gland: a report of seven cases and review of the literature. *J Neurol Neurosurg Psychiatry* 52: 991–5.

Knight RSG, Fielder AR, Firth JL (1986) Benign intracranial hypertension: visual loss and optic nerve sheath fenestration. *J Neurol Neurosurg Psychiatry* 49: 243–50.

Kobayashi T, Kida Y, Mori Y, Hasegawa T (2005) Long-term results of gamma knife surgery for the treatment of craniopharyngioma in 98 consecutive cases. *J Neurosurg* 103 (6 Suppl): 482–8.

Koh S, Turkel SB, Baram TZ (1997) Cerebellar mutism in children: report of six cases and potential mechanisms. *Pediatr Neurol* 16: 218–9.

Konczak J, Schoch B, Dimitrova A, et al. (2005) Functional recovery of children and adolescents after cerebellar tumour resection. *Brain* 128: 1428–41.

Kortmann RD, Timmermann B, Taylor RE, et al. (2003a) Current and future strategies in radiotherapy of childhood low-grade glioma of the brain. Part I: Treatment modalities of radiation therapy. *Strahlenther Onkol* 179: 509–20.

Kortmann RD, Timmermann B, Taylor RE, et al. (2003b) Current and future strategies in radiotherapy of childhood low-grade glioma of the brain. Part II: Treatment-related late toxicity. *Strahlenther Onkol* 179: 585–597.

Krauss JK, Nobbe F, Wakhloo AK, et al. (1992) Movement disorders in astrocytomas of the basal ganglia and the thalamus. *J Neurol Neurosurg Psychiatry* 55: 1162–7.

Kreiger PA, Okada Y, Simon S, et al. (2005) Losses of chromosomes 1p and 19q are rare in pediatric oligodendrogliomas. *Acta Neuropathol* 109: 387–92.

Krontiris TG (1995) Oncogenes. *N Engl J Med* 333: 303–6.

Kuenzle C, Weissert M, Roulet E (1994) Follow-up of optic pathway gliomas in children with neurofibromatosis type 1. *Neuropediatrics* 25: 295–300.

Kulkantrakorn K, Awwad EE, Levy B, et al. (1997) MRI in Lhermitte–Duclos disease. *Neurology* 48: 725–31.

Kumar R, Singh S (2005) Childhood choroid plexus papilloma: operative complications. *Childs Nerv Syst* 21: 138–43.

Kwon S, Koo J, Lee S (2001) Clinical spectrum of reversible posterior leukoencephalopathy syndrome. *Pediatr Neurol* 24: 361–4.

Lamy C, Mas JL, Varet B, et al. (1991) Postradiation lower motor neuron syndrome presenting as monomelic amyotrophy. *J Neurol Neurosurg Psychiatry* 54: 648–9.

Lee AC, Ou Y, Lee WK, Wong YC (2003) Paraneoplastic limbic encephalitis masquerading as chronic behavioural disturbance in an adolescent girl. *Acta Paediatr* 92: 506–9.

Lefton DR, Pinto RS, Silvera VM, et al. (2000) Radiologic features of pediatric thalamic and hypothalamic tumors. *Crit Rev Diagn Imaging* 41: 237–78.

Lehtinen SS, Huuskonen UE, Harila-Saari AH, et al. (2002) Motor nervous system impairment persists in long-term survivors of childhood acute lymphoblastic leukemia. *Cancer* 94: 2466–73.

Lellouch-Tubiana A, Boddaert N, Bourgeois M, et al. (2005) Angiocentric neuroepithelial tumor (ANET): a new epilepsy-related clinicopathological entity with distinctive MRI? *Brain Pathol* 15: 201–206.

Lena G, Genitori L, Molina J, et al. (1990) Choroid plexus tumors in children. Review of 24 cases. *Acta Neurochir* 106: 68–72.

Lesniak MS, Klem JM, Weingart J, Carson BS (2004) Surgical outcome following resection of contrast-enhanced pediatric brainstem gliomas. *Pediatr Neurosurg* 39: 314–22.

Lessell S, Rosman NP (1986) Permanent visual impairment in childhood pseudotumor cerebri. *Arch Neurol* 43: 801–4.

Levisohn L, Cronin-Golomb B, Schmahmann JD (2000) Neuropsychological consequences of cerebellar tumour resection in children: cerebellar cognitive affective syndrome in a paediatric population. *Brain* 123: 1041–50.

Levy B, Bollaert PE, Nace L, Larcan A (1995) Intracranial hypertension and adult respiratory distress syndrome: usefulness of tracheal gas insufflation. *J Trauma* 39: 799–801.

Lewis MB (1999) Cyclosporine toxicity after chemotherapy. Cyclosporine causes reversible posterior leukoencephalopathy syndrome. *BMJ* 319: 54–5.

Liang L, Korogi Y, Sugahara T, et al. (2002) MRI of intracranial germ-cell tumours. *Neuroradiology* 44: 382–8.

Lin HM, Teitell MA (2005) Second malignancy after treatment of pediatric Hodgkin disease. *J Pediatr Hematol Oncol* 27: 28–36.

Listernick R, Darling C, Greenwald M, et al. (1995) Optic pathway tumors in children: the effect of neurofibromatosis type 1 on clinical manifestations and natural history. *J Pediatr* 127: 718–22.

Listernick R, Ferner RE, Piersall L, et al. (2004) Late-onset optic pathway tumors in children with neurofibromatosis 1. *Neurology* 63: 1944–6.

Listernick R, Ferner RE, Liu GT, GutmaNn DH (2007) Optic pathways gliomas in neurofibromatosis-1: controversies and recommendations. *Ann Neurol* 61: 189–98.

Lok C, Viseux V, Avril MF, et al. (2005) Brain magnetic resonance imaging in patients with Cowden syndrome. *Medicine* 84: 129–36.

LoMonaco M, Milone M, Batocchi AP, et al. (1992) Cisplatin neuropathy: clinical course and neurophysiological findings. *J Neurol* 239: 199–204.

Lu S, Ahn D, Johnson G, et al. (2004) Diffusion-tensor MR imaging of intracranial neoplasia and peritumoral edema: introduction of the tumor infiltration index. *Radiology* 232: 221–8.

Lund E, Hamborg-Pedersen B (1984) Computed tomography of the brain following prophylactic treatment with irradiation therapy and intraspinal methotrexate in children with acute lymphoblastic leukemia. *Neuroradiology* 26: 351–8.

Lustig PH, Post SR, Srivannaboon K, et al. (2003) Risk factors for the development of obesity in children surviving brain tumors. *J Clin Endocrinol Metab* 88: 611–6.

Luyken C, Blumcke I, Fimmers R, et al. (2004) Supratentorial gangliogliomas: histopathologic grading and tumor recurrence in 184 patients with a median follow-up of 8 years. *Cancer* 101: 146–55.

Lyons MK, Kelly PJ (1991) Posterior fossa ependymomas: report of 30 cases and review of the literature. *Neurosurgery* 28: 659–65.

Macaya A, Roig M, Fernandez JM, Boronat M (1988) Pseudotumor cerebri, spinal and radicular pain and hyporeflexia: a clinical variant of the Guillain–Barré syndrome? *Pediatr Neurol* 4: 120–1.

MacCollin M (1995) CNS Young Investigator Award Lecture: Molecular analysis of the neurofibromatosis 2 tumor suppressor. *Brain Dev* 17: 231–8.

MacDonald JV, Klump TE (1986) Intraspinal epidermoid tumors caused by lumbar puncture. *Arch Neurol* 43: 936–9.

Mack EE, Wilson CB (1993) Meningiomas induced by high-dose cranial irradiation. *J Neurosurg* 79: 28–31.

MacLean WE, Noll RB, Stehbens JA, et al. (1995) Neuropsychological effects of cranial irradiation in young children with acute lymphoblastic leukemia 9 months after diagnosis. The Children's Cancer Group. *Arch Neurol* 52: 156–60.

Mallouh AA (1989) Nasopharyngeal Hodgkin's disease with intracranial extension in a child. *Med Pediatr Oncol* 17: 174–7.

Mahmoud HH, Rivera GK, Hancock ML, et al. (1993) Low leukocyte counts with blast cells in cerebrospinal fluid of children with newly diagnosed acute lymphoblastic leukemia. *N Engl J Med* 329: 314–9.

Maiuri F, Iaconetta G, Esposito M (2006) Neurological picture. Recurrent episodes of sudden tetraplegia caused by an anterior cervical arachnoid cyst. *J Neurol Neurosurg Psychiatry* 77: 1185–6.

Mandera M, Marcol W, Bierzynska-Macyszyn G, Kluczewska E (2003) Pineal cyts in childhood. *Childs Nerv Syst* 19: 750–5.

Martinez-Lage JF, Casas C, Fernández MA, et al. (1994) Macrocephaly, dystonia, and bilateral temporal arachnoid cysts: glutaric aciduria type 1. *Childs Nerv Syst* 10: 198–203.

Martinez-Lage JF, Perz-Espejo MA, Esteban JA, Poza M (2002) Thalamic tumors: clinical presentation. *Childs Nerv Syst* 18: 405–11.

Massimino M, Spreafico F, Cefalo G, et al. (2002) High response rate to cisplatin/etoposide regimen in childhood low-grade glioma. *J Clin Oncol* 20: 2409–16.

Massimino M, Gandola L, Giangaspero F, et al. (2004) Hyperfractionated radiotherapy and chemotherapy for childhood ependymoma: final results of the first prospective AIEOP (Associazione Italiana di Ematologia-Oncologia Pediatria) study. *Int J Radiat Oncol Biol Phys* 58: 1336–45.

Massimino M, Gandola L, Luksch R, et al. (2005) Sequential chemotherapy, high-dose thiotepa, circulating progenitor cell rescue, and radiotherapy for childhood high-grade glioma. *Neuro Oncol* 7: 41–8.

Merchant TE (2002) Current treatment of childhood ependymoma. *Oncology* 16: 629–42, 644; discussion 645–6, 648.

Merchant TE, Mulhern RK, Krasin MJ, et al. (2004) Preliminary results from a phase II trial of conformal radiation therapy and evaluation of radiation-related CNS effects for pediatric patients with localized ependymoma. *J Clin Oncol* 22: 3156–69.

Mewasingh LD, Kadhim H, Christophe C, et al. (2003) Nonsurgical cerebellar mutism (anarthria) in two children. *Pediatr Neurol* 28: 59–63.

Millichap JG (1997) Temporal lobe arachnoid cyst–attention deficit disorder syndrome: role of the electroencephalogram in diagnosis. *Neurology* 48: 1435–9.

Minns RA, ed. (1991) *Problems of Intracranial Pressure in Childhood. Clinics in Developmental Medicine No. 113/114.* London: Mac Keith Press.

Miozzo M, Dalprà L, Riva P, et al. (2000) A tumor suppressor locus in familial and sporadic chordoma maps to 1p36. *Int J Cancer* 87: 68–72.

Mitchell WG, Fishman LS, Miller JH, et al. (1991) Stroke as a late sequela of cranial irradiation for childhood brain tumors. *J Child Neurol* 6: 128–33.

Mittal R, Mottl H, Nemec J (2005) Acute transient cerebral toxicity associated with administration of high-dose methotrexate. *Med Princ Pract* 14: 202–4.

Mohn A, Schoof E, Fahlbusch R, et al. (1999) The endocrine spectrum of arachnoid cysts in childhood. *Pediatr Neurosurg* 31: 316–21.

Molloy PT, Bilaniuk LT, Vaughan SN, et al. (1995) Brainstem tumors in patients with neurofibromatosis type 1: a distinct clinical entity. *Neurology* 45: 1897–902.

Mori K, Aoki A Yamamoto T, et al. (2001) Aggressive decompressive surgery in patients with massive hemispheric embolic cerebral infarction associated with severe brain swelling. *Acta Neurochir* 143: 483–91; discussion 491–2.

Mottolese C, Stan H, Hermier M, et al. (2001) Intracystic chemotherapy with bleomycin in the treatment of craniopharyngiomas. *Childs Nerv Syst* 17: 724–30.

Mottolese C, Szathmari A, Berlier P, Hermier M (2005) Craniopharyngiomas: our experience in Lyon. *Childs Nerv Syst* 21: 790–8.

Mukai K, Seljeskog EL, Dehner LP (1986) Pituitary adenomas in patients under 20 years old. A clinicopathological study of 12 cases. *J Neurooncol* 4: 79–89.

Muller HL, Emser A, Faldum A, et al. (2004a) Longitudinal study on growth and body mass index before and after diagnosis of childhood craniopharyngioma. *J Clin Endocrinol Metab* 89: 3298–305.

Muller HL, Gebhardt U, Etavard-Gorris N, et al. (2004b) Prognosis and sequela in patients with childood craniopharygioma — results of HIT-ENDO and update on KRANIOPHARYNGEOM 2000. *Klin Padiatr* 216: 343–8.

Munoz A, Barkovich JA, Mateos F, Simon R (2002) Symptomatic epidural lipomatosis of the spinal cord in a child: MR demonstration of spinal cord injury. *Pediatr Radiol* 32: 865–8.

Murphy MA, Fabinyi GCA, Berkovic SF, et al. (1995) Seizure outcome and pathological findings following temporal lobectomy in patients with complex partial seizures and foreign tissue lesions seen only on MRI. *J Clin Neurosci* 1: 38–41.

Muzumdar D, Goel A (2001) Posterior cranial fossa dermoid in association with craniovertebral and cervical spinal anomaly: report of two cases. *Pediatr Neurosurg* 35: 158–61.

Nagaraja S, Powell T, Griffiths PD, Wilkinson ID (2004) MR imaging and spectroscopy in Lhermitte–Duclos disease. *Neuroradiology* 46: 355–8.

Nagib MG, O'Fallon MT (1997) Myxopapillary ependymoma of the conus medullaris and filum terminale in the pediatric age group. *Pediatr Neurosurg* 26: 2–7.

Nagib MG, O'Fallon MT (2000) Lateral ventricle choroid plexus papilloma in childhood: management and complications. *Surg Neurol* 54: 366–72.

Naidich TP, McLone DG, Radkowski MA (1985–86) Intracranial arachnoid cysts. *Pediatr Neurosci* 12: 112–22.

Nelson DR, Yuh WT, Wen BC, et al. (1990) Cerebral necrosis simulating an intraparenchymal tumor. *AJNR* 11: 211–2.

Neumann HP, Eggert HR, Weigel K, et al. (1989) Hemangioblastomas of the central nervous system. A 10-year study with special reference to von Hippel–Lindau syndrome. *J Neurosurg* 70: 24–30.

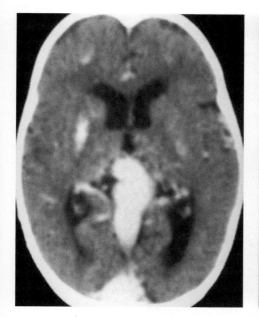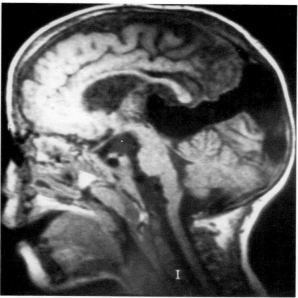

Fig. 14.3. Arteriovenous aneurysm of the vein of Galen. *(Left)* CT showing large venous drainage channel and abnormal veins draining the malformation. Note calcification of central grey matter indicative of hypoxia resulting from vascular steal through the malformation. *(Right)* T$_1$-weighted MRI, median sagittal cut showing marked dilatation of the ampulla of Galen draining into the sagittal sinus through an abnormal ascending venous trunk. Note 'void' appearance, indicating high flow within the venous channel, and moderate external hydrocephalus. (Courtesy Prof. F Brunelle, Hôpital des Enfants Malades, Paris.)

hydrocephalus (usually both internal and external, often moderate or arrested), Parinaud syndrome, mental retardation and other features are common. An occasional patient will present with a pseudodegenerative, progressive deterioration, apparently due to ischaemia resulting from steal by the fistula. Such patients may have extensive calcification in the brain (Chuang 1989).

CT and MRI will demonstrate the malformation, and angiography will allow for a detailed study of the feeding and draining vessels, which is necessary for any form of treatment. MRI is useful for determining the exact topography, especially of venous drainage channels, and permits evaluation of the ventricular system and parenchyma.

Treatment starts with anticongestive, cardiotonic drugs. Lasjaunias et al. (1989a) and Rodesch et al. (1994) prefer to defer attempts at curative treatment until the cardiac situation is stable, usually between 2 and 6 months of age. Reduction in the flow through the fistula is best performed by interventional radiological techniques (Edwards et al. 1988, Hoffman 1989, Lasjaunias et al. 1991a). The best results are obtained in mural fistulae but embolization of other forms is sometimes possible. Lasjaunias et al. (2006) treated 216 of their 317 cases by embolization: 23 died (10.6%); 20 had severe and 30 mild to moderate mental retardation; and 143 had normal development at follow-up. Early shunting of hydrocephalus may be associated with subependymal haemorrhage or increased ventricular dilatation and should probably be deferred until after treatment of the malformation (Lasjaunias et al. 1989a). Surgical attack by transtentorial (Hoffman 1989) or other approaches can be used in older patients but is not indicated in most cases.

SINGLE-HOLE ARTERIOVENOUS FISTULAE
These are an uncommon type of AVM, usually located in a hemisphere, and may be important in infants and in fetuses. Weon et al. (2005) reviewed 41 cases with a mean age at presentation of 24 months, 4 of which were diagnosed in utero. The most common clinical presentation was cardiac insufficiency (13/41) followed by seizures (10/41) and macrocrania (6/41). Venous ectasia and pial venous stenosis were the most frequent angiographic features. Eleven of their patients had hereditary haemorrhagic telangiectasia. Results of embolization, performed in 35 children, were satisfactory with a low mortality (2 patients) and neurological morbidity, stabilization in 31 patients, and complete exclusion of the lesion in 14 cases.

CAVERNOUS ANGIOMAS (CAVERNOMAS)
In cavernous angiomas of the brain, abnormal dilated blood vessels are clustered together so tightly that they are not separated by neural tissue. These vessels are usually but not always thin-walled and capacious. They are often calcified and contain haemosiderin deposits lying within the connective tissue that separates the vessels. They form well-limited masses in the parenchyma but may have a subarachnoid component (Rorke 1989). Cavernomas can be sporadic or genetically determined with an autosomal dominant inheritance. In the latter case they are often but not necessarily multiple. At least three loci are known on chromosomes 7q, 7p and 3q, and the corresponding genes – *KRIT1*, *MGC4507* and *PCD10* – have been identified (Denier et al. 2004a,b; Bergametti et al. 2005). The protein coded for by the *KRIT1* gene localizes in vascular endothelium,

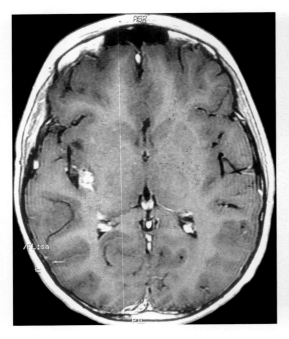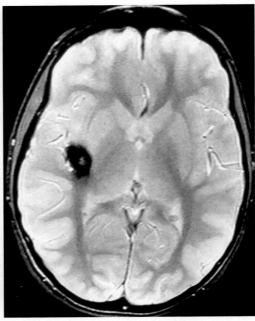

Fig. 14.4. Cavernous angioma in a child. (a) MRI T$_1$ sequence after gadolinium enhancement shows contrast uptake of the lesion. (b) T$_2$ sequence shows area of void signal due to the long relaxation time resulting from the paramagnetic effect of haemosiderin deposition.

astrocytes and pyramidal neurons of the adult human cortex (Guzeloglu-Kayisli et al. 2004). No obvious phenotypic differences are apparent. Denier et al. (2004a) found the three genes were responsible for 40%, 20% and 40% of cases respectively, but there seem to be large variations in different populations. There is only a weak genotype–phenotype correlation; it seems that the CCM3 mutation is more often associated withn haemorrhage and has an earlier onset in childhood (Denier et al. 2006). The proportions of sporadic and familial forms may also be variable (Laurans et al. 2003). Within *KRIT1*-affected families, the age at diagnosis varied from 2 to 72 years; nearly half the carriers were asymptomatic by age 50 and over, and 5 individuals aged 27–48 years had negative MRI studies. Sporadic cases induced by radiation therapy have been reported (Noel et al. 2002).

The most common manifestations of cavernous angiomas in the large series of Denier et al. were seizures (in 55% of patients) and hemiplegia (32%). Neurological disturbances often appear acutely. Epilepsy was present in two thirds of cases in another seies (Kattapong et al. 1995). Seizures may appear at any age from infancy to adulthood (Mottolese et al. 2001). The seizures are partial in type and are often difficult to control. Focal motor deficits, sometimes fluctuating, are a less common manifestation (Simard et al. 1986, Requena et al. 1991). They are probably related to episodes of minor bleeding. Major bleeding is less common. Headache and psychiatric manifestations are relatively common. MRI is the most powerful diagnostic means. Mathieson et al. (2003) reviewed the features of 68 cases and their surgical treatment.

CT shows small areas of calcification in about half the cases, combined with changes in density varying from oedematous to haematoma-like. Enhancement may be only moderate and patchy.

The MRI features of cavernous malformations are distinctive (Zimmerman et al. 1991) and consist of well-defined lesions with a central focus of mixed signal intensity surrounded by a rim of void signal due to the paramagnetic effect of haemosiderin, which becomes more evident on T$_2$-weighted images because of its long relaxation time (Fig. 14.4). Gradient echo sequences are significantly more sensitive and reveal many more lesions than T$_2$ sequences (Denier et al. 2004b). Angiography may be normal or reveals an avascular mass, and cavernous angiomas are the most common type of angiographically cryptic malformations. Multiple cavernomas are common and can involve any area.

Cavernous angiomas involve the posterior fossa structures or the brainstem in 15% of cases (Zimmerman et al. 1991; Kattapong et al. 1995; Di Rocco et al. 1997, 2000).

The natural history of cavernomas is incompletely defined. Cavernous angiomas may enlarge and clinically they may mimic a tumour. Appearance of new lesions has been observed in some cases and the disorder may well be progressive (Kattapong et al. 1995). The course of familial forms has been studied by Labauge et al. (2000) who followed 40 patients with cavernomas and found evidence of changes in the lesions in 28 of these, bleeding in 21 and appearance of new lesions in 23, indicating the evolutivity of the condition. However, a more benign prognosis has been suggested (Churchyard et al. 1992).

Multiple cutaneous and cavernous angiomas in infants may rarely be part of a syndrome of neonatal miliary haemangiomatosis (Heudes et al. 1990) that includes CNS involvement in 30% of cases, and of genetic syndromes featuring hepatic and

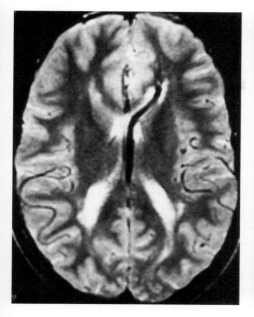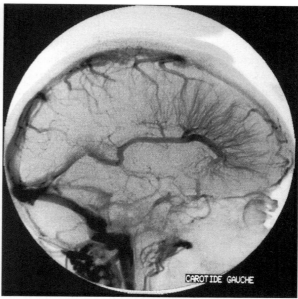

Fig. 14.5. So-called venous angioma of the left frontal region. *(Left)* MRI shows a large vessel, as indicated by a 'void' signal, running from the left frontal horn to the midline and back to the region of the vein of Galen. *(Right)* Digitalized angiography shows the vessel to be a large vein emptying into the vein of Galen. Veins from the anterior left frontal lobe drain into the abnormal venous trunk instead of the sagittal sinus. This represents abnormal venous drainage rather than an angioma.

retinal cavernous haemangiomas or limb reduction defects (Filling-Katz et al. 1992, Drigo et al. 1994) in addition to cerebral lesions.

Operative treatment is recommended for patients with epilepsy and progressive focal deficit, provided the lesion is accessible, and gives excellent results. Fine-beam radiotherapy has also been used. The attitude when facing a silent lesion is still uncertain, and surgery to eliminate the risk of massive haemorrhage is controversial for deep lesions. For multiple lesions, it seems that surgical resection of accessible lesions that have been responsible for symptoms or are clearly progressive is justified. Other lesions must be regularly monitored by MRI. Family members should be examined for the presence of asymptomatic lesions.

CAPILLARY TELANGIECTASIAS

Capillary telangiectasias, like cavernous angiomas, consist of endothelium-lined sinusoidal capillaries of various sizes. They are related to, and sometimes associated with, cavernous angiomas (Clatterbuck et al. 2001) from which they differ by the presence of normal intervening neural tissue. They are predominantly located in the posterior fossa, especially the brainstem, less commonly the cerebellum (McCormick 1984).

Telangiectasias represent another type of cryptic vascular malformation and are often asymptomatic. They may rarely rupture producing intracranial haematoma or subarachnoid haemorrhage (Howard 1986), especially in the brainstem and cerebellum (Bland et al. 1994). They are now more often diagnosed by their MRI characteristics, which include focal areas of hyperintensity on T_2-weighted spin-echo sequences, hypointensity on T_2-weighted gradient-echo images, and enhancement after contrast on T_1 images (Scaglione et al. 2001, Attal et al. 2003).

VENOUS ANGIOMAS

These are a developmental anomaly rather than a neoplasm; they have no arterial component (Nomura et al. 2006). They consist of a radiating array of enlarged subcortical or periventricular veins that drain centripetally into a dilated venous trunk (Olson et al. 1984) (Fig. 14.5). These lesions are better termed venous pseudoangiomas (Lasjaunias et al. 1991b). Venous angiomas are the most common of all intracranial vascular malformations. Sarwar and McCormick (1978) found they constituted 63% of 165 vascular malformations in a study of 4069 consecutive autopsies. Garner et al. (1991) found 50 venous angiomas, 33 cavernomas and 17 AVMs in an MRI study of 8200 subjects. They are mainly located to the cerebellum and the frontal lobe. They rarely cause bleeding unless they are associated with a cavernous angioma or there is venous obstruction in their drainage system. Migraine-like headache is not uncommon, except, perhaps, when the lesion is located in the posterior fossa. The MRI appearance is highly suggestive with images of radiating vessels usually draining into an enlarged venous channel. They are associated with functional circulatory changes (increased blood flow and volume, prolonged mean transit time) that can be demonstrated by MRI but are not necessarily associated with symptoms (Camacho et al. 2004). They are frequently discovered incidentally, and surgical excision should be considered only for those venous malformations from which bleeding has occurred (Martin and Edwards 1989).

RARE CONGENITAL ANGIODYSPLASIAS

Multiple angiomas of the CNS infrequently accompany multiple peripheral and visceral angiomas. They may be complicated by heart failure, hydrocephalus or meningitis. They can be transmitted as a dominant trait (Leblanc et al. 1996).

In diffuse meningocerebral angiodysplasia the whole cerebral surface is covered by densely packed, dilated, tortuous vessels (Jellinger et al. 1966). The relationship of such cases with Sturge–Weber disease on the one hand and with the diffuse cerebromeningeal noncalcifying angiomatosis of Divry and van Bogaert (Chapter 3) is unclear.

A diffuse vascular dysplasia may be responsible for the cases of leukodystrophy, with cyst formation recently reported by Labrune et al. (1996).

INTRACRANIAL ARTERIAL ANEURYSMS

Aneurysms are dilated segments of an artery with thinned walls. The frequency of aneurysms in childhood is much lower than that of AVMs but they may have a greater tendency to rupture, though rarely in prepubertal patients. However, in one large series they were responsible for 40% of spontaneous intracranial haemorrhages before age 20 years (Sedzimir and Robinson 1973). Contrary to aneurysms in adults, acquired factors such as hypertension, smoking and alcohol consumption are not important in children. Arterial hypertension plays a role in their genesis and rupture as shown by their occurrence in patients with coarctation of the aorta and other causes of hypertension. Five to 40 per cent of cases of dominant polycystic kidney disease are associated with cerebral aneurysms. Aneurysms are also, but less commonly, a complication of Marfan syndrome and of Ehlers–Danlos syndrome type IV (Brisman et al. 2006). In children, most arterial aneurysms are either congenital or dissecting aneurysms. Lasjaunias et al. (2005) found 33 cases of dissecting aneurysm and 16 saccular aneurysms in a series of 75 aneurysms in 59 children under 15 years of age. Other causes include infections and genetic factors. Aneurysms may be familial in 8% of cases (Schievink et al. 1995, Wang et al. 1995). A defect of collagen III may be an aetiological factor in some cases but was not found to be a common cause in two large series (Kuivaniemi et al. 1993, Schievink et al. 1994a). Aneurysms are present in 10% of patients with polycystic kidney disease (Gabow 1993). Association with Marfan syndrome and with multiple malformations has been reported (ter Berg et al. 1987). Aneurysms may follow a closed head injury or surgical operation; traumatic aneurysms represent 14–39% of paediatric aneurysms (Ventureyra and Higgins 1994).

SACCULAR ANEURYSMS

In children and adolescents, saccular neurysms are frequently found at the bifurcation of the internal carotid artery; in children, however, they are often more distal than in adults and are found in unusual locations such as the posterior circulation (Allison et al. 1998). Most seem to be congenital (Østergaard 1991). Large or giant aneurysms are also common, and the saccular type is less frequent than in adults. Allison et al. (1998) found that 44% of aneurysms in children and adolescents were in the vertebrobasilar circulation and that 40% were large or giant in size.

Haemorrhagic stroke is the presenting manifestation in most patients and may occur as early as 5 months of age. It may be preceded by premonitory symptoms such as severe focal headache, meningeal signs, transient neurological deficits or cranial nerve palsies. Such pseudotumoural features were present in almost half the cases of Meyer et al. (1989). Seizures may also be the first clinical manifestation of aneurysms. Complex partial seizures (Tanaka et al. 1994) are common. All children suspected of intracranial haemorrhage should undergo imaging studies. MRI and MRA have considerably facilitated the diagnosis (Fasulakis and Andronikou 2003). Imaging usually demonstrates subarachnoid or parenchymal haemorrhage and localizes the aneurysm in many cases as a mass lesion or a void area; it may demonstrate the presence of multiple lesions, while MRA will inform the surgeon on the status of collateral circulation and of the circle of Willis. Prenatal diagnosis of basilar artery aneurysm by ultrasound examination has been reported (Muszynski et al. 1994).

Treatment is by surgery (clipping) or by endovascular embolization (coiling). Coiling currently seems to be preferred in adults because of its lower morbidity and mortality (Johnston et al. 2000). A few cases can benefit from unusual techniques such as wrapping.

The mortality rate of bleeding aneurysms is of the order of 25%, and residual neurological disability is not rare. Results of elective surgery are often favourable. Operation at the time of bleeding is much more hazardous because of the possibility of vascular spasm, and the best timing of surgery remains disputed.

FUSIFORM ANEURYSMS

Fusiform aneurysms, also termed giant serpentine aneurysms or dolichoectasic cranial arteries (Nishizaki et al. 1986), are a relatively common form of giant aneurysm. Common sites of dolichoectasia include the bifurcation of the internal carotid artery and the vertebrobasilar artery, which may be affected in as many as 53% of cases (Peerless et al. 1989). Bleeding occurs in over one third of cases, but focal neurological deficits, sometimes fluctuating, or thrombosis are the most frequent manifestations, and a significant proportion are asymptomatic. Surgical treatment for selected cases can give favourable results.

MYCOTIC ANEURYSMS

Mycotic aneurysms are a classic complication of bacterial endocarditis. They can result from local invasion of intracranial vessels by adjacent infections, especially septic cavernous thrombophlebitis (Andrews et al. 1989). The most frequent aetiological agent is *Staphylococcus aureus* (Abbassioun et al. 1985). Fungal infections are a rare cause. The cornerstone of treatment of mycotic aneurysms is the prolonged administation of antimicrobial drugs. Surgical therapy is controversial.

DISSECTING ANEURYSMS

In the large series of Lasjanunias et al. (2005), dissecting aneurysms accounted for a majority of cases of aneurysmal arteriopathy in children. They are a significant cause of ischaemic stroke (Chabrier et al. 2003). Most dissecting lesions were encountered in the vertebrobasilar sytem. They can manifest with bleeding or thrombosis even in young children. Lasjaunias et al. (2005) identify two types: acute segmental arterial tear without thrombosis manifested by acute subarachnoid bleeding, and subacute focal dissection with partial thrombosis or mural haematoma, usually without haemorrhage. The former type would require aggressive therapy. It is not clear whether the presence of aneurysmal dilatation in the latter cases is distinct from the dissection often responsible for ischaemic strokes and requires a different treatment (see below).

SPINAL VASCULAR MALFORMATIONS
The most common vascular malformations occurring in relation to the spinal cord are AVMs. Telangiectasias, cavernous malformations and aneurysms are very rare. Spinal AVMs and fistulae are uncommon in children but may be seen even in infants. Arteriovenous fistulae can be an early manifestation of hereditary haemorrhagic telangiectasia in infants (Krings et al. 2005).

Dural spinal AVMs belong to several subtypes. Type I arteriovenous fistulae associated with venous hypertension can result in ischaemic myelopathy; type 2 fistulae are revealed by haemorrhage in the same manner as arteriovenous pial anomalies; in other forms, bleeding may involve extraneural tissue (Ferch et al. 2001).

Clinical manifestations of spinal vascular malformations include subarachnoid haemorrhage, myelopathy and radiculopathy. Symptoms may appear suddenly and may fluctuate with exercise, posture and temperature. Local pain is an important diagnostic cue in patients with subarachnoid haemorrhage, and in unexplained cases it is important to explore the cord. Cutaneous angioma is sometimes associated (Chapter 3). The diagnosis rests on MRI and spinal angiography (Koenig et al. 1989). Treatment is by surgery or embolization. The outcome depends on the site and type of the lesions.

Acute or subacute myelopathy with ascending necrosis of the spinal cord (subacute necrotizing myelitis or Foix–Alajouanine syndrome) is actually the result of thrombosis and venous hypertension in patients with dural arteriovenous fistulae (Criscuolo et al. 1989, Hurst et al. 1995, Jellema et al. 2006).

SUBARACHNOID AND OTHER INTRACRANIAL HAEMORRHAGES
Not all cases of subarachnoid haemorrhage are explained by detectable vascular malformations. In one series, no lesion was found in as many as 31% of cases (Hourihan et al. 1984). Whatever the aetiology, subarachnoid haemorrhage may interfere with vascularization of the brain, although this is mainly observed in cases of malformations and is uncommon in 'spontaneous' subarachnoid haemorrhage.

'Spontaneous' intracranial haematomas are probably caused by small vascular malformations that are destroyed or collapsed by the haemorrhage they induced. It is therefore essential in cases of apparently spontaneous subarachnoid haemorrhage or haematoma to repeat angiography or imaging some time after the acute episode as a causal AVM may then have become detectable.

Such haematomas mainly affect the cerebral hemispheres but they occasionally occur in the cerebellum or brainstem. In the latter case, the clinical picture may simulate multiple sclerosis, although a rapidly fatal course is more usual.

Intracranial haematomas show a variable appearance on MRI at various times because the methaemoglobin they contain is in different phases of chemical breakdown (Gomori et al. 1988). In 321 patients younger than 20 years reviewed by Sedzimir and Robinson (1973) the recurrence rate was 41% and the mortality rate 28%.

Suh et al. (2001) observed 28 infants under 2 years of age with subarachnoid bleeding. Causative lesions included AVMs, dural in 4, arteriovenous fistulae in 3, aneurysms in 2, developmental venous anomalies in 2, vein of Galen malformation in 1, and other types in 3. A majority of cases suffered intracranial haematomas and/or intraventricular haemorrhage.

Repeated bleeding in the subarachnoid space can cause *superficial haemosiderosis*, which is rare in children (Fearnley et al. 1995). Surgical treatment may be possible (Schievink et al. 1998). Progressive neurological impairment is associated with repeatedly xanthochromic CSF. High-field MRI may show marginal zones of hypointensity. Recurrent haemorrhage can be the result of a bleeding spinal haemangioma (Naranjo et al. 1987), which should be sought when no cranial lesion is found.

OTHER VASCULAR ANOMALIES
Variants of intracranial vessels are found in 15% of MRA studies (Koelfen et al. 1995). Congenital absence of one (Ito et al. 2005) or both carotid arteries (Schlenska 1986) is usually unaccompanied by clinical manifestations, and this also applies to absence or hypoplasia of the vertebral arteries. Other abnormalities of the carotid artery such as cervical stenosis or buckling have been implicated as causal factors of acute acquired hemiplegia. However, such abnormalities are mostly coincidental findings (Togay-Isikay et al. 2005). Various anomalies of the circle of Willis, such as direct origin of the posterior cerebral artery from the carotid artery, are not rare (Koelfen et al. 1995). Abnormalities of cervical or intracranial arteries may be associated with abnormalities of the aorta and other systemic vessels, facial angiomas and cerebellar hypoplasia, and are part of the PHACE (or PHACES) syndrome that also features cardiac, ocular and neurological defects (Chapter 3). Persistence of anastomotic arteries at the base of the brain, such as the trigeminal, acoustic and hypoglossal arteries, may occur as normal variants (Resche et al. 1980) but are frequent with PHACE syndrome. Their association with saccular aneurysm or spontaneous subarachnoid haemorrhage has been reported but may be coincidental. *Hypoplasia* of one or several vessels is often asymptomatic (Giuffre and Sherkat 2000). Bojinova et al. (2000) collected 205 cases in children 3–14 years, involving the carotid artery in 41.9% of cases, the middle cerebral artery in 54.1%, and the basilar or anterior cerebral arteries in the remaining cases. Tortuosity, kinking and coiling of arteries (carotids) is probably not associated with an increased incidence of stroke (Togay-Isikay et al. 2005). Symptomatic cases manifested with transient ischaemic accidents in 21%, cerebral infarct in 17%, and seizures in 56%. These may in fact be unrelated to the anomalies. Progressive hemispheral atrophy was a rare manifestation.

Vascular steal from the CNS as a result of the stenosis of a subclavian artery is a rare occurrence. The same phenomenon may be observed following Blalock–Taussig type anastomoses.

Abnormalities of the veins or sinuses resulting in increased sinusal pressure and consequent hydrocephalus are rare. Affected children may have extensive collateral circulation. Angiography can show stenosis or absence of segments of sinuses; and reflux into veins after contrast injection into the sagittal sinus is prominent. Treatment by venous bypass graft from the transverse sinus to the jugular vein has been shown to control hydrocephalus (Sainte-Rose et al. 1984).

OCCLUSIVE ARTERIAL DISEASE

Cerebrovascular occlusion can affect both arteries and cranial sinuses or cerebral veins. It may result from thrombosis or from migration of emboli, most frequently of cardiac origin. In the majority of cases, vascular occlusion is a sudden event or or at least produces rapidly developing clinical manifestations. The term 'stroke', which may be either haemorrhagic or ischaemic, is defined as a clinical syndrome of rapidly developed clinical signs of focal or global disturbance of cerebral function lasting more than 24 hours or leading to death, with no obvious cause other than of vascular origin. Only ischaemic stroke is considered in this section. Similar events lasting less than 24 hours are termed transient ischaemic attacks.

The annual incidence of stroke in childhood is approximately 1.2–3/100,000. Schoenberg et al. (1978) reported an annual incidence of 2.52 cases per 100,000 children in Rochester, Minnesota, equating, pro rata, to approximately half the incidence of brain tumours in children in the USA. Haemorrhagic strokes in that series were slighly more common (55%) than ischaemic ones. Similar figures have been obtained in Sweden (Eeg-Olofsson and Ringheim 1983), whereas Giroud et al. (1997), in a study of 54 children found that ischaemic strokes were more common (57% vs 43%). Blom et al. (2003) recorded incidence rates of 1.5–3.0/100,000.

Neonatal stroke is more common than previously thought, and is disussed below.

MECHANISMS AND PATHOLOGY
Arterial occlusion can result from cerebral embolism or from thrombosis. Irrespective of the cause, cerebral infarction results. When obstruction involves one of the larger cerebral arteries, infarction may involve both the cortex and underlying white matter. In haemorrhagic infarction, the involved area is congested and stippled with petechial haemorrhages. In pale infarct, the tissue appears pale, usually with a significant amount of swelling. In the centre of the infarcted region there is massive necrosis of all tissue components, while the damage becomes progressively less severe toward the periphery of the infarct. During the first hours of acute ischaemia, damage in this peripheral part (so-called 'penumbra') is reversible with re-establishment of blood flow. Emergency treatment at this time is therefore imperative. The area of penumbra is not shown by CT

or standard MRI but gives a high signal with water-diffusion MRI.

After a few hours polymorphonuclear infiltration is found, replaced within 4–5 days by mononuclear phagocytes. Eventually, astrocytes develop and lay down a fibre network with resulting retraction and sclerosis of cortical convolutions (ulegyria). The area of greatest damage may become cystic, leaving a cavity within the brain that is often improperly called 'porencephaly' (Chapter 2).

The vulnerability of the brain to even brief periods of ischaemia is well known. Swelling of brain tissue can increase the lesion by compressing capillaries, thus preventing revascularization from collateral sources, the 'no-reflow phenomenon' in which complex factors are implicated. In contrast with ischaemia within the infarcted territory, there is increased blood flow around the lesion, the so-called 'luxury perfusion' that is demonstrable by neuroimaging and brain scan. The role of lactic acid and of other abnormal metabolites in the sequence of events that leads to ischaemia and infarction has been extensively discussed (Plum 1983).

The causes of thrombosis or emboli are extremely variable (see below) but in many cases they remain undetermined.

CLINICAL FEATURES
The clinical features in most cases do not differ, irrespective of whether the infarction results from thrombosis or embolism. In general, ischaemic stroke of thrombotic origin has a less sudden onset than haemorrhagic stroke, takes longer to develop and and may be preceded by regressive similar incidents. In some cases, the aetiology or circumstances of occurrence suggest a particular mechanism. For example, the presence of bacterial endocarditis or valvular heart disease favours embolism, whereas a 'stuttering' onset of the clinical manifestations is more suggestive of thrombosis. A history of cervical trauma is suggestive of dissection of the carotid or vertebral arteries (Garg et al. 1993, Garg and DeMyer 1995)

Essentially, occlusive vascular disease manifests by the sudden appearance of neurological deficit in the territory of one major cerebral vessel, most commonly acute onset hemiplegia (Lanska et al. 1991). In some patients – 23% of cases in the study of Abram et al. (1996) – ischaemic strokes are preceded, usually by about a week, by episodes of transient hemiplegia lasting from one to several hours that may be accompanied by other deficits such as visual field defects, abnormal movements or aphasia. Symptoms and signs of intracranial hypertension may be present with large strokes and may require emergency treatment. *Dysphasia* is present in right-sided hemiplegia when the cortex is affected (Cranberg et al. 1987). It has also been observed in some cases of infarcts restricted to the capsulo-putamino-caudate area (Ferro et al. 1982, Dusser et al. 1986). The dysphasia tends to be mainly expressive in type in children under 8–10 years of age. However, aphasia is uncommon in young children and, when present before age of 2, it is often manifested as mutism. The term acute hemiplegia of childhood is sometimes used to designate only those cases in which no aetiology is found after

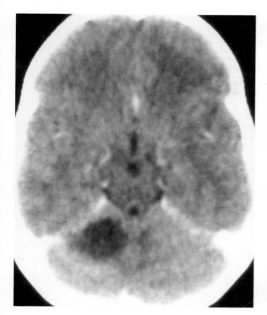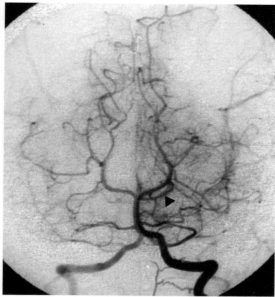

Fig. 14.6. Cerebellar infarct localized to the right hemisphere. *(Left)* CT showing area of hypodensity in right cerebellar hemisphere. *(Right)* Vertebral arteriography showing absence of injection of right superior cerebellar artery. *Arrow* indicates opposite superior cerebellar artery. (15-year-old boy with sudden appearance of right cerebellar syndrome that progressively subsided over the following months.)

full investigation. The anterior circulation is by far the most commonly affected so that the typical picture of ischaemic stroke in children is that of acute hemiplegia, but cases of hemiplegia of vascular origin are distributed throughout childhood and adolescence whereas postconvulsive hemiplegias are concentrated in the first three years of life. Onset is at any age, most commonly before 6 years.

In one large series of acquired hemiplegias (Aicardi et al. 1969), 27% of the cases of acquired hemiplegia in childhood were not preceded by convulsive seizures, and most of those were thought to be due to vascular occlusions. Contrariwise, only occasional cases of demonstrated vascular occlusion are preceded by status epilepticus, although isolated fits may occur in up to a quarter of the cases of cerebral infarction in the territory of the middle cerebral artery at onset of the hemiplegia. Yang et al. (1995) found that 36 of 56 patients with stroke suffered at least one seizure, and these were reccurent in 21. However, seizures were rare when imaging did not show cortical involvement. Differences among various series likely result from heterogeneity of the cases referred to various centres. Fever may precede the onset of vascular hemiplegia, although it is more common with postconvulsive cases. A search for prodromal features such as headache, cervical pain, ipsilateral Horner syndrome or a history of transient ischaemic episodes preceding hemiplegia may help uncover particular causes such as dissection.

In all acquired hemiplegias, weakness is maximal immediately after onset and flaccidity is the rule (Isler 1984). Spasticity and pyramidal tract signs appear later. The degree of recovery is extremely variable. A substantial recovery can be expected to take place during the first two or three weeks, and further slow progress

may continue for several months. Involuntary movements of athetoid type or frank disturbances are rare.

The topography of the infarcts responsible for acquired hemiplegia is variable. Table 14.1 shows the arteries involved, the corresponding territories of infarction, and the main clinical features. However, the topography and extent of infarction depend on several factors in addition to the vessel involved, such as the quality of collateral and systemic circulation, and individual anatomical variations. The location of infarct may also vary with the aetiology. Ischaemic strokes in the basal ganglia are more often idiopathic than superficial ones (Dusser et al. 1986, Kappelle et al. 1989). Stroke can affect any arterial territory. Involvement of the internal capsule and lenticular nuclei has been said to be rare, but in fact they are involved in approximately half the cases (Dusser et al. 1986). Angiography may be difficult to interpret or even normal in capsuloputaminal strokes.

Involvement of the posterior circulation is much rarer than that of the carotid arteries and their branches. Echenne et al. (1983) reviewed 36 cases and only a few more cases have been added since. Many of the cases of vertebrobasilar occlusive diseases have been associated with trauma responsible for dissection (Garg et al. 1993), which may also occur spontaneously (Sturzenegger 1995, Khurana et al. 1996), with cervical spine abnormalities (Ross et al. 1987, Phillips et al. 1988) or with vascular malformations. All the causes of stroke can be found, and 'idiopathic' cases are frequent. More limited occlusions may affect only one cerebellar artery (Chatkupt et al. 1987), with resulting cerebellar infarcts (Fig. 14.6). However, lateral medullary syndrome has been observed with vertebral artery thrombosis (Klein et al. 1976). Thalamic infarction may be due to proximal obstruction

TABLE 14.1
Main syndromes of arterial occlusion

Artery involved	Area of ischaemia	Clinical features	References
Internal carotid artery (ICA)	Whole territory of MCA or only part of it. Rarely both territories of MCA and ACA	Hemiplegia proportional, aphasia if dominant hemisphere. Partial involvement with only incomplete hemiplegia is not rare	Bogousslavsky and Caplan (1995)
Middle cerebral artery (MCA)	Convexity of hemispheres, except paramedial aspect of occipital lobe. Insula, part of temporal lobe, internal capsule and basal ganglia, orbital aspect of frontal lobe	Hemiplegia with upper limb predominance. Hemianopsia, aphasia if dominant hemisphere	Golden (1985), VanDongen et al. (1985)
Anterior cerebral artery (ACA)	Mesial aspect of hemispheres. Paramedian part of the convexity. Anterior part of internal capsule and of basal ganglia[1]	Hemiplegia predominating in lower limb	Golden (1985)
Anterior choroidal artery (AChA)	Optic tract; posterior limb of internal capsule; cerebral peduncle; pallidum; variable involvement of thalamus and caudate; lateral geniculate body	Hemiplegia, visual field defects, dysarthria, sometimes ataxia[2]	Begousslavsky et al. (1986), Decroix et al. (1986), Helgason et al. (1986), Helgason (1988)
Posterior cerebral artery (PCA)	Lower part of temporal lobe, posterior part of thalamus, subthalamic nuclei	Homonymous hemianopsia, ataxia, hemiparesis, vertigo, cerebellar (peduncular) tremor[2]	Castaigne et al. (1973)
Basilar artery (BA)	Whole or part of PCA territory (uni- or bilateral). Brainstem nuclei and tracts. May involve cerebellar arteries	Variable manifestations (see text)	Echenne et al. (1983)
Superior cerebellar artery (SCA)	Upper brainstem, superior cerebellar peduncles, dentate nucleus, upper cerebellar cortex	Vertigo, ataxia of limbs or trunk, tremor, pontine signs (cranial nerves V, VII and VIII)[2]	Golden (1985)
Anterior inferior cerebellar artery (AICA)	Central brainstem, flocculus and adjacent part of cerebellar hemisphere	Idem	Idem
Posterior inferior cerebellar artery (PICA) or vertebral artery and PICA	Roof nuclei of 4th ventricle, lateral medulla, lower aspect of cerebellum	Lateral medullary syndrome, vertigo, nystagmus, ipsilateral ataxia, sensory loss, contralateral Horner syndrome[2]	Barth et al. (1993)
Thalamostriate arteries and other penetrating branches	Caudate, putamen, internal capsule	Hemiplegia, motor, sensory or mixed. No hemianopsia. Language disturbances. Sometimes bilateral thalamic involvement	Kappelle et al. (1989), Garg and DeMyer (1995)
	Subcortical white matter of hemispheres or brainstem	Lacunar syndrome including pure, sensory or motor hemisyndrome, ataxia, hemiparesis, mesencephalothalamic syndrome, abulia with IIIrd nerve palsy or paralysis of vertical gaze, locked-in syndrome, dementia[2]	Kappelle (1989), Moulin et al. (1995)

[1]Infarction of the recurrent artery of Heubner, a branch of the ACA, may involve the anterior striatum and tip of thalamus and be responsible for paralysis of the upper limb variably associated with other symptoms of ACA involvement (Miller et al. 2000).
[2]Ataxic hemiplegia can also occur with mass lesions (Bendheim and Berg 1981). Responsible lesions typically are in the basis pontis but may also be in the internal capsule or in the corona radiata (Ichikawa et al. 1982, Hellweg-Larsen et al. 1988).

of one vertebral artery in the neck (Garg et al. 1993, Garg and DeMyer 1995, Garg and Edwards-Brown 1995). The clinical picture of vertebrobasilar occlusion includes vomiting, ataxia, tremor, hemiplegia, vertigo, ocular motor palsies, quadriplegia, dysarthria, nystagmus and lower cranial nerve involvement (Mehler 1988). Disturbances of consciousness, opisthotonic attacks and respiratory disturbances have been reported (Echenne et al. 1983). Although some reports mention the occurrrence of tonic–clonic attacks, these are probably not true epileptic seizures (Ropper 1988). More limited infarcts can give rise to isolated ataxia and to abnormal ocular motility or to disturbances of consciousness and of language. *Bilateral thalamic infarction* can be due to a single

thalamoperforate artery obstruction (Garg and DeMyer 1995). Dementia may follow strokes in the mesencephalon and diencephalon. Occlusive accidents in the posterior circulation are often preceded by repeated episodes of vertebrobasilar insufficiency, days, weeks or even months before the definitive attack. Compression of the vertebral artery by head rotation may be responsible for transient ischaemic attacks (Garg and Edwards-Brown 1995).

IMAGING FEATURES
The imaging appearance of arterial occlusion is dependent both on the size of the infarct and on the delay between onset of stroke and examinations (Raybaud et al. 1985). CT and even MR

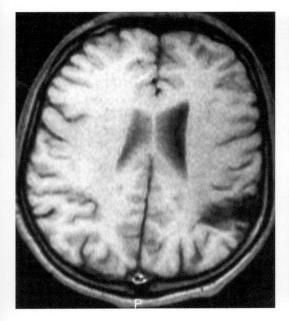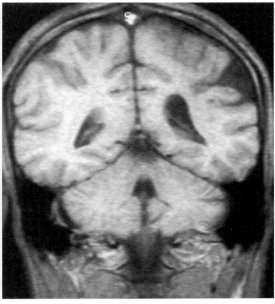

Fig. 14.7. Old infarct in a posterior branch of the left middle cerebral artery in 16-year-old boy who suddenly developed right hemiplegia at age 20 months in the course of a febrile illness. (There was minimal residual hemiparesis). T_1-weighted MRI scans show a triangular defect in the parietal cortex penetrating into the white matter. Note relatively small left hemisphere.

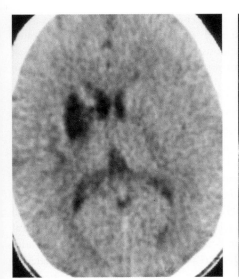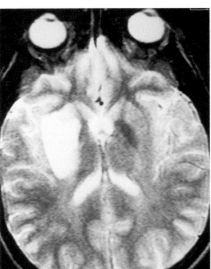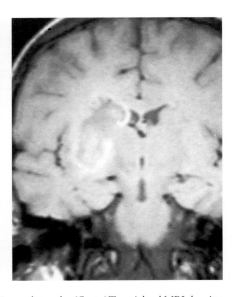

Fig. 14.8. Lacunar infarct in 14-year-old boy. *(Left)* CT showing lacuna in the right caudate nucleus and internal capsule. *(Centre)* T_1-weighted MRI showing large area of high signal probably corresponding to oedema. *(Right)* T_2-weighted MRI showing large area of low signal in right hemisphere, lined by high signal perhaps due to mild bleeding.

scans obtained within the first 10–24 hours are normal, but water-diffusion MRI can demonstrate extensive abnormal signal that may regress in part or totally (Warach et al. 1995). Later, there is an area of decreased attenuation with ill-defined borders, which extends, becomes better defined and reaches its peak over the next few days. This low-density area is accompanied by a variable mass effect that peaks in 2–3 days.

Most infarcts do not enhance on contrast injection during the first week. In children, however, early enhancement is not uncommon even after 24–48 hours. Enhancement mostly involves the cortical grey matter and appears as an undulating ribbon following brain convolutions. Later, the infarct appears as a depressed, triangular scar (Fig. 14.7).

Small lacunar infarcts often do not enhance on contrast injection and may remain undetectable by CT but are usually visible on T_2-weighted MRI (Inagaki et al. 1992). The largest lacunae, such as those that involve the putamen or pallidum, may sometimes take up contrast. Haemorrhages within the infarcted area may appear during the first week of the course.

MRI reveals even small ischaemic areas, giving a low-intensity signal in T_1-weighted sequences and an intense signal of probable oedematous nature in T_2-weighted sequences. Haemorrhage may best be seen on T_1-weighted MRI at the periphery of the infarct (Fig. 14.8).

Since the advent of modern neuroimaging, conventional angiography is not required in most cases for diagnosis of infarction. Indeed, lacunar infarcts are generally unaccompanied by visible vascular abnormalities, because involved vessels are too small and too variable in appearance for angiography to permit a definite diagnosis (Kappelle et al. 1989). For patients with unexplained strokes, angiography is in my opinion still indicated to rule in or out intrinsic vascular disease such as fibromuscular dysplasia and dissection and to recognize cases with multiple vascular lesions of the moyamoya type. This is important for prognostic and therapeutic reasons. MRA may not be adequate for this purpose as it gives information on flow rather than on vascular structure. On the other hand it gives some dynamic information on tissue perfusion. Reperfusion of thrombosed vessels may occur as early as two days after a stroke (Isler 1984), which may explain the frequency of normal angiograms in childhood strokes. Recent technical advances in MRA are described by Husson et al. (2002) and Husson and Lasjaunias (2004). Parker et al. (1998) reviewed the results and specific indications of different imaging methods. MRA permits assessment of flow more than of vascular walls. It is not precise enough to demonstrate subtle vascular abnormalities such as arterial stenosis or mural irregularities. New CT angiography (spiral CT) techniques are promising. Digital subtraction angiography by intravenous route may be sufficient for the detection of relatively large multiple lesions but precise analysis still requires the use of the arterial route. MRI can show clearly dissection of neck and intracranial arteries as a cause of infarct (Zuber et al. 1993). Water-diffusion MRI and perfusion-weighted MRI now permit earlier diagnosis of stroke and better evaluation of the infarcted and penumbra areas thus allowing refinement of the diagnosis and especially a more accurate determination of the prognosis (Sakoh et al. 2001). Spectroscopy using 1H-MR has also been used for the same purpose (Imamura et al. 2004).

Transcranial and duplex/Doppler ultrasound examination is a noninvasive and valuable method allowing visualization of arterial anomalies and, with refined technique, assessment of functional characteristics of circulation within a given vessel (Sturzenegger 1995).

DIFFERENTIAL DIAGNOSIS

Acquired vascular hemiplegia should be distinguished from the multiple other causes of acute hemiplegia. The differentiation from acute postconvulsive hemiplegia (HHE syndrome) that is only rarely due to vascular thrombosis (Chapters 7, 15) is usually easy. CT and MR images are totally different as they show initially swelling and decreased density of a whole hemisphere without preferential involvement of any vascular territory, later followed by hemiatrophy of the brain (Kataoka et al. 1988).

Hemiplegic migraine (Chapter 16) may be difficult to distinguish from arterial occlusion and may, in rare cases, be the cause of a stroke. In cardiac patients, acquired hemiplegia may also result from venous thrombosis or from brain abcess, the latter only after 2–3 years of age (Chapter 22). In case of doubt, it is reasonable to place all such children on antibiotic therapy, which may be discontinued after one week if abcess is ruled out. Tumours, especially of the brainstem, may result in rapidly acquired hemiplegia (Chapter 13). In contrast, some infarcts develop progressively and mimic a mass lesion (Chatkupt et al. 1987). Epileptic seizures and other paroxysmal events can produce transient hemiplegia that is not usually difficult to distinguish from vascular hemiplegia, except at the very onset (Chapter 16). Haemorrhagic stroke has been discussed above.

Transient ischaemic attacks are uncommon in children but can occur in patients with arterial stenosis of any cause or as a prodromal event in cases of dissection or thrombosis. They are marked by short-lived hemiplegia, hemianopia or hemisensory deficits. Acute but transitory attacks of hemiparesis that occur in children with insulin-dependent diabetes mellitus (Chapter 22) may represent a diagnostic challenge. Neuroimaging does not demonstrate infarction, and the hemiplegia resolves in 24–48 hours. Such attacks are different from the actual strokes that may occur in young diabetics during episodes of ketoacidosis. Occlusion of the posterior cerebral artery occurred in an 8-year-old diabetic girl with marked cerebral oedema as a result of improper treatment of ketoacidosis and was probably due to compression of the artery against the tentorial edge (personal case) (see also Chapter 16).

OUTCOME AND PROGNOSIS

The outcome of acquired occlusive disease depends in large part on the cause of the vascular disorder (see below). The prognosis is guarded if there is a detectable disorder of the brain vascular tree such as moyamoya disease or fibromuscular dysplasia. In a Swiss register of 80 children who were followed up for 2 years (Steinlin et al. 2005), 4 died within 6 months, but the overall mortality rate was relatively low. However, neuropsychological problems were found on follow-up in 25 of 33 children, and 6 children had an IQ <85 (Pavlovic et al. 2006). Transient cerebral arteriopathies, possibly of inflammatory origin (Chabrier et al. 1998) (see below), may be a common cause with a generally favourable outcome.

Vascular accidents without known cause recur only uncommonly (8–10%) even after prolonged follow-up. However, Abram et al. (1996) encountered 16 recurrences in a series of 42 children with idiopathic stroke, and Brankovic-Sreckovic et al. (2004) reported 7 recurrences in 36 children followed up for 5.5 years. In the study of Sträter et al. (2002), the recurrence rate after a median follow-up of 44 months was 6.6% and was possibly related to prothrombic abnormalities. In most cases, the outcome and the frequency of later recurrences depend on multiple factors, among which the importance of prothrombic disorders is currently emphasized (Chan and DeVeber 2000, Lanthier et al. 2000, Sträter et al. 2002). If no such cause is present (i.e. in idiopathic arterial occlusion), the outcome prognosis is more favourable.

The prognosis seems to be better for ischaemic arterial strokes in neonates, with a recurrence rate of less than 2% (Kurnik et al. 2003).

Motor sequelae are frequent, although total recovery is possible. Most nonrecurrent vascular hemiplegias show significant motor improvement, and total recovery may occur in over half the cases. In the series of Dusser et al. (1986), only 5 of 14 such patients had persisting weakness. However, even moderate or mild hemiparesis is a severerely disabling condition from a psychological point of view. Lacunar infarcts often have a favourable motor outcome (Dusser et al. 1986, Inagaki et al. 1992). In less favourable cases, the persistence of hemiplegia may be complicated by secondary dystonia (Dusser et al. 1986). Dystonia is a common complication and may emerge long after the appearance of hemiplegia (Pettigrew and Jankovic 1985). In the series of Pavlovic et al. (2006), 16 of the 33 children followed up for 2 years or more had a good outcome. The mean IQ level was 94 (Performance IQ 93, Verbal IQ 102), but 6 children had an IQ of less than 85 and school performance was often affected. Bilateral occlusion is exceptional (Shirane et al. 1992).

Intelligence is often unaffected by arterial occlusive accidents except if they are multiple or recurrent or in the case of large infarcts occurring in young infants, especially in congenital heart disease. Epileptic seizures are relatively uncommon. In one series (Aicardi et al. 1969), only 2 of 28 patients developed seizures and 25 were of normal intelligence. A poor outcome can be predicted if the hemiplegia persists after a month if the infarct is cortical rather than subcortical and with bilateral disease (Abram et al. 1996).

TREATMENT

The acute treatment remains in dispute. However, emergency intervention is essential. Determination of the cause is important in orientating therapy. Anticoagulation with heparin (especially low molecular weight heparin) followed by warfarin derivatives does not seem to increase the risk of haemorrhage within the infarcted area. Whether it is capable of limiting the volume of infarct when given early remains to be seen but it tends to be generally recommended in patients with arterial abnormalities or a thrombotic tendency. Aspirin treatment is generally indicated although few decisive data are available. Strepto/urokinase therapy has been found to be effective in adult stroke. Anticoagulation may be indicated when there are vascular abnormalities such as dissection producing secondary embolic strokes (Khurana et al. 1996) or abnormal blood coagulation. Antihypertensive treatment is indicated in some cases of extensive infarcts and may include heroic measures such as extensive decompressive craniotomies.

CAUSES AND RISK FACTORS

Occlusive vascular diseases have multiple causes that differ with the type of vessels involved and with the aetiology. In general, two categories of factors are at play: (1) arrest or severe decrease of the blood flow due to parietal disease or to obstruction of the intra-

TABLE 14.2
Haematological and coagulation factors that can play an aetiological role in arterial or venous strokes in childhood*

Protein S deficiency
Protein C deficiency
Factor V Leiden mutation
Plasminogen deficiency
Heparin cofactor II deficiency
Prothrombin G 20210A mutation
Antithrombin deficiency
Dysfibrinogenaemia
Factor XII deficiency
Antifactor V
High lipoprotein (a)
Antiphospholipid antibodies, anticardiolipin antibodies, lupus anticoagulant
Iron deficiency anaemia
Polycythaemia
Platelet disorders
Elevated blood lipoprotein
Hypertriglyceridaemia
Hyperhomocystinaemia
Methylenetetrahydrofolate reductase mutation G677T

*Data from Chan and deVeber (2000), Chan et al. (2003), Ganesan et al. (2003), Barnes et al. (2004), Kirkham and Hogan (2004), Lynch et al. (2005).

luminal blood flow (e.g. by arrest of a migrating clot or foreign bodies such as fat or air bubbles); (2) in situ thrombosis or severely decreased flow that may result from abnormal dynamics of the blood circulation or from decreased fluidity or increased coagulability of the blood itself. However, it is difficult to attribute vascular occlusions to any single factor as multiple causes are often operative. Parietal abnormalities and thrombophilic factors are usually jointly active. Thrombophilic factors are found in a high proportion of cases with arterial ischaemic strokes (20–50%) and sinovenous thrombosis (33–99%) (Barnes et al. 2004, Kirkham and Hogan 2004), but their role probably requires the presence of other factors in a multifactorial aetiology (Chan and deVeber 2000, Ganesan et al. 2003) (Table 14.2).

Because of the intrication of multiple factors, attempts at classification have been based on different parameters such as pathogenesis (Chabrier et al. 2000) or aetiology (Sträter et al. 2002). Wraige et al. (2005) have proposed an aetiological classification of ischaemic stroke into eight subtypes applicable to children: sickle cell disease; cardioembolic; moyamoya; cervical dissection; steno-occlusive cerebral arteriopathy; other determined aetiologies; multiple probable/possible aetiologies; undetermined aetiology. The proportion of the various causes depends on the populations studied and the date of study. In a review of 198 cases in nine published series (Wraige et al. 2005) the most common causes were sickle cell disease in 8.7%, cardiac embolism in 13.2%, moyamoya syndrome in 7.9%, arterial dissection in 4.7%, and cerebral arteriopathies in 6.9%. In the recent series of Bowen et al. (2005), aetiology remained undetermined in 6 of the 27 cases, while dissection was found in 5, coagulopathy in 4, embolism in 4, moyamoya in 3, sickle cell disease in 3, vasculitis in 3, and other causes in 3. The frequency of idiopathic stroke varies with the extent of the investigations performed. Recent work suggests that truly idiopathic strokes are relatively uncommon

TABLE 14.3
Main causes of arterial occlusion and stroke in childhood

Cardiac diseases

Congenital cyanotic heart disease	Tyler and Clark (1957), Freedom (1989)
Right-to-left shunts	Pellicer et al. (1992)
Rheumatic heart disease	Isler (1984)
Endocarditis	Salgado et al. (1989)
Myocarditis	Asinger et al. (1989)
Cardiac myoxoma	Cerebral Embolism Task Force (1986), Ricci (2003)
Prosthethic valves	Riela and Roach (1993)
Mistral valve prolapse	Jackson et al. (1984)
Disorders of rhythm	Zapson et al. (1995)

Vascular dysplasias

Moyamoya syndrome	
Idiopathic	This chapter
Acquired	Scott et al. (2004)
Neurofibromatosis type 1	Chapter 3
Fibromuscular dysplasia	Chiu et al. (1996)
Williams syndrome	Ardinger et al. (1994)
Dissecting aneurysm	Lasjaunias et al. (2005)
Weber–Rendu–Osler disease	Chapter 3

Inflammatory vascular diseases

Periarteritis nodosa	Chapter 11
Lupus erythematosus	Chapter 11
Takayasu arteritis	Ozen et al. (2007)
Kawasaki disease	Suda et al. (2003)
Other vasculitides	Moore (1989), Barron et al. (1993)
Schönlein–Henoch purpura	Chapter 11
Transient cerebral arteriopathy	Chabrier et al. (1998)

Connective tissue disorders

Pseudoxanthoma elasticum	Viljoen (1988)
Ehlers–Danlos syndrome (type IV)	North et al. (1995)
Defects in collagen III	Pope et al. (1981)
Marfan syndrome	Svensson et al. (2002)
COL4A1 deficit and porencephaly	Chapter 7

Other vascular diseases

CADASIL	Chabriat et al. (1995a,b)
Arterial hypertension	Wright and Mathews (1996)
Sneddon syndrome	Chapter 3
Antiphospholipid antibodies	Chan and deVeber (2000)
Anticardiolipin antibodies	Chan and deVeber (2000)
Other thrombotic factors	Ganesan et al. (2003)
Degos disease	Rosemberg et al. (1988)
Dissection of carotid, vertebral and intracranial arteries	Schievink et al. (1995), Fullerton et al. (2001)

Haematological diseases

Haemoglobinopathies	Adams (1995), Steen et al. (2003a,b)
Polycythaemia	Riela and Roach (1993)
Leukaemia and treatment	Schobess et al. (2004)
Coagulopathies	See Table 14.2
Iron deficiency anaemia	Hartfield et al. (1997)

Metabolic diseases

Mitochondrial encephalopathy with stroke-like episodes (MELAS)	Chapter 8
Sulfite oxidase deficiency	Riela and Roach (1993)
Disorders of glycosylation (CDG)	Chapter 8
Fabry disease	Chapter 8
Ammonia cycle disorders	Sperl et al. (1997)
Propionic and methylmalonic acidaemias	Haas et al. (1995)

Infectious diseases

Bacterial meningitides	Chapter 10
Tuberculous meningitis	Chapter 10
Viral diseases	
Varicella	Lanthier et al. (2005)
Herpes zoster	Lanthier et al. (2005)
AIDS	Narayan et al. (2002)
Coxsackie A9	Roden et al. (1975)
Parvovirus B19	Guidi et al. (2003)
Fungal disease, esp. mucormycosis	Ryan et al. (2001)
Cervical infections	Waterman et al. (2007)
Lymphadenopathy	Tagawa et al. (1985)
Cat scratch disease	Selby and Walker (1979)
Necrotizing fasciitis	Bush et al. (1984)
Ear and mastoid infections	Sébire et al. (2005)
Lemierre syndrome	Duong and Wenger (2005)

Tumours

Direct invasion or compression by tumour or leukaemic infiltrates	Packer et al. (1985)
L-asparaginase toxicity	Barron et al. (1992)
Methotrexate-induced thrombosis	Hanefeld and Riehm (1980)

Trauma and toxic causes

Head injury including minor trauma	Isler (1984), Debehnke and Singer (1991)
Trauma to vertebral artery	Garg and Edwards-Brown (1995)
Trauma to carotid artery	Schievink et al. (1994b), Patel et al. (1995)
Catheterization of temporal and other arteries	Prian et al. (1978)
Cranial irradiation of tumours	Mitchell et al. (1991)
Fat embolism	
Traumatic	
Non-traumatic including intravenous fat infusions	Barson and Chiswick (1978)
Nasal decongestants	Montalban et al. (1989)
Cocaine abuse	Mangiardi et al. (1988)
Wasp sting	Romano et al. (1989)
Solvent abuse	Parker et al. (1984)

Miscellaneous

Nephrotic syndrome	Igarashi et al. (1988)
Migraine	Riikonen and Santavuori (1994)
Familial hemiplegic migraine	Chabriat et al. (1995a)
Livedo reticularis	Chapter 3

---

when full investigation is carried out. The course of cerebral arteriopathies was recently studied in 43 cases (Danchaivijitr et al. 2006). Evidence for progression of the arterial disease was found in 12 patients, 3 of whom had recurrences. Eleven cases showed chronic stable arteriopathy. Improvement of imaging was observed within 6 monhs in 6 children who received a diagnosis of transient cerebral arteriopathy, and 17 additional patients

were assigned to the same category on clinical criteria. None of these 24 had recurrences. Twelve of these 24 children had a recent history of chicken-pox.

The main causes of ischaemic stroke in children are indicated in Table 14.3 and some of the most frequent are dealt with in more detail below. I will study consecutively cardiac causes and abnormalities (primary or secondary) of the arterial tree.

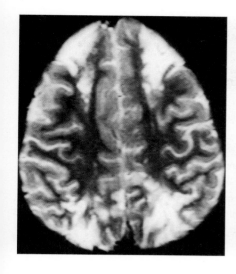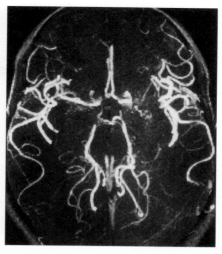

Fig. 14.12. Sickle-cell anaemia. *(Far left)* T$_2$-weighted MRI showing bilateral areas of ischaemia in both frontal and parietal areas. *(Left)* MR angiography showing abnormal flow in both middle cerebral arteries, predominantly on the left (right side of picture). Note development of collateral circulation. (Courtesy Dr F Kirkham, Great Ormond Street Hospital, London.)

Clinically, neurological complications are mainly due to vascular disease and include strokes, TIAs and haemorrhage. However, other neurological complications are possible including meningitis, coma, sinovenous thrombosis and reversible leukoencephalopathy due to hypertension, and seizures that occur in 12–14% of children with sickle cell disease (Prengler et al. 2005). Strokes occur in 20–30% of patients; they usually become apparent before age 5 years, presenting with headaches, seizures and behavioural disturbances. Strokes are recurrent if untreated in two thirds of cases. These are less common with sickle cell–haemoglobin C disease (Fabian and Peters 1984). In addition, silent infarcts are common (Adams 1995). Steen et al. (2003b) systematically looked for brain injury in 146 children with sickle cell disease assessed by MRI and MRA at 10.5 years of age. They found MRI abnormalities in 46% and vasculopthy by MRA in 64% of studied children. MR abnormalities included cystic infarction, encephalomalacia, atrophy and leukoencephalopathy. MRA revealed vascular abnormalities ranging from mild tortuosity and dilatation to severe stenosis and occlusion. Rarely, neurological symptoms appear in patients with sickle cell trait, often at times of stress, but mild abnormalities of cerebral vessels have been found in some heterozygotes for the sickle cell trait (Steen et al. 2003).

Vascular occlusions occur most frequently in children 2–5 years of age and can be precipitated by sickle cell crises. However, a significant proportion of infarctions remain silent (Adams 1995). When clinical stroke occurs, focal or generalized seizures are common. Hemiplegia or other focal neurological deficits are the main findings. They may be transient or irreversible. Multiple lesions are the rule (Fig. 14.12) and eventually may result in dementia, epilepsy and pseudobulbar syndrome. Intracranial haemorrhage is uncommon in children but has a high mortality rate. Additional independent risk factors include prior TIAs, low haemoglobin concentration, recent acute chest syndrome, increased blood pressure and certain haplotypes.

Sickle cell disease is a prime consideration in children of African origin with neurological symptoms, even though these occur only uncommonly as a first manifestation. The diagnosis is confirmed by demonstration of the abnormal haemoglobin. The extent of brain damage is best evaluated by MRI, which may show one or several areas of hypodensity or atrophy or both. Diffusion and perfusion MRI can confirm the abnormalities of brain perfusion (Kirkham et al. 2001, Prengler et al. 2005). There is a good correspondence between the results of MRI and the clinical evidence of ischaemic damage. Glauser et al. (1995) found that 12 of 13 patients with a normal MRI were neurologically intact and had no history of acute neurological event. Armstrong et al. (1996) identified MRI abnormalities in 17.9% of 194 children. Those with a silent infarct, often located in border zone distribution on MRI, performed significantly worse on cognitive tests than children without MRI anomaly (DeBaun et al. 1998). Those with a history of clinical stroke did worse than those with only MRI changes. Conventional angiography is not recommended. MRA shows stenosis often affecting several large or medium-size arteries so that the development of a moyamoya pattern is frequent. Multiple aneurysms have been reported (Overby and Rothman 1985) but are not seen before 15 years of age. Transcranial measurement of time-averaged blood flow velocity in the distal carotids and major cerbral arteries by Doppler ultrasonography reliably shows high blood flow velocity and correlates well with angiographic data (Adams 1995). Abnormal velocities are correlated with the occurrence of neurological complications including strokes and seizures (Prengler et al. 2006) and may be predictive of the occurrence of stroke (Adams et al. 2001).

The *acute treatment of vascular accidents* in patients with known sickle cell includes prompt hydration, immediate administration of oxygen to maintain a saturation of 96–99%, and immediate transfusion of packed red cells to correct any anaemia of less than 10 g/dL and reduce haemoglobin S level to below 30%. CT or MRI should be performed to exclude intracranial haemorrhage and the possibilty of associated anomaly such as dissection or sinovenous thrombosis (Kirkham and DeBaun 2004).

Prevention of recurrences is the next step. Recurrent strokes can be prevented by regular transfusions to maintain the level of haemoglobin A above 60% (Prohovnik et al. 1989, Pegelow et al. 1995). This regime significantly reduces the frequency of further strokes and of other accidents such as acute chest syndrome or other vaso-occlusive events. Hankins et al. (2005a) found that the incidence of acute chest syndrome decreased from 1.3 to 0.1 episode per patient per year. Transfusions also improve the growth of treated children and their overall physical strength (Wang et al. 2005). The major problem is iron overload, in addition to the practical problem of repeated transfusions. Rare complications such as intracranial haemorrhage associated with hypertension in overly transfused patients have been reported (Prohovnik et al. 1989), and a similar syndrome has been seen in thalassaemic patients after multiple blood transfusions (Wazi et al. 1978). The duration of treatment is not established, but recurrences have been observed on discontinuation of transfusions after three years, and lifelong therapy may be needed, so a safer and more practical prophylactic treatment is being looked for. Hydroxyurea therapy has been shown to stimulate the synthesis of fetal haemoglobin, to improve the anaemia and to allow for a significant decrease in the frequency of transfusions (de Montalembert et al. 1997, Teixeira et al. 2003). Long-term treatment appears to be safe and effective (Hankins et al. 2005b). However, a significant proportion of patients have no or only a weak response, and the actual value of this drug as well as the very long-term tolerance remain to be determined. Hyperventilation during EEG should be avoided as it may produce stroke (Allen et al. 1976), but apnoea has also been associated with this complication (Robertson et al. 1988).

Thrombophilic factors
These include antithrombin, protein C, protein S, plasminogen, factor V Leiden, prothrombin gene G20210A, dysfibrinogenaemia, antifactor V, antiphospholipid antibodies including lupus anticoagulant and anticardiolipin antibodies (Levine et al. 1990), hyperhomocystinaemia and elevated protein (a), and an additional role may be played by elevated lipoprotein, polycythaemia, iron deficiency anaemia and platelet disorders. Strokes of arterial origin have been reported with protein C and S deficiency (van Kuijck et al. 1994, Schöning et al. 1994, Simioni et al. 1994, Kennedy et al. 1995) and with resistance to activated protein C (Nowak-Göttl et al. 1996). High levels of triglycerides, low LDL (low density lipoprotein) cholesterol and depressed HDL (high density lipoprotein) cholesterol were found in one third of the cases of Abram et al. (1996). Whether and how often thrombophilic factors play a directly causal role, however, is still unclear (Barnes et al. 2004). Heller et al. (2003) pointed out that only protein C deficiency, which may be secondary to the stroke and should be verified 6 months later (Dusser et al. 1988), had an independent association with venous thrombosis. Factor V Leiden mutation, which is the most frequent hereditary cause of venous thrombosis (Svensson and Dahlbäck 1994, Nowak-Göttl et al. 1996), may also be a cause of arterial thrombosis in infants and even during late fetal life (Thorarensen et al. 1997). Hartfield et al. (1997) have suggested that iron deficiency anaemia may be a significant aetiological factor of stroke and reported 6 cases, 3 of them with arterial infarcts. The primary antiphospholipid syndrome has been found in a significant number of children with cerebrovascular ischaemic events (Angelini et al. 1994, Schöning et al. 1994), and even in infants, but its significance is variably appreciated (Göbel 1994, Takanashi et al. 1995). An association with the human leukocyte antigen HLA B51 has been reported (Mintz et al. 1992).

The role of prothrombic factors is probably less important in cases of arterial thrombosis than in those of venous thrombosis (Chan and deVeber 2000).

Thrombophilic factors appear to be more a favouring underlying condition than the sole cause, and they act mostly in combination with the presence of another disorder.

Other risk factors
These include neurocutaneous disorders, especially neurofibromatosis type 1, Down syndrome, trauma, and bacterial or viral infections. Genetic factors are probably at play but have not been precisely characterized (Kirkham and Hogan 2004). Connective tissue disease may also be a cause (North et al. 1995). In about one third to one half of the cases, no risk factor is present.

SPECIAL PROBLEMS
Arterial occlusion of traumatic origin
This affects mostly the carotid arteries in the neck and the main lesion is dissection (see above). Hemiplegia can result from injury of the carotid artery, vertebral artery or intracranial vessels due to stretching of the artery or dissection. Direct cervical trauma and even mild or trivial trauma to the head and neck sustained during exercise and sports may induce thrombosis of the carotid artery.

Trauma with long bone fracture can result in traumatic fat embolism that may provoke coma and/or focal neurological disturbances (Jacobson et al. 1986). Fat embolism may also complicate cardiopulmonary bypass surgery, pancreatitis, osteomyelitis and intravenous infusion of lipids (Table 14.3).

Children who fall with a blunt object in their mouth (Pearl 1987) and those with penetrating or even blunt neck injuries can sustain injuries to the carotid artery. The onset of symptoms is often delayed for hours or days. Hemiparesis or other focal deficits may be transitory or persistent. Any child with a penetrating wound of the neck or trauma to the tonsillar fossa should be closely observed for neurological signs. Exploration of the vessel by ultrasound and especially by MRA should be considered to detect and determine the presence and type of injury (Ofer et al. 2001). Surgery may be indicated in case of tearing or major damage. Preventive anticoagulation may be considered in case of doubt even though the efficacy of preventive treatment has not been proved (Samson 1989). Arterial dissection is probably the cause in most cases.

Surgical trauma may result in hemiplegia: infarction of the anterior choroidal artery territory, the so-called 'manipulation' hemiplegia, is a rare complication of anterior temporal lobectomy (Helgason et al. 1987).

Traumatic carotid–jugular fistulae are a rare complication of trauma. Iatrogenic trauma may cause cerebral thrombosis. This has been reported following temporal artery catheterization (Prian et al. 1978), and I have observed a few cases of cerebral infarction following catheterization for congenital cardiac disease.

X-irradiation of the brain may cause arterial stenosis and ischaemic accidents that may be transient or leave permanent residua. In some cases, anastomosis between the extracerebral and intracerebral arterial systems may be considered if the stenosis is limited to one segment with normal peripheral branches.

Spinal arterial occlusions
Spontaneous occlusions of spinal arteries leading to infarction of the spinal cord are uncommon. They are often the manifestation of an underlying vascular malformation.

Direct or indirect injuries to the spinal arteries are reviewed in Chapter 12. Spinal damage is a rare complication of surgery for the repair of coarctation of the aorta and may result in complete paraplegia or lesser degrees of weakness. It is related to the duration of aortic occlusion and to circulatory factors. Similar problems may occur with surgery of the sympathetic chain or vertebrae. Paraplegia of vascular mechanism is a rare complication of catheterization of the umbilical artery or of injections of drugs into this vessel (Dulac and Aicardi 1975). The *spinal artery syndrome* can occur in children. The clinical features include an abrupt or rapid onset of paraplegia associated with disturbances of superficial sensation with a clear-cut upper level, with characteristic dissociation between severely altered superficial sensation and preserved deep sensation (Blennow and Starck 1987). This results from preservation of the posterior half of the cord, which is supplied by the posterior spinal arteries, while the spinocerebellar fasciculi are involved. The syndrome is observed after surgery of the aorta or posterior mediastinum, or following severe hypotensive episodes compromising circulation in the anterior spinal arteries.

PERINATAL STROKE

Perinatal stroke (see also Chapter 1) may be due either to ischaemia of arterial origin or to venous thrombosis. These are studied below.

ISCHAEMIC ARTERIAL STROKE
Ischaemic arterial stroke has been increasingly reported in recent years (Lee et al. 2005b, Schulzke et al. 2005, Steinlin et al. 2005). The causes, presentation and outcome of perinatal stroke are different to those in older children. Risk factors are not precisely known. Boys appear to be more frequently affected than girls (Golomb et al. 2004). Prothrombotic factors are often present but rarely as the sole finding (Chalmers 2005, Steinlin et al. 2005). The importance of perinatal difficulties and of gravidic factors has been variably assessed (Steinlin et al. 2005). Lee et al. (2005a) compared 40 newborn infants with stroke diagnosed on the basis of MRI with 120 random controls. Most affected infants were born at term and there was a moderate excess of primiparity, of

fetal heart rate abnormalities, of a prolonged second stage of labour and of emergency caesarian section. Independent risk factors significantly linked to stroke included a history of infertility, pre-eclampsia, prolonged rupture of the membranes and chorioamnionitis. Stroke can, however, occur with a normal pre- and perinatal history.

The middle cerebral artery territory is involved in most cases. The posterior cerebral artery was affected in only 3 of 47 cases reported by Cowan et al. (2005), and the anterior cerebral artery in only 1.

Clinical symptoms commonly appear during the first few days of life, usually before 48 hours. In fact, fetal stroke has been demonstrated in a few cases (Ozduman et al. 2004, Verdu et al. 2005). The clinical picture in most neonates is marked by seizures that are usually focal and occur repeatedly in the same fixed location. They were present in 19 of 23 neonates with arterial ischaemic stroke in the study of Steinlin et al. (2005), in which only 30 out of 80 infants had abnormalities of muscle tone. Motor deficit is not always apparent at this period and hemiplegia often becomes apparent only after several months; some infants remain asymptomatic.

The diagnosis is established by imaging. Ultrasonography, which is easy to perform in the nursery, can show abnormalities in most cases. In a study of 43 infants by Cowan et al. (2005), their presence was identified in 29 early and 37 late examinations. However, small lesions can be missed.

MRI is the technique of choice, and water-diffusion MRI may be useful. Using this technique, De Vries et al. (2005) were able to predict the functional outcome as a function of the topography and number of abnormalities. Involvement of the posterior limb of the internal capsule indicates the likelihood of hemiparesis. Boardman et al. (2005) found that areas of abnormal signal could involve the white matter in the internal capsule, the cerebral peduncle or the motor cortex. When all three areas were affected, hemiplegia was later present, but not when only one or two areas were abnormal. Involvement of the basal ganglia was not followed by the development of dystonia. Hemiparesis was usually of mild to moderate degree and was absent altogether in a substantial proportion (56%) of patients. However, in the large study of Lee et al. (2005b) only 7 out of 46 patients had a normal outcome. Spastic cerebral palsy was found in 23 infants after 2 months of age, epilepsy in 15, delayed language in 10 and behavioural abnormalities in 9. Predictors of sequelae were large size of the infarct, involving both cortical areas and basal ganglia, and delayed clinical presentation without clinical symptoms in the neonatal period. Likewise, Golomb et al. 2007) found that 55 of their 111 patients had associated disabilities, in particular epilepsy and mental retardation. This is in contrast with the De Vries et al. study (Chapter 1), in which more than half of children had normal development.

STROKES OF VENOUS ORIGIN
These are frequent in the neonatal period (deVeber et al. 2001) and are discussed below with venous occlusion in later childhood and adolescence.

TABLE 14.4
Main causes of cranial sinovenous thrombosis*

Cause	Preferential age of occurrence	References
Septic thrombosis	Any age	
Otitis media and mastoiditis		Southwick et al. (1986), Sébire et al. (2005)
Paranasal sinusitis		Soga et al. (2001)
Cutaneous infections (head and face)		Southwick et al. (1986)
Purulent meningitis		Chapter 10
Metastatic infections		Southwick et al. (1986)
Sepsis	Neonates	Barron et al. (1992)
Aseptic thrombosis		
Debilitating disorders, chronic	Childhood	deVeber et al. (2001)
Diabetes mellitus		Chapter 22
Lupus erythematosus		Uziel et al. (1995)
Inflammatory bowel disease		Sébire et al. (2005)
Behçet disease		Alper et al. (2001)
Nephrotic syndrome		Igarashi et al. (1988)
Other chronic diseases		This chapter
Heart disease		
Cyanotic		
Congenital disease	Infants	Chapter 22
Cardiac failure	Any age	Chapter 22
Haematological disorders and malignancies	Infants and children	
Leukaemia and myeloproliferative disorders		deVeber et al. (2001), Schobess et al. (2004)
Iron deficiency anaemia		Hartfield et al. (1997)
Haemolytic anaemias and haemoglobinopathies		See Table 14.3
Prothrombotic conditions	Any age	See Table 14.3
Acute dehydration		deVeber et al. (2001)
Central venous catheterization and ventriculocardiac shunts	Children	deVeber et al. (2001), Sébire et al. (2005)
Other (predisposing) factors	Children and adolescents	
Pregnancy		Bousser et al. (1985)
Hormonal contraception		Martinelli et al. (1998)
Recent head trauma		See Table 14.3
Recent surgery		See Table 14.3

*Several factors are often operative in the same patient.

OCCLUSIVE VENOUS DISEASE, THROMBOSIS OF CEREBRAL VEINS AND DURAL SINUSES

The incidence of venous thrombosis has been estimated to be 0.67 per 100,000 children per year (deVeber et al. 2001) and may well be higher as the diagnosis is being increasingly made due to improved imaging techniques and because of the realization that the condition can be life-threatening and cause long-term neurological deficits and treatment is possible and effective (Chan et al. 2003, Heller et al. 2003).

The causes of sinovenous thrombosis in children differ from those in adults, and in newborn infants from those in older children. Among neonates, which comprised 69 of the 160 cases studied by deVeber et al. (2001), acute systemic illnesses including dehydration were the most common aetiological factors, being present in 84%. An abnormal prothrombic state was also more common than in older patients. In older children, infections, especially of ear or sinuses, and chronic conditions such as cancer and haematological diseases were the predominant causes. Indwelling central venous catheters are also a frequent cause of

sinovenous thrombosis (Gebara et al. 1995, Chan et al. 2003). Infections remain a common factor even in recent series (Sébire et al. 2005) (Table 14.4). Septic thrombosis may complicate otitis media and mastoiditis, infections of paranasal sinuses and facial infections. Although its frequency has decreased, infection was still responsible for 4 of 15 cases of thrombosis in older children in one series (Barron et al. 1992) and they remain a major cause of venous thrombosis. Mastoiditis was a cause in 20 of the 42 patients of Sébire et al., and other infections in 10 of them.

Aseptic or primary thrombosis is a common complication of congenital cyanotic heart disease, in which it occurs preferentially in patients over 2–3 years of age with a haematocrit of more than 70%, and in association with dehydration. It may be difficult to distinguish from strokes of arterial origin. Alterations in haemodynamics such as dehydration, shock or heart failure, diabetic ketoacidosis and chronic debilitating conditions may be responsible.

Haematological disorders such as leukaemia or thrombocytosis (Haan et al. 1988), or a hypercoagulable state such as results from the use of certain drugs, especially 4-L-asparaginase (Barron

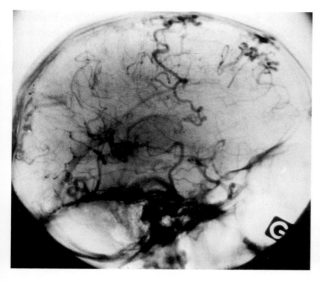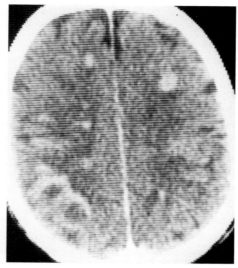

Fig. 14.13. Idiopathic thrombosis of the sagittal sinus in 13-year-old boy. *(Left)* Angiogram showing absence of opacification of sagittal sinus. Note stagnation of contrast in veins of hemispheral convexity. *(Right)* CT showing areas of hypodensity and haemorrhage in upper part of both hemispheres.

et al. 1992), or from diseases such as the nephrotic syndrome, are important causes in older children. Lupus erythematosus may be a cause (Uziel et al. 1995), and the possible responsibility of antiphospholipid antibodies has been considered (Göbel 1994). Idiopathic cases occur (Konishi et al. 1987). Oral contraceptives, which are increasingly used by adolescent girls, may be a factor in some of these cases but with low-dose oestrogen agents have not been shown to be associated with increased risk. Pregnancy is known to predispose to venous thrombosis.

In newborns, perinatal complications and sepsis play a significant role (Barron et al. 1992) but many cases appear to be idiopathic (Shevell et al. 1989, Rivkin et al. 1992). Prothrombotic factors are present in betwen 30% and 75% of cases. They are more frequent in newborns than in in older children (Table 14.4).

The clinical picture of venous thrombosis is variable and non-specific. Most patients, especially neonates, present acutely with seizures. In older children, headache, disturbances of consciousness, visual disturbances including papilloedema, and focal signs such as seizures, hemiparesis, hemianopia or aphasia should suggest the diagnosis when they complicate a febrile illness or another predisposing condition. Some cases, especially of isolated sinus thrombosis, present with isolated intracranial hypertension, the so-called pseudotumour cerebri (Chapter 13), whereas with cortical vein thrombosis that produces haemorrhagic infarcts convulsions and focal signs are usually present. A dramatic picture of septic thrombosis with rigors and high spiking fever is now rare. When it involves the cavernous sinus, proptosis, ophthalmoplegia and papilloedema with high ICP may be associated (Soga et al. 2001). *Thrombosis of the deep cerebral veins and straight sinus* can produce profound disturbances of consciousness, dystonia and opisthotonus, seizures and ocular signs as a result of infarction of the thalami and deep grey and white structures.

In infants, and especially in neonates, dural sinus or cerebral

vein thrombosis is mainly manifested by seizures and/or lethargy (Rivkin et al. 1992). Seizures were present in 3 of 7 cases studied by Rivkin et al. and in 15 of 17 cases reported by Shevell et al. (1989). Paucisymptomatic cases are common and the diagnosis often goes unrecognized. The CSF is often xanthochromic or haemorrhagic.

Angiography demonstrates well obliteration or filling defects in the sinuses (McArdle et al. 1987) but has now been replaced by CT and MRI in most cases. CT can show areas of low density and an abnormal visibility of the sinuses on unenhanced scans (Brant-Zawadzki et al. 1982, d'Avella et al. 1984). The empty delta sign is a filling defect within the posterior part of the sagittal sinus on contrast-enhanced scans. Although it may be mimicked by early division of the sagittal sinus, it is a fairly reliable sign (Virapongse et al. 1987). MRI is much more precise; it can demonstrate absence of flow void in the major sinuses and may show spontaneous opacity of the affected sinuses or cerebral veins. MRA is the method of choice. Localization of the thrombosis was superficial in 86% and deep in 38% of the 160 cases reviewed by deVeber et al. (2001). The MRI findings pass through three successive stages: absence of flow void, with low signal in T_2-weighted sequences in the first 1–5 days, then increasing T_1 and T_2 signal from the sinuses between days 6 and 15, progressively returning to normal in 3–4 months; recanalization may occur (Grossman et al. 1993, Isensee et al. 1994, Perkin 1995). Thrombosis of cortical veins in the deep system may be quite difficult to evidence and may require conventional angiography (Sébire et al. 2005).

The diagnosis has been made considerably easier by modern neuroimaging techniques. Infarcts are found in about half the cases; they may be haemorrhagic and then visible on T_1-weighted sequences, and multiple haemorrhagic areas may be present in the deep white matter bilaterally (Fig. 14.13). Non-haemorrhagic infarcts appear as areas of low T_1 and high T_2 signal. Imaging can show filling defects in the sinuses.

A fluctuating course is not unusual. Evolution depends on the extent and location of parenchymal damage, which is often haemorrhagic in type (Konishi et al. 1987). When parenchymal involvement is absent or modest the outcome is generally favourable. This was the case in the newborn infants studied by Shevell et al. (1989) and Rivkin et al. (1992), but Barron et al. (1992) found sequelae only in neonates. Even extensive lesions involving the territory of the deep cerebral veins may regress without sequelae (Forsting et al. 1989), although such cases are usually severe and sometimes lethal. Mortality was 8% in the series of deVeber et al. (2001) and 5/42 in that of Sébire et al. (2005). Neurological sequelae and cognitive difficulties remained in approximately one quarter to one third of patients. Chronic pseudotumour cerebri is not rare. It was found in 12 of 37 survivors in the latter study, and was regularly associated with later cognitive problems and sometimes with epilepsy and visual or neurological sequelae. Predictors of adverse neurological outcome included seizures and the presence of infarcts.

The treatment of sinus and cerebral vein thrombosis is still disputed. Heparin therapy has been recommended in recent studies. It was given to 22 of 42 neonates and children deVeber's study and to 25 of 42 in Sébire's. In no case did the treatment aggravate the condition or increase the size of infarcts even when these were haemorrhagic. No comparative study is available but clinical impression is favourable (deVeber et al. 2001) and this therapy is being increasingly used. In addition, anticonvulsive treatment is indicated, and control of intracranial hypertension is important. In some cases, lumboperitoneal shunt may be necessary for persistent intracranial hypertension. Thrombolytic treatment with urokinase or streptokinase has sometimes been used (Isensee et al. 1994, Perkin 1995). Direct thrombolysis by injection in the sagittal sinus has been used in infants (Higashida et al. 1989). General treatment includes antibiotics for septic cases, control of seizures, and reduction of high ICP, which may be obtained by the use of dexamethasone.

Thrombosis of the superior vena cava or of both jugular veins induced by indwelling catheters can result in intracranial hypertension or hydrocephalus that usually stabilizes spontaneously (Chapters 13, 22).

NEUROLOGICAL COMPLICATIONS OF ARTERIAL HYPERTENSION

Neurological symptoms are a frequent feature of high blood pressure in children and they may be the first manifestation of an unrecognized hypertension. Measurement of blood pressure should be systematic in all children with neurological problems.

HYPERTENSIVE ENCEPHALOPATHY
This disorder is characterized by multiple arteriolar dilatations with disturbance of the blood–brain barrier and consequent disseminated areas of oedema. Headache, seizures, disturbances of consciousness, and cortical blindness or blurred vision are the main clinical features (Kandt et al. 1995, Wright and Mathews 1996). Hemiplegia, focal seizures, brainstem signs and symptoms suggestive of a mass lesion have been observed in some patients (Del Giudice and Aicardi 1979). Blindness and paraplegia have been recorded (Hulse et al. 1979). Papilloedema is often present and is of great diagnostic value especially when accompanied by stellate retinopathy and narrow, abnormal arteries. The EEG shows diffuse slow-wave activity sometimes alternating with episodes of seizure. Paroxysmal complexes reminiscent of those in herpes encephalitis have been reported (Del Giudice and Aicardi 1979). In many cases neuroimaging shows the so-called *reversible posterior leukoencephalopathy* (Singhi et al. 2002, Lamy et al. 2004) with increased signal predominating in the white matter of occipital and parietal regions but also often involving the cortex, and occasionally being seen in the anterior part of the brain (Kandt et al. 1995). This is more clearly demonstrated using FLAIR sequences. The abnormalities disappear after reduction of the high blood pressure except in rare cases (Prasad et al. 2003). MRI demonstrates focal symmetrically increased signal intensity in white matter and cortex with occipital lobe involvement in each case on T_2-weighted sequences.

Hypertensive encephalopathy requires emergency treatment with antihypertensive and anticonvulsant drugs. When high blood pressure is corrected there is clinical recovery, and complete resolution of the abnormal images is observed in a few weeks. The frequent affectation of the occipital cortex accounts for the visual manifestations such as cortical blindness. Renal disease, especially pyelonephritis, is the most common cause of hypertensive encephalopathy and should be systematically searched for. Hemiplegia may, in a few patients, be a manifestation of hypertension. In an occasional such case, CT has shown a 'fibre-splitting' haemorrhage of the internal capsule (Brett 1997). Clinical symptoms include disturbances of consciouness and vision, headaches and seizures. These originate primarily from the occipital lobes (Bakshi et al. 1998). A variant with swelling and MRI abnormalities of the brainstem has been reported (Kitagushi et al. 2005). Posterior leukoencephalopathy may not be due to hypertension but result instead from cytotoxic therapy for cancer or immunological disorders, especially cyclosporine and tacrolimus (Norman et al. 2007) or from renal or immunological disease. Infants can be affected (Arroyo et al. 2003, Tam et al. 2004).

FACIAL PARALYSIS AND HYPERTENSION
The association of facial palsy with hypertension is well recognized in children and adolescents. Facial palsy occurs only with severe hypertension and may be the presenting manifestation of high blood pressure. Its onset usually coincides with a rise in blood pressure, whereas it tends to disappear when the pressure is lowered. Palsy may last weeks to months and may be recurrent (Harms et al. 2000). According to Brett (1997), 11% of children with hypertension develop facial palsy and 11% of peripheral lower facial palsies in children are caused by hypertension. Haemorrhage within the nerve sheath may be the cause of paralysis. Thomke et al. (2002) proposed that it could be the manifestation of small pontine infarct.

COMPLICATIONS OF HYPOTENSIVE TREATMENT

Hulse et al. (1979) reported severe neurological problems at the time of reduction of long-standing arterial hypertension in 3 children. All 3 patients developed optic nerve infarction with permanent loss of vision, and 1 child had, in addition, ischaemic transverse myelopathy. This serves to emphasize that lowering of blood pressure should be cautiously conducted in patients with established hypertensive disorder. Sudden reduction of hypertension such as may occur in newborn infants with bronchopulmonary dysplasia following the use of captopril can produce seizures and focal neurological deficits (Perlman and Volpe 1989).

REFERENCES

Abbassioun K, Amirjamshidi A, Rahmat H (1985) Bilateral mycotic aneurysms of the intracavernous carotid artery. *Neurosurgery* 16: 235–7.

Abe M, Kjellberg RN, Adam RD (1989) Clinical presentations of vascular malformations of the brain stem: comparison of angiographically positive and negative types. *J Neurol Neurosurg Psychiatry* 52: 167–75.

Abram HS, Knepper LE, Warty VS, Painter MJ (1996) Natural history, prognosis and lipid abnormalities of idiopathic ischemic childhood stroke. *J Child Neurol* 11: 276–82.

Adams RJ (1995) Sickle cell disease and stroke. *J Child Neurol* 10: 75–6.

Adams RJ, McKie VC, Carl EM, et al. (2001) Long-term stroke risk in children with sickle cell disease screened with transcranial Doppler. *Ann Neurol* 42: 699–704.

Aicardi J, Amsili J, Chevrie JJ (1969) Acute hemiplegia in infancy and childhood. *Dev Med Child Neurol* 11: 162–73.

Allen JP, Imbus CE, Powars DR, Haywood LJ (1976) Neurologic impairment induced by hyperventilation in children with sickle cell anemia. *Pediatrics* 58: 124–6.

Allison JW, Davis PC, Sato Y, et al. (1998) Intracranial aneurysms in infants and children. *Pediatr Radiol* 28: 223–9.

Alper G, Yilmaz Y, Ekinci G, Kose O (2001) Cerebral vein thrombosis in Behçet's disease. *Pediatr Neurol* 25: 332–5.

Anderson KA, Burbach JA, Fenton LJ, et al. (1985) Idiopathic arterial calcification of infancy in newborn siblings with unusual light and electron microscopic manifestations. *Arch Pathol Lab Med* 109: 838–42.

Andrews BT, Hudgins RJ, Edwards MSB (1989) Mycotic aneurysms in children. In: Edwards MSB, Hoffman HJ, eds. *Cerebral Vascular Disease in Children and Adolescents.* Baltimore: Williams & Wilkins, pp. 275–82.

Angelini L, Ravelli A, Caporali R, et al. (1994) High prevalence of antiphospholipid antibodies in children with idiopathic cerebral ischemia. *Pediatrics* 94: 500–3.

Ardinger RH, Rose DF, Caporali R, et al. (1994) Cerebrovascular stenoses with cerebral infarction in a child with Williams syndrome. *Am J Med Genet* 51: 200–2.

Armstrong FD, Thompson RJ, Wang W, et al. (1996) Cognitive functioning and brain magnetic resonance imaging in children with sickle cell disease. *Pediatrics* 97: 864–70.

Arroyo HA, Gañez LA, Fejerman N (2003) [Posterior reversible encephalopathy in infancy.] *Rev Neurol* 37: 506–11 (Spanish).

Arroyo HA, Russo RA, Rugilo C (2005) Cerebral vasculitis. *Rev Neurol* 42: 176–86.

Asinger RW, Dyken ML, Fisher M, et al. (1989) Cardiogenic brain embolism. The second report of the Cerebral Embolism Task Force. *Arch Neurol* 46: 727–43.

Attal P, Vilgrain V, Brancatelli G, et al. (2003) Telangiectatic focal nodular hyperplasia: US, CT, and MR imaging findings with histopathologic correlation in 13 cases. *Radiology* 220: 465–72.

Aviv RI, Benseler SM, Silverman ED, et al. (2006) MR imaging and angiography of primary CNS vasculitis of childhood. *AJNR* 27: 192–9.

Bakshi R, Bates W, Mechtler LL, et al. (1998) Occipital lobe seizures as a major manifestation of reversible posterior leukoencephalopathy syndrome: magnetic resonance findings. *Epilepsia* 39: 295–9.

Barnes C, Newall F, Furmedge I, et al. (2004) Arterial ischaemic stroke in children. *J Paediatr Child Health* 40: 384–7.

Barron TF, Gusnard DA, Zimmerman RA, Clancy MR (1992) Cerebral venous thrombosis in neonates and children. *Pediatr Neurol* 8: 112–6.

Barron TF, Ostrov BE, Zimmermann RA, Packer RJ (1993) Isolated angiitis of CNS: treatment with pulse cyclophosphamide. *Pediatr Neurol* 9: 73–5.

Barson AJ, Chiswick ML (1978) Fat embolism in infancy after intravenous fat infusions. *Arch Dis Child* 53: 218–23.

Barth A, Bogousslavsky J, Regli F (1993) The clinical and topographic spectrum of cerebellar infarcts: a clinical–magnetic resonance imaging correlation study. *Ann Neurol* 33: 451–6.

Bendheim PE, Berg BO (1981) Ataxic hemiparesis from a midbrain mass. *Ann Neurol* 9: 405–7.

Benseler SM, deVeber G, Hawkins C, et al. (2005) Angiography-negative primary central nervous system vaculitis in children: a newly recognized inflammatory central nervous system disease. *Arthritis Rheum* 52: 2159–64.

Benseler SM, Silverman E, Aviv RI, et al. (2006) Primary central nervous system vasculitis in children. *Arthritis Rheum* 54: 1291–7.

Bergametti F, Denier G, Labauge P, et al. (2005) Mutations in the programmed cell death 10 gene cause cerebral cavernous malformations. *Am J Hum Genet* 76: 42–51.

Bland LI, Lapham LW, Ketonen L, Okawara SH (1994) Acute cerebellar hemorrhage secondary to capillary telangiectasia in an infant. A case report. *Arch Neurol* 51: 1151–4.

Blennow G, Starck L (1987) Anterior spinal artery syndrome: report of seven cases in childhood. *Pediatr Neurosci* 13: 33–7.

Blom I, De Schryver EL, Kappelle LJ, et al (2003) Prognosis of haemorrhagic stroke in childhood: a long-term follow-up study. *Dev Med Child Neurol* 45: 233–9.

Boardman JP, Ganesan V, Rutherford MA, et al. (2005) Magnetic resonance image correlates of hemiparesis after neonatal and childhood middle cerebral artery stroke. *Pediatrics* 115: 321–6.

Bodensteiner JB, Hille MR, Riggs JE (1992) Clinical features of vascular thrombosis following varicella. *Am J Dis Child* 146: 100–2.

Boet R, Poon WS, Chan MS, Yu SC (2001) Childhood posterior foassa pial–dural arteriovenous fistula treated by endovascular occlusion. *Childs Nerv Syst* 17: 681–4.

Bogousslavsky J, Caplan L, eds. (1995) *Stroke Syndromes.* Cambridge: Cambridge University Press.

Bogousslavsky J, Regli F, Delaloye B, et al. (1986) [Hemiataxia and ipsilateral sensory deficit. Infarct in the territory of the anterior choroidal artery. Crossed cerebellar diaschisis.] *Rev Neurol* 142: 671–6 (French).

Bojinova V, Dimova P, Belopitova L (2000) Clinical manifestations of cerebrovascular hypoplasias in childhood. *J Child Neurol* 15: 166–71.

Bousser MG, Chiras J, Bories J, Castaigne P (1985) Cerebral venous thrombosis: a review of 38 cases. *Stroke* 16: 199–213.

Bowen MD, Burak CR, Barron TF, et al. (2005) Childhood ischemic stroke in a nonurban population. *J Child Neurol* 20: 194–7.

Brankovic-Sreckovic V, Milic-Rasic V, Jovic N, et al. (2004) The recurrence risk of ischemic stroke in childhood. *Med Princ Pract* 13: 153–8.

Brant-Zawadzki M, Chang GY, McCarty GE (1982) Computed tomography in dural sinus thrombosis. *Arch Neurol* 39: 446–7.

Brett EM (1997) Vascular disorders of the nervous system in childhood. In: Brett EM, ed. *Paediatric Neurology, 3rd edn.* Edinburgh: Churchill Livingstone, pp. 571–88.

Brisman JL, Song JK, Newell DW (2006) Cerebral aneurysms. *N Engl J Med* 355: 928–39.

Buis DR, Van den Berg R, Lycklama G, et al. (2004) Spontaneous regression of brain arteriovenous malformation—a clinical study and review of the literature. *J Neurol* 251: 1375–82.

Bush JK, Givner LB, Whitaker SH, et al. (1984) Necrotizing fasciitis of the parapharyngeal space with carotid artery occlusion and acute hemiplegia. *Pediatrics* 73: 343–7.

Caekebeke JFV, Peters ACB, Vandvik B, et al. (1990) Cerebral vasculopathy associated with primary varicella infection. *Arch Neurol* 47: 1033–5.

Camacho A, Villarejo A, de Aragon AM, et al. (2001) Spontaneous carotid and vertebral dissection in children. *Pediatr Neurol* 25: 250–3.

Camacho DI, Smith JK, Gimme JD, et al. (2004) Atypical MR imaging perfusion in developmental venous anomalies. *AJNR* 25: 1549–52.

Castaigne P, Lhermitte F, Gautier JC, et al. (1973) Arterial occlusion in the vertebro-basilar system. A study of 44 patients with post-mortem data. *Brain* 96: 133–54.

Celli P, Ferrante L, Palma L (1984) Cerebral arteriovenous malformations in children. Clinical features and outcome of treatment in children and adults. *Surg Neurol* 22: 43–9.

Cerebral Embolism Task Force (1986) Cardiogenic brain embolism. *Arch Neurol* 43: 71–84.

Chabriat H, Tournier-Lasserve E, Vahedi K, et al. (1995a) Autosomal dominant migraine with MRI white-matter abnormalities mapping to the CADASIL locus. *Neurology* 45: 1086–91.

Chabriat H, Vahedi K, Iba-Zizen MT, et al. (1995b) Clinical spectrum of CADASIL: a study of 7 families. *Lancet* 346: 934–9.

Chabrier S, Rodesch J, Lasjaunias P, et al. (1998) Transient cerebral arteriopathy: a disorder recognized by serial angiograms in children with stroke. *J Child Neurol* 13: 27–32.

Chabrier S, Husson B, Lasjaunias P, et al. (2000) Stroke in childhood: outcome and recurrence risk in 59 patients. *J Child Neurol* 15: 290–4.

Chabrier S, Lasjaunias P, Husson B, et al. (2003) Ischaemic stroke from dissection of the craniocervical arteries: Report of 12 patients. *Eur J Paediatr Neurol* 7: 39–42.

Chalhub EG, De Vivo DC, Siegel BA, et al. (1977) Coxsackie A9 focal encephalitis associated with acute infantile hemiplegia and porencephaly. *Neurology* 27: 574–9.

Chalmers EA (2005) Perinatal stroke: risk factors and management. *Br J Haematol* 130: 333–43.

Chan AK, deVeber G (2000) Prothrombotic disorders and ischemic stroke in children. *Semin Pediatr Neurol* 7: 301–8.

Chan AK, deVeber G, Monagle P, et al. (2003) Venous thrombosis in children. *J Thromb Haemost* 1: 1443–55.

Chatkupt S, Epstein LG, Rappaport R, Koenigsberger MR (1987) Cerebellar infarction in children. *Pediatr Neurol* 3: 363–6.

Chisholm CA, Kuller JA, Katz VL, McCoy MC (1996) Aneurysm of the vein of Galen: prenatal diagnosis and perinatal management. *Am J Perinatol* 13: 503–6.

Chiu NC, DeLong GR, Heinz ER (1996) Intracranial fibromuscular dysplasia in a 5-year-old child. *Pediatr Neurol* 14: 262–4.

Chuang S (1989) Vascular diseases of the brain in children. In: Edwards MSB, Hoffman HJ, eds. *Cerebral Vascular Disease in Children and Adolescents.* Baltimore: Williams & Wilkins, pp. 69–93.

Churchyard A, Khangure M, Grainger K (1992) Cerebral cavernous angioma: a potentially benign condition? Successful treatment in 16 cases. *J Neurol Neurosurg Psychiatry* 55: 1040–5.

Clatterbuck RE, Elmaci I, Rigamonti D (2001) The juxtaposition of a capillary telangiectasia, cavernous malformation, and developmental venous anomaly in the brainstem of a single patient: case report. *Neurosurgery* 49: 1246–50.

Cognard C, Casasco A, Toevi M, et al. (1998) Dural arteriovenous fistulas as a cause of intracranial hypertension due to impairment of cranial venous outflow. *J Neurol Neurosurg Psychiatry* 65: 308–16.

Cowan F, Mercuri E, Groenendaal F, et al. (2005) Does cranial ultrasound imaging identify arterial cerebral infarction in term neonates? *Arch Dis Child Fetal Neonatal Ed* 90: F252–6.

Cranberg LD, Filley CM, Hart EJ, Alexander MP (1987) Acquired aphasia in childhood: clinical and CT investigations. *Neurology* 37: 1165–72.

Crawford PM, West CR, Chadwick DW, Shaw MDM (1986) Arteriovenous malformations of the brain: natural history in unoperated patients. *J Neurol Neurosurg Psychiatry* 49: 1–10.

Criscuolo GR, Oldfield EH, Doppman JL (1989) Reversible acute and subacute myelopathy in patients with dural arteriovenous fistulas. Foix–Alajouanine syndrome reconsidered. *J Neurosurg* 70: 354–9.

Danchaivijitr N, Cox TC, Saunders DE, Ganesan V (2006) Evolution of cerebral arteriopathies in childhood arterial ischemic stroke. *Ann Neurol* 59: 620–6.

d'Avella D, Russo A, Santoro G, et al. (1984) Diagnosis of superior sagittal sinus thrombosis by computerized tomography. Report of two cases. *J Neurosurg* 61: 1129–31.

Debehnke DJ, Singer JI (1991) Vertebrobasilar occlusion following minor trauma in an 8-year-old boy. *Am J Emerg Med* 9: 49–51.

Decroix JP, Graveleau P, Masson M, Cambier J (1986) Infarction in the territory of the anterior choroidal artery. A clinical and computerized tomographic study of 16 cases. *Brain* 109: 1071–85.

DeBaun MR, Schatz J, Siegel MJ, et al. (1998) Cognitive screening examinations for silent cerebral infarcts in sickle cell disease. *Neurology* 50: 1678–82.

Del Giudice E, Aicardi J (1979) Atypical aspects of hypertensive encephalopathy in childhood. *Neuropediatrics* 10: 150–7.

de Montalembert M, Belloy M, Bernaudin F, et al. (1997) Three-year follow-up of hydroxyurea treatment in severely ill children with sickle cell disease.

The French Study Group on Sickle Cell Disease. *J Pediatr Hematol Oncol* 19: 313–8.

Denier C, Goutagny S, Labauge P, et al. (2004a) Mutations within the MCG 4607 gene cause cerebral cavernous malformations. *Am J Hum Genet* 74: 326–37.

Denier C, Labauge P, Brunereau J, et al. (2004b) Clinical features of cerebral cavernous malformation patients with KRIT1 mutations. *Ann Neurol* 55: 213–20.

Denier C, Labauge P, Bergametti F, et al. (2006) Genotype–phenotype correlations in cerebral cavernous malformations patients. *Ann Neurol* 60: 550–6.

deVeber G, Andrew M, Adams C, et al. (2001) Cerebral sinovenous thrombosis in children. *N Engl J Med* 345: 417–23.

De Vries LS, Van der Grond J, Van Haastert JC, Groenendaal F (2005) Prediction of outcome in new-born infants with arterial ischaemic stroke using diffusion-weighted magnetic resonance imaging. *Neuropediatrics* 36: 12–20.

Di Rocco C, Iannelli A, Tamburrini G (1997) Cavernous angiomas of the brain stem in children. *Pediatr Neurosurg* 27: 92–9.

Di Rocco C, Tamburrini G, Rollo M (2000) Cerebral arteriovenous malformations in children. *Acta Neurochir* 142: 145–56.

Drigo P, Mammi I, Battistella PA, et al. (1994) Familial cerebral, hepatic, and retinal cavernous angioma: a new syndrome. *Childs Nerv Syst* 10: 205–9.

Drolet BA, Dohl M, Golomb MR, et al. (2006) Early stroke and cerebral vasculopathy in children with facial hemangiomas and PHACE association. *Pediatrics* 117: 259–64.

Duffau H, Lopes M, Janosevic V, et al. (1999) Early rebleeding from intracranial dural arteriovenous fistulas: report of 20 cases and review of the literature. *J Neurosurg* 90: 78–84.

Dulac O, Aicardi J (1975) [Paraplegia complicating umbilical artery catheterization.] *Arch Fr Pediatr* 32: 659–64 (French).

Duong M, Wenger J (2005) Lemierre syndrome. *J Pediatr Emerg Care* 21: 589–93.

Dusser A, Goutières F, Aicardi J (1986) Ischemic strokes in children. *J Child Neurol* 1: 131–6.

Dusser A, Boyer-Neumann C, Wolf M (1988) Temporary protein C deficiency associated with cerebral arterial thrombosis in childhood. *J Pediatr* 113: 849–51.

Echenne B, Gras M, Astruc J, et al. (1983) Vertebrobasilar arterial occlusion in childhood. Report of a case and review of the literature. *Brain Dev* 5: 577–81.

Edwards MSB, Hieshima GB, Higashida RT, Halbach VV (1988) Management of vein of Galen malformations in the neonate. *Int Pediatr* 3: 184–8.

Eeg-Olofsson O, Ringheim Y (1983) Stroke in children: clinical characteristics and prognosis. *Acta Paediatr Scand* 72: 391–6.

Essig M, Wenz F, Schoenberg SO, et al. (2000) Arteriovenous malformations: assessment of gliotic and ischemic changes with fluid-attenuated inversion–recovery MRI. *Invest Radiol* 35: 689–94.

Fabian RH, Peters BH (1984) Neurological complications of hemoglobin SC disease. *Arch Neurol* 41: 289–2.

Fasulakis S, Andronikou S (2003) Comparison of MR angiography and conventional angiography in the investigation of intracranial arteriovenous malformations and aneurysms in children. *Pediatr Radiol* 33: 378–84.

Fearnley JM, Stevens JM, Rudge P (1995) Superficial siderosis of the central nervous system. *Brain* 118: 1051–66.

Ferch RD, Morgan MK, Sears WR (2001) Spinal arteriovenous malformations: a review with case illustrations. *J Clin Neurosci* 8: 299–304.

Ferro JM, Martins IP, Castro-Caldas FPA (1982) Aphasia following right striato-insular infarction in a left-handed child: a clinico-radiological study. *Dev Med Child Neurol* 24: 173–8.

Filling-Katz MR, Levin SW, Patronas NJ, Katz NNK (1992) Terminal transverse limb defects associated with familial cavernous angiomatosis. *Am J Med Genet* 42: 346–51.

Forman HP, Levin S, Stewart B, et al. (1989) Cerebral vasculitis and hemorrhage in an adolescent taking diet pills containing phenylpropanolamine: case report and review of literature. *Pediatrics* 83: 737–41.

Forsting M, Krieger D, Seier U, Hacke W (1989) Reversible bilateral thalamic lesions caused by primary internal cerebral vein thrombosis: a case report. *J Neurol* 236: 484–6.

Freedom RM (1989) Cerebral vascular disorders of cardiovascular origin in infants and children. In: Edwards MSB, Hoffman HJ, eds. *Cerebral Vascular Disease in Children and Adolescents.* Baltimore: Williams & Wilkins, pp. 423–8.

Fujiwara J, Nakahara S, Enomoto T, et al. (1996) The effectiveness of O_2 administration for transient ischemic attacks in moyamoya disease in children. *Childs Nerv Syst* 12: 69–75.

Fukuyama Y, Osawa M, Kanai M (1992) Moyamoya disease (syndrome) and the Down syndrome. *Brain Dev* 14: 254–6.

Fullerton H, Johnson SC, Smith WS (2001) Arterial dissection and stroke in children. *Neurology* 57: 1155–60

Fults D, Kelly DL (1984) Natural history of arteriovenous malformations of the brain: a clinical study. *Neurosurgery* 15: 658–62.

Fung LW, Thompson D, Ganesan V (2005) Revascularization surgery for paediatric moyamoya: a review. *Childs Nerv Syst* 21: 358–64.

Furlan AJ, Breuer AC (1984) Central nervous system complications of open heart surgery. *Stroke* 15: 912–5.

Gabow PA (1993) Autosomal dominant polycystic kidney disease. *N Engl J Med* 329: 332–42.

Ganesan V, Chong WK, Cox TC, et al. (2002) Posterior circulation stroke in childhood: risk factors and recurrence. *Neurology* 59: 1552–6.

Ganesan V, Prengler M, McShane MA, et al. (2003) Investigation of risk factors in children with arterial ischemic stroke. *Ann Neurol* 53: 167–73.

Garcia-Monaco R, De Victor D, Mann C, et al. (1991a) Congestive cardiac manifestations from cerebrocranial arteriovenous shunts. Endovascular management in 30 children. *Childs Nerv Syst* 7: 48–52.

Garcia-Monaco R, Rodesch G, Terbrugge K, et al. (1991b) Multifocal dural arteriovenous shunts in children. *Childs Nerv Syst* 7: 425–31.

Garel C, Azarian M, Lasjaunias P, Luton D (2005) Pial arteriovenous fistulas: dilemmas in prenatal diagnosis, counselling and postnatal treatment. Report of three cases. *Ultrasound Obstet Gynecol* 26: 293–6.

Garg BP, DeMyer WE (1995) Ischemic thalamic infarction in children: clinical presentation, etiology, and outcome. *Pediatr Neurol* 13: 46–9.

Garg BP, Edwards-Brown MK (1995) Vertebral artery compression due to head rotation in thalamic stroke. *Pediatr Neurol* 12: 162–4.

Garg BP, Ottinger CJ, Smith RR, Fishman MA (1993) Strokes in children due to vertebral artery trauma. *Neurology* 43: 2555–8.

Garner TB, Curling OD, Kelly DL, Laster DW (1991) The natural history of intracranial venous angiomas. *J Neurosurg* 75: 715–22.

Gauvrit JY, Leclerc X, Oppenheim C, et al. (2005) Three-dimensional dynamic MR digital subtraction angiography using sensitivity encoding for the evaluation of intracranial arterivenuos malformations: a preliminary study. *AJNR* 26: 1525–31.

Gebara BM, Goetting MG, Wang AM (1995) Dural sinus thrombosis complicating subclavian vein catheterization: treatment with local thrombolysis. *Pediatrics* 95: 138–40.

Giroud M, Lemerle M, Madinier G, et al. (1997) Stroke in children under 16 years of age. Clinical and etiological differences with adults. *Acta Neurol Scand* 96: 401–6.

Giuffre R, Sherkat S (2000) Maldevelopmental pathology of the vertebral artery in infancy and childhood. *Childs Nerv Syst* 18: 627–32.

Glauser TA, Siegel MJ, Lee BC, et al. (1995) Accuracy of neurologic examination and history in detecting evidence of MRI-diagnosed cerebral infarctions in children with sickle cell hemoglobinopathy. *J Child Neurol* 10: 88–92.

Göbel U (1994) Inherited or acquired disorders of blood coagulation in children with neurovascular complications. *Neuropediatrics* 25: 4–7.

Golden GS (1985) Stroke syndromes in childhood. *Neurol Clin* 3: 59–65.

Golomb MR, Dick PT, MacGregor DL, et al. (2004) Neonatal arterial ischemic stroke and cranial sinus venous thrombosis are more commonly diagnosed in boys. *J Child Neurol* 19: 493–7.

Golomb MR, Saha C, Garg BP, et al. (2007) Association of cerebral palsy with other disabilities in children with perinatal arterial ischemic stroke. *Pediatr Neurol* 37: 245–9.

Gomori JM, Grossman RI, Hackney DB, et al. (1988) Variable appearance of subacute intracranial hematomas on high-field spin-echo MR. *Am J Roentgenol* 150: 171–8.

Gordon N, Isler W (1989) Childhood moyamoya disease. *Dev Med Child Neurol* 31: 103–7.

Greenwood RD (1984) Mitral valve prolapse. Incidence and clinical course in a pediatric population. *Clin Pediatr* 23: 318–20.

Griffiths PD, Hoggard N, Warren DJ, et al. (2000) Brain arteriovenous malformations: assessment with dynamic MR digital subtraction angiography. *AJNR* 21: 1892–9.

Grossman RJ, Bruce DA, Zimmerman RA, et al. (1984) Vascular steal associated with vein of Galen aneurysm. *Neuroradiology* 26: 381–6.

Grossman RJ, Novak G, Patel M, et al. (1993) MRI in neonatal dural sinus thrombosis. *Pediatr Neurol* 9: 235–8.

Grosso S, Mostardini R, Venturi C, et al. (2002) Recurrent torticollis caused by dissecting vertebral artery aneurysm in a pediatric patient: results of endovascular treatment by use of coil embolization: case report. *Neurosurgery* 50: 204–7.

Guazzo EP, Xuereb JH (1994) Spontaneous thrombosis of an arteriovenous malformation. *J Neurol Neurosurg Psychiatry* 57: 1410–2.

Guidi B, Bergonzini P, Crisi G, et al. (2003) Case of stroke in a 7-year-old male after parvovirus B19 infection. *Pediatr Neurol* 28: 69–71.

Guzeloglu-Kayisli O, Amankulor NM, Voorhees J, et al. (2004) KRIT1/cerebral cavernous malformation 1 protein localizes in vascular endothelium, astrocytes, and pyramidal cells in the adult human cerebral cortex. *Neurosurgery* 54: 943–9.

Haan J, Caekebeke JFV, Van der Meer FJM, Wintzen AR (1988) Cerebral venous thrombosis as presenting sign of myeloproliferative disorders. *J Neurol Neurosurg Psychiatry* 51: 1219–20.

Hallam DK, Russell EJ (1998) Imaging of angiographically occult cerebral vascular malformations. *Neuroimaging Clin N Am* 8: 323–47.

Haas RH, Marsden DL, Capistrano-Estrada S, et al. (1995) Acute basal ganglia infarction in propionic acidemia. *J Child Neurol* 10: 18–22.

Hamilton MG, Spetzler RE (1994) The prospective application of a grading system for arteriovenous malformations. *Neurosurgery* 34: 2–7.

Hanefeld F, Riehm H (1980) Therapy of acute lymphoblastic leukaemia in childhood: effects on the nervous system. *Neuropädiatrie* 11: 3–16.

Hankins J, Jeng M, Harris S, et al. (2005a) Chronic transfusion therapy for children with sickle cell disease and recurrent acute chest syndrome. *J Pediatr Hematol Oncol* 27: 158–61.

Hankins JS, Ware RE, Rogers ZR, et al. (2005b) Long-term hydroxyurea therapy for infants with with sickle cell anemia: the HUSOFT extension study. *Blood* 106: 2269–75.

Harms MM, Rotteveel JJ, Kar NC, Gabreëls FJ (2000) Recurrent alternating facial paralysis and malignant hypertension. *Neuropediatrics* 31: 318–20.

Hartfield DS, Lowry NS, Keene DL, Yager JY (1997) Iron deficiency: a cause of stroke in infants and children. *Pediatr Neurol* 16: 50–3.

Helgason CM (1988) A new view of anterior choroidal artery territory infarction. *J Neurol* 235: 387–91.

Helgason CM, Caplan LR, Goodwin J, Hedges T (1986) Anterior choroidal artery-territory infarction. Report of cases and review. *Arch Neurol* 43: 681–6.

Helgason CM, Bergen D, Bleck TP, et al. (1987) Infarction after surgery for focal epilepsy: manipulation hemiplegia revisited. *Epilepsia* 28: 340–5.

Heller C, Heinecken A, Junker R, et al. (2003) Cerebral venous thrombosis in children: a multifactorial origin. *Circulation* 106: 1362–7.

Helweg-Larsen S, Larsson H, Henriksen O, Sorensen PS (1988) Ataxic hemiparesis: three different locations of lesions studied by MRI. *Neurology* 38: 1322–4.

Heros RC, Korosue K, Diebold PM (1990) Surgical excision of arteriovenous malformations: late results. *Neurosurgery* 25: 570–8.

Heudes AM, Boullie MC, Lauret P, Mallet E (1990) [Neonatal miliary haemangioma.] *Arch Fr Pediatr* 47: 135–8 (French).

Higashida RT, Helmer E, Halbach VV, Hieshima GB (1989) Direct thrombolytic therapy for superior sagittal sinus thrombosis. *AJNR* 10: 54–6.

Hladky J-P, Lejeune J-P, Blond S, et al. (1994) Cerebral arteriovenous malformations in children: report on 62 cases. *Childs Nerv Syst* 10: 328–33.

Hoffman HJ (1989) Malformations of the vein of Galen. In: Edwards MSB, Hoffman HJ, eds. *Cerebral Vascular Disease in Children and Adolescents.* Baltimore: Williams & Wilkins, pp. 239–46.

Horton DP, Ferriero DM, Mentzer WC (1995) Nontraumatic fat embolism syndrome in sickle cell anemia. *Pediatr Neurol* 12: 77–80.

Hosain SA, Hughes JT, Forem SL, et al. (1994) Use of a calcium channel blocker (nicardipine HCl) in the treatment of childhood moyamoya disease. *J Child Neurol* 9: 378–80.

Hourihan M, Gates PC, McAllister VL (1984) Subarachnoid hemorrhage in childhood and adolescence. *J Neurosurg* 60: 1163–6.

Howard RS (1986) Brainstem haematoma due to presumed cryptic telangiectasia. *J Neurol Neurosurg Psychiatry* 49: 1241–5.

Hulse JA, Taylor DS, Dillon MJ (1979) Blindness and paraplegia in severe childhood hypertension. *Lancet* 2: 553–6.

Humphreys RP (1989) Infratentorial arteriovenous malformations. In: Edwards MSD, Hoffman HJ, eds. *Cerebral Vascular Disease in Children and Adolescents.* Baltimore: Williams & Wilkins, pp. 309–20.

Hurst RW, Kenyon LC, Lavi E, et al. (1995) Spinal dural arteriovenous fistula: the pathology of venous hypertensive myelopathy. *Neurology* 45: 1309–13.

Husson B, Lasjaunias P (2004) Radiological approach to disorders of arterial brain infarcts: a comparison between MRA and and contrast angiography. *Pediatr Radiol* 34: 10–5.

Husson B, Rodesch G, Lasjaunias P, et al. (2002) Magnetic resonance angiography in childhood arterial brain infarcts: a comparison study with contrast angiography. *Stroke* 33: 1280–5.

Huttenlocher PR, Moohr JW, Johns L, Brown FD (1984) Cerebral blood flow in sickle cell cerebrovascular disease. *Pediatrics* 73: 615–21.

Ichikawa K, Tsutsumishita A, Fujioka A (1982) Capsular ataxic hemiparesis. A case report. *Arch Neurol* 39: 585–6.

Igarashi M, Roy S, Stapleton FB (1988) Cerebrovascular complications in children with nephrotic syndrome. *Pediatr Neurol* 4: 362–5.

Imaizumi T, Hayashi K, Saito K, et al. (1998) Long-term outcomes of pediatric moyamoya disease monitored to adulhood. *Pediatr Neurol* 18: 321–5.

Imamura A, Matsuo N, Ariki M, et al. (2004) MR imaging on 1H-MR spectroscopy in a case of cerebral infarction with transient cerebral arteriopathy. *Brain Dev* 20: 535–8.

Inagaki M, Koeda T, Takeshita K (1992) Prognosis and MRI after ischemic stroke of the basal ganglia. *Pediatr Neurol* 8: 104–8.

Isensee C, Reul J, Thron A (1994) Magnetic resonance imaging of thrombosed dural sinuses. *Stroke* 25: 29–34.

Ishikawa T, Houkin K, Kamiyama T, et al (1997) Effect of surgical revascularization on outcome in patients with pediatric moyamoya disease. *Stroke* 28: 1170–3.

Isler W (1984) Stroke in childhood and adolescence. *Eur Neurol* 23: 421–4.

Ito S, Miyazaki H, Iino N, et al (2005) Unilateral agenesis and hypoplasia of the internal carotid artery: a report of three cases. *Neuroradiology* 47: 311–5.

Izawa M, Hayashi M, Chernov M, et al. (2005) Long-term complications after gamma knife surgery for arteriovenous malformations. *J Neurosurg* 102 Suppl: 34–7.

Jackson AC, Boughner DR, Barnett HJM (1984) Mitral valve prolapse and cerebral ischemic events in young patients. *Neurology* 34: 784–7.

Jacobson DM, Terrence CF, Reinmuth OM (1986) The neurologic manifestations of fat embolism. *Neurology* 36: 847–51.

Jansen JN, Donker AJM, Luth WJ, Smit ME (1990) Moyamoya disease associated with renovascular hypertension. *Neuropediatrics* 21: 44–7.

Jellema K, Tijssen CC, van Gijn J (2006) Spinal dural areriovenous fistulas: a congestive myelopathy that initially mimics a peripheral nerve disorder. *Brain* 129: 3150–64.

Jellinger K, Kucsko L, Seitelberger F (1966) [Diffuse meningo-cerebral angiodysplasia with hypoplasiogenic isthmus stenosis in a newborn infant.] *Beitr Pathol Anat* 133: 41–72 (German).

Johnston SC, Wilson CB, Halbach VV, et al. (2000) Endovascular and surgical treatment of unruptured cerebral aneurysms: comparison of risks. *Ann Neurol* 48: 11–9.

Joy JL, Carlo JR, Vélez-Borrás JR (1989) Cerebral infarction following herpes zoster: the enlarging clinical spectrum. *Neurology* 39: 1640–3.

Kandt RS, Caoili AQ, Lorentz WB, Elster AD (1995) Hypertensive encephalopathy in children: neuroimaging and treatment. *J Child Neurol* 10: 236–9.

Kappelle LJ, Willemse J, Ramos LMP, Van Gijn J (1989) Ischaemic stroke in the basal ganglia and internal capsule in childhood. *Brain Dev* 11: 283–92.

Kataoka K, Okuno T, Mikawa H, Hojo H (1988) Cranial computed tomographic and electroencephalographic abnormalities in children with post-convulsive hemiplegia. *Eur Neurol* 28: 279–84.

Kattapong VJ, Hart BL, Davis LE (1995) Familial cerebral cavernous angiomas: clinical and radiologic studies. *Neurology* 45: 492–7.

Kennedy CR, Warner G, Kai M, Chisholm M (1995) Protein C deficiency and stroke in early life. *Dev Med Child Neurol* 37: 723–30.

Khurana DS, Bonnemann CG, Dooling EC, et al. (1996) Vertebral artery dissection: issues in diagnosis and management. *Pediatr Neurol* 14: 255–8.

Kirkham FJ, DeBaun MR (2004) Stroke in children with sickle cell disease. *Curr Treat Options Neurol* 6: 357–75.

Kirkham FJ, Hogan AM (2004) Risk factors for arterial ischemic stroke in childhood. *CNS Spectr* 9: 454–64.

Kirkham FJ, Calamante F, Bynevelt M, et al. (2001) Perfusion magnetic resonance abnormalities in patients with sickle cell disease. *Ann Neurol* 49: 477–85.

Kitaguchi H, Tomimata H, Miki Y, et al. (2005) A brainstem variant of posterior leukoencephalopathy syndrome. *Neuroradiology* 47: 652–6.

Klein RA, Snyder RD, Schwarz HJ (1976) Lateral medullary syndrome in a child. Arteriographic confirmation of vertebral artery occlusion. *JAMA* 235: 940–1.

Koelfen W, Wentz U, Freund M, Schultze C (1995) Magnetic resonance angiography in 140 neuropediatric patients. *Pediatr Neurol* 12: 31–8.

Koenig E, Thron A, Schrader V, Dichgans J (1989) Spinal arteriovenous malformations and fistulae: clinical, neuroradiological and neurophysiological findings. *J Neurol* 236: 260–6.

Kondziolka D, Humphreys RP, Hoffman HJ, et al. (1992) Arteriovenous malformations of the brain in children: a forty-year experience. *Can J Neurol Sci* 19: 40–5.

Konishi Y, Kuriyama M, Sudo M, et al. (1987) Superior sagittal thrombosis in infancy. *Pediatr Neurol* 3: 222–5.

Konovalov AN, Pitskhelauri DI, Arutionnov NV (2002) Surgical treatment of thrombosed vein of Galen aneurysm. *Acta Neurochir* 144: 909–15.

Krings T, Ozanne A, Chng SM, et al. (2005) Neurovascular phenotypes in hereditary hemorrhagic telangiectasia patients according to age. Review of 50 consecutive patients aged 1 day–60 years. *Neuroradiology* 47: 711–20.

Kuivaniemi H, Prockop DJ, Wu Y, et al. (1993) Exclusion of mutations in the gene for type III collagen (COL3AI) as a common cause of intracranial aneurysms or cervical artery dissections. Results from sequence analysis of the coding sequences of type III collagen from 55 unrelated patients. *Neurology* 43: 2652–8.

Kurnik K, Kosch A, Strater R, et al. (2003) Recurrent thromboembolism in infants and children suffering from symptomatic neonatal arterial stroke: a prospective follow-up study. *Stroke* 34: 2892–3.

Kurul S, Cakmakçi H, Kovanlikaya A, Dirik E (2001) The benign course of carotid–cavernous fistula in a child. *Eur J Radiol* 39: 77–9.

Labauge P, Brunereau I, Levy C, et al. (2000) The natural history of familial cerebral cavernomas: a retrospective MRI study of 40 patients. *Neuroradiology* 42: 327–32.

Labrune P, Lacroix C, Goutières F, et al. (1996) Extensive brain calcifications, leukodystrophy, and formation of parenchymal cysts: a new progressive disorder due to diffuse cerebral microangiopathy. *Neurology* 46: 1297–301.

Lamy C, Oppenheimer C, Meder JF, Max JL (2004) Neuroimaging in posterior leukoencephalopathy syndrome. *J Neuroimaging* 14: 89–96.

Lanska MJ, Lanska DJ, Horwitz SJ, Aram DM (1991) Presentation, clinical course, and outcome of childhood stroke. *Pediatr Neurol* 7: 333–41.

Lanthier S (2002) Primary angiitis of the central nervous system in children: 10 cases proven by biopsy. *J Rheumatol* 29: 1575–6.

Lanthier S, Carmant L, David M, et al. (2000) Stroke in children: the coexistence of multiple risk factors predicts poor outcome. *Neurology* 54: 371–8.

Lanthier S, Lortie A, Michaud J, et al. (2001) Isolated angiitis of the CNS in children. *Neurology* 56: 837–42.

Lanthier S, Armstrong D, Domi T, deVeber G (2005) Post-varicella arteriopathy of childhood: natural history of vascular stenosis. *Neurology* 64: 660–3.

Larsen PD, Hellbusch LC, Lefkowitz DH, Schaefer GB (1997) Cerebral arteriovenous malformation in three successive generations. *Pediatr Neurol* 17: 74–6.

Lasjaunias P, Lopez-Ibor L, Abanou A, Halimi P (1984) Radiological anatomy of the vascularization of cranial dural arteriovenous malformations. *Anat Clin* 6: 87–99.

Lasjaunias P, Rodesch G, Pruvost P, et al. (1989a) Treatment of vein of Galen aneurysmal malformation. *J Neurosurg* 70: 746–50.

Lasjaunias P, Rodesch G, Terbrugge K, et al. (1989b) Vein of Galen aneurysmal malformations. Report of 36 cases managed between 1982 and 1988. *Acta Neurochir* 99: 26–37.

Lasjaunias P, Garcia-Monaco R, Rodesch G, et al. (1991a) Vein of Galen malformation. Endovascular management of 43 cases. *Childs Nerv Syst* 7: 360–7.

Lasjaunias P, Terbrugge K, Rodesch G, et al. (1991b) [True and false cerebral venous malformations. Venous pseudo-angiomas and cavernous hemangiomas.] *Neurochirurgie* 35: 132–9 (French).

Lasjaunias P, Hui, F., Zerah, M., et al. (1995) Cerebral arteriovenous malformations in children. Management of 179 consecutive cases and review of the literature. *Childs Nerv Syst* 11: 66–79.

Lasjaunias P, Wuppalapati S, Alvarez H, et al (2005) Intracranial aneurysms in children aged under 15 years: review of 59 consecutive children with 75 aneurysms. *Childs Nerv Syst* 21: 437–50.

Lasjaunias PL, Chng SM, Sachet M, et al (2006) The management of vein of Galen aneurismal malformations. *Neurosurgery* 59 (5 Suppl 3): S184–94; erratum 2007 60 (4 Suppl 2): 393.

Laurans MS, DiLuna ML, Shin D, et al. (2003) Mutational analysis of 206 families with cavernous malformations. *J Neurosurg* 99: 38–43.

Leblanc R, Melanson D, Wilkinson RD (1996) Hereditary neurocutaneous angiomatosis. Report of four cases. *J Neurosurg* 86: 1135–42.

Le Coz P, Woimant F, Rougemont D, et al. (1988) [Benign cerebral angiopathies and phenylpropanolamine.] *Rev Neurol* 144 : 295–300.

Lee J, Croen LA, Backstrand KH, et al. (2005a) Maternal and infant characteristics associated with perinatal arterial stroke in the infant. *JAMA* 293: 723–9.

Lee J, Croen LA, Lindan C, et al. (2005b) Predictors of outcome in perinatal arterial stroke: a population-based study. *Ann Neurol* 58: 303–8.

Leis AA, Butler IJ (1987) Infantile herpes zoster ophthalmicus and acute hemiparesis following intrauterine chickenpox. *Neurology* 37: 1537–8.

Lemme-Plaghos L, Kucharczyk W, Brant-Zawadzki M, et al. (1986) MRI of angiographically occult vascular malformations. *Am J Roentgenol* 146: 1223–8.

Levine SR, Welch KMA (1988) Cocaine and stroke. *Stroke* 19: 779–83.

Levine SR, Deegan MJ, Futrell N, Welch KMA (1990) Cerebrovascular and neurologic disease associated with antiphospholipid antibodies: 48 cases. *Neurology* 40: 1181–9.

Loeffler IS, Rossitch E, Siddon R, et al. (1990) Role of stereotactic radiosurgery with a linear accelerator in treatment of intracranial arteriovenous malformations and tumors in children. *Pediatrics* 85: 774–82.

Lynch JK, Han CJ, Nee LE, Nelson KE (2005) Prothrombic factors in children with stroke or porencephaly. *Pediatrics* 116: 442–53.

Maity A, Shu HK, Tan JE, et al. (2004) Treatment of pediatric arteriovenous malformations with linear accelerator-based stereotactic radiosurgery: the University of Pennsylvania experience. *Pediatr Neurosurg* 40: 207–14.

Mangiardi JR, Daras M, Geller ME, et al. (1988) Cocaine-related hemorrhage: report of nine cases and review. *Acta Neurol Scand* 77: 177–80.

Martin NA, Edwards MSB (1989) Supratentorial arteriovenous malformations. In: Edwards MBS, Hoffman HJ, eds. *Cerebral Vascular Disease in Children and Adolescents.* Baltimore: Williams & Wilkins, pp. 283–308.

Martinelli I, Sacchi E, Landi G, et al. (1998) High risk of cerebral-vein thrombosis in carriers of a prothrombin-gene mutation and in users of oral contraceptives. *N Engl J Med* 338: 1793–7.

Maruyama K, Kawahara N, Shin M, et al. (2005) The risk of hemorrhage after radiosurgery for cerebral arteriovenous malformations. *N Engl J Med* 352: 146–53.

Mathieson T, Elner G, Kihlstrom I (2003) Deep and brainstem cavernomas: a consecutive eight-year series. *J Neurosurg* 99: 1115–7.

McArdle CB, Mirfakhraee M, Amparo EG, Kulkarni MV (1987) MR imaging of transverse/sigmoid dural sinus and jugular vein thrombosis. *J Comput Assist Tomogr* 11: 831–8.

McCormick WF (1984) Pathology of vascular malformations of the brain. In: Wilson CB, Stein BM, eds. *Intracranial Arteriovenous Malformations.* Baltimore: Williams & Wilkins, pp. 44–63.

Mehler ME (1988) The neuro-ophthalmologic spectrum of the rostral basilar artery syndrome. *Arch Neurol* 45: 966–71.

Mendelow AD, Erfurth A, Grossart K, McPherson P (1987) Do cerebral arteriovenous malformations increase in size? *J Neurol Neurosurg Psychiatry* 50: 980–7.

Meyer FB, Sundt TM, Fode NC, et al. (1989) Cerebral aneurysms in childhood and adolescence. *J Neurosurg* 70: 420–5.

Miller SP, O'Gorman AM, Shevell ML (2000) Recurrent artery of Heubner infarction in infancy. *Dev Med Child Neurol* 42: 344–6.

Mineharu Y, Takanaka K, Yamakawa H, et al (2006) Inheritance pattern of familial moyamoya disease: autosomal dominant mode and genetic imprinting. *J Neurol Neurosurg Psychiatry* 77: 1025–9.

Mintz M, Epstein LG, Koenigsberger MR (1992) Idiopathic childhood stroke is associated with human leucocyte antigen (HLA)-B51. *Ann Neurol* 31: 675–7.

Mitchell WG, Fishman LS, Miller JH, et al. (1991) Stroke as a late sequela of cranial irradiation for childhood brain tumors. *J Child Neurol* 6: 128–33.

Montalban J, Ibanez L, Rodriguez C, et al. (1989) Cerebral infarction after excessive use of nasal decongestants. *J Neurol Neurosurg Psychiatry* 52: 541–2.

Moore PM (1989) Diagnosis and management of isolated angiitis of the central nervous system. *Neurology* 39: 167–73.

Morales E, Pineda C, Martínez-Lavín M (1991) Takayasu's arteritis in children. *J Rheumatol* 18: 1081–4.

Morita A, Meyer FB, Nichols DA, Patterson MC (1995) Childhood dural arteriovenous fistulae of the posterior dural sinuses: three case reports and literature review. *Neurosurgery* 37: 193–9.

Mottolese C, Hermier M, Stan H, et al. (2001) Central nervous system cavernomas in the pediatric age group. *Neurosurg Rev* 24: 55–71.

Moulin T, Bogousslavsky J, Chopard JL, et al. (1995) Vascular ataxic hemiparesis: a re-evaluation. *J Neurol Neurosurg Psychiatry* 58: 422–7.

Murphy MJ (1985) Long-term follow-up of seizures associated with cerebral arteriovenous malformations. Results of therapy. *Arch Neurol* 42: 477–9.

Muszynski CA, Carpenter RJ, Armstrong DL (1994) Prenatal sonographic detection of basilar aneurysms. *Pediatr Neurol* 10: 70–2.

Nakaji P, Spetzler RF (2005) Indications for surgical treatment of arteriovenous malformations. *Neurosurg Clin N Am* 16: 365–6.

Namba R, Toda M, Kuroda S, et al. (2005) Sequence analysis and bioinformatic analysis of chromosome 17q25 in familial moyamoya disease. *Childs Nerv Syst* 21: 62–8.

Naranjo IC, Rieger JS, Gonzalez RM, et al. (1987) Recurrent subarachnoid haemorrhage due to spinal haemangioma. *J Neurol Neurosurg Psychiatry* 50: 1722–3.

Narayan P, Samuels OB, Barrow DL (2002) Stroke and pediatric human immunodeficiency virus infection. Case report and review of the literature. *Pediatr Neurol* 37: 158–63.

Nishizaki T, Tamaki N, Takeda N, et al. (1986) Dolichoectatic basilar artery: a review of 23 cases. *Stroke* 17: 1277–81.

Noel L, Christmann D, Jacques C, et al. (2002) [Intracerebral radiation-induced cavernous angiomas.] *J Neuroradiol* 29: 49–56 (French).

Nomura S, Kato S, Ishihara H, et al. (2006) Association of intra- and extradural developmental venous anomalies, so-called venous angiomas and sinus pericranii. *Childs Nerv Syst* 22: 428–31.

Norman JK, Parke JT, Wilson DA, McNall-Knapp RY (2007) Reversible posterior leukoencephalopathy syndrome in children undergoing induction therapy for acute lymphoblastic leukemia. *Pediatr Blood Cancer* 49: 198–203.

Norman MG, Becker LE (1974) Cerebral damage in neonates resulting from arteriovenous malformation of the vein of Galen. *J Neurol Neurosurg Psychiatry* 37: 252–8.

North KN, Whiteman DAH, Pepin MG, Byers PH (1995) Cerebrovascular complications in Ehlers–Danlos syndrome type IV. *Ann Neurol* 38: 960–4.

Nowak-Göttl U, Koch HG, Aschka I, et al. (1996) Resistance to activated protein C (APCR) in children with venous or arterial thromboembolism. *Br J Haematol* 92: 992–8.

Ofer A, Nitecki SS, Braun J, et al. (2001) CT angiography of the carotid arteries in trauma to the neck. *Eur J Vasc Endovasc Surg* 21: 401–7.

Olson E, Gilmor RL, Richmond B (1984) Cerebral venous angiomas. *Radiology* 151: 97–104.

Overby MC, Rothman AS (1985) Multiple intracranial aneurysm in sickle cell anemia. *J Neurosurg* 62: 430–4.

Østergaard JR (1991) Aetiology of intracranial saccular aneurysms in childhood. *Br J Neurosurg* 5: 575–80.

Oyesiku NM, Gahm NH, Goldman RL (1988) Cerebral arteriovenous fistulae in the Klippel–Trenaunay–Weber syndrome. *Dev Med Child Neurol* 30: 245–51.

Ozduman K, Pober BR, Barnas P, et al. (2004) Fetal stroke. *Pediatr Neurol* 30: 151–62.

Ozen S, Duzova A, Bakkaloglu A, et al. (2007) Takayasu arteritis in children: preliminary experience with cyclophosphamide induction and corticosteroids followed by methotrexate. *J Pediatr* 150: 72–6.

Packer RJ, Rorke LB, Lange BJ, et al. (1985) Cerebrovascular accidents in children with cancer. *Pediatrics* 76: 194–201.

Parker MJ, Tarlow MJ, Milne-Anderson J (1984) Glue sniffing and cerebral infarction. *Arch Dis Child* 59: 675–7.

Parker DL, Tsuruda JS, Goodrich KC, et al. (1998) Contrast-enhanced magnetic resonance angiography of cerebral vessels. A review. *Invest Radiol* 33: 560–72.

Pascual-Castroviejo I, Pascual-Pascual SI (2002) Congenital vascular malformations in childhood. *Semin Pediatr Neurol* 9: 254–73.

Patel H, Smith RR, Garg BP (1995) Spontaneous extracranial carotid artery dissection in children. *Pediatr Neurol* 13: 55–60.

Patsalides AD, Wood LV, Atac GK, et al. (2002) Cerebrovascular disease in HIV-infected pediatric patients. *Am J Roentgenol* 10: 103–6.

Pavlovic J, Kaufmann F, Boltshauser E, et al. (2006) Neuropsychological problems after paediatric stroke: two year follow-up of Swiss children. *Neuropediatrics* 37: 13–9.

Pearl PL (1987) Childhood stroke following intraoral trauma. *J Pediatr* 10: 574–5.

Peerless SJ, Nemoto S, Drake CG (1989) Giant intracranial aneurysms in children and adolescents. In: Edwards MSB, Hoffman HJ, eds. *Cerebral Vascular Disease in Children and Adolescents*. Baltimore: Williams & Wilkins, pp. 255–73.

Pegelow CH, Adams RJ, McVie V, et al. (1995) Risk of recurrent stroke in patients with sickle cell disease treated with erythrocyte transfusions. *J Pediatr* 126: 896–9.

Pellicer A, Cabañas F, Garcia-Alix A, et al. (1992) Stroke in neonates with cardiac right-to-left shunt. *Brain Dev* 14: 381–5.

Pellock JM, Kleinman PK, McDonald BM, Wixson D (1980) Childhood hypertensive stroke with neurofibromatosis. *Neurology* 30: 656–9.

Perkin GD (1995) Cerebral venous thrombosis: developments in imaging and treatment. *J Neurol Neurosurg Psychiatry* 59: 1–3 (editorial).

Perlman JM, Volpe JJ (1989) Neurologic complications of captopril treatment of neonatal hypertension. *Pediatrics* 83: 47–52.

Perret G, Nishioka H (1966) Report on the cooperative study of intracranial aneurysms and subarachnoid hemorrhage. Section VI. Arteriovenous malformations. An analysis of 545 cases of cranio-cerebral arteriovenous malformations and fistulae reported to the cooperative study. *J Neurosur* 25: 467–90.

Perrini P, Scollato A, Cellerini M, et al. (2004) Results of surgical and endovascular treatment of intracranial microarteriovenous malformations with emphasis on superselective angiography. *Acta Neurochir* 146: 755–66.

Pettigrew LC, Jankovic J (1985) Hemidystonia: a report of 22 patients and a review of the literature. *J Neurol Neurosurg Psychiatry* 48: 650–7.

Phillips PC, Lorensten KJ, Shropshire LC, Ahn HS (1988) Congenital odontoid aplasia and posterior circulation stroke in childhood. *Ann Neurol* 23: 410–3.

Pierot L, Gobin P, Cognard C, et al. (1992) [Intracranial dural arteriovenous fistulas. Clinical aspects, radiological investigations and therapeutic modalities.] *Rev Neurol* 150: 444–51 (French).

Pierot L, Cognard C, Spelle L (2004) [Cerebral arteriovenous malformations: evaluation of the haemorrhagic risk and its morbidity.] *J Neuroradiol* 31: 369–75.

Plum F (1983) What causes infarction in ischemic brain? The Robert Wartenberg lecture. *Neurology* 33: 222–33.

Pope FM, Nicholls AC, Narcisi P, et al. (1981) Some patients with cerebral aneurysms are deficient in type III collagen. *Lancet* 1: 973–5.

Prasad N, Gulati S, Gupta RK (2003) Is reversible posterior leukoencephalopathy with severe hypertension completely reversible in all patients? *Pediatr Nephrol* 18: 1161–6.

Prengler M, Pavlakis SG, Prohovnik I, Adams RJ (2002) Sickle cell disease: neurological complications. *Ann Neurol* 51: 543–52.

Prengler M, Pavlakis SG, Boyd S, et al. (2005) Sickle cell disease: ischemia and seizures. *Ann Neurol* 58: 290–302.

Prengler M, Pavlakis SG, Boyd S, et al. (2006) Sickle cell disease and electroencephalogram hyperventilation. *Ann Neurol* 59: 214–5.

Prian GW, Wright GB, Rumack CM, O'Meara OP (1978) Apparent cerebral embolization after temporal artery catheterization. *J Pediatr* 93: 115–8.

Prohovnik I, Pavlakis SG, Piomelli S, et al. (1989) Cerebral hyperemia, stroke and transfusion in sickle cell disease. *Neurology* 39: 344–8.

Pruvost P, Lasjaunias P, Rodesch G, et al. (1989) [Benign pulsatile cranial bruit in children: à propos of 6 cases.] *Arch Fr Pediatr* 46: 579–82 (French).

Raupp S, van Rooij WJ, Sluzewski M, Tijssen CC (2003) Type 1 cerebral dural arteriovenous fistulas of the lateral sinus: clinical features in 24 patients. *Eur J Neurol* 11: 489–91.

Raybaud CA, Livet MO, Jiddane M, Pinsard N (1985) Radiology of ischemic strokes in children. *Neuroradiology* 27: 567–78.

Requena I, Arias M, López-Ibor L, et al. (1991) Cavernomas of the central nervous system: clinical and neuroimaging manifestations in 47 patients. *J Neurol Neurosurg Psychiatry* 54: 590–4.

Resche F, Resche-Perrin I, Robert R, et al. (1980) [The hypoglossal artery. Report of a case. Review of the literature.] *J Neuroradiol* 7: 27–43 (French).

Ribai P, Liesnard C, Rodesch G, et al. (2003) Transient cerebral arteriopathy in infancy associated with enteroviral infection. *Eur J Paediatr Neurol* 7: 73–5.

Ricci S (2003) Embolism from the heart in the young patient: a short review. *Neurol Sci* 24 (Suppl 1): S13–4.

Riela AR, Roach ES (1993) Etiology of stroke in children. *J Child Neurol* 8: 201–20.

Riikonen R, Santavuori P (1994) Hereditary and acquired risk factors for childhood stroke. *Neuropediatrics* 25: 227–33.

Rivkin MJ, Anderson ML, Kaye EM (1992) Neonatal idiopathic cerebral venous thrombosis: an unrecognized cause of transient seizures or lethargy. *Ann Neurol* 32: 51–6.

Robertson PL, Aldrich MS, Hanash SM, Golstein GW (1988) Stroke associated with obstructive sleep apnea in a child with sickle cell anemia. *Ann Neurol* 23: 614–6.

Roden VJ, Cantor HE, O'Connor DM, et al. (1975) Acute hemiphegia of childhood associated with Coxsackie A9 viral infection. *J Pediatr* 86: 56–8.

Rodesch G, Lasjaunias P, Terbrugge K, Burrows P (1988) [Intracranial arteriovenous vascular lesions in children. Role of endovascular techniques, apropos of 44 cases.] *Neurochirurgie* 34: 293–303 (French).

Rodesch G, Hui F, Alvarez H, et al. (1994) Prognosis of antenatally diagnosed vein of Galen aneurysmal malformations. *Childs Nerv Syst* 10: 79–83.

Rodesch G, Malherbe V, Alvarez H, et al. (1995) Nongalenic cerebral arteriovenous malformations in neonates and infants. Review of 26 consecutive cases (1982–1992). *Childs Nerv Syst* 11: 231–41.

Romano JT, Riggs JE, Bodensteiner JB, Gutmann L (1989) Wasp sting-associated occlusion of the supraclinoid internal carotid artery: implications regarding the pathogenesis of moyamoya syndrome. *Arch Neurol* 46: 607–8.

Ropper AH (1988) "Convulsions" in basilar artery occlusion. *Neurology* 38: 1500–1.

Rorke LB (1989) Pathology of cerebral vascular disease in children and adolescents. In: Edwards MSB, Hoffman HJ, eds. *Cerebral Vascular Diseases in Children and Adolescents*. Baltimore: Williams & Wilkins, pp. 95–136.

Rosembeg S, Lopes MB, Sotto MN, Graudenz MS (1988) Childhood Degos disease with prominent neurological symptoms: case report of a clinicopathological case. *J Child Neurol* 3: 43–6.

Rosenbloom S, Edwards MSB (1989) Dural arteriovenous malformations. In: Edwards MSB, Hoffman HJ, eds. *Cerebral Vascular Disease in Children and Adolescents*. Baltimore: Williams & Wilkins, pp. 343–65.

Ross CA, Curnes JT, Greenwood RS (1987) Recurrent vertebrobasilar embolism in an infant with Klippel–Feil anomaly. *Pediatr Neurol* 3: 181–3.

Ross IB, Shevell MI, Montes JL, et al. (1994) Encephaloduroarteriosynangiosis (EDAS) for the treatment of childhood moyamoya disease. *Pediatr Neurol* 10: 199–204.

Ruano R, Benachi A, Aubry MC, et al. (2003) Perinatal three-dimensional color power Doppler ultrasonography of vein of Galen aneurysms. *J Ultrasound Med* 22: 1357–62.

Ryan M, Yeao S, Maguire M, et al. (2001) Rhinocerebral mucormycosis in a child with lymphoblastic leukaemia. *Eur J Paediatr* 160: 235–8.

Sainte-Rose C, LaCombe J, Pierre-Kahn A, et al. (1984) Intracranial venous sinus hypertension: cause or consequence of hydrocephalus in infants? *J Neurosurg* 60: 727–36.

Sainte-Rose C, Oliveira R, Puget S, et al. (2006) Multiple bur hole surgery for the treatment of moyamoya disease in children. *J Neurosurg* 105 (6 Suppl): 437–43.

Sakoh M, Østergaard L, Gjedde A, et al. (2001) Prediction of tissue survival after middle cerebral artery occlusion based on the changes in the apparent diffusion of water. *J Neurosurg* 95: 450–8.

Sakurai K, Horiuchi Y, Ikeda H, et al. (2004) A novel susceptibility locus for moyamoya disease on chromosome 8q23. *Am J Hum Genet* 49: 278–81.

Salgado AN, Furlan AJ, Keys TF, et al. (1989) Neurologic complications of endocarditis: a 12-year experience. *Neurology* 39: 173–8.

Samson D (1989) Traumatic lesions of the cerebral vasculature. In: Edwards MSB, Hoffman HJ, eds. *Cerebral Vascular Disease in Children and Adolescents*. Baltimore: Williams & Wilkins, pp. 195–201.

Sarwar M, McCormick WF (1978) Intracerebral venous angioma: case report and review. *Arch Neurol* 35: 323–5.

Scaglione C, Salvi F, Riguzzi P, et al. (2001) Symptomatic unruptured capillary telangiectasia of the brain stem: report of three cases and review of the literature. *J Neurol Neurosurg Psychiatry* 71: 390–3.

Schievink WI, Piepgras DG, Earnest F, Gordon H (1991) Spontaneous carotid–cavernous fistulae in Ehlers–Danlos syndrome type IV. *J Neurosurg* 74: 991–8.

Schievink WI, Michels VV, Piepgras DG (1994a) Neurovascular manifestations of heritable connective tissue disorders. A review. *Stroke* 25: 889–903.

Schievink WI, Mokri B, Piepgras DG (1994b) Spontaneous dissections of cervicocephalic arteries in childhood and adolescence. *Neurology* 44: 1607–12.

Schievink WI, Schaid DJ, Michels VV, Piepgras DG (1995) Familial aneurysmal subarachnoid hemorrhage: a community-based study. *J Neurosurg* **83**: 426–9.

Schievink WI, Apostolides PJ, Spetzler RF (1998) Surgical treatment of superficial siderosis associated with spinal arteriovenous malformation. Case report. *J Neurosurg* **89**: 1029–31.

Schlenska GK (1986) Absence of both internal carotid arteries. *J Neurol* **233**: 263–6.

Schobess R, Kempf-Bielack B, Schwabe D, et al. (2004) Thrombosis in children with hematologic malignancies. *Rev Clin Exp Hematol* **8**: E2.

Schoenberg BS, Mellinger JF, Schoenberg DG (1978) Cerebrovascular disease in infants and children: a study of incidence, clinical features, and survival. *Neurology* **28**: 763–8.

Schöning M, Klein R, Krägeloh-Mann I, et al. (1994) Antiphospholipid antibodies in cerebrovascular ischemia and stroke in childhood. *Neuropediatrics* **25**: 8–14.

Schulzke S, Weber P, Luetschg J, Fahnenstich H (2005) Incidence and diagnosis of unilateral arterial cerebral infarction in newborn infants. *J Perinat Med* **33**: 170–5.

Scott RM, Smith JL, Robertson RL, et al. (2004) Long-term outcome in children with moyamoya syndrome after cranial revascularization by pial synangiosis. *J Neurosurg* **100** (2 Suppl Pediatrics): 142–9.

Sébire G, Tabarki B, Saunders DE, et al. (2005) Cerebral venous sinus thrombosis in children: risk factors, presentation, diagnosis and outcome. *Brain* **128**: 477–89.

Sedzimir CB, Robinson J (1973) Intracranial hemorrhage in children and adolescents. *J Neurosurg* **38**: 269–73.

Seko Y (2007) Giant cell and Takayasu arteritis. *Curr Opin Rheumatol* **19**: 39–43.

Selby G, Walker GL (1979) Cerebral arteritis in cat scratch disease. *Neurology* **29**: 1413–8.

Seol HJ, Wang KC, Kim SK, et al (2006) Familial occurrence of moyamoya disease: a clinical study. *Childs Nerv Syst* **22**: 1143–8.

Sheth RD, Bodensteiner JB (1995) Progressive neurologic impairment from an arteriovenous malformation vascular steal. *Pediatr Neurol* **13**: 352–4.

Shevell MI, Silver K, O'Gorman AM, et al. (1989) Neonatal dural sinus thrombosis. *Pediatr Neurol* **5**: 161–5.

Shirane R, Sato S, Yoshimoto T (1992) Angiographic findings of ischemic stroke in children. *Childs Nerv Syst* **8**: 432–6.

Silber MH, Sandok BA, Earnest F (1987) Vascular malformations of the posterior fossa: clinical and radiologic features. *Arch Neurol* **44**: 965–9.

Simard JM, Garcia-Bengochea F, Ballinger WE, et al. (1986) Cavernous angioma: a review of 126 collected and 12 new clinical cases. *Neurosurgery* **18**: 162–72.

Simioni P, Battistella PA, Drigo P, et al. (1994) Childhood stroke associated with familial protein S deficiency. *Brain Dev* **16**: 241–5.

Singhi P, Subramanian C, Jan V, et al. (2002) Reversible brain lesions in childhood hypertension. *Acta Paediatr* **91**: 1005–7.

Slovut DP, Olin JW (2005) Fibromuscular dysplasia. *Curr Treat Options Cardiovasc Med* **7**: 159–69.

Soga Y, Oka K, Sato M, et al. (2001) Cavernous sinus thrombophlebitis caused by sphenoid sinusitis—report of an autopsy case. *Clin Neuropathol* **20**: 101–5.

Southwick FS, Richardson EP, Swartz MN (1986) Septic thrombosis of the dural venous sinuses. *Medicine* **65**: 82–106.

Sperl W, Felber S, Skladal D, Wermuth B (1997) Metabolic stroke in carbamyl phosphate synthetase deficiency. *Neuropediatrics* **28**: 229–34.

Statham P, Macpherson P, Johnston R, et al. (1990) Cerebral radiation necrosis complicating stereotactic radiosurgery for arteriovenous malformation. *J Neurol Neurosurg Psychiatry* **53**: 476–9.

Steen RG, Hankins GM, Wang WC, et al. (2003a) Prospective brain imaging evaluation of children with sickle cell trait: initial observation. *Radiology* **228**: 208–15.

Steen RG, Xiong X, Langston JW, Helton KJ (2003b) Brain injury in children with sickle cell disease: prevalence and etiology. *Ann Neurol* **54**: 559–63.

Steiger HJ, Hanggi D, Schmid-Elsaesser R (2005) Cranial and spinal dural arteriovenous malformations and fistulas: an update. *Acta Neurochir Suppl* **94**: 115–22.

Stein BM, Mohr JP (1988) Vascular malformations of the brain. *N Engl J Med* **319**: 368–70.

Steinberg GK, Fabrikant JI, Marks MP, et al. (1990) Stereotactic heavy-charged-particle Bragg-peak radiation for intracranial arteriovenous malformations. *N Engl J Med* **323**: 96–101.

Steiner L (1986) Radiosurgery in cerebral arteriovenous malformations. In: Flamm E, Fein J, eds. *Textbook of Cerebrovascular Surgery, vol. 4.* New York: Springer, pp. 1161–215.

Steinlin M, Pfister I, Pavlovic J, et al. (2005) The first three years of the Swiss Neuropaediatric Stroke Registry (SNPSR): a population-based study of incidence, symptoms and risk factors. *Neuropediatrics* **36**: 90–7.

Sträter R, Vielhaber H, Kassenbohmer R, et al. (1999) Genetic risk factors of thrombophilia in ischaemic childhood stroke of cardiac origin. A prospective ESPED survey. *Eur J Pediatr* **158** Suppl 3: S122–5.

Sträter R, Becker S, von Eckardstein A, et al. (2002) Prospective assessment of risk factors for recurrent stroke during childhood—a 5-year follow-up study. *Lancet* **360**: 1540–5.

Sturzenegger M (1995) Spontaneous internal carotid artery dissection: early diagnosis and management in 44 patients. *J Neurol* **242**: 231–8.

Suda K, Matsumura M, Ohta S (2003) Kawasaki disease complicated by cerebral infarction. *Cardiol Young* **13**: 101–5.

Suh DC, Alvarez H, Battacharya JS, et al. (2001) Intracranial haemorrhage within the first two years of life. *Acta Neurochir* **143**: 997–1004.

Svensson PJ, Dahlbäck B (1994) Resistance to activated protein C as a basis for venous thrombosis. *N Engl J Med* **330**: 517–22.

Svensson LG, Nadolny EM, Kimmel WA (2002) Multimodal protocol influence on stroke and neurocognitive deficit prevention after ascending/arch aortic operations. *Ann Thorac Surg* **74**: 2040–6.

Tagawa T, Mimaki T, Yabuuchi H, et al. (1985) Bilateral occlusions in the cervical portion of the internal carotid arteries in a child. *Stroke* **16**: 896–8.

Takanashi J, Sugita K, Miyazato S, et al. (1995) Antiphospholipid antibody syndrome in childhood strokes. *Pediatr Neurol* **13**: 323–6.

Tam CS, Galanos J, Seymour JF, et al. (2004) Reversible posterior leukoencephalopathy syndrome complicating cytotoxic chemotherapy for hematologic malignancies. *Am J Hematol* **77**: 72–6.

Tanaka K, Hirayama K, Hattori H, et al. (1994) A case of cerebral aneurysm associated with complex partial seizures. *Brain Dev* **16**: 233–7.

Tatemichi TK, Prohovnik I, Mohr JP, et al. (1988) Reduced hypercapnic vasoreactivity in moya moya disease. *Neurology* **38**: 1575–81.

Teixeira SM, Cortellazzi LC, Grotto HZ (2003) Effect of hydroxyurea on G gamma chain fetal hemoglobin synthesis by sickle-cell disease patients. *Braz J Med Biol Res* **36**: 1289–92.

ter Berg HWM, Bijlsma JB, Willemse J (1987) Familial occurrence of intracranial aneurysms in childhood: a case report and review of the literature. *Neuropediatrics* **18**: 227–30.

Thomke F, Urban PP, Marx JJ, et al. (2002) Seventh nerve palsies may be the only sign of a small pontine infarct in diabetic and hypertensive patients. *J Neurol* **249**: 1556–62.

Thorarensen O, Ryan S, Hunter J, Younkin DP (1997) Factor V Leiden mutation: an unrecognized cause of hemiplegic cerebral palsy, neonatal stroke, and placental thrombosis. *Ann Neurol* **42**: 372–5.

Togay-Isikay C, Kim J, Betterman K, et al. (2005) Carotid artery tortuosity, kinking, coiling; stroke risk factor, marker, or curiosity? *Acta Neurol Belg* **105**: 68–72.

Troffkin NA, Graham GB, Berkmen T, Wakhloo AK (2003) Combined transvenous and transarterial embolization of a tentorial–incisural dural arteriovenous malformation followed by primary stent placement in the associated stenotic straight sinus. Case report. *J Neurosurg* **99**: 579–83.

Tyler HR, Clark DB (1957) Cerebrovascular accidents in patients with congenital heart disease. *AMA Arch Neurol Psychiatry* **77**: 483–9.

Uziel Y, Laxer RM, Blaser S, et al. (1995) Cerebral vein thrombosis in childhood systemic lupus erythematosus. *J Pediatr* **126**: 722–7.

Vanderzant C, Bromberg M, Macguire A, McCune WJ (1988) Isolated small-vessel angiitis of the central nervous system. *Arch Neurol* **45**: 683–7.

Van Damme H, Sakalihasan N, Limet R (1999) Fibromuscular dysplasia of the internal carotid artery. Personal experience with 13 cases and literature review. *Acta Chir Belg* **99**: 163–8.

van Diemen-Steenvoorde R, van Nieuwenhuizen O, De Klerk JBC, Duran M (1990) Quasi-moyamoya disease and heterozygosity for homocystinuria in a five-year old girl. *Neuropediatrics* **21**: 110–2.

VanDongen HR, Loonen CB, VanDongen KJ (1985) Anatomical basis for acquired fluent aphasia in children. *Ann Neurol* **17**: 306–9.

van Kuijck MAP, Rotteveel JJ, van Oostrom CG, Novakova I (1994) Neurological complications in children with protein C deficiency. *Neuropediatrics* **25**: 16–9.

Ventureyra EC, Higgins MJ (1994) Traumatic intracranial aneurysms in childhood and adolescence. Case reports and review of the literature. *Childs Nerv Syst* **10**: 361–79.

Verdu A, Cazorla MR, Moreno JC, Casado LF (2005) Prenatal stroke in a neonate heterozygous for factor V Leiden mutation. *Brain Dev* 27: 451–4.

Viljoen DN (1988) Pseudoxanthoma elasticum (Grönblad–Stanberg syndrome). *J Med Genet* 25: 488–90.

Virapongse C, Cazenave C, Quisling R, et al. (1987) The empty delta sign: frequency and significance in 76 cases of dural sinus thrombosis. *Radiology* 162: 779–85.

Wakamoto H, Kume A, Nakano N, Negao H (2006) Benign angiopathy of the central nevous system associated with phenytoin intoxication. *Brain Dev* 28: 336–8.

Wallace RC, Bourekas EC (1998) Brain arteriovenous malformations. *Neuroimaging Clin N Am* 8: 883–9.

Wang PS, Longstreth WE, Koepsell TD (1995) Subarachnoid hemorrhage and family history. A population-based case–control study. *Arch Neurol* 52: 202–4.

Wang WC, Morales KH, Scher CD, et al. (2005) Effect of long-term transfusion on growth in children with sickle cell anemia: results of the STOP trial. *J Pediatr* 147: 244–7.

Warach S, Gaa J, Siewert B, et al. (1995) Acute human stroke studied by whole brain echo planar diffusion-weighted magnetic resonance imaging. *Ann Neurol* 37: 231–41.

Warren DJ, Hoggerd N, Walton J, et al. (2001) Cerebral arteriovenous malformations: comparison of novel magnetic resonance angiographic techniques and conventional catheter angiography. *Neurosurgery* 48: 973–82.

Watanabe K, Negoro T, Maehara M, et al. (1990) Moyamoya disease presenting with chorea. *Pediatr Neurol* 6: 40–2.

Waterman JA, Balbi HJ, Vaysman D, et al. (2007) Lemierre syndrome: a case report. *Pediatr Emerg Care* 23: 103–5.

Wazi P, Na-Nakorn S, Poutrakal P (1978) A syndrome of hypertension, convulsion and cerebral haemorrhage in thalassaemic patients after multiple blood transfusions. *Lancet* 1: 602–4.

Weon YC, Yoshida Y, Sachet M, et al. (2005) Supratentorial cerebral arteriovenous fistulas (AVFs) in children: review of 41 cases with 63 non choroidal single-hole AVFs. *Acta Neurochir* 147: 17–31.

Willinsky RA, Lasjaunias P, Terbrugge K, Burrows P (1990) Multiple cerebral arteriovenous malformations (AVMs). Review of our experience from 203 patients with cerebral vascular lesions. *Neuroradiology* 32: 207–10.

Wraige E, Pohl MR, Ganesan V (2005) A proposed classification for subtypes of arterial ischaemic stroke in children. *Dev Med Child Neurol* 47: 252–6.

Wright RR, Mathews KD (1996) Hypertensive encephalopathy in childhood. *J Child Neurol* 11: 193–6.

Yang JS, Park YD, Hartlage PL (1995) Seizures associated with stroke in childhood. *Pediatr Neurol* 12: 136–8.

Yokoyama K, Asano Y, Murakawa T, et al. (1991) Familial occurrence of arteriovenous malformation of the brain. *J Neurosurg* 74: 585–9.

Yoshida Y, Weon YC, Sachet M, et al. (2004) Posterior cranial fossa single-hole arteriovenous fistulae in children: 14 consecutive cases. *Neuroradiology* 46: 474–81.

Younger DS, Hays AP, Brust JCM, Rowland LP (1988) Granulomatous angiitis of the brain: an inflammatory reaction of diverse etiology. *Arch Neurol* 45: 514–8.

Zapson DS, Riviello JJ, Bagwell S (1995) Supraventricular tachycardia leading to stroke in childhood. *J Child Neurol* 10: 239–41.

Zimmerman RS, Spetzler RF, Lee KS, et al. (1991) Cavernous malformations of the brain stem. *J Neurosurg* 75: 32–9.

Zuber M, Meary E, Meder JF, Mas JL (1993) Magnetic resonance imaging and dynamic CT scan in cerebral artery dissections. *Stroke* 25: 576–81.

PART VII

PAROXYSMAL DISORDERS

Alexis Arzimanoglou and Jean Aicardi

Paroxysmal phenomena represent the single most common neurological problem in childhood. Evidence from general practice suggests lifetime prevalence of about 20 per 1000 for single or repeated paroxysmal attacks and 17 per 1000 for recurrent seizures (Goodridge and Shorvon 1983). Ross et al. (1980) and Ross and Peckham (1983) found that 6.7% of a British national cohort had experienced at least one episode of altered consciousness. However, paroxysmal disorders form a highly heterogeneous group of conditions with completely different mechanisms, causes, outcomes and management, and epileptic attacks represent only one portion of all paroxysmal episodes. In the series referred to above, epilepsy was thought to account for 4.1% of cases, while febrile convulsions, breath-holding attacks, faints or other paroxysmal events accounted for the remaining 2.6%.

Whatever the figures, the essential fact is that acute transient loss of consciousness with or without other manifestations is not necessarily due to epilepsy, and it may be difficult to differentiate epileptic seizures from attacks of other origin. Jeavons (1983) has indicated that 30% of patients referred to his epilepsy clinic did not have epilepsy, an experience shared by many investigators (see Stephenson 1990).

The main reasons for misdiagnosis of nonepileptic events as epilepsy are that paroxysmal attacks are brief and usually witnessed only by parents or caregivers, and that, between attacks, most such children have no abnormal clinical manifestations or signs. All too often, physicians attempt to determine the nature of an ictal event by studying interictal status, whether clinically or by laboratory examination, rather than trying to gather the maximum descriptive information about the event itself. This is, clearly, a logical error, as there is no necessary relationship between, say, the presence of abnormal EEG potentials, and the nature of the event. Thus a child with a rolandic spike focus may have had a syncope or faint, even though the presence of EEG paroxysms increases the probability of a diagnosis of epilepsy. As

emphasized by Stephenson (1990), detailed description of the clinical event is all-important and "the diagnosis is as good as the history". No amount of interictal information, technical or otherwise, will replace a missing description. The rate of misdiagnosis by itself is a strong argument for specialist care of epilepsy (Chadwick and Smith 2002). The advances in and increased choice of pharmacological and other treatments further support this case. In a recent study estimating the financial costs of epilepsy misdiagnosis in the NHS in England and Wales, 92,000 people were found to have been misdiagnosed in 2002. The estimated annual medical costs were £29 million, while total costs could reach up to £138 million a year (Juarez-Garcia et al. 2006).

In this part, seizures of epileptic mechanism (Chapter 15) and nonepileptic events (Chapter 16) will be discussed separately; however, in reality the distinction may be very unclear. "The term epileptic seizure refers to sudden change in the electrical activity of the brain, usually accompanied by subjective or objective changes in behaviour. Non-epileptic seizures are sudden changes in objective or subjective behaviour which do not have at their root an independent sudden change in the electrical activity of the brain" (Stephenson 1990). However, the changes in electrical activity *during attacks* are only seldom actually demonstrated in the individual patient and are therefore surmised rather than observed. Moreover, a 'nonepileptic' change in behaviour, e.g. a tonic motor discharge during an hypoxic attack, may well also originate from some sort of abnormal brain activity such as a discharge of tonigenic neurons liberated from inhibition by higher (cortical) structures. What distinguishes such an activity from some epileptic seizures such as tonic spasms is difficult to establish in electrophysiological terms, in the absence of an ictal EEG record.

Even though the distinction between epileptic and nonepileptic events may be theoretically and practically unclear, in general, experienced clinicians can recognize the epileptic 'flavour' of an attack by observing a seizure and even by examining patient history.

REFERENCES

Chadwick D, Smith D (2002) The misdiagnosis of epilepsy. *BMJ* **324**: 495–6.

Goodridge DMG, Shorvon SD (1983) Epileptic seizures in a population of 6000. *BMJ* **287**: 641–7.

Jeavons PM (1983) Non-epileptic attacks in childhood. In: Rose FC, ed. *Research Progress in Epilepsy.* London: Pitman, pp. 224–30.

Juarez-Garcia A, Stokes T, Shaw B, et al. (2006) The costs of epilepsy misdiagnosis in England and Wales. *Seizure* **15**: 598–605.

Ross EM, Peckham CS (1983) Seizure disorder in the National Child Development Study. In: Rose FC, ed. *Research Progress in Epilepsy.* London: Pitman, pp. 46–59.

Ross EM, West PB, Butler NR (1980) Epilepsy in childhood: findings from the National Child Development Study. *BMJ* **1**: 207–10.

Stephenson JBP (1990) Fits and Faints. *Clinics in Developmental Medicine No. 109.* London: Mac Keith Press.

15

EPILEPSY AND OTHER SEIZURE DISORDERS

Alexis Arzimanoglou and Jean Aicardi

Epilepsy is neither a disease nor a syndrome, but rather a symptom of multiple causes, genetic or lesional, representing a very significant part of neurology, and can thus be present in an extreme variety of conditions and circumstances. It is clearly impossible to provide exhaustive coverage of all its manifestations within the confines of this chapter, and the reader is referred to publications by Arzimanoglou et al. (2004), Roger et al. (2005) and Engel and Pedley (2007). Epileptic seizures represent its most characteristic but not its sole manifestation, and interictal abnormalities may also represent an important part of its semiology. This applies to EEG manifestations as well as to clinical disturbances, especially neurological, cognitive and behavioural ones that may be present interictally.

DEFINITIONS

Epileptic seizures are transient clinical events that result from abnormal and excessive activity of synchronized, more or less extensive populations of cerebral neurons. This abnormal activity results in *paroxysmal disorganization* of one or several brain functions, manifested by positive, excitatory phenomena (motor, sensory, psychic) or negative phenomena (such as loss of awareness, of muscle tone or of language), or by a mixture of the two. The clinical events that constitute epileptic seizures can be extremely diverse, and no single manifestation is essential. A detailed description of the ictal event is the cornerstone of accurate diagnosis.

The EEG events that underlie the seizure constitute the epileptic discharge, which in some cases may remain without clinical expression or have only subtle clinical consequences, referred to as 'subclinical seizures' (Gastaut 1973). The seizure discharge and/or clinical seizure may remain localized or be expressed bilaterally over most of the cortical surface – the so-called 'generalized seizure'. In this chapter the term 'seizure' is used in its etymological sense (from 'to seize') and applied to both epileptic and nonepileptic events (Stephenson 1990), although it is more often reserved for seizures of epileptic mechanism.

Epileptic seizures may occur as a result of intercurrent events such as fever, hypoglycaemia or acute CNS infections (*occasional seizures*), or recur spontaneously without a known precipitant (*unprovoked epileptic seizures that, when repeated, constitute epilepsy*). The dividing line between isolated (or occasional provoked) and unprovoked epileptic seizures is not always evident. In fact isolated (occasional) seizures can have a recognizable cause, or they can apparently be unprovoked. On the other hand, for all seizures, factors that precipitate the attack and factors that contribute to arresting it must exist. Some precipitating factors, such as intermittent photic stimulation, certain sounds, or lack of sleep, are known. However, many more precipitating factors are as yet unknown or only imperfectly described, while still others are only suspected. Stress, psychological factors and fatigue are probably responsible for precipitating a sizeable proportion of epileptic seizures, but the exact nature of these stimuli and their mechanisms of action in producing epilepsy remain unexplored. A certain degree of confusion is also due to the fact that the terms 'provoked' and 'triggered' are sometimes used as if they were interchangeable. As discussed by Pohlmann-Eden et al. (2006), provoking factors include fever, head injury, excessive alcohol intake, withdrawal from alcohol or drugs, hypoglycaemia, electrolyte disturbance, brain infection, ischaemic stroke, intracranial haemorrhage and proconvulsive drugs. Seizures that follow severe psychological stress or considerable sleep deprivation are not considered as 'acute symptomatic' but instead 'triggered' by these factors in susceptible individuals with an underlying epilepsy disorder. Reflex seizures are also considered to be triggered by a given stimulus (stroboscopic lights, reading, etc.). In fact, most seizures likely have a multifactorial origin.

Epilepsy is on the contrary defined as an enduring condition, or rather a group of conditions, in which epileptic seizures occur repeatedly without a detectable cause (Gastaut 1973) as a result of either structural brain damage or an intrinsic functional propensity to have epileptic seizures. For epidemiological purposes, the term epilepsy is often used for at least two seizures not occurring in a single episode. In clinical practice it is used for a lasting, 'chronic' condition. Epilepsy may be more than the repetition of seizures (Aicardi 1997, Beckung and Uvebrant 1997). Subclinical epileptic activity, when prolonged, can probably disorganize many brain functions and be responsible for transient or lasting cognitive and behavioural disturbances (Tassinari et al. 1992, Beckung and Uvebrant 1997, Arzimanoglou et al. 2005).

Convulsions are attacks of involuntary muscle contractions, either sustained (tonic convulsions) or interrupted (clonic convulsions). In principle, convulsions may be either epileptic or non-

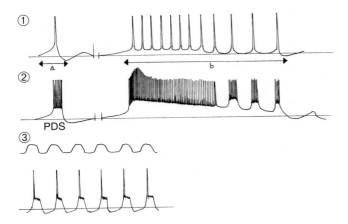

Fig. 15.1. Schematic representation of relationship between EEG discharges and cortical intracellular events in partial or secondarily generalized seizure.

1. EEG: *(a)* interictal spikes; *(b)* seizure discharge with tonic followed by clonic phases.

2. Intracellular events: paroxysmal depolarization shift (PDS) corresponds to EEG spike *(a)*. Transition to seizure is marked by failure to develop inhibitory potential thus allowing persistent depolarization and discharge.

3. In generalized spike–wave discharges, strong inhibitory potentials, probably of thalamic origin, follow each spike and correspond to the slow component. The oscillation in the thalamocortical circuit prevents continuous cortical neuron discharge.

epileptic in nature. However, the term is traditionally used to designate occasional epileptic seizures, such as febrile seizures, on the one hand because occasional seizures are almost exclusively marked by motor phenomena, and on the other because the term has come to convey the idea of benignity and avoids the use of the dreaded word 'epilepsy'. Nevertheless, the clinician must still remember that most infantile convulsions are indeed epileptic seizures.

MECHANISMS OF EPILEPTIC SEIZURES

The epileptic discharge, which is the basic electrophysiological feature of epileptic seizures, typically consists of rhythmical and high-amplitude oscillations of electrical potential that can usually be recorded from the scalp on the EEG but may, in some cases, remain undetectable even on the surface of the brain, depending on the volume of brain involved, its geometry and the manner of propagation (Bancaud and Talairach 1975). It is the most direct evidence of the abnormal, excessive neuronal activity postulated by Hughlings Jackson as the origin of epilepsy. The scalp or cortical epileptic discharge is related both to the abnormal behaviour of individual neurons and to the excessive synchronization of a large cellular population. As shown schematically in Figure 15.1, the EEG spikes correspond to the summation of field potentials that are themselves the direct consequence of intracellular events. The most remarkable of these, in seizures of focal origin, is an enormous increase in the size of membrane depolarization induced by excitatory postsynaptic potentials, the *paroxysmal depolarization shift*. This corresponds to a spike on the interictal EEG record, at a threshold level of affected neurons, and

it is followed by prolonged increased after-polarization. When a seizure occurs, this hyperpolarization disappears so that repetitive bursting goes unchecked. This, in turn, recruits neighbouring neurons that discharge synchronously.

In generalized seizures, different mechanisms may be operative, but in the case of convulsive attacks, all involve sustained membrane depolarization. The mechanism of nonconvulsive seizures such as absences, on the other hand, involves a succession of excitatory and inhibitory potentials (Snead 1995). The EEG slow wave apparently reflects GABA-mediated increased inhibition, which, together with enhanced excitation, helps to produce and maintain a *state of epileptic hypersynchrony*. Low-threshold calcium currents in reticular thalamic pacemaker neurons seem to be responsible for driving the hypersynchronous spike-and-wave discharge of absence epilepsy. Gloor and Fariello (1988) postulated that primary generalized epilepsy is characterized by a diffusely hyperexcitable cortex, so that an epileptic discharge can be triggered by excitation of the thalamic reticular system induced by the thalamocortical input, and thus both the cortex and subcortical structures are necessary for its genesis.

Detailed study of the mechanisms responsible for the generation of epileptic discharges is beyond the scope of this book (for reviews, see Jones 2006, Najm et al. 2006b).

The enhanced excitability of the brain may conceivably result from genetically determined chemical imbalance between excitatory and inhibitory neurotransmitters, from inbuilt subtle changes in cortical circuitry, or from the action of a localized lesion. In this regard, the possible influence of abnormally discharging neurons on the rest of the brain has attracted considerable attention. Focal subclinical stimulation of neuronal groups becomes increasingly effective with properly repeated stimulations and eventually may result in generalized seizures (Moshé and Ludvig 1988). The relevance of this 'kindling' phenomenon for human epilepsy, however, is still undetermined, although it may be a factor in the emergence of secondary foci (Morrell 1989).

Decreased inhibitory mechanisms are thought to play an important role in epilepsy, and the main cortical inhibitory neurotransmitter, gamma-aminobutyric acid (GABA), has been extensively studied. The GABA hypothesis has been at the origin of major therapeutic efforts and of the development of important antiepileptic drugs.

Current research is also directed to the study of *excitatory neurotransmitters* such as glutamate and aspartate, an excess of which could account for the local or generalized enhanced cortical excitability (Najm et al. 2006b). Changes in the receptors of both excitatory (glutamate and aspartate) and inhibitory (GABA) neurotransmitters probably play a major role in the modulation of cortical excitability, and their differential rate of maturation with age may explain the changing susceptibility to epilepsy at various ages (Moshé 1987, Johnston 1996, Holmes 1997).

Whatever the mechanisms involved, brain maturation plays a critical role in the susceptibility to seizures and in their clinical expression. The morphological, electrophysiological and biochemical bases of brain maturation in relation to seizures are being actively explored (Jensen 1999, Ben-Ari 2006).

TABLE 15.1
Main causes of occasional epileptic seizures

Cause	References
Fever due to extracranial infections (febrile convulsions)	This chapter
Intracranial infections	
Bacterial	
Meningitis, brain abcess, empyema	Chapter 10
Septic venous thrombosis	Chapters 1, 10, 14
Viral: viral meningitis, encephalitis	Chapter 10
Fungal or parasitic	Chapter 10
Parainfectious encephalopathies	
Reye syndrome	Chapter 10
Other acute encephalopathies of obscure origin	Lyon et al. (1961)
Haemorrhagic shock	Harden et al. (1991)
Metabolic disturbances	
Hypocalcaemia and hypomagnesaemia	
Hypoglycaemia	
Hyponatraemia	Chapters 1, 22
Inappropriate secretion of ADH	
Water intoxication	
Inadequate rehydratation	
Hypernatraemia	Chapter 22
Consequence of vascular collapse due to dehydration	
Consequence of rapid correction of sodium levels	
Inborn errors of metabolism (especially during episodes of decompensation)	Chapter 8
Intoxications	
Endogenous	
Uraemia, renal dialysis	Chapter 22
Hepatic encephalopathy	Chapter 22
Diabetic ketoacidosis	Greene et al. (1990)
Hypertensive encephalopathy	Del Giudice and Aicardi (1979)
Renal disease	
Acute nephritis (may be paucisymptomatic)	Del Giudice and Aicardi (1979)
Haemolytic–uraemic syndrome	Chapter 22
Head trauma	
Early epileptic seizures	Chapter 12
Extradural/subdural haematoma	This chapter
Brain contusion	Chapter 12
Acute cerebral hypoxia	
Cardiac arrest	Aubourg et al. (1985)
Drowning	Chapter 12
Acute vascular collapse	Chapter 12
Cerebrovascular accidents	Chapter 14
Arterial occlusion (thrombosis or embolism)	Chapter 14
Venous thrombosis	Chapter 14
Haemorrhage from vascular malformations	Murphy (1985)
Burns encephalopathy	Mohnot et al. (1982)

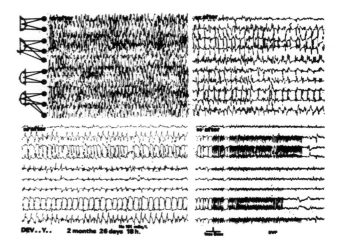

Fig. 15.2. Generalized epileptic seizure (in 2-month-old infant with hypernatraemia). Tonic discharge *(top left)*, followed by clonic discharge *(top right, continued bottom left)*. Trace at *bottom right* was recorded at slow paper speed and shows termination of seizure.

The EEG features of this seizure are slightly atypical, e.g. the rhythm of the tonic discharge is not the same over both hemispheres. This is common in infants, in whom typical generalized seizures are rare.

They can be due to acute brain conditions, such as acute structural brain damage resulting from trauma, metabolic disturbances or infections, which can occur in children without any predisposition to seizures. More commonly, however, a special predisposition to seizures, likely to be largely of genetic origin and often age-dependent, is present that renders the individual susceptible to the action of specific stimuli, of which the most common example is febrile seizures. However, there is not an absolute opposition between the two groups of occasional seizures from an aetiological viewpoint. Structural lesions precipitate seizures more frequently in patients with a family history of epilepsy than in the general population, and the same may apply to other causes, e.g. acute meningitis.

Epilepsy (as a chronic disorder) can also be due exclusively to genetic factors or chronic brain damage (congenital or acquired), or to various combinations of these (Berkovic et al. 1987).

The epilepsies are usually divided into idiopathic, symptomatic and cryptogenic cases. *Idiopathic epilepsies* are those in which no detectable brain lesion or abnormality is present; *symptomatic epilepsies* are those resulting from brain abnormalities or acquired damage; *cryptogenic epilepsies* are those for which an organic cause is probable but cannot be demonstrated. The frequency of this last category tends to decrease as refinements to the methods of investigation are made.

Genetic factors are of predominant importance in those epilepsies that are not associated with neurological abnormalities (idiopathic epilepsies) but may also play a role in epilepsies associated with demonstrable brain damage (Ottman 1989, 2005).

The role and mode of inheritance are variable with the type of epilepsy, and known genetic data will be indicated for each epilepsy syndrome (Table 15.2). Monofactorial origin has been demonstrated in the past 20 years to be the cause of some genetic

AETIOLOGY OF SEIZURE DISORDERS

Occasional epileptic seizures, as defined above, can be provoked by a host of intercurrent events (Table 15.1) such as fever, hypoglycaemia, metabolic imbalance or acute diseases. They almost always present as generalized convulsive seizures (Fig. 15.2).

TABLE 15.2
Identified genes for epilepsy*

Epilepsy syndrome	Seizure types	Locus	Gene		(Dys)function
GEFS+; Dravet	Febrile, absence, myoclonic, tonic–clonic, focal	2q24	SCN1A	Sodium channel α1 subunit	Somatodendritic sodium influx
GEFS+; BFNIC	Febrile, afebrile, generalized tonic and tonic–clonic	2q24	SCN2A	Sodium channel α2 subunit	Fast sodium influx initiation and propagation of action potential
GEFS+	Febrile, absence, tonic–clonic, myoclonic	19q13	SCN1B	Sodium channel β1 subunit	Coadjuvate and modulate α subunit
AD JME	Tonic–clonic, myoclonic, absence	5q34	GABRA1	GABA_A α1 receptor α1 subunit	Partial inhibition of GABA-activated currents
FS; CAE; GEFS+	Febrile, absence, tonic-clonic, myoclonic, clonic, focal	5q31	GABRG2	GABA_A receptor γ2 subunit	Rapid inhibition of GABAergic neurons
GEFS+	Febrile and afebrile seizures	1p36	GABRD	GABA_A receptor δ2 subunit	Decreased GABAA receptor current amplitudes
JME	Tonic–clonic, myoclonic	6p12–p11	EFHC1	Protein with an EF-hand motif	Reduced mouse hippocampal induced apoptosis
JME	Tonic–clonic, myoclonic	6p21	BRD2 (RING3)	Nuclear transcriptional regulator	?
BFNC	Neonatal convulsions	20q13	KCNQ2	Potassium channel	M current interacts with KCNQ3
BFNC	Neonatal convulsions	8q24	KCNQ3	Potassium channel	M current interacts with KCNQ2
BFNIC + familial hemiplegic migraine	Infantile convulsions	1q23	ATP1A2	Na+, K+ ATPase pump	Dysfunction of ion transportation
IGE	Tonic–clonic, myoclonic, absence	3q26	CLCN2	Voltage gated-chloride channel	Neuronal chloride efflux
ADNFLE	Sleep-related focal seizures	20q13	CHRNA4	Acetylcholine receptor α4 subunit	Nicotinic current modulation; interacts with β2 subunit
ADNFLE	Sleep-related focal seizures	8q	CHRNA2	Acetylcholine receptor α2 subunit	Nicotinic current modulation; interacts with β2 and β4 subunits
ADNFLE	Sleep-related focal seizures	1p21	CHRNB2	Acetylcholine receptor β2 subunit	Nicotinic current modulation; interacts with α4 subunit
ADPEAF	Focal seizures with auditory or visual hallucinations	10q24	LGI1	Leucine-rich, glioma-inactivated	Disregulates homeostasis, interactions between neurons and glia?
Generalized epilepsy and paroxysmal dyskinesia		10q22	KCNMA1	Calcium-sensitive potassium (BK) channel	Increase in Ca++ sensitivity, rapid repolarization of action potentials

*Modified from Arzimanoglou et al. (2004), Guerrini (2006).

Abbreviations: AD = autosomal dominant; ADNFLE = autosomal dominant nocturnal frontal lobe epilepsy; ADPEAF = autosomal dominant partial epilepsy with auditory features; BFNC = benign familial neonatal convulsions; BFNIC = benign familial neonatal–infantile convulsions; CAE = childhood absence epilepsy; Dravet syndrome = severe myoclonic epilepsy of infancy; FS = febrile seizures; GABA = gamma-aminobutyric acid; GEFS+ = generalized epilepsy with febrile seizures plus [GEFS+ is included under the heading 'syndromes' for convenience; as discussed in the text the term covers a variety of epilepsy syndromes and/or types of seizures found in a family and is not defined with the same (electroclinical) criteria as the majority of epilepsy syndromes]; IGE = idiopathic generalised epilepsy; JME = juvenile myoclonic epilepsy.

syndromes, and rapid progress is being made in the molecular genetics of childhood epilepsy (for reviews, see Battaglia and Guerrini 2005, Duron et al. 2005, Gardiner 2005, Heron et al. 2007). Only a small proportion of the cases (1–2%) can be attributed to single-locus traits such as tuberous sclerosis or to metabolic errors. Epilepsy syndromes with a monogenic dominant transmission, described below, include benign neonatal convulsions (Leppert et al. 1989), benign infantile seizures (Vigevano et al. 1992, Echenne et al. 1994), and familial frontal (Scheffer et al. 1995a), mesial and lateral (Berkovic et al. 1996, Andermann and Kobayashi 2005) temporal lobe epilepsy syndromes.

The role of genetic factors is not limited to these relatively rare cases. A number of genes have been found to be operative in the genesis of epilepsy outside the monogenic forms. More complex inheritance is much more common (Turnbull et al. 2005) even though dominant inheritance has been suggested for epilepsies with 3 Hz spike–wave activity and possibly applies to some forms of photosensitive epilepsy (Doose and Waltz 1993). Doose and Baier (1987) had suggested that certain EEG traits (e.g. photosensitivity or spontaneous spike–wave paroxysms) could be inherited independently and that the combination of such EEG traits (and probably other factors) might account for the inherited propensity to various forms of epilepsy. Complex inheritance (multifactortial inheritance) even accounts for some syndromes once thought to be dominant, e.g. in juvenile myoclonic epilepsy, for which a dominant gene had been indicted

TABLE 15.9
Main causes of infantile spasms (West syndrome)

Neurocutaneous syndromes
Tuberous sclerosis
Neurofibromatosis
Sturge–Weber syndrome
Incontinentia pigmenti
Ito disease
Linear naevus syndrome

Brain malformations
Aicardi syndrome
Agyria–pachygyria
Congenital perisylvian syndrome
Holoprosencephaly
Hemimegalencephaly
Heterotopias, cortical dysplasias and other migration disorders
Down syndrome
Fragile X chromosome

Metabolic and degenerative diseases
Phenylketonuria
Nonketotic hyperglycinaemia
Hyperornithinaemia–hyperammonaemia–homocitrullinaemia (HHH
  syndrome)
Leigh disease
Pyridoxine dependency
Degenerative diseases of unknown cause (poliodystrophy, leukodystrophy)
Mitochondrial disorders
Biotinidase deficiency
Menkes disease
Carbohydrate-deficient glycoprotein (CDG) syndrome type IV
PEHO syndrome (progressive encephalopathy with oedema,
  hypsarrhythmia and optic atrophy)
X-linked infantile spasms

Infectious disorders
Fetal infections especially cytomegalovirus

Toxic
Sequelae of neonatal hypoglycaemia
Lithium toxicity

Hypoxic–ischaemic encephalopathy
Prenatal, perinatal and postnatal
Cerebral infarcts
Near-drowning

Cardiac surgery with hypothermia

Trauma and haemorrhage

Brain tumours (rarely)

Neonatal haemangiomatosis

The term cryptogenic does not exclude the presence of a lesion, thus blurring the distinction between the two categories. With the latter definition, cryptogenic spasms account for only 10–15% of cases, but these are much more likely than symptomatic cases to run a favourable course. Some investigators (Vigevano et al. 1993, Dulac and Tuxhorn 2005) describe an *idiopathic group* of infantile spasms with a good prognosis and peculiar clinical and EEG features. However, Haga et al. (1995) and Watanabe et al. (2001) were unable to differentiate aetiological groups on the sole basis of clinical or EEG (ictal or interictal) features. *Symptomatic spasms* are most commonly due to brain dysgenesis and neurocutaneous syndromes (mainly

tuberous sclerosis) (Vigevano et al. 1994a, Arzimanoglou et al. 2004, Dulac and Tuxhorn 2005). Gross malformations include lissencephaly, pachygyria, diffuse subcortical heterotopias and agenesis of the corpus callosum, especially Aicardi syndrome (see Chapter 2). Tuberous sclerosis accounts for 10–20% of cases. Focal cortical dysplasias (Chugani et al. 1990, 1996; Robain and Vinters 1994; Chugani and Conti 1996) may be the single most important cause of infantile spasms. Chronic congenital and acquired lesions account for the majority of remaining symptomatic cases (Cowan and Hudson 1991). Metabolic diseases are uncommonly causative. Infantile spasms are also observed in chromosomal disorders associated with epilepsy (Battaglia and Guerrini 2005).

West syndrome is usually sporadic, except when due to metabolic disorders. Genetically determined forms are uncommon. X-linked cases are mainly due to mutations in the *ARX* gene (Suri 2005) and may be associated with other abnormalities, some of which are congenital. Other cases due to mutations at chromosome Xp11p11–Xpter (Claes et al. 1997) and in the *CDLK5* gene (Weaving et al. 2004) have been reported. Spasms are also a feature of the PEHO syndrome of peripheral oedema, hypsarrhythmia and optic atrophy (Chapter 9). From a pathological point of view, a majority of autopsied cases of infantile spasms are due to prenatal factors. Meencke and Gerhard (1985) found no detectable pathology in only 11% of 107 cases. Most cases are related to diffuse lesions, but unilateral lesions, in particular cystic softenings in the middle artery territory (so-called porencephalic cysts) (Palm et al. 1988), may be responsible for infantile spasms that are not necessarily of poor prognosis (Alvarez et al. 1987, Cusmai et al. 1988).

The *treatment* of West syndrome is not yet agreed upon universally. Most conventional anticonvulsant drugs are ineffective. So far, only corticosteroids or ACTH and vigabatrin have been generally recognized as effective in recent reviews such as the Cochrane review (Hancock et al. 2003) and the American Academy of Neurology Practice parameters (Mackay et al. 2004). Other agents, e.g. topiramate, lamotrigine, valproate, pyridoxine and zonisamide, and non-pharmacological methods have been found useful by some authors (for reviews, see Arzimanoglou et al. 2004, Dulac and Tuxhorn 2005). All studies underscore the need for well designed, prospective studies with larger numbers of participants, taking into account the underlying aetiology and having a long follow-up.

• *Hormonal treatment.* ACTH and corticosteroids are both used. The modalities of *ACTH therapy* have been extremely variable. ACTH doses used vary from 10 to 40 units of natural hormone or 0.1–0.5 mg/kg as tetracosactide. Corticosteroids including prednisolone at 2–10 mg/kg, hydrocortisone at 5–20 mg/kg/day and dexamethasone at 0.3–0.5 mg/kg/day have been used alone or in various combinations with ACTH. Only a few controlled studies and even fewer compararative studies have been performed (Glaze et al. 1988, Mackay et al. 2004).

One controlled comparative study of tetracosactide vs prednisolone found ACTH to be more effective in a small number of patients, producing remission in 13 of 15 infants as against 4 of 14 receiving prednisolone (Baram et al. 1996). In contrast, the recent large controlled United Kingdom Infantile Spasms Study (UKISS; Lux et al. 2005) did not find any superiority of one product over the other. High-dose ACTH (150 IU/kg/day) had not been found more effective than low dosage (20 IU/kg/day) in another study (Hrachovy et al. 1994), and two low-dose regimes of tetracosactide showed no difference between the lower and higher dosages (Kondo et al. 2005). Various other protocols are currently available (review in Arzimanoglou et al. 2004). Heiskala et al. (1996) proposed individualizing progressive ACTH therapy, starting with a dose of 3 IU/kg/day and progressively increasing to a maximum of 12 IU/kg/day if no response is obtained. The clinical impression is that some cases may respond selectively to either agent.

Corticosteroids obviate the need for injection and shorten hospitalization, and many clinicians continue to use steroids for this reason. However, ACTH might be preferred if its superiority were confirmed in more convincing, larger studies. The mode of action of both agents is unknown. Duration of treatment is no less variable, from 3–4 weeks to several months. Our own practice is to use hormonal treatment for short periods of the order of 4–6 weeks.

ACTH or steroid therapy controls the spasms in 50–70% of cases and normalizes or improves the EEG in a slightly lower proportion. Relapses occur in 20–35% of patients. The long-term effect of therapy is less striking (Riikonen 1996, Gaily et al. 1999, Goh et al. 2005), with normal cognitive development in about 25–30% and an additional 10–15% with only mild impairment, but is better in cryptogenic cases where the proportions are respectively 50% and 25%. Seizures persist in approximately half the patients. They commonly present with the characteristics of the Lennox–Gastaut syndrome, but partial seizures are also observed.

Side effects of ACTH or corticosteroids are frequent and may be severe including hypertension, infections and metabolic disturbances. In addition to the classical side effects of corticosteroids, brain shrinkage is usually observed (Konishi et al. 1992). Neuroimaging assessment of patients is therefore best performed before starting treatment.

• *Antiepileptic agents. Vigabatrin* has been shown to be efficacious in several studies (for reviews, see Arzimanoglou et al. 2004, Dulac and Tuxhorn 2005). In doses of 100–150 mg/day it can control the spasms in approximately 50–60% of cases usually in less than a week (Aicardi et al. 1996). Its effect on EEG abnormalities is slower than that of corticosteroids. In a comparative study with hormonal treatment as first-line therapy (Vigevano and Cilio 1997), vigabatrin was more effective than ACTH as treatment for infantile spasms due to cerebral malformations or tuberous sclerosis, whereas ACTH proved more effective in perinatal hypoxic–ischaemic injury cases. The efficacy of the two drugs was similar in cryptogenic cases. Disappearance of interictal EEG abnormalities occurred sooner in patients randomized to ACTH than in those who received vigabatrin as initial therapy.

In the multicentre randomized controlled UKISS trial (O'Callaghan et al. 2004, Lux et al. 2005, Riikonen 2005), proportions with no spasms on days 13 and 14 were: 40 (73%) of 55 infants assigned hormonal treatments (prednisolone 21/30, tetracosactide 19/25) and 28 (54%) of 52 infants assigned vigabatrin (difference 19%, 95% CI 1–36%, p=0.043). Two infants allocated to tetracosactide and one allocated to vigabatrin received prednisolone. Adverse events were reported in 30 (55%) of 55 infants on hormonal treatments and 28 (54%) of 52 infants on vigabatrin. When the same groups of patients were assessed at 12–14 months of age (Lux et al. 2005), the absence of spasms at final clinical assessment was similar in each treatment group [hormone 41/55 (75%) vs vigabatrin 39/51 (76%)]. Neurodevelopment was also evaluated in this follow-up study, using the Vineland Adaptive Behaviour Scales (VABS). Mean scores did not differ significantly [hormone 78.6 (SD 16.8) vs vigabatrin 77.5 (SD 12.7)]; except for infants with no identified underlying aetiology, in whom the mean VABS score was higher in those allocated to hormone treatment than in those allocated to vigabatrin.

Vigabatrin seems highly effective in spasms due to tuberous sclerosis (Chiron et al. 1990, 1997) and is currently the drug of choice in such cases (Aicardi et al. 1996), whereas hormonal treatment is still advised by some (Riikonen 2005) in cryptogenic cases. However, interpretation of differences is not easy, and initial use of vigabatrin is still preferred by the present authors because of its rapid action (efficacy on seizures can be evaluated in less than a week in many cases) and the good immediate tolerance of the drug. Suggested dose is 100–150 mg/kg/day. In cases where vigabatrin remains without effect after a few days, trial steroid treatment is the next choice (Arzimanoglou et al. 2004).

The most worrying side effect of vigabatrin is constriction of the visual field, which occurs in up to 30–50% of adult patients and may not regress. Its frequency has varied considerably among series. Vanhatalo et al. (2002) found that 17 (18.5%) of 91 children exposed to the agent had restriction of the temporal field. There was a positive correlation between field loss and duration and dose of treatment. The shortest duration of vigabatrin treatment associated with visual field constriction was 15 months, and the lowest total dose 914 g. Hammoudi et al. (2005) found that contrast sensitivity and visual acuity were reduced in a series of 28 children. The severity of the defect is usually mild, and it seems unlikely that short-term treatment (less than 6 months) will produce a severe defect, so we believe the balance of risks in a severe condition like infantile spasms still favours the use of the drug.

Recurrences are not rare with either hormonal or vigabatrin therapy, and the optimal duration of treatment is yet to be defined.

Other forms of treatment for infantile spasms include the *benzodiazepines*, especially *nitrazepam*. These are sometimes effective against clinical spasms (Chamberlain 1996) but their effect on the EEG abnormalities is limited. One comparative study found no difference between nitrazepam and hormonal treatment (Dreifuss et al. 1986) but most authors regard this treatment as less effective than steroids.

TABLE 15.10
Syndromes related to infantile spasms

Syndrome	Clinical features	EEG features	Aetiological factors
Neonatal myoclonic encephalopathy[1] (early myoclonic encephalopathy)	Erratic myoclonus and partial seizures from the first days of life. Infantile spasms appear secondarily. Severe course with death in first year in 50% of cases	Suppression–burst pattern later evolving into atypical hypsarrhythmia	Unknown. Familial cases known
Glycine encephalopathy[1] (nonketotic hyperglycinaemia)	Same features, death within 1 month in 50% of cases	Idem	Enzyme defect (Chapter 8)
Early infantile epileptic encephalopathy (Ohtahara syndrome)	Tonic spasms from the first days of life. Partial seizures sometimes	Idem	Brain malformations + unknown
Periodic lateralized spasms	Repetitive lateralized spasms often following a partial seizure	Asymmetrical slow complexes following a localized discharge with superimposed fast rhythms	Mainly brain malformations

[1]These two entities may be regarded as belonging to the same electroclinical syndrome.

Sodium valproate in high doses (100–200 mg/kg/day) has produced good results for some investigators (Siemes et al. 1988, Prats et al. 1991, Ohtsuka et al. 1994), with control of the spasms in 40–65% of cases.

The *prognosis* of infantile spasms with ACTH/steroids or vigabatrin treatment depends on aetiology, and better results are obtained in cryptogenic (or idiopathic) cases with a completely normal development before the spasms. The occurrence of previous seizures, of neurological signs and of major MRI abnormalities are predictors of a poor outcome. Koo et al. (1993) found average developmental quotients of 71 in 17 cryptogenic cases and 48 in 40 symptomatic cases. Fifty-one per cent of patients had other seizures and these were significantly associated with a symptomatic aetiology and a poor cognitive outcome. The eventual effect of treatment choices on global developmental outcome was never properly assessed. One of the main difficulties for such studies derives from the various aetiologies at the origin of West syndrome.

• *Surgical resection* of localized brain areas of cortical dysplasia thought to be responsible for the spasms has been performed (Chugani et al. 1990, Shields et al. 1992, Chugani and Pinard 1994, Jonas et al. 2005, Kang et al. 2006) and may be indicated as early treatment in selected cases, particularly when a clearly identifiable dysplastic lesion is detectable by MRI or in cases with hemimegalencephaly.

Delimitation of the abnormal cortex is usually by MRI but some cases may be detectable only by positron emission tomography (PET – Chugani et al. 1996), or by single photon emission computed tomography (SPECT – Miyazaki et al. 1994). However, transient PET abnormalities, especially during the period of active hypsarrhythmia, have been found (Watanabe et al. 1994), and the relationship between PET anomalies and the causes and outcome of the syndrome is currently unclear (Watanabe 1996). Identification of, and possible preventive treatment

for infants with neonatal difficulties at risk of developing infantile spasms have been attempted (Okumura and Watanabe 2001).

Syndromes closely related to infantile spasms (Table 15.10)
These include *neonatal myoclonic encephalopathy* (Aicardi 1990, Arzimanoglou et al. 2004), *Ohtahara syndrome* or early infantile epileptic encephalopathy (EIEE) (Ohtahara et al. 1987) and the *syndrome of periodic spasms* described by Gobbi et al. (1987). This last syndrome can be observed at any age and is almost always due to brain malformations or extensive brain damage.

Neonatal (or early) myoclonic encephalopathy (EME) is an extremely severe condition of very early onset, characterized by partial or fragmentary erratic myoclonus from birth, massive hypotonia, and often the late occurrence of repetitive tonic spasms. The EEG consistently shows a suppression–burst pattern, characterized by a succession of bursts of paroxysmal activity separated by episodes of flat or low-amplitude tracing. The course is severe, neurological development remains absent or rudimentary, and death supervenes in about half the cases, most often in the first year of life (Aicardi and Ohtahara 2005). Non-ketotic hyperglycinaemia is a major cause.

Early infantile epileptic encephalopathy (EIEE), also known as *Ohtahara syndrome* (Aicardi and Ohtahara 2005), is characterized by a very early onset, frequent tonic spasms, and a suppression–burst EEG pattern. It is closely related to infantile spasms, of which it may be regarded as a neonatal form. It usually does not feature myoclonus, and is compatible with survival with neurological and mental sequelae.

All three syndromes are of lesional or metabolic origin and share a poor prognosis. Although EIEE is thought to be mostly due to brain malformations and EME to metabolic disorders, there are many exceptions to that rule and migration disorder has been shown to be a cause of myoclonic encephalopathy (Du Plessis et al. 1993).

Moreover, cases of glycine encephalopathy may present with

severe neonatal encephalopathy but without myoclonic phenomena, suggesting that there is no strict relationship between aetiology and clinical features (Aicardi and Ohtahara 2005). Thus the separation between EIEE and neonatal myoclonic encephalopathy may be artificial (Lombroso 1990), and EIEE may be an early form of infantile spasms.

Dentato-olivary dysplasia (Harding and Boyd 1991) is a rare cause of neonatal tonic seizures and possibly of infantile spasms. The prognosis is very poor and the diagnosis is possible only at autopsy. One familial case is known (Harding and Copp 1997).

Lennox–Gastaut and related syndromes
The Lennox–Gastaut syndrome (LGS) includes patients with epilepsy starting mainly between 1 and 7 years of age, who present with variable proportions of tonic, atonic and myoclonic seizures resulting in multiple falls and atypical absences, and whose interictal EEGs contain bilateral, though not necessarily symmetrical, slow (<2.5 Hz) spike–wave activity. The limits of LGS are variably understood by different investigators who use diverse criteria for its definition and for its separation from related syndromes such as the myoclonic epilepsies (for a discussion on the nosology of the syndrome, see Aicardi and Levy Gomes 1988, 1989; Arzimanoglou et al. 2004).

Most investigators now accept the definition proposed by Beaumanoir and colleagues (Beaumanoir and Dravet 1992, Beaumanoir and Blume 2005), i.e. of a syndrome of multiple seizure types with interictal slow spike–waves, spikes and bursts of 10–20 Hz spikes during sleep, most often associated with mental retardation.

The seizures of LGS include 'core' seizures (myoatonic and tonic, atypical absences and episodes of nonconvulsive status epilepticus) that can be variably associated with less characteristic attacks such as tonic–clonic, partial or unilateral seizures.

Tonic seizures are encountered in 55–92% of cases. Clinically, they are marked by body stiffening involving mainly the axial and proximal limb muscles, with extension more commonly than flexion of the trunk, lower limbs and arms. They may be limited to the trunk and neck, with opening of the eyes and, frequently, apnoea. They sometimes consist only of eye opening with mild 'stretching' movements. Their duration does not exceed 30 seconds and is often no more than 10 seconds. Even in such cases, the contraction is clearly tonic, resulting in sustained clinical and electromyographic muscle activity (Aicardi and Levy Gomes 1988). The *ictal EEG* shows a generalized discharge of fast activity (≥10 Hz) of increasing or high amplitude (Beaumanoir and Dravet 1992, Arzimanoglou et al. 2004, Beaumanoir and Blume 2005), sometimes followed by a few spike–wave complexes. Similar discharges of brief duration without clinical manifestations are recorded during slow sleep. Tonic seizures are often nocturnal but their manifestations in sleep may be so mild as to go unnoticed (Aicardi and Levy Gomes 1988, Yaqub 1993, Beaumanoir and Blume 2005).

Atonic seizures occur in 26–56% of LGS patients. They consist of abrupt muscle relaxation and are a common cause of falls in such children, although tonic and myoclonic attacks can also result in falls. These represent a major practical problem as they often cause injuries not easily prevented by wearing a helmet. The mechanisms of falls are often unclear when no polygraphic recording is available, so the noncommittal term of *astatic seizure* should be preferred. Most atonic seizures are associated with loss of consciousness, and it is not clear whether they are purely atonic or are associated with tonic phenomena. Most have the same EEG concomitants as tonic seizures. Thus, they seem to differ from pure atonic seizures associated with bursts of spike–wave activity as observed in the myoclonic–astatic epilepsies (Oguni et al. 1993, 1996, 2001a).

True myoclonic seizures may be seen in up to 28% of cases and may also be associated with falls. The type of seizure observed depends on the age of onset of LGS. In cases of early onset, tonic seizures predominate, whereas myoclonic jerks and absences are more frequent in late-onset cases (Chevrie and Aicardi 1972, 1996).

Atypical absences are present in 17–60% of patients. Although their onset and termination may be more progressive than in typical absences (see below), they are marked by the same interruption of awareness and responsiveness with only mild motor components (stiffness, hypotonia, simple automatisms) and their recognition depends on the clinical context and the EEG concomitants. These are sometimes ictal slow spike–waves, difficult to distinguish from interictal spike–waves, but more often fast discharges similar to those associated with tonic seizures.

Episodes of nonconvulsive status epilepticus are frequent (Dravet et al. 1986, Beaumanoir et al. 1988) and may last several days or even weeks. They may be responsible for the alternation of good and bad periods with considerable changes in reaction time and mental activity. The most common type is characterized by the alternation of tonic attacks and episodes of confused behaviour, often with erratic myoclonic activity of the face and upper limbs, and may last from hours to weeks (Arzimanoglou et al. 2004).

The interictal EEG of patients with LGS shows a diffuse slow spike–wave pattern, with slow blunted spikes followed by irregular 1–2 Hz slow waves of variable amplitude, usually on a slow, irregular background tracing. They may be asymmetrical and are often unaccompanied by obvious clinical manifestations. They show little or no response to hyperventilation or photic stimulation but are activated during drowsiness and slow sleep (Aicardi and Levy Gomes 1988). During non-REM sleep, runs of 10–20 Hz rhythms of a few seconds duration characteristically occur and probably represent subclinical or minimal tonic seizures (Fig. 15.5). At the same stage, slow spike–wave complexes are frequently replaced by polyspike–wave complexes.

Mental retardation is present before onset of seizures in 20–60% of cases (Arzimanoglou et al. 2006). The proportion of patients with retardation increases with the passing of time, rising to 90% five years after onset (Chevrie and Aicardi 1972). Clear loss of skills is observed in some patients. Psychotic symptoms are often present.

The *aetiology* of LGS is heterogeneous. Brain damage plays an important role, whereas genetic factors are regarded as less important. Up to two thirds of cases may result from a demonstrable brain abnormality or occur in patients with previous develop-

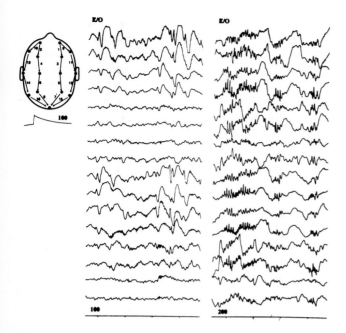

Fig. 15.5. Lennox–Gastaut syndrome. EEG findings in a child with multiple seizure types, but particularly tonic attacks and atypical absences. *(Left)* The portion of waking record shows sharp waves and slow components at around 2–2.5/sec over the anterior half of the head. *(Right)* A burst of 10–12/sec spiky components is seen during sleep associated with spontaneous eye opening. (Courtesy Dr S Boyd, Great Ormond Street Hospital, London.)

mental delay, and these are termed *symptomatic*. A significant proportion of LGS cases follow infantile spasms, with a gradual transition, and are due to the same brain insults that produce the infantile spasms. Brain malformations, however, are less common in LGS, and LGS has been only exceptionally recorded in the course of Aicardi syndrome and of lissencephaly. Focal or multifocal abnormalities of cortical development are frequent, and cases of band heterotopia and of bilateral perisylvian syndromes are on record (Chapter 2). Tuberous sclerosis and less common neurocutaneous syndromes, such as linear naevus sebaceus and Ito hypomelanosis (personal cases), may be responsible. Acquired destructive lesions are also less common. Metabolic diseases are exceptional, although LGS due to Leigh encephalomyelopathy has been recorded (Matsuishi et al. 1985). Rare cases of LGS secondary to brain tumours are known (Honda et al. 1985).

A proportion of cases have no obvious recognized cause and are considered *cryptogenic*. The occurrence of LGS in patients with unilateral lesions has led to attempts at distinguishing 'true' LGS from bilateral secondary synchrony (Gastaut and Zifkin 1988). In fact, cases of secondary bilateral synchrony fulfil the usual criteria for the diagnosis of LGS, although it may be important to recognize them because of the possibility of surgery. PET studies have recognized several metabolic patterns (focal, multifocal or diffuse) that may correspond to different mechanisms (Chugani et al. 1987, Iinuma et al. 1987, Theodore et al. 1987). Their practical significance is still unclear as the criteria for the diagnosis of LGS varied with the series.

Diagnosis of LGS is not difficult if strict criteria are used. However, differentiation of LGS from some other syndromes associated with falls may be problematic (for discussion, see Aicardi 1996), particularly at the early stages of the disorder or if tonic seizures are not yet part of the clinical picture (Arzimanoglou et al. 2004). A real problem may be posed by the rare cases of 'atypical benign epilepsy of children' (Aicardi and Levy Gomes 1992) or pseudo-Lennox syndrome (Hahn 2000), in which repeated falls and diffuse paroxysmal EEG activity during sleep may suggest LGS. Such cases may run a relatively benign course and it is important to recognize them.

The *prognosis* of LGS is poor (Arzimanoglou 2003). Approximately 80% of patients continue to have seizures and, due to their seizures or mental deterioration, only a very few patients are able to live independent lives. The outcome is especially poor for patients with brain damage, early onset of seizures or antecedents of infantile spasms, and where mental retardation was present before the initial seizures. Less than 10% of patients have a normal intellectual level. It has proved difficult to distinguish such cases from those with less favourable outcome, although a later age of onset, a positive response to hyperventilation and a higher incidence of 3 Hz spike–wave complexes have some prognostic value. Cases with such features were termed 'intermediate petit mal' but the separation of such a subgroup seems debatable as the criteria of diagnosis were similar to those of LGS in general. In typical cases the clinical pattern changes with age. At between 15 and 20 years of age the overall seizure frequency usually diminishes. Atypical absences and drop attacks may become rare but all other types of seizures, including tonic seizures in sleep, persist. In older patients tonic seizures during sleep are probably underreported by the parents (Arzimanoglou et al. 2004, Beaumanoir and Blume 2005).

The *treatment* of LGS is difficult. Among conventional antiepileptic drugs, combinations of sodium valproate and a benzodiazepine are least unsatisfactory, but all such drugs may be worth trying in individual patients. Carbamazepine is deemed satisfactory by some clinicians for partial and tonic seizures but it has no effect on, or may perhaps even aggravate, other types of seizures. Because of its lack of interactions with other antiepileptic drugs (AEDs), vigabatrin has been used with some measure of success, particularly in LGS patients combining focal seizures with the core seizures of the syndrome. Lamotrigine is reported to be efficacious (Motte et al. 1997) especially against atonic seizures and is probably the best treatment now available, often in association with sodium valproate. Felbamate, particularly when used in accordance with existing recommendations and close monitoring, may still be considered, despite possible toxicity, as it is often effective (Pellock et al. 2006). Topiramate was also shown to be effective in some cases (Sachdeo et al. 1999). Interestingly, combinations of drugs are often required as individual drugs may have a specific activity against only certain types of seizures. Most treatments are based on clinical wisdom or uncontrolled studies, and only very few, including felbamate, topiramate and lamotrigine, are based on controlled studies (Glauser and Morita 2001, Hancock and Cross 2003). A good knowledge of AED interactions is required, and usually these children are better treated by child neurologists specialized in epilepsy. The recent Cochrane review (Hancock and Cross 2003) also concluded that the optimum treatment for LGS remains uncertain, and no study to date has shown any one drug to be highly efficacious. Until further research has been undertaken, clinicians will need to continue to consider each patient individually, taking into account the potential benefit of each therapy weighed against the risk of adverse effects.

Because of the high rate of drug failure, other methods may be worth trying. The *ketogenic diet* has given good short-term effects (Kinsman et al. 1992) despite practical difficulties due to unpalatability and side effects. However, Kinsman and colleagues have been able to maintain the treatment for one or two years, controlling seizures in half their patients. Interestingly, they claim that the diet can be withdrawn after two years without recurrence of the seizures. *Steroids* are used mainly to tide the patient over bad periods of very active epilepsy or status. Intravenous immunoglobulins have been advocated but have not been properly tested. *Thyrotropin-releasing hormone* (Matsumoto et al. 1987) has been used mainly in Japan. *Vagus nerve stimulation* may also be an alternative, and *resective surgery* has been used in a few cases with cortical dysplasia. In selected cases *callosotomy* was tried for the control of seizures with falls, which represent the most incapacitating type of seizure (see below in section on treatment issues).

Dravet syndrome
This syndrome was initially described by Charlotte Dravet as *severe myoclonic epilepsy of infants*. Although it does often feature myoclonic phenomena, only uncommonly are these the first manifestation of the syndrome. As suggested by clinical observations (Veggiotti et al. 2001), recent progress in molecular genetics has confirmed that Dravet syndrome is part of a continuum of severe epilepsies of infancy that may or may not feature additional generalized tonic–clonic seizures, focal seizures, atypical absences and myoclonias. Dravet syndrome can be considered as the most severe end of the spectrum of epilepsy syndromes described as 'GEFS *plus*' (see p. 606).

In over 80% of cases, Dravet syndrome is due to new mutations in the sodium channel gene *SCN1A* (Claes et al. 2001). More than 100 de novo mutations have been described (Mulley et al. 2005), most frequently truncating mutations, but also splice site, deletion and missense mutations. In the remaining 20%, no mutations of the *SCNA1* gene are present. Two familial cases of *GABRG2* mutations have been reported. Recently, Depienne et al. (2006) reported somatic and germline mosaicism in the transmitting asymptomatic parents in two families with more than one case of Dravet syndrome.

Onset, usually between 4 and 10 months of age, is characterized by clonic seizures, often unilateral and prolonged, precipitated by fever in 75% of cases. Such seizures recur several times, at short intervals (usually less than two months). The initial development appears normal. During the second or third year, other types of seizure appear including partial seizures, atypical

absences, myoclonic jerks and episodes of nonconvulsive status. At the same time, slowing of cognitive development becomes evident. Pyramidal tract signs and ataxia often evolve. Interictal EEG recordings are generally normal during the first months of the disease despite the frequent seizures. From the second year of life, EEG does not show slow spike–wave complexes but rather bursts of fast spike–wave complexes, often in association with multifocal spikes. Photosensitivity is present in 25% of patients, and self-precipitation of seizures is not rare. The long-term outcome is poor. The seizures persist mainly as tonic–clonic attacks, and myoclonic seizures tend to disappear. Mental retardation of variable degree is constant (Oguni et al. 2001b, Dravet and Bureau 2005).

In some patients, generalized or unilateral clonic seizures, often precipitated by mild fever or even by hot baths, are the prominent or even the sole seizure type, whereas the brief seizures may not be in the forefront and may not always include myoclonic attacks, which, in any case, are seldom the most striking seizure form. Several investigators have described such cases as variants of severe myoclonic epilepsy (Ogino et al. 1989, Watanabe et al. 1989), epilepsy with hemi-grand mal and high-amplitude EEG slow waves (Doose 1992) or as idiopathic epilepsy of infancy (Ebach et al. 2005). Such forms have been grouped (Oguni et al. 2001a, Fukuma et al. 2004) as 'borderline cases' of severe myoclonic epilepsy. The course of such cases seems to be similar to that of the typical form, although it may be less severe. Some of these atypical forms have been shown to be due to mutations of the *SCNA1* gene but often different from those in the typical forms, especially as truncating mutations are rare (Claes et al. 2001, Fujiwara et al. 2003, Fukuma et al. 2004). The same gene can also be responsible for other epilepsy syndromes including epilepsy with myoclonic astatic seizures and some cases reported within GEFS *plus* families (see p. 606) (Ebach et al. 2005). Harkin et al. (2007) reviewed 90 cases of 'epileptic encephalopathy' with *SCN1A* mutations: 52 had typical Dravet syndrome; 25 atypical forms; 6 had cryptogenic generalized epilepsy, 4 had cryptogenic focal epilepsy, 2 had myoclonic–astatic epilepsy and 1 had Lennox–Gastaut syndrome, broadening the range of expression of the gene.

Berkovic et al. (2006) identified *SCN1A* mutations in 11 of 14 patients with *alleged vaccine encephalopathy*. Clinical–molecular correlation showed mutations in 8 cases with phenotypes of Dravet syndrome, in 3 of 4 cases with borderline Dravet syndrome, but not in 2 cases with Lennox–Gastaut syndrome. These findings, although they need replication, provide a substantial alternative explanation that these disorders of early childhood, which many are convinced are caused by vaccinations, may have an entirely different unrelated cause.

The *therapy* of severe myoclonic epilepsy is disappointing, although occasional cases with a satisfactory outcome using large doses of sodium valproate have been reported. Recently, stiripentol (Chiron 2007) was granted orphan drug status in the European Union for the treatment of Dravet syndrome, following a study where it was used in combination with sodium valproate and clobazam (Chiron et al. 2000). The interactions of stiripentol with a large number of other drugs need to be carefully taken into account. Although complete control was rarely reached, this association seems to reduce both the frequency and the duration of convulsive episodes. In the past, vigabatrin gave good results in patients with an attenuated myoclonic component of the syndrome. Finally, topiramate gave promising results in open studies and should probably be prescribed early in the course of the disease (Dravet and Bureau 2005). Topiramate and stiripentol seem to be easily and safely associated (Kröll-Seger et al. 2006). Lamotrigine was reported to have an aggravating effect in young children with Dravet syndrome (Guerrini et al. 1998b).

EPILEPSIES OF INFANCY AND EARLY CHILDHOOD WITH PREDOMINANTLY MYOCLONIC SEIZURES

Epilepsies that consist mainly of true myoclonic seizures – i.e. seizures marked clinically by very brief shock-like muscle contractions and, electrically, by fast spike–wave or polyspike–wave complexes – occur in infancy and early childhood (Aicardi 1996, Guerrini and Aicardi 2003, Arzimanoglou et al. 2004). Such epilepsies are often confused with Lennox-Gastaut syndrome because of the frequent repetition of brief attacks that may produce multiple falls, the presence of spike–wave discharges in both groups, and the frequent association of mental retardation or deterioration with the seizures. However, the clinical and EEG manifestations of the myoclonic epilepsies differ from those of LGS, and the outlook for control of seizures and mental development may not be the same.

Myoclonic seizures consist of sudden, lightning-like muscle contractions that may involve the whole body (massive myoclonic attacks) or be limited to the upper limbs, the face or the eyelids. The jerks are usually symmetrical but may be unilateral or even localized to small muscle groups. *Ictal EEG* shows polyspike–wave paroxysms. Ictal electromyography demonstrates an extremely brief muscle contraction followed by a period of inactivity lasting 100–350 ms. When this period is relatively long, muscle resolution may become clinically evident, resulting in a myoatonic seizure (Oguni et al. 1994, 1997). Occasionally, only the atonic phase is detectable, the so-called *'negative myoclonus'* (Guerrini and Aicardi 2003). Clinically, atonia of variable intensity and duration often follows the myoclonic jerk. When generalized and long enough, it results in falls (drop-attacks), and the differentiation of atonic from myoclonic seizures may therefore be clinically impossible. Myoclonic–astatic epilepsy may thus be considered only as a variant of myoclonic epilepsy in which the atonic component is particularly obvious.

The *nosology* of the myoclonic epilepsies remains confused. The International Classification identifies three major groups: severe myoclonic epilepsy or Dravet syndrome (Dravet et al. 1986, 1992a, 2005) (see above), benign myoclonic epilepsy (Dravet et al. 1992, Dravet and Bureau 2005), and epilepsy with myoclonic–astatic seizures (Doose 1992) to which unclassifiable cases should be added.

Benign myoclonic epilepsy of infancy
Benign myoclonic epilepsy (BME) is characterized by brief myoclonic seizures, spontaneous or provoked by noise or contact, starting between the ages of 4 months and 3 years in otherwise neurodevelopmentally normal children, predominantly in boys (Dravet et al. 1992, 2005). Myoclonic seizures are the only type of seizures present, with the exception of rare simple febrile convulsions in some. The interictal EEG, including sleep organization, is normal, and spontaneous spike–wave discharges are rare. Myoclonias are associated with an EEG discharge, in the form of fast generalized spike–wave or polyspike–waves at more than 3 Hz, lasting the same time as the myoclonias.

The course is benign with a good response to monotherapy with sodium valproate and, when indicated, the association of ethosuximide or a benzodiazepine. Treatment is usually maintained for 3 or 4 years. A number of affected children, however, have mild learning difficulties or mild retardation. In fact, the benign prognosis of this form is far from constant as more than 10% of patients end up with behavioural and some cognitive difficulties (Dravet and Bureau 2005).

It is not clear whether the term 'benign myoclonic epilepsy' should be limited to cases with only myoclonic seizures. Aicardi and Levy Gomes (1989) reported on 19 young children, mainly boys with a high frequency of familial antecedents of seizures, who had infrequent tonic–clonic seizures and/or brief absences in addition to frequent myoclonic jerks and a relatively favourable outcome. Such cases suggest the existence of a spectrum of non-lesional, probably genetically determined, myoclonic epilepsies.

In some infants, seizures are precipitated by sudden exteroceptive or proprioceptive stimuli. This *'touch' or reflex myoclonic epilepsy* (Ricci et al. 1995) seems to have an excellent prognosis and treatment may be avoided. Cases similar to BME may also occur in older children, and BME can be considered as the early expression of idiopathic generalized epilepsy (Arzimanoglou et al. 2004), the infantile equivalent of juvenile myoclonic epilepsy as suggested by Dravet and Bureau (2005).

The genetics of BME are unknown. Cases are rare and no family cases of BME have been described. Arzimanoglou et al. (1996) described a family in which the proband had epilepsy with myoclonic–astatic seizures and his younger brother experienced a typical BME with excellent outcome.

Myoclonic–astatic epilepsy
Myoclonic–astatic epilepsy (probably more appropriately *epilepsy with myoclonic–astatic seizures*) is perhaps better regarded as a category of generalized non-lesional myoclonic epilepsies rather than as a discrete syndrome (Guerrini and Aicardi 2003, Arzimanoglou et al. 2004, Guerrini et al. 2005). The term 'myoclonic–astatic' was first used by Doose et al. (1970) in a paper on 'centrencephalic myoclonic–astatic petit mal' and further developed in by Doose and Baier (1987) in a paper entitled 'Genetic factors in epilepsies with primarily generalized minor seizures.' It was initially defined as a form of genetically determined, non-lesional generalized epilepsy, and probably included cases that are now termed severe or benign myoclonic epilepsy as well as cases fulfiling the current concept of myoclonic–astatic epilepsy (Guerrini and Aicardi 2003).

HEAD DROP

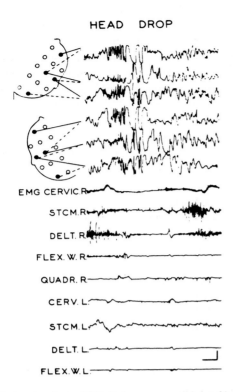

EMG CERVIC.R

STCM.R

DELT.R

FLEX. W. R

QUADR. R

CERV. L

STCM. L

DELT. L

FLEX.W.L

Fig. 15.6. Atonic seizure. EEG discharge starts with brief burst of fast rhythm, followed by a few spike–wave complexes and by slow waves. EMG trace shows disappearance of normal tonic activity during EEG discharge in posterior cervical muscles (CERVIC.R), sternomastoid (STCM.R) and deltoid (DELT.R) on right side. (Courtesy Dr J Roger, Centre Saint Paul, Marseille.)

Onset is later than for BME or Dravet syndrome, usually between 1 and 5 years of age, and it is seen more often in boys. It is characterized clinically by the predominance of purely myoclonic and/or myo-astatic seizures (Fig. 15.6); the seizures may result in falls or produce only a series of head drops and/or sagging at the knees when brief. Other types of seizures are often associated, including generalized tonic–clonic attacks, atypical absences and episodes of nonconvulsive status epilepticus. Tonic seizures are not prominent but they occurred relatively frequently in some series (Kaminska et al. 1999, Oguni et al. 2001a). The latter authors found them to be present in up to two thirds of their cases. Astatic seizures (drop attacks) may have different mechanisms (myoclonic, astatic or tonic) that are indistinguishable without polygraphic recording. Tonic seizures may be more frequent in children with an unfavourable outcome, but they are also observed in almost 30% of cases with a favourable outcome (Kaminska et al. 1999).

The EEG shows fast (≥3 Hz) generalized spike–wave or polyspike–wave discharges of short duration (usually less than 4–5 seconds). Doose emphasized the presence of biparietal theta rhythms.

Remission within a few years with normal cognition is possible in almost 60% of the cases (Oguni et al. 2001a, Guerrini et al. 2005). However, at onset, falls may prove difficult to

control. They can produce injuries and represent a serious practical problem. Some patients run an unfavourable course with frequent seizures and learning difficulties (20%) or mental retardation (20%), but the outcome is unpredictable at the onset of the disease.

The effectiveness of antiepileptic drugs is variable. Sodium valproate is considered the first choice drug or, if needed, a combination of sodium valproate and lamotrigine. Ethosuximide, for myoclonic seizures and absences, or benzodiazepines, particularly clobazam, can prove effective. Finally, topiramate and levetiracetam can be interesting alternatives. Carbamazepine, vigabatrin, oxcarbazepine and gabapentin should be avoided (Arzimanoglou et al. 2004, Guerrini et al. 2005).

Unclassified forms
A number of cases of myoclonic epilepsies in infancy and early childhood remain unclassified, and intermediate forms between the different syndromes exist (Arzimanoglou et al. 2004). They must be distinguished from other syndromes with frequent brief attacks and repeated falls, especially Lennox–Gastaut syndrome. The term 'myoclonic–astatic epilepsy' is still not well-delineated, clinically or by EEG, is only arbitrarily and with difficulty separated from other myoclonic forms and might apply to many of the myoclonic epilepsies. Degenerative myoclonic epilepsies with a progressive course are studied in Chapter 9.

FOCAL EPILEPSIES OF INFANCY AND EARLY CHILDHOOD
Focal epilepsies can start at any age. In this chapter they are mainly dealt with in the section dealing with seizures and syndromes of late childhood and adolescence, and are only briefly discussed here. A large proportion of seizures that occur in the first two years of life cannot be categorized into a recognized epilepsy syndrome (Korff and Nordli 2006). A majority of such seizures are probably partial ones, even though their clinical manifestations may not obviously point to a focal origin. Features of partial seizures may include version of the head and eyes or focal tonic contraction, but seizures with generalized vasomotor phenomena or diffuse tonic changes may have a focal origin, as shown by the EEG (Duchowny 1987, Rathgeb et al. 1998, Watanabe et al. 2005). Evaluation of the state of consciousness is obviously very difficult in this age range (Acharya et al. 1997).

Most such seizures, especially focal attacks, are due to gross brain damage (Chevrie and Aicardi 1977, 1979; Cavazzuti et al. 1984). Duchowny (1987, 1992) reported on 14 infants with complex partial seizures due to gross brain damage whose main ictal features were head version and body stiffening, very much like most cases of partial seizures of infants. Generalized seizures, which are rare in this age group, may have a better outlook in the absence of gross brain pathology (Chevrie and Aicardi 1978). The recent development of high-definition neuroimaging techniques has facilitated the early detection in infants of small lesions (cortical dysplasias, dysembryoplastic neuroepithelial tumours, gangliogliomas and tuberous sclerosis related lesions) at the origin of focal seizures, which are often surgically treatable despite the young age of the patients. Treatment of lesional epilepsies will be further discussed in a later section of this chapter, as more data are available on epilepsies of late childhood and adolescence. However, it is important to underscore here the possibility of focal epilepsies in infancy due to identifiable small lesions, as this may influence treatment choices. Whether early surgery of such lesions might modify the overall epilepsy and cognitive outcome of these children is currently under evaluation.

Other specific syndromes of partial seizures in infancy have been described. A rare syndrome of *partial migratory seizures in infancy with malignant outcome* (Coppola et al. 1995) is characterized by very frequent partial seizures of multiple origin and neurological deterioration leading rapidly to death. Although this syndrome has been described as a progressive condition, similar features may be obtained with fixed or progressive encephalopathies with several causes (Ishii et al. 2002).

BENIGN EPILEPSY SYNDROMES OF INFANCY
Recognition of benign epilepsy syndromes in infants is important, as their prognosis is much better than that usually attached to seizures in this age range. Their frequency is not known and may be variable depending on ethnic origin.

Watanabe et al. (1987) described the cases of 9 infants with complex partial seizures that ran a favourable course as 'benign complex partial epilepsy of infancy'. They later described a second group of 7 children who developed secondarily generalized seizures with focal onset (Watanabe 1996). More recently, Okumura et al. (2006) reviewed 33 cases and grouped them all under the term of *benign partial epilepsy in infancy*. Seizures had their onset before 6 months of age in 26 cases and were infrequent (average of 7 seizures). They often occurred in clusters and could be focal with alteration of consciousness, secondarily generalized or both. Seizures stopped before the age of 18 months in all cases, although a few infants later experienced febrile seizures. Seventeen of the infants had a family history of seizures. Several syndromes sharing similar characteristics have been reported (for reviews, see Vigevano and Bureau 2005, Chahine and Mikati 2006).

Vigevano et al. (1992, 1994b) first descibed a *syndrome of familial benign partial seizures of infants*. This syndrome is dominantly inherited and has its onset after the neonatal period. The interictal EEG is usually normal. In a few infants, small-amplitude spikes during sleep were reported, and these cases are sometimes considered a specific syndrome (Coppola et al. 1995, 2006). The diagnosis in all cases rests on a history of similar events in relatives, consistent with an autosomal dominant transmission. In an as yet undefined proportion of cases, choreo-athetotic movements supervene in the same patients several months or years after disappearance of the convulsions (Szepetowski et al. 1997, Swoboda et al. 2000) and respond well to carbamazepine.

Focal infantile convulsions are linked to several loci on chromosomes including 19q and 16 but no genes are yet characterized (see Table 15.2). The form with movement disorder seems consistently linked to centromeric chromosome 16 (Striano et al. 2006). Berkovic et al. (2004) observed an intermediate form be-

tween neonatal and infantile seizures, termed *infantile–neonatal convulsions*, caused by a mutation in the gene encoding the voltage-gated sodium channel a2 subunit (*SCN2A*) on chromosome 2q24 (Heron et al. 2002).

Caraballo et al. (2003) in a study of 64 cases of infantile seizures found no clinical differences between genetic and apparently non-genetic infantile convulsions. It remains to be determined whether the clinically similar benign syndromes of infantile seizures belong to the same or to different entities.

Benign seizures were also described in Oriental patients and recently in European infants in association with benign diarrhoeal disease (Lee et al. 1993, Komori et al. 1995, Imai et al. 1999). A syndrome of *benign infantile focal epilepsy with midline spikes and waves during sleep* was first described by Bureau and Maton (1998) and later refined by Capovilla et al. (2006). Seizures occurred in wakefulness or sleep, with onset characterized by some combination of staring, psychomotor arrest, stiffening of the arms, and loss of consciousness, and, in all, cyanosis, particularly of the face. Seizure duration ranged from 1 to 5 minutes. EEG during wakefulness consistently showed no abnormalities, while during sleep diphasic spikes of low or medium voltage followed by a bell-shaped slow wave of higher voltage were recorded. Morphologically, they are readily discernable from physiological sleep vertex spikes. Seizures usually stop before the age of 4 years and treatment is usually not necessary.

FEBRILE CONVULSIONS
Febrile convulsions are epileptic seizures precipitated by fever that is not due to an intracranial infection or other definable CNS cause and are not preceded by afebrile seizures. Febrile convulsions are the single most common problem in paediatric neurology, with a total incidence of 2–5% of children under 5 years of age in Western countries and up to about 8% in Japan. Excellent reviews of the topic are available (Nelson and Ellenberg 1981, Wallace 1988, Baram and Shinnar 2002).

Aetiology
Genetic factors are important in the causation of febrile convulsions, and there is a high incidence of a family history of febrile convulsions varying between 17% and 31% in first-degree relatives. Most studies suggest a polygenic mode of transmission (Rich et al. 1987). An autosomal dominant pattern, however, may be at play in probands with three or more episodes (Anderson et al. 1988) and in some families with multiple affected members and a tendency to long-lasting seizures (see also discussion on GEFS plus, p. 606). The genes responsible for febrile convulsions are probably distinct from those that cause afebrile seizures (see Table 15.2). Only a small proportion of children with febrile convulsions have a first-degree relative with epilepsy (Berg et al. 1992). Febrile seizures may precede some forms of epilepsy such as absences, rolandic epilepsy and Lennox–Gastaut syndrome, but the frequency of such an occurrence is poorly known (Arzimanoglou et al. 2004), and the overall risk of later epilepsy into the third decade of life remains increased following febrile convulsions (Hauser 1992). The genetic predisposition to febrile

convulsions is age-dependent. Febrile convulsions are rare before the age of 5–6 months, and 85% of children have had their first seizure by 4 years with a median age of 17–23 months. They occur mostly between 6 months and 4 years of age: 60% occur under 2 years, 20% between 2 and 3 years, and in only 20% is the first occurrence after age 3 years. Occurrence of febrile convulsions before the age of 6 months should suggest the possibility of meningitis.

The fever responsible for febrile seizures is usually high (>38.5°C) and has the same causes as other fevers in the same age group, including immunizations (Millichap and Millichap 2006). One exception may be *exanthema subitum*, which is associated with a higher incidence of seizures, varying between 8% and 13% (Asano et al. 1994). Gastroenteritis, on the other hand, is a relatively rare cause for the degree of temperature (Berg et al. 1995). Seizures usually occur early in the course of a fever and are actually the first symptom in 25–42% of cases. An earlier onset is noted in girls and in children with complex seizures (Wallace 1988).

Prenatal and perinatal factors do not play an important role in causation (Nelson and Ellenberg 1990), even though they may adversely influence the prognosis with regard to later afebrile seizures. Some delay in passing early milestones may be slightly more frequent than in the general population (Wallace 1988). The only predictors of febrile convulsions are a fever >40.5°C and a family history of febrile seizures (Bethune et al. 1993, Berg et al. 1995).

Clinical features
The great majority of febrile convulsions are brief, bilateral clonic or tonic–clonic seizures. Unilateral seizures occur in about 4% of patients. These are often prolonged seizures lasting 30 minutes or more (Nelson and Ellenberg 1981). Seizures lasting more than 15 minutes, unilateral seizures, and those followed by a Todd paralysis are termed *complicated febrile convulsions* and have a higher risk (up to 50%) of being followed by epilepsy. However, most cases of epilepsy subsequent to febrile convulsions occur after brief (so-called simple) febrile convulsions, just because these are overwhelmingly frequent and despite their lower attendant risk of epilepsy (about 1%).

Febrile convulsions lasting 30 minutes or more are one type of status epilepticus and may leave sequelae if allowed to go untreated (Aicardi and Chevrie 1976, Viani et al. 1987, Phillips and Shanahan 1989). These include the *hemiconvulsion–hemiplegia–epilepsy syndrome* (Arzimanoglou and Dravet 2003, Chauvel and Dravet 2005), now rare in developed countries.

The role of long-lasting febrile convulsions in the genesis of partial epilepsy, especially the syndrome of mesial temporal epilepsy with hippocampal sclerosis, remains disputed. However, MRI studies have shown evidence of acute swelling of the hippocampus in the days following a long febrile convulsion (VanLandigham et al. 1998, Scott et al. 2003) and the later development of hippocampal atrophy and sclerosis in patients with intractable temporal lobe epilepsy and a history of prolonged febrile seizures (Kuks et al. 1993, Holthausen 1994, Harvey et

al. 1995, Cendes et al. 2005), and there are strong arguments in favour of a causal relationship. Thus, vigorous treatment of febrile status is imperative, as shown by the persistence of sequelae in areas where emergency treatment is not available and febrile seizures are allowed to go untreated for hours.

Most cases of prolonged febrile convulsions occur during the first 18 months of life and especially before the age of 12 or 13 months. After 2 years of age, the risk of status epilepticus decreases (Aicardi and Chevrie 1983, Arzimanoglou et al. 2004). The role of developmental malformations in the aetiology of temporal lobe seizures following febrile convulsions may also be considered, either as explaining the whole sequence of the febrile seizures that are followed by unprovoked seizures or as a factor determining the localization and severity of the febrile convulsions. The latter would then constitute a 'second hit' in the full sequence leading to hippocampal sclerosis.

EEG tracings recorded within a week of a febrile convulsion may be abnormally slow for a few days in approximately one third of patients. Epileptic EEG activitiy is found in about one third of children with febrile convulsions that are prospectively followed, whether in the form of rolandic spike foci or bilateral spike–wave bursts (Kajitani et al. 1981, Sofijanov et al. 1992). However, the real figures may be lower because hypnagogic bursts, frequent in this age bracket, can be misdiagnosed as actual paroxysms. Such abnormalities are poorly correlated with the later occurrence of epilepsy (Sofijanov et al. 1992). In particular, they are exceptional in children below 18 months of age who are particularly at risk of recurrences and of the development of afebrile seizures (Viani et al. 1987), whereas they occur in up to 50% of 4-year-olds who are at much lower risk. Therefore, *the EEG has no place in the management of febrile convulsions.*

Differential diagnosis
The differential diagnosis of febrile convulsions includes primarily seizures with infections of the CNS (meningitis and encephalitis). In CNS infections, there is almost always an abnormal CSF. Green et al. (1993) found that in none of 115 children who had convulsions with meningitis was the disease occult. However, such cases are known to occur (Heijbel et al. 1980), so lumbar puncture is advised in children below 18 months and especially below 6 months of age. Lumbar puncture is also indicated in children with long-lasting or otherwise atypical convulsions and in those who fail to recover full consciousness promptly. *Herpes encephalitis* often manifests itself initially in infants with febrile partial seizures and may pose a real problem. Millner and Puchhammer-Stöckl (1993) found a positive polymerase chain reaction for herpes simplex virus in 5 cases regarded as complicated febrile convulsions. Two of these patients had no cells in their CSF. In such cases, MRI can be of considerable value by showing signal alterations in a localized or multifocal distribution. Differentiation of acute convulsive encephalopathies from febrile seizures may be difficult when the CSF is normal. Indeed, the distinction is sometimes made only *a posteriori*, cases with sequelae not being regarded as febrile convulsions. However, cases of febrile convulsions with sequelae do exist and are important in

assessing the prognosis of febrile seizures. Likewise, it is very difficult to separate febrile seizures from 'true' epileptic seizures precipitated by fever as there is a large overlap between these categories. Dravet syndrome starting with prolonged unilateral febrile seizures may be difficult to diagnose early. Repetition of long-lasting seizures within a short period (<2 months) may be suggestive. Nonepileptic paroxysmal events are frequent in febrile children. They include primarily febrile syncopes ('anoxic seizures') (Stephenson 1990); febrile delirium and rigors can also be mistaken for febrile convulsions.

Prognosis

The prognosis of febrile convulsions is generally extremely favourable. Approximately 60–70% of children have only one episode of febrile convulsions and most of the remaining will have two or three seizures. Only 9% of patients experience more than three episodes. Three quarters of the recurrences take place during the year following the first seizure, and the risk of severe recurrence is quite low (Nelson and Ellenberg 1981, Annegers et al. 1990, Van Esch et al. 1996).

The risk of recurrences is greater in children who have seizures in the first two hours of fever or with temperature below 40°C, in those with a family history of febrile or afebrile seizures, in children under 1 year of age, and in those who have had already two or more episodes. Complex febrile seizures are also a predictor of a higher risk of recurrence (Offringa et al. 1994, Baram and Shinnar 2002).

The risk of developing afebrile seizures is of the order of 2–5%. It is low in children with simple seizures occurring after age 1 year but increases at a younger age. The presence of previous developmental or neurological abnormality, a family history of epilepsy, and complex febrile convulsions (Verity et al. 1993) each increase the risk of developing afebrile seizures, which reaches up to 50% when all three unfavourable factors are present (Annegers et al. 1990).

The majority of epilepsies following febrile convulsions are primary generalized epilepsies with tonic–clonic attacks, often with only a few seizures (Wallace 1991, Camfield et al. 1994). Such cases mainly follow brief, uncomplicated febrile convulsions (Aicardi and Chevrie 1976) and are relatively common. The afebrile seizures are mostly infrequent and generally tend to disappear by 9–10 years of age (Arzimanoglou et al. 2004).

Partial epilepsy with focal seizures may be observed following long-lasting unilateral seizures (Aicardi and Chevrie 1976, 1983), although the frequency of this remains disputed. Whether afebrile seizures are a direct consequence of febrile convulsions is debated, but the fact that such seizures are observed following febrile convulsions is well established

The neurodevelopmental prognosis of febrile convulsions is excellent, except in patients who develop epilepsy, some of whom develop learning difficulties. This illustrates the tendency of complications to occur in association and is often the case with accidental prolongation of an episode of febrile convulsions. Some such children may have had a previous subclinical brain lesion before the febrile seizure with the result that it was long-lasting and localized. This is in agreement with the relatively high incidence of abnormal pre- and perinatal history found in several studies (Chevrie and Aicardi 1975, Wallace 1988).

Treatment

Brief febrile convulsions do not require any treatment except that of the causative febrile illness (Baram and Shinnar 2002). Simple measures such as removal of excess blankets and physical cooling are usually recommended. However, there is no evidence that antipyretic agents are effective in the prevention of febrile convulsions (Uhari et al. 1995). Hospitalization is unnecessary for uncomplicated febrile convulsions if adequate surveillance is possible. In case of doubt, a 12-hour hospitalization is sufficient. Long-lasting episodes should be vigorously treated (see Table 15.13 for the treatment of status epilepticus), as they may be associated with later epilepsy and sequelae, especially when they occur before 1 year of age. Parents and caretakers have to be instructed on how to rapidly use rectal diazepam (at a dose of 0.5–1 mg/kg) for acute febrile episodes lasting more than 2–3 minutes. Other routes of administration (nasal or buccal midazolam) are also under evaluation (McIntyre et al. 2005).

Continuous prophylactic treatment of recurrences is not generally advised (Consensus Developmental Panel 1980) but may be indicated when factors of high risk are present. Our own practice is to treat systematically infants below 1 year of age; treatment for patients with complex febrile seizures may be indicated, although there is no proof that it prevents the occurrence of later epilepsy (Nelson and Ellenberg 1981, Shinnar and Berg 1996). Phenobarbitone (30–40 mg/kg/day) that reaches a blood level of around 15 μg/mL is reasonably safe, although concern has been expressed about the effects of the drug on IQ levels (Farwell et al. 1990). The significance of the small IQ loss observed remains uncertain. Sodium valproate reduces the recurrence rate to a similar extent (Wallace 1988).

Although it has been shown that prophylactic treatment with either phenobarbitone or sodium valproate reduces the frequency of recurrences by about two thirds (Wallace 1988), the balance of risks and advantages of this practice is generally thought not to be in favour of prophylactic therapy. The American Academy of Pediatrics Practice Parameter Committee recently reached a similar conclusion and stated that the potential toxicity associated with antiepileptic therapy outweighs the relatively minor risks associated with simple febrile seizures. Thus, long-term treatment is not recommended (Baumann and Duffner 2000).

Intermittent prophylaxis with oral diazepam is effective provided large enough doses are used (0.5 mg/kg t.i.d.) (Autret et al. 1990, Rosman et al. 1993, Knudsen 1996). However, efficacy is limited by the early occurrence of seizures, which may be the first symptom of fever – as was the case in 25% of patients in the series reported by Wolf et al. (1977). Knudsen et al. (1996) reported on a cohort of 289 children with febrile convulsions who had been randomized in early childhood to either intermittent prophylaxis (diazepam at fever) or no prophylaxis (diazepam at seizures) and followed up 12 years later. Children with simple and complex febrile convulsions had the same benign outcome. The long-term prognosis in terms of subsequent epilepsy and neurological, motor, intellectual, cognitive and scholastic ability was not influenced by the type of treatment applied in early childhood. They concluded that it was "as good to interrupt as to prevent" a febrile seizure and thought that prophylactic treatment at the time of fever should be reserved for special cases. Intermittent treatment of fever with acetaminophen alone (Bethune et al. 1993) or combined with low-dose diazepam (Uhari et al. 1995) is not effective.

GENERALIZED EPILEPSY WITH FEBRILE SEIZURES *PLUS*

The term 'generalized epilepsy with febrile seizures *plus*' (GEFS *plus*, or GEFS+) was first used by Scheffer and Berkovic (1997) to describe "a genetic disorder with heterogeneous clinical phenotypes". The description was based on the recognition that in one large Anglo-Australian extended family, febrile seizures, often of unusual duration or severity, and afebrile generalized seizures of various types appeared to be transmitted as a dominant genetic character. Simple febrile seizures constituted the most common manifestation. However, these often tended to occur beyond the usual upper limit of 6 years, and the term 'febrile seizures *plus*' was proposed for children with febrile seizures persisting after the age of 6 years.

Afebrile seizures, mainly generalized tonic–clonic ones, but in some cases, myoclonic attacks, myoclonic-astatic epilepsy or even episodes of status epilepticus occurred in some pedigree members. The pattern of inheritance was autosomal dominant. Although GEFS+ is named after the occurrence of generalized tonic–clonic seizures, these are not the only type of attacks that are observed. Indeed, in some individual cases, such attacks may be absent altogether. More often they are associated with other seizure types. The very term of 'syndrome' may not be appropriate to designate the condition as it is not characterized by the "non-fortuitous association of signs and symptoms in one individual patient but by its genetic nature indicated by the familial occurrence and by the demonstration of the same genes in affected persons of GEFS+ families in some cases" (Arzimanoglou 2007). Other authors reported that patients within the GEFS+ spectrum may present with partial seizures like temporal lobe epilepsy (Abou-Khalil et al. 2001) associated or not with hippocampal sclerosis. The fact that GEFS+ is linked to mutations in genes coding for sodium channels and GABA-A receptors suggests that this 'genetic syndrome' belongs to the 'channelopathies'. The mechanism for the phenotypic variability in GEFS+ families is uncertain.

A locus for the GEFS+ spectrum was mapped to chromosome 19q13, where the voltage-gated sodium channel ,1 subunit gene (*SCN1B*) had been assigned. A second mutation in *SCN1A*, which encodes for the alpha-1 subunit of the same sodium channel, with linkage to chromosome 2q24–33, was found in patients with a similar picture. Claes et al. (2001) found different mutations of this gene in 7 children with Dravet syndrome (see above). The GABA-A receptor gamma-2 subunit gene, *GABRG2* (5q31), is also involved in the pathogenesis of GEFS+, confirming locus

heterogeneity for this spectrum of epilepsy phenotypes (Bananni et al. 2004; for a review, see also Baulac et al. 2004).

SEIZURES AND SYNDROMES OF LATE CHILDHOOD AND ADOLESCENCE

Several of the epilepsy syndromes of infants and young children may persist or have their onset later in life, and there is no abrupt separation between the two age groups. They can manifest with generalized (absences, myoclonic, tonic–clonic seizures) or focal seizures. Focal non-idiopathic epilepsies having presented earlier in life with just a few, easily controlled, seizures may present later with recurrence of seizures or an increase in frequency.

Most epilepsy syndromes of later childhood and adolescence are unassociated with gross brain damage, and genetic factors probably play a prominent role at their origin. As a result, affected children are usually normal from both cognitive and neurological points of view, and the prognosis is generally better than that of early-onset epilepsies, in which brain lesions are the most common cause.

SYNDROMES OF LATE CHILDHOOD AND ADOLESCENCE WITH PREDOMINANTLY TYPICAL ABSENCES

The International Classification recognizes two varieties of absences: *typical* and *atypical*. To avoid confusion when discussing seizure phenomenology, Lüders et al. (1999) suggested the term *'dialeptic seizures'*, underscoring the fact that a further distinction between 'typical' and 'atypical' absences can be made only when EEG findings or a more precise syndromic diagnosis become available.

Typical absences are a well-defined type of seizures with a striking EEG correlate. They are characterized by the sudden suppression or marked decrease of consciousness, with abolition of awareness, responsiveness and memory recording (Arzimanoglou et al. 2004, Hirsch and Panayiotopoulos 2005). They can be *simple* or *complex*. Simple typical absences last 5–15 seconds in 90% of cases (Penry et al. 1975) and usually do not involve motor phenomena, except for possible mild jerking of eyelids and minor changes in muscle tone. The onset and termination of a typical absence are relatively abrupt: this is of value to differentiate absences from focal seizures with alteration of consciousness and minimal motor symptoms. The same also applies to the lack of a postictal phase of impaired awareness and/or fatigue (Penry et al. 1975). In *complex typical absences*, more marked motor components (increased or decreased muscle tone), simple automatisms (Penry et al. 1975) and autonomic phenomena accompany the loss of consciousness and the duration of the attack is often longer. As discussed below, the degree of consciousness impairment is variable depending on the epilepsy syndrome of which the typical absences are a part (Panayiotopoulos et al. 1989).

The EEG in typical absences, whether simple or complex, shows rhythmical bursts of spike–wave complexes at a rhythm of 2.5–3.5 Hz that are bilateral, synchronous and symmetrical with abrupt onset and termination (Fig. 15.7). Less ryhthmical discharges may be seen, especially during sleep, and some degree of

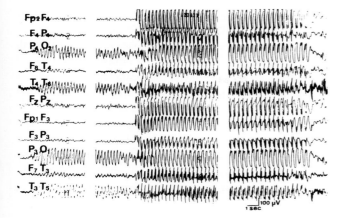

Fig. 15.7. Typical absence attack in a 6-year-old girl. The absence is preceded by a run of 3 Hz slow waves without spikes in the posterior leads over both sides.

asymmetry is present in 9% of cases (Loiseau et al. 2002). EEG variants are observed in some absence syndromes (Panayiotopoulos et al. 1989, Hirsch and Panayiotopoulos 2005). The interictal records are often normal, but brief bursts of irregular spike–wave complexes are seen in 30% of patients. Posterior 3 Hz slow waves are present in 10–20% of children with typical absences.

Hyperventilation is highly effective in precipitating typical absences and can be performed safely during the outpatient clinics in the absence of cerebral vascular disorder (to be avoided in the presence of moyamoya disease). In an untreated child a negative test makes the diagnosis of absences unlikely. About 10–20% of children with absences may respond to light stimulation, and these may be more likely to develop grand mal attacks. These cases may belong to syndromes different from childhood absence epilepsy (Hirsch and Panayiotopoulos 2005).

Absences should be distinguished from inattention and daydreaming, from tics and from abnormal head movements and stereotypies. Distinction from complex focal seizures may be difficult. The brief duration of attacks, their frequent repetition and the lack of a postictal phase are all important features, but an EEG with ictal recording is necessary for final diagnosis. The differentiation from atypical absences rests on the EEG aspect and on the different history, often with other types of attacks in addition to absences. Atypical absences are mainly observed in Lennox–Gastaut syndrome and some forms of polymorphic epilepsy. Absences due to frontal lobe damage result from posttraumatic atrophy or even from tumours (Ferrie et al. 1995).

The occurrence of typical absences as the predominant or exclusive type of seizure in a patient defines absence epilepsy. Several *syndromes of absence epilepsy* are recognized. These include absence epilepsy of childhood, absence epilepsy of adolescence, absences in juvenile myoclonic epilepsy, myoclonic or clonic absences and some rarer syndromes (Panayiotopoulos 1998, 2002).

Childhood absence epilepsy
Childhood absence epilepsy (CAE), also called *pyknolepsy* or (incorrectly) petit mal, has its onset between the ages of 3 and 8 years, although rare cases can manifest as early as the first year of life (Aicardi 1995, Chaix et al. 2003). It is more common in girls than in boys. The absences occur many times daily and constitute the first manifestation of epilepsy, although febrile convulsions may have taken place in infancy. Affected children are normal between the attacks, and so is the interictal EEG, although brief bursts of spike–wave complexes without clinical absence may be recorded. The absences do not include prominent clonic or atonic phenomena but simple automatisms and complex absences are not rare (Loiseau and Duché 1995, Loiseau et al. 2002). The loss of consciousness is marked, and the eyes open during the discharge (Panayiotopoulos 1994b, 1998). In typical cases no neuroimaging study is useful, as there is no appreciable brain pathology, while a family history of seizures is relatively frequent. The occurrence of several cases of absence in the same lineage is not rare (Loiseau and Duché 1995) and polygenic inheritance appears likely.

Treatment with sodium valproate, ethosuximide or lamotrigine is usually effective (Arzimanoglou et al. 2004, Hirsch and Panayiotopoulos 2005). For refractory cases, an association of two drugs may be effective. In some resistant cases, benzodiazepines (especially clobazam) may control otherwise intractable attacks. Typical absence attacks do not respond to many AEDs including carbamazepine, oxcarbazepine, vigabatrin, gabapentin and phenytoin, which in some cases may increase seizure frequency or facilitate the occurrence of myoclonias.

The outlook of CAE is favourable. However, absences may persist in adulthood in a small proportion of cases, and generalized tonic–clonic seizures develop in about 10–30% of patients followed into adulthood, though they are infrequent and easily treatable in most cases (Loiseau et al. 1983). Wirrell et al. (1996) showed that only 65% of children presenting with CAE had remission of their epilepsy. Forty-four per cent of those without remission had developed juvenile myoclonic epilepsy (JME). At the time of diagnosis, remission was difficult to predict accurately in most patients. Development of generalized tonic–clonic seizures or myoclonic seizures during AED treatment was ominous, predicting both lack of remission of CAE and progression to JME. Trinka et al. (2004) reported similar figures.

The educational achievements are often less than optimal. Socioprofessional outlook for CAE is less favourable than that of rolandic epilepsy, and affected individuals often fare less well than their cognitive level would normally allow (Loiseau et al. 1983).

Juvenile absence epilepsy
Juvenile absence epilepsy occurs in patients beyond the age of 9–10 years, although the borderline between childhood and juvenile types is not clearly demarcated. Absences in adolescents are usually less frequently repeated than those in children, and they often cluster in the hour following awakening. Loss of consciousness is less profound than in pyknolepsy (Panayiotopoulos et al. 1994b, 1998), and in some cases the absences are hardly detectable even by the patient.

Other types of seizures, especially generalized tonic–clonic seizures, are associated in 90% of cases, and in some youngsters myoclonic seizures are also present. In the latter cases the absences may be especially mild and often are limited to infraclinical discharges, so some investigators regard absences associated with JME as a distinct syndrome that may have its onset in early childhood and last into adulthood (Panayiotopoulos 1989, 1998). The EEG of juvenile absences either is identical to that of childhood absences or may contain faster spike–wave activity at 4–5 Hz (Janz et al. 1994).

Typical absences may also occur in *juvenile myoclonic epilepsy*. They can precede the apppearance of others types of seizures (Martinez-Juarez et al. 2006). Such cases might be a subgroup of JME and might be responsible for some of the cases of absences that evolve into adult epilepsies and may also be resistant to drug treatment (Panayiotopoulos 2002).

Juvenile absences, generalized tonic–clonic seizures on awakening and JME, often associated as a triad, constitute the group of *primary generalized epilepsy of adolescence*. The associated tonic–clonic seizures and sometimes the absences tend to persist into adulthood.

Treatment choices are similar to those in CAE. However, ethosuximide cannot be used as monotherapy as it may control absence seizures but has no effect on eventual generalized tonic–clonic seizures. Treatment needs to be maintained for long periods, and particularly for female patients issues related to future contraception or pregnancy must be taken into account when choosing the most appropriate antiepileptic drug.

Other syndromes featuring typical absences
The rare syndrome of *epilepsy with myoclonic absences* (clonic absences) is characterized by a specific seizure type, the myoclonic absences (Bureau and Tassinari 2005). Clinically, the intensity of the clonic jerking that affects the upper and often the lower limbs is distinctive. The EEG expression is without specificity as polygraphic recordings show a bilateral rhythmic spike–wave discharge at 3 Hz as in typical absences. Rare cases may have their onset during the first year of life but mean age at onset is 7 years. The course is variable. Some cases develop mental retardation and may evolve to Lennox–Gastaut syndrome, while others respond well to treatment and run a benign course (Manonmani and Wallace 1994, Bureau and Tassinari 2005). Some children develop tonic seizures. The classical treatment combines sodium valproate with ethosuximide or lamotrigine. Benzodiazepines may also be of some help.

Others less well-defined syndromes of absence epilepsy include cases of absences preceded by generalized tonic–clonic seizures other than febrile convulsions (Dieterich et al. 1985) that generally have an unfavourable outcome, *eyelid myoclonia with absences* (Jeavons syndrome) which is essentially a form of myoclonic epilepsy (see below), and *perioral myoclonia with absences*, which may prove drug resistant (Hirsch and Panayiotopoulos 2005). The individualization of some of these syndromes remains debated (Arzimanoglou et al. 2004). Very slight absences, often unrecognized even by the patient and sometimes revealed only by associated rare tonic–clonic seizures, have been termed *phantom absences* (Panayiotopoulos 2002).

Absences associated with brain damage are rare (Ferrie et al. 1995). They may be related to either diffuse lesions or focal damage (Fig. 15.8), especially to the mediobasal frontal lobe. A focal component (clinical and/or EEG) may be present. In most cases the association is probably coincidental.

The genetics of epilepsies featuring typical absences (see Table 15.2) are imperfectly understood. Typical CAE appears to be genetically unrelated to JME, and linkage to chromosome 6p has been excluded. Photosensitive cases seem to be genetically distinct, often with a dominant inheritance, and some may be genetically related to JME (Bianchi et al. 1995). Rare cases of absences linked to definite mutations are on record (Hirose et al. 2005, Ito et al. 2005).

SYNDROMES OF LATE CHILDHOOD AND ADOLESCENCE WITH PREDOMINANTLY GENERALIZED TONIC–CLONIC SEIZURES
Generalized tonic–clonic seizures may be generalized from the start and are often a manifestation of idiopathic epilepsy. They may also represent the secondary generalization of a partial seizure that is traditionally termed the 'aura' of the generalized attack. These two types may be difficult to separate clinically, although their aetiological significance is different (Arzimanoglou et al. 2004, Hirsch et al. 2006a).

Generalized tonic–clonic seizures comprise a stereotyped succession of events, beginning with a tonic contraction of the entire musculature with respiratory blockade resulting in cyanosis and loss of consciousness. After 10–30 seconds, the tonic phase gives way to clonic jerks that progressively slow down and become increasingly violent. After 30–60 seconds, muscular relaxation occurs. The patient remains unconscious for variable durations. Tongue-biting and urinary or, rarely, double incontinence are frequent manifestations but they are by no means specific and can be seen with nonepileptic seizures (Stephenson 1990). From the EEG viewpoint, generalized tonic–clonic seizures are characterized by the succession of a fast (≥10 Hz) rhythm of increasing amplitude that becomes fragmented during the clonic phase, converting to single spike–wave complexes. A flat tracing follows the clonic phase and is rapidly replaced by slow waves that progressively decrease to merge with interictal tracing. The EEG may show generalized spike–wave complexes, sometimes with a positive response to photic stimulation. Even in patients with typical bilateral paroxysms, lateralizing manifestations such as version or circling activity are sometimes present (Gastaut et al. 1986, Lancman et al. 1994). Although usually easy to diagnose, some idiopathic generalized seizures may exhibit focal features and raise a diagnostic problem with focal epilepsies (Ferrie 2005) and/or with some symptomatic epilepsies (Oguni 2005).

Secondarily generalized tonic–clonic seizures can be of two varieties (Theodore et al. 1994). In some cases, the initial partial seizure is clinically manifest, with localized motor, sensory or other phenomena. In other cases, the seizure seems to be gener-

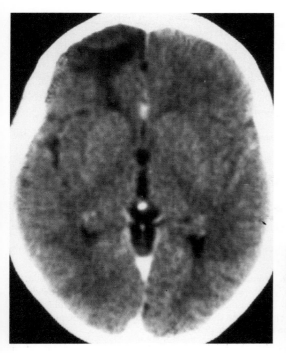

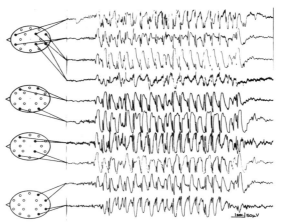

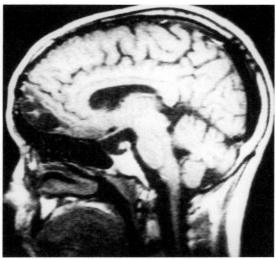

Fig. 15.8. Secondary bilateral synchrony in 15-year-old girl operated on at age 9 years for craniopharyngioma. Intractable epilepsy since operation with generalized tonic seizures (often starting with head turning to left side) and absence attacks, sometimes associated with head turning. *(Top right)* EEG showing absence with bilateral synchronous spike–wave activity. *(Above)* CT showing right frontal lesion. *(Bottom right)* Sagittal MRI showing anterior and inferior location of frontal lobe lesion. (Following removal of anterior frontal lobe, there was total disappearance of all seizures, persisting 19 months postoperatively.)

alized from the start and only ictal EEG recordings demonstrate the existence of an initial, clinically silent, focal discharge. When no ictal records are available, the presence of a stable interictal spike focus – present in 20–40% of patients with tonic–clonic seizures (Arzimanoglou et al. 2004) – is indirect evidence for secondarily generalized attacks. Such seizures are usually the expression of a localized brain lesion but may also occur with nonlesional epilepsies.

Atypical tonic–clonic seizures are very common in childhood: the clonic phase may be extremely brief and EEG activity is not always synchronous or symmetrical. In some children the tonic phase is too brief to be noted.

Generalized tonic–clonic seizures occur with a number of epilepsy syndromes, so they are not particularly helpful for classification and diagnosis. Indeed, when they occur in association with other seizures in the same patient, the latter are considered more characteristic. For example, in this age range, the association of typical absences will evoke the diagnosis of *juvenile absence epilepsy* (see above), while the presence of myoclonic jerks will evoke *juvenile myoclonic epilepsy* (see below).

Syndromes with secondarily generalized seizures will be discussed in detail in the section on focal epilepsies (see below).

Epilepsy with grand mal seizures on awakening

Epilepsies with exclusively or predominantly generalized tonic–clonic seizures have also been classified according to their relationship to the sleep–waking cycle: awakening grand mal; grand mal of sleep; and diffuse (or of random distribution) grand mal (Janz 1994, Wolf 2002, Genton et al. 2005, Fernandez and Salas-Puig 2007). The only relatively well-defined syndrome in this category is *awakening grand mal*, considered as a form of idiopathic generalized epilepsy. However, the diagnosis of this condition is difficult as a strict relation to awakening is necessary for the diagnosis, and the number of attacks necessary for diagnosis is arbitrary. Janz (1994) stated that the diagnosis should be accepted only if 90% of seizures occur in the half-hour following awakening, whereas Wolf (2002) requires that the clear majority of seizures occur either in the first two hours after awakening. Andermann and Berkovic (2001) suggest that the three syndromes of awakening grand mal, juvenile myoclonic epilepsy and juvenile absences can be regarded as variants of a broader epilepsy syndrome termed *primary generalized epilepsy*.

Triggering factors such as sleep deprivation, photic stimulation, and excessive alcohol intake have been identified, and counselling of the patients is important. The pharmacological sensitivity is probably similar to other idiopathic generalized epilepsies (valproate, lamotrigine, topiramate or levetiracetam), but controlled studies are lacking. Duration of treatment is unknown and can only be decided on an individual basis.

SYNDROMES OF LATE CHILDHOOD AND ADOLESCENCE WITH PREDOMINANTLY MYOCLONIC SEIZURES

In some epilepsies of late childhood and adolescence, myoclonias constitute a predominant, if not exclusive, proportion of the seizures. The epilepsies characterized by marked myoclonic phenomena in this age range are, in most cases, idiopathic in origin. A strong genetic predisposition to convulsive disorders is very common (Arzimanoglou et al. 2004). A phenomenon that is more typical of older children and adolescents is a succession of myoclonic jerks often culminating in a generalized tonic–clonic seizure (*clonic–tonic–clonic seizure*). Myoclonic attacks in this setting differ in outlook and therapy from what is oberved in Lennox–Gastaut or Dravet syndrome, discussed in the previous section. Properly recognizing the different types of seizures is important and involves not only careful questioning of parents but also the use of polygraphy and/or video–EEG when indicated.

The precise determination of the other seizure types that often accompany myoclonic attacks is also important, as the associated seizures are critical for classifying the myoclonic epilepsies.

Epilepsy syndromes with prominent myoclonus can be divided into four main categories: (a) those in which the seizures associated with the myoclonus are mainly absence attacks (epilepsy with myoclonic absences and eyelid myoclonia with absences); (b) those in which myoclonic attacks are induced electively by intermittent photic stimulation (see under Stimulus-sensitive epilepsies, p. 624); (c) those with onset in adolescence, in which grand mal attacks are the main type of seizures but which may also feature absence attacks (i.e. juvenile myoclonic epilepsy, discussed below); (d) those with onset in a wide age range spanning from late childhood to well into adulthood, and which are mostly familial, with prominent rhythmic distal myoclonus, as well as generalized jerks, and tonic–clonic and focal seizures in some patients. Duron et al. (2005) have reviewed extensively the frequency of different seizure types in generalized epilepsy syndromes, their age dependency and the temporal profile of seizures.

Juvenile myoclonic epilepsy (JME)

JME (also referred to as *myoclonic epilepsy of adolescence* or *Janz syndrome*) is the most frequent and well-defined syndrome of idiopathic geneneralized epilepsy. Onset is between 12 and 18 years of age (Delgado-Escueta and Enrile-Bacsal 1984, Janz 1989) but may occur outside this age range. The condition was sometimes termed 'myoclonic petit mal' or 'impulsive petit mal', which is confusing as it is clearly different from absence epilepsy. It occurs in 5–11% of adolescents with epilepsy. The myoclonic jerks affect mainly the shoulders and arms, and uncommonly the lower extremities. They may be asymmetrical and even unilateral (Genton et al. 1994, Janz 1994). Consciousness is usually preserved, but the involuntary movements often result in the patient

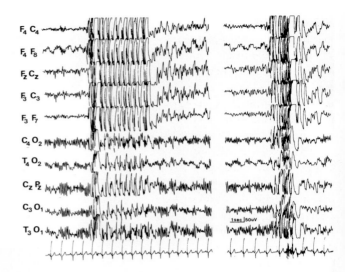

Fig. 15.9. Juvenile myoclonic epilepsy (Janz syndrome). Traces at left show fast (4 Hz) spike–wave discharge with initial polyspikes (no clinical correlate). Those at right show myoclonic jerk (note myographic artefact on ECG channel) and discharge of polyspike on EEG. (Reproduced by permission from Aicardi 1986.)

throwing whatever s/he happens to be holding at the time.

The jerks occur mainly after awakening and may be single shocks or serial jerks that rarely amount to myoclonic status. Ninety per cent of patients have associated generalized tonic–clonic seizures. The latter may sometimes supervene following a series of jerks, a sequence referred to as clonic–tonic–clonic seizure. Fifteen to 30 per cent of patients also have absence attacks. The complex relationship between the various idiopathic generalized epielpsies is discussed by Thomas et al. (2005).

The typical ictal EEG consists of a burst of spikes of high frequency followed by one or several slow waves (Fig. 15.9). Similar polyspike–wave complexes may be present interictally. Focal EEG features may be present in up to 20% of cases (Panayiotopoulos 1994a). Sleep deprivation and often photic stimulation can trigger seizures.

About 80% of patients respond well to sodium valproate therapy, but treatment should be prolonged, probably indefinitely. In women with JME, future pregnancy issues should be taken into account when choosing the most appropriate AED (Tomson and Battino 2005). In resistant cases benzodiazepines are worth trying. Lamotrigine has also been used with variable effect, including aggravation or absence of control of myoclonic jerks in some cases. Topiramate and zonisamide are interesting alternatives. A randomized double-blind control study showed clear efficacy of levetiracetam for the control of myoclonic jerks in JME (Vedru et al. 2005).

A particular profile of pharmacosensitivity of JME, similar to that of other idiopathic generalized epilepsies, has been pointed out by Thomas et al. (2006) who stressed the potential for seizure aggravation observed by the use of phenytoin, and especially of carbamazepine, which could even precipitate myoclonic status. A very important factor is preventing those seizures that are precipitated by sleep deprivation, by eliminating those factors that may hinder physiological sleep.

Response to treatment is excellent or good, with complete control in approximately 80–90% of cases, and spontaneous remission is said to be very rare. Seizure relapse after discontinuation of medication is, on the other hand, frequent, even after many years of seizure control, but can be delayed for several years in some cases (Thomas et al. 2005).

Diagnosis is usually easy. However, rare progressive myoclonus epilepsies (Chapter 9), like Lafora disease and some cases of Unverricht–Lundborg disease, should be ruled out, as at onset they may mimic JME. Subsequent worsening of the myoclonic syndrome, appearance of slow background EEG activity and cognitive deterioration suggest the possibility of a progressive disorder (Arzimanoglou et al. 2004).

Genetic factors play a considerable role in the causation of this syndrome (see Table 15.2). Several linkage studies have been performed (review in Thomas et al. 2005), and linkage to the short arm of chromosome 6 or the long arm of chromosome 15 have been suggested. The results of family studies are often contradictory, mainly concerning the mode of transmission. At present a polygenic model is considered the most probable (Bate and Gardiner 1999), and might account for the ambiguous and contradictory results of linkage studies that relied on simple, mendelian models of transmission. This polygenic model would include a common core of genes that induce the lowering of the epileptogenic threshold in idiopathic generalized epilepsies, the specific expression of JME being the consequence of the implication of one or several other genes (Sander et al. 2000).

Eyelid myoclonia with absences
This disorder is characterized by the very frequent occurrence of eyelid jerks with upwards deviation of the eyes, that may be associated with a brief and mild loss of awareness (Jeavons 1982, Appleton et al. 1993, Panayiotopoulos 1998). The EEG shows discharges of polyspike–wave complexes of short duration (<6 seconds) and there is marked photosensitivity. Treatment, with sodium valproate or other AEDs indicated in idiopathic generalized epilepsies, is effective but probably has to be maintained into adulthood.

Other myoclonic syndromes
These include late cases similar to 'benign myoclonic' epilepsy of infancy but with a late onset up to 5–6 years of age (Guerrini et al. 1994a) and self-induced photomyoclonic seizures (see p. 624).

An autosomal dominant association of cortical tremor, myoclonus and epileptic seizures has been reported in many Japanese and European families with different acronyms, currently known as *familial adult myoclonic epilepsy*. Striano et al. (2005) reviewed the familial cases presenting this clinical picture and concluded that they are the same clinical entity even if genetically heterogeneous, with Japanese families linked to 8q24 and Italian ones to 2p11.1–q12. A third locus could also be involved, and sporadic cases with similar characteristics have also been reported.

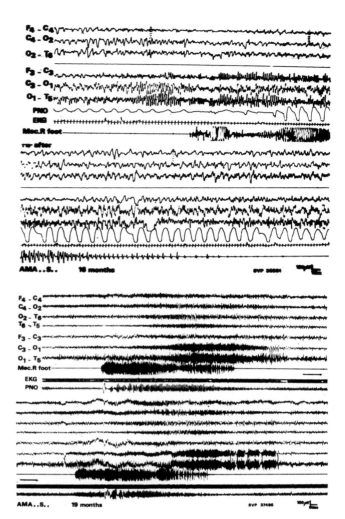

Fig. 15.10. Focal (or partial) epileptic seizure. *(Top)* Onset of spike discharge in left occipitotemporal region (O_1–T_5). Note secondary apnoea (PNO = pneumographic recording) and secondary onset of tonic followed by clonic activity in right lower limb (Mec. R foot = mechanographic recording of right foot movements). *(Bottom)* Slow paper speed recording, same patient, showing another seizure. Note temporal discrepancy between EEG discharge (again starting at O_1–T_5) and clinical seizure (Mec. R foot).

EPILEPSY SYNDROMES OF LATE CHILDHOOD AND ADOLESCENCE WITH FOCAL (PARTIAL) SEIZURES
Focal (partial) epileptic seizures are defined as seizures that have their onset in a neuronal population limited to one part of a cerebral hemisphere (Fig. 15.10). Partial seizures in children are not necessarily indicative of the presence of a localized brain lesion, focal seizures as a manifestation of an idiopathic epilepsy being very frequent in this age range. The symptomatology of non-idiopathic forms may be similar, but the combination of various elements, both clinical and EEG features, enables diagnosis (Kahane et al. 2005).

Focal seizures of lesional origin are caused mainly by dysplastic lesions (including developmental tumours) and by destructive lesions of pre-, peri- or postnatal origin. The extent of the causal lesion largely determines the outcome. Large lesions of prenatal origin may involve several lobes and raise formidable problems of treatment. However, even relatively small lesions may have a noxious effect on overall brain function and be responsible for behavioural and/or cognitive deterioration through poorly understood mechanisms. Early resection of lesions whenever possible may prevent a progressive course.

Two main categories of partial seizures were recognized by the ILAE (Commission on Classification and Terminology 1989) depending on the presence or absence of impairment of consciousness. Consciousness is defined operationally as awareness and responsiveness (Commission on Classification and Terminology 1981). Seizures with impairment of awarenesss and/or responsiveness were termed *complex partial seizures*; those without impaired consciousness were termed *simple partial seizures*. Although the concept is debatable (Gloor 1986), this scheme has been widely used even in recent publications. The ILAE classification states that both forms can evolve into generalized seizures, and that simple partial seizures can evolve into the complex form. Currently, the trend is to use more descriptive terms without necessarily attributing to them a pathophysiological value (Lüders et al. 1993, 1999; Engel 2001; Arzimanoglou et al. 2004), because loss of consciousness is related to a wider diffusion of the discharge rather than to a different origin. If the diffusion is restricted, the clinical expression is a simple partial seizure; when the discharge diffuses the 'simple' partial seizure constitutes the aura of the 'complex partial' attack.

Recognizing the focal origin of a seizure by obtaining a detailed description of the ictal clinical phenomena is of primary importance as it will orientate investigation priorities and treatment choices. The next important step is to differentiate, on the basis of clinical examination and EEG data, purely 'functional' (idiopathic) from lesional (non-idiopathic) epilepsies and orientate, when applicable, neuroimaging investigations. The latter should be orientated taking into account the topographic hypotheses suggested by clinical semiology.

The various types of seizures have been listed in Tables 15.5 and 15.6. Their clinical expression will reflect the origin and/or propagation of the epileptic discharge.

The partial epilepsies of childhood can be conveniently divided into two groups: the idiopathic focal epilepsies and the non-idiopathic forms.

IDIOPATHIC FOCAL EPILEPSY SYNDROMES
Rolandic epilepsy
Rolandic epilepsy (benign partial epilepsy of childhood with centro-temporal spikes; BECTS) is the most common syndrome of idiopathic partial epilepsy in childhood and one of the best-defined epilepsy syndromes. Fifteen to 25 per cent of school-age children with epilepsy are affected (Heijbel et al. 1975, Dalla Bernardina et al. 2005). The syndrome is often thought to be genetically determined but whether a dominant or a multifactorial transmission is responsible remains undecided, although the latter seems more likely (see Table 15.2). Recently, studies in twins (Vladlamundi et al. 2006) have cast doubt on a genetic origin and suggest the pobable importance of acquired factors. The issue is compounded by the fact that fewer than 10% of children with

rolandic spikes have seizures, and the EEG trait seems to be what is inherited. Foci of characteristic rolandic sharp waves are thus frequently encountered in children without epilepsy and their diagnostic value, when isolated, is limited.

The age of onset is almost always between 2 and 13 years, with rare cases recorded as early as 1 year. The typical seizures are 'simple' partial seizures, therefore without impairment of consciousness. They are mainly motor in expression, although buccal or labial paraesthesiae are common, and they preferentially involve the face and oropharyngeal musculature, with resulting salivation and/or speech arrest. Individual seizures are brief (30–60 seconds). Sixty to 80 per cent of seizures occur while the patient is asleep or upon awakening. Secondary generalization occurs in 20% of patients, mainly in the middle part of the night, while motor seizures tend to occur on falling asleep or awakening. Postictal transient paresis (Todd paralysis) can be observed. Most children have only rare seizures, and the response to antiepileptic drugs is good, indicating a low epileptogenicity of the focus, which remains clinically silent in over 90% of cases (Arzimanoglou et al. 2004, Dalla Bernardina et al. 2005).

All patients with rolandic epilepsy have a normal neurological examination, and most make normal neurodevelopmental progress. However, language difficulties of mild to moderate severity have been observed, and a number of articles discuss cognition issues in BECTS (Staden et al. 1998, Deonna 2000, Saint-Martin et al. 2001a, Pinton et al. 2006). In a case–control study, Weglage et al. (1997) frequently found visuomotor and spatial difficulties in children with centrotemporal spikes.

The typical and necessary *EEG abnormality* for the diagnosis of rolandic epilepsy is the presence of a special type of focal epileptiform discharges – a focal negative diphasic slow spike, of medium to high voltage, followed by a slow wave located in the centro-temporal areas with possible diffusion to the adjacent regions – appearing on a normal background activity. A more posterior predominance is often observed in younger individuals. These discharges may occur in isolation or in brief runs (Fig. 15.11). A temporary disappearance and migration of paroxysms from one hemisphere to the other is frequently observed. The field distribution is a horizontal dipole (positivity in the frontal area and maximum negativity in the rolandic region). Activation by sleep is constant. Localization over the upper rolandic area is also possible but the middle area is not involved (Legarda et al. 1994). However, unusual localizations are not infrequent (Wirrell et al. 1995) and the shape of the spikes is more important for their definition than their precise topography. Yet, paroxysms quite similar in shape to those found in benign partial epilepsy may rarely exist in epilepsies due to brain injury (Gobbi et al. 1989, Santanelli et al. 1989, Ambrosetto 1992). As reported by several authors (for a review, see Dalla Bernardina et al. 2005), the most striking finding of centro-temporal spikes is the significant increase in their frequency during drowsiness and through all stages of sleep. In approximately 30% of children they appear only during sleep.

The *outcome* of rolandic epilepsy in terms of seizures is excellent. Up to 25% of children have only one seizure and most

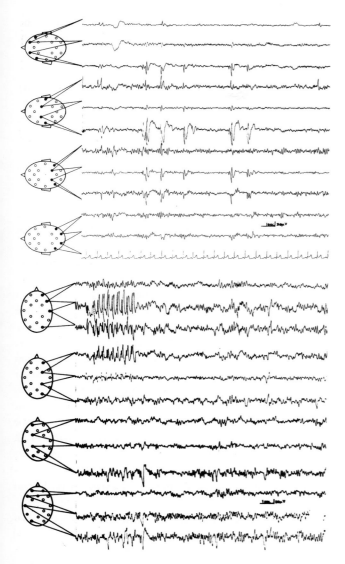

Fig. 15.11. Benign partial epilepsy with centrotemporal spikes. *(Top)* Left-sided focus in an 8-year-old boy. *(Bottom)* Right-sided focus with runs of repetitive rolandic spikes and waves in right centrotemporal region in a 6-year-old boy. In both cases the paroxysmal activity is clearly localized to the lower rolandic, midtemporal electrodes.

have only a few attacks; whilst in some patients seizures are frequent, this does not appear to alter the outcome. Recurrences after the age of 16 years are exceptional (Loiseau et al. 1988). Occasional generalized tonic–clonic seizures have been observed in a few adult patients after the resolution of rolandic epilepsy, and a few cases of status epilepticus have also been reported. Prognosis for school and social functioning is good (Loiseau et al. 1983) despite the possible difficulties mentioned above.

Several investigators have reported on *atypical aspects of benign partial epilepsy* (Aicardi and Chevrie 1982, Fejerman et al. 2000, Saint-Martin et al. 2001a). In a few children with rolandic foci and occasional focal nocturnal seizures, atonic and/or myoclonic seizures, often grouped in clusters and repeated many times daily, may occur, and have been termed *atypical benign*

partial epilepsy (Aicardi 2000, Fejerman et al. 2000) or pseudo-Lennox syndrome (Hahn et al. 2001) on account of the atonic seizures and intense EEG anomalies. Atonic attacks are particularly prominent and may occur several dozen times daily, often with falls. The clusters may last 2–3 weeks and be separated by periods of months. The sleep EEG of such children is very much like that of cases of continuous spike–waves during slow sleep (Aicardi and Chevrie 1982, Aicardi and Levy Gomes 1992), and the awaking EEG shows multiple bilateral discharges of spike–wave complexes. Such patients often receive an erroneous diagnosis of Lennox–Gastaut syndrome, because of the falls and the intense paroxysmal activity during sleep. Although the course of this syndrome may be favourable with spontaneous remission before the age of 10 years and after two or more clusters, cases with a more severe outcome are known (Hahn et al. 2001). Cognitive and behavioural abnormalities can persist but have not been studied in detail.

The exact nosological situation of this syndrome is not yet established (Deonna et al. 1986) but it clearly belongs to the spectrum of epilepsies with continuous spike-waves during sleep (CSWS). The atonic episodes may represent partial or secondarily generalized negative myoclonus. Such episodes have been reported in patients with benign partial epilepsy treated with carbamazepine (Caraballo et al. 1989). However, many patients with this syndrome have not received this drug (Aicardi and Levy Gomes 1992).

Episodes of *opercular status epilepticus* involving the face, tongue and pharyngo-laryngeal structures have been reported (Saint-Martin et al. 1999). They are accompanied by rhythmical spike–wave discharges, the spikes being synchronous with the facial jerks. During these episodes, pseudobulbar symptoms such as drooling and dysarthria may be observed (Roulet et al. 1989, Boulloche et al. 1990, Deonna et al. 1993, Fejerman et al. 2000) and true aphasia has been noted occasionally (Roulet et al. 1989). Some such episodes have required steroids for control (Fejerman and Di Blasi 1987).

Scheffer et al. (1995b) observed *severe and permanent speech dyspraxia* and difficulties of orobuccal movements in several members of a family with an autosomal dominant inheritance and possible anticipation, and Guerrini et al. (1999) reported the occurrence of paroxysmal dystonia in the form of writer's cramp and ataxia as an autosomal recessive syndrome, but this condition is different from the usual benign type. Recently, Roll et al. (2006) have identified the Xq22 gene *SRPX2* as being responsible for rolandic seizures associated with oral and speech dyspraxia and mental retardation.

Idiopathic occipital epilepsies
The occipital epilepsies of childhood form a heterogeneous group (Covanis et al. 2005). The most common type is an idiopathic and benign epilepsy initially described by Panayiotopoulos and now called *Panayiotopoulos-type occipital epilepsy* or *Panayiotopoulos syndrome*. Such cases have their onset between 1 and 10 years, with a maximum incidence around 3–4 years, in developmentally normal children. Seizures are generally infrequent and

mostly occur during sleep. They are marked mainly by eye deviation with disturbances of awareness that are difficult to assess in sleep. Autonomic symptoms are often prominent, especially vomiting. The seizures most often last a few minutes, although in up to 44% of cases (Ferrie et al. 1997) they may last from several minutes to several hours with vomiting, unconsciousness and eye deviation. In the latter case they may easily be mistaken for a coma of toxic or metabolic origin (Panayiotopoulos 1989, 2000; Kivity and Lerman 1992) or may mimic emergency abdominal problems. Long-lasting seizures may end with prolonged unilateral convulsions. Atypical cases may manifest as syncopes that are difficult to differentiate from cardiac or vasovagal episodes. Visual symptoms are rare. Postictal headache is frequent. Interictal EEG may show various types of spikes, usually localized to or predominating in the occipital area uni- or bilaterally, but may occasionally be normal. This activity is decreased or arrested by visual fixation. Such cases may constitute the most common benign epilepsy syndrome under the age of 5 years and are probably related to rolandic epilepsy. The limits of the syndrome are not entirely defined: clinically, some atypical manifestations such as syncopes and lasting coma may be misleading; from the EEG point of view, the localization and appearance of the paroxysmal activity may be quite variable with predominant extra-occipital paroxysms in 10% of cases (Panayiotopoulos 2002). This form often seems benign, although occasional atypical cases have been reported (Ferrie et al. 2002, Kikumoto et al. 2006).

Another syndrome, known as *Gastaut-type benign occipital epilepsy*, is characterized by the occurrence of partial seizures with predominantly visual symptoms, associated with the presence, over one or both occipital areas, of continuous, more or less rhythmical, spike–wave activity that is arrested or considerably lessened by eye-opening. Onset is usually between 3 and 9 years (Gobbi and Guerrini 1998). The visual seizures may consist of negative phenomena (transient loss of vision) or of positive symptoms, mainly simple visual hallucinations of colours and/or geometric shapes (Aso et al. 1987, Thomas et al. 2003). Nonvisual seizures may also be the presenting or sole symptom (Panayiotopoulos et al. 1989). Postictal headache, often migrainous, occurs in around one third of cases of benign occipital epilepsy.

The *outcome* of the syndromes of idiopathic occipital epilepsy is good. However, 'benign' cases may be difficult to distinguish from cases in brain-damaged children (Newton and Aicardi 1983, Dalla Bernardina et al. 1993).

Idiopathic partial photosensitive epilepsy is a rare third type of occipital epilepsy (Guerrini et al. 1994b, 1995). Seizures are characterized by visual phenomena. They are often long lasting with a slow progression of the visual abnormalities. The syndrome is usually responsive to treatment and has a favourable outcome.

Recently described idiopathic focal epilepsies
In the past few years, several new syndromes predominantly characterized by focal seizures and apparently not associated with brain lesions have been reported. Some of these are genetically transmitted (Picard et al. 2000), mostly in a dominant manner,

and a few of the responsible genes have been identified. In the majority, however, evidence of a genetic transmission rests on pedigree studies, and in many cases a genetic origin has not been convincingly demonstrated.

The most important of these newly described syndromes are *autosomal dominant nocturnal frontal epilepsy* and *familial temporal lobe epilepsy*, the latter being reported only in adults. *Familial epilepsy with multiple foci* (Scheffer et al. 1998), *familial temporal lobe epilepsy with and without auditory symptoms* and *autosomal dominant rolandic epilepsy with speech dyspraxia* have been observed in rare families (Andermann and Kobayashi 2005).

• *Autosomal dominant nocturnal frontal lobe epilepsy (ADNFLE).* This disorder is characterized by brief nocturnal motor seizures with hyperkinetic or tonic manifestations, frequently of a hypermotor type. Patients often experience an aura (fear, forced thinking) and usually remain conscious throughout the events. Seizures are brief and are mainly tonic or dystonic in character. They often recur in clusters of several attacks in one night, especially on dozing or shortly before awakening. The epilepsy can begin at any age but usually in childhood and seems to last through adult life, with considerable variations in severity. Interictal EEG studies may be unhelpful. In some cases, focal theta or delta rhythms or sharp waves are recorded in the frontal area. Ictal EEG may also be uncharacteristic or be blurred by movement artifacts. Most cases respond to carbamazepine, but up to 30% of cases may be difficult to control. Neuroimaging is normal. Scheffer et al. (1995a) described 47 affected persons in five families and other cases have been reported since (see Picard et al. 2000). The disorder shows an autosomal dominant inheritance with a high penetrance.

Diagnosis may be difficult with some types of parasomnias and with pseudoseizures. Dystonic attacks are probably identical to those described as nocturnal dystonia by Lugaresi et al. (1986). The nosological situation of ADNFLE and related cases remains partly unsettled. Mutations in the gene coding for the alpha or beta subunits of the neuronal nicotinic acetylcholine receptor have been found in some families (see Table 15.2). However, demonstration of a genetic origin has not been brought about for many cases, and the possibility remains of sporadic cases and/or phenocopies. Small areas of dysplasia, escaping MRI diagnosis, may produce a similar picture, and the presence of such lesions remains plausible in some cases. The localization of the epileptogenic area has not often been confirmed, and although a frontal location is probable, various areas within and outside the frontal lobe can be at the origin of similar seizures (Arzimanoglou et al. 2004). Recently, Ryvlin et al. (2006) reported cases with similar semiology that proved to be of insular origin.

• *Familial temporal lobe epilepsy.* Berkovic et al. (1996) described idiopathic cases in adults with a dominant transmission and a favourable course and with symptoms suggestive of mesial temporal epilepsy. At the time of writing, no case has been described in children. Again this 'syndrome' is defined by genetic data, as the clinical and EEG features do not seem to differ significantly from those of more common temporal lobe epilepsies. Even though interrogations still persist, the realization that not all cases of temporal lobe epilepsy are due to brain damage and are likely to be intractable is clearly of great significance in terms of prognosis and investigations.

A second type of familial temporal lobe epilepsy with dominant inheritance is characterized by the presence of *auditory ictal symptoms* (Ottman et al. 1995, Cendes et al. 2005). This syndrome presents as a relatively mild epilepsy characterized by focal seizures with usually elementary auditory hallucinations, often generaliezd tonic–clonic seizures and familial dominant character. In some cases other symptoms, especially ictal dysphasia, occur (Bisulli et al. 2004, Ottman et al. 2004). Response to drugs is usually, but not invariably, good. A gene (*LTI1/epitempin*), mapped to chromosome 10q, is responsible for some cases. However, other cases are not linked to this locus, and sporadic cases are on record (Bisulli et al. 2004).

NON-IDIOPATHIC FOCAL EPILEPSY SYNDROMES

Under the term 'non-idiopathic focal epilepsies' we refer to all focal epilepsies known or suspected to be the result of a brain lesion or abnormality. The terms 'symptomatic' and 'probably symptomatic' or 'cryptogenic' are also used in the literature. As opposed to the much better defined category of idiopathic focal epilepsies, non-idiopathic focal epilepsies are a very heterogeneous group of conditions with respect to aetiology, pathology and clinical presentations (Arzimanoglou et al. 2004, Kahane et al. 2005). The clinical expression of lesion-related epilepsies may not differ from the seizure expression of an idiopathic form.

Only a few reasonably well-defined syndromes can be individualized among the epilepsies of lesional origin (e.g. mesio-temporal epilepsy). The so-called topographic syndromes (frontal, temporal, parietal and occipital epilepsies) designate in fact very large anatomical regions involved in a given epileptic seizure. But, even within a same lobe, clinical semiology may differ and the interictal or ictal EEG abnormalities are not a constant feature. Furthermore, dominant clinical symptoms may sometimes be the result of seizure propagation and do not necessarily reflect the origin of the ictal event. Consequently, the definition (and description) of the various focal non-idiopathic epilepsies is essentially based on description of the seizures and the eventual presence of interictal abnormalities. As a result, the causes and the prognosis often have to be determined on the basis of an individual combination of signs and symptoms, and on the results of multiple investigations, among which neuroimaging holds a prominent place.

Accurate description of the semiology of focal seizures is important for a correct clinical diagnosis and for attempting a *topographic diagnosis*, especially when surgical treatment can be an option. The characteristics of clinical manifestations as well as the ictal and interictal EEG features can help to localize the origin of a seizure to a particular cortical area. However, it should always be kept in mind that an epileptic seizure is a dynamic process that is not stationary but propagates to neighbouring and distant areas by both normal and abnormal (facilitated) pathways.

Similarly, the relationship between the location of a lesion and that of the resulting epileptic discharge is complex, and there is no absolute concordance between them. With these reservations in mind, some elements of localization can be tentatively indicated. What follows is a very brief description of the main characteristics of so-called *topographic syndromes*.

Partial seizures of lesional origin are caused mainly by dysplastic lesions (including developmental tumours) and by destructive lesions of pre-, peri- or postnatal origin. The extent of the causal lesion largely determines the outcome. Large lesions of prenatal origin may involve several lobes and raise formidable problems of treatment. However, even relatively small lesions may have a noxious effect on overall brain function and may be responsible for behavioural and/or cognitive deterioration through poorly understood mechanisms. Early resection of lesions whenever possible may prevent a progressive course.

Frontal lobe seizures

Frontal lobe epilepsies (FLEs) account for only 10–20% of patients in surgical series, but the incidence in non-surgical patient cohorts seems to be much higher. The typical clinical presentation of seizures includes contralateral clonic movements, uni- or bilateral tonic motor activity and complex automatisms (Chauvel et al. 1992, Kellinghaus and Luders 2004). Seizures tend to be nocturnal, frequently repeated, of brief duration and with only a brief or no postictal manifestation. Complex motor automatisms (hypermotor seizures) include thrashing of the extremities, body rocking and bicycling leg movements. The yield of surface EEG may be limited due to the difficulty in detection of mesial or basal foci, and the patient may be misdiagnosed as having non-epileptic events. In addition, in patients with mesial frontal foci the epileptiform discharges may be mislateralized ('paradoxical lateralization'). The advent of sophisticated neuroimaging techniques, particularly MRI with epilepsy-specific sequences, has made it possible to delineate the epileptogenic lesion and detect a specific aetiology in an increasing number of patients. Small tumours or dysplasias are the most frequently encountered aetiologies.

Salanova et al. (1995b) studied 150 seizures manifested by 24 adolescent and adult patients. Symptoms and signs could be clustered into three groups:

(1) *Supplementary motor area group (n=9).* When the seizure discharges involved the supplementary motor area and adjacent frontal lobe, consciousness was preserved despite unresponsiveness due to motor phenomena. A sensory aura could be reported but the manifestations were predominantly motor with tonic contraction of one or both arms, sometimes with a classical 'fencing' attitude, version of the head, bilateral tonic extension of the trunk or neck and vocalization. These motor manifestations, often mistaken for generalized seizures or for pseudoseizures, also occur in children (Bass et al. 1995, Laskowitz et al. 1995) and are usually symptomatic of a mesial frontal or precentral frontal lesion.

(2) *Focal motor group (n=7).* When seizures arose in the vicinity of the frontal eye field, patients experienced unilateral, face

and/or arm clonic seizures, speech arrest, blinking and head rotation. Preservation of consciousness was an almost constant feature.

(3) *Complex partial seizures group (n=8).* In 5 of these patients, the seizure started by 'staring' or 'looking ahead'. Partial or complete unresponsiveness was present in all. Even though unilateral or bilateral arm tonic posture was similar to that of patients with supplementary motor area seizures, this symptom was never observed at onset of the attack. Oroalimentary automatisms also occurred rarely and were observed towards the end of the seizure.

In much younger children, motor features are common but the characteristics may differ. Fogarasi et al. (2001) analysed 111 videotaped seizures from 14 patients aged 3–81 months (mean, 30 months) and with FLE related to focal cortical dysplasia. Ictal events were categorized into behavioural, consciousness, autonomic and sensory features, as well as motor patterns, which included tonic, clonic, epileptic spasm and myoclonic seizure components. Patients had a high seizure frequency, up to 40 attacks per day, often presenting in clusters. Mean duration of seizures was short (29 seconds), and in nearly half of the patients they started in sleep. The most common seizure components were motor manifestations, mostly tonic–clonic seizures, and epileptic spasms. Behavioural change was frequent, and hypermotor seizures were not seen. In 5 patients, motor features were contralateral to the epileptic focus, including 2 children with asymmetric epileptic spasms. Secondarily generalized tonic–clonic seizures were not recorded, but had been reported in the history of 2 patients. Complex motor automatisms were not seen, whereas oral automatisms appeared in 3 young children.

The same group (Fogarasi et al. 2005) analysed 177 seizures from 35 children (aged 11 months to 12 years) with extratemporal epilepsy (FLE compared to posterior cortex epilepsy) selected by postoperative seizure-free outcome. Twenty patients had FLE, and 15 had posterior cortex epilepsy (PCE). Patients from both groups had daily seizures without significant differences in frequency but with higher nocturnal dominance in children with FLE ($p<0.05$). Visual aura, nystagmus, and versive seizure were observed exclusively in the PCE group, whereas somatosensory aura and hypermotor seizures appeared only in FLE. Tonic seizures were significantly more frequent in FLE ($p<0.01$). Myoclonic seizures, epileptic spasms, psychomotor seizures, atonic seizures, oral and manual automatisms, as well as vocalization and eye deviation appeared in both groups without significant differences in their frequency. The study showed that, especially in infants and preschool children, the characteristic features described in adults' extra-temporal epilepsies were frequently missing.

Children with FLE are particularly at risk of misdiagnosis (Fusco et al. 1990, Stores et al. 1991) because of their unusual clinical features and frequent lack of EEG abnormalities. Automatisms do not involve oroalimentary movements but are gestural, complex and often violent with rocking, kicking and dystonic activity. The bizarre appearance of these seizures often suggests a diagnosis of pseudoseizures, the more so as screaming, shouting and the utterance of abusive language are frequent features.

FLE clinical and EEG features have been compared to mesial temporal lobe epilepsy (MTLE) characteristics in a population of 56 children (FTLE = 39; MTLE = 17) who underwent video–EEG monitoring for presurgical evaluation (Lawson et al. 2002). In FLE, seizures were significantly briefer, more frequent, and predominantly during sleep, and had differing motor characteristics. The rates of bilateral epileptiform interictal and ictal EEG abnormalities were significantly higher in FLE, and a nonlesional MRI was significantly more common in FLE.

Seizures from the central region

Seizures involving the central region, which includes the portion of the cortex surrounding the rolandic sulcus corresponding to the primary sensorimotor cortex, feature a jacksonian march or very narrowly localized clonic or tonic motor phenomena, which are evidence favouring the primary involvement of the rolandic strip. Concomitant sensations of tingling, a feeling of electricity and loss of muscle tone are common. Reflex activation of simple motor seizures by sudden contact or the contraction of specific muscles is observed in some patients. Facial buccolingual, tonic–clonic contractures with aphemia, swallowing, salivation and masticatory movements that are often accompanied by sensory symptoms, including tongue sensations of crawling, stiffness or coldness, gustatory hallucinations, and/or laryngeal symptoms, point to the involvement of the lowermost part of the perirolandic strip in the upper bank of the sylvian fissure (Lombroso 1967, Loiseau and Beaussart 1973, Wieser and Williamson 1993). More extensive insular involvement is accompanied by vegetative symptoms, which may be digestive, urogenital, cardiovascular or respiratory. These manifestations are easily misinterpreted as being of temporal lobe origin.

Temporal lobe seizures

Seizures originating in the temporal lobe are thought to account for the large majority of cases of seizures with alteration of consciousness. However, alteration of consciousness may be even more common with extratemporal seizures, especially in children (Fusco et al. 1990; Chauvel et al. 1992; Williamson et al. 1993a,b). Seizures with and without alteration of consciousness often coexist in the same patient. Attacks are usually prolonged, lasting 1–2 minutes. Autonomic manifestations, psychic and sensory symptoms represent the whole or only the onset (aura) of a more complex episode evolving into alteration of consciousness (Bancaud 1987).

Partial seizures of temporal lobe origin in children are generally similar to those in adults (Kotagal et al. 1987, Devinsky et al. 1988) but tend to have an atypical and minimal expression in younger children with progression to a more characteristic picture with increasing age (Brockhaus and Elger 1995, Fogarasi et al. 2002, Villanueva and Serratosa 2005). Analysis of video recordings of 29 children aged 18 months to 16 years with temporal lobe epilepsy (TLE) (Brockhaus and Elger 1995) showed that clinical features of temporal lobe seizures can be misleading in younger children, including symmetrical motor phenomena of the limbs, postures similar to frontal lobe seizures in adults,

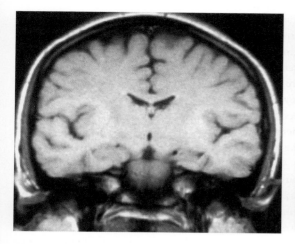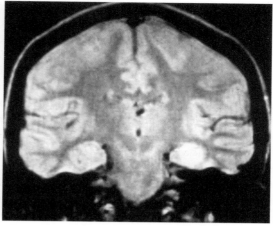

Fig. 15.12. Sclerosis of the left hippocampus in 14-year-old girl who had an episode of right-sided status epilepticus at age 14 months and developed partial complex seizures consistent with a left temporal lobe origin from 4 years of age. *(Left)* T₁-weighted MRI showing global atrophy of left temporal lobe and a markedly shrunken hippocampus. *(Right)* T₂-weighted MRI showing intense signal in left hippocampal area.

and head nodding as in infantile spasms. Fogarasi et al. (2002) reached a similar conclusion by performing a video analysis of 83 seizures from 15 children (aged 11–70 months). Parallel with age, the frequency of motor components decreased, and in 5 of 11 children older than 3 years, motor features were totally absent.

In infants and children under 2 years of age, tonic posturing and head rotation are often the initial and dominant manifestations. The duration of seizures is usually longer than that of absences (60–120 seconds) and they are followed by a period of confusion and/or of intense tiredness. Onset is often with behavioural arrest and staring. Oroalimentary automatisms tend to predominate in young children (Duchowny 1987) and include licking, lip-smacking, chewing or swallowing movements, while in older children, gestural automatisms such as fingering or fumbling with clothes are also frequent (Holmes 1986, Wyllie et al. 1993, Fogarasi et al. 2002). In young children, the most common aura is an epigastric sensation often associated with fear. In older children, temporal lobe seizures may be preceded by auras with affective or other psychic phenomena such as hallucinations or illusions affecting various sensory modalities (see Arzimanoglou et al. 2004).

TLEs can be schematically divided into those mainly implicating *mesio-temporal structures* and those of *lateral* (or neocortical) origin.

The *mesial temporal lobe syndrome* is defined not only on a topographic criterion, the MRI evidence of hippocampal involvement (Fig. 15.12) but also on clinical, EEG and evolutive features (Cendes et al. 2005). The syndrome frequently occurs in patients with a history of complex febrile convulsions in infancy, especially long-lasting unilateral attacks, reported in at least 40% of cases and followed by a second phase of latency, of variable duration. Focal seizures mark the third phase of chronic epilepsy, which often appears during the second half of the first decade; however, an earlier onset is not unusual with focal epilepsy starting within a few years after the initial febrile seizures (Abou-Khalil et al.

1993, Williamson et al. 1993a, Harvey et al. 1995). This "roller coaster course" (Berg et al. 2006) of TLE probably explains the very long delays in recognizing the intractable character of this epilepsy syndrome and in envisaging the possibilities for surgical treatment (Arzimanoglou et al. 2005).

Seizures are marked by behavioural arrest and staring followed by automatisms involving especially the oroalimentary muscles (lip-smacking, licking, swallowing). A significant proportion of these automatisms are, in fact, conscious (Munari et al. 1994, Ebner et al. 1995). Dystonic posturing of the arm contralateral to the discharging temporal lobe is often seen (Kotagal et al. 1989), while simple automatisms may occur in the ipsilateral arm.

The EEG usually shows an interictal anterior temporal spike focus or sometimes a paroxysmal theta rhythm (Gastaut et al. 1985), while ictal EEG shows a focal discharge that may diffuse to the contralateral temporal lobe.

MRI shows atrophy of the hippocampus, loss of its internal structure and increased T₂ signal (Jackson et al. 1990, Cross et al. 1993, Cendes et al. 2005). Recent research brought evidence supporting the suggestion that hippocampal sclerosis may be a progressive disorder (Fuerst et al. 2003) and that progressive volume loss in the mesial temporal lobe in relation to duration of epilepsy is probably not limited to the hippocampus but affects the entorhinal cortex and the amygdala (Bernasconi et al. 2005).

PET scan with fluorodeoxyglucose shows local hypometabolism. SPECT shows reduced blood flow to the mesial temporal lobe interictally and increased fixation during the seizure (Harvey et al. 1993a, 1995).

The outcome of this syndrome following surgery is often good (Abou-Khalil et al. 1993). More than two thirds of patients with drug-resistant TLE will be free of disabling seizures with continued medical treatment after temporal resection. Of those, almost one third will achieve complete discontinuation of AEDs (Schmidt and Loscher 2003).

In a prospective randomized study (Wiebe et al. 2001), 80 adult patients with TLE were randomly assigned to surgery (40 patients) or treatment with antiepileptic drugs for one year (40 patients). At one year, the number of patients who were free of seizures impairing awareness was 23 in the surgical group but just 3 in the medical group (p<0.001), clearly showing that surgery was superior to prolonged medical therapy. Patients in the surgical group had fewer seizures impairing awareness and a significantly better quality of life (p<0.001 for both comparisons) than those in the medical group. Four patients had adverse effects of surgery, and one patient in the medical group died.

Most studies on epilepsy surgery of intractable TLE concern adult patients with a long history of epilepsy, and randomized trials are rare (Engel et al. 2003, Schmidt et al. 2004). Extrapolation of these data to children is debatable. Prospective studies are necessary to characterize benign mesial TLE with hippocampal sclerosis, define its incidence and prevalence relevant to the severe form, and determine whether the benign and severe forms represent two different pathophysiological conditions, or a spectrum of a single condition (Wieser 2004). Such a differentiation is of extreme importance particularly when discussing evolution, not only in terms of seizures but also in terms of socio-cognitive development (Arzimanoglou et al. 2005). For patients who are compromised by such seizures, referral to an epilepsy surgery centre should be strongly considered early in the course of the disorder since, based on retrospective cohort data in children, failure of a first AED trial accurately predicts refractory TLE at 2 years after onset (Dlugos et al. 2001).

Another syndrome that is very similar in clinical expression is produced by *small mesial developmental tumours* (Wyllie et al. 1993, Raymond et al. 1994, Arzimanoglou et al. 2004). Such patients have no antecedent history. Wyllie et al. (1993) emphasized that, contrary to mesial temporal sclerosis in which the ictal and interictal EEG anomalies are usually localized to the anterior temporal area, the EEG is often diffusely abnormal in small tumours whose diagnosis rests on MRI.

Patients with focal cortical dysplasia represent a heterogeneous group. Different age at epilepsy onset and transient responsiveness to AEDs may reflect different dynamics in epileptogenicity of the underlying FCD. Dual pathology, rather frequent in children (Mohamed et al. 2001), may be associated with different pathological mechanisms in patients with and without febrile seizures (Fauser et al. 2006). Recent studies have emphasized the role of neuronal glial tumours especially *gangliogliomas* and *developmental neuroepithelial tumours* in the causation of chronic epilepsy that may remain monosymptomatic in the form of recurrent partial seizures for many years. Taylor-type cortical dysplasias are another frequent cause. All these lesions are highly epileptogenic, and related epilepsy is resistant to drugs in most cases.

A number of temporal lobe seizures in children may arise from the *basal temporal lobe* rather than from the mesial temporal lobe (Duchowny et al. 1994). Such seizures are marked by behavioural arrest followed by automatisms that begin several seconds after seizure onset. Propagation of seizures with *mesio-basal onset* is rapid and mainly to the contralateral hippocampus, but some attacks spread to the cingulate gyrus or to the orbital and lateral frontal cortex.

Lateral (or neocortical) temporal origin is often characterized by auditory or complex perceptual visual hallucinations, illusions, a dreamy state or vertiginous symptoms. Impairment of consciousness may begin with motor arrest, or staring, followed by oroalimentary automatisms. However, automatisms may appear while the patient is still responsive or when consciousness is fluctuating. Amnesia for the ictal event is the rule after alteration of consciousness but may be present even when the patient had apparently remained conscious. According to Blume et al. (1993) and Munari et al. (1994), the neocortex is responsible for many features of all temporal lobe seizures. Post-ictal confusion and, in small children, post-ictal sleep are frequent. Temporal lobe seizures of neocortical origin are less frequent than limbic attacks.

In general, localization of focal seizures to a particular cortical area is difficult, and distinction between temporal lobe and frontal lobe origin only on the basis of clinical symptoms may be impossible (Manford et al. 1996a).

Sensory (parietal lobe) seizures
Symptoms produced by ictal involvement of the parietal lobe may be difficult to diagnose (Salanova et al. 1995a), especially in children, as they are mostly subjective and may be overshadowed by symptoms produced by contiguous central, temporal and occipital cortex. Somatosensory seizures may have a jacksonian march (Mauguière and Courjon 1978). They are often associated with motor phenomena.

Focal seizures arising from the parietal lobe are characterized by positive or negative somatosensory symptoms, rarely pain (Young et al. 1986, Trevathan and Cascino 1988, Ho et al. 1994), or by nausea or an intra-abdominal sensation, illusions of movement or loss of awareness of a part of the body (asomatognosia – especially with non-dominant hemisphere involvement), vertigo or disorientation in space. Receptive or conductive language impairment (with dominant hemisphere involvement) and postural or rotatory movements may also be seen, and visual symptoms may appear with involvement of the parieto-temporo-occipital junction. Inferior parietal involvement may be accompanied by contralateral or ipsilateral rotatory movements with posturing of the limbs contralateral to the involved hemisphere. Visual illusions, such as macropsia or micropsia or metamorphopsia suggest involvement of the posterior parietal cortex or parieto-temporo-occipital junction.

Occipital lobe seizures
Symptoms of occipital lobe involvement are mainly subjective and they may be overshadowed by manifestations resulting from spread to contiguous cortex. Epileptic discharges affecting the primary visual cortex are characterized by elementary visual phenomena, which may be either positive (flashes, phosphenes, rotating colours) or, less frequently, negative (scotomata, hemianopsia, amaurosis). Location is in the hemifield contralateral to the lobe involved. With discharges located more anteriorly,

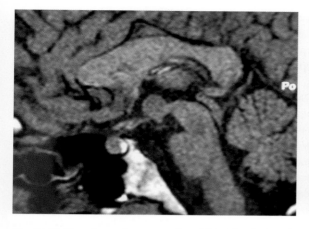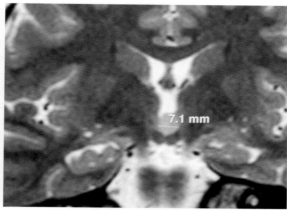

Fig. 15.13. Hypothamus hamartoma in a child with gelastic epilepsy. *(Left)* MRI, sagittal cut showing small mass arising from the floor of the third ventricle developing mainly upwards into the ventricle. *(Right)* Coronal cut. The tumour is seen at the lowermost part of the third ventricle; its density is slightly lower than that of the grey matter.

conjugate deviation of the head and eyes (version) is common. Version is not necessarily contralateral. The deviation of the eyes may be periodically interrupted by brief jerks that return the eyes to the primary position, the so-called 'epileptic nystagmus'. Additional manifestations include eyelid flutter or forced closure of the eyelids and a sensation of eye-pulling (Salanova et al. 1992, Williamson et al. 1992).

SOME SPECIAL EPILEPSY SYNDROMES OF LESIONAL ORIGIN

A syndrome of *gelastic seizures* (giggling attacks) of early onset (often in the first year and usually before 2 years of age) is associated with the occurrence of a *hamartoma of the hypothalamus* (Fig. 15.13). The seizures are frequently repeated and highly resistant to treatment (Berkovic et al. 1988, Arzimanoglou et al. 2003, Mullatti 2003). They are associated with cognitive and mental abnormalities that often begin at the same time as secondary generalization of seizures (Berkovic et al. 2003). Precocious puberty is a frequent feature. The seizure discharge may arise from the tumour itself, and surgical excision, when possible, may control the seizures (Kahane et al. 2003). Surgical deconnection or removal has given good results, and radiosurgery techniques are under evaluation (Fohlen et al. 2003; Polkey 2003a,b).

Cerebellar hamartomas may produce repeated brief attacks of tonic facial contraction of early onset, similar to the facial hemispasm of adults (Al-Shahwan et al. 1996). Harvey et al. (1996) and Arzimanoglou et al. (1999) showed that these may correspond to a typical epileptic EEG discharge within the lesion.

Abnormalities of cortical development (see Table 15.4) represent the most frequent cause of focal non-idiopathic epilepsies and nearly 40% of drug-resistant ones. A detailed review of these lesional epilepsies is beyond the scope of this chapter. Excellent detailed publications provide an overview of the topic (Guerrini et al. 2003).

The *syndrome of occipital epilepsy associated with uni- or bilateral occipital calcifications* (Fig. 15.14) may run a benign course (De Marco and Lorenzin 1990) or a more severe one with secondarily generalized seizures and mental deterioration (Tiacci et al. 1993, Gobbi et al. 1988, Gobbi 2005). Such cases are closely reminiscent of Sturge–Weber syndrome without cutaneous angioma, and similar vascular abnormalities have been reported (Bye et al. 1993) but are inconstant (Toti et al. 1996). However, there is only minimal or no atrophy of the brain, and enlargement of the choroid plexus and abnormal deep venous drainage is not seen. Most if not all cases of epilepsy with occipital calcification are associated with *coeliac disease*, and are probably of lesional nature, although their expression may be reduced to villous atrophy of the intestinal mucosa (Gobbi 2005). The relationship between the coeliac disease and the calcification is not understood.

OCCASIONAL SEIZURES

Occasional seizures may rarely occur with acute febrile diseases in older children. They can also occur in a well child or adolescent without fever (Aicardi 1994). *Isolated afebrile seizures in adolescents* are relatively common. Seizures may be generalized or focal. About half such seizures remain single as an isolated cluster lasting less than 36 hours (Loiseau and Louiset 1992, Capovilla et al. 2001). For that reason, treatment of the first afebrile seizure is not recommended unless specific reasons militate for immediate therapy. Isolated convulsions are especially apt to occur in adolescents during stress and sleep deprivation (Caraballo et al. 2004) have emphasized that seizures in adolescents usually do not recur when the EEG is normal. This *syndrome of partial benign epileptic seizures in teenagers* accounted, in their experience, for 24% of all partial seizures beginning in adolescence. The course is benign, but distinction from lesional cases is difficult and neuroimaging studies are required.

OTHER UNUSUAL EPILEPTIC SEIZURES

Epileptic seizures can disturb all brain functions, and a wide variety of ictal phenomena have been reported.

Abdominal epilepsy is characterized by attacks of epigastric or periumbilical pain and/or by repeated episodes of unexplained

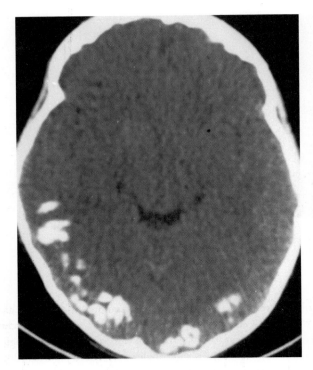

Fig. 15.14. Epilepsy with bilateral occipital calcification in 6-year-old boy with visual seizures. There was no facial naevus, and neither CT nor MRI (with gadolinium enhancement) showed any evidence of pial angioma. This case is similar to those reported by Gobbi *et al.* (1988).

vomiting. However, epilepsy is rarely the cause of the syndrome of recurrent abdominal pain and periodic vomiting, which is probably more often a manifestation of migraine (Arzimanoglou et al. 2004). In real cases of abdominal epilepsy, loss of consciousness is a feature.

Seizures limited to vomiting (ictus emeticus) occur rarely (Kramer et al. 1988, Thomas and Zifkin 1999, Shuper and Goldberg-Stern 2004). Other autonomic phenomena that can be the sole or main manifestation of a seizure include cardiac arrest (Kiok et al. 1986, Smaje et al. 1987), ictal arrhythmias (Gilchrist 1985), and apnoea and cyanosis (Southall et al. 1987, Donati et al. 1995, Hewertson et al. 1996). *Unusual visual attacks* may affect eye movements with ictal gaze deviation or epileptic nystagmus (Thurston et al. 1985) and ictal blindness (Barry et al. 1985). Pain as a seizure phenomenon is rare (Young et al. 1986, Trevathan and Cascino 1988). Shuddering attacks in children have been reported by Holmes and Russman (1986), and isolated disturbances of memory (Gallassi et al. 1988) and of sleep with repeated nocturnal awakenings (Peled and Lavie 1986) have also been mentioned.

SEIZURES AND SYNDROMES OF THE NEONATAL PERIOD

Seizures occurring during the first 28 days of life are a major problem of neonatal neurology. Seizures in the first trimester raise similar issues. Distinguishing epileptic from non-epileptic motor phenomena and autonomic signs in the newborn infant remains

difficult despite the increasing use of video–EEG techniques that has certainly reduced the number of errors (overdiagnosis of epileptic seizures or delay of diagnosis and treatment of true epileptic seizures) (Arzimanoglou and Aicardi 2001).

NEONATAL SEIZURES
Clinical features
The main types of neonatal seizures are shown in Table 15.11. Only some behavioural phenomena classically described as neonatal seizures are regularly associated with rhythmical EEG discharges (Mizrahi and Kellaway 1987, Scher and Painter 1990), similar to those in older patients. These events include *focal clonic seizures*, which are always partial with a fixed or shifting location (migratory seizures), and multifocal seizures which often demonstrate asynchronism between the various foci that discharge at different rhythms, either simultaneously or in succession. *Generalized tonic–clonic seizures* are exceptional in this age group; only familial neonatal convulsions have been associated with an EEG activity reminiscent of that observed at later ages (Hirsch et al. 1993, Ronen et al. 1993). *Myoclonic seizures* are also unusual. *Tonic seizures* and subtle or 'minimal' seizures that include such phenomena as oral or ocular movements, grimacing, eye opening, blinking or staring, pedalling or boxing movements, and, rarely, isolated apnoea (Watanabe et al. 1982a, Donati et al. 1995) are the most common types.

A large group of behavioural phenomena, often regarded as seizures on a clinical basis, are not regularly associated with EEG discharges (Fig. 15.15). These include a majority of the tonic (generalized or partial) and 'subtle' seizures. Scher et al. (1993a) were able to demonstrate paroxysmal EEG correlates in only 17% of their patients with subtle seizures. Such phenomena can often be elicited by stimulation, the severity varying with the intensity of stimulation, and they may demonstrate temporal or spatial summation (Mizrahi and Kellaway 1987). Those authors proposed that they do not represent epileptic seizures but rather 'release' phenomena related to disinhibition of brainstem structures resulting from cortical damage.

Although this concept seems essentially sound, it should be observed that *absence of an EEG discharge on the scalp is no proof of the nonepileptic nature of an event* (Volpe 1989, Lombroso 1996). Undoubted epileptic seizures without EEG correlates are known to exist. The problem is further complicated by the fact that EEG seizure discharges without clinical seizures are frequent in neonates (Clancy et al. 1988, Scher and Painter 1990), most commonly following repeated seizures treated with anticonvulsants but also, less frequently, in untreated infants. Brief discharges lasting less than 10 seconds ('brief intermittent rhythmic discharges' or BIRDs) (Scher et al. 1993a,b) are frequent in the EEG of newborn infants and are not associated with clinical seizure activity. As a result, the definition of neonatal seizures is still imprecise and, consequently, their incidence is poorly known. Figures quoted vary from 0.15% to 1.4% (Arzimanoglou et al. 2004).

Both term and preterm infants may be affected. Seizures in preterm infants have a limited expression and purely EEG dis-

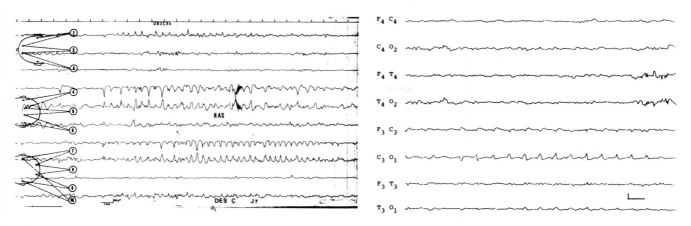

Fig. 15.15. Neonatal seizures. *(Left)* Well-formed EEG discharges occurring independently over two closely spaced areas of right hemisphere in term baby. *(Right)* Rhythmic discharge of low amplitude over posterior left hemisphere in preterm neonate. (Reproduced by permission from Aicardi 1986.)

TABLE 15.11
Features of the main types of neonatal seizures

Type of seizures	Clinical features	Ictal paroxysmal EEG discharges
Generalized tonic–clonic	Tonic contraction followed by a few jerks. Seen only with benign familial neonatal convulsions	Present in most cases
Generalized tonic	Sustained symmetrical posturing of neck and trunk sometimes provoked by stimulation	Rarely present
Focal clonic	Rhythmical jerks, focal or multifocal (in this case often asynchronous). Not suppressed by restraint	Almost always present
Focal tonic	Sustained posturing of single limb, sustained eye deviation not suppressed by restraint	Present in some cases
Myoclonic	Arrhythmical, nonrepetitive jerks, generalized, focal or fragmentary	Present in 80% of cases
Subtle or minimal seizures or motor automatisms	Roving eye movements, blinking, grimacing, sucking, chewing, thrusting tongue movements, swimming, boxing or cycling movements, suppressed by restraint and precipitated by stimulation when nonepileptic	Seldom present

charges are especially common (Scher et al. 1993a,b).

Neonatal seizures rarely occur as isolated events. Most frequently, brief seizures occur repeatedly over a period of a few hours or days (Clancy and Legido 1987, Scher et al. 1993b, Bye and Flanagan 1995) and tend to subside, even without treatment, after 24–96 hours. The mean duration of individual seizures was 14.2 minutes for term infants and 3.1 minutes for preterm babies in the study by Scher et al. (1993b), but the difference was the result of the frequency of status in term infants and its rarity in preterm babies.

Ictal EEG discharges may consist of focal rhythmic spikes or sharp wave forms at variable frequencies (from alpha to delta) or of discharges of sharp waves (Tharp 1981, Holmes 1985, Lombroso 1996) (Fig. 15.15). Such discharges may be found in both term and preterm infants (Radvanyi-Bouvet et al. 1985, Legido et al. 1988).

Neonatal seizures should be distinguished from *tremors* and *jitteriness*, which are extremely common but are periodic movements at a rhythm of 5–6 per second that can be suppressed by restraint or repositioning (Kramer and Harel 1994, Fernandez-Alvarez and Aicardi 2001) and have a favourable outcome; from *benign neonatal sleep myoclonus* (Chapter 16); and from some vegetative phenomena such as *nonepileptic apnoea*. The most difficult issue is to decide whether atypical seizures with suggestive clinical manifestations but unassociated with EEG paroxysms should be regarded as epileptic in nature. The problem remains unsolved in some cases.

Clinical recognition of nonepileptic phenomena in neonates is, however, often possible. Important diagnostic clues include the ability to elicit abnormal phenomena by stimulation, whether tactile or otherwise; the demonstration that spatial or temporal summation of stimuli is effective; and the ability to prevent or interrupt abnormal events by restraint. More importantly, the clinician must consider the neurological context within which the paroxysmal phenomena are observed (Arzimanoglou and Aicardi 2001).

TABLE 15.12
Main causes of neonatal seizures

Hypoxic–ischaemic encephalopathy (may produce both clearly epileptic attacks and seizures probably nonepileptic in nature)

Intracranial haemorrhage
  Subarachnoid haemorrhage (clonic seizures in term infants 1–5 days of age)
  Intraventricular haemorrhage (mainly tonic seizures and episodes of apnoea without EEG correlates, occasionally typical EEG discharges)
  Intracerebral haematoma (fixed localized clonic seizures)

Intracranial infections
  Bacterial meningitis and/or abcess
  Viral meningoencephalitis

Cerebral malformations
  Myoclonic and focal tonic seizures, infantile spasms, others

Metabolic causes
  Hypocalcaemia (clonic, multifocal seizures)
  Hypoglycaemia
  Hyponatraemia
  Inborn errors of amino acids or organic acids and NH$_3$ metabolism (often atypical, mostly unassociated with EEG discharges)
  Molybdenum cofactor deficiency
  Bilirubin encephalopathy (atypical, no EEG discharges)
  Pyridoxine dependency
  Biotinidase deficiency
  Carbohydrate-deficient glycoprotein syndrome

Toxic or withdrawal seizures (probably not true epileptic seizures in most cases)

Familial neonatal convulsions (clonic localized, shifting seizures with EEG correlates)

'Benign' neonatal seizures of unknown origin ('fifth-day fits')
  Clonic and apnoeic seizures with typical EEG correlates

Aetiology

The main causes of neonatal seizures are listed in Table 15.12. In fact, many seizures associated with intracranial haemorrhage or with inborn errors of metabolism are probably not epileptic, and the same applies to *hypoxic–ischaemic encephalopathy (HIE)* even though this still represents a common cause of neonatal seizures (Levene and Trounce 1986). It seems possible that many infants with HIE have already suffered harm in utero, as shown by the frequency of prenatal placental damage (Burke and Tannenberg 1995, Scher 2003), and that the perinatal events may not have played a significant role.

The seizures of HIE occur within the first 24–48 hours of life. They are regularly associated with other manifestations of the disease such as apathy and coma (Chapter 1). The associated EEG in severe cases is of the inactive or discontinuous type ('*tracé paroxystique*').

Localized arterial infarction has emerged as an important cause of localized, fixed, clonic seizures (Levy et al. 1985). Scher et al. (1993a) found such infarctions in 58% of their cases of EEG-confirmed neonatal seizures (Chapter 4).

Infections are mainly of viral origin. However, the frequency of meningitis and encephalitis is high enough to justify lumbar puncture whenever there is no obvious other cause.

Hypocalcaemia and hypoglycaemia (Cornblath and Schwartz 1991) are much less common but treatable conditions (Chapter 1). Late hypocalcaemia due to high phosphorus load in artificial milk feeds is now rarely seen, and currently observed cases are often associated with cardiac disease and have a guarded prognosis (Lynch and Rust 1994). Early hypocalcaemia is usually associated with other problems, so another cause for the seizures should be sought in such patients. De Vivo et al. (1991) have described a *defect of glucose transport* across the blood–brain barrier caused by the genetic absence of the GLUT1 protein, which results in severe hypoglycorrhachia manifested by isolated seizures without hypoglycaemia. The onset is usually towards the end of the first month of life but truly neonatal cases do occur (Chapter 1).

Rare metabolic causes include pyridoxine dependency (Chapters 8, 22), spongiform encephalopathy with low activity of Na/K pumps (Renkawek et al. 1992), pyridoxal-dependent seizures and familial folinic acid-responsive seizures (Hyland et al. 1995, Baxter 2002, Wolf et al. 2005). Cases of neonatal seizures resistant to pyridoxine but responsive to pyridoxal phosphate have been reported (Wang et al. 2005).

Epileptic seizures related to hereditary metabolic disorders are usually combined with widespread neurological dysfunction. A key factor is the early appearance of symptoms, following a symptom-free period of a few hours or days, particularly if otherwise unexplained (no antenatal or prenatal history). The diversity of causes calls for rigorous analysis of symptoms and of biological samples in the interest of rapid diagnosis and the most appropriate treatment (Livet et al. 2005). Seizure types are rarely specific for a particular metabolic disorder, and neither are EEG findings (Wolf et al. 2005).

Seizures in infants born to mothers addicted to narcotics or barbiturates are probably often nonepileptic in nature but the EEGs have only rarely been recorded in such cases. Their prognosis appears to be favourable (Doberczak et al. 1988).

Seizures due to cerebral malformations are often infantile spasms or myoclonic in type. Neonatal convulsions without detectable cause are not uncommon (Painter et al. 1986, Aicardi 1991).

The current aetiological profile and neurodevelopmental outcome of seizures in term newborn infants was recently reported (Tekgul et al. 2006). Eighty-nine term infants with clinical neonatal seizures were evaluated in the newborn period and at 12–18 months. Aetiology was found in 77 infants. Global cerebral hypoxia–ischaemia, focal cerebral hypoxia–ischaemia, and intracranial haemorrhage were most common. Neonatal mortality was 7%, and 28% of the survivors had poor long-term outcome. Association between seizure aetiology and outcome was strong, with cerebral dysgenesis and global hypoxia–ischaemia associated with poor outcome. A normal neonatal period/early infancy neurological examination was associated with uniformly favourable outcome at 12–18 months; abnormal examination lacked specificity. Normal/mildly abnormal neonatal EEG had a favourable outcome, particularly if neonatal neuroimaging was normal. Moderate/severely abnormal EEG and multifocal/diffuse cortical or primarily deep grey matter lesions had a worse outcome. In the current era of neonatal intensive care mortality associated with neonatal seizures has declined, although long-term neurodevelopmental morbidity remains unchanged. Seizure aetiology and background EEG patterns remain powerful prognostic factors.

SYNDROMES OF THE NEONATAL AND EARLY INFANTILE PERIOD

Only a few well-defined syndromes have been recognized in newborn infants.

Benign familial neonatal convulsions (BFNC) are dominantly inherited. The most frequently implicated gene is located on chromosome 20q (Leppert et al. 1989, Malafosse et al. 1994) and codes for the KCNQ2 potassium channel (Singh et al. 1998), but rare cases are linked to chromosome 8 on a gene for KCNQ3 (Ryan et al. 1991, Charlier et al. 1998). In other cases no linkage to either locus has been found (Plouin 1994).

The onset of seizures is within 2–15 days of birth. Seizures recur for a few days then stop. Later relapses have been observed in 14% of cases (for a review, see Plouin and Anderson 2005). The seizures appear generalized (Hirsch et al. 1993, Ronen et al. 1993), although partial attacks have been reported (Aso and Watanabe 1992, Bye 1994). The phenotype is variable, some members of affected families presenting other forms such as febrile convulsions or generalized epilepsies (Berkovic et al. 1994). Rare cases of apparently recessively inherited neonatal seizures are on record (Schiffmann et al. 1991). The diagnosis rests on a history of similar events in relatives, consistent with an autosomal dominant transmission. A mutation of the SCNA2 sodium channel subunit has been found in a subtype in which onset of seizures may be either neonatal or infantile (see below). An overview of phenotypic, functional and mutational variations in BFNC can be seen in the Utah study of 17 families with *KCNQ2* mutations (Singh et al. 2003). In two members of one family, the phenotype extended beyond neonatal seizures and included rolandic seizures, and a subset of families has onset of seizures in infancy. A case of BFNC that evolved to rolandic epilepsy was reported by Coppola et al. (2003).

A slightly later onset was observed in a few families and named *benign familial infantile convulsions (BFIC)*, characterized by partial seizures, with or without secondary generalization, occurring mostly in clusters, and with an onset age ranging from 3 to 9 months. Patients typically have normal psychomotor development at seizure onset and a favourable outcome (Vigevano et al. 1992, Chahine and Mikati 2006). The condition is genetically heterogeneous and loci were identified on chromosomes 19q12–13.1 and 16p12–q12, allelic to infantile convulsions and choreoathetosis. Subsequently, mutations were identified in the gene encoding the voltage-gated sodium channel a2 subunit (SCN2A) on chromosome 2q24 (Heron et al. 2002) in two families affected by neonatal and infantile seizures (*benign familial neonatal–infantile convulsions*) and confirmed in six other families investigated by the same group (Berkovic et al. 2004). The relevance of chromosome 16 locus in BFIC was confirmed in a recent study of 16 families (Striano et al. 2006).

Benign non-familial neonatal convulsions (Plouin and Anderson 2005), also known as 'fifth day seizures', consist of repeated seizures mainly clonic or apnoeic in type with onset between 3 and 7 days of age. The interictal neurological state and EEG are normal, although the latter may show peaked theta rhythm (so-called *théta pointu alternant*) (Plouin 1994). In general, seizures of late onset (after 3 days) without known cause tend to have a favourable outcome (Lombroso 1996).

A *syndrome of focal neonatal convulsions and stroke* is less well defined. However, this possibility is suggested by the occurrence in the 2nd to 7th day of age of repeated focal clonic seizures that remain localized to the same restricted part of the body. The diagnosis can be confirmed by neuroimaging that demonstrates the presence of an infarction involving mostly the territory of the middle cerebral artery. The overall prognosis is favourable but a hemiplegia persists in about half the cases.

Severe neonatal or infantile epilepsies with suppression–burst pattern (early infantile epileptic encephalopathy with suppression–bursts or Ohtahara syndrome and early neonatal myoclonic encephalopathy) are discussed in the section on infantile and early childhood epilepsies.

Prenatal seizures have been demonstrated by ultrasonography (Landy et al. 1989, Du Plessis et al. 1993). They may occur with pyridoxine dependency and with some brain malformations (Du Plessis et al. 1993).

PROGNOSIS

The prognosis in neonatal seizures is mainly determined by their cause (Volpe 1989, Lombroso 1996, Tekgul et al. 2006). The possible role of the seizures themselves in generating or increasing brain damage remains disputed (Volpe 1989, Lombroso 1996, Scher 2003). Although some aggravating effect of seizures is likely, the occurrence of seizures of long duration without sequelae, such as those of hypocalcaemia or of familial seizures, suggests that the role of paroxysmal activity (Lombroso 1996) is less important than its causes.

The worst outcome is for seizures due to *brain dysplasias*, followed by hypoxic–ischaemic encephalopathy and neonatal infections, with a high mortality rate and a high incidence of later epilepsy, mental retardation and cerebral palsy (Holden et al. 1982; Watanabe et al. 1982b; Lombroso 1983b, 1996). The prognosis for some metabolic seizures (late hypocalcaemia) is very good and that for seizures of unknown cause with onset after the second day of life is also largely favourable (Arzimanoglou and Aicardi 2001). In a series of patients with electroencephalographically confirmed seizures (Legido et al. 1988), the mortality was 32.5% and sequelae were found in 55.5% of survivors (Legido et al. 1988). Late epilepsy occurs in 10–26% of patients but may be as high as 81% when brain malformation is the cause. The prognostic value of the interictal EEG for neurodevelopment has been repeatedly emphasized (Lombroso 1983b, Scher and Beggarly 1989).

TREATMENT

Symptomatic treatment is imperative in addition to treatment of the cause of seizures. It includes maintenance of a free airway and of the vital constants (cardiac rate, blood pressure, etc.) and specific therapy whenever indicated (e.g. in late hypocalcaemia, hypomagnesaemia and some cases of hypoglycaemia). A *trial of pyridoxine*, and when available of pyridoxal phosphate, should be made. A single dose of 100 mg for all neonates is usually given, but too large doses should be avoided as hypotonia and apnoea may result (Kroll 1985).

Antiepileptic drug treatment commonly uses phenobarbitone or phenytoin. Large loading doses are usually recommended (phenytoin, a single i.v. dose of 20 mg/kg, not to be repeated – further doses can be administered under control of blood level; phenobarbitone, 20–25 mg/kg/day i.v. – some authors use doses as high as 30–120 mg/kg/day in 10 mg/kg boluses every 30 minutes), provided ventilatory support is available (Crawford et al. 1988). However, anticonvulsant agents may have deleterious effects on the neonatal brain (Mikati et al. 1994) and their efficacy is not established. Painter et al. (1999) found that the apparent effectiveness of phenobarbitone and phenytoin was the same. More importantly, they found that seizure frequency decreased on treatment mainly when a decreasing trend had been observed previously, and that the drugs failed to prevent the onset of subsequent seizures, to delay the time to onset of recurrent seizures, or to attenuate the severity of recurrence. It has also long been known that antiepileptic agents often eliminate the clinical expression of the seizure but leave unaffected the ictal EEG discharge.

Benzodiazepines, especially lorazepam, may be satisfactory as a first-line or even as the only treatment (Deshmukh et al. 1986, Hakeem and Wallace 1990), and are favoured as first-line treatment by Lombroso (1983b). A recent retrospective and non-randomized study (Castro Conde et al. 2005) demonstrated complete electrical control with midazolam in 13 nonresponders to phenobarbitone and phenytoin, and encountered no adverse reactions. Our own practice is to use benzodiazepines as first drugs, which often avoids the use of other drugs. Lidocaine and paraldehyde are used by some. Maintenance treatment should be carefully monitored as most AEDs are slowly metabolized in the neonatal period with a consequent risk of accumulation. In fact, prolonged treatment of neonatal seizures is probably not warranted except in the case of major structural brain abnormalities, as neonatal seizures have a strong tendency to be short-lasting (Hellström-Westas et al. 1995).

Many uncertainties continue to surround the treatment of neonatal seizures (Sankar and Painter 2005). The two most commonly used medications, phenobarbitone and phenytoin, were introduced as anticonvulsants in 1914 and 1938 respectively. Little was known then about the control of cellular and network excitability or how the developing brain is physiologically distinct from the mature brain. Phenobarbitone and phenytoin had been used to treat seizures in the adult human, and were handed down for use in infants and children. The choice of phenobarbitone or phenytoin likely rests on the availability of those agents in parenteral dosage forms for preterm infants and the relative comfort level of treating physicians (Sankar and Painter 2005). Data are scarce concerning newer AEDs. A recent Cochrane review (Booth and Evans 2004) concluded that at present there is little evidence from randomized controlled trials to support the use of any of the anticonvulsants currently used in the neonatal period. In the literature, there remains a body of opinion that seizures should be treated because of the concern that seizures in themselves may be harmful, although this is only supported by relatively low-grade evidence. Development of safe and effective treatment strategies relies on future studies of high quality (randomized controlled trials with methodology that assures validity) and of sufficient size to have the power to detect clinically important reductions in mortality and severe neurodevelopmental disability in addition to any short-term reduction in seizure burden (see also Clancy 2006).

No guidelines have been proposed for the treatment of benign familial neonatal convulsions. In older generations probably no treatment was given (Plouin and Anderson 2005). Phenobarbitone, sodium valproate or phenytoin are the drugs usually used, over a period of 3–6 months.

STIMULUS-SENSITIVE EPILEPSIES

The precipitation of seizures by specific stimuli is found in many epilepsy syndromes, both idiopathic and symptomatic. Also called 'reflex epilepsies', they would be considered as a discrete syndrome only if a patient had solely or predominantly precipitated seizures, which is rare (Wolf et al. 2004, Wolf and Inoué 2005). A certain degree of confusion is also due to the fact that the terms 'provoked' and 'triggered' are sometimes used as if they were interchangeable (Pohlmann-Eden et al. 2006). Aird (1983) indicated that 40 seizure-precipitating mechanisms are known. These include tension states, alteration of the level of attention or of consciousness, sleep (Baldy-Moulinier 1986), psychological factors and hydration state.

PHOTOSENSITIVE EPILEPSIES
Epileptic seizures triggered by photic (intermittent) stimulation can be observed with various epilepsy syndromes and do not constitute a separate syndrome (Harding and Jeavons 1994). Photosensitivity is especially frequent in adolescents with idiopathic generalized epilepsy (Harding and Jeavons 1994), in eyelid myoclonia with absence, and in some types of myoclonic epilepsy (Newmark and Penry 1979, Guerrini et al. 1995). Self-provocation is not rare in such patients. The role of television is emphasized by Harding and Jeavons (1994) and Kasteleijn-Nolst Trenité et al. (2002), although other investigators found it limited (Mayr et al. 1987). Among the factors provoking paroxysmal discharges some seem crucial: the frequency of the TV screen (the 100 Hz screen seems significantly safer than the 50 Hz), the distance from the screen (100 cm safer than 50 cm), and, particularly for the 50 Hz screen, the specific pattern of the images and the act of playing (Badinand-Hubert et al. 1998). Provocation by video games (Maeda et al. 1990, Ferrie et al. 1994, Graf et al. 1994) is also possible, though computer screens are only rarely a causal factor. This problem, as well as that of pattern-sensitive epilepsy, was studied in detail by Harding and Jeavons (1994).

The treatment of photosensitive epilepsy may be with AEDs only, especially sodium valproate. Additional measures may include the use of polarized glasses as well as precautions when watching television; drug therapy may not be necessary if the patient can avoid the stimulus by appropriate measures such as watching TV at a distance of 2–3 m and wearing dark glasses. *Self-induced photogenic or pattern-induced seizures* (Harding and Jeavons 1994) are difficult to control. Fenfluramine has been used in such cases together with antiepileptic agents, with some measure of success (Aicardi 1994).

STARTLE EPILEPSY AND MOVEMENT-INDUCED SEIZURES

Startle epilepsy is relatively common in children with congenital brain damage (Arzimanoglou et al. 2004). Many patients have congenital hemiparesis but others have diffuse brain damage including Down syndrome. Attacks are usually tonic, involving one or both sides, and follow the startle reaction induced by sudden unexpected stimuli (Chauvel et al. 1992). Sound is often particularly effective but proprioceptive or exteroceptive stimuli can also be the cause and some patients may respond electively to particular stimuli. Most cases have their onset in infancy and many patients have mild to severe mental retardation. However, Manford et al. (1996b) found that about half the patients with the condition have normal intelligence and a normal neurological profile, and these cases may be associated with cortical dysplasia rather than destructive lesions. Treatment is with anticonvulsant drugs but the occurrence of startle seizures usually announces a difficult-to-treat epilepsy. Such seizures should be distinguished from excessive startle disease and from paroxysmal dystonias (Chapter 16). *Touch epilepsy* (Ricci et al. 1995) and movement-induced epilepsy are rarer than startle epilepsy.

OTHER 'REFLEX' EPILEPSIES

A host of specific stimuli can induce seizures. These include sound, music, and complex and sometimes specific mental activities (Wilkins and Lindsay 1985). Eating epilepsy (Fiol et al. 1986) may occur with temporal lobe lesions. Reading epilepsy is a well-defined syndrome but is rare in childhood (Wolf 1994, Wolf and Inoué 2005). Seizures induced by immersion in hot water (bathing epilepsy) (Roos and Van Dijk 1988) should be distinguished from syncopes (Stephenson 1990), which are probably more common. Other uncommon precipitating factors have been reviewed by Wilkins and Lindsay (1985), Aicardi (1994), Arzimanoglou et al. (2004) and Wolf et al. (2004).

STATUS EPILEPTICUS

Status epilepticus (SE) is defined as "an epileptic seizure that is sufficiently prolonged or repeated at sufficiently brief intervals so as to produce an unvarying and enduring epileptic condition" (Gastaut 1973). There are two major categories of status epilepticus: *convulsive status* that may be generalized or localized, and *nonconvulsive status*, which can be divided in turn into partial nonconvulsive status and generalized nonconvulsive status, also improperly known as 'petit mal status'. Electrical status epilepticus during slow sleep is a separate category, included for discussion in this section.

CONVULSIVE STATUS EPILEPTICUS

TONIC–CLONIC STATUS

Convulsive SE may present as a succession of tonic–clonic seizures without recovery of consciousness between individual attacks, or as a single, prolonged, convulsive seizure, most often of a purely clonic type. The duration necessary to diagnose SE is variably estimated (Shorvon 1994, DeLorenzo et al. 1999, Lowenstein et al. 1999). The difficulties for a universally accepted definition based on duration derive directly from the fact that in everyday clinical practice, a treatment is applied to all seizures lasting longer than 5 or 10 minutes, while changes in metabolism and vital functions usually appear after 30 minutes or more. If a duration component should be included in the definition of status – to be used for the evaluation of new drugs or for epidemiological studies – this should be the minimum duration (10 minutes) after which medical care is usually applied (Arzimanoglou et al. 2004). Care should be taken not to include the postictal period. Lowenstein et al. (1999) discussed the need for a revised, more operational, definition of SE. The findings by Theodore et al. (1994), who evaluated the overall duration of the convulsive part of a 'typical' isolated seizure as being slightly more than 1 minute and rarely in excess of 2 minutes, support the operational definition for status proposed by Lowenstein et al. (1999).

Exclusively or predominantly unilateral seizures are more common in childhood than bilateral status (Aicardi and Chevrie 1983). In most patients, clonic jerks may wax and wane in intensity and the involved territory may vary from moment to moment as does the rhythm of the jerks, which, generally, are not synchronous in the affected segments.

Convulsive SE is often preceded by a *premonitory stage of serial seizures*, during which treatment is particularly effective (Shorvon 1994, Pellock et al. 2004). *Established status* can be divided into an *early or compensated stage* during which physiological mechanisms are sufficient to meet the metabolic demands and cerebral tissue is protected from hypoxic or metabolic damage, and a *stage of decompensation* when compensatory mechanisms break down and brain damage may occur. As the duration of status increases, the clinical seizures tend to become less conspicuous, eventually evolving into coma with minimal jerks or without visible movements, while autonomic changes become more prominent with resulting respiratory and circulatory impairment, often associated with hyperthermia.

The *EEG features* of convulsive SE are variable. Generalized paroxysmal activity as described in adults (Treiman 1993, Shorvon 1994) is less common in children than asymmetrical slow waves irregularly interspersed by spikes and sharp waves. In cases of prolonged SE, episodes of 'flattening' of the EEG frequently occur. *Periodic generalized or lateralized epileptiform discharges* may be seen in very long episodes and indicate a poor prognosis (Garg et al. 1995).

The term *focal or partial convulsive status epilepticus* applies only to those cases in which convulsive activity remains localized to a restricted segment on one side of the body without generalization or diffusion to the whole of the affected side. When segmental myoclonic jerks are continuous, the condition is known as *epilepsia partialis continua*. In such instances, intermittent somatomotor seizures may start from the area of the body that is involved by permanent myoclonus; this association defines the *Kojewnikow syndrome*.

Convulsive SE is a major complication of epilepsy and remains a dangerous condition, even though its prognosis has improved over the past few decades. The pathogenesis of SE and of its consequences has been extensively studied (see Brown and Hussain 1991a; Shorvon 1994; Wasterlain and Treiman 2006). It involves multiple factors that include progressive hypoxia, substrate failure, ATP depletion and intracellular acidosis. These, in turn, eventually produce a fall in cardiac output, hyperkalaemia, metabolic acidosis and cerebral oedema, all of which participate in the genesis of sequelae, which, however, rarely appear after episodes of status lasting less than 90–120 minutes (Aicardi and Chevrie 1983). The role of excitotoxicity due to excessive activation of the excitatory neurotransmitters, especially glutamate (glutamate cascade), with consequent massive influx of Ca^{++} ions in neurons producing apoptosis or cell necrosis is now considered as the essential noxious phenomenon and has received considerable attention. Blocking the excitotoxic cascade in status may become an important method for neuroprotection (see corresponding chapters in Wasterlain and Treiman 2006).

Systemic factors also play an important role in the production of sequelae. However, it seems that the epileptic activity itself, in the absence of systemic complications, can generate brain lesions, especially in the temporal lobe (Holmes 2002, Lado et al. 2002, Wasterlain and Treiman 2006), probably at least in part by a mechanism of glutamate-induced excitotoxic damage.

The *incidence* of SE ranges from 3% to 16% of all patients with epilepsy (Hauser 1994, Wu et al. 2006) in childhood series of epilepsy. Contrary to the situation that prevails in adults, status is often the first epileptic seizure in infants and children. This was the case for 77% of the 239 patients of Aicardi and Chevrie (1970). Similarly, 24% of all children with a first afebrile seizure before the age of 10 years, seen in Minneapolis (Hauser 1983), presented with SE. Status is especially common during the first 2 years of life, and approximately 75–85% of cases occur before the age of 5 years (Aicardi and Chevrie 1970). In older children, after the age of 3 years, the annual frequency remains stable at around 3–5% until the age of 15 (Aicardi and Chevrie 1970). The overall incidence of SE has not seemed to decline. A prospective population-based study performed by the North London Status Epilepticus in Childhood Surveillance Study (NLSTEPSS) group enrolled 226 children, 176 of whom had a first ever episode of convulsive SE (Chin et al. 2006). Ninety-eight children (56%) were neurologically healthy before their first ever episode, and 56 (57%) of those children had had a prolonged febrile seizure. Eleven (12%) of the children with their first ever febrile convulsive SE had acute bacterial meningitis. A conservative estimation of 1-year recurrence of convulsive SE was 16% (10–24%). Case fatality was 3% (2–7%).

Status epilepticus can be *symptomatic*, resulting from underlying CNS diseases that may be acute, such as trauma, vascular collapse, electrolyte disorders, meningitis or encephalitis, or pro-

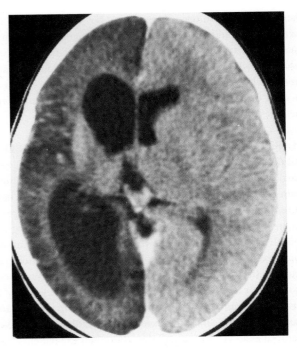

Fig. 15.16. Hemiconvulsion–hemiplegia–epilepsy (HHE) syndrome. CT of 6-year-old girl who had febrile status epilepticus at age 11 months, localized on left side and lasting several hours, followed by permanent hemiplegia. Overall atrophy of right hemisphere and dilatation of whole right ventricle; marked hypodensity of right hemisphere and shift of midline to right. This image is virtually pathognomonic of HHE syndrome and probably corresponds to postconvulsive 'hemiatrophia cerebri'.

gressive such as brain tumours or progressive encephalopathies; *remote symptomatic*, due to chronic nonprogressive brain lesions such as glial scars or late sequelae of infectious or anoxic events; or *cryptogenic*, occurring at the onset of the epilepsy or in the course of a recurring seizure disorder (Hauser 1993). In this case, interruption of treatment is often a precipitating event. It may also represent an occasional seizure, in practice mostly a febrile seizure that fails to stop for unknown reasons. Such cases differ from common febrile seizures only in duration, not in nature. Currently, it appears that a large majority of cases of status observed in industrialized countries are of symptomatic origin especially in infants. The dramatic decrease in the frequency of cryptogenic status probably results in large part from a better and more prompt treatment of epilepsy and of incipient febrile status. The improved outlook for status should not lead to underestimation of the potential risks or failure to instigate immediate vigorous therapy.

A once common syndrome of convulsive SE is the *hemiconvulsion–hemiplegia or H-H syndrome* (Gastaut et al. 1960, Arzimanoglou and Dravet 2003), characterized by the occurrence, in the course of a febrile disease in a child of less than 4 years of age, of prolonged clonic seizures with a marked unilateral predominance, followed by a long-lasting hemiplegia. After one to several years, partial epilepsy, with seizures originating in the hemisphere contralateral to the hemiplegia, often occurs (hemiconvulsion–hemiplegia–epilepsy or HHE syndrome), and 85% of affected children have mental retardation. CT and MRI are

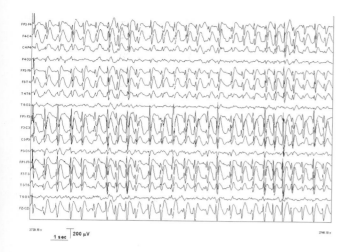

Fig. 15.17. Continuous spike–wave in slow sleep in an 8-year-old boy with atonic seizures and mental deterioration.

disappears, with some recovery of cognitive function. Morikawa et al. (1985) found identifiable brain pathology in 20–30% of cases, and Gaggero et al. (1995) demonstrated areas of reduced blood flow by SPECT corresponding to the most actively discharging brain areas in 4 of their 10 cases. Guerrini et al. (1998c) reported on children with ESESS associated with unilateral focal polymicrogyria, and similar cases have been reported since by other authors (e.g. Caraballo et al. 1999). These results suggest that the syndrome is heterogeneous and not infrequently caused by multifocal pathological abnormalities. Another organic cause is hydrocephalus, which may be related to thalamic injury (Guzzetta et al. (2005). Ethosuximide and corticosteroids may have some efficacy but treatment is often disappointing. Some investigators claim satisfactory results with sulthiame (Gross-Selbeck 1995, Lerman and Lerman-Sagie 1995) or short cycles of high doses of benzodiazepines (De Negri et al. 1993). ACTH steroids are, in fact, the most commonly used agents and are considered effective, although only anecdotal evidence is available. Treatment is usually for prolonged periods (months or even years). Recognition of electrical SE is of great importance as the syndrome is a cause of partially treatable cognitive deterioration. It is, therefore, essential to obtain a sleep EEG in such cases, even in the absence of clinical seizures.

Landau–Kleffner syndrome
Landau–Kleffner syndrome (LKS), a condition also called 'epileptic aphasia', presents a similar paroxysmal sleep EEG activity. This is defined as acquired aphasia, often but not always predominantly receptive in type, with intense paroxysmal EEG activity, usually more intense in sleep. Awake tracings show uni- or bilateral spike foci often over the temporal lobes (Hirsch et al. 1990, 2006b; Beaumanoir 1992; Maquet et al. 1995). There may be a correlation between the intensity of paroxysmal activity, especially during sleep, and language deterioration. In such cases, there is a rapid or progressive loss of language abilities that often involves mainly verbal auditory discrimination. Approximately

80% of children have seizures. Most often, these are focal and are not severe. Occasionally, they are atypical absences and are frequently repeated. In most cases, the epilepsy and the EEG abnormalities disappear before age 15 years (Dulac et al. 1983, Rossi et al. 1999, Hommet et al. 2000).

The outlook for language is poor and most patients still have language difficulties as adults, even though severity is variable from almost no verbal ability to mild or moderate deficits in verbal communication (Bishop 1985, Deonna et al. 1989).

Similar EEG activity involving other brain areas may be responsible for disturbance of other functions. Hirsch et al. (1995) reported apraxia associated with continuous parietal EEG paroxysms and suggested the mechanism was the same as that of LKS. Neville and Boyd (1995) suggested that epilepsy may manifest as a gait disorder that responds to corticosteroid treatment.

LKS is highly heterogeneous (Deonna et al. 1977, Hirsch et al. 1990, Maquet et al. 1995). Some children have predominant disturbances in expressive language or complex patterns of language disturbance. Others do not exhibit the pattern of continuous spike–wave discharges during sleep, and occasionally patients may have severe persisting epilepsy.

The mechanism of the syndrome is unclear. PET studies have given heterogeneous results (Maquet et al. 1990, Rintahaka et al. 1995, De Tiège et al. 2004, Luat et al. 2005). Magnetoencephalographic spikes originated in the left auditory area in one study (Paetau et al. 1992), and various techniques also point to this area (Morrell et al. 1995). There is evidence to suggest that the paroxysmal EEG abnormality itself may be responsible for the aphasia. Both LKS and CSWSS are examples of *epileptic encephalopathy*, illustrating the effects of 'subclinical' discharges on brain function, and a confirmation that epilepsy is not limited to seizures may have more pervasive effects. Indeed, some cases of LKS also manifest more diffuse dysfunction, for example in frontal lobe mechanisms (Roulet et al. 1991, Hirsch et al. 1995), and transient deficits in various localized brain functions such as anterior opercular syndrome (Roulet et al. 1989, Boulloche et al. 1990) have also been linked to intense, localized, paroxysmal EEG activity.

Treatment of the condition is disappointing. Anticonvulsant agents usually fail to abolish the paroxysmal activity or to improve language, although some success has been reported with the drugs used in CSWSS. Corticosteroids or ACTH treatment is an accepted practice but has to be continued for one year or more (Lerman et al. 1991, Hirsch et al. 1995). There are no controlled clinical trials investigating therapeutic options for LKS. Only open-label data are available. Early diagnosis and initiation of prompt medical treatment appear to be important to achieving better long-term prognosis. Several antiepileptic drugs have been reported to be beneficial, including valproic acid, diazepam, ethosuximide, clobazam and clonazepam. Reports on the efficacy of lamotrigine, sulthiame, felbamate, nicardipine, vigabatrin, levetiracetam, vagal nerve stimulation and a ketogenic diet are few and more experience is needed. Carbamazepine and possibly phenobarbitone and phenytoin have been reported to occasionally exacerbate the syndrome (Mikati and Shamseddine 2005).

Only anecdotal reports are available and the relationship between treatment and language improvement, although it is generally accepted, has not been proved. The same applies to surgical treatment by multiple temporal transections (Morrell et al. 1989, Devinsky et al. 1994, Morrell et al. 1995, Robinson et al. 2001).

INVESTIGATIONS IN PATIENTS WITH EPILEPSY

Epileptic seizures are transient clinical events. Consequently, the identification of an attack as epileptic mainly depends upon reports from the patient and/or other witnesses. History taking is the most important 'investigation' for the diagnosis of epilepsy, if medical errors, in terms of both diagnosis and treatment choices, are to be avoided. The mainstay of the diagnosis is a good eyewitness account of the episode, but this information may not be available, may be incomplete, misleading or rather vague, and may not correspond to the definition of the various epileptic seizures or syndromes. The results of the additional investigations like the EEG may be noninformative, may provide information that is difficult to interpret, or may seem to be contradictory to the clinical data.

The first step, following a first paroxysmal event reported by the patient or their family, is to obtain a precise description and make an hypothesis about the epileptic or non-epileptic nature of the event. The accuracy of the diagnosis of epilepsy varies from a misdiagnosis rate of 5% in a prospective childhood epilepsy study in which the diagnosis was made by a panel of three experienced paediatric neurologists (Stroink et al. 2003) to at least 23% in a British population-based study (Scheepers et al. 1998), and may be even higher in everyday practice. The level of experience of the treating physician plays an important role. The EEG may be helpful but one should be reluctant to make a diagnosis of epilepsy mainly on the EEG findings without a reasonable clinical suspicion based on the history. Being aware of the possibility of interobserver variation and inaccuracy, adopting a systematic approach to the diagnostic process, and timely referral to specialized care may be helpful to prevent misdiagnosis (Van Donselaar et al. 2006).

History taking usually requires more than one session because new memories and questions may arise after the first questioning. The family needs to be informed about the importance of focal clinical signs if present, and about all other elements that can provide clues for diagnosis and treatment. The parents should be encouraged to provide a home videotape, an invaluable source of information. A detailed description of the clinical paroxysmal events, performed in a methodical and comprehensive manner, is mandatory.

The physician must be familiar with the various types of generalized seizures, their main features and characteristics, and their pattern of appearance. For example, typical absences usually occur several times a day; infantile spasms usually occur in clusters; atypical absences are rarely the sole type of seizure in a patient; and tonic seizures are usually encountered in non-idio-pathic forms of epilepsy. The difference between generalized tonic-clonic seizures and secondarily generalized seizures must be clearly understood. Before accepting that a seizure is a primarily generalized one, any focal sign preceding the tonic–clonic phase must be carefully sought. A number of practical consequences, in terms of both diagnostic investigations and treatment, will directly result from this first diagnostic step.

The *age of the patient* at onset of the epilepsy is another essential consideration in diagnosis. Several epilepsy syndromes are strongly age-dependent. Consequently, age consideration will provide valuable clues for a precise syndromic diagnosis.

A complete neurological and general examination will provide other vital diagnostic elements. It should involve especially the skin, the eyes, the search for focal neurological signs and a rapid assessment of the patient's competence both cognitively and socially. History taking should include questioning about the life history of the patient, from birth and early development, past major diseases, school cursus and socio-professional situation.

Although history taking is the cornerstone of diagnosis in epilepsy, and physical examination may give essential clues, technical developments have added considerably to our knowledge in this field and may be of great clinical importance. EEG and neuroimaging are the main investigations performed but functional neuroimaging and biochemical investigations are indicated in selected cases.

The Quality Standards Subcommittee of the American Academy of Neurology recommends routine EEG as part of the diagnostic evaluation; other studies such as laboratory evaluations and neuroimaging studies are recommended as based on specific clinical circumstances (Hirtz et al. 2000). The EEG is important for diagnosis and differential diagnosis but of little help in the determination of a cause. Neuroimaging is essential for the latter purpose. Functional neuroimaging (PET or SPECT) seems to be especially useful in conjunction with other methods for research of a focal origin to the seizures when surgery is contemplated.

ELECTROENCEPHALOGRAPHY

An EEG is systematically recorded in children with seizure disorders, with the exception of febrile convulsions. It may identify specific interictal or ictal abnormalities that are associated with an increased epileptogenic potential and/or correlate with a seizure disorder. In general, an EEG, like any other investigation, should be required only when some sort of hypothesis has been formulated. It is essential that the recording technique is correct and that someone with paediatric EEG experience interprets the records, as the EEG profoundly changes with the age of patients, both in terms of background tracing and in the type of abnormalities expected. The reader is referred to the specialized EEG literature (Daly and Pedley 1990, Blume and Kalbara 1995, Mizrahi et al. 2004, Kaminska et al. 2005, Crespel et al. 2006) for details.

The EEG is of no value in patients with febrile convulsions and in many cases of occasional seizures. It is rarely indicated as an emergency investigation (suspicion of neonatal seizures; suspicion of infantile spasms; suspicion of non-convulsive SE; coma of undetermined aetiology; confusional state; neurological signs suggesting a localized brain insult). In patients with already diagnosed epilepsy, systematic repetition of the EEG every time they present to an emergency department following a seizure is useless (Arzimanoglou et al. 2004). Following a first unprovoked seizure the quantity of expected information from the EEG is too low to affect treatment recommendations in most patients (Gilbert and Buncher 2000).

The information obtained must be interpreted in conjunction with the clinical history. A normal EEG, even if repeated, does not exclude the diagnosis of epilepsy, nor does an abnormal or even a paroxysmal tracing establish it. The diagnostic yield of the interictal EEG can be increased if the conditions for its realization and/or the techniques applied are based upon a syndromic diagnostic hypothesis (e.g. sleep deprivation EEG when suspecting juvenile myoclonic epilepsy).

ROUTINE EEG

The 'routine' EEG of infants and young children should systematically include a sleep record. Standard activation procedures such as hyperventilation and photic stimulation should be included, and eventually adapted to the diagnostic hypothesis (e.g. investigating the spectrum of photosensitivity when suspecting a stimulus-sensitive epilepsy or reaction to low-frequency photic stimulation when suspecting a progressive myoclonic epilepsy).

In occasional cases, the EEG tracings may suggest an aetiology (e.g. the presence of a slow-wave focus may indicate a focal lesion; localized subclinical EEG discharges may suggest a focal cortical dysplasia). The lateralizing and localizing value of the EEG has been extensively discussed. Although a consistently focal EEG focus is of considerable value, diffuse paroxysmal EEG abnormalities are not rare in children with focal lesions, especially cortical malformations and developmental tumours (Kahane et al. 2005), and should be kept in mind as not contraindicating the possibility of surgery.

The prognostic significance of the EEG is sometimes clear-cut. Such tracings as slow spike–wave complexes or multifocal spikes with abnormally slow background indicate the likelihood of an unfavourable outlook. Likewise, in some studies at least, an abnormal EEG before discontinuation of therapy is associated with a high recurrence rate (Shinnar et al. 1990, 1994).

In general, however, the EEG is not an essential guide to therapy. The presence of EEG paroxysms is not in itself an indication to drug treatment nor a necessary contraindication to its discontinuation. In rolandic epilepsy, for example, the EEG usually normalizes several months to years after cessation of seizures. The greater or lesser paroxysmal EEG activity is rarely, if ever, an indication for stepping up or reducing therapy, except possibly in the case of some epileptic encephalopathies in which there are arguments (but no certainty) for trying to suppress or diminish the EEG epileptic activity.

OTHER EEG TECHNIQUES

In addition to hyperventilation, intermittent photic stimulation

and brief sleep, which are routinely employed, *prolonged sleep studies* are of great interest under certain circumstances. All-night sleep records are particularly useful in such epilepsy syndromes as the Landau–Kleffner syndrome, and atypical partial benign epilepsy, or when continuous spike–waves of slow sleep are suspected. Sleep EEG is essential for recording nocturnal seizures, e.g. in frontal lobe epilepsy. Nap recordings may be sufficient in many cases and should be privileged in children (Peraita-Adrados et al. 2001). Prolonged monitoring is also of value for the surveillance of neonates with seizures and in cases of encephalopathies as often there is a EEG/clinical dissociation.

Cassette recordings (*ambulatory EEG monitoring*) are a useful technique in cases in which the clinical history and sleep EEG are not sufficient to establish or rule out the diagnosis of epilepsy and in which seizures are frequent enough to make their occurrence likely during a 24- or 48-hour period. Distinction between true and pseudoseizures is one of the best indications for this technique. It also facilitates sleep recording in older children who may not easily fall asleep in the laboratory.

Video–EEG recordings (either of short duration conducted in the laboratory or of long duration during hospitalization) has become an essential tool for diagnosis and treatment. Its main indication is the recording of ictal phenomena for differential diagnosis and for a better syndromic diagnosis. Interictal activity can also be registered for a longer duration and correlated to the behavioural status of the child.

Digital EEG acquisition and storage in a format for subsequent remontaging and filtering have improved the speed with which interpretable ictal recordings may be obtained over paper recordings.

Telemetric EEG monitoring combined with neuropsychological tests has shown that isolated discharges or even single spikes may be associated with transient cognitive dysfunction (Arts et al. 1988). Their presence does not signify that treatment should be systematically prescribed. Indications to treat with AEDs, the choic of the drug to be prescribed and the duration of treatment trial can be evaluated only on a case-by-case basis and in collaboration with a pediatric epileptologist (Arzimanoglou et al. 2004).

Video–EEG monitoring of both ictal and interictal activity is absolutely required before considering surgery. However, particularly in this setting, video–EEG monitoring is of very limited added value if not accompanied by close observation by experienced personnel (medical or paramedics) who will test the patient during seizures looking for signs and symptoms of localizing value such as a transient aphasia, a limb dystonia, a visual field defect or a memory defect.

Other EEG techniques, discussion of which is beyond the scope of this book, include semi-invasive (sphenoidal or ethmoidal electrodes, foramen ovale electrodes) and invasive techniques (extradural, subdural or depth electrode recordings).

NEUROIMAGING IN EPILEPSY
STRUCTURAL NEUROIMAGING
Although abnormalities on neuroimaging are seen in up to one

third of children with a first seizure, most of these abnormalities do not influence immediate treatment or management decisions such as the need for hospitalization or further investigations. Hirtz et al. (2000) reported that imaging results significantly contributed to further clinical management in an average of only about 2% of patients. In the majority of these cases imaging had been performed because the seizure was focal or there were specific clinical findings in addition to the occurrence of a seizure. Thus, there is insufficient evidence to support a recommendation at the level of guidelines for the use of routine neuroimaging, i.e. imaging performed for which having had a first nonfebrile seizure in a child is the sole indication.

Factors to be considered for the realization of a *non-urgent neuroimaging study* include the age of the child, the need for sedation to perform the study, the EEG results, a history of head trauma, and other clinical circumstances such as a family history of epilepsy. MRI should be seriously considered in any child with a significant cognitive or motor impairment of unknown aetiology, unexplained abnormalities on neurological examination, a seizure of focal onset with or without secondary generalization, or an EEG that is not typical of benign partial epilepsy of childhood or primary generalized epilepsy, and in children under 1 year of age (King et al. 1998, Hirtz et al. 2000).

Emergency neuroimaging following a first seizure is justified only when the physical and/or neurological examinations suggest a serious condition that may require immediate intervention. Indications include a postictal focal deficit that does not quickly resolve or where consciousness has not returned to baseline within several hours after the seizure. The possible effects of emergency medication used to treat the seizure must be taken into consideration.

In children with an established diagnosis of epilepsy, MRI is clearly preferable to CT (Commission on Neuroimaging 1997). CT may have special indications, especially for demonstrating calcifications that are better visualized than with MRI. However, CT/MRI are not indicated in children with only typical generalized epilepsy of the idiopathic type (childhood absence epilepsy and juvenile myoclonic epilepsy) or partial benign epilepsy with classical rolandic focus. Difficulties of interpretation may arise especially when intense convulsive activity is present (Kramer et al. 1987, Yaffe et al. 1995) and excellent quality imaging is mandatory. Special techniques such as 3D acquisition and high-resolution MRI should be used (Bergin et al. 1995), particularly when investigating focal epilepsies.

There are two major indications for performing MRI: (i) as part of the diagnostic screening in patients with epilepsy associated with an underlying neurological disorder (this indication particularly applies to cases with an epileptic encephalopathy, suspicion of a metabolic or degenerative disorder, etc.); (ii) all cases of non-idiopathic focal epilepsy (see also Duncan 1997).

Particularly in non-idiopathic focal epilepsies, poor low-field image quality could miss subtle abnormalities despite interpretation by experienced neuroradiologists (Knake and Grant 2006). Consequently, MRI should be performed on a state-of-the-art 1.5- or 3-T scanner. The possibility of using different planes of imaging is of considerable value for the detection of

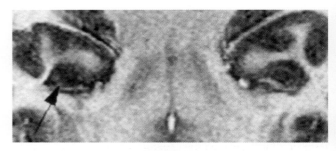
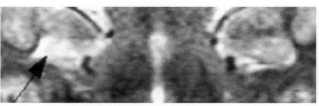

Fig. 15.18. MRI of both hippocampi of a patient with mesial temporal sclerosis showing details that can be obtained with high-resolution techniques. *(Top)* Right hippocampus *(arrow)* is of almost normal size but internal structure cannot be made out. *(Bottom)* Increased T$_2$ signal in external part of right hippocampus *(arrow)*. (Courtesy Dr G Jackson, Melbourne, Australia.)

small lesions such as cortical dysplasias, small indolent tumours and hippocampal sclerosis. Several sequences should be used, including fluid attenuated inversion recovery (FLAIR), thin cuts, 3D acquisition, reformatting in different planes and gadolinium enhancing.

The diagnosis of hippocampal sclerosis by MRI rests on a decreased size of the Ammon horn on one side, on increased T$_2$ signal and on loss of the internal structure of the hippocampus (Jackson et al. 1990; Cendes et al. 1993a,b) (Fig. 15.18). This lesion is highly correlated with the occurrence of partial seizures of temporal lobe origin (Raymond et al. 1994, Cendes et al. 1995, Cendes 2005). A careful search for additional anomalies is indicated in cases of hippocampal sclerosis, especially with a view to detection of dual pathology (for example coexistence of a cortical dysplasia).

It is our practice not to recommend neuroimaging studies for children with classical idiopathic generalized epilepsies (absence epilepsy, juvenile myoclonic epilepsy) or for children with typical rolandic epilepsy. Contrariwise, imaging is in order for children with all other types of seizures or for any patient with atypical epilepsy. In children with non-idiopathic focal epilepsy that resists AED treatment, we repeat the MRI investigation using high-resolution techniques. Informing the neuroradiologist about the suspected topography of the epileptogenic zone is mandatory.

FUNCTIONAL NEUROIMAGING AND OTHER TECHNIQUES OF INVESTIGATION
Functional imaging studies using radiotracers, such as positron emission tomography and single-photon-emission computed tomography, are performed to identify or confirm the ictal focus in preparation for surgery, to identify eloquent cortical regions to be spared during epilepsy surgery, and to investigate the patho-

physiology of partial and generalized seizure disorders (for detailed reviews, see Duncan 1997, Gaillard 2006).

Positron emission tomography (PET) allows for the measurement of regional variations in glucose metabolism using ^{18}FDG (fluoro-deoxyglucose), to map cerebral blood flow by means of ^{15}O-labelled water and ^{11}C-flumazenil to quantify benzodiazepines receptors. The basic aspects and limitations of the technique, the various other radiopharmaceuticals that have been tested in epilepsy, the sensitivity of the different types of PET investigations, and the practical utility of PET imaging in pre-surgical assessment of partial epilepsies have been recently reviewed (Mauguière and Ryvlin 2004).

Because of its slow time resolution, PET does not allow ictal studies but does permit evaluation of interictal glucose metabolism, and a correlation has been shown to exist between lesions and hypometabolic areas (Chugani et al. 1987, Theodore et al. 1992). In children with infantile spasms and normal MRI, PET may evidence regional metabolic abnormalities that could guide removal of the suspected epileptogenic zone (Chugani et al. 1988). In some children, however, the metabolic abnormalities seen at the onset of infantile spasms may resolve with time and thus may represent a functional state that is potentially reversible (Itomi et al. 2002).

In children with tuberous sclerosis, the PET tracer [^{11}C]methyl-L-tryptophan (AMT) has been said to be selectively taken up by epileptogenic tubers (Chugani et al. 1998), which could allow differentiation from nonepileptogenic tubers in the interictal state and facilitate presurgical evaluation (Kagawa et al. 2005). [^{11}C]AMT uptake is also enhanced in focal cortical dysplasia (Fedi et al. 2003, Juhasz et al. 2003). PET studies in Lennox–Gastaut and Landau–Kleffner syndromes have yielded mixed results (for a review, see Gaillard 2006).

Single photon emission computed tomography (SPECT) has a lower spatial resolution than PET, but the use of ^{99m}TC-HMPAO permits the study of ictal events when injected during a seizure as it is immediately taken up by active cells, while scanning can be performed 4–6 hours after injection (Harvey et al. 1993a,b; Newton et al. 1995). Interictal SPECT gives results generally similar to those of PET, e.g. decreased localized uptake in the region of origin of seizures, although its accuracy is far from perfect (Cross et al. 1997). Ictal SPECT compared with an interictal investigation demonstrated regional hyperperfusion in 67–90% of patients (Gaillard 2006) that in a majority of patients correlated with the ictal focus. Such a correlation has been validated with simultaneous intracranial EEG (Spanaki et al. 1999). Seizure localization using ictal SPECT was also reported in children with intractable epilepsy (Harvey et al. 1993a,b; Cross et al. 1995). False localization is reported in 3–4% of studies, most probably because of seizure propagation, particularly following late injection times. Subtraction techniques with MRI coregistration improve postictal SPECT localization of seizure foci (O'Brien et al. 2004). The main technical limitation of this technique derives from the fact that in order for an ictal SPECT study to be useful, the ligand must be injected during the very first seconds of the seizure, which demands a constant surveillance during

video–EEG investigations.

Functional magnetic resonance imaging (fMRI) is based on the fact that oxygenated haemoglobin gives a different MR signal to that of deoxyhaemoglobin, and that the increased blood flow to actively discharging neurons results in increased signal. The resulting increased oxyhaemoglobin/deoxyhaemoglobin ratio (Morris et al. 1994, Detre et al. 1995), permits localization of areas of active brain regardless of whether the activity is normal, e.g. voluntary movements, or abnormal, e.g. epileptic. Functional MRI may have a dual role: (1) to localize epileptic foci by identifying regional blood flow changes that accompany partial seizures; and (2) to map the brain areas such as the motor circonvolution or language areas that must be respected surgically. Several studies indicate that fMRI language paradigms reliably identify hemispheric dominance for language, including bilateral and right-hemisphere language representation in adults and in children 5 years of age and older (for reviews, see Gaillard 2006, Pelletier et al. 2007). This technique may eventually replace more invasive methods such as intracarotid injection of amytal to determine language lateralization (the Wada test) or other essential functions (Pelletier et al. 2007).

Other techniques that are being assessed include *magneto-encephalography (MEG)*, as well as various computerized methods of signal interpretation and EEG topographic studies (e.g. *dipole models*). MEG registers magnetic brain activity with a high spatio-temporal resolution. It allows for the placement of magnetic spike sources on a conventional MR scan, the so-called magnetic source imaging, so that the locus of epileptiform activity can be determined. Since distortion of magnetic fields by the skin, skull and CSF is negligible, the technique, while still expensive, offers an almost undistorted view of brain activity and offers promising possibilities for focus localization and presurgical functional mapping in patients with epilepsy (Rampp and Stefan 2007). MEG spike clusters are corroborated now by intraoperative invasive subdural grid monitoring that shows good correlation in the majority of cases. Another important role of MEG relates to the mapping of critical regions of brain function using known paradigms for speech, motor, sensory, visual and auditory brain cortex. When linked to standard neuronavigation devices, MEG brain mapping can be helpful to the neurosurgeon approaching nonlesional epilepsy cases or lesional cases where the safest and most direct route to the surgical disease can be selected. As paradigms for brain mapping improve and as MEG software upgrades become more sensitive to analysing all types of spike sources, MEG might play an increasingly important role in paediatric neurosurgery, especially for the child with intractable epilepsy (Grondin et al. 2006). Equivalent dipole modeling is another relatively novel technique for the spatio-temporal analysis of scalp voltage fields. Although an imperfect representation of spike or seizure sources, proper interpretation of dipole models can lead to a better characterization of their location and propagation. Modern techniques of 3-D MRI reconstruction and realistic head models have both improved localization accuracy and provided a means of displaying results in an image of the individual's brain (Ebersole and Hawes-Ebersole 2007).

TREATMENT OF EPILEPTIC SEIZURES AND EPILEPSIES

The management of epilepsy is not limited to the prescription of drugs but in complicated cases requires considerable time, competences, and technical and human resources. In many 'ordinary' cases it still requires careful attention, and specialist neurological advice should be sought in most, if not all, cases before starting treatment. The impact of epilepsy on the life of the child and the family group is considerable, and the education and support of parents, counselling and help with educational problems, and management of behavioural difficulties may be even more important than drug therapy of seizures.

EDUCATION AND SUPPORT OF PARENTS

Because the impact of the diagnosis of epilepsy is not only – or not even essentially – concerned with the rational aspects but has also to take into account myths, misunderstandings and prejudices that are traditionally associated with seizure disorders, an adapted yet full explanation should be given to the patient and family. The false idea that epilepsy is a disease in its own right should be dispelled, and the fact that epileptic seizures are only a symptom of many types of brain dysfunction, some of which are quite benign, should be thoroughly explained. False but firmly entrenched ideas, e.g. that all epilepsies are life-long conditions or are related to psychiatric disorders, should be discussed and dispelled, as should the frequently expressed fear that brain tumours or other serious brain disorders are a common cause (Brett 1997, Arzimanoglou et al. 2004). All of this information cannot usually be given in one session, and repeated interviews are required.

Full explanation of the aims of therapy, its shortcomings and possible side effects, is imperative, as is an indication of the probable duration of treatment and of the difficulties that may be encountered when discontinuing it. This is essential for the establishment of a confident relationship between patient and physician (Aicardi and Taylor 1998).

It is extremely important to give the parents precise ideas about what their child can do and what restrictions of activity are warranted. Such restrictions should be limited to a reasonable minimum, with the knowledge that some risks are unavoidable. Swimming is possible with adequate one-to-one supervision. The use of a bicycle (except on safe roads), and especially of a motorbike, is one of the most difficult problems and can be solved only individually and often imperfectly.

EDUCATIONAL, LEARNING AND BEHAVIOUR PROBLEMS

Although the majority of children with epilepsy do not have learning difficulties or basic behavioural problems, one fifth to one third of them do, at least in part as a result of the CNS lesions responsible for their epileptic seizures (Sillanpää 1992, 2004; Beghi et al. 2006). Conversely, 20% of children with mental retardation also have epilepsy, and one third of these also have cerebral palsy (Forsgren et al. 1990).

Various educational and behavioural difficulties are present in many children with epilepsy but without mental retardation. The prevalence of psychiatric disorder is several times higher in epileptic children than in the general population (Freilinger et al. 2006, Austin and Caplan 2007). The reason for this association is not clear, as assessment of social and other factors suggests that it is not explained by differences in sex, age, presence of physical disability or low intelligence.

Underachievement at school is significantly more common in children with epilepsy than in the general population (Seidenberg et al. 1986, Arts et al. 2004, Hermann and Seidenberg 2007). This is certainly a consequence of the limited intellectual abilities in some children. Bourgeois et al. (1983), Rodin et al. (1986) and Aldenkamp et al. (1990), among others, have shown that some children with epileptic seizures develop intellectual difficulties for which the disease, the treatment and socioeducational factors may all be partly responsible. However, an undue number of patients with various types of epilepsy, even well controlled, discontinue educational training prematurely. Over one third of patients with absence epilepsy in one series were overqualified for their job (Olsson and Campenhausen 1992). This may indicate low self-esteem and/or low parental expectations (Levin et al. 1988, Collings 1990). Sillanpää (1990) showed that professional underachievement was common in adult patients who had had epilepsy starting in childhood, even when their IQ was normal. Loiseau et al. (1983) have shown that children with absence epilepsy do less well, in terms of social and professional achievement, than would be expected from their IQ and the relative benignity of their epilepsy, whereas children with benign partial epilepsy have a completely normal outlook from this point of view. The reasons for such differences are obscure. Considerable attention has been given to the interference of infraclinical EEG discharges with learning or other mental processes that may involve attention or concentration but may also interfere specifically with specialized tasks (Arts et al. 1988; Kasteleijn-Nolst Trenité et al. 1988, 1990; Aldenkamp et al. 1992; Arzimanoglou et al. 2005; Deonna and Roulet-Perez 2005). However important subclinical discharges may be, they are unlikely to account for all the behavioural and learning difficulties of many children with epilepsy. Feelings of inadequacy and specialized neuropsychological deficits are clearly correlated with aggressive behaviour, poorer school performance, and having fewer friends and fewer interests (Hermann 1982, Viberg et al. 1987), but the exact mechanisms need further research. Careful assessment and often remedial help may be needed on an individual basis. In an overwhelming majority of children with isolated epilepsy, regular schooling is possible, and special schools for epileptic patients are rarely – if ever – justified for patients without other neurodevelopmental problems.

DRUG TREATMENT
GENERAL PRINCIPLES
Drug treatment is the major form of therapy for the vast majority of children with seizure disorders. The main drugs currently available are shown in Table 15.14 and the main pharmacokinetic

Drug	Indication	Total daily dose*	No of daily doses
Carbamazepine[1]	Focal seizures, generalized tonic–clonic seizures[2]	10–20 mg/kg	2
Sodium valproate, valproic acid[1]	Generalized tonic–clonic and focal seizures; myoclonic seizures; absences; idiopathic generalized epilepsies	20–50 mg/kg	2
Lamotrigine[3]	Focal and secondarily generalized seizures; primary generalized and myoclonic seizures, absence seizures, Lennox–Gastaut syndrome	On enzyme inducer = 5–15 mg/kg/day On sodium valproate = 1–5 mg/kg/day	2
Levetiracetam[4]	Focal and secondarily generalized seizures; primary generalized and myoclonic seizures	40–60 mg/kg	
Gabapentin	Focal and secondarily generalized seizures[2]	20–50 mg/kg	2–3
Topiramate	Partial and secondarily generalized seizures; myoclonic seizures; Lennox–Gastaut syndrome	Adults 200–800 mg; children 1–5 mg/kg[6]	2
Vigabatrin	Infantile spasms, refractory focal seizures[2]	40–100 mg/kg (up to 150 mg/kg for infantile spasms)	2
Felbamate[5]	Lennox–Gastaut syndrome; refractory partial seizures	Up to 45 mg/kg	3–4
Zonisamide	Focal and generalized seizures	5–15 mg/kg	2
Ethosuximide	Absences and myoclonic seizures	20–40 mg/kg	1–2
Clonazepam	All forms	0.05–0.2 mg/kg	2–3
Clobazam	All forms, including Landau–Kleffner syndrome	0.25–1.0 mg/kg	2
Stiripentol	Dravet syndrome		2
Phenytoin	Generalized convulsive seizures, focal seizures	8–10 mg/kg <3 yrs; 4–7 mg/kg >3 yrs	2
Phenobarbitone	Generalized convulsive seizures, focal seizures	3–5 mg/kg <5 yrs; 2–3 mg/kg >5 yrs	2 or 1
Primidone	Generalized convulsive seizures, focal seizures	10–20 mg/kg	2
Diazepam[6]	All forms, mainly status epilepticus and febrile seizures	0.25–1.5 mg/kg; i.v. 0.1–0.3 mg/kg; rectally 0.5–1 mg/kg	
Nitrazepam	Infantile spasms, myoclonic epilepsies	0.25–1.0 mg/kg	2
Lorazepam[6]	Status epilepticus	0.05 mg/kg i.m. or i.v.	
Midazolam[6]	Status epilepticus	0.1–0.2 mg/kg i.m.	
Acetazolamide	Absence seizures, grand mal and partial seizures	10 mg/kg 0–1 yr; 20–30 mg/kg 1–15 yrs	2
ACTH	Infantile spasms, Lennox–Gastaut syndrome, severe myoclonic epilepsy, resistant partial epilepsy	0.1–10 IU/kg	
Corticosteroids	Infantile spasms, Lennox–Gastaut syndrome, severe myoclonic epilepsy, resistant partial epilepsy; Landau–Kleffner syndrome and CSWSS	2 mg/kg (prednisolone); 10–15 mg/kg (hydrocortisone)	

*Oral administration unless otherwise noted (i.v. = intravenously, i.m. = intramusculary).
[1]Slow release preparation available.
[2]May aggravate myoclonic and absence seizures.
[3]Progressive increase in dose especially important.
[4]Oral, liquid and i.v. preparations available.
[5]For refractory cases only.
[6]For acute treatment of status.

data in Table 15.15. In addition to first-line drugs, favourable results are occasionally obtained with such agents as clorazepate (Naidu et al. 1986, Fujii et al. 1987), bromides (Steinhof and Kruse 1992) and sulthiame (Lerman and Lerman-Sagie 1995, Ben-Zeev et al. 2004), as well as with other 'minor' agents (Levy et al. 2002).

A number of wide-spectrum AEDs have been developed during the last 20 years, including lamotrigine, levetiracetam, topiramate, felbamate and zonisamide. Others, such as oxcarbazepine, gabapentine, vigabatrin, pregabalin and tiagabine, are indicated for the control of focal seizures. Controlled data in children are usually lacking, and the drugs are often used out of licence on the basis of data extrapolated from studies in adults.

Unconventional agents such as ACTH and corticosteroids are extremely potent drugs for the treatment not only of infantile spasms but also of other types of resistant epilepsy, especially when cognitive and/or major behavioural disturbances appear. They deserve a full trial (2–4 weeks or more) in such cases.

The *mode of action of AEDs* is beyond the scope of this book (for reviews, see Levy et al. 2002, Wyllie et al. 2006) and still imperfectly known. The main steps in the processing of AEDs are shown in Fig. 15.19. Steps from absorption through entry and

TABLE 15.15
Main pharmacokinetic data on anticonvulsant drugs

Drug	Oral availability (%)	T_{max}* (hr)	% protein bound	Apparent volume of distribution (L/kg)	Elimination half-life (hr)	Route of elimination	Therapeutic range (mg/L)	(mmol/L)	Remarks
Phenobarbitone	80–100	2–10	50	0.51–0.57	37–73[1]	Hepatic metabolism	10–30	45–130	Enzyme inducer
Phenytoin	80–95	4–12	90	0.5–0.7	9–40	Saturable hepatic metabolism	10–20	40–80	Zero order kinetics makes small change of dosage result in wide changes of level; numerous interactions
Carbamazepine	70–80	2–10	60–80	0.8–1.6	8–24[2] 24–46[3]	Hepatic metabolism, active metabolite (10,11 epoxide)	4–12	17–50	Autoinduction common; induction of other drug metabolism; multiple interactions
Primidone	90–100	0.5–4	10–20	0.4–0.8	5–10	Hepatic metabolism, active metabolites (PEMA** + phenobarbitone) 40% excreted unchanged	5–12	25–50	Metabolized to PEMA** and phenobarbitone
Ethosuximide	90–100	1–4	0	0.6–0.9	20–40	Hepatic metabolism, 25% excreted unchanged	40–100	300–750	Not an enzyme inducer
Sodium valproate	100	1–3	90	0.10–0.20	7–15	Hepatic metabolism, active metabolites (PEMA** + phenobarbitone) 40% excreted unchanged	50–100	345–690	Not an enzyme inducer; mildly inhibits oxidative metabolism; full pharmacological action may require weeks
Clonazepam	90	1–3	80–90	2.1–4.3	20–30	Hepatic metabolism	Not established		
Clobazam	90	1–3	90	0.7–1.6	10–30	Hepatic metabolism, active metabolites (PEMA** + phenobarbitone) 40% excreted unchanged	Not established		
Diazepam	75	1–2	95	1.1–1.8	10–20	Hepatic metabolism, active metabolites (PEMA** + phenobarbitone) 40% excreted unchanged	0.15–0.25	0.52–0.87	
Vigabatrin	60–80	1–4	0	0.6–0.10	5–7[4]	Excreted largely unchanged	Not established		No drug interaction
Lamotrigine	98	2–3	55	0.9–1.3	12	5% hepatic in enzyme-induced patients, 25% in patients on sodium valproate	Not established		Elimination inhibited by sodium valproate, increased by enzyme inducers
Levetiracetam	>95%	1.3	0	0.5–0.7	5–7	Renal	Not established		No drug interaction
Gabapentin	51–72	2–3	0	0.57	5–7	>90% renal	Not established		No drug interaction
Felbamate	>90	2–6	22–25	0.7–0.8	2–6	90% renal	Not established		Inhibits elimination of valproate, carbamazepine epoxide, phenytoin and phenobarbitone
Topiramate	80	2	13–17	Not known	21	70% renal, 30% metabolized	Not established		Phenytoin, carbamazepine decrease levels by 40%, sodium valproate by 14%

*T_{max} = time to peak plasma level after administration of single dose.
**PEMA = phenylethylmalonamide.
[1]Half-life may exceed 100 hours in the first two weeks of life.
[2]Half-life in patients receiving the dose chronically, when autoinduction has developed, or receiving other inducing agents.
[3]Half-life in patients receiving the drug as monotherapy; before development of induction.
[4]Not significant as the drug binds irreversibly to glutamate-transaminase thus increasing brain GABA level, therefore the important half-life is that or restoration of enzyme level.

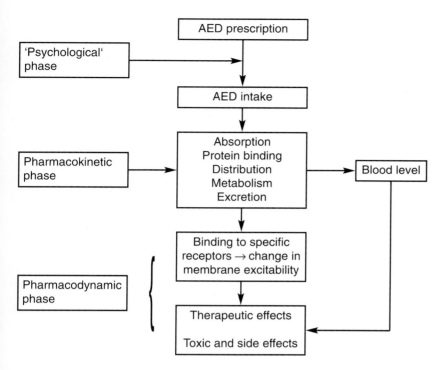

Fig. 15.19. Schematic representation of the successive steps from prescription of antiepileptic drugs (AEDs) to their clinical effects. Note that some toxic or side effects may be due solely to their presence in blood (*e.g.* skin rashes, liver or kidney toxicity, interference with other drugs) while others (*e.g.* drowsiness, ataxia) necessitate, like their therapeutic effect, their presence at brain sites.

distribution into the brain constitute the pharmacokinetics of a drug. Considerable knowledge has accumulated over the past two decades about the pharmacokinetics of AEDs, especially in children (Dodson and Pellock 1993, Kearns et al. 2003, Booth and Evans 2004). Later steps with resulting changes in neuronal excitability constitute the pharmacodynamic phase of drug action. Initial pharmacokinetic steps (from absorption to brain entry) are reflected in the blood levels of a drug. It has been shown that the blood levels of AEDs are more closely related to brain levels than to the dosage ingested, which is the rationale for their determination. However, blood levels are only one link in the chain of processes that take place between ingestion of a drug and its therapeutic and other effects, and their relationship to brain levels and to levels at the receptors are not necessarily close. Such discrepancies are frequent with sodium valproate and can also occur with carbamazepine (Suzuki et al. 1991, Scheyer et al. 1994). Some children handle anticonvulsant drugs in an atypical manner, and in such cases special studies of their metabolism may be indicated (Gilman et al. 1994).

PRACTICAL INDICATIONS AND MODALITIES
Instigation of treatment
Instigation of an antiepileptic treatment is a serious decision that requires a firm diagnosis of epilepsy. Consequently, drug therapy should not be initiated for children with paroxysmal events of uncertain origin (Arzimanoglou et al. 2004), for those with a

single seizure (unless it is of a type observed only in chronic epilepsies) or for those with epileptic EEG abnormalities without clear-cut clinical manifestations (Hirtz et al. 2000, Arts et al. 2004, Beghi 2007). Likewise, preventive drug treatment for patients with potentially epileptogenic brain lesions is of unproven value and is best avoided as it may result in years of useless drug therapy (Shinnar and Berg 1996).

The problem posed by children with paroxysmal EEG discharges associated with clinical nonparoxysmal manifestations such as behavioural or cognitive difficulties is delicate. There exist arguments to support a role for EEG paroxysms in such cases (Nicolai et al. 2006), especially when they are intense and prolonged. Treatment is clearly indicated for some syndromes of severe deterioration such as CSWSS or the Landau–Kleffner syndrome, even though there is only anecdotal evidence of efficacy. In fact, these syndromes are often resistant to conventional treatment, and the response to any form of therapy is very difficult to assess. Most clinicians are not inclined to treat children with learning difficulties or attention deficit solely because of EEG anomalies. In fact, treatment decisions need to be evaluated on an individual basis and preferably by a child neurologist with experience in childhood epilepsies.

Children who have had two or more seizures or those with a first seizure predictably announcing chronic epilepsy are candidates for drug treatment. Some investigators, however, tend to withhold treatment for patients with infrequent seizures that are

TABLE 15.16
Epilepsy syndromes and choice of antiepileptic drugs*

Idiopathic generalized epilepsies

Childhood absence epilepsy
First choice: sodium valproate, ethosuximide
Second choice: association with lamotrigine

Juvenile absence epilepsy
First choice: sodium valproate, lamotrigine
Second choice: association with lamotrigine or topiramate or levetiracetam

Juvenile myoclonic epilepsy
First choice: sodium valproate, levetiracetam
Second choice: association with lamotrigine or topiramate or levetiracetam

Remark: Avoid treatment with oxcarbazepine or carbamazepine

Idiopathic partial epilepsies
First choice: abstinence if possible (depending on age, frequency and duration of seizures)
Second choice: benzodiazepines, preferably clobazam
Third choice: sodium valproate or gabapentin or sulthiame
Remark: Aggravation has been reported in cases of rolandic epilepsy and related syndromes (Landau–Kleffner; CSWSS) when using carbamazepine or oxcarbazepine. However, this is not a constant feature and these drugs are frequently used, particularly in occipital idiopathic epilepsies (Panayiotopoulos and Gastaut types)

Symptomatic partial epilepsies
First choice: lamotrigine, gabapentin, sodium valproate, oxcarbazepine, carbamazepine, levetiracetam
Second choice: topiramate
Third choice: association of two AEDs
Remark: All AEDs, with the exception of ethosuximide, are indicated for the treatment of focal seizures. Choice depends on tolerance, experience of the treating physician and local legal authorization issues

Epileptic encephalopathies

Infantile spasms and West syndrome
First choice: vigabatrin
Second choice: ACTH or hydrocortisone
Third choice: Benzodiazepines (nitrazepam), sodium valproate ↗

Dravet syndrome
First choice: sodium valproate
Second choice: association of sodium valproate, clobazam and stiripentol
Third choice: topiramate usually in association with one or two of the above
Remark: Avoid treatment with lamotrigine, phenobarbitone or carbamazepine, particularly at the early stages of the disorder

Epilepsies with myoclonic–astatic seizures (Doose and related syndromes)
First choice: sodium valproate
Second choice: association of sodium valproate and lamotrigine, particularly if tonic–clonic seizures predominate, or association of sodium valproate and levetiracetam or ethosuximide when myoclonic or astatic seizures predominate
Third choice: topiramate
Remark: Avoid treatment with oxcarbazepine or carbamazepine

Lennox–Gastaut syndrome
First choice: sodium valproate
Second choice: association of sodium valproate and lamotrigine or lamotrigine and topiramate
Third choice: Association of clobazam; association of felbamate
Remark: Avoid the association of more than three AEDs; steroids may be useful to tide-up during periods of aggravation

Syndrome of continuous spike–wave during slow sleep (CSWSS) and related disorders
First choice: benzodiazepines, particularly clobazam, or sulthiame
Second choice: association of benzodiazepines and ethosuximide or sodium valproate
Third choice: Prednisone or hydrocortisone
Remark: Avoid carbamazepine and oxcarbazepine

*Lack of controlled studies for the use of AEDs in children often obliges one to off-licence drug use. The table summarizes the experience of the authors without necessarily taking into account local legal authorizations for the use of AEDs.

---

of limited expression and/or occur at socially 'convenient' times. The decision to start treatment depends heavily on the patient's and parents' lifestyle and preferences when seizures are relatively rare (Beghi 2007).

Choice of drug(s)
The choice of drug(s) depends, in the first place, on the epilepsy syndrome, or at least on the type of seizure experienced by the patient (Arzimanoglou 2002). Table 15.16 indicates the order of preference for the usual AEDs in the most frequent types of childhood epilepsy. Any choice is of necessity arbitrary, in part because neither the efficacy nor the unwanted effects of any drug are entirely predictable (Arzimanoglou et al. 2004). Selection of the first drug often depends critically on the toxicity, side effects and specific handling of any particular drug, because the effectiveness of several different drugs is often comparable. This does not apply to absence attacks and many myoclonic seizures for which mostly sodium valproate, ethosuximide, levetiracetam and the benzodiazepines are active. Comparative studies both in adults (Mattson et al. 1992, Richens et al. 1994) and in children

(Verity et al. 1995, de Silva et al. 1996) have failed to show significant differences in the efficacy of conventional drugs (phenobarbitone, phenytoin, carbamazepine, sodium valproate) used as monotherapy for partial or generalized convulsive seizures. These results do not exclude the possibility of some agents being more effective than others in subsets of patients or in individual cases.

There is evidence that some agents work better in generalized forms of epilepsy or have a wide spectrum of activity for the control of both focal and generalized seizures (sodium valproate, lamotrigine, levetiracetam, topiramate, zonisamide) while others are more indicated for focal seizures (carbamazepine, gabapentine, oxcarbazepine, vigabatrin). There is also evidence that some agents may aggravate rather than improve some forms of epilepsy (e.g. carbamazepine for idiopathic generalized epilepsies or syndromes with predominantly myoclonic seizures or typical absences, lamotrigine in some cases of Dravet syndrome). However, while this applies for the initial choice of drugs, in resistant cases with tonic–clonic seizures applying too strict rules may be counterproductive.

In many instances the likelihood of side effects will be a critical factor in the selection of a drug. Major side effects are rare (see below), but even relatively mild side effects should be taken into account as their impact on everyday life may be considerable. Thus, given the choice between carbamazepine, phenobarbitone and phenytoin, the first agent will be preferred because it is much easier to handle than phenytoin and it does not produce the behavioural disturbances or effects on cognition attributed to phenobarbitone, or the 'minor' side effects such as gingival hyperplasia and hirsutism that are so common with phenytoin. Such side effects may indeed be of consequence by making physically obvious the difference that mythically separates patients with epilepsy from other children. New generation AEDs have shown a clearly better short- and long-term tolerability than older antiepileptic agents and should be preferred as a first choice.

Monotherapy versus polytherapy

Giving only one drug is associated with fewer and less confusing side effects than polypharmacy and avoids the problem of drug interactions. Therefore, treatment should almost always be started with a single agent. Seventy to 90 per cent of newly diagnosed, common forms of epilepsy can be controlled with monotherapy (Forsythe and Sills 1984, Brodie 1990).

Drug combinations should be used only after single drugs in correct dosages have failed for a period long enough to make an adequate assessment. In case of failure of a drug, progressive substitution by other agents should precede the use of combined therapy. The value of adding a second drug is uncertain. Approximately 10–15% of patients so treated have improved seizure control, but a few patients may deteriorate and there is a tendency to increasing side effects.

Combinations of more than two drugs are rarely indicated (Aicardi and Shorvon 1998). No consensus exists on the number of monotherapy trials that should be attempted before combination therapy is introduced. The authors believe that at least two appropriate AEDs at the maximally tolerated dose must be tried. Evidence from open clinical trials in adolescents and adults (Kwan and Brodie 2000b, 2001) has shown that full control of seizures is only rarely obtained from a third drug when the first two have failed. This probably applies to children as well. However, the occurrence of two types of seizures in the same patient (e.g. Lennox–Gastaut syndrome or Dravet syndrome) that require different therapy (Aird et al. 1984, Perucca and Levy 2002) sometimes justifies the early introduction of combination therapy. Even in such cases, however, the use of some modern drugs with a large spectrum of action (e.g. valproate, lamotrigine, levetiracetam, topiramate) may obviate the need for polytherapy (Arzimanoglou 2002).

MODE OF ADMINISTRATION

In principle, the use of more than two doses per day is to be avoided except in cases of very resistant epilepsy treated with drugs of short half-life. Some drugs, e.g. phenobarbitone, vigabatrin or lamotrigine, may be given in a single evening dose. Sodium valproate can also be used as a single dose in adolescents, which

improves the compliance and seems to be effective for the control of primary generalized epilepsies (Covanis and Jeavons 1980).

A gradual increase or decrease in dosage on initiation or withdrawal of any drug is an essential rule. The first or successive drug should be introduced at low dosage and increased gradually until control is obtained or the limit of tolerance reached. This is especially important with lamotrigine as the frequency of rashes is higher with rapid introduction. Slow withdrawal is also important for barbiturates, vigabatrin and felbamate, whose discontinuation may induce status epilepticus when a first drug has failed. However, in the common epilepsies of childhood, withdrawal over 4–8 weeks did not seem to be associated with a higher recurrence rate (Dooley et al. 1996).

When a first drug has failed and another drug is being introduced, the first agent should be withdrawn progressively. It should be remembered that achievement of a stable drug level requires approximately four times the plasma half-life. The time to reach stable levels may be much longer as the dose is usually gradually increased and as phenomena of induction progressively modify (usually shorten) the apparent half-life of drugs.

Monitoring of anticonvulsant drug therapy

Regular clinical supervision is the only essential measure. Special attention should be given to the search for side effects such as diplopia or vertigo that some patients come to consider as normal phenomena. Digestive disturbances, drowsiness or language expression disturbances should also be considered carefully. However, most of these adverse events are transitory and early discontinuation of a drug can be avoided in most cases, provided that the patient is informed beforehand and titration is slow.

Monitoring of blood cell counts is probably useless with regular drugs except for defensive purposes (Camfield et al. 1986), and the same applies to tests of hepatic function as moderate leukopenia and elevation of transaminases are common and do not herald the appearance of hepatic failure or pancytopenia.

In evaluating the efficacy of any drug regimen, clinical judgement based on seizure recurrences is fundamental. It is relatively easy in patients with frequent, regularly repeated seizures (e.g. in absence epilepsy) but it becomes long and difficult in patients with rare seizures or in those whose seizures occur irregularly or in clusters, and may require several months or more. This difficulty must not lead one to forget that the end-point of treatment is the control of seizures, not a normal EEG or a 'therapeutic' blood level.

Monitoring the blood levels of AEDs is not routinely indicated. It is useless in children with epilepsies that are well controlled on regular or low-dosage monotherapy. Many patients are seizure-free with blood levels well below the published ranges, and modification of dosage to obtain 'therapeutic' levels is ineffective (Woo et al. 1988) and increases the risk of side effects. Likewise, discontinuation of a drug because its level is 'subtherapeutic' can result in seizure relapse (Richens 1982). Conversely, in resistant cases, the dose should be pushed to the limit of clinical tolerance, regardless of blood levels.

Blood level determinations are useful to check patients' compliance; to confirm suspected toxicity in infants or in children with mental retardation, in whom diagnosis may be difficult; and to detect blood interactions in patients on polypharmacy. They are also indicated for patients on phenytoin therapy as the therapeutic ratio (i.e. the margin of safety) of this drug is low and, especially, in uncontrolled cases and in the case of 'breakthrough' seizures in previously well-controlled children (Aicardi 1994). Blood levels are useless with some drugs (vigabatrin, levetiracetam) and of dubious value with others, e.g. sodium valproate, whose levels are poorly correlated to clinical effects.

Interpretation of blood levels is not always straightforward, especially in cases of drug interactions (Levy et al. 2002); for drugs whose binding to protein may vary with resultant change in levels of free, unbound, drug; and for those that have active metabolites, such as carbamazepine, as the rate of formation of the metabolite is not constant and the blood level not measured routinely.

Unwanted effects of antiepileptic drugs

Side effects of antiepileptic drugs are common (Table 15.17) and extensive reviews are available (Levy et al. 2002, Kothare and Kaleyias 2007). The most common side effects are transient and occur at the beginning of treatment. These include mainly digestive disturbances, drowsiness and dizziness. All antiepileptic agents may – albeit rarely – produce side effects that seriously hamper the patient's activities. These side effects range from acute intoxication with disturbances of consciousness (Larrieu et al. 1985; Zaret and Cohen 1986; Weaver et al. 1988; Meador 1994, 2001; Martin et al. 1999) or, exceptionally, death (Stone and Lange 1986, Murphy et al. 1987, Leestma et al. 1997) to subtle chronic toxicity with protean manifestations (McLeod et al. 1978, Dravet et al. 1980, Joyce and Gunderson 1980, Karas et al. 1982, McLachlan 1987, Pellock 1987, Appleton et al. 1990, Weig and Pollack 1993, Gerber et al. 2000), and to apparently minor but sometimes psychologically and socially disabling effects such as acne, excessive weight gain (Egger and Brett 1981, Dinesen et al. 1984, DeToledo et al. 1997), or weight loss (Potter et al. 1997). Allergic or idiosyncratic reactions are also common, and these may rarely be responsible for fatalities (Gilhus and Matte 1986, Browne et al. 1988, Kaufman et al. 1997, Schlienger et al. 1998, Fernández-Calvo et al. 2000). Based on the underlying mechanisms, idiosyncratic reactions can be differentiated thus: (1) immune-mediated hypersensitivity reactions, which may range from benign skin rashes to serious conditions such as drug-related rash with eosinophilia and systemic symptoms; (2) reactions involving unusual nonimmune-mediated individual susceptibility, often related to abnormal production or defective detoxification of reactive cytotoxic metabolites (as in valproate-induced liver toxicity); and (3) off-target pharmacology, whereby a drug interacts directly with a system other than that for which it is intended, an example being some types of AED-induced dyskinesias. Although no AED is free from the potential of inducing idiosyncratic reactions, the magnitude of risk and the most common manifestations vary from one drug to another, a

consideration that impacts on treatment choices (Zaccara et al. 2007).

The cognitive effects of anticonvulsants (Aldenkamp et al. 1993; Meador 1994, 2001; Aldenkamp 2001) are particularly worrying, and no drug appears to be completely exempt from unfavourable cognitive or behavioural effects, even though these may be more marked with some agents (e.g. phenobarbitone, topiramate) than with others (e.g. sodium valproate, carbamazepine, lamotrigine or gabapentin). The relative effects of the newer AEDs have yet to be fully determined. No cognitive effects were found with lamotrigine in one study (Smith et al. 1993), and several studies using quality-of-life measures reported a beneficial effect of lamotrigine on patient perception of psychological well-being (Smith et al. 1993, Brodie et al. 1995). In 25 healthy adults participating in a double-blind randomized crossover design study, lamotrigine produced significantly fewer cognitive and behavioural effects than did carbamazepine (Meador 2001). Psychomotor slowing, language problems and difficulty with memory are reported with topiramate (Martin et al. 1999, Bootsma et al. 2006). The word-finding difficulty seen in both children and adults is unique to topiramate (Meador 2001).

Finally, the possibility of teratogenicity when treatment is prolonged to the reproductive age must be taken into account when long-term treatment is being prescribed to female adolescents (Morrell 2002, Tettenborn et al. 2002). The older AEDs (benzodiazepines, phenytoin, phenobarbitone, carbamazepine and valproate) are associated with a risk of major fetal malformations, including cleft lip and palate and cardiac defects. The incidence of these major malformations in infants born to mothers taking AEDs is 4–6%, compared with 2–4% for the general population. Neural tube defects occur in 1–2% of infants exposed to valproate and in 0.5–1% of those exposed to carbamazepine (Rosa 1991, Omtzigt et al. 1992). The UK Epilepsy and Pregnancy Register (Morrow et al. 2006) showed that only 4.2% of live births to women with epilepsy had a major congenital malformation (MCM). The MCM rate for polytherapy exposure was greater than for monotherapy exposure. Polytherapy regimens containing valproate had significantly more MCMs than those not containing valproate. For monotherapy exposures, carbamazepine was associated with the lowest risk of MCM (Morrow et al. 2006).

All authors agree that the risks of malformations are highest in those fetuses exposed to multiple AEDs and in those exposed to higher doses. Little information regarding effects of newer AEDS on the developing human fetus is yet available. For some, substantial data are accumulating (Tennis et al. 2002, Hunt et al. 2006), but more than 2000 prospective pregnancies are needed to detect a drug effect that occurs in 4–8% of exposed fetuses (Morrell 2002). The teratogenic potential of AEDs will be better defined when the results of the currently ongoing global prospective registries become available (Beghi et al. 2001, EURAP Study Group 2006, Vajda et al. 2006, Cunnington et al. 2007). The majority of patients with epilepsy maintain seizure control during pregnancy.

Clinicians following adolescent girls for their epilepsy must

TABLE 15.17
Main side effects and toxicity of anticonvulsant drugs*

Drug	Side effects	Severe toxicity
Phenobarbitone	*Drowsiness* *Aggression* *Sleep disturbances* *Hyperactivity* Osteomalacia Rashes	Aplastic anaemia Stevens–Johnson syndrome Rheumatism
Phenytoin	*Ataxia* Anorexia Nausea Acne *Nystagmus* *Gum hypertrophy* *Hirsutism* Megaloblastic anaemia Osteomalacia Reduced IgA Depression Neuropathy	Orofacial dyskinesia Anaemia *Lupus-like syndrome* Pseudolymphoma Stevens–Johnson syndrome Hepatitis Encephalopathy
Primidone	*Drowsiness* Dizziness Nausea Vomiting *Personality change* Diplopia Ataxia Rashes	Agranulocytosis Lupus-like syndrome Thrombocytopenia
Carbamazepine	*Diplopia* *Dizziness* *Ataxia* Nausea Hyponatraemia Rashes (5–10%)	Orofacial dyskinesia Cardiac arrhythmia Hepatotoxicity Lupus-like syndrome Pseudolymphoma

Sodium valproate	*Anorexia*
	Nausea
	Vomiting
	Hair loss
	Weight gain
	Tremor
	Drowsiness
	Thrombocytopenia
	Hyperammonaemia
	  (usually mild)
		Hepatotoxicity
		  (especially in children
		  with mental retardation
		  <3 yrs of age who may
		  have underlying disorder)[1]
		Pancreatitis
		Stupor, encephalopathy

Lamotrigine	Drowsiness Behavioural changes *Rashes*	*Stevens–Johnson syndrome*

Drug	Side effects	Severe toxicity
Ethosuximide	Anorexia Nausea *Vomiting* Drowsiness *Headache* Hiccups Rashes	*Lupus-like syndrome* Aplastic anaemia Psychosis
Clonazepam/ clobazam	*Fatigue* *Ataxia* *Hyperkinetic* *syndrome* *Aggression* *Drowsiness* *Hypersalivation*[2] *Bronchorrhoea*[2] *Muscle weakness*	Psychosis Thrombocytopenia
Vigabatrin	Drowsiness Hyperactivity Aggression Weight gain	Psychosis Depression
Gabapentin	Headache Dizziness	None
Felbamate	Drowsiness Nausea	Aplastic anaemia Hepatic failure (can be lethal)
Topiramate	Loss of appetite Weight loss Slurring of speech Difficulty concentrating	None
Levetiracetam	Transient somnolence Nervousness Behavioural changes	None
Zonisamide	Somnolence Dizziness Anorexia	Nephrolithiasis (rare) Rash (rare)

*Features in *italics* are frequent or clinically important.

[1]Metabolic diseases can be revealed by administration of sodium valproate (Coulter 1991).

[2]These complications may be responsible for severe aspiration and even sudden death (Murphy et al. 1987) in infants and children with mental retardation. This may be due to cricopharyngeal muscle incoordination, which has also been reported with nitrazepam (Wyllie et al. 1986).

be aware that the malformations associated with AEDs are all generated in the first trimester of pregnancy and that neural tube defects are formed by day 28 after conception. Pre-conception counselling is thus essential. Modifications of the ongoing treatment should take place before conception to allow optimal therapy with the lowest possible dose, preferably of monotherapy. The type(s) of seizures must be taken into account. For example, if generalized tonic–clonic seizures in a patient with juvenile myoclonic epilepsy are well controlled with an average dose of lamotrigine but some myoclonic jerks persist, not adding any other medication, at least until the end of the first trimester, might be preferable.

In some cases, AEDs may produce a paradoxical increase in seizure frequency (Guerrini et al. 1998a, 2002c; Perucca et al. 1998). Carbamazepine is contraindicated in patients with absence epilepsy and juvenile myoclonic epilepsy (Shorvon et al. 1978, Callahan and Noetzel 1992), but in some cases its use might be necessary for the control of tonic–clonic seizures resistant to other available drugs. It should also be used with caution in patients with a mixed seizure disorder, particularly in those with a combination of atonic, tonic–clonic, myoclonic and atypical absence seizures and generalized bilateral EEG discharges (Perucca et al. 1998). Vigabatrin or gabapentin may be responsible for an increase in the frequency of typical absences and/or myoclonias. An aggravating effect has been reported when lamotrigine is administered in young children with Dravet syndrome (Guerrini et al. 1998b). The aggravation of absence or myoclonic seizures with the use of phenytoin has also been reported, but the overall number of cases is lower than that recorded with carbamazepine.

In view of the problems associated with chronic treatment with AEDs (Oxley et al. 1983, Herranz et al. 1988, Schmidt 1989, Aldenkamp et al. 1993, American Academy of Pediatrics Committee on Drugs 1995), much depends on the intelligent cooperation of the patient and his or her family and on their understanding of the problems posed by the disorder. Therefore, the nature of the problem should be explained in simple terms, and the necessity for prolonged supervision should be made clear. Treatment is a reasonable compromise between benefits and toxicity (i.e. between control of seizures and side effects), and that essential aspect should be understood by families.

It is important to warn parents at the outset of initiating anticonvulsant medication that modifying the dosage to find the best dose for the individual child is often necessary and that trying a different or additional medication if the first drug fails to control seizures is also not uncommon. This may help parents to accept later changes with less anxiety and fewer doubts about the competence of their physician than if they are not warned from the beginning.

NON-DRUG MEDICAL TREATMENTS
KETOGENIC DIET
The ketogenic diet has long been in use for the treatment of children with severe epilepsies (Freeman et al. 2007). Although the mechanism of action of the diet is obscure, a high concentration of ketone bodies in the blood is necessary for its effectiveness. Various types of ketogenic diets are available, using either medium-chain triglycerides or conventional 4:1 or 3:1 diet. Although the diet is unpalatable, its taste and appearance can be made acceptable (Freeman et al. 1994). Side effects include diarrhoea, growth failure and, in some children, renal stones and severe episodes of acidosis. These may be life threatening, and fatalities have occurred, especially when acetazolamide was used concomitantly with the diet (Prasad et al. 1996), so this drug should be discontinued two weeks before starting the diet. Elevated levels of cholesterol have occasionally been observed in treated children, and the long-term effects of the drug are as yet poorly documented. The short-term beneficial effect of the diet is indisputable for several types of seizures including myoclonic seizures (Caraballo et al. 2006), the Lennox–Gastaut syndrome (Schwartz et al. 1989a,b) and some cases of resistant partial or generalized seizures (Kossoff et al. 2006). Kinsman et al. (1992) were able to control the seizures completely in 17 of 58 children (29%) and obtained a 50% decrease of frequency in a further 22 (38%). Improvement in awareness may be an additional benefit. The diet has been maintained for two years or more in some childen, and the effect is said to persist after discontinuation in patients treated for a year or more. However, the drop-out rate is high, and in some children the effect of the diet is only transient. Long-term

studies are in progress; it now appears that a trial of ketogenic diet is reasonable for at least some refractory epilepsies. Education of parents is all-important and a team approach is essential for optimal results (Kossoff et al. 2007). However, trials have been uncontrolled so the evidence is largely anecdotal and assessment of risks and benefits requires further study.

SURGICAL TREATMENT OF EPILEPSY
Although approximately 70% of patients respond satisfactorily to drugs, resistant cases especially in children are not rare. A sizeable number of these can potentially be controlled by surgical treatment, as shown by experience in adults. Paediatric surgical data are also encouraging and no different from the adult surgical outcome data (Lindsay et al. 1979, Gilliam et al. 1997, Wylliet et al. 1998, Mathern et al. 1999, Bittar et al. 2002, Schmidt et al. 2004). Successful surgical therapy would appear particularly desirable for children and deserves to be considered more liberally and earlier than is now customary (Engel 1996, Arzimanoglou et al. 2004, Cross et al. 2006). It would constitute a definitive treatment, not only preventing the possible harmful consequences on the brain of repeated seizures and the psychosocial problems resulting from interference of epilepsy with everyday life and education, but also by permitting the use of smaller dosages for AEDs or even their discontinuation (Aicardi 1997). In spite of these potential advantages, the utilization of epilepsy surgery in children is yet to realize its full potential (Lachhwani 2005). Although epilepsy surgery programmes have been launched in most major paediatric centres, the interval between onset of the disease and surgery is still extremely long, often more than 15 or 20 years. Unfortunately, such delays remain true even for well-defined epilepsy syndromes such as mesio-temporal epilepsy (Berg et al. 2003). In one randomized controlled trial, Wiebe et al. (2001) compared surgical versus medical treatment for temporal lobe epilepsy in adults, showing that seizure control and quality of life were significantly better with surgery than with medical treatment.

The most obvious and probably still strongest arguments against surgery are cultural and psychological. Information on surgical possibilities is poorly diffused among general practitioners and even neurologists and child neurologists. Lack of knowledge, concern or outright fear regarding surgery may contribute to the delay. The roller-coaster course that some forms of epilepsy appear to take with remission followed by intractability followed by remission and so forth may also make it difficult to know when a patient's condition is truly intractable and has vanishingly small to no hope of ever achieving seizure control with medication (Berg et al. 2006). Additional factors are the poorly known natural history of many childhood epilepsies, varied aetiologies, and the fact that the few available reports often discuss together both lesional and MRI-negative focal epilepsies, epilepsies with multiple lesions or diffuse EEG abnormalities, and rare epileptic encephalopathies. At least for focal epilepsies, there may often be a prolonged period over which the natural history of the disorder evolves, and it may not follow a linear path. Finally, as a field, we need to work on meaningful approaches to recognizing intractable epilepsy and identifying those at highest risk as soon as possible (Berg et al. 2003).

The development of several new and very useful AEDs during the last two decades was inevitably an additional factor that increased delays to presurgical evaluation. Finally, specialized centres are still rare, so access to specialized advice may be difficult to obtain early in the course of the disorder.

In recent years, an increasing bulk of available knowledge provides strong arguments in favour of the view that surgery for epilepsy is a realistic early therapeutic option for an increasing number of children. It is now realized that procrastination in the hope that several drug trials may permit full control of epilepsy is not justified. There is mounting evidence, both in adults (Kwan and Brodie 2000a) and in children (Camfield et al. 1997, Berg et al. 2001, Arts et al. 2004), that drug-resistant epilepsy can be predicted successfully after the failure of only one or two well-chosen antiepileptic drugs. The presence of a lesion, especially hippocampal sclerosis, a dysplastic lesion or dual pathology, is an additional prognostic factor suggesting resistance to drugs (Semah et al. 1998). Consequently, multiple AED trials in children who are favourable surgical candidates are likely to be futile (Lachhwani 2005). Every new drug regimen not only delays a definitive surgical procedure but also continues to expose the young patient to a significant risk of morbidity (and mortality) from ongoing seizures, not to mention direct detrimental effects on cognitive development (Vasconcellos et al. 2001, Nolan et al. 2003, Aldenkamp et al. 2005, Laurent and Arzimanoglou 2006) and long-term adverse effects of AEDs (see above).

Another major step that facilitated early access to surgery has resulted from the development of new and powerful neuroimaging techniques (MRI, PET, SPECT, fMRI, MEG) that nowadays permit precise definition of the type and operability of epileptogenic lesions. Futher development of video–EEG techniques as well as of depth electrodes by multidisciplinary groups, and of neurosurgical tools and techniques, also contributed to the current change of views regarding epilepsy surgery in children. This better capacity to identify localized lesions or neurophysiological anomalies has also led to the revision of some traditional concepts. It is becoming increasingly clear that epilepsies formerly considered generalized may indeed be due to localized, if more or less extensive, lesions, some of which may be amenable to surgery (Aicardi 1997). This applies, for example, to many cases of infantile spasms and possibly to other syndromes with diffuse or multifocal features (Madhavan et al. 2007). Epilepsy surgery may be successful for selected children and adolescents with a congenital or early-acquired brain lesion, despite abundant generalized or bilateral epileptiform discharges on EEG (Wyllie et al. 2007).

Indications, contraindications and types of available surgical treatment

Most surgical techniques are intended to remove the epileptogenic tissue that is responsible for initiation and spread of the seizure discharge. Criteria for surgical removal of epileptogenic tissue include refractoriness of seizures, a severity sufficient to interfere with everyday life, signs of cognitive deterioration related to active epilepsy, clinical and other evidence pointing to a localized brain area, and the possibility of removing such an area without producing unacceptable functional sequelae.

Several operations are available for the treatment of epilepsy, and these can be schematically grouped into two major categories: (1) resective surgery, in which the object is to remove the cortical neuronal pool that is responsible for generation of the seizures, thereby obtaining full seizure control; and (2) palliative or functional surgery, which aims not at complete seizure control but rather to interrupt or limit the propagation of the seizure discharges, thus limiting their clinical manifestations and consequences.

Resective surgery can range from small cortical resections to hemispherectomy. Palliative surgery (Polkey 2003a) is mostly represented by *callosotomy*, whether of the anterior half or two thirds of this structure or complete. Other palliative techniques include *vagus nerve stimulation*, which requires placement of a stimulator under the skin. In this technique, an electrode is wrapped around the left vagus nerve, so that adjustable pulsed stimuli can be applied. In children, the results are encouraging with reduced seizure frequency, particularly in the epileptic encephalopathies (Polkey 2003a,b; Alexopoulos et al. 2006; Benifla et al. 2006). The role of *gamma-knife radiosurgery* in the treatment of cortical–subcortical cavernous angiomas and hypothalamic hamartomas is undergoing evaluation (Régis et al. 2007). Another technique that is still experimental, almost exclusively in adult patients, is *deep brain stimulation* (Chabardes et al. 2002, Benabid et al. 2003), the results of which are still too recent to draw conclusions.

The majority of candidates for epilepsy surgery, in both children and adults, belong to the syndromic category of focal non-idiopathic epilepsies (Hirsch and Arzimanoglou 2004, Kahane et al. 2005). The requirements for resective surgery in children with partial epilepsy vary with the type of resection considered. Three basic requirements apply to almost all cases: (a) the epileptogenic area must be localized to a territory whose removal is contemplated; (b) no other *independent* epileptogenic area exists in those areas that are not included in the planned resection, and (c) any possible deficit resulting from resection must be acceptable (Arzimanoglou et al. 2004). Current experience confirms that complete resection of the epileptogenic area is the major condition for a satisfactory surgical result. The possibilities for resective surgery depend upon the location of the ictal onset zone, its relationship with adjacent functional brain areas and the availability of convergent data that point to a single location. Epilepsy surgery mandates a multidisciplinary approach that requires special skills and often sophisticated instruments and materials that cannot be improvised. A global evaluation of risks and expected benefits is always required. All decisions require close collaboration between the epilepsy team, the patient and the family. With the exception of high-quality MRI and video–EEG recording of seizures, the need to perform any other complementary presurgical investigation should be evaluated on an individual basis (Engel 1993, 1996; Tuxhorn et al. 1997; Lüders and Comair 2001).

Particularly in children, the clinical expression of epilepsy may sometimes be misleading, as paroxysmal events may present as generalized seizures despite having a focal onset. The spectrum of surgical possibilities for early-onset epilepsy has tended to widen rapidly and to include not only other focal epilepsies but also more difficult types. This is because developmental lesions that are the major cause of infantile epilepsy are often poorly localized, involve extensive brain areas and require extensive operations (e.g. hemispherotomy). Surgery is also used for progressive conditions such as Rasmussen's encephalitis (Bien et al. 2005), Sturge–Weber syndrome (Arzimanoglou et al. 2000, Bourgeois et al. 2007) or tuberous sclerosis (Jansen et al. 2007).

Presurgical evaluation of children
Presurgical evaluation has the same bases in children as it does in adults. Detailed consideration of the existing methods is beyond the scope of this book, and the reader is referred to the extensive literature available (e.g. Lüders and Comair 2001, Kahane et al. 2005). The presurgical assessment of a patient is a stepwise process. Detailed history taking and precise definition of the clinical seizure pattern (in terms of both symptoms and sequence of events) are indispensable. The importance of the EEG has been repeatedly emphasized. In some lesional cases interictal EEG and high-quality structural neuroimaging may prove sufficient to suggest the region to be resected. In a number of other cases, both lesional and MRI-negative, combined video–EEG recording is an integral and essential part of the evaluation. Congruence among the results of the clinical history and the definition of seizure pattern, the neuropsychological evaluation and neuroradiology, scalp EEG (interictal and ictal), and, in selected cases, other supporting tests (e.g. ictal or interictal SPECT and PET, functional MRI) has to be sought as any discordance in the results of the various investigation methods considerably decreases the chances of a good outcome. Intracranial EEG recording remains the gold standard for the localization and definition of the extent of the epileptogenic zone, particularly for MRI-negative cases or when the limits of the lesion cannot be clearly identified by structural neuroimaging. The method to be used (grids, strips, stereotactically implanted depth electrodes) depends on the preoperative hypothesis and the experience of the epilepsy surgery team.

All available data must be reviewed and analysed by an experienced multidisciplinary group. Prospective studies are still needed to evaluate the long-term cognitive evolution of children operated on early for their epilepsy.

SOME PROGNOSTIC ASPECTS OF EPILEPSY

The prognosis of seizure disorders varies widely with the epilepsy syndrome, its aetiology and associated manifestations, and with the age of patients. Therefore, studies that do not specify the type of children observed are of limited value. They may be only an indication of the overall fate of children with epilepsy if the referral of patients is not too selective or biased.

However, a brief overview of some prognostic aspects of the epilepsies of children in general (the risk of recurrence after a first seizure; the risk of relapse after discontinuation of drug therapy; the problem of intractable epilepsy; the social and educational outcome of epilepsy; the risk of sudden death in adolescents and young adults) may be of interest as it provides at least some idea of the magnitude of the problems raised by epileptic disorders, particularly those with convulsive seizures, and of the needs of the community with regard to those individuals and their families. Furthermore, studies of the global prognosis of childhood epilepsy have shown that certain factors (e.g. frequency of seizures, presence or absence of neurological or mental deficits, type of seizure, duration of seizures) have a strong correlation with the outcome of epilepsy. Such factors have a predictive value, not only for unclassified cases of epilepsy but also for some cases belonging to well-defined syndromes.

RISK OF RECURRENCE AFTER A FIRST UNPROVOKED SEIZURE

Several studies (Annegers et al. 1986; Boulloche et al. 1989; Shinnar et al. 1990, 1996, 2000; Berg et al. 1998; Haut et al. 2007) give figures for generalized tonic–clonic seizures that vary from 25% to 54%. Most recurrences occur within one year of the first seizure. Such studies suggest that treatment of a first seizure, although effective (First Seizure Trial Group 1993, Beghi 2007), is not indicated as half the children will remain seizure-free. Risk factors for recurrences include an abnormal neurodevelopmental state and, in some studies, a young age (<4 years) at first seizure, a family history of epilepsy, and an abnormal EEG (Shinnar et al. 1994). The recurrence risk in this study was 25% at 24 months with an idiopathic first seizure and a normal EEG, 34% when the EEG was abnormal but nonepileptiform, and 54% with epileptiform abnormalities. An early age of onset (<2 years) is strongly associated with resistant epilepsies. However, this mainly results from the inclusion of cases of epileptic encephalopathies. When these are excluded, the recurrence rate for infants is the same as for older children (Camfield et al. 1993).

These figures apply only to cases of isolated seizures or epilepsies. When neurological signs and/or mental retardation are present, the risk of recurrence is much higher. In a longitudinal study of 246 children, Sillanpää (1993) found that the likelihood of a 5-year terminal remission after 35 years of follow-up was 80% in idiopathic epilepsy, 69% in cryptogenic epilepsy, and only 56% in symptomatic cases. While 77% of patients with normal neurological and intellectual status reached a 5-year terminal remission, the proportion dropped to 50% for patients with mental retardation, to 46% for those with cerebral palsy, and to 29% when both mental retardation and cerebral palsy were present. Even a minor neurological abnormality significantly decreased the probability of a remission. However, Cockerell et al. (1997) in a large population of both children and adults with newly diagnosed epilepsy found a 3-year remission rate of 86% and a 5-year remission rate of 68% after a 9-year follow-up.

In a study aimed at defining the prospects of newly diagnosed childhood epilepsy, assessing the dynamics of its course, identifying relevant variables and developing models to assess the individual prognosis, Arts et al. (2004) evaluated 453 children with newly diagnosed epilepsy followed for 5 years. Terminal remission at 5 years (TR5) was compared with terminal remission at 2 years (TR2) and with the longest remission during follow-up. Variables defined at intake and at 6 months of follow-up were analysed for their prognostic relevance. Three hundred and forty-five children (76%) had a TR5 >1 year, 290 (64%) >2 years and 65 (14%) had not had any seizure during the entire follow-up. Out of 108 children (24%) with TR5 <1 year, 27 actually had intractable seizures at 5 years. Medication was started in 388 children (86%). In 227 of these (59%), AEDs could be withdrawn. A TR5 >1 year was attained by 46% on one AED, by 19% on a combination of two AEDs, and by 9% on all additional AED regimes. Almost 60% of the children treated with a second or additional AED regime had a TR5 >1 year. Variables predicting the outcome at intake were aetiology, history of febrile seizures and age. For intake and 6-month variables combined, sex, aetiology, postictal signs, history of febrile seizures and TR at 6 months were significant. The course of the epilepsy was constantly favourable in 51%, steadily poor in 17%, improving in 25% and deteriorating in 6%. Intractability was, in part, only a temporary phenomenon. The outcome at 5 years in this cohort of children with newly diagnosed epilepsy was favourable in 76%; 64% were off medication at that time. Almost a third of the children had a fluctuating course; improvement was clearly more common than deterioration.

To provide evidence as to whether different patterns of evolution of drug resistance and remission exist, a prospective, long-term population-based study of 144 patients, followed on average for 37.0 years (SD 7.1, median 40.0, range 11–42) since their first seizure before the age of 16 years, was performed by Sillanpää and Schmidt (2006a). Nearly half of the patients with childhood-onset epilepsy entered terminal remission without relapse, and one fifth after relapse. One third had a poor long-term outcome in terms of persistent seizures after remission or without any remission ever.

RISK OF RELAPSE AFTER DISCONTINUATION OF TREATMENT

Several reports have concluded that the risk of relapse is relatively low in children who remain seizure-free for two or three years on therapy (Bouma et al. 1987, Arts et al. 1988, Ehrhardt and Forsythe 1989, Aldenkamp et al. 1993, Shinnar et al. 1994). Figures varied between 12% and 42%, again suggesting that discontinuation of therapy after two years is probably possible in many common types of epilepsy. Dooley et al. (1996) found that the recurrence rate was no higher with discontinuation of treatment one year after the last seizure than after two years, and Tennison et al. (1994) found no difference in recurrence rate between a 6-week and a 9-month weaning period. Similar results were obtained in a prospective study by the Medical Research Council (1991).

The long-term outcome with respect to seizure relapse after planned discontinuation of AEDs in seizure-free patients was evaluated in the longitudinal population-based study of 148 patients from the onset of their epilepsy to an average follow-up of 37 years (Sillanpää and Schmidt 2006b). During the study, AEDs were completely discontinued in 90 patients. Seizure relapse after AED discontinuation was observed in 33 (37%) of these patients at an average follow-up of 32 years. Among 8 of the 33 patients who elected to restart AEDs, two achieved 5-year terminal remission, but only 10–19 years after restarting treatment. The other 6 patients never achieved this long remission, and 2 of the 6 never entered a 5-year remission period during follow-up. Factors associated with failure to reach remission were symptomatic aetiology and localization-related epilepsy.

INTRACTABLE EPILEPSY

Intractable epilepsy is usually defined as epilepsy with seizures that have remained uncontrolled, despite 'relevant' therapy (Juul-Jensen 1968). This definition is highly imprecise because what constitutes adequate therapy is variably appreciated, and the level of control of epilepsy and the appreciation of impact of eventual side effects are individual and depend on the way of the life of the patient and his/her own judgement. Some cases are indeed inadequately treated rather than intractable epilepsies for medical or patient-related reasons, and it is therefore essential to look for factors associated with apparent intractibility such as unrecognized progressive causal disease, precipitating factors and treatment irregularities. Misdiagnosis of the type of epilepsy resulting in the use of an inappropriate drug – e.g. ethosuximide for focal seizures, carbamazepine for myoclonic seizures – or failure to recognize that the patient's seizures are not epileptic in nature but rather psychogenic or cardiocirculatory are other common causes of apparent intractability (Aicardi and Shorvon 1998).

Even 'true' intractability is a graduated rather than an all-or-nothing phenomenon, as partial control is sometimes possible and can help the patients, although studies have shown that the best quality of life is achieved with complete seizure control (Birbeck et al. 2002, Spencer et al. 2007).

In fact, the concept of 'intractability' is defined in no single way. Individual studies use different definitions, creating difficulties for comparisons of results across studies. Within a single prospective study of 613 children in Connecticut with newly diagnosed epilepsy (1993–1997), six different published definitions or indicators for intractability were applied and compared (Berg and Kelly 2006). All definitions were assessed at various times within the first 5 years after diagnosis, with the exact timing reflecting how they were used in their initial reports. Depending on the specific definition, the epilepsy of 9–24% of children was considered intractable. All definitions were strongly associated with remission status as of last follow-up and with longer-term outcome. The authors rightly concluded that no single preferred definition of intractable epilepsy exists and that consideration should be given to whether a single definition will suit all purposes or whether different types of definitions are needed for different purposes.

In general, about 20–30% of real epilepsies are resistant to drug therapy. Intractable epilepsies include many of the 'catastrophic syndromes' or epileptic encephalopathies such as Lennox–

Gastaut syndrome or Dravet syndrome, and cases of focal seizures, mainly those of lesional origin. The molecular and cellular mechanisms underlying drug resistance are still unknown (Sisodiya 2005, Remy and Beck 2006).

Particularly for focal non-idiopathic epilepsies, natural evolution is variable thus making it often difficult to decide at what point and after how many trials of mono- and polytherapy this epilepsy should be considered intractable. Clearly when other therapeutic options – especially resective surgery – are available and have a good prospect of success, medical therapy should probably not be prolonged for more than one or two years or even less in case of deterioration. However, not all epilepsies resistant to medical therapy are amenable to surgery, and in those cases various drug regimens will be tried for much longer periods.

Predictors of intractability include infantile spasms, remote symptomatic epilepsy, a history of status epilepticus, neonatal seizures and microcephaly (Berg et al. 1996). To determine prospectively when in the course of epilepsy intractability becomes apparent, Berg et al. (2006) analysed the data from a prospective cohort of 613 children followed for a median of 9.7 years. Epilepsy syndromes were grouped: focal, idiopathic, catastrophic, and other. Intractability was defined in both a stringent (two drugs failed, and one seizure/month, on average, for 18 months) and in a looser way (failure of two drugs). Delayed intractability was defined as three or more years after epilepsy diagnosis. Eighty-three children (13.8%) met the stringent definition and 142 (23.2%) met the two-drug definition. Intractability depended on syndrome (p<0.0001): 26 children (31.3%) meeting the stringent definition and 39 (27.5%) meeting the two-drug definition had delayed intractability. Intractability was delayed more often in focal than in catastrophic epilepsy (stringent: 46.2% vs 14.3%, p=0.003; two-drug: 40.3% vs 2.2%, p≤0.0001). Early remission periods preceded delayed intractability in 65.4–74.3% of cases. After becoming intractable, 20.5% subsequently entered remission and 13.3% were seizure free at last contact. These findings help explain why surgically treatable epilepsies may take 20 years or longer before referral to surgery.

SOCIAL AND EDUCATIONAL OUTCOME

The educational level of persons with epilepsy as a group is much lower than that of the general population. In a long-term study of adults with childhood-onset epilepsy, Sillanpää (1992) found that approximately one third of 176 patients had received less than primary education and 37% only primary education. Only 18% went to secondary school and 9% graduated. Three per cent had a university degree. The proportion of patients with a driving licence (61%), of those married or having a stable relationship (65%), of those having children (49.5%) were all significantly lower than in random matched controls. The proportion who were unemployed (9.1%) was higher. Patients with active epilepsy did signficantly less well than those who had been in remission for five years or more.

Another study from Finland (Koponen et al. 2007) explored social functioning and psychological well-being in a population-based cohort of epilepsy patients compared to matched controls

identified through the National Registry of Social Insurance Institution. The age at onset of epilepsy was significantly associated with the level of further education, and the level of seizure control with the employment status. Patients with epilepsy and a lower level of basic education had also significantly lower level of further education, employment, and fewer social relations. Some differences in psychological well-being were also seen in those who had passed a matriculation examination when compared to matched controls. The most important conclusion of the study was the fact that in young adults with well-controlled epilepsy and successful basic education, social functioning is comparable with that of healthy peers, suggesting that social and educational support during the time of basic education may be crucial to favourable intellectual, functional, and social development later in life. Both professional and informal support is needed in addition to conventional treatment of epilepsy.

All the above figures reflect, in part, the presence of complicating factors such as neurological impairment, learning difficulties and mental retardation. However, even patients without complicating factors tend to do less well than the general population in terms of professional and social adjustment (Loiseau et al. 1983). This is probably due, in part, to school absenteeism, low expectations from parents and teachers, rejection by peers, and practical problems (e.g. lack of driving licence). Many such factors reflect prejudice and ill-informedness of the public and patients themselves about their condition and could be improved by a better awareness.

RISK OF SUDDEN DEATH IN YOUNG PEOPLE WITH EPILEPSY

Mortality rates are increased in people with epilepsy (Nilsson et al. 1997, Shackleton et al. 1999). A recent review of published series (Shackleton et al. 2002) showed that the mortality risk in patients with epilepsy is dependent on source population of patients. Within the different source populations, considerable unexplained variance remains. Hence no uniform summary estimate for the elevated mortality can be determined.

In a series devoted exclusively to childhood epilepsy, mortality during the first 10 years after onset was 5.7%, and another 2.9% of the patients died between 11 and 12 years after onset (Kurokawa et al. 1982). Trevathan et al. (1997) reported that 4% of their epileptic population died before 11 years of age. An Australian study found a mortality rate of 3 per 1000 individuals, compared with 0.23 per 1000 in control children (Harvey et al. 1993c). Mortality was found to be higher in those epilepsies with an onset before the age of 1 year, in symptomatic epilepsy and in infantile spasms than in epilepsies with grand mal seizures.

Excess mortality is also present in population-based studies. In a review of the literature, Harvey et al. (1993c) found the mean estimate of death in epileptic children younger than 15 years was approximately 5 per 1,000 children. Children with secondary epilepsy accounted for 94% of all deaths. In a prospective community cohort of 613 children (Berg et al. 2004), symptomatic aetiology and epileptic encephalopathy were independently associated with mortality. The overall standardized mortality ratio for the cohort was 7.54. In children with symptomatic epilepsy, the standardized mortality ratio was 33.46 (95% CI, 18.53–60.43), and in those with nonsymptomatic epilepsy, it was 1.43 (95% CI, 0.36–5.73). These results suggest that children with epilepsy have an increased risk of death and that most deaths occur in children with severe underlying conditions and are not directly related to the occurrence of seizures.

By and large, the overall mortality among patients of all ages is two to three times that of the general population (O'Donoghue and Sander 1997). Although the causes of death are quite variable, sudden unexpected death, accidents and suicide deserve special consideration.

Suicide is considered to be one of the most important causes of death contributing to the increased mortality of persons with epilepsy. In a case–control study (Nilsson et al. 2002) there was a ninefold increase in risk of suicide with mental illness and a 10-fold increase in relative risk with the use of antipsychotic drugs. The profile of the epilepsy patient who commits suicide that emerges from this study was a patient with early onset, particularly onset during adolescence (but not necessarily severe epilepsy), psychiatric illness, and perhaps inadequate neurological follow-up.

Sudden unexpected death in epilepsy patients (SUDEP) refers to cases in which autopsy fails to reveal an anatomic or toxicological cause of death. SUDEP mainly occurs in adolescents and young adults and constitutes a significant cause of mortality in this age group. The rate is around 1 per 1000 patients per year (Nashef et al. 1995) so the issue clearly warrants continued investigation. A retrospective study from Australia (Opeskin et al. 2000) examined 15,751 autopsy records covering a 6 year period; 357 cases had epilepsy, 50 of which (14%) were classified as SUDEPs. The SUDEP rate was approximately 1 per 3000 individuals with epilepsy per year. This study suggested the following positive associations: young age, tonic–clonic seizures, seizure frequency greater than 10 per year, duration of epilepsy >10 years, mental retardation, psychiatric disease and alcohol abuse. The role of factors such as AED compliance, psychotropic drug prescription and recent unusually stressful life events was less clear. These observations support the hypothesis that seizures are the mechanism of many cases of SUDEP. The associations observed were largely in agreement with previous studies.

The mechanisms of sudden death in epilepsy are obscure. Asphyxia and cardiac dysrhythmias are likely factors. However, impressive apnoeic seizures with major cyanosis do not necessarily suggest a bad prognosis. Hewertson et al. (1994) reported a benign outcome in four of six infants and children with such events. Ryvlin et al. (2006b) discussed the pathophysiology and potential prevention of SUDEP. According to the authors, ictal arrhythmias may represent a more prevalent cause of SUDEP than previously thought. No clear recommendations have emerged from the literature regarding the most appropriate therapeutic strategies to prevent the event, apart from the supervision at night of patients with refractory epilepsy (Langan et al. 2005).

The question of whether to discuss the risk of SUDEP, and when to discuss it, with patients who have epilepsy is a major issue. As for all other issues related to epilepsy treatment and care, the discussion of SUDEP should be considered on a case-by-case basis. It should take into account the wishes of the patient to talk about it and the possibility of applying specific protective measures (e.g. night surveillance for drug-resistant cases, arguments in favour of better compliance).

REFERENCES

Abou-Khalil B, Andermann E, Andermann F, et al. (1993) Temporal lobe epilepsy after prolonged febrile convulsions: excellent outcome after surgical treatment. *Epilepsia* **34**: 878–83.

Abou-Khalil B, Ge Q, Delai R, et al. (2001). Partial and generalized epilepsy with febrile seizures plus and a novel SCN1A mutation. *Neurology* **57**: 2265–72.

Acharya JN, Wyllie E, Lüders HO, et al. (1997) Seizure symptomatology in infants with localization-related epilepsy. *Neurology* **48**: 189–96.

Aicardi J (1990) Neonatal myoclonic encephalopathy and early infantile epileptic encephalopathy. In: Wasterlain CG, Vert P, eds. *Neonatal Seizures.* New York: Raven Press, pp. 41–9.

Aicardi J (1991) Neonatal seizures. In: Dam M, Gram L, eds. *Comprehensive Epileptology.* New York: Raven Press, pp. 99–112.

Aicardi J (1994) Syndromic classification in the management of childhood epilepsy. *J Child Neurol* **9** Suppl 2: 14–8.

Aicardi J (1995) Typical absences in the first two years of life. In: Duncan J, Panayiotopoulos C, eds. *Typical Absences and Related Epileptic Syndromes.* London: Churchill Communication Europe, pp. 284–8.

Aicardi J (1996) Epileptic syndromes with onset in early childhood. In: Wallace SJ, ed. *Epilepsy in Children.* London: Chapman & Hall, pp. 247–74.

Aicardi J (1997) Paediatric epilepsy surgery: how the view has changed. In: Tuxhorn I, Holthausen H, Boenigk H, eds. *Paediatric Epilepsy Syndromes and their Surgical Treatment.* London: John Libbey, pp. 3–7.

Aicardi J (2000) Atypical semiology of rolandic epilepsy in some related syndromes. *Epil Disord* **2** Suppl. 1: S5–9.

Aicardi J, Chevrie JJ (1970) Convulsive status epilepticus in infants and children. *Epilepsia* **11**: 187–97.

Aicardi J, Chevrie JJ (1976) Febrile convulsions: neurological sequelae and mental retardation. In: Brazier MAB, Coceani F, eds. *Brain Dysfunction in Infantile Febrile Convulsions.* New York: Raven Press, pp. 247–57.

Aicardi J, Chevrie JJ (1982) Atypical benign partial epilepsy of childhood. *Dev Med Child Neurol* **24**: 281–92.

Aicardi J, Chevrie JJ (1983) Consequences of status epilepticus in infants and children. *Adv Neurol* **34**: 115–25.

Aicardi J, Levy Gomes A (1988) The Lennox–Gastaut syndrome: clinical and electroencephalographic features. In: Niedermeyer E, Degen D, eds. *The Lennox–Gastaut Syndrome.* New York: Alan R Liss, pp. 25–46.

Aicardi J, Levy Gomes A (1989) The myoclonic epilepsies of childhood. *Cleve Clin J Med* **56** Suppl: S34–9.

Aicardi J, Levy Gomes A (1992) Clinical and EEG symptomatology of the "genuine" Lennox–Gastaut syndrome and its differentiation from other forms of epilepsy of early childhood. In: Degen R, ed. *The Benign Localised and Generalised Epilepsies of Early Childhood, vol. 6.* Amsterdam: Elsevier, pp. 179–86.

Aicardi J, Ohtahara S (2005) Severe neonatal epilepsies with suppression–burst pattern. In: Roger J, Bureau M, Dravet C, et al., eds. *Epileptic Syndromes in Infancy, Childhood and Adolescence. 4th edn.* London: John Libbey Eurotext, pp. 39–50.

Aicardi J, Shorvon S (1998) Intractable epilepsy. In: Engel J, Pedley TA, eds. *Epilepsy: a Comprehensive Textbook, vol. 2.* New York: Lippincott–Raven, pp. 1325–31.

Aicardi J, Taylor DC (1998) History and physical examination. In: Engel J, Pedley TA, eds. *Epilepsy: a Comprehensive Textbook, vol. 1.* New York: Lippincott-Raven, pp. 805–10.

Aicardi J, Mumford JP, Dumas C, Wood S (1996) Vigabatrin as initial therapy for infantile spasms: a European retrospective survey. Sabril IS Investigator and Peer Review Groups. *Epilepsia* **37**: 638–42.

Aird RB (1983) The importance of seizure-inducing factors in the control of refractory forms of epilepsy. *Epilepsia* **24**: 567–83.

Aird RB, Masland RL, Woodbury DM (1984) *The Epilepsies—a Critical Review.* New York: Raven Press.

Aldenkamp AP (2001) Effects of antiepileptic drugs on cognition. *Epilepsia* 42 Suppl 1: 46–9; discussion 50–1.

Aldenkamp AP, Alpherts WC, Dekker MJ, Overweg J (1990) Neuropsychogical aspects of learning disabilities in epilepsy. *Epilepsia* 31 Suppl 4: S9–20.

Aldenkamp AP, Gutter T, Beun AM (1992) The effect of seizure activity and paroxysmal electroencephalographic discharges on cognition. *Acta Neurol Scand Suppl* 140: 111–21.

Aldenkamp AP, Alpherts WC, Blennow G, et al. (1993) Withdrawal of antiepileptic medication in children—effects on cognitive function: the multicenter Holmfrid study. *Neurology* 43: 41–50.

Aldenkamp AP, Weber B, Overweg-Plandsoen WC, et al. (2005) Educational underachievement in children with epilepsy: a model to predict the effects of epilepsy on educational achievement. *J Child Neurol* 20: 175–80.

Aldenkamp A, Vigevano F, Arzimanoglou A, Covanis A (2006) Role of valproate across the ages. Treatment of epilepsy in children. *Acta Neurol Scand Suppl* 184: 1–13.

Alexopoulos AV, Kotagal P, Loddenkemper T, et al. (2006) Long-term results with vagus nerve stimulation in children with pharmacoresistant epilepsy. *Seizure* 15: 491–503.

Alldredge BK, Wall DB, Ferriero DM (1995) Effect of prehospital treatment on the outcome of status epilepticus in children. *Pediatr Neurol* 12: 213–6.

Al-Shahwan SA, Singh B, Riela AR, Roach ES (1996) Hemisomatic spasms in children. *Neurology* 44: 1332–3.

Alvarez N, Hartford E, Doubt C (1981) Epileptic seizures induced by clonazepam. *Clin Electroencephalogr* 12: 57–65.

Alvarez N, Shinnar S, Moshe SL (1987) Infantile spasms due to unilateral cerebral infarcts. *Pediatrics* 79: 1024–6.

Ambrosetto G (1992) Unilateral opercular macrogyria and benign childhood epilepsy with centrotemporal (rolandic) spikes: report of a case. *Epilepsia* 33: 499–503.

American Academy of Pediatrics Committee on Drugs (1995) Behavioural and cognitive effects of anticonvulsant therapy. *Pediatrics* 96: 538–40.

Andermann F, Berkovic SF (2001) Idiopathic generalized epilepsy with generalized and other seizures in adolescence. *Epilepsia* 42: 317–20.

Andermann F, Kobayashi E (2005) Genetic focal epilepsies: state of the art and pathways to the future. *Epilepsia* 46: 61–7.

Andermann F, Rasmussen TR, Villemure JG (1992) Hemispherectomy: results for control of seizures in patients with hemiparesis. In: Lüders H, ed. *Epilepsy Surgery*. New York: Raven Press, pp. 625–32.

Anderson VE, Wilcox KJ, Hauser WA, et al. (1988) A test of autosomal dominant inheritance in febrile convulsions. *Epilepsia* 29: 705–6 (abstract).

Annegers JF, Shirts SB, Hauser WA, Kurland LT (1986) Risk of recurrence after an initial unprovoked seizure. *Epilepsia* 27: 43–50.

Annegers JF, Blakley SA, Hauser WA, Kurland LT (1990) Recurrence of febrile convulsions in a population-based cohort. *Epilepsy Res* 5: 209–16.

Antozzi C, Franceschetti S, Filippini G, et al. (1995) Epilepsia partialis continua associated with NADH-coenzyme Q reductase deficiency. *J Neurol Sci* 129: 152–61.

Appleton RE, Farrell K, Applegarth DA, et al. (1990) The high incidence of valproate hepatotoxicity in infants may relate to familial metabolic defects. *Can J Neurol Sci* 17: 145–8.

Appleton RE, Panayiotopoulos CP, Acomb BA, Beirne M (1993) Eyelid myoclonia with typical absences: an epilepsy syndrome. *J Neurol Neurosurg Psychiatry* 56: 1312–6.

Appleton RE, Sweeney A, Choonara I, et al. (1995) Lorazepam versus diazepam in the acute treatment of epileptic seizures and status epilepticus. *Dev Med Child Neurol* 37: 682–8.

Armstrong DD (2005) Epilepsy-induced microarchitectural changes in the brain. *Pediatr Dev Pathol* 8: 607–14.

Arts WF, Visser LH, Loonen MC, et al. (1988) Follow-up of 146 children with epilepsy after withdrawal of antiepileptic therapy. *Epilepsia* 29: 244–50.

Arts WF, Brouwer OF, Peters AC, et al. (2004) Course and prognosis of childhood epilepsy: 5-year follow-up of the Dutch study of epilepsy in childhood. *Brain* 127: 1774–84.

Arzimanoglou A (2002) Treatment options in pediatric epilepsy syndromes. *Epileptic Disord* 4: 217–25.

Arzimanoglou A (2003) Prognosis of Lennox–Gastaut syndrome. In: Jallon P, ed. *Prognosis of Epilepsies*. Paris: John Libbey Eurotext, pp. 277–88.

Arzimanoglou A (2007) Generalized epilepsy with febrile seizures plus. In: MedLink Neurology (online at: www.medlink.com).

Arzimanoglou A, Aicardi J (2001) Seizure disorders of the neonate and infant. In: Levine MI, Chevenak FA, Whittle M, eds. *Fetal and Neonatal Neurol-*

ogy and Neurosurgery. London: Churchill Livingstone, pp. 647–56.

Arzimanoglou A, Dravet C (2006) Hemiconvulsion–hemiplegia–epilepsy syndrome. Online at: http://www.ilae-epilepsy.org/Visitors/Centre/ctf/hemiconvulsion.html.

Arzimanoglou A, Prudent M, Salefranque F (1996) [Myoclonic–astatic epilepsy and benign myoclonic epilepsy of infancy in the same family: some reflections on the classification of the epilepsies.] *Epilepsies* 8: 307–15 (French).

Arzimanoglou AA, Salefranque F, Goutières F, Aicardi J (1999) Hemifacial spasm or subcortical epilepsy? *Epileptic Disord* 1: 121–5.

Arzimanoglou AA, Andermann F, Aicardi J, et al. (2000) Sturge–Weber syndrome: indications and results of surgery in 20 patients. *Neurology* 55: 1472–9.

Arzimanoglou AA, Hirsch E, Aicardi J (2003) Hypothalamic hamartoma and epilepsy in children: illustrative cases of possible evolutions. *Epileptic Disord* 5: 187–99.

Arzimanoglou A, Guerrini R, Aicardi J (2004) *Aicardi's Epilepsy in Children, 3rd edn*. Philadelphia: Lippincott, Williams & Wilkins.

Arzimanoglou A., Aldenkamp A, Cross H, et al. (2005) *Cognitive Dysfunction in Children with Temporal Lobe Epilepsy. Progress in Epileptic Disorders, vol. 1*. Paris: John Libbey Eurotext.

Arzimanoglou A, Laurent A, de Schonen S (2006) Nonidiopathic focal epilepsies: methodological problems for a comprehensive neuropsychological evaluation. *Epilepsia* 47 Suppl 2: 91–5.

Asano Y, Yoshikawa T, Suga S, et al. (1994) Clinical features of infants with primary human herpesvirus 6 infection (exanthema subitum, roseola infantum). *Pediatrics* 93: 104–8.

Aso K, Watanabe K (1992) Benign familial neonatal convulsions: generalized epilepsy? *Pediatr Neurol* 8: 226–8.

Aso K, Watanabe K, Negoro T, et al. (1987) Visual seizures in children. *Epilepsy Res* 1: 246–53.

Austin JK, Caplan R (2007) Behavioral and psychiatric comorbidities in pediatric epilepsy: toward an integrative model. *Epilepsia* 48: 1639–51.

Autret E, Billard C, Bertrand P, et al. (1990) Double-blind randomized trial of diazepam versus placebo for prevention of recurrences of febrile seizures. *J Pediatr* 117: 490–4.

Badinand-Hubert N, Bureau M, Hirsch E, et al. (1998) Epilepsies and video games: results of a multicentric study. *Electroencephalogr Clin Neurophysiol* 107: 422–7.

Baldy-Moulinier M (1986) Inter-relationships between sleep and epilepsy. In: Pedley TA, Meldrum BS, eds. *Recent Advances in Epilepsy, vol. 3*. Edinburgh: Churchill Livingstone, pp. 37–55.

Bancaud J (1987) Clinical symptomatology of epileptic seizures of temporal origin. *Rev Neurol* 143: 392–400.

Bancaud J, Talairach J (1975) Macro-stereo-electroencephalography in epilepsy. In: *Handbook of EEG and Clinical Neurophysiology, vol. 10B*. Amsterdam: Elsevier, pp. 3–10.

Baram TZ (2003) Long-term neuroplasticity and functional cosequences of single and recurrent early-life seizures. *Ann Neurol* 54: 701–5.

Baram T, Shinnar S (2002) *Febrile Seizures*. New York, Academic Press.

Baram TZ, Mitchell WG, Tournay A, et al. (1996) High-dose corticotropin (ACTH) versus prednisone for infantile spasms: a prospective, randomized, blinded study. *Pediatrics* 97: 375–9.

Barkovich AJ, Kuzniecky RI, Jackson GD, et al. (2005) A developmental and genetic classification for malformations of cortical development. *Neurology* 65: 1873–87.

Barry E, Sussman NM, Bosley TM, Harner RN (1985) Ictal blindness and status epilepticus amauroticus. *Epilepsia* 26: 577–84.

Bass WT, Lewis DW (1995) Neonatal segmental myoclonus associated with hyperglycorrhachia. *Pediatr Neurol* 13: 77–9.

Bass N, Wyllie E, Comair Y, et al. (1995) Supplementary sensorimotor area seizures in children and adolescents. *J Pediatr* 126: 537–44.

Bate L, Gardiner M (1999) Genetics of inherited epilepsies. *Epileptic Disord* 1: 7–19.

Battaglia A, Guerrini R (2005) Chromosomal disorders associated with epilepsy. *Epileptic Disord* 7: 181–92.

Bauer J, Stefan H, Huk WJ, et al. (1989) CT, MRI and SPECT neuroimaging in status epilepticus with simple partial and complex partial seizures: case report. *J Neurol* 236: 296–9.

Baulac M, De Grissac N, Hasboun D, et al. (1998) Hippocampal developmental changes in patients with partial epilepsy: magnetic resonance imaging and clinical aspects. *Ann Neurol* 44: 223–33.

Baulac S, Gourfinkel-An I, Nabbout R, et al. (2004) Fever, genes, and epilepsy. *Lancet Neurol* **3**: 421–30.

Baumann RJ, Duffner PK (2000) Treatment of children with simple febrile seizures: the AAP practice parameter. American Academy of Pediatrics. *Pediatr Neurol* **23**: 11–7.

Baxter P (2002) Pyridoxine dependent and pyridoxine responsive seizures. In: Baxter P, ed. *Vitamin Responsive Conditions in Paediatric Neurology. International Review of Child Neurology Series.* London: Mac Keith Press for the International Child Neurology Association, pp. 109–165.

Beaumanoir A (1992) The Landau–Kleffner syndrome. In: Roger J, Bureau M, Dravet C, et al., eds. *Epileptic Syndromes in Infancy, Childhood and Adolescence. 2nd edn.* London: John Libbey, pp. 231–43.

Beaumanoir A, Blume W (2005) The Lennox–Gastaut syndrome. In: Roger J, Bureau M, Dravet C, et al., eds. *Epileptic Syndromes in Infancy, Childhood and Adolescence. 4th edn.* Paris: John Libbey Eurotext, pp. 125–48.

Beaumanoir A, Dravet C (1992) The Lennox–Gastaut syndrome. In: Roger J, Bureau M, Dravet C, et al., eds. *Epileptic Syndromes in Infancy, Childhood and Adolescence, 2nd edn.* London: John Libbey, pp. 115–32.

Beaumanoir A, Foletti G, Magistris M, Volanschi D (1988) Status epilepticus in the Lennox–Gastaut syndrome. In: Niedermeyer E, Degen R, eds. *The Lennox–Gastaut Syndrome.* New York: Alan R Liss, pp. 283–99.

Beckung E, Uvebrant P (1997) Hidden dysfunction in childhood epilepsy. *Dev Med Child Neurol* **39**: 72–9.

Beghi E (2007) Treatment of first unprovoked seizure. In: Ryvlin P, Beghi E, Camfield P, Hesdorffer D, eds. *From First Unprovoked Seizure to Newly Diagnosed Epilepsy. Progress in Epileptic Disorders, vol. 3.* Paris: John Libbey Eurotext, pp. 156–68.

Beghi E, Annegers JF; Collaborative Group for the Pregnancy Registries in Epilepsy (2001) Pregnancy registries in epilepsy. *Epilepsia* **42**: 1422–5.

Beghi M, Cornaggia CM, Frigeni B, Beghi E (2006) Learning disorders in epilepsy. *Epilepsia* **47** Suppl 2: 14–8.

Bellman MH, Ross EM, Miller DL (1983) Infantile spasms and pertussis immunisation. *Lancet* **1**: 1031–4.

Benabid AL, Vercueil L, Benazzouz A, et al. (2003) Deep brain stimulation: what does it offer? *Adv Neurol* **91**: 293–302.

Ben-Ari Y (2006) Basic developmental rules and their implications for epilepsy in the immature brain. *Epileptic Disord* **8**: 91–102.

Benifla M, Rutka JT, Logan W, Donner EJ (2006) Vagal nerve stimulation for refractory epilepsy in children: indications and experience at The Hospital for Sick Children. *Childs Nerv Syst* **22**: 1018–26.

Ben-Zeev B, Watemberg N, Lerman P, et al. (2004) Sulthiame in childhood epilepsy. *Pediatr Int* **46**: 521–4.

Berg AT, Kelly MM (2006) Defining intractability: comparisons among published definitions. *Epilepsia* **47**: 431–6.

Berg AT, Shinnar S, Hauser WA, et al. (1992) A prospective study of recurrent febrile seizures. *N Engl J Med* **327**: 1122–7.

Berg AT, Shinnar S, Shapiro ED, et al. (1995) Risk factors for a first febrile seizure: a matched case–control study. *Epilepsia* **36**: 334–41.

Berg AT, Levy SR, Novotny EJ, Shinnar S (1996) Predictors of intractable epilepsy in childhood: a case–control study. *Epilepsia* **37**: 24–30.

Berg AT, Darefsky AS, Holford TR, Shinnar S (1998) Seizures with fever after unprovoked seizures: an analysis in children followed from the time of a first febrile seizure. *Epilepsia* **39**: 77–80.

Berg AT, Shinnar S, Levy SR, et al. (2001) Early development of intractable epilepsy in children: a prospective study. *Neurology* **56**: 1445–52.

Berg AT, Langfitt J, Shinnar S, et al. (2003) How long does it take for partial epilepsy to become intractable? *Neurology* **60**: 186–90.

Berg AT, Shinnar S, Testa FM, et al. (2004) Mortality in childhood-onset epilepsy. Arch Pediatr Adolesc Med 158: 1147–52.

Berg AT, Vickrey BG, Testa FM, et al. (2006) How long does it take for epilepsy to become intractable? A prospective investigation. *Ann Neurol* **60**: 73–9.

Bergin PS, Fish DR, Shorvon SD, et al. (1995) Magnetic resonance imaging in partial epilepsy: additional abnormalities shown with the fluid attenuated inversion recovery (FLAIR) pulse sequence. *J Neurol Neurosurg Psychiatry* **58**: 439–43.

Berkovic SF, Scheffer IE (1997) Epilepsies with single gene inheritance. *Brain Dev* **19**: 13–8.

Berkovic SF, Andermann F, Andermann E, Gloor P (1987) Concept of absence epilepsies: discrete syndromes or biological continuum? *Neurology* **37**: 993–1000.

Berkovic SF, Andermann F, Melanson D, et al. (1988) Hypothalamic hamar-

tomas and ictal laughter: evolution of a characteristic epileptic syndrome and diagnostic value of magnetic resonance imaging. *Ann Neurol* **23**: 429–39.

Berkovic SF, Kennerson ML, Howell RA, et al. (1994) Phenotypic expression of benign familial neonatal convulsions linked to chromosome 20. *Arch Neurol* **51**: 1125–8.

Berkovic SF, McIntosh A, Howell RA, et al. (1996) Familial temporal lobe epilepsy: a common disorder identified in twins. *Ann Neurol* **40**: 227–35.

Berkovic SF, Arzimanoglou A, Kuzniecky R, et al. (2003) Hypothalamic hamartoma and seizures: a treatable epileptic encephalopathy. *Epilepsia* **44**: 969–73.

Berkovic SF, Heron SE, Giordano L, et al. (2004) Benign familial neonatal–infantile seizures: characterization of a new sodium channelopathy. *Ann Neurol* **55**: 550–7.

Berkovic SF, Harkin L, McMahon JM, et al. (2006) De-novo mutations of the sodium channel gene SCN1A in alleged vaccine encephalopathy: a retrospective study. *Lancet Neurol* **5**: 488–92.

Bernasconi N, Natsume J, Bernasconi A (2005) Progression in temporal lobe epilepsy: differential atrophy in mesial temporal structures. *Neurology* **65**: 223–8.

Besag FMC, Wallace SJ, Dulac O, et al. (1995) Lamotrigine for treatment of epilepsy in children. *J Pediatr* **127**: 991–7.

Bethune P, Gordon K, Dooley J, et al. (1993) Which child will have a febrile seizure? *Am J Dis Child* **147**: 35–9.

Bianchi A, Italian League Against Epilepsy Collaborative Group (1995) Study of concordance of symptoms in families with absence epilepsies. In: Duncan JS, Panayiotopoulos CP, eds. *Typical Absences and Related Epileptic Syndromes.* London: Churchill Communications Europe, pp. 328–37.

Bien CG, Widman G, Urbach H, et al. (2002) The natural history of Rasmussen's encephalitis. *Brain* **125**: 1751–9.

Bien CG, Granata T, Antozzi C, et al. (2005) Pathogenesis, diagnosis and treatment of Rasmussen encephalitis: a European consensus statement. *Brain* **128**: 454–71.

Birbeck GL, Hays RD, Cui X, Vickrey BG (2002) Seizure reduction and quality of life improvements in people with epilepsy. *Epilepsia* **43**: 535–8.

Bishop DVM (1985) Age of onset and outcome in 'acquired aphasia with convulsive disorder' (Landau–Kleffner syndrome). *Dev Med Child Neurol* **27**: 705–12.

Bisulli F, Tinuper P, Avoni P, et al. (2004) Idiopathic partial epilepsy with auditory features (IPEAF): a clinical and genetic study of 53 sporadic cases. *Brain* **127**: 1343–52.

Bittar RG, Rosenfeld JV, Klug GL, et al. (2002) Resective surgery in infants and young children with intractable epilepsy. *J Clin Neurosci* **9**: 142–6.

Blume WT, Borghesi J, Lemieux JF (1993) Interictal indices of temporal seizure origin. *Ann Neurol* **34**: 703–9.

Blume WT, Kalbara M (1995) *Atlas of Adult Electroencephalography.* New York: Raven Press.

Bonanni P, Malcarne M, Moro F, et al. (2004) Generalized epilepsy with febrile seizures plus (GEFS+): clinical spectrum in seven Italian families unrelated to SCN1A, SCN1B and GABRG2 mutations. *Epilepsia* **45**: 149–58.

Booth D, Evans DJ (2004) Anticonvulsants for neonates with seizures. *Cochrane Database Syst Rev* (4): CD004218.

Bootsma HP, Aldenkamp AP, Diepman L, et al. (2006) The effect of antiepileptic drugs on cognition: patient perceived cognitive problems of topiramate versus levetiracetam in clinical practice. *Epilepsia* **47** Suppl 2: 24–7.

Boulloche J, Leloup P, Mallet E, et al. (1989) Risk of recurrence after a single, unprovoked, generalized tonic–clonic seizure. *Dev Med Child Neurol* **31**: 626–32.

Boulloche J, Husson A, Le Luyer B, Le Roux P (1990) [Dysphagia, speech disorders and centrotemporal spike–waves.] *Arch Fr Pediatr* **47**: 115–7.

Bouma P, Peters ACB, Arts RJHM, et al. (1987) Discontinuation of antiepileptic therapy: a prospective study in children. *J Neurol Neurosurg Psychiatry* **50**: 1579–83.

Bourgeois B, Prensky AL, Palkes HS, et al. (1983) Intelligence in epilepsy: a prospective study in children. *Ann Neurol* **14**: 438–44.

Bourgeois M, Crimmins DW, de Oliveira RS, et al. (2007) Surgical treatment of epilepsy in Sturge–Weber syndrome in children. J *Neurosurg* **106** (1 Suppl): 20–8.

Brett EM (1997) Epilepsy and convulsions. In: Brett EM, ed. *Paediatric Neurology, 3rd edn.* Edinburgh: Churchill Livingstone, pp. 333–95.

Brockhaus A, Elger CE (1995) Complex partial seizures of temporal lobe origin in children of different age groups. *Epilepsia* **36**: 1173–81.

Brodie MJ (1990) Established anticonvulsants and treatment of refractory epilepsy. *Lancet* **336**: 350–4.

Brodie MJ, Richens A, Yuen AW (1995) Double-blind comparison of lamotrigine and carbamazepine in newly diagnosed epilepsy. UK Lamotrigine/ Carbamazepine Monotherapy Trial Group. *Lancet* 345: 476–9; erratum 662.

Brown JK, Hussain IHMI (1991a) Status epilepticus. I: Pathogenesis. *Dev Med Child Neurol* 33: 3–17.

Brown JK, Hussain IHMI (1991b) Status epilepticus. II: Treatment. *Dev Med Child Neurol* 33: 97–109.

Browne TR, Szabo GK, Evans JE, et al. (1988) Carbamazepine increases phenytoin serum concentration and reduces phenytoin clearance. *Neurology* 38: 1146–50.

Bruton CJ (1988) *The Neuropathology of Temporal Lobe Epilepsy. Maudsley Monograph No. 31.* Oxford: Oxford University Press.

Bureau M (1995) Continuous spikes and waves during slow sleep (CSWS): definition of the syndrome. In: Beaumanoir A, Bureau M, Deonna T, et al., eds. *Continuous Spikes and Waves During Slow Sleep, Electrical Status Epilepticus During Slow Sleep. Acquired Epileptic Aphasia and Related Conditions. Mariani Foundation Paediatric Neurology Series no. 3.* London: John Libbey, pp. 17–26.

Bureau M, Maton B (1998) Valeur de l'EEG dans le prognostic précoce des épilepsies partielles non idiopathiques de l'enfant. In: Bureau M, Kahane P, Munari C, eds. *Épilepsies Partielles Graves Pharmacorésistantes de l'Enfant: Stratégies Diagnostiques et Traitements Chirurgicaux.* Montrouge: John Libbey Eurotext, pp. 67–78.

Bureau M, Tassinari CA (2005) The syndrome of myoclonic absences. In: Roger J, Bureau M, Dravet C, et al., eds. *Epileptic Syndromes in Infancy, Childhood and Adolescence. 4th edn.* Paris: John Libbey Eurotext, pp. 337–44.

Burke CJ, Tannenberg AE (1995) Prenatal brain damage and placental infarction—an autopsy study. *Dev Med Child Neurol* 37: 555–62.

Bye AME (1994) Neonate with benign familial neonatal convulsions: recorded generalized and focal seizures. *Pediatr Neurol* 10: 164–5.

Bye AME, Flanagan D (1995) Spatial and temporal characteristics of neonatal seizures. *Epilepsia* 36: 1009–16.

Bye AME, Andermann F, Robitaille Y, et al. (1993) Cortical vascular abnormalities in the syndrome of celiac disease, bilateral occipital calcifications, and folate deficiency. *Ann Neurol* 34: 399–403.

Callahan DJ, Noetzel MJ (1992) Prolonged absence status epilepticus associated with carbamazepine therapy, increased intracranial pressure, and transient MRI abnormalities. *Neurology* 42: 2198–201.

Camfield C, Camfield P, Smith E, Tibbles JA (1986) Asymptomatic children with epilepsy: little benefit from screening for anticonvulsant-induced liver, blood, or renal damage. *Neurology* 36: 838–41.

Camfield C, Camfield P, Smith B, et al. (1993) Outcome of childhood epilepsy: a population-based study with a simple predictive scoring system for those treated with medication. *J Pediatr* 122: 861–8.

Camfield PR, Camfield C, Gordon K, Dooley J (1994) What types of epilepsy are preceded by febrile seizures? A population-based study of children. *Dev Med Child Neurol* 36: 887–92.

Camfield PR, Camfield CS, Gordon K, Dooley JM (1997) If a first antiepileptic drug fails to control a child's epilepsy, what are the chances of success with the next drug? *J Pediatr* 131: 821–4.

Capovilla G, Gambardella A, Romeo A, et al. (2001) Benign partial epilepsies of adolescence: a report of 37 new cases. *Epilepsia* 42: 1549–52.

Capovilla G, Beccaria F, Montagnini A (2006) Benign focal epilepsy in infancy with vertex spikes and waves during sleep. Delineation of the syndrome and recalling as "benign infantile focal epilepsy with midline spikes and waves during sleep" (BIMSE). *Brain Dev* 28: 85–91.

Caraballo R, Fontana E, Michelizza B, et al. (1989) Carbamazepina, "assenze atipiche", "crise atoniche", e stato di Po continua del sonno (POCB). *Boll Lega Ital Contra Epilessia* 66/67: 379–81.

Caraballo R, Cersósimo RO, Fejerman N (1999) A particular type of epilepsy in children with congenital hemiparesis associated with unilateral polymicrogyria. *Epilepsia* 40: 865–71.

Caraballo R, Cersósimo RO, Espeche A, Fejerman N (2003) Benign familial and non-familial seizures: a study of 64 patients. *Epileptic Disord* 5: 45–9.

Caraballo R, Cersósimo RO, Fejerman N (2004) Benign focal seizures of adolescence: a prospective study. *Epilepsia* 45: 1600–3.

Caraballo RH, Cersósimo RO, Sakr D, et al. (2006) Ketogenic diet in patients with myoclonic–astatic epilepsy. *Epileptic Disord* 8: 151–5.

Carrazana EJ, Lombroso CT, Mikati M, et al. (1993) Facilitation of infantile spasms by partial seizures. *Epilepsia* 34: 97–109.

Cascino GD (1993) Nonconvulsive status epilepticus in adults and children. *Epilepsia* 34 Suppl 1: S21–8.

Cascino GD, Andermann F, Berkovic SF, et al. (1993) Gelastic seizures and hypothalamic hamartomas: evaluation of patients undergoing chronic intracranial EEG monitoring and outcome of surgical treatment. *Neurology* 43: 747–50.

Castro Conde JR, Hernández Borges AA, Doménech Martínez E, et al. (2005) Midazolam in neonatal seizures with no response to phenobarbital. *Neurology* 64: 876–9.

Cavazzuti GB, Ferrari P, Lalla M (1984) Follow-up study of 482 cases with convulsive disorders in the first year of life. *Dev Med Child Neurol* 26: 425–37.

Cendes F (2005) Progressive hippocampal and extrahippocampal atrophy in drug resistant epilepsy. *Curr Opin Neurol* 18: 173–7.

Cendes F, Andermann F, Dubeau F, et al. (1993a) Early childhood prolonged febrile convulsions, atrophy and sclerosis of mesial structures, and temporal lobe epilepsy: an MRI volumetric study. *Neurology* 43: 1083–7.

Cendes F, Andermann F, Gloor P, et al. (1993b) Atrophy of mesial structures in patients with temporal lobe epilepsy: cause or consequence of repeated seizures? *Ann Neurol* 34: 795–801.

Cendes F, Cook MJ, Watson C, et al. (1995) Frequency and characteristics of dual pathology in patients with lesional epilepsy. *Neurology* 45: 2058–64.

Cendes F, Kobayashi E, Lopes-Cendes I (2005) Familial temporal lobe epilepsy with auditory features. *Epilepsia* 46 Suppl 10: 50–60.

Chabardes S, Kahane P, Minotti L, et al. (2002) Deep brain stimulation in epilepsy with particular reference to the subthalamic nucleus. *Epileptic Disord* 4 Suppl 3: S83–93.

Chahine LM, Mikati MA (2006) Benign pediatric localization-related epilepsies: Part I. Syndromes in infancy. *Epileptic Disord* 8: 169–83.

Chaix Y, Daquin G, Monteiro F, et al. (2003) Absence epilepsy with onset before age three years: a heterogeneous and often severe condition. *Epilepsia* 44: 944–9.

Chamberlain MC (1996) Nitrazepam for refractory infantile spasms and the Lennox–Gastaut syndrome. *J Child Neurol* 11: 31–4.

Chamberlain JM, Altieri MA, Futterman C, et al. (1997) A prospective, randomized study comparing intramuscular midazolam with intravenous diazepam for the treatment of seizures in children. *Pediatr Emerg Care* 13: 92–4.

Charlier C, Singh NA, Ryan SG, et al. (1998). A pore mutation in a novel KQT-like potassium channel gene in an idiopathic epilepsy family. *Nat Genet* 18: 53–5.

Chassoux F, Devaux B, Landré E, et al. (2000) Stereoelectroencephalography in focal cortical dysplasias: a 3D approach delineating the dysplastic cortex. *Brain* 123: 1733–51.

Chauvel P, Dravet C (2005) The HHE syndrome. In: Roger J, Bureau M, Dravet C, et al., eds. *Epileptic Syndromes in Infancy, Childhood and Adolescence. 4th edn.* London: John Libbey Eurotext, pp. 277–93.

Chauvel P, Delgado-Escueta AV, Halgren E, Bancaud J (1992) *Frontal Lobe Seizures and Epilepsies.* New York: Raven Press.

Chevrie JJ, Aicardi J (1972) Childhood epileptic encephalopathy with slow spike–wave. A statistical study of 80 cases. *Epilepsia* 13: 259–71.

Chevrie JJ, Aicardi J (1975) Duration and lateralization of febrile convulsions. Etiological factors. *Epilepsia* 16: 781–9.

Chevrie JJ, Aicardi J (1977) Convulsive disorders in the first year of life. Etiologic factors. *Epilepsia* 18: 489–98.

Chevrie JJ, Aicardi J (1978) Convulsive disorders in the first year of life. Neurologic and mental outcome and mortality. *Epilepsia* 19: 67–74.

Chevrie JJ, Aicardi J (1979) Convulsive disorders in the first year of life. Persistence of epileptic seizures. *Epilepsia* 20: 643–9.

Chevrie JJ, Aicardi J, Goutières F (1987) Epilepsy in childhood mitochondrial encephalomyopathies. In: Wolf P, Dam M, Janz D, Dreifuss F, eds. *Advances in Epileptology. XVIth Epilepsy International Symposium.* New York: Raven Press, pp. 181–4.

Chin RF, Neville BG, Peckham C, et al. (2006) Incidence, cause, and short-term outcome of convulsive status epilepticus in childhood: prospective population-based study. *Lancet* 368: 222–9.

Chinchilla D, Dulac O, Robain O, et al. (1994) Reappraisal of Rasmussen's syndrome with special emphasis on treatment with high doses of steroids. *J Neurol Neurosurg Psychiatry* 57: 1325–33.

Chiron C (2007) Stiripentol. *Neurotherapeutics* 4: 123–5.

Chiron C, Dulac O, Luna D, et al. (1990) Vigabatrin in infantile spasms. *Lancet* 335: 363–364 (letter).

Chiron C, Dumas C, Jambaque I, et al. (1997) Randomized trial comparing vigabatrin and hydrocortisone in infantile spasms due to tuberous sclerosis. *Epilepsy Res* **26**: 389–95.

Chiron C, Marchand MC, Tran A, et al. (2000) Stiripentol in severe myoclonic epilepsy in infancy: a randomised placebo-controlled syndrome-dedicated trial. STICLO study group. *Lancet* **356**: 1638–42.

Chugani DC, Chugani HT, Muzik O, et al. (1998) Imaging epileptogenic tubers in children with tuberous sclerosis complex using alpha-[11C]methyl-L-tryptophan positron emission tomography. *Ann Neurol* **44**: 858–66.

Chugani HT, Conti JR (1996) Etiologic classification of infantile spasms in 140 cases: role of positron emission tomography. *J Child Neurol* **11**: 44–8.

Chugani HT, Pinard JM (1994) Surgical treatment. In: Dulac O, Chugani HT, Dalla Bernardina B, eds. *Infantile Spasms and West Syndrome*. Philadelphia: WB Saunders, pp. 257–64.

Chugani HT, Mazziota JC, Engel J, Phelps ME (1987) The Lennox–Gastaut syndrome: metabolic subtypes determined by 2-deoxy-2 18F fluoro-D-glucose positron emission tomography. *Ann Neurol* **21**: 4–13.

Chugani HT, Shields WD, Shewmon DA, et al. (1990) Infantile spasms: I. PET identifies focal cortical dysgenesis in cryptogenic cases for surgical treatment. *Ann Neurol* **27**: 406–13.

Chugani HT, Da Silva E, Chugani DC (1996) Infantile spasms: III. Prognostic implications of bitemporal hypometabolism on positron emission tomography. *Ann Neurol* **39**: 643–9.

Claes L, Del-Favero J, Ceulemans B, et al. (2001) De novo mutations in the sodium-channel gene SCN1A cause severe myoclonic epilepsy of infancy. *Am J Hum Genet* **68**: 1327–32.

Claes S, Devriendt K, Lagae L, et al. (1997) The X-linked infantile spasms syndrome (MIM 308350) maps to Xp11.4–Xpter in two pedigrees. *Ann Neurol* **42**: 360–4.

Clancy RR (2006) Summary proceedings from the neurology group on neonatal seizures. *Pediatrics* **117**: S23–7.

Clancy RR, Legido A (1987) The exact ictal and interictal duration of electroencephalographic neonatal seizures. *Epilepsia* **28**: 537–41.

Clancy RR, Legido A, Lewis D (1988) Occult neonatal seizures. *Epilepsia* **29**: 256–61.

Cockerell OC, Rothwell J, Thompson PD, et al. (1996) Clinical and physiological features of epilepsia partialis continua. Cases ascertained in the UK. *Brain* **119**: 393–407.

Cockerell OC, Johnson AL, Sander JWAS, Shorvon SD (1997) Prognosis of epilepsy: a review and further analysis of the first nine years of the British National General Practice Study of Epilepsy, a prospective population-based study. *Epilepsia* **38**: 31–46.

Collings JA (1990) Psychosocial well-being and epilepsy: an empirical study. *Epilepsia* **31**: 418–26.

Commission on Classification and Terminology of the International League against Epilepsy (1981) Proposal for revised clinical and electroencephalographic classification of epileptic seizures. *Epilepsia* **22**: 489–501.

Commission on Classification and Terminology of the International League against Epilepsy (1989) Proposal for revised classification of epilepsies and epileptic syndromes. *Epilepsia* **30**: 389–99.

Commission on Neuroimaging of the International League Against Epilepsy (1997) Recommendations for neuroimaging of patients with epilepsy. *Epilepsia* **38**: 1255–6.

Consensus Development Panel (1980) Febrile seizures: long-term management of children with fever-associated seizures. *Pediatrics* **66**: 1009–12.

Coppola G, Plouin P, Chiron C, et al. (1995) Migrating partial seizures in infancy: a malignant disorder with developmental arrest. *Epilepsia* **36**: 1017–24.

Coppola G, Castaldo P, Miraglia del Giudice E, et al. (2003) A novel KCNQ2 K+ channel mutation in benign neonatal convulsions and centrotemporal spikes. *Neurology* **61**: 131–4.

Coppola G, Veggiotti P, Del Giudice EM, et al. (2006) Mutational scanning of potassium and chloride channels in malignant migrating partial seizures in infancy. *Brain Dev* **28**: 76–9.

Cornblath M, Schwartz R (1991) *Disorders of Carbohydrate Metabolism in Infancy*, 3rd edn. Oxford: Blackwell.

Cornford ME, McCormick GF (1997) Adult-onset temporal lobe epilepsy associated with smoldering herpes simplex 2 infection. *Neurology* **48**: 425–30.

Coulter DL (1991) Carnitine, valproate and toxicity. *J Child Neurol* **6**: 7–14.

Covanis A, Jeavons PM (1980) Once-daily sodium valproate in the treatment of epilepsy. *Dev Med Child Neurol* **22**: 202–4.

Covanis A, Ferrie CD, Koutroumanidis M, et al. (2005) Panayiotopoulos syndrome and Gastaut type idiopathic childhood occipital epilepsy. In: Roger J, Bureau M, Dravet C, et al., eds. *Epileptic Syndromes in Infancy, Childhood and Adolescence. 4th edn.* London: John Libbey Eurotext, pp. 227–53.

Cowan LD, Hudson LS (1991) The epidemiology and natural history of infantile spasms. *J Child Neurol* **6**: 355–64.

Crawford TO, Mitchell WG, Fishman LS, Snodgrass SR (1988) Very high-dose phenobarbital for refractory status epilepticus in children. *Neurology* **38**: 1035–40.

Crespel A, Gélisse P, Bureau M, Genton P (2006) *Atlas of Electroencephalography. Vol. 2: The Epilepsies, EEG and Epileptic Syndromes*. Paris: John Libbey Eurotext.

Cross JH, Jackson GD, Neville BGR, et al. (1993) Early detection of abnormalities in partial epilepsy using magnetic resonance. *Arch Dis Child* **69**: 104–9.

Cross JH, Gordon I, Jackson GD, et al. (1995) Children with intractable focal epilepsy: ictal and interictal 99TcM HMPAO single photon emission computed tomography. *Dev Med Child Neurol* **37**: 673–81.

Cross JH, Gordon I, Connelly A, et al. (1997) Interictal 99Tc(m) HMPAO SPECT and 1H MRS in children with temporal lobe epilepsy. *Epilepsia* **38**: 338–45.

Cross JH, Jayakar P, Nordli D, et al. (2006) Proposed criteria for referral and evaluation of children for epilepsy surgery: recommendations of the Subcommission for Pediatric Epilepsy Surgery. *Epilepsia* **47**: 952–9.

Cunnington M, Ferber S, Quartey G; International Lamotrigine Pregnancy Registry Scientific Advisory Committee (2007) Effect of dose on the frequency of major birth defects following fetal exposure to lamotrigine monotherapy in an international observational study. *Epilepsia* **48**: 1207–10.

Cusmai R, Dulac O, Diebler C (1988) [Focal lesions in infantile spasms.] *Neurophysiol Clin* **18**: 235–41 (French).

Dalla Bernardina B, Watanabe K (1994) Interictal EEG: variations and pitfalls. In: Dulac O, Chugani HT, Dalla Bernardina B, eds. *Infantile Spasms and West Syndrome*. Philadelphia: WB Saunders, pp. 63–81.

Dalla Bernardina B, Fontana E, Sgrò V, et al. (1992) Myoclonic epilepsy ('myoclonic status') in non-progressive encephalopathies. In: Roger J, Bureau M, Dravet C, et al., eds. *Epileptic Syndromes in Infancy, Childhood and Adolescence. 2nd edn.* London: John Libbey, pp. 89–96.

Dalla Bernardina B, Fontana E, Cappellaro O, et al. (1993) The partial occipital epilepsies in childhood. In: Andermann F, Beaumanoir H, Mira L, et al., eds. *Occipital Seizures and Epilepsies in Children*. London: John Libbey, pp. 173–81.

Dalla Bernardina B, Sgrò V, Fejerman N (2005) Epilepsy with centro-temporal spikes and related syndromes. In: Roger J, Bureau M, Dravet C, et al., eds. *Epileptic Syndromes in Infancy, Childhood and Adolescence. 4th edn.* London: John Libbey Eurotext, pp. 203–225.

Dalla Bernardina B, Fontana E, Osanni E, et al. (2007) Epileptic spasms: interictal patterns. In: Guzzetta F, Dalla Bernardina B, Guerrini R, eds. *Progress in Epileptic Spasms and West Syndrome. Progress in Epileptic Disorders no. 4.* Paris: John Libbey Eurotext, pp. 43–60.

De Lanerolle NC, Lee TS (2005) New facets of the neuropathology and molecular profile of human temporal lobe epilepsy. *Epilepsy Behav* **7**: 190–203.

Del Brutto OH, Santibañez R, Noboa CA, et al. (1992) Epilepsy due to neurocysticercosis: analysis of 203 patients. *Neurology* **42**: 389–92.

Delgado-Escueta AV, Enrile-Bacsal F (1984) Juvenile myoclonic epilepsy of Janz. *Neurology* **34**: 285–94.

DeLorenzo RJ, Garnett LK, Towne AR, et al. (1999) Comparison of status epilepticus with prolonged seizure episodes lasting from 10 to 29 minutes. *Epilepsia* **40**: 164–9.

DeMarco P, Lorenzin G (1990) Growing bilateral occipital calcifications and epilepsy. *Brain Dev* **12**: 342–4.

De Negri M, Baglietto MG, Biancheri R (1993) Electrical status epilepticus in childhood: treatment with short cycles of high-dosage benzodiazepine (preliminary note). *Brain Dev* **15**: 311–2.

Deonna T (2000) Rolandic epilepsy: neuropsychology of the active epilepsy phase. *Epileptic Disord* **2** Suppl 1: S59–61.

Deonna T, Roulet-Perez E, eds. (2005) *Cognitive and Behavioural Disorders of Epileptic Origin in Children. Clinics in Developmental Medicine no. 168.* London: Mac Keith Press.

Deonna T, Beaumanoir A, Gaillard P, Assal G (1977) Acquired aphasia in childhood with seizure disorder: a heterogeneous syndrome. *Neuropädiatrie* **8**: 263–73.

Deonna T, Ziegler AL, Despland PA (1986) Combined myoclonic–astatic and "benign" focal epilepsy of childhood ("atypical benign partial epilepsy of childhood"). A separate syndrome? *Neuropediatrics* **17**: 144–51.

Deonna T, Peter C, Ziegler AL (1989) Adult follow-up of the acquired aphasia–epilepsy syndrome in childhood. Report of 7 cases. *Neuropediatrics* **20**: 132–8.

Deonna T, Roulet E, Fontan D, Marcoz JP (1993) Speech and oromotor deficits of epileptic origin in benign partial epilepsy of childhood with rolandic spikes (BPERS). Relationship to the acquired aphasia–epilepsy syndrome. *Neuropediatrics* **24**: 83–7.

Depienne C, Arzimanoglou A, Trouillard O, et al. (2006) Parental mosaicism can cause recurrent transmission of SCN1A mutations associated with severe myoclonic epilepsy of infancy. *Hum Mutat* **27**: 389.

Deshmukh A, Wittert W, Schnitzler E, Mangurten HH (1986) Lorazepam in the treatment of refractory neonatal seizures: a pilot study. *Am J Dis Child* **140**: 1042–4.

de Silva M, MacArdle B, McGowan M, et al. (1996) Randomised comparative monotherapy trial of phenobarbitone, phenytoin, carbamazepine and sodium valproate for newly diagnosed childhood epilepsy. *Lancet* **347**: 709–13.

De Tiège X, Goldman S, Laureys S, et al. (2004) Regional cerebral glucose metabolism in epilepsies with continuous spikes and waves during sleep. *Neurology* **63**: 853–7.

DeToledo JC, Toledo C, DeCerce J, Ramsay RE (1997) Changes in body weight with chronic, high-dose gabapentin therapy. *Ther Drug Monit* **19**: 394–6.

Detre JA, Sirven JI, Alsop DC, et al. (1995) Localization of subclinical ictal activity by functional magnetic resonance imaging: correlation with invasive monitoring. *Ann Neurol* **38**: 618–24.

Devinsky O, Kelley K, Porter RJ, Theodore WH (1988) Clinical and electroencephalographic features of simple partial seizures. *Neurology* **38**: 1347–52.

Devinsky O, Perrine K, Vazquez B, et al. (1994) Multiple subpial transections in the language cortex. *Brain* **117**: 255–65.

De Vivo DC, Trifiletti RR, Jacobson RI, et al. (1991) Defective glucose transport across the blood–brain barrier as a cause of persistent hypoglycorrhachia, seizures and developmental delay. *N Engl J Med* **325**: 703–9.

Dieckmann RA (1994) Rectal diazepam for prehospital pediatric status epilepticus. *Ann Emerg Med* **23**: 216–24.

Diehl B, Najm I, Mohamed A, et al. (2002) Interictal EEG, hippocampal atrophy, and cell densities in hippocampal sclerosis and hippocampal sclerosis associated with microscopic cortical dysplasia. *J Clin Neurophysiol* **19**: 157–62.

Dieterich E, Doose H, Baier WK, Fichsel H (1985) Long-term follow-up of childhood epilepsy with absences. II: Absence epilepsy with initial grand mal. *Neuropediatrics* **16**: 155–8.

Di Mario FJ, Clancy RR (1988) Paradoxical precipitation of tonic seizures by lorazepam in a child with atypical absence seizures. *Pediatr Neurol* **4**: 249–51.

Dinesen H, Gram L, Andersen T, Dam M (1984) Weight gain during treatment with valproate. *Acta Neurol Scand* **70**: 65–9.

Dlugos DJ, Sammel MD, Strom BL, Farrar JT (2001) Response to first drug trial predicts outcome in childhood temporal lobe epilepsy. *Neurology* **57**: 2259–64.

Doberczak TM, Shanzer S, Cutler R, et al. (1988) One-year follow-up of infants with abstinence associated seizures. *Arch Neurol* **45**: 649–53.

Dobyns WB, Kuzniecky R (2006) Malformations of cortical development and epilepsy. In: Wyllie E, Gupta A, Lachhwani DK, eds. *The Treatment of Epilepsy*, 4th edn. Philadelphia: Lippincott, Williams & Wilkins, pp. 37–53.

Dodson WE, Pellock JM, eds. (1993) Pediatric Epilepsy: *Diagnosis and Therapy*. New York: Demos.

Donat JF, Wright FS (1991a) Seizures in series: similarities between seizures of the West and Lennox–Gastaut syndromes. *Epilepsia* **32**: 504–9.

Donat JF, Wright FS (1991b) Simultaneous infantile spasms and partial seizures. *J Child Neurol* **6**: 246–50.

Donat JF, Wright FS (1991c) Unusual variants of infantile spasms. *J Child Neurol* **6**: 313–8.

Donati F, Schäffler L, Vassella F (1995) Prolonged epileptic apneas in a newborn: a case report with ictal EEG recording. *Neuropediatrics* **26**: 223–5.

Dooley J, Gordon K, Camfield P, et al. (1996) Discontinuation of anticonvulsant therapy in children free of seizures for 1 year: a prospective study. *Neurology* **46**: 969–74.

Doose H (1992) Myoclonic astatic epilepsy of early childhood. In: Roger J, Bureau M, Dravet C, et al., eds. *Epileptic Syndromes in Infancy, Childhood and Adolescence. 2nd edn.* London: John Libbey, pp. 103–14.

Doose H, Baier WK (1987) Genetic factors in epilepsies with primarily generalized minor seizures. *Neuropediatrics* **18** Suppl 1: 1–64.

Doose H, Waltz S (1993) Photosensitivity—genetics and clinical significance. *Neuropediatrics* **24**: 249–55.

Doose H, Gerken H, Leonhardt R, et al. (1970) Centrencephalic myoclonic–astatic petit mal. Clinical and genetic investigation. *Neuropadiatrie* **2**: 59–78.

Dravet C, Bureau M (2005) Benign myoclonic epilepsy in infancy. Roger J, Bureau M, Dravet C, et al., eds. *Epileptic Syndromes in Infancy, Childhood and Adolescence. 4th edn.* London: John Libbey Eurotext, pp. 77–88.

Dravet C, Dalla Bernardina B, Mesdjian E, et al. (1980) [Paroxysmal dyskinesia during treatment with diphenylhydantoin.] *Rev Neurol* **136**: 1–14 (French).

Dravet C, Natale O, Magaudda A, et al. (1986) [Status epilepticus in the Lennox–Gastaut syndrome.] *Rev Electroencephalogr Neurophysiol Clin* **15**: 361–8 (French).

Dravet C, Bureau M, Roger J (1992) Benign myoclonic epilepsy in infants. In: Roger J, Bureau M, Dravet C, et al., eds. *Epileptic Syndromes in Infancy, Childhood and Adolescence, 2nd edn.* London: John Libbey, pp. 67–74.

Dravet C, Bureau M, Oguni H, et al. (2005) Severe myoclonic epilepsy in infancy (Dravet syndrome). In: Roger J, Bureau M, Dravet C, et al., eds. *Epileptic Syndromes in Infancy, Childhood and Adolescence. 4th edn.* London: John Libbey Eurotext, pp. 89–113.

Dreifuss F, Farwell J, Holmes G, et al. (1986) Infantile spasms: comparative trial of nitrazepam and corticotropin. *Arch Neurol* **43**: 1107–10.

Duchowny MS (1987) Complex partial seizures of infancy. *Arch Neurol* **44**: 911–4.

Duchowny MS (1992) The syndrome of partial seizures in infancy. *J Child Neurol* **7**: 66–9.

Duchowny MS, Harvey AS (1996) Pediatric epilepsy syndromes: an update and critical review. *Epilepsia* **37** Suppl 1: S26–40.

Duchowny MS, Jayakar P, Resnik T, et al. (1994) Posterior temporal epilepsy: electroclinical features. *Ann Neurol* **35**: 427–31.

Dulac O, Tuxhorn I (2005) Infantile spasms and West syndrome. In: Roger J, Bureau M, Dravet C, et al., eds. *Epileptic Syndromes in Infancy, Childhood and Adolescence. 4th edn.* London: John Libbey Eurotext, pp. 53–72.

Dulac O, Billard C, Arthuis M (1983) [Electroclinical and developmental aspects of epilepsy in the aphasia–epilepsy syndrome.] *Arch Fr Pediatr* **40**: 299–308 (French).

Duncan JS (1997) Imaging and epilepsy. *Brain* **120**: 339–77.

Du Plessis AJ, Kaufmann WE, Kupsky WJ (1993) Intrauterine-onset myoclonic encephalopathy associated with cerebral cortical dysgenesis. *J Child Neurol* **8**: 164–70.

Durner M (1994) Genetics of juvenile myoclonic epilepsy. In: Wolf P, ed. *Epileptic Seizures and Syndromes.* London: John Libbey, pp. 169–79.

Duron RM, Medina MT, Martinez-Suarez E, et al. (2005) Seizures of idiopathic generalized epilepsies. *Epilepsia* **46** Suppl 9: 34–47.

Ebach K, Joos H, Doose H, et al. (2005) SCN1A mutation analysis in myoclonic astatic epilepsy and severe idiopathic generalized epilepsy of infancy with generalized tonic clonic seizures. *Neuropediatrics* **36**: 210–3.

Ebersole JS, Hawes-Ebersole S (2007) Clinical application of dipole models in the localization of epileptiform activity. *J Clin Neurophysiol* **24**: 120–9.

Ebner A, Dinner DS, Noachtar S, Lüders H (1995) Automatisms with preserved responsiveness: a lateralizing sign in psychomotor seizures. *Neurology* **45**: 61–4.

Echenne B, Humbertclaude V, Rivier F, et al. (1994) Benign infantile epilepsy with autosomal dominant inheritance. *Brain Dev* **16**: 108–11.

Egger J, Brett EM (1981) Effects of sodium valproate in 100 children with special reference to weight *BMJ (Clin Res Ed)* **283**: 577–81.

Egli M, Mothersill I, O'Kane M, O'Kane F (1985) The axial spasm—the predominant type of drop seizure in patients with secondary generalized epilepsy. *Epilepsia* **26**: 401–15.

Ehrhardt P, Forsythe WI (1989) Prognosis after grand mal seizures: a study of 187 children with three-year remissions. *Dev Med Child Neurol* **31**: 633–9.

Engel J (1993) *Surgical Treatment of the Epilepsies, 2nd edn.* New York: Raven Press.

Engel J (1996) Surgery for seizures. *N Engl J Med* **334**: 647–52.

Engel J (2001) A proposed diagnostic scheme for people with epileptic seizures and with epilepsy: report of the ILAE Task Force on Classification and Terminology, International League Against Epilepsy (ILAE). *Epilepsia* 42: 796–803.

Engel J (2006) Report of the ILAE classification core group. *Epilepsia* 47: 1558–68.

Engel J, Pedley TA, eds. (2007) *Epilepsy: a Comprehensive Textbook, 2nd edn.* Philadelphia: Lippincott, Williams & Wilkins.

Engel J, Wiebe S, French J, et al. (2003) Practice parameter: temporal lobe and localized neocortical resections for epilepsy: report of the Quality Standards Subcommittee of the American Academy of Neurology, in association with the American Epilepsy Society and the American Association of Neurological Surgeons. *Neurology* 60: 538–47.

Erba G, Browne TR (1983) Atypical absence, myocloic, atonic and tonic seizures and the "Lennox–Gastaut syndrome". In: Browne TR, Feldman RG, eds. *Epilepsy: Diagnosis and Management.* Boston: Little Brown, pp. 75–94.

EURAP Study Group (2006) Seizure control and treatment in pregnancy: observations from the EURAP epilepsy pregnancy registry. *Neurology* 66: 354–60.

Farwell JR, Lee YJ, Hirtz DG, et al. (1990) Phenobarbital for febrile seizures: effects on intelligence and on seizure recurrence. *N Engl J Med* 322: 364–9.

Fauser S, Huppertz HJ, Bast T, et al. (2006) Clinical characteristics in focal cortical dysplasia: a retrospective evaluation in a series of 120 patients. *Brain* 129: 1907–16.

Fedi M, Reutens DC, Andermann F, et al. (2003) Alpha-[11C]-methyl-L-tryptophan PET identifies the epileptogenic tuber and correlates with interictal spike frequency. *Epilepsy Res* 52: 203–13.

Fejerman N, Di Blasi AM (1987) Status epilepticus of benign partial epilepsies in children: report of two cases. *Epilepsia* 28: 351–8.

Fejerman N, Caraballo R, Tenembaum SN (2000). Atypical evolutions of benign localization-related epilepsies in children: are they predictable? *Epilepsia* 41: 380–90.

Fernandez LB, Salas-Puig J (2007) Pure sleep seizures: risk of seizures while awake. *Epileptic Disord* 9: 65–70.

Fernandez-Alvarez E, Aicardi J (2001) *Movement Disorders in Children. International Review of Child Neurology Series.* London: Mac Keith Press for the International Child Neurology Association.

Fernández-Calvo C, Olascoaga J, Resano A, Urcola J, Tuneu A, Zubizarreta J (2000) [Lyell syndrome associated with lamotrigine.] *Rev Neurol* 31: 1162–4 (Spanish).

Ferrie CD (2005) Idiopathic generalized epilepsies imitating focal epilepsies. *Epilepsia* 46 Suppl 9: 91–5.

Ferrie CD, De Marco P, Grünewald RA, et al. (1994) Video game induced seizures. *J Neurol Neurosurg Psychiatry* 57: 925–31.

Ferrie CD, Giannakodimos S, Robinson RO, Panayiotopoulos CP (1995) Symptomatic typical absence seizures. In: Duncan JC, Panayiotopoulos CP, eds. *Typical Absences and Related Epileptic Syndromes.* London: Churchill Communications Europe, pp. 241–52.

Ferrie CD, Beaumanoir A, Guerrini R, et al. (1997) Early-onset benign occipital seizure susceptibility syndrome. *Epilepsia* 38: 285–93.

Ferrie CD, Koutroumanidis M, Rowlinson S, et al. (2002) Atypical evolution of Panayiotopoulos syndrome: a case report. *Epileptic Disord* 4: 35–42.

Fiol ME, Leppik IE, Pretzel K (1986) Eating epilepsy: EEG and clinical study. *Epilepsia* 27: 441–5.

First Seizure Trial Group (1993) Randomized clinical trial on the efficacy of antiepileptic drugs in reducing the risk of relapse after a first unprovoked tonic–clonic seizure. *Neurology* 43: 478–83.

Fogarasi A, Janszky J, Faveret E, et al. (2001) A detailed analysis of frontal lobe seizure semiology in children younger than 7 years. *Epilepsia* 42: 80–5.

Fogarasi A, Jokeit H, Faveret E, et al. (2002) The effect of age on seizure semiology in childhood temporal lobe epilepsy. *Epilepsia* 43: 638–43.

Fogarasi A, Tuxhorn I, Hegyi M, Janszky J (2005) Predictive clinical factors for the differential diagnosis of childhood extratemporal seizures. *Epilepsia* 46: 1280–5.

Fohlen M, Lellouch A, Delalande O (2003) Hypothalamic hamartoma with refractory epilepsy: surgical procedures and results in 18 patients. *Epileptic Disord* 5: 267–73.

Forsgren L, Edvinsson SO, Blomquist HK, et al. (1990) Epilepsy in a population of mentally retarded children and adults. *Epilepsy Res* 6: 234–48.

Forsythe WI, Sills MA (1984) One drug for childhood grand mal: medical audit for three-year remissions. *Dev Med Child Neurol* 26: 742–8.

Francione S, Vigliano P, Tassi L, et al. (2003) Surgery for drug resistant partial

epilepsy in children with focal cortical dysplasia: anatomical–clinical correlations and neurophysiological data in 10 patients. *J Neurol Neurosurg Psychiatry* 74: 1493–501.

Freeman JM, Kelly MT, Freeman J (1994) *The Epilepsy Diet Treatment: an Introduction to the Ketogenic Diet.* New York: Demos Vermande.

Freeman JM, Kossoff EH, Hartman AL (2007) The ketogenic diet: one decade later. *Pediatrics* 119: 535–43.

Freilinger M, Reisel B, Reiter E, et al. (2006) Behavioral and emotional problems in children with epilepsy. *J Child Neurol* 21: 939–45.

Fuerst D, Shah J, Shah A, Watson C (2003) Hippocampal sclerosis is a progressive disorder: a longitudinal volumetric MRI study. *Ann Neurol* 53: 413–6.

Fujii T, Okuno T, Go T, et al. (1987) Clorazepate therapy for intractable epilepsy. *Brain Dev* 9: 288–91.

Fujiwara T, Sugawara T, Mazaki-Miyazaki E, et al. (2003) Mutations in the sodium channel alpha subunit type 1 (SNC1A) in intractable epilepsies with frequent tonic–clonic seizures. *Brain* 126: 531–46.

Fukuma G, Oguni H, Shirasaka Y, et al. (2004) Mutations of neuronal voltage-gated Na+ channel alpha 1 subunit gene SCN1A in core severe myoclonic epilepsy in infancy (SMEI) and in borderline SMEI (SMEB). *Epilepsia* 45: 140–8.

Fusco L, Iani C, Faedda MT, et al. (1990) Mesial frontal lobe epilepsy: a clinical entity not sufficiently described. *J Epilepsy* 3: 123–35.

Fusco L, Bertini E, Vigevano F (1992) Epilepsia partialis continua and neuronal migration anomalies. *Brain Dev* 14: 323–8.

Gaggero R, Caputo M, Fiorio P, et al. (1995) SPECT and epilepsy with continuous spike waves during slow-wave sleep. *Childs Nerv Syst* 11: 154–60.

Gaillard WD (2006) Metabolic and functional neuroimaging. In: Wyllie E, Gupta A, Lachhwani DK, eds. *The Treatment of Epilepsy, 4th edn.* Philadelphia: Lippincott, Williams & Wilkins, pp. 1041–58.

Gaily EK, Shewmon DA, Chugani HT, Curran JG (1995) Asymmetric and asynchronous infantile spasms. *Epilepsia* 36: 873–82.

Gaily E, Appelqvist K, Kantola-Sorsa E, et al. (1999) Cognitive deficits after cryptogenic infantile spasms with benign seizure evolution. *Dev Med Child Neurol* 41: 660–4.

Gallassi R, Morreale A, Lorusso S, et al. (1988) Epilepsy presenting as memory disturbances. *Epilepsia* 29: 624–9.

Gardiner M (2005) Genetics of idiopathic generalized epilepsies. *Epilepsia* 46 Suppl 9: 15–20.

Garg BP, Patel H, Markand ON (1995) Clinical correlation of periodic lateralized epileptiform discharges in children. *Pediatr Neurol* 12: 225–9.

Gastaut H (1973) *Dictionary of Epilepsies. Part I: Definitions.* Geneva: World Health Organization.

Gastaut H (1982) A new type of epilepsy: benign partial epilepsy of childhood with occipital spike–waves. *Clin Electroencephalogr* 13: 12–22.

Gastaut H, Zifkin BG (1988) Secondary bilateral synchrony and Lennox–Gastaut syndrome. In: Niedermeyer E, Degen R, eds. *The Lennox–Gastaut Syndrome.* New York: Alan R Liss, pp. 221–42.

Gastaut H, Poirier F, Payan H, et al. (1960) HHE syndrome: hemiconvulsions–hemiplegia–epilepsy. *Epilepsia* 1: 418–47.

Gastaut H, Santanelli PK, Salinas Jara M (1985) Une activité EEG intercritique spécifique d'une variété particulière d'épilepsie temporale. Le rythme théta temporal épileptique. *Rev Electroencephalogr Neurophysiol Clin* 15: 113–20.

Gastaut H, Aguglia U, Tinuper P (1986) Benign versive or circling epilepsy with bilateral 3-cps spike-and-wave discharges in late childhood. *Ann Neurol* 19 : 301–3.

Genton P, Salas Puig X, Tunon A, et al. (1994) Juvenile myoclonic epilepsy and related syndromes: clinical and neurophysiological aspects. In: Malafosse A, Genton P, Hirsch E, et al., eds. *Idiopathic Generalized Epilepsies.* London: John Libbey, pp. 253–65.

Genton P, Gonzalez-Sanchez M, Thomas P (2005) Epilepsy with grand mal on awakening. In: Roger J, Bureau M, Dravet C, et al. (eds) *Epileptic Syndromes in Infancy, Childhood and Adolescence. 4th edn.* Montrouge: John Libbey Eurotext, pp. 389–94.

Gerber PE, Hamiwka L, Connolly MB, Farrell K (2000) Factors associated with behavioral and cognitive abnormalities in children receiving topiramate. *Pediatr Neurol* 22: 200–3.

Gilbert DL. Buncher CR (2000) An EEG should not be obtained routinely after first unprovoked seizure in childhood. *Neurology* 54: 635–41.

Gilchrist JM (1985) Arrhythmogenic seizures: diagnosis by simultaneous EEG/ECG recording. *Neurology* 35: 1503–6.

Gilhus NE, Matre R (1986) Carbamazepine effects on mononuclear blood cells in epileptic patients. *Acta Neurol Scand* 74: 181–5.

Gilliam F, Wyllie E, Kashden J, et al. (1997) Epilepsy surgery outcome: Comprehensive assessment in children. *Neurology* 48: 1368–74.

Gilman JT, Duchowny M, Jayakar P, Resnick TJ (1994) Medical intractability in children evaluated for epilepsy surgery. *Neurology* 44: 1341–3.

Glauser TA, Morita DA (2001) Encephalopathic epilepsy after infancy. In: Pedlock JM, Dodson WE, Bourgeois B, eds. *Pediatric Epilepsy: Diagnosis and Therapy.* New York: Demos, p. 201–18.

Glaze DG, Hrachovy RA, Frost JD, et al. (1988) Prospective study of outcome of infants with infantile spasms treated during controlled studies of ACTH and prednisone. *J Pediatrics* 112: 389–96.

Gloor P (1986) Consciousness as a neurological concept in epileptology: a critical review. *Epilepsia* 27 Suppl 2: S14–26.

Gloor P, Fariello RG (1988) Generalized epilepsy: some of its cellular mechanisms differ from those of focal epilepsy. *Trends Neurosci* 11: 63–8.

Gobbi G (2005) Coeliac disease, epilepsy and cerebral calcifications. *Brain Dev* 27: 189–200.

Gobbi G, Guerrini R (1998) Childhood epilepsy with occipital spikes and other benign localization-related epilepsies. In: Engel J, Pedley TA, eds. *Epilepsy: A Comprehensive Textbook, vol. 3.* New York: Lippincott-Raven, pp. 2315–26.

Gobbi G, Bruno L, Pini A, et al. (1987) Periodic spasms: an unclassified type of epileptic seizure in childhood. *Dev Med Child Neurol* 29: 766–75.

Gobbi G, Sorrenti G, Santucci M, et al. (1988) Epilepsy with bilateral occipital calcifications: a benign onset with progressive severity. *Neurology* 38: 913–20.

Gobbi G, Tassinari CA, Roger J, et al. (1989) [Electrencephalographic findings in severe symptomatic partial epilepsies in childhood.] *Neurophysiol Clin* 19: 209–18 (French).

Goh S, Kwiatkowski DJ, Dorer DJ, Thiele EA (2005) Infantile spasms and intellectual outcomes in children with tuberous sclerosis complex. *Neurology* 65: 235–8.

Goodridge DMG, Shorvon SD (1983) Epileptic seizures in a population of 6000. *BMJ* 287: 641–7.

Gorman DG, Shields WD, Shewmon DA, et al. (1992) Neurosurgical treatment of refractory status epilepticus. *Epilepsia* 33: 546–9.

Graf WD, Chatrian GE, Glass ST, Knauss TA (1994) Video game-related seizures: a report on 10 patients and a review of the literature. *Pediatrics* 93: 551–6.

Green SM, Rothrock SG, Clem KS, et al. (1993) Can seizures be the sole manifestation of meningitis in febrile children? *Pediatrics* 92: 527–34.

Greenberg DA, Delgado-Escueta AV, Maldonado HM, Widelitz H (1988) Segregation analysis of juvenile myoclonic epilepsy. *Genet Epidemiol* 5: 81–94.

Grondin R, Chuang S, Otsubo H, et al. (2006) The role of magnetoencephalography in pediatric epilepsy surgery. *Childs Nerv Syst* 22: 779–85.

Gross-Selbeck G (1995) Treatment of "benign" partial epilepsies of childhood, including atypical forms. *Neuropediatrics* 26: 45–50

Guerrini R (2006) Epilepsy in children. *Lancet* 367: 499–524.

Guerrini R, Aicardi J (2003) Epileptic encephalopathies with myoclonic seizures in infants and children (severe myoclonic epeilpesy and myoclonic astatic epilepsy). *J Clin Neurophysiol* 20: 449–51.

Guerrini R, Carrozzo R (2001) Epilepsy and genetic malformations of the cerebral cortex. *Am J Med Genet* 106: 160–73.

Guerrini R, Filippi T (2005) Neuronal migration disorders, genetics, and epileptogenesis. *J Child Neurol* 20: 287–99.

Guerrini R, Dravet C, Gobbi G, et al. (1994a) Idiopathic generalized epilepsies with myoclonus in infancy and childhood. In: Malafosse A, Genton P, Hirsch F, et al., eds. *Idiopathic Generalized Epilepsies: Clinical, Experimental and Genetic Aspects.* London: John Libbey, pp. 267–80.

Guerrini R, Ferrari AR, Battaglia A, et al. (1994b) Occipitotemporal seizures with ictus emeticus induced by intermittent photic stimulation. *Neurology* 44: 253–9.

Guerrini R, Dravet C, Genton P, et al. (1995) Idiopathic photosensitive occipital lobe epilepsy. *Epilepsia* 36: 883–91.

Guerrini R, Andermann F, Canapicchi R, et al., eds. (1996) *Dysplasias of Cerebral Cortex and Epilepsy.* New York: Lippincott–Raven.

Guerrini R, Belmonte A, Genton P (1998a) Antiepileptic drug-induced worsening of seizures in children. *Epilepsia* 39 Suppl 3: S2–10.

Guerrini R, Dravet C, Genton P, et al. (1998b) Lamotrigine and seizure aggravation in severe myoclonic epilepsy. *Epilepsia* 39: 508–12.

Guerrini R, Genton P, Bureau M, et al. (1998c) Multilobar polymicrogyria, intractable drop attack seizures and sleep-related electrical status epilepticus. *Neurology* 51: 504–12.

Guerrini R, Bonanni P, Nardocci N, et al. (1999) Autosomal recessive rolandic epilepsy with paroxysmal exercise-induced dystonia and writer's cramp: delineation of the syndrome and gene mapping to chromosome 16p12–11.2. *Ann Neurol* 45: 344–52.

Guerrini R, Sicca F, Parmeggiani L (2003) Epilepsy and malformations of the cerebral cortex. *Epileptic Disord* 5 Suppl 2: S9–26.

Guerrini R, Sicca F, Parmeggiani L (2005) Genetic malformations of the cerebral cortex and epilepsy. *Epilepsia* 46 Suppl 1: 32–7.

Guzzetta F, Crisafulli A, Isaya Crinó M (1993) Cognitive assessment of infants with West syndrome: how useful is it for diagnosis and prognosis? *Dev Med Child Neurol* 35: 379–87.

Guzzetta F, Frisone MF, Ricci D, et al. (2002) Development of visual attention in West syndrome. *Epilepsia* 43: 1106–9.

Guzzetta F, Battaglia D, Veredice C, et al. (2005) Early thalamic injury with epliepsy and continuous spike–wave during slow sleep. *Epilepsia* 46: 889–900.

Guzzetta F, Dalla Bernardina B, Guerrini R (2007) *Progress in Epileptic Spasms and West Syndrome. Progress in Epileptic Disorders, vol. 4.* Paris: John Libbey Eurotext.

Haga Y, Watanabe K, Negoro T, et al. (1995) Do ictal, clinical, and electroencephalographic features predict outcome in West syndrome? *Pediatr Neurol* 13: 226–9.

Hahn A (2000) Atypical benign partial epilepsy/pseudo-Lennox syndrome. *Epileptic Disord* 2 Suppl 1: S23–8.

Hahn A, Pistohl J, Neubauer BA, Stephani U (2001) Atypical 'benign' partial epilepsy or pseudo-Lennox syndrome. Part 1: Symptomatology and long-term prognosis. *Neuropediatrics* 32: 1–8.

Hakeem VF, Wallace SJ (1990) EEG monitoring of therapy for neonatal seizures. *Dev Med Child Neurol* 32: 858–64.

Hammoudi DS, Lee SS, Madison G, et al. (2005) Reduced visual function associated with infantile spasms on vigabatrin. *Invest Ophthalmol Vis Sci* 46: 514–20.

Hancock E, Cross H (2003) Treatment of Lennox–Gastaut syndrome. *Cochrane Database Syst Rev* (3): CD003277.

Hancock E, Osborne J, Milner P (2003) Treatment of infantile spasms. *Cochrane Database Syst Rev* (3): CD001770.

Harding BN, Boyd SG (1991) Intractable seizures from infancy can be associated with dentato-olivary dysplasia. *J Neurol Sci* 104: 157–65.

Harding BN, Copp JA (1997) Malformations. In: Graham DL, Lantos PL, eds. *Greenfield's Neuropathology, 6th edn.* London: Arnold, pp. 397–533.

Harding GFA, Jeavons PM (1994) *Photosensitive Epilepsy. New Edition. Clinics in Developmental Medicine no. 133.* London: Mac Keith Press.

Harkin LA, McMahon JM, Iona X, et al. (2007) The spectrum of SCN1A-related infantile epileptic encephalopathies. *Brain* 130: 843–52.

Hart Y (2004) Rasmussen's encephalitis. *Epileptic Disord* 6: 133–44.

Hart YM, Cortez M, Andermann F, et al. (1994) Medical treatment of Rasmussen's syndrome (chronic encephalitis and epilepsy): effect of high-dose steroids or immunoglobulins in 19 patients. *Neurology* 44: 1030–6.

Hart YM, Andermann F, Fish DN, et al. (1997) Chronic encephalitis and epilepsy in adults and adolescents. *Neurology* 48: 418–24.

Harvey AS, Bowe JM, Hopkins IJ, et al. (1993a) Ictal 99mTc-HMPAO single photon emission computed tomography in children with temporal lobe epilepsy. *Epilepsia* 34: 869–77.

Harvey AS, Hopkins IJ, Bowe JM, et al. (1993b) Frontal lobe epilepsy: clinical seizure characteristics and localization with ictal 99mTc-HMPAO SPECT. *Neurology* 43: 1966–80.

Harvey AS, Nolan T, Carlin JB (1993c) Community-based study of mortality in children with epilepsy. *Epilepsia* 34: 597–603.

Harvey AS, Grattan-Smith JD, Desmond PM, et al. (1995) Febrile seizures and hippocampal sclerosis: frequent and related findings in intractable temporal lobe epilepsy of childhood. *Pediatr Neurol* 12: 201–6.

Harvey AS, Jayakar P, Duchowny M, et al. (1996) Hemifacial seizures and cerebellar ganglioglioma: an epilepsy syndrome of infancy with seizures of cerebellar origin. *Ann Neurol* 40: 91–8.

Hauser WA (1983) Status epilepticus: frequency, etiology, and neurological considerations *Adv Neurol* 34: 3–14.

Hauser WA (1992) Seizure disorders: the changes with age. *Epilepsia* 33 Suppl 4: S6–14.

Hauser WA (1994) The prevalence and incidence of convulsive disorders in children. *Epilepsia* 35 Suppl 2: S1–6.

Haut SR, O'Dell C, Shinnar S (2007) Risk factors for developing epilepsy after a first unprovoked seizure. In: Ryvlin P, Beghi E, Camfield P, Hesdorffer

D, eds. *From First Unprovoked Seizure to Newly Diagnosed Epilepsy. Progress in Epileptic Disorders, vol. 3.* Paris: John Libbey Eurotext, pp. 37–48.

Heijbel J, Blom S, Bergfors PG (1980) Simple febrile convulsions. A prospective incidence study and an evaluation of investigations initially needed. *Neuropediatrics* 11: 45–56.

Heiskala H, Riikonen R, Santavuori P, et al. (1996) West syndrome: individualized ACTH therapy. *Brain Dev* 18: 456–60.

Hellström-Westas L, Blennow G, Lindroth M (1995) Low-risk of seizure recurrence after early withdrawal of anti-epileptic treatment in the neonatal period. *Arch Dis Child* 72: 97–101.

Henry TR, Drury I, Brunberg JA, et al. (1994) Focal cerebral magnetic resonance changes associated with partial status epilepticus. *Epilepsia* 35: 35–41.

Hermann BP (1982) Neuropsychological functioning and psychopathology in children with epilepsy. *Epilepsia* 23: 545–54.

Hermann B, Seidenberg M (2007) Epilepsy and cognition. *Epilepsy Curr* 7: 1–6.

Heron SE, Crossland KM, Andermann E, et al. (2002) Sodium-channel defects in benign familial neonatal–infantile seizures. *Lancet* 360: 851–2.

Heron SE, Scheffer IE, Berkovic SF, et al. (2007) Channelopathies in idiopathic epilepsy. *Neurotherapeutics* 4: 295–304.

Herranz JL, Armijo JA, Arteaga R (1988) Clinical side effects of phenobarbital, primidone, phenytoin, carbamazepine, and valproate during monotherapy in children. *Epilepsia* 29: 794–804.

Hewertson J, Poets CF, Samuels MP, et al. (1994) Epileptic seizure-induced hypoxemia in infants presenting with apparent life-threatening events. *Pediatrics* 94: 148–56.

Hewertson J, Boyd SG, Samuels MP, et al. (1996) Hypoxaemia and cardiorespiratory changes during epileptic seizures in young children. *Dev Med Child Neurol* 38: 511–22.

Hirose S, Mitsudome A, Okada M, et al. (2005) Genetics of idiopathic epilepsies. *Epilepsia* 46 Suppl 1: 38–43.

Hirsch E, Arzimanoglou A (2004) [Children with drug-resistant partial epilepsy: criteria for the identification of surgical candidates.] *Rev Neurol* 160 Spec No 1: 5S210-9 (French).

Hirsch E, Panayiotopoulos CP (2005) Childhood absence epilepsy and related syndromes. In: Roger J, Bureau M, Dravet C, et al., eds. *Epileptic Syndromes in Infancy, Childhood and Adolescence. 4th edn.* London: John Libbey Eurotext, pp. 315–35.

Hirsch E, Marescaux C, Maquet P, et al. (1990) Landau–Kleffner syndrome: a clinical and EEG study of five cases. *Epilepsia* 31: 756–67.

Hirsch E, Velez A, Sellal F, et al. (1993) Electroclinical signs of benign neonatal familial convulsions. *Ann Neurol* 34: 835–41.

Hirsch E, Maquet P, Metz-Lutz MN, et al. (1995) The eponym 'Landau–Kleffner syndrome' should not be restricted to childhood-acquired aphasia with epilepsy. In: Beaumanoir A, Bureau M, Deonna T, et al., eds. *Continuous Spikes and Waves During Slow Sleep. Electrical Status Epilepticus During Slow Sleep. Acquired Epileptic Aphasia and Related Conditions. Mariani Foundation Paediatric Neurology Series no. 3.* London: John Libbey, pp. 57–64.

Hirsch E, Andermann F, Chauvel P, et al., eds. (2006a) *Generalized Seizures: From Clinical Phenomenology to Underlying Systems and Networks. Progress in Epileptic Disorders no. 2.* Paris: John Libbey Eurotext.

Hirsch E, Valenti MP, Rudolf G, et al. (2006b) Landau–Kleffner syndrome is not an eponymic badge of ignorance. *Epilepsy Res* 70 Suppl 1: S239–47.

Hirtz D, Ashwal S, Berg A, et al. (2000) Practice parameter: evaluating a first nonfebrile seizure in children. *Neurology* 55: 616–23.

Ho SS, Berkovic SF, Newton MR, et al. (1994) Parietal lobe epilepsy: clinical features and seizure localization by ictal SPECT. *Neurology* 44: 2277–84.

Holden KR, Mellits ED, Freeman JM (1982) Neonatal seizures. I: Correlation of prenatal and perinatal events with outcomes. *Pediatrics* 70: 165–76.

Holmes GL (1985) Neonatal seizures. In: Pedley TA, Meldrum BS, eds. *Recent Advances in Epilepsy, vol. 1.* Edinburgh: Churchill Livingstone, pp. 207–37.

Holmes GL (1986) Partial seizures in children. *Pediatrics* 77: 725–31.

Holmes GL (1997) Epilepsy in the developing brain: lesions from the laboratory and clinic. *Epilepsia* 38: 12–30.

Holmes GL (2002) Seizure-induced neuronal injury: animal data. *Neurology* 59 Suppl 5: S3–6.

Holmes GL, Russman BS (1986) Shuddering attacks: evaluation using electroencephalographic frequency modulation radiotelemetry and videotape monitoring. *Am J Dis Child* 140: 72–3.

Holthausen H (1994) Febrile convulsions, mesial temporal sclerosis and temporal lobe epilepsy. In: Wolf P, ed. *Epileptic Seizures and Syndromes.* London: John Libbey, pp. 449–67.

Hommet C, Billard C, Barthez MA, et al. (2000) Continuous spikes and waves during slow sleep (CSWS): outcome in adulthood. *Epileptic Disord* 2: 107–12.

Honda K, Shinomiya N, Nomura Y, et al. (1985) Effects of neurosurgical treatment on diffuse slow spike and wave complex: a case of left frontal mass lesion with diffuse slow spike and wave complex (DSSW). *Brain Dev* 7: 496–9.

Hrachovy RA, Frost JD, Glaze DG (1994) High-dose, long-duration versus low-dose, short-duration corticotropin therapy for infantile spasms. *J Pediatr* 124: 803–6.

Hunt S, Craig J, Russell A, et al. (2006) Levetiracetam in pregnancy: preliminary experience from the UK Epilepsy and Pregnancy Register. *Neurology* 67: 1876–9.

Hyland K, Buist NRM, Powell SR (1995) Folinic acid responsive seizures: a new syndrome? *J Inherit Metab Dis* 18: 177–81.

Iinuma K, Yanai K, Yanagisawa T, et al. (1987) Cerebral glucose metabolism in five patients with Lennox–Gastaut syndrome. *Pediatr Neurol* 3: 12–8.

Ikeno T, Shigematsu H, Miyakoshi M, et al. (1985) An analytic study of epileptic falls. *Epilepsia* 26: 612–21.

Imai K, Otani K, Yanagihara K, et al. (1999) Ictal video–EEG recording of three partial seizures in a patient with the benign infantile convulsions associated with mild gastroenteritis. *Epilepsia* 40: 1455–8.

Inoue Y, Fujiwara T, Matsuda K, et al. (1997) Ring chromosome 20 and nonconvulsive status epilepticus. A new epileptic syndrome. *Brain* 120: 939–53.

Ishii K, Oguni H, Hayashi K, et al. (2002) Clinical study of catastrophic infantile epilepsy with focal seizures. *Pediatr Neurol* 27: 369–77.

Ito M, Ohmori I, Nakahori T, et al. (2005) Mutation screen of GABRA1, GABRA2 ahd GABRG2 gene in Japanese patients with absence seizures. *Neurosci Lett* 383: 220–4.

Itomi K, Okumura A, Negoro T, et al. (2002) Prognostic value of positron emission tomography in cryptogenic West syndrome. *Dev Med Child Neurol* 44: 107–11.

Jackson GD, Berkovic SF, Tress BM, et al. (1990) Hippocampal sclerosis can be reliably detected by magnetic resonance imaging. *Neurology* 40: 1869–75.

Jansen FE, van Huffelen AC, Algra A, van Nieuwenhuizen O (2007) Epilepsy surgery in tuberous sclerosis: a systematic review. *Epilepsia* 48: 1477–84.

Janz D (1989) Juvenile myoclonic epilepsy—epilepsy with impulsive petit mal. *Cleve Clin J Med* 56 Suppl: S23–33.

Janz D (1994) Pitfalls in the diagnosis of grand mal on awakening. In: Wolf P, ed. *Epileptic Seizures and Syndromes.* London: John Libbey, pp. 213–20.

Janz D, Beck-Mannagetta G, Spröder B, Waltz S (1994) Childhood absence epilepsy (pyknolepsy) and juvenile absence epilepsy: one or two syndromes? In: Wolf P, ed. *Epileptic Seizures and Syndromes.* London: John Libbey, pp. 115–26.

Jawad S, Oxley J, Wilson J, Richens A (1986) A pharmacodynamic evaluation of midazolam as an antiepileptic compound. *J Neurol Neurosurg Psychiatry* 49: 1050–4.

Jayakar P, Seshia SS (1991) Electrical status epilepticus during slow-wave sleep: a review. *J Clin Neurophysiol* 8: 299–311.

Jeavons PM (1982) Myoclonic epilepsies: therapy and prognosis. In: Akimoto H, Kazamatsuri H, Seino M, Ward AA, eds. *Advances in Epileptology. XIIIth Epilepsy International Symposium.* New York: Raven Press, pp. 141–4.

Jeavons PM (1983) Non-epileptic attacks in childhood. In: Rose FC, ed. *Research Progress in Epilepsy.* London: Pitman, pp. 224–30.

Jensen FE (1999) Acute and chronic effects of seizures in the developing brain: experimental models. *Epilepsia* 40 Suppl 1: S51–8; discussion S64–6.

Johnston MV (1996) Developmental aspects of epileptogenesis. *Epilepsia* 37 Suppl 1: S2–9.

Jonas R, Asarnow RF, LoPresti C, et al. (2005) Surgery for symptomatic infant-onset epileptic encephalopathy with and without infantile spasms. *Neurology* 64: 746–50.

Jones SW (2006) Basic cellular neurophysiology. In: Wyllie E, Gupta A, Lachhwani DK, eds. *The Treatment of Epilepsy, 4th edn.* Philadelphia: Lippincott, Williams & Wilkins, pp. 67–89.

Joyce RP, Gunderson CH (1980) Carbamazepine-induced orofacial dyskinesia. *Neurology* 30: 1333–4.

Juhasz C, Chugani DC, Muzik O, et al. (2003) Alpha-methyl-L-tryptophan PET detects epileptogenic cortex in chidren with intractable epilepsy. *Neurology* 60: 960–8.

Juul-Jensen P (1968) Frequency of recurrence after discontinuance of anticonvulsant therapy in patients with epileptic seizures. A new follow-up study after 5 years. *Epilepsia* 9: 11–6.

Kagawa K, Chugani DC, Asano E, et al. (2005) Epilepsy surgical outcome in children with tuberous sclerosis complex evaluated with alpha-[11c]methyl-L-tryptophan positron emission tomography (PET). *J Child Neurol* **20**: 429–38.

Kahane P, Ryvlin P, Hoffmann D, et al. (2003) From hypothalamic hamartoma to cortex: what can be learnt from depth recordings and stimulation? *Epileptic Disord* **5**: 205–17.

Kahane P, Arzimanoglou A, Bureau M, Roger J (2005) Non-idiopathic partial epilepsies of childhood. In: Roger J, Bureau M, Dravet C, et al., eds. *Epileptic Syndromes in Infancy, Childhood and Adolescence. 4th edn.* London: John Libbey Eurotext, pp. 255–75.

Kajitani T, Ueoka K, Nakamura M, Kumanomidou Y (1981) Febrile convulsions and rolandic discharges. *Brain Dev* **3**: 351–9.

Kaminska A, Ickowicz A, Plouin P, et al. (1999) Delineation of cryptogenic Lennox–Gastaut syndrome and myoclonic astatic epilepsy using multiple correspondence analysis. *Epilepsy Res* **36**: 15–29.

Kaminska A, Moutard ML, Plouin P, Soufflet C (2005) *L'EEG en Pédiatrie.* Paris: John Libbey Eurotext.

Kang HC, Jung da E, Kim KM, et al. (2006) Surgical treatment of two patients with infantile spasms in early infancy. *Brain Dev* **28**: 453-7.

Karas BJ, Wilder BJ, Hammond EJ, Bauman AW (1982) Valproate tremors. *Neurology* **32**: 428–32.

Kasteleijn-Nolst Trenité DG, Bakker DJ, Binnie CD, et al. (1988) Psychological effects of subclinical epileptiform EEG discharges. I: Scholastic skills. *Epilepsy Res* **2**: 111–6.

Kasteleijn-Nolst Trenité DG, Siebelink BM, Berends SGC, et al. (1990) Lateralized effects of subclinical epileptiform EEG discharges on scholastic performance in children. *Epilepsia* **31**: 740–6.

Kasteleijn-Nolst Trenité DG, Martins de Silva A, Ricci S, et al. (2002) Video games are exciting; a European study of video game-induced seizures and eplepsy. *Epileptic Disord* **4**: 121–8.

Kaufman DW, Kelly JP, Anderson T, et al. (1997) Evaluation of case reports of aplastic anemia among patients treated with felbamate. *Epilepsia* **38**: 1265–9.

Kearns GL, Abdel-Rahman SM, Alander SW, et al. (2003) Developmental pharmacology—drug disposition, action, and therapy in infants and children. *N Engl J Med* **349**: 1157–67.

Kellinghaus C, Lüders HO (2004) Frontal lobe epilepsy. *Epileptic Disord* **6**: 223–39.

Kikumoto K, Yoshinaga H, Oka M, et al. (2006) EEG and seizure exacerbation induced by carbamazepine in Panayiotopoulos syndrome. *Epileptic Disord* **8**: 53–6.

King MA, Newton MR, Jackson GD, et al. (1998) Epileptology of first seizure presentation: a clinical, electroencephalographic and magnetic resonance imaging study of 300 consecutive patients. *Lancet* **352**: 1007–11.

Kinsman SL, Vining EPG, Quaskey SA, et al. (1992) Efficacy of the ketogenic diet for intractable seizure disorders: review of 58 cases. *Epilepsia* **33**: 1132–6.

Kiok MC, Terrence CF, Fromm GH, Lavine S (1986) Sinus arrest in epilepsy. *Neurology* **36**: 115–6.

Kivity S, Lerman P (1992) Stormy onset prolonged loss of consciousness in benign childhood epilepsy with occipital paroxysms. *J Neurol Neurosurg Psychiatry* **55**: 45–8.

Knake S, Grant PE (2006) Magnetic resonance imaging techniques in the evaluation of epilepsy surgery. In: Wyllie E, Gupta A, Lachhwani DK, eds. *The Treatment of Epilepsy, 4th edn.* Philadelphia: Lippincott, Williams & Wilkins, pp. 1009–29.

Knudsen FU (1996) Febrile seizures: treatment and outcome. *Brain Dev* **18**: 438–49.

Knudsen FU, Paerregaard A, Andersen R, Andresen J (1996) Long term outcome of prophylaxis for febrile convulsions. *Arch Dis Child* **74**: 13–8.

Komori H, Wada M, Eto M, et al. (1995) Benign convulsions with mild gastroenteritis: a report of 10 recent cases detailing clinical varieties. *Brain Dev* **17**: 334–7.

Kondo Y, Okumura A, Watanabe K, et al. (2005) Comparison of two low dose ACTH therapies for West syndrome: their efficacy and side effect. *Brain Dev* **27**: 326–30.

Konishi Y, Yasujima M, Kuriyama M, et al. (1992) Magnetic resonance imaging in infantile spasms: effects of hormone therapy. *Epilepsia* **33**: 304–9.

Koo B, Hwang PA, Logan WJ (1993) Infantile spasms: outcome and prognostic factors of cryptogenic and symptomatic groups. *Neurology* **43**: 2322–7.

Koponen A, Seppälä U, Eriksson K, et al. (2007) Social functioning and psychological well-being of 347 young adults with epilepsy only—population-based, controlled study from Finland. *Epilepsia* **48**: 907–12.

Korff CM, Nordli DR (2006) The clinical–electrographic expression of infantile seizures. *Epilepsy Res* **70** Suppl 1: S116–31.

Kossoff EH, McGrogan JR, Bluml RM, et al. (2006) A modified Atkins diet is effective for the treatment of intractable pediatric epilepsy. *Epilepsia* **47**: 421–4.

Kossoff EH, Turner Z, Bergey GK (2007) Home-guided use of the ketogenic diet in a patient for more than 20 years. *Pediatr Neurol* **36**: 424–5.

Kotagal P, Rothner AD, Erenberg G, et al. (1987) Complex partial seizures of childhood onset. *Arch Neurol* **44**: 1177–80.

Kotagal P, Lüders H, Morris HH, et al. (1989) Dystonic posturing in complex partial seizures of temporal lobe onset: a new lateralizing sign. *Neurology* **39**: 196–201.

Kothare SV, Kaleyias J (2007) The adverse effects of antiepileptic drugs in children. *Expert Opin Drug Saf* **6**: 251–65.

Kramer RE, Lüders H, Lesser RP, et al. (1987) Transient focal abnormalities of neuroimaging studies during focal status epilepticus. *Epilepsia* **28**: 528–32.

Kramer RE, Lüders H, Goldstick LP, et al. (1988) Ictus emeticus: an electro-clinical analysis. *Neurology* **38**: 1048–52.

Kroll JS (1985) Pyridoxine for neonatal seizures: an unexpected danger. *Dev Med Child Neurol* **27**: 377–9.

Kröll-Seger J, Portilla P, Dulac O, Chiron C (2006) Topiramate in the treatment of highly refractory patients with Dravet syndrome. *Neuropediatrics* **37**: 325–9.

Kuks JBM, Cook MJ, Fish DR, et al. (1993) Hippocampal sclerosis in epilepsy and childhood febrile seizures. *Lancet* **342**: 1391–4.

Kurokawa T, Fung KC, Hanai T, Goya N (1982) Mortality and clinical features in cases of death among epileptic children. *Brain Dev* **4**: 321–5.

Kuzniecky R, Powers R (1993) Epilepsia partialis continua due to cortical dysplasia. *J Child Neurol* **8**: 386–8.

Kuzniecky R, Andermann F, Melanson D, et al. (1988) Focal cortical myoclonus and rolandic cortical dysplasia: clarification by magnetic resonance imaging. *Ann Neurol* **23**: 317–25.

Kwan P, Brodie MJ (2000a) Early identification of refractory epilepsy. *N Engl J Med* **342**: 314–9.

Kwan P, Brodie MJ (2000b) Epilepsy after the first drug fails: substitution or add-on? *Seizure* **9**: 464–8.

Kwan P, Brodie MJ (2001) Effectiveness of first antiepileptic drug. *Epilepsia* **42**: 1255–60.

Lachhwani DK (2005) Pediatric epilepsy surgery: lessons and challenges. *Semin Pediatr Neurol* **12**: 114–8.

Lado FA, Lauretta EC, Moshé SL (2002) Seizure-induced hippocampal damage in the mature and immature brain. *Epileptic Disord* **4**: 83–97.

Lahat E, Goldman M, Barr J, et al. (2000) Comparison of intranasal midazolam with intravenous diazepam for treating febrile seizures in children: prospective randomised study. *BMJ* **321**: 83–6.

Lancman ME, Asconapé JJ, Golimstok A (1994) Circling seizures in a case of juvenile myoclonic epilepsy. *Epilepsia* **35**: 317–8.

Landy HJ, Khoury AN, Heyl PS (1989) Antenatal ultrasonographic diagnosis of fetal seizure activity. *Am J Obstet Gynecol* **161**: 308.

Langan Y, Nashef L, Sander JW (2005) Case–control study of SUDEP. *Neurology* **64**: 1131–3.

Larrieu JL, Lagueny A, Julien J (1985) [State of confusion induced by valproic acid and reversed after administration of clonazepam.] *Rev Electroencephalogr Neurophysiol Clin* **15**: 179–84 (French).

Laskowitz DT, Sperling MR, French JA, O'Connor MJ (1995) The syndrome of frontal lobe epilepsy: characteristics and surgical management. *Neurology* **45**: 780–7.

Laurent A, Arzimanoglou A (2006) Cognitive impairments in children with nonidiopathic temporal lobe epilepsy. *Epilepsia* **47** Suppl 2: 99–102.

Lawson JA, Cook MJ, Vogrin S, et al. (2002) Clinical, EEG, and quantitative MRI differences in pediatric frontal and temporal lobe epilepsy. *Neurology* **58**: 723–9.

Lawson JA, Birchansky S, Pacheco E, et al. (2005) Distinct clinicopathologic subtypes of cortical dysplasia of Taylor. *Neurology* **64**: 55–61.

Lee WL, Low PS, Rajan U (1993) Benign familial infantile epilepsy. *J Pediatr* **123**: 588–90.

Leestma JE, Annegers JF, Brodie MJ, et al. (1997) Sudden unexplained death in epilepsy: observations from a large clinical development program. *Epilepsia* **38**: 47–55.

Legarda S, Jayakar P, Duchowny M, et al. (1994) Benign rolandic epilepsy: high central and low central subgroups. *Epilepsia* **35**: 1125–9.

Legido A, Clancy RR, Berman PH (1988) Recent advances in the diagnosis, treatment and prognosis of neonatal seizures. *Pediatr Neurol* **4**: 79–86.

Leppert M, Anderson VE, Quattlebaum T, et al. (1989) Benign familial neonatal convulsions linked to genetic markers on chromosome 20. *Nature* **337**: 647–8.

Lerman P, Lerman-Sagie T (1995) Sulthiame revisited. *J Child Neurol* **10**: 241–2.

Lerman P, Lerman-Sagie T, Kivity S (1991) Effect of early corticosteroid therapy for Landau–Kleffner syndrome. *Dev Med Child Neurol* **33**: 257–60.

Levene MI, Trounce JQ (1986) Cause of neonatal convulsions: towards a more precise diagnosis. *Arch Dis Child* **61**: 78–87.

Levin R, Banks S, Berg B (1988) Psychosocial dimensions of epilepsy: a review of the literature. *Epilepsia* **29**: 805–16.

Levy RH, Mattson RH, Meldrum BS, Perucca E, eds. (2002) *Antiepileptic Drugs, 5th edn.* New York: Lippincott, Williams & Wilkins.

Levy SR, Abroms IF, Marshall PC, Rosquette EE (1985) Seizures and cerebral infarction in the full-term newborn. *Ann Neurol* **17**: 366–70.

Lindsay J, Ounsted C, Richards P (1979) Long-term outcome in children with temporal lobe seizures. III: Psychiatric aspects in childhood and adult life. *Dev Med Child Neurol* **21**: 630–6.

Liu Z, Mikati M, Holmes GL (1995) Mesial temporal sclerosis: pathogenesis and significance. *Pediatr Neurol* **12**: 5–16.

Livet MO, Aicardi J, Plouin P, et al. (2005) Epilepsies in inborn errors of metabolism. In: Roger J, Bureau M, Dravet C, et al., eds. *Epileptic Syndromes in Infancy, Childhood and Adolescence. 4th edn.* London: John Libbey Eurotext, pp. 423–40.

Livingston JH, Brown JK (1987) Non-convulsive status epilepticus resistant to benzodiazepines. *Arch Dis Child* **187**: 41–4.

Logroscino G, Hesdorffer DC, Cascino GD, et al. (2002) Long-term mortality after a first episode of status epilepticus. *Neurology* **58**: 537–41.

Loiseau P, Beaussart M (1973) The seizures of benign childhood epilepsy with Rolandic paroxysmal discharges. *Epilepsia* **14**: 381–9.

Loiseau P, Duché B (1995) Childhood absence epilepsy. In: Duncan JS, Panayiotopoulos CP, eds. *Typical Absences and Related Epileptic Syndromes.* London: Churchill Communications Europe, pp. 152–60.

Loiseau P, Louiset P (1992) Benign partial epilepsies of adolescence. In: Roger J, Bureau M, Dravet C, et al., eds. *Epileptic Syndromes in Infancy, Childhood and Adolescence. 2nd edn.* London: John Libbey, pp. 343–5.

Loiseau P, Pestre M, Dartigues JF, et al. (1983) Long-term prognosis in two forms of childhood epilepsy: typical absence seizures and epilepsy with rolandic (centrotemporal) EEG foci. *Ann Neurol* **13**: 642–8.

Loiseau P, Duché B, Cordova S, et al. (1988) Prognosis of benign childhood epilepsy with centrotemporal spikes: a follow-up study of 168 patients. *Epilepsia* **29**: 229–35.

Loiseau P, Panayiotopoulos CP, Hirsch E (2002) Childhood absence epilepsy and related syndromes. In: Roger J, Bureau M, Dravet C, et al., eds. *Epileptic Syndromes in Infancy, Childhood and Adolescence. 3rd edn.* London: John Libbey, pp. 286–303.

Lombroso CT (1967) Sylvian seizures and midtemporal spike foci in children. *Arch Neurol* **17**: 52–9.

Lombroso CT (1983a) A prospective study of infantile spasms: clinical and therapeutic correlations. *Epilepsia* **24**: 135–58.

Lombroso CT (1983b) Prognosis in neonatal seizures. *Adv Neurol* **34**: 101–13.

Lombroso CT (1990) Early myoclonic encephalopathy, early infantile epileptic encephalopathy, and benign and severe infantile myoclonic epilepsies: a critical review and personal contributions. *J Clin Neurophysiol* **7**: 380–408.

Lombroso CT (1996) Neonatal seizures: a clinician's overview. *Brain Dev* **18**: 1–28.

Lombroso CT, Fejerman N (1977) Benign myoclonus in early infancy. *Ann Neurol* **1**: 138–43.

Lowenstein DH, Bleck T, Macdonald RL (1999) It's time to revise the definition of status epilepticus. *Epilepsia* **40**: 120–2.

Luat AF, Asano E, Juhász C, et al. (2005) Relationship between brain glucose metabolism positron emission tomography (PET) and electroencephalography (EEG) in children with continuous spike-and-wave activity during slow-wave sleep. *J Child Neurol* **20**: 682–90.

Lüders H, Comair YG (2001) *Epilepsy Surgery, 2nd edn.* Philadelphia: Lippincott, Williams & Wilkins.

Lüders H, Burgess R, Noachtar S (1993) Expanding the International Classification of Seizures to provide localization information. *Neurology* **43**: 1650–5.

Lüders H, Acharya J, Baumgartner C, et al. (1998) Semiological seizure classification. *Epilepsia* **34**: 1006-13.

Lüders HO, Acharya J, Baumgartner C, et al. (1999) A new epileptic seizure classification based exclusively on ictal semiology. *Acta Neurol Scand* **99**: 1137–41.

Lugaresi E, Cirignotta F, Montagna P (1986) Nocturnal paroxysmal dystonia. *J Neurol Neurosurg Psychiatry* **49**: 375–80.

Lux AL, Osborne JP (2004) A proposal for case definitions and outcome measures in studies of infantile spasms and West syndrome: consensus statement of the West Delphi group. *Epilepsia* **45**: 1416–28.

Lux AL, Edwards SW, Hancock E, et al. (2005) The United Kingdom Infantile Spasms Study (UKISS) comparing hormone treatment with vigabatrin on developmental and epilepsy outcomes to age 14 months: a multicentre randomised trial. *Lancet Neurol* **4**: 712–7.

Lynch BJ, Rust AS (1994) Natural history of neonatal hypocalcemic and hypomagnesemic seizures. *Pediatr Neurol* **11**: 23–7.

Mackay MT, Weiss SK, Adams-Webber T, et al. (2004) Practice parameter: medical treatment of infantile spasms: report of the American Academy of Neurology and the Child Neurology Society. *Neurology* **62**: 1668–81.

Madhavan D, Schaffer S, Yankovsky A, et al. (2007) Surgical outcome in tuberous sclerosis complex: a multicenter survey. *Epilepsia* **48**: 1625–8.

Maeda Y, Kurokawa T, Sakamoto K, et al. (1990) Electroclinical study of video-game epilepsy. *Dev Med Child Neurol* **32**: 493–500.

Malafosse A, Beck C, Bellet H, et al. (1994) Benign infantile familial convulsions are not an allelic form of the benign familial neonatal convulsions gene. *Ann Neurol* **35**: 479–82.

Manford M, Fish DR, Shorvon SD (1996a) An analysis of clinical seizure patterns and their localizing value in frontal and temporal lobe epilepsies. *Brain* **119**: 17–40.

Manford M, Fish DR, Shorvon SD (1996b) Startle provoked epileptic seizures: features in 19 patients. *J Neurol Neurosurg Psychiatry* **61**: 151–6.

Manonmani V, Wallace SJ (1994) Epilepsy with myoclonic absences. *Arch Dis Child* **70**: 288–90.

Maquet P, Hirsch E, Dive D, et al. (1990) Cerebral glucose utilization during sleep in Landau–Kleffner syndrome: a PET study. *Epilepsia* **31**: 778–83.

Maquet P, Hirsch E, Metz-Lutz MN, et al. (1995) Regional cerebral glucose metabolism in children with deterioration of one or more cognitive functions and continuous spike-and-wave discharges during sleep. *Brain* **118**: 1497–520.

Marks DA, Kim J, Spencer DD, Spencer SS (1995) Seizure localization and pathology following head injury in patients with uncontrolled epilepsy. *Neurology* **45**: 2051–7.

Martin R, Kuzniecky R, Ho S, et al. (1999) Cognitive effects of topiramate, gabapentin, and lamotrigine in healthy young adults. *Neurology* **52**: 321–7.

Martinez-Juarez IE, Alonso ME, Medina MT, et al. (2006) Juvenile myoclonic epilepsy syndromes: family studies and long-term follow-up. *Brain* **129**: 1269–80.

Mathern GW, Babb TL, Mischel PS, et al. (1996) Childhood generalized and mesial temporal epilepsies demonstrate different amounts and patterns of hippocampal neuron loss and mossy fibre synaptic reorganization. *Brain* **119**: 965–87.

Mathern GW, Giza CC, Yudovin S, et al. (1999) Postoperative seizure control and antiepileptic drug use in pediatric epilepsy surgery patients: the UCLA experience, 1986–1997. *Epilepsia* **40**: 1740–9.

Matsuishi T, Yoshino M, Tokunaga O, et al. (1985) Subacute necrotizing encephalomyelopathy (Leigh disease): report of a case with Lennox–Gastaut syndrome. *Brain Dev* **7**: 500–4.

Matsumoto A, Kumagai T, Takeuchi T, et al. (1987) Clinical effects of thyrotropin-releasing hormone for severe epilepsy in childhood: a comparative study with ACTH therapy. *Epilepsia* **28**: 49–55.

Mattson RH, Cramer JA, Collins JF (1992) A comparison of valproate with carbamazepine for the treatment of complex partial seizures and secondarily generalized tonic–clonic seizures in adults. The Department of Veterans Affairs Epilepsy Cooperative Study No. 264, Group D. *N Engl J Med* **327**: 765–71.

Mauguière F, Courjon J (1978) Somatosensory epilepsy: a review of 127 cases. *Brain* **101**: 307–32.

Mauguière F, Ryvlin P (2004) The role of PET in presurgical assessment of partial epilepsies. *Epileptic Disord* **6**: 193–215.

Mayr N, Wimberger D, Pichler H, et al. (1987) Influence of television on photosensitive epileptics. *Eur Neurol* **27**: 201–8.

McBride MC, Dooling EC, Oppenheimer EY (1981) Complex partial status epilepticus in young children. *Ann Neurol* 9: 526–30.

McIntyre J, Robertson S, Norris E, et al. (2005) Safety and efficacy of buccal midazolam versus rectal diazepam for emergency treatment of seizures in children: a randomised controlled trial. *Lancet* 366: 205–10.

McLachlan RS (1987) Pseudoatrophy of the brain with valproic acid monotherapy. *Can J Neurol Sci* 14: 294–6.

McLeod DC, Rhule D, Kitrenos JG, Hunt SN (1978) Use of a pharmacy technologist to manage technicians' activities. *Am J Hosp Pharm* 35: 1393–4.

Meador KJ (1994) Cognitive side effects of antiepileptic drugs. *Can J Neurol Sci* 21: S12-6.

Meador KJ (2001) Cognitive effects of epilepsy and of antiepileptic medications. In: Wyllie E, ed. *The Treatment of Epilepsy, 3rd edn.* Philadelphia: Lippincott, Williams & Wilkins, pp. 1215–25.

Medical Research Council Antiepileptic Drug Withdrawal Study Group (1991) Randomised study of antiepileptic drug withdrawal in patients in remission. *Lancet* 337: 1175–80.

Meencke HJ, Gerhard C (1985) Morphological aspects of aetiology and the course of infantile spasms (West-syndrome). *Neuropediatrics* 16: 59–66.

Meldrum BS (1978) Physiological changes during prolonged seizures and epileptic brain damage. *Neuropadiatrie* 9: 203–12.

Meldrum BS (1983) Metabolic factors during prolonged seizures and their relation to nerve cell death. *Adv Neurol* 34: 261–75.

Mikati MA, Shamseddine AN (2005) Management of Landau–Kleffner syndrome. *Paediatr Drugs* 7: 377–89.

Mikati MA, Holmes GL, Chronopoulos A, et al. (1994) Phenobarbital modifies seizure-related brain injury in the developing brain. *Ann Neurol* 36: 425–33.

Millichap JG, Millichap JJ (2006) Role of viral infections in the etiology of febrile seizures. *Pediatr Neurol* 35: 165–72.

Millner MM, Puchhammer-Stöckl E (1993) Herpes simplex virus encephalitis and febrile convulsions: contribution of polymerase chain reaction and magnetic resonance imaging. *Ann Neurol* 34: 503 (abstract).

Miyazaki M, Hashimoto T, Fujii E, et al. (1994) Infantile spasms: localized cerebral lesions on SPECT. *Epilepsia* 35: 988–92.

Mizrahi EM, Kellaway P (1987) Characterization and classification of neonatal seizures. *Neurology* 37: 1837–44.

Mizrahi EM, Hrachovy RA, Kellaway P (2004) *Atlas of Neonatal Electroencephalography, 3rd edn.* Philadelphia: Lippincott, Williams & Wilkins.

Mohamed A, Wyllie E, Ruggieri P, et al. (2001) Temporal lobe epilepsy due to hippocampal sclerosis versus medial temporal lobe tumors. *Neurology* 56: 1643–9.

Morikawa T, Seino M, Osawa T, Yagi K (1985) Five children with continuous spike–wave discharges during sleep. In: Roger J, Dravet C, Bureau M, et al., eds. *Epileptic Syndromes in Infancy, Childhood and Adolescence.* London: John Libbey, pp. 205–12.

Morrell F (1989) Variation of human secondary epileptogenesis. *J Clin Neurophysiol* 6: 227–75.

Morrell M (2002) Antiepeleptic drug use in women. In: Levy RH, Mattson RH, Meldrum BS, et al., eds. *Antiepeleptic Drugs, 5th edn.* Philadelphia: Lippincott, Williams & Wilkins, pp. 132–48.

Morrell F, Whisler WW, Bleck TP (1989) Multiple subpial transection: a new approach to the surgical treatment of focal epilepsy. *J Neurosurg* 70: 231–9.

Morrell F, Whisler WW, Smith MC, et al. (1995) Landau–Kleffner syndrome. Treatment with subpial intracortical transection. *Brain* 118: 1529–46.

Morris GL, Mueller WM, Yetkin FZ, et al. (1994) Functional magnetic resonance imaging in partial epilepsy. *Epilepsia* 35: 1194–8.

Morrow J, Russell A, Guthrie E, et al. (2006) Malformation risks of antiepileptic drugs in pregnancy: a prospective study from the UK Epilepsy and Pregnancy Register. *J Neurol Neurosurg Psychiatry* 77: 193–8.

Moshé SL (1987) Epileptogenesis and the immature brain. *Epilepsia* 28 Suppl 1: S3–15.

Moshé SL, Ludvig N (1988) Kindling. In: Pedley TA, Meldrum BS, eds. *Recent Advances in Epilepsy, vol. 4.* Edinburgh: Churchill Livingstone, pp. 21–44.

Motte J, Trevathan E, Arvidsson JF, et al. (1997) Lamotrigine for generalized seizures associated with the Lennox–Gastaut syndrome. Lamictal Lennox–Gastaut Study Group. *N Engl J Med* 337: 1807–12; erratum 1998 339: 851–2.

Mullatti N (2003) Hypothalamic hamartoma in adults. *Epileptic Disord* 5: 201–4.

Mulley JC, Scheffer IE, Harkin LA, et al. (2005) Susceptibility genes for complex epilepsy. *Hum Mol Genet* 14 Spec No 2: R243–9.

Munari C, Tassi L, Kahane P, et al. (1994) Analysis of clinical symptomatology during stereo-EEG recorded mesiotemporal lobe seizurres. In: Wolf P, ed. *Epileptic Seizures and Syndromes.* London: John Libbey, pp. 335–7.

Murphy JV, Sawasky F, Marquardt KM, Harris DJ (1987) Deaths in young children receiving nitrazepam. *J Pediatr* 111: 145–7.

Musumeci SA, Elia M, Ferrir R, et al. (1995) A further family with epilepsy, dementia and yellow teeth: the Kohlschütter syndrome. *Brain Dev* 17: 133–8.

Naidu S, Gruener G, Brazis D (1986) Excellent results with chlorazepate in recalcitrant childhood epilepsies. *Pediatr Neurol* 2: 18–22.

Najm I, Duvernoy H, Schuele S (2006a) Hippocampal anatomy and hippocampal sclerosis. In: Wyllie E, Gupta A, Lachhwani DK, eds. *The Treatment of Epilepsy, 4th edn.* Philadelphia: Lippincott, Williams & Wilkins, pp. 58–68.

Najm I, Möddel G, Janigro D (2006b) Mechanisms of epileptogenesis and experimental models of seizures. In: Wyllie E, Gupta A, Lachhwani DK, eds. *The Treatment of Epilepsy, 4th edn.* Philadelphia: Lippincott, Williams & Wilkins, pp. 91–102.

Nashef L, Fish DR, Garner S, et al. (1995) Sudden death in epilepsy: a study of incidence in a young cohort with epilepsy and learing difficulty. *Epilepsia* 36: 1187–94.

Nelson KB, Ellenberg JH, eds. (1981) *Febrile Seizures.* New York: Raven Press.

Nelson KB, Ellenberg JH (1990) Prenatal and perinatal antecedents of febrile seizures. *Ann Neurol* 27: 127–31.

Neville BGR, Boyd SG (1995) Selective epileptic gait disorder. *J Neurol Neurosurg Psychiatry* 58: 371–3.

Newmark ME, Penry JK (1979) *Photosensitivity and Epilepsy. A Review.* New York: Raven Press.

Newton MR, Berkovic SF, Austin MC, et al. (1995) SPECT in the localisation of extratemporal and temporal seizure foci. *J Neurol Neurosurg Psychiatry* 59: 26–30.

Newton R, Aicardi J (1983) Clinical findings in children with occipital spike–wave complexes suppressed by eye-opening. *Neurology* 33: 1526–9.

Nicolai J, Aldenkamp AP, Arends J, et al. (2006) Cognitive and behavioral effects of nocturnal epileptiform discharges in children with benign childhood epilepsy with centrotemporal spikes. *Epilepsy Behav* 8: 56–70.

Nilsson L, Ahlbom A, Farahmand BY, et al. (2002) Risk factors for suicide in epilepsy: a case control study. *Epilepsia* 43: 644–51.

Nilsson L, Tomson T, Farahmand BY, et al. (1997) Cause-specific mortality in epilepsy: a cohort study of more than 9,000 patients once hospitalized for epilepsy. *Epilepsia* 38: 1062–8.

Nolan MA, Redoblado MA, Lah S, et al. (2003) Intelligence in childhood epilepsy syndromes. *Epilepsy Res* 53: 139–50.

O'Brien TJ, So EL, Cascino GD, et al. (2004) Subtraction SPECT coregistered to MRI in focal malformations of cortical development: localization of the epileptogenic zone in epilepsy surgery candidates. *Epilepsia* 45: 367–76.

O'Callaghan FJ, Verity CM, Osborne JP (2004) The United Kingdom Infantile Spasms Study comparing vigabatrin with prednisolone or tetracosactide at 14 days: a multicentre, randomised controlled trial. *Lancet* 364: 1773–8.

O'Donoghue MF, Sander JW (1997) A historical perspective on the mortality associated with chronic epilepsy. *Acta Neurol Scand* 96: 138–41.

Offringa M, Bossuyt PMM, Lubsen J, et al. (1994) Risk factors for seizure recurrence in children with febrile seizures: a pooled analysis of individual patient data from five studies. *J Pediatr* 124: 574–84.

Ogino T, Ohtsuka Y, Yamatogi Y, et al. (1989) The epileptic syndrome sharing common features during early childhood with severe myoclonic epilepsy in infancy. *Jpn J Psychiatry Neurol* 43: 479–81.

Oguni H (2005) Symptomatic epilepsies imitating idiopathic generalized epilepsies. *Epilepsia* 46 Suppl 9: 84–90.

Oguni H, Imaizumi Y, Uehara T, et al. (1993) Electroencephalographic features of epileptic drop attacks and absence seizures: a case study. *Brain Dev* 15: 226–30.

Oguni H, Mukahira K, Oguni M, et al. (1994) Video–polygraphic analysis of myoclonic seizures in juvenile myoclonic epilepsy. *Epilepsia* 35: 307–16.

Oguni H, Uehara T, Imai K, Osawa M (1996) Atonic epileptic drop attacks associated with generalized spike-and-slow wave complexes: video–polygraphic study in two patients. *Epilepsia* 38: 813–8.

Oguni H, Mukahira K, Uehara T, et al. (1997) Electrophysiological study of myoclonic seizures in children. *Brain Dev* 19: 279–84.

Oguni H, Fukuyama Y, Tanaka T, et al. (2001a) Myoclonic–astatic epilepsy of early childhood: clinical and EEG analysis of myoclonic–astatic seizures, and discusssions on the nosology of the syndrome. *Brain Dev* 23: 757–64.

Oguni H, Hayashi K, Awaya T, et al. (2001b) Severe myoclonic epilepsy in infants—a review based on the Tokyo Women's Medical University series of 84 cases. *Brain Dev* 23: 736–48.

Ohtahara S, Ohtsuka Y, Yamatogi Y, Oka E (1987) The early-infantile epileptic encephalopathy with suppression–burst: developmental aspects. *Brain Dev* 9: 371–6.

Ohtsuka Y, Murashima I, Oka E, Ohtahara S (1994) Treatment and prognosis of West syndrome. *J Epilepsy* 7: 279–84.

Okumura A, Watanabe K (2001) Clinico-electrical evolution of pre-hypsarrhythmic stage: towards prediction and prevention of West syndrome. *Brain Dev* 23: 483–7.

Okumura A, Watanabe K, Negoro T, et al. (2006) The clinical characterizations of benign partial epilepsy in infancy. *Neuropediatrics* 37: 359–63.

Olsson I, Campenhausen G (1992) Social adjustment in young adults with absence epilepsy. *Epilepsia* 33: 325–329.

Omtzigt JG, Los FJ, Grobbee DE, et al. (1992) The risk of spina bifida aperta after first-trimester exposure to valproate in a prenatal cohort. *Neurology* 42 Suppl 5: 119–25.

Opeskin K, Harvey AS, Cordner SM, Berkovic SF (2000) Sudden unexpected death in epilepsy in Victoria. *J Clin Neurosci* 7: 34–7.

Ottman R (1989) Genetics of the partial epilepsies: a review. *Epilepsia* 30: 107–11.

Ottman R, Risch N, Hauser WA, et al. (1995) Localization of a gene for partial epilepsy to chromosome 10q. *Nat Genet* 10: 56–60.

Ottman R, Winawer MR, Kalachikov S, et al. (2004) LGI1 mutations in autosomal dominant partial epilepsy with auditory features. *Neurology* 62: 1120–6.

Ottman R (2005) Analysis of genetically complex epilepsies. *Epilepsia* 46 Suppl 10: 7-14.

Oxley J, Janz D, Meinhardi H, eds. (1983) *Chronic Toxicity of Antiepilepectic Drugs*. New York: Raven Press.

Pachatz C, Fusco L, Vigevano F (1999) Benign myoclonus of infancy. *Epileptic Disord* 1: 53–61.

Paetau R, Kasola M, Karhu J, et al. (1992) Magnetoencephalographic localization of epileptic cortex—impact on surgical treatment. *Ann Neurol* 32: 106–9.

Painter MJ, Bergman I, Crumrine P (1986) Neonatal seizures. *Pediatr Clin North Am* 33: 91–109.

Painter MJ, Scher MS, Stein AD, et al. (1999) Phenobarbital compared with phenytoin for the treatment of neonatal seizures. *N Engl J Med* 341: 485–9.

Palm DG, Brandt M, Korinthenberg R (1988) West syndrome and Lennox–Gastaut syndrome in children with porencephalic cysts. In: Niedermeyer E, Degen R, eds. *The Lennox–Gastaut Syndrome*. New York: Alan R Liss, pp. 419–26.

Palmini A, Andermann F, Olivier A, et al. (1991) Focal neuronal migration disorders and intractable partial epilepsy: results of surgical treatment. *Ann Neurol* 30: 750–7.

Panayiotopoulos CP (1989) Benign childhood epilepsy with occipital paroxysms: a 15-year prospective study. *Ann Neurol* 26: 51–6.

Panayiotopoulos CP (1994a) Juvenile myoclonic epilepsy: an underdiagnosed syndrome. In: Wolf P, ed. *Epileptic Seizures and Syndromes*. London: John Libbey, pp. 221–30.

Panayiotopoulos CP (1994b) The clinical spectrum of typical absence seizures and absence epilepsies. In: Malafosse A, Genton P, Hirsch E, et al., eds. *Idiopathic Generalized Epilepsies: Clinical, Experimental and Genetic Aspects*. London: John Libbey, pp. 75–85.

Panayiotopoulos CP (1998) Absence epilepsies. In: Engel J, Pedley TA, eds. *Epilepsy: a Comprehensive Textbook, vol. 3*. New York: Lippincott-Raven, pp. 2327–46.

Panayiotopoulos CP (2000) Benign childhood epileptic syndrome with occipital spikes: new classification proposed by the International League Against Epilepsy. *J Child Neurol* 15: 548–52.

Panayiotopoulos CP (2002) *Panayiotopoulos Syndrome: A Common and Benign Epileptic Syndrome*. London: John Libbey.

Panayiotopoulos CP, Obeid T, Waheed G (1989) Differentiation of typical absence seizures in epileptic syndromes—a video EEG study of 225 seizures in 20 patients. *Brain* 112: 1039–56.

Parent JM, Lowenstein DH (1994) Treatment of refractory generalized status epilepticus with continuous infusion of midazolam. *Neurology* 44: 1837–40.

Peled R, Lavie P (1986) Paroxysmal awakenings from sleep associated with excessive daytime somnolence: a form of nocturnal epilepsy. *Neurology* 36: 95–8.

Pelletier I, Sauerwein HC, Lepore F, et al. (2007) Non-invasive alternatives to the Wada test in the presurgical evaluation of language and memory functions in epilepsy patients. *Epileptic Disord* 9: 111–26.

Pellock JM (1987) Carbamazepine side effects in children and adults. *Epilepsia* 28 Suppl 3: S64–70.

Pellock JM, Faught E, Leppik IE, et al. (2006) Felbamate: consensus of current clinical experience. *Epilepsy Res* 71: 89–101.

Pellock JM, Marmarou A, DeLorenzo R (2004) Time to treatment in prolonged seizure episodes. *Epilepsy Behav* 5: 192–6.

Penry JK, Porter RJ, Dreifuss FE (1975) Simultaneous recording of absence seizures with video tape and electroencephalography. A study of 374 seizures in 48 patients. *Brain* 98: 427–40.

Peraita-Adrados R, Gutierrez-Solana L, Ruiz-Falco ML, Garcia-Penas JJ (2001) Nap polygraphic recordings after partial sleep deprivation in patients with suspected epileptic seizures. *Neurophysiol Clin* 31: 34–9.

Perucca E, Levy RH (2002) Combination therapy and drug interactions. In: Levy RH, Mattson RH, Meldrum BS, Perucca E, eds. *Antiepileptic Drugs, 5th edn*. Philadelphia; Lippincott, Williams & Wilkins, pp. 96–102.

Perucca E, Gram L, Avanzini G, Dulac O (1998) Antiepileptic drugs as a cause of worsening seizures. *Epilepsia* 39: 5–17.

Petit J, Roubertie A, Inoue Y, Genton P (1999) Non-convulsive status in the ring chromosome 20 syndrome: a video illustration of 3 cases. *Epileptic Disord* 1: 237–41.

Phillips SA, Shanahan RJ (1989) Etiology and mortality of status epilepticus in children. A recent update. *Arch Neurol* 46: 74–6.

Picard F, Baulac P, Kahane P, et al. (2000) Dominant partial epilepsies: a clinical, electrophysiological and genetic study of 19 European families. *Brain* 123: 1247–62.

Pinton F, Ducot B, Motte J, et al. (2006) Cognitive functions in children with benign childhood epilepsy with centrotemporal spikes (BECTS). *Epileptic Disord* 8: 11–23.

Plouin P (1994) Benign idiopathic neonatal convulsions (familial and non-familial). Open questions about these syndromes. In: Wolf P, ed. *Epileptic Seizures and Syndromes*. London: John Libbey, pp. 193–202.

Plouin P, Anderson VE (2005) Benign familial and non-familial neonatal seizures. In: Roger J, Bureau M, Dravet C, et al., eds. *Epileptic Syndromes in Infancy, Childhood and Adolescence. 4th edn*. London: John Libbey Eurotext, pp. 3–15.

Plouin P, Dulac O (1994) Other types of seizures. In: Dulac O, Chugani HT, Dalla Bernardina B, eds. *Infantile Spasms and West Syndrome*. Philadelphia: WB Saunders, pp. 52–62.

Pohlmann-Eden B, Beghi E, Camfield C, Camfield P (2006) The first seizure and its management in adults and children. *BMJ* 332: 339–42.

Polkey CE (2003a) Alternative surgical procedures to help drug-resistant epilepsy – a review. *Epileptic Disord* 5: 63–75.

Polkey CE (2003b) Resective surgery for hypothalamic hamartoma. *Epileptic Disord* 5: 281–6.

Porter RJ, Penry JK (1983) Petit mal status. *Adv Neurol* 34: 61–7.

Potter D, Edwards KR, Norton J (1997) Sustained weight loss associated with 12-month topiramate therapy *Epilepsia* 38 Suppl 8: 97 (abstract).

Prasad AN, Stafstrom CF, Holmes GH (1996) Alternative epilepsy therapies: the ketogenic diet, immunogloblins, and steroids. *Epilepsia* 37 Suppl 1: S81–95.

Prats JM, Garaizar C, Rua MJ, et al. (1991) Infantile spasms treated with high doses of sodium valproate: initial response and follow-up. *Dev Med Child Neurol* 33: 617–25.

Radvanyi-Bouvet MF, Vallecalle MH, Morel-Kahn F, et al. (1985) Seizures and electrical discharges in premature infants. *Neuropediatrics* 16: 143–8.

Rampp S, Stefan H (2007) Magnetoencephalography in presurgical epilepsy diagnosis. *Expert Rev Med Devices* 4: 335–47.

Rasmussen T, Andermann F (1989) Update on the syndrome of "chronic encephalitis" and epilepsy. *Cleve Clin J Med* 56 (Suppl): S181–4.

Raspall-Chaure M, Chin RF, Neville BG, Scott RC (2006) Outcome of paediatric convulsive status epilepticus: a systematic review. *Lancet Neurol* 5: 769–79.

Rathgeb JP, Plouin P, Sohfflet C, et al. (1998) Le cas particulier des crises partielles du nourrisson: semiologie électroclinique. In: *Épilepsies Partielles Graves Pharmacorésistantes de l'Enfant: Stratégies Diagnostiques et Traitements Chirurgicaux*. Montrouge: John Libbey Eurotext, pp. 122–34.

Raymond AA, Fish DR, Stevens JM, et al. (1994) Association of hippocampal sclerosis with cortical dysgenesis in patients with epilepsy. *Neurology* 44: 1841–5.

Raymond AA, Fish DR, Sisokiya S, Alsanjari N, et al. (1995) Abnormalities of gyration, heterotopias, tuberous sclerosis, focal cortical dysplasia, microdysgenesis, dysembryoplastic neuroepithelial tumour and dysgenesis of the archicortex in epilepsy. Clinical, EEG and neuroimaging features in 100 adult patients. *Brain* **118**: 629–60.

Regis J, Scavarda D, Tamura M, et al. (2007) Gamma knife surgery for epilepsy related to hypothalamic hamartomas. *Semin Pediatr Neurol* **14**: 73–9.

Remy S, Beck H (2006) Molecular and cellular mechanisms of pharmacoresistance in epilepsy. *Brain* **129**: 18–35.

Renkawek K, Renier WO, De Pont JJHM, et al. (1992) Neonatal status convulsions, spongiform encephalopathy and low activity of Na+/K+ ATPase in the brain. *Epilepsia* **33**: 58–64.

Ricci S, Cusmai R, Fusco L, Vigevano F (1995) Reflex myoclonic epilepsy in infancy: a new age-dependent idiopathic epileptic syndrome related to startle reaction. *Epilepsia* **36**: 342–8.

Rich SS, Annegers JF, Hauser WA, Anderson VE (1987) Complex segregation analysis of febrile convulsions. *Am J Hum Genet* **41**: 249–57.

Richens A (1982) Clinical pharmacology and medical treatment. In: Laidlaw J, Richens A, eds. *A Textbook of Epilepsy, 2nd edn.* Edinburgh: Churchill Livingstone, pp. 292–348.

Richens A, Davidson DLW, Cartlidge NEF, et al. (1994) A multicentre comparative trial of sodium valproate and carbamazepine in adult onset epilepsy. *J Neurol Neurosurg Psychiatry* **57**: 682–7.

Riikonen R (1982) A long-term follow-up study of 214 children with the syndrome of infantile spasms. *Neuropediatrics* **13**: 14–23.

Riikonen R (1996) Long-term otucome of West syndrome: a study of adults with a history of infantile spasms. *Epilepsia* **37**: 367–72.

Riikonen R (2005) The latest on infantile spasms. *Curr Opin Neurol* **18**: 91–5.

Riikonen R, Amnell G (1981) Psychiatric disorders in children with earlier infantile spasms. *Dev Med Child Neurol* **23**: 747–60.

Rintahaka PJ, Chugani HT, Sankar R (1995) Landau–Kleffner syndrome with continuous spikes and waves during slow-wave sleep. *J Child Neurol* **10**: 127–33.

Robain O, Vinters HV (1994) Neuropathologic studies. In: Dulac O, Chugani HT, Dalla Bernardina B, eds. *Infantile Spasms and West Syndrome.* Philadelphia: WB Saunders, pp. 99–117.

Robinson RO, Baird G, Robinson G, et al. (2001) Landau–Kleffner syndrome: course and correlates with outcome. *Dev Med Child Neurol* **43**: 243–7.

Rodin EA, Schmaltz S, Twitty G (1986) Intellectual functions of patients with childhood-onset epilepsy. *Dev Med Child Neurol* **28**: 25–33.

Roger J, Bureau M, Dravet C, et al., eds. (2005) *Epileptic Syndromes in Infancy, Childhood and Adolescence. 4th edn.* Montrouge: John Libbey Eurotext.

Roll P, Rudolf G, Pereira S, et al. (2006) SRPX2 mutations in disorders of language cortex and cognition. *Hum Mol Genet* **15**: 1195–207.

Ronen GM, Rosales TO, Connolly M, et al. (1993) Seizure characteristics in chromosome 20 benign familial neonatal convulsions. *Neurology* **43**: 1355–60.

Roos RAC, Van Dijk JG (1988) Reflex-epilepsy induced by immersion in hot water: case report and review of the literature. *Eur Neurol* **28**: 6–10.

Rosa FW (1991) Spina bifida in infants of women treated with carbamazepine during pregnancy. *N Engl J Med* **324**: 674–7.

Rosman NP, Colton T, Labazzo J, et al. (1993) A controlled trial of diazepam administered during febrile illnesses to prevent recurrence of febrile seizures. *N Engl J Med* **329**: 79–84.

Ross EM, Peckham CS (1983) Seizure disorder in the National Child Development Study. In: Rose FC, ed. *Research Progress in Epilepsy.* London: Pitman, pp. 46–59.

Ross EM, West PB, Butler NR (1980) Epilepsy in childhood: findings from the National Child Development Study. *BMJ* **1**: 207–10.

Rossi PG, Parmeggiani A, Posar A, et al. (1999) Landau–Kleffner syndrome (LKS): long-term follow-up and links with electrical status epilepticus during sleep (ESES). *Brain Dev* **21**: 90–8.

Roulet E, Deonna T, Despland PA (1989) Prolonged intermittent drooling and oromotor dyspraxia in benign childhood epilepsy with centrotemporal spikes. *Epilepsia* **30**: 564–8.

Roulet E, Deonna T, Gaillard F, et al. (1991) Acquired aphasia, dementia, and behavior disorder with epilepsy and continuous spike and waves during sleep in a child. *Epilepsia* **32**: 495–503.

Russo GL, Tassi L, Cossu M, et al. (2003) Focal cortical resection in malformations of cortical development. *Epileptic Disord* 5 Suppl 2: S115–23.

Ryan SG, Wiznitzer M, Hollman C, et al. (1991) Benign familial neonatal convulsions: evidence for clinical and genetic heterogeneity. *Ann Neurol* **29**: 469–73.

Ryvlin P, Minotti L, Demarquay G, et al. (2006a) Nocturnal hypermotor seizures, suggesting frontal lobe epilepsy, can originate in the insula. *Epilepsia* **47**: 755–65.

Ryvlin P, Montavont A, Kahane P (2006) Sudden unexpected death in epilepsy: from mechanisms to prevention. *Curr Opin Neurol* **19**: 194–9.

Sachdeo RC, Glauser TA, Ritter F, et al. (1999) A double-blind, randomized trial of topiramate in Lennox–Gastaut syndrome. Topiramate YL Study Group. *Neurology* **52**: 1882–7.

Sagar HJ, Oxbury JM (1987) Hippocampal neuron loss in temporal lobe epilepsy: correlation with early childhood convulsions. *Ann Neurol* **22**: 334–40.

Saint-Martin AD, Petiau C, Massa L, et al. (1999) Idiopathic rolandic epilepsy with 'interictal' facial myoclonia and oromotor deficit: a longitudinal EEG and PET study. *Epilepsia* **40**: 614–20.

Saint-Martin AD, Carcangiu R, Arzimanoglou A, et al. (2001a) Semiology of typical and atypical rolandic epilepsy: a video–EEG analysis. *Epileptic Disord* **3**: 173–82.

Salanova V, Andermann F, Olivier A, et al. (1992) Occipital lobe epilepsy: electroclinical manifestations, electrocorticography, cortical stimulation and outcome in 42 patients treated between 1930 and 1991. Surgery of occipital lobe epilepsy. *Brain* **115**: 1655–80.

Salanova V, Andermann F, Rasmussen T, et al. (1995a) Parietal lobe epilepsy. Clinical manifestations and outcome in 82 patients treated surgically between 1929 and 1988. *Brain* **118**: 607–27.

Salanova V, Morris HH, Van Ness P, et al. (1995b) Frontal lobe seizures: electroclinical syndromes. *Epilepsia* **36**: 16–24.

Sander T, Schulz H, Saar K, et al. (2000) Genome search for susceptibility loci of common idiopathic generalised epilepsies. *Hum Mol Genet* **9**: 1465–72.

Sankar FR, Painter MJ (2005) Neonatal seizures: after all these years we still love what doesn't work. *Neurology* **64**: 776–7.

Santanelli P, Bureau M, Magaudda A, et al. (1989) Benign partial epilepsy with centrotemporal (or rolandic) spikes and brain lesion. *Epilepsia* **30**: 182–8.

Sarnat HB, Flores-Sarnat L (2004) Integrative classification of morphology and molecular genetics in central nervous system malformations. *Am J Med Genet A* **162**: 386–92.

Scheepers B, Clough P, Pickles C (1998) The misdiagnosis of epilepsy: findings of a population study. *Seizure* **7**: 403–6.

Scheffer IE, Berkovic SF (1997) Generalized epilepsy with febrile seizures plus. A genetic disorder with heterogeneous clinical phenotypes. *Brain* **120**: 479–501.

Scheffer IE, Bhatia KP, Lopes-Cendes I, et al. (1995a) Autosomal dominant nocturnal frontal lobe epilepsy. A distinctive clinical disorder. *Brain* **118**: 61–73.

Scheffer IE, Jones L, Pozzebon M, et al. (1995b) Autosomal dominant rolandic epilepsy and speech dyspraxia: a new syndrome with anticipation. *Ann Neurol* **38**: 633–42.

Scheffer IE, Phillips HA, O'Brien CE, et al. (1998) Familial partial epilepsy with variable foci: a new partial epilepsy syndrome with suggestion of linkage to chromosome 2. *Ann Neurol* **44**: 890–9.

Scher MS (2003) Prenatal contibutions to epilepsy: lessons from the bedside. *Epileptic Disord* **5**: 77–91.

Scher MS, Beggarly M (1989) Clinical significance of focal periodic discharges in neonates. *J Child Neurol* **4**: 175–85.

Scher MS, Painter MJ (1990) Electroencephalographic diagnosis of neonatal seizures: issues of diagnostic accuracy, clinical correlation and survival. In: Wasterlain CG, Vert P, eds. *Neonatal Seizures.* New York: Raven Press, pp. 15–25.

Scher MS, Aso K, Beggarly ME, et al. (1993a) Electrographic seizures in preterm and full-term neonates: clinical correlates, associated brain lesions, and risk for neurologic sequelae. *Pediatrics* **91**: 128–34.

Scher MS, Hamid MY, Steppe DA, et al. (1993b) Ictal and interictal electrographic seizure durations in preterm and term neonates. *Epilepsia* **34**: 284–8.

Scheyer RD, During MJ, Spencer DD, et al. (1994) Measurement of carbamazepine and carbamazepine epoxide in the human brain using in vivo microdialysis. *Neurology* **44**: 1469–72.

Schiffman R, Shapira Y, Ryan SG (1991) An autosomal recessive form of benign familial neonatal seizures. *Clin Genet* **40**: 467–70.

Schlienger RG, Knowles SR, Shear NH (1998) Lamotrigine-associated anticonvulsant hypersensitivity syndrome. *Neurology* **51**: 1172–5.

Schmidt D (1989) Adverse effects of antiepileptic drugs in children. The relevance of drug interaction. *Cleve Clin J Med* **56** Suppl Pt 1: S132–9; discussion S147–9.

Schmidt D, Loscher W (2003) How effective is surgery to cure seizures in drug-resistant temporal lobe epilepsy? *Epilepsy Res* **56**: 85–91.

Schmidt D, Baumgartner C, Loscher W (2004) The chance of cure following surgery for drug-resistant temporal lobe epilepsy. What do we know and do we need to revise our expectations? *Epilepsy Res* **60**: 187–201.

Schwartz RH, Boyes S, Ainsley-Green A (1989a) Metabolic effects of three ketogenic diets in the treatment of severe epilepsy. *Dev Med Child Neurol* **31**: 152–60.

Schwartz RH, Eaton J, Bower BD, Ainsley-Green A (1989b) Ketogenic diets in the treatment of epilepsy: short-term clinical effects. *Dev Med Child Neurol* **31**: 145–51.

Scott RC, King MD, Gadian DG, et al. (2003) Hippocampal abnormalities after prolonged febrile convulsion: a longitudinal MRI study. *Brain* **126**: 2551–7.

Seidenberg M, Beck N, Geisser M, et al. (1986) Academic achievement of children with epilepsy. *Epilepsia* **27**: 753–9.

Semah F, Picot MC, Adam C, et al. (1998) Is the underlying cause of epilepsy a major prognostic factor for recurrence? *Neurology* **51**: 1256–62.

Shackleton DP, Westendorp RG, Trenite DG, Vandenbroucke JP (1999) Mortality in patients with epilepsy: 40 years of follow up in a Dutch cohort study. *J Neurol Neurosurg Psychiatry* **66**: 636–40.

Shackleton DP, Westendorp RG, Kasteleijn-Nolst Trenite DG, et al. (2002) Survival of patients with epilepsy: an estimate of the mortality risk. *Epilepsia* **43**: 445–50.

Shewmon DA (1994) Ictal aspects with emphasis on unusual variants. In: Dulac O, Chugani HT, Dalla Bernardina B, eds. *Infantile Spasms and West Syndrome.* Philadelphia: WB Saunders, pp. 36–51.

Shields WD, Shewmon DA, Chugani HT, Peacock WJ (1992) Treatment of infantile spasms: medical or surgical? *Epilepsia* **33** Suppl 4: S26–31.

Shinnar S, Berg AT (1996) Does antiepileptic drug therapy prevent the development of "chronic epilepsy"? *Epilepsia* **37**: 701–8.

Shinnar S, Berg AT, Moshé SL, et al. (1990) Risk of recurrence following a first unprovoked seizure in childhood: a prospective study. *Pediatrics* **85**: 1076–85.

Shinnar S, Berg AT, Moshé SL, et al. (1994) Discontinuing antiepileptic drugs in children with epilepsy: a prospective study. *Ann Neurol* **35**: 534–45.

Shinnar S, Berg AT, Moshé SL, et al. (1996) The risk of seizure recurrence after a first unprovoked afebrile seizure in childhood: an extended follow-up. *Pediatrics* **98**: 216–25.

Shinnar S, Pellock JM, Moshé SL, et al. (1997) In whom does status epilepticus occur: age-related differences in children. *Epilepsia* **38**: 907–14.

Shinnar S, Berg AT, O'Dell C, et al. (2000) Predictors of multiple seizures in a cohort of children prospectively followed from the time of their first unprovoked seizure. *Ann Neurol* **48**: 140–7.

Shorvon S (1994) *Status Epilepticus: its Clinical Features and Treatment in Children and Adults.* Cambridge: Cambridge University Press.

Shorvon SD, Chadwick D, Galbraith AW, Reynolds EH (1978) One drug for epilepsy. *BMJ* **1**: 474–6.

Shuper A, Goldberg-Stern H (2004) Ictus emeticus (ictal vomiting). *Pediatr Neurol* **31**: 283–6.

Siemes H, Spohr HL, Michael T, Nau H (1988) Therapy of infantile spasms with valproate: results of a prospective study. *Epilepsia* **29**: 553–60.

Sillanpää M (1990) Children with epilepsy as adults: outcome after 30 years of follow-up. *Acta Paediatr Scand Suppl* **368**: 1–78.

Sillanpää M (1992) Epilepsy in children: prevalence, disability, and handicap. *Epilepsia* **33**: 444–9.

Sillanpää M (1993) Remission of seizures and predictors of intractability in long-term follow-up. *Epilepsia* **34**: 930–6.

Sillanpää M (2004) Learning disability: occurrence and long-term consequences in childhood-onset epilepsy. *Epilepsy Behav* **5**: 937–44.

Sillanpää M, Schmidt D (2006a) Natural history of treated childhood-onset epilepsy: prospective, long-term population-based study. *Brain* **129**: 617–24.

Sillanpää M, Schmidt D (2006b) Prognosis of seizure recurrence after stopping antiepileptic drugs in seizure-free patients: A long-term population-based study of childhood-onset epilepsy. *Epilepsy Behav* **8**: 713–9.

Singh NA, Charlier C, Stauffer D, et al. (1998) A novel potassium channel gene, KCNQ2, is mutated in an inherited epilepsy of newborns. *Nat Genet* **18**: 25–9.

Singh NA, Westenskow P, Charlier C, et al. (2003) KCNQ2 and KCNQ3 potassium channel genes in benign familial neonatal convulsions: expansion of the functional and mutation spectrum. *Brain* **126**: 2726–37.

Sisodiya SM (2004) Malformations of cortical development: burdens and insights from important causes of human epilepsies. *Lancet Neurol* **3**: 29–38.

Sisodiya SM (2005) Genetics of drug resistance. *Epilepsia* **46** Suppl 10: 33–8.

Smaje JC, Davidson C, Teasdale GM (1987) Sino-atrial arrest due to temporal lobe epilepsy. *J Neurol Neurosurg Psychiatry* **50**: 112–3.

Smith D, Baker G, Davies G, et al. (1993) Outcomes of add-on treatment with lamotrigine in partial epilepsy. *Epilepsia* **34**: 312–22.

Snead OC (1995) Basic mechanisms of generalized absence seizures. *Ann Neurol* **37**: 146–57.

Sofijanov N, Emoto S, Kuturec M, et al. (1992) Febrile seizures: clinical characteristics and initial EEG. *Epilepsia* **33**: 52–7.

Southall DP, Stebbens V, Abraham N, Abraham L (1987) Prolonged apnoea with severe arterial hypoxaemia resulting from complex partial seizures. *Dev Med Child Neurol* **29**: 784–9.

Spanaki MV, Zubal IG, MacMullan J, Spencer SS (1999) Periictal SPECT localization verified by simultaneous intracranial EEG. *Epilepsia* **40**: 267–74.

Spencer SS, Berg AT, Vickrey BG, et al. (2007) Health-related quality of life over time since resective epilepsy surgery. *Ann Neurol* **62**: 327–34.

Staden UF, Isaacs E, Boyd SG et al. (1998) Language dysfunction in children with rolandic epilepsy. *Neuropediatrics* **29**: 242–8.

Steinhoff BJ, Kruse R (1992) Bromide treatment of pharmaco-resistant epilepsies with general tonic–clonic seizures: a clinical study. *Brain Dev* **14**: 144–9.

Stephenson JBP (1990) *Fits and Faints. Clinics in Developmental Medicine no. 109.* London: Mac Keith Press.

Stephenson JBP, King MD (1989) *Handbook of Neurological Investigations in Children.* London: Butterworth.

Stone S, Lange LS (1986) Syncope and sudden unexpected death attributed to carbamazepine in a 20-year-old epileptic. *J Neurol Neurosurg Psychiatry* **49**: 1460–1.

Stores G, Zaiwalla Z, Bergel N (1991) Frontal lobe complex partial seizures in children: a form of epilepsy at particular risk of misdiagnosis. *Dev Med Child Neurol* **33**: 998–1009.

Striano P, Zara F, Striano S (2005) Autosomal dominant cortical tremor, myoclonus and epilepsy: many syndromes, one phenotype. *Acta Neurol Scand* **111**: 211–7.

Striano P, Lispi ML, Gennaro E, et al. (2006) Linkage analysis and disease models in benign familial infantile seizures: a study of 16 families. *Epilepsia* **47**: 1029–34.

Stroink H, Van Donselaar CA, Geerts AT, et al. (2003) The accuracy of the diagnosis of paroxysmal events in children. *Neurology* **60**: 979–82.

Suri M (2005) The phenotypic spectrum of ARX mutations. *Dev Med Child Neurol* **47**: 133–7.

Sutula TP (2004) Mechanisms of epilepsy progression: current theories and perspectives from neuroplasticity in adulhood and development. *Epilepsy Res* **60**: 161–71.

Sutula TP, Hagen J, Pitkonen A (2003) Do epileptic seizures damage brain? *Curr Opin Neurol* **16**: 189–95.

Sutula T, Cascino G, Cavazos J, et al. (1989) Mossy fiber synaptic reorganization in the epileptic human temporal lobe. *Ann Neurol* **26**: 321–30.

Suzuki Y, Cox S, Hayes J, Walson PD (1991) Carbamazepine age–dose ratio relationship in children. *Ther Drug Monit* **13**: 201–8.

Swoboda KJ, Soong BW, McKenna C, et al. (2000) Paroxysmal kinesigenic dyskinesia and infantile convulsions. Clinical linkage studies. *Neurology* **55**: 224–30.

Szepetowski P, Rochette J, Berquin P, et al. (1997) Familial infantile convulsions and paroxysmal choreoathetosis: a new neurological syndrome linked to the pericentric region of chromosome 16. *Am J Hum Genet* **61**: 889–98.

Tassi L, Colombo N, Garbelli L, et al. (2002) Focal cortical dysplasia: neuropathological subtypes, EEG, neuroimaging and surgical outcome. *Brain* **125**: 1718–32.

Tassinari CA, Bureau M, Dravet C, et al. (1992) Epilepsy with continuous spikes and waves during slow sleep, otherwise described as ESES (epilepsy with electrical status epilepticus during slow sleep). In: Roger J, Bureau M, Dravet C, et al., eds. *Epileptic Syndromes in Infancy, Childhood and Adolescence. 2nd edn.* London: John Libbey, pp. 245–56.

Taylor DC, Falconer MA, Bruton DJ, et al. (1971) Focal dysplasia of the cerebral cortex in epilepsy. *J Neurol Neurosurg Psychiatry* **34**: 369–87.

Tekgul H, Gauvreau K, Soul J, et al. (2006) The current etiologic profile and neurodevelopmental outcome of seizures in term newborn infants. *Pediatrics* **117**: 1270–80.

Tennis P, Eldridge RR; International Lamotrigine Pregnancy Registry Scientific Advisory Committee (2002) Preliminary results on pregnancy outcomes in women using lamotrigine. *Epilepsia* **43**: 1161–7.

Tennison M, Greenwood R, Lewis D, Thorn M (1994) Discontinuing antiepileptic drugs in children with epilepsy. A comparison of a six-week and a nine-month taper period. *N Engl J Med* **330**: 1407–10.

Tettenborn B, Genton P, Polson D (2002) Epilepsy and women's issues: an update. *Epileptic Disord* **4** Suppl 2: S23–31.

Tharp BR (1981) Neonatal and pediatric electroencephalography. In: Aminoff MJ, ed. *Electrodiagnosis in Clinical Neurology.* Edinburgh: Churchill Livingstone, pp. 67–117.

Theodore WH, Rose D, Patronas N, et al. (1987) Cerebral glucose metabolism in the Lennox–Gastaut syndrome. *Ann Neurol* **21**: 14–21.

Theodore WH, Sato S, Kufta C, et al. (1992) Temporal lobectomy for uncontrolled seizures: the role of positron emission tomography. *Ann Neurol* **32**: 789–94.

Theodore WH, Porter RJ, Albert P, et al. (1994) The secondarily generalized tonic–clonic seizure: a videotape analysis. *Neurology* **44**: 1403–7.

Thomas P, Zifkin BG (1999) Pure photosensitive ictus emeticus. *Epileptic Disord* **1**: 47–50.

Thomas P, Beaumanoir A, Genton P, et al. (1992) 'De novo' absence status of late onset: report of 11 cases. *Neurology* **42**: 104–10.

Thomas P, Arzimanoglou A, Aicardi J (2003) Benign idiopathic occipital epilepsy: report of a case of the late (Gastaut) type. *Epileptic Disord* **5**: 57–9.

Thomas P, Genton P, Gelisse P, Wolf P (2005) Juvenile myoclonic epilepsy. In: Roger J, Bureau M, Dravet C, et al., eds. *Epileptic Syndromes in Infancy, Childhood and Adolescence. 4th edn.* London: John Libbey Eurotext, pp. 367–88.

Thomas P, Valton L, Genton P (2006) Absence and myoclonic status epilepticus precipitated by antiepileptic drugs in idiopathic generalized epilepsy. *Brain* **129**: 1281–92.

Thurston SE, Leigh RJ, Osorio I (1985) Epileptic gaze deviation and nystagmus. *Neurology* **35**: 1518–21.

Tiacci C, D'Alessandro P, Cantisani TA, et al. (1993) Epilepsy with bilateral occipital calcifications: Sturge–Weber variant or a different encephalopathy? *Epilepsia* **34**: 528–39.

Tomson T, Battino D (2005) Teratogenicity of antiepileptic drugs: state of the art. *Curr Opin Neurol* **18**: 135–40.

Toti P, Balestri P, Cano M, et al. (1996) Celiac disease with cerebral calcium and silica deposits. *Neurology* **46**: 1088–92.

Treiman DM (1993) Generalized convulsive status epilepticus in the adult. *Epilepsia* **34** Suppl 1: S2–11.

Treiman DM, Walker MC (2006) Treatment of seizure emergencies: convulsive and non-convulsive status epilepticus. *Epilepsy Res* **68** Suppl 1: 77–82.

Trevathan E, Cascino GD (1988) Partial epilepsy presenting as focal paroxysmal pain. *Neurology* **38**: 329–30.

Trevathan E, Murphy CC, Yeargin-Ilsopp M (1997) Death among children with epilepsy in Atlanta. *Epilepsia* **38** Suppl 8: 248–9.

Trinka E, Baumgartner S, Unterberger I, et al. (2004) Long-term prognosis for childhood and juvenile absence epilepsy. *J Neurol* **251**: 1235–41.

Turnbull J, Lohi H, Kearney JA, et al. (2005) Sacred disease secrets revealed: the genetics of human epilepsy. *Hum Mol Genet* **14** Special No 2: 2491–500.

Tuxhorn I, Holthausen H, Boenigk H, eds. (1997) *Paediatric Epilepsy Syndromes and their Surgical Treatment.* London: John Libbey.

Uhari M, Rantala H, Vainionpää L, Kurttila R (1995) Effect of acetaminophen and of low intermittent doses of diazepam on prevention of recurrences of febrile seizures. *J Pediatr* **126**: 991–5.

Vajda FJ, Hitchcock A, Graham J, et al. (2006) Foetal malformations and seizure control: 52 months data of the Australian Pregnancy Registry. *Eur J Neurol* **13**: 645–54.

Van Donselaar CA, Stroink H, Arts WF; Dutch Study Group of Epilepsy in Childhood (2006) How confident are we of the diagnosis of epilepsy? *Epilepsia* **47** Suppl 1: 9–13.

Van Esch A, Ramlal RI, van Steesel-Moll HA, et al. (1996) Outcome after febrile status epilepticus. *Dev Med Child Neurol* **38**: 19–24.

Vanhatalo S, Nousiainen I, Eriksson K, et al. (2002) Visual field constriction in 91 Finnish children treated with vigabatrin. *Epilepsia* **43**: 748–56.

VanLandingham KE, Heinz ER, Cavazos JE, Lewis DV (1998) Magnetic resonance imaging evidence of hippocampal injury after prolonged focal febrile convulsions. *Ann Neurol* **43**: 413–26.

Vasconcellos E, Wyllie E, Sullivan S, et al. (2001) Mental retardation in pediatric candidates for epilepsy surgery: the role of early seizure onset. *Epilepsia* **42**: 268–74.

Vedru P, Wajgt A, Schiemann Delgado J, Noachtar S (2005) Efficacy and safety of levetiracetam 3000mg/d as adjunctive treatment in adolescents and adults suffering from idiopathic generalized epilepsy with myoclonic seizures. *Epilepsia* **46** Suppl 6: 56–7.

Veggiotti P, Cardinali S, Montalenti E, et al. (2001) Generalized epilepsy with febrile seizures plus and severe myoclonic epilepsy in infancy: a case report of two Italian families. *Epileptic Disord* **3**: 29–32.

Verity CM, Ross EM, Golding J (1993) Outcome of childhood status epilepticus and lengthy febrile convulsions: findings of national cohort study. *BMJ* **307**: 225–8.

Verity CM, Hosking G, Easter DJ (1995) A multicentre comparative trial of sodium valproate and carbamazepine in paediatric epilepsy. The Paediatric EPITEG Collaborative Group. *Dev Med Child Neurol* **37**: 97–108.

Viani F, Beghi E, Romeo A, van Lierde A (1987) Infantile febrile status epilepticus: risk factors and outcome. *Dev Med Child Neurol* **29**: 495–501.

Viberg M, Blennow G, Polski B (1987) Epilepsy in adolescence: implications for the development of personality. *Epilepsia* **28**: 542–6.

Vigevano F, Bureau M (2005) Idiopathic and/or benign localization-related epilepsies in infants and young children. In: Roger J, Bureau M, Dravet C, et al., eds. *Epileptic Syndromes in Infancy, Childhood and Adolescence. 4th edn.* London: John Libbey Eurotext, pp. 171–8.

Vigevano F, Cilio MR (1997) Vigabatrin versus ACTH as first-line treatment for infantile spasms: a randomized prospective study. *Epilepsia* **38**: 270–4.

Vigevano F, Fusco L, Di Capua M, et al. (1992) Benign infantile familial convulsions. *Eur J Pediatr* **151**: 608–12.

Vigevano F, Fusco L, Cusmai R, et al. (1993) The idiopathic form of West syndrome. *Epilepsia* **34**: 743–6.

Vigevano F, Fusco L, Ricci S, et al. (1994a) Dysplasias. In: Dulac O, Chugani HT, Dalla Bernardina B, eds. *Infantile Spasms and West Syndrome.* London: WB Saunders, pp. 178–91.

Vigevano F, Santanelli R, Fusco L, et al. (1994b) Benign infantile familial convulsions. In: Malafosse A, Genton P, Hirsch E, et al., eds. *Idiopathic Generalized Epilepsies: Clinical, Experimental and Genetic Aspects.* London: John Libbey, pp. 45–9.

Vigevano F, Fusco L, Pachatz T (2001) Neurophysiology of spasms. *Brain Dev* **23**: 467–72.

Vigevano F, Fusco L, Lo Russo G, Broggi G, eds. (2003) Abnormalities of cortical development and epilepsy. *Epileptic Disord* **5** Suppl 2.

Villanueva V, Serratosa JM (2005) Temporal lobe epilepsy: clinical semiology and age at onset. *Epileptic Disord* **7**: 83–90.

Ville D, Kaminska A, Bahi-Buisson N, et al. (2006) Early pattern of epilepsy in the ring chromosome 20 syndrome. *Epilepsia* **47**: 543–9.

Vining EPG, Freeman JM, Brandt J, et al. (1993) Progressive unilateral encephalopathy of childhood (Rasmussen's syndrome): a reappraisal. *Epilepsia* **34**: 639–50.

Vining EPG, Freeman JM, Pillas DJ, et al. (1997) Why would you remove half a brain? The outcome of 58 children after hemispherectomy. The Johns Hopkins experience: 1968 to 1996. *Pediatrics* **100**: 163–71.

Vinters HV, Wasterlain CG (1996) Pathology of childhood epilepsy. In: Wallace SJ, ed. *Epilepsy in Children.* London: Chapman & Hall, pp. 87–107.

Volpe JJ (1989) Neonatal seizures: current concepts and classification. *Pediatrics* **84**: 422–8.

Wallace SJ (1988) *The Child with Febrile Seizures.* Guildford: Butterworth.

Wallace SJ (1991) Epileptic syndromes linked with previous history of febrile seizures. In: Fukuyama Y, Kamoshita S, Ohtsuka C, Suzuki Y, eds. *Modern Perspectives of Child Neurology.* Tokyo: Japanese Society of Child Neurology, pp. 175–81.

Wang HS, Kuo MF, Chou ML, et al. (2005) Pyridoxal phosphate is better than pyridoxine for controlling idiopathic intractable epilepsy. *Arch Dis Child* **90**: 512–5.

Wasterlain C, Treiman D (2006) *Status Epilepticus: Mechanisms and Management.* Massachusetts: MIT Press.

Watanabe K (1996) Recent advances and some problems in the delineation of epileptic syndromes in children. *Brain Dev* **18**: 423–37.

Watanabe K, Hara K, Miyazaki S, et al. (1982a) Apneic seizures in the newborn. *Am J Dis Child* **136**: 980–4.

Watanabe K, Kuroyanagi M, Hara K, Miyazaki S (1982b) Neonatal seizures and subsequent epilepsy. *Brain Dev* **4**: 341–6.

Watanabe K, Yamamoto N, Negoto T, et al. (1987) Benign complex partial epilepsies in infancy. *Pediatr Neurol* **3**: 208–11.

Watanabe K, Negoro T, Aso K (1993) Benign partial epilepsy with secondary generalized seizures in infancy. *Epilepsia* **34**: 635–8.

Watanabe K, Negoro T, Aso K, et al. (1994) Clinical, EEG and positron emission tomography features of childhood onset epilepsy with localized cortical dysplasia detected by magnetic resonance imaging. *J Epilepsy* **7**: 108–16.

Watanabe K, Negoro T, Okumura A (2001) Symptomatology of infantile spasms. *Brain Dev* **23**: 453–66.

Watanabe K, Okumura A, Aso K, Duchowny M (2005) Non-idiopathic localization-related epilepsies in infants and young children. In: Roger J, Bureau M, Dravet C, et al., eds. *Epileptic Syndromes in Infancy, Childhood and Adolescence. 4th edn.* London: John Libbey Eurotext, pp. 181–200.

Watanabe M, Fujiwara T, Terauchi N, et al. (1989) Intractable grand mal epilepsy developed in the first year of life. In: Manelis J, Bental E, Loeber JN, Dreifuss FE, eds. *Advances in Epileptology, vol. 17. The XVIIth Epilepsy International Symposium.* New York: Raven Press, pp. 327–329.

Weaver DF, Camfield P, Fraser A (1988) Massive carbamazepine overdose: clinical and pharmacologic observations in five episodes. *Neurology* **38**: 755–9.

Weaving LS, Christodoulou J, Williamson Sl, et al. (2004) Mutations in the CDKL5 gene cause a severe developmental disorder with infantile spasms and mental retatardation. *Am J Hum Genet* **75**: 1079–93.

Weglage J, Demsky A, Pietsch M, Kurlemann G (1997) Neuropsychological, intellectual, and behavioral findings in patients with centrotemporal spikes with and without seizures. *Dev Med Child Neurol* **39**: 646–51.

Weig SG, Pollack P (1993) Carbamazepine-induced heart block in a child with tuberous sclerosis and cardiac rhabdomyoma: implications for evaluation and follow-up. *Ann Neurol* **34**: 617–9.

Wiebe S, Blume WT, Girvin JP, et al. (2001) A randomized, controlled trial of surgery for temporal-lobe epilepsy. *N Engl J Med* **345**: 311–8.

Wieser HG; ILAE Commission on Neurosurgery of Epilepsy (2004) ILAE Commission Report. Mesial temporal lobe epilepsy with hippocampal sclerosis. *Epilepsia* **45**: 695–714.

Wieser HG, Williamson PD (1993) Ictal semiology. In: Engel J, ed. *Surgical Treatment of the Epilepsies, 2nd edn.* New York: Raven Press, pp. 161–71.

Wilkins A, Lindsay J (1985) Common forms of reflex epilepsy: physiological mechanisms and techniques for treatment. In: Pedley TA, Meldrum BS, eds. *Recent Advances in Epilepsy, vol. 2.* Edinburgh: Churchill Livingstone, pp. 239–71.

Williamson PD, Thadani VM, Darcey TM, et al. (1992) Occipital lobe epilepsy: clinical characteristics, seizure spread patterns, and results of surgery. *Ann Neurol* **31**: 3–13.

Williamson PD, French JA, Thadani VM, et al. (1993a) Characteristics of medial temporal lobe epilepsy: II. Interictal and ictal scalp electroencephalography, neuropsychological testing, neuroimaging, surgical results and pathology. *Ann Neurol* **34**: 781–7.

Williamson PD, Spencer DD, Spencer SS, et al. (1993b) Complex partial seizures of frontal lobe origin. *Ann Neurol* **18**: 497–504.

Wirrell EC, Camfield PR, Gordon KE, et al. (1995) Benign rolandic epilepsy: atypical features are very common. *J Child Neurol* **10**: 455–8.

Wirrell EC, Camfield CS, Camfield PR, et al. (1996) Long-term prognosis of typical childhood absence epilepsy: remission or progression to juvenile myoclonic epilepsy. *Neurology* **47**: 912–8.

Wolf NI, Bast T, Surtees R (2005) Epilepsy in inborn errors of metabolism. *Epileptic Disord* **7**: 67–81.

Wolf P (1994) Reading epilepsy. In: Wolf P, ed. *Epileptic Seizures and Syndromes.* London: John Libbey, pp. 67–73.

Wolf P (2002) Epilepsy with grand mal on awakening. In: Roger J, Bureau M, Dravet C, et al., eds. *Epileptic Syndromes in Infancy, Childhood and Adolescence. 3rd edn.* London: John Libbey, pp. 357–67.

Wolf P, Inoue Y (2005) Complex reflex epilepsies: reading epilepsy and praxis induction. In: Roger J, Bureau M, Dravet C, et al., eds. *Epileptic Syndromes in Infancy, Childhood and Adolescence. 4th edn.* London: John Libbey Eurotext, pp. 347–58.

Wolf P, Inoué Y, Zifkin B, eds. (2004) *Reflex Epilepsies: Progress in Understanding.* Paris: John Libbey Eurotext.

Wolf SM, Carr A, Davis DC, et al. (1977) The value of phenobarbital in the child who has had a single febrile seizure: a controlled prospective study. *Pediatrics* **59**: 378–85.

Woo E, Chan YM, Yu YL, et al. (1988) If a well stabilized epileptic patient has a subtherapeutic antiepileptic drug level, should the dose be increased? A randomized prospective study. *Epilepsia* **29**: 129–39.

Wu JY, Koh S, Sankar R (2006) Status epilepticus in infancy and childhood. In: Wasterlain C, Treiman D, eds. *Status Epilepticus: Mechanisms and Management.* Cambridge, MA: MIT Press, pp. 113–23.

Wyllie E, Lüders H, Morris HH, et al. (1986) The lateralizing significance of versive head and eye movements during epileptic seizures. *Neurology* **36**: 606–11.

Wyllie E, Chee M, Granström ML, et al. (1993) Temporal lobe epilepsy in early childhood. *Epilepsia* **34**: 859–68.

Wyllie E, Comair YG, Kotagal P, et al. (1998) Seizure outcome after epilepsy surgery in children and adolescents. *Ann Neurol* **44**: 740–8.

Wyllie E, Gupta A, Lachhwani DK, eds. (2006) *The Treatment of Epilepsy, 4th edn.* Philadelphia: Lippincott, Williams & Wilkins.

Wyllie E, Lachhwani DK, Gupta A, et al. (2007) Successful surgery for epilepsy due to early brain lesions despite generalized EEG findings. *Neurology* **69**: 389–97.

Yaffe K, Ferriero D, Barkovich AJ, Rowley H (1995) Reversible MRI abnormalities following seizures. *Neurology* **45**: 104–8.

Yaqub BA (1993) Electroclinical seizures in Lennox–Gastaut syndrome. *Epilepsia* **34**: 120–7.

Young GB, Barr HWK, Blume WT (1986) Painful epileptic seizures involving the second sensory area. *Ann Neurol* **19**: 412 (letter).

Zaccara G, Franciotta D, Perucca E (2007) Idiosyncratic adverse reactions to antiepileptic drugs. *Epilepsia* **48**: 1223–44.

Zaret BS, Cohen RA (1986) Reversible valproic acid-induced dementia: a case report. *Epilepsia* **27**: 234–40.

16
PAROXYSMAL DISORDERS OTHER THAN EPILEPSY

Epilepsy is the most important of the paroxysmal neurological disorders of childhood but a host of other paroxysmal conditions are observed in children. Indeed, the diagnosis of epilepsy is often made wrongly in the presence of paroxysmal events. An incorrect diagnosis of epilepsy was made in 20–30% of children referred to one epilepsy clinic (Jeavons 1983), in 27 of 124 children (22%) reported by Desai and Talwar (1992), and in 10–20% of children according to Metrick et al. (1991). Such figures reflect a common experience (Aicardi 2003). Because an incorrect label of epilepsy all too often has profound consequences on a child's life, such misdiagnoses must be avoided. The present chapter reviews the most common nonepileptic paroxysmal conditions that cause faints and other turns.

ANOXIC SEIZURES

So-called 'anoxic' seizures are due to cortical hypoxic failure of energy metabolism as a result of anoxia or hypoxia. They may occur in many circumstances: bradycardia of less than 40 beats per minute, tachycardia of more than 150 beats per minute, asystole of more than 4 seconds, systolic pressure <50 mmHg or venous O_2 pressure <20 mmHg.

Cortical hypoxia results in loss of consciousness and of postural tone. When severe, liberation of tonigenic brainstem centres from corticoreticular inhibition causes decorticate rigidity and/or opisthotonus. Increasing degrees of cortical hypoxia produce slowing of frequency of the dominant cortical rhythms, followed by complete flattening of the EEG tracing, which corresponds to the tonic phase. With correction of hypoxia, slow waves reappear and may be synchronous with a few jerks of the limbs before resumption of normal EEG activity (Gastaut 1974, Stephenson 1990).

Anoxic seizures can be due to several different mechanisms (Table 16.1), several of which may be operative in the same patient or even in the same attack (Stephenson 1990).

REFLEX SYNCOPES AND FAINTS

A syncope is a sudden loss of consciousness and of postural tone associated with a cutting off of energy substrates to the brain usually through a decrease in cerebral perfusion by oxygenated blood, due to reduction in cerebral blood flow or to a drop of the oxygen content, or to a combination of both. Low perfusion is usually the consequence of a cardioinhibitory mechanism mediated through the vagus nerve or of a vasodepressor mechanism with variable vagal accompaniment (*vasovagal or neurocardiogenic syncope*). Rarely it results from primary cardiac events. In faints, the loss of consciousness is generally preceded by sensations of light-headedness, weakness or a feeling of things going far away, and the loss of tone is progressive, the patient slowly slumping to the ground. Occasionally, the loss of posture is abrupt with a sudden fall. In such cases the tip of the tongue may be cut, though true tongue-biting with lateral laceration occurs only exceptionally (Stephenson 1990, Lempert et al. 1994). Urinary incontinence is not uncommon and does not indicate an epileptic mechanism. The diagnosis of syncope rests essentially on the circumstances of occurrence, which include emotional stimuli or stress, a standing posture, especially in a confined atmosphere, or minor pain. In some individuals faints are regularly provoked by the same stimulus such as getting into or out of a bath (Stephenson 1990, Patel et al. 1994), combing one's hair (Lewis and Frank 1993) or stretching (Pelekanos et al. 1990). During the attack, the patient is pale, the eyes may be deviated vertically and the pulse may be slow.

In some cases, a *true epileptic attack can be induced* by the hypoxia resulting from a syncope (Aicardi et al. 1988, Battaglia et al. 1989, Stephenson 1990). Such instances have been termed *anoxic–epileptic seizures* (Stephenson 1990, Horrocks et al. 2005) and may be of long duration resulting in episodes of status epilepticus (Battaglia et al. 1989).

Alternatively, cardiac arrhythmias can occasionally result from an epileptic discharge involving cardioregulatory efferents. Such a phenomenon (*epileptic–anoxic seizure*) may play a role in sudden death of epileptic patients (Oppenheimer et al. 1990, Stephenson 1990, Stephenson et al. 2004). The epileptic nature of such attacks may be difficult to diagnose.

Many syncopes have an abrupt onset; clonic movements occur in perhaps 50% of cases and incontinence in 10% (Stephenson 1990). Syncopes can occur in the sitting and even in the supine position, they may be preceded by hallucinatory phenomena, and postictal confusion may be observed, thus making distinction from an epileptic seizure difficult. Vasovagal syncopes are mostly a benign phenomenon even though they can

TABLE 16.1
Possible mechanisms of anoxic seizures

Breath-holding with prolonged expiratory apnoea (Southall et al. 1985) and ventilatory/perfusion mismatch or intrapulmonary shunting (Southall et al. 1990) responsible for cyanosis

Obstructive apnoea especially awake apnoea associated with gastrointestinal reflux (Spitzer et al. 1984)

Suffocation
  Self-suffocation or strangulation
  Induction of anoxic seizure in an infant by an adult (Munchausen syndrome by proxy or Meadow syndrome)

Valsalva manoeuvre
  May play a role in breath-holding
  May be exclusive mechanism in some self-induced syncopes (Gastaut 1980)

Cardiac disease
  Valvular (aortic stenosis)
  Congenital cyanotic heart disease (Daniels et al. 1987)
  Ventricular tachyarrhythmias
  Sick sinus syndrome (Gordon 1994b)

Fainting and reflex anoxic seizures
  May alternate with 'true' breath-holding

Other circulatory syncopes
  Vagovagal syncope (Woody and Kiel 1986)
  'Hypervagism' (Stephenson 1990)
  Carotid sinus disorders

Brain compression
  Chiari malformation (Stephenson 1990)
  Brainstem tumours (Southall et al. 1987)

generate considerable anxiety. Reassurance is usually sufficient therapy, and only for frequently repeated attacks may atropine treatment be justified.

Vasovagal syncopes are often familial in nature (Camfield and Camfield 1990, Cooper et al. 1994) but do not obey mendelian rules of inheritance.

Syncopes may occur electively in *febrile children* and such accidents are apt to be mistaken for febrile convulsions. The oculocardiac reflex produces a lasting slowing of the heart rate and may induce a fit identical to the patient's usual attack. This mechanism is not universally accepted, as a strong oculocardiac reflex does not exclude the possibility of a febrile convulsion.

One reported cause of fainting and loss of consciousness is the use of niaprazine, an antihistaminic drug. Loss of consciousness is associated with hypotonia and pallor, is of brief duration and occurs within 30 minutes of absorption in most cases (Bodiou and Bavoux 1988). Severe cases are rare (Auduy 1988).

BREATH-HOLDING SPELLS
Breath-holding spells occur in about 4% of all children below the age of 5 years. There are two major forms, the cyanotic and the pallid types (Lombroso and Lerman 1967). The mechanisms of the two forms are different, and most 'pallid breath-holding attacks', such as occur when a child bumps her/his head and almost immediately loses consciousness, are best regarded as reflex hypoxic syncopes precipitated by painful stimuli or emotion (Stephenson 1990, Breningstall 1996).

Cyanotic breath-holding attacks are provoked by fright, pain, anger or frustration. The child cries vigorously then holds her/his breath in expiration. This results in cyanosis and eventually culminates in loss of consciousness and limpness. The latter may be followed by brief body stiffening before respiration resumes and the attack ends. Polygraphic recordings have shown a sequence of slowing of the EEG tracing with bradycardia such as one would expect in the overshoot phase of a Valsalva manoeuvre. Despite their frightening appearance, breath-holding spasms are harmless (Gordon 1987). The mechanism of cyanotic breath-holding spells is still imperfectly known (DiMario and Burleson 1993). Oxygen desaturation and reduction of cerebral blood flow because of increased intrathoracic pressure with decreased venous return play a role. However, cyanosis develops with surprising rapidity and an intrapulmonary right-to-left shunt seems likely as a result of imperfect matching of ventilation to perfusion (Breningstall 1996). Gastaut (1974) made the distinction between breath-holding spells and sobbing spasms or sobbing syncopes in which the child would "sob intensely and intractably for a long period of time (1–3 minutes)" before losing consciousness. Exceptional cases of breath-holding attacks resulting in death have been associated with severe underlying conditions (Southall et al. 1990). Such exceptions do not modify the benign prognosis of the condition.

Pallid breath-holding attacks may exist in isolation or alternate with the cyanotic form in the same child. They accounted for 19% of cases in the study by Lombroso and Lerman (1967). In this type, which is often precipitated by pain, especially from a bump on the head, the children lose consciousness following a minimum of crying or no crying at all. Pallor is marked and stiffening is the rule. In many such patients, the attack is associated with a period of asystole (*cardio-inhibitory syncope*) that can also be induced by compression of the eyeballs (Lombroso and Lerman 1967, Stephenson 1980). Urinary incontinence is not rare in this form. The mechanism is reflex cardioinhibition resulting in cardiac standstill with a consequent hypoxic attack. On the EEG tracings, the tonic attack is associated with flattening of the record that follows a run of slow waves. A few clonic jerks are not infrequently observed following the tonic attack (Fig. 16.1). Pallid breath-holding attacks are more frequently mistaken for epilepsy than the cyanotic forms. The diagnosis rests as much on the fact that all attacks are precipitated by an adequate stimulus as on the seizure description, which may be difficult to distinguish by history from an epileptic seizure. Indeed, they may be responsible for *anoxic–epileptic seizures* (Stephenson 1990, Stephenson et al. 2004, Horrocks et al. 2005). The outlook for this form is also favourable, and explanation and reassurance that the attacks produce no harm and will cease is often followed by a marked diminution of their frequency. Rarely is psychiatric help needed, and no drug treatment is necessary or effective (Gordon 1987). Exceptionally, cardiac pacing has been needed (Wilson et al. 2005).

UNUSUAL TYPES OF REFLEX SYNCOPES
Self-induced reflex syncopes are rare but may pose difficult

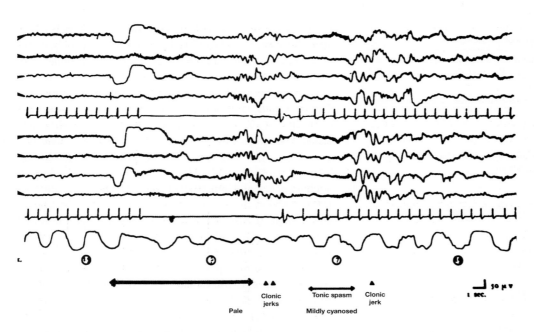

Clonic
jerks

Pale

Tonic spasm

Mildly cyanosed

Clonic
jerk

30 μV

1 sec.

Fig. 16.1. Anoxic seizure induced by pressure on the eyeballs. Ocular pressure was applied at the first horizontal arrow, resulting in cardiac asytole with appearance, after a few seconds, of slow waves on the EEG. The patient turned pale and had two clonic jerks. Later, the EEG flattened while the boy became mildly cyanosed and a tonic spasm occurred (second horizontal arrow). Following resumption of cardiac contractions, slow waves reappeared on the EEG and a further clonic jerk was observed. (Courtesy Prof. H Gastaut, Hôpital de la Timone, Marseilles.)

diagnostic problems. Such attacks are seen in psychotic patients with mental retardation (Gastaut et al. 1987) and are usually mistaken for absences or drop-attacks. The children stop breathing and inflate their chest or abdomen, producing a Valsalva manoeuvre. After a few seconds, they turn pale with a vacant look and a loss of tone that may be limited to the neck or involve also the lower limbs with resultant fall. The same phenomenon is frequently seen in girls with Rett syndrome where it alternates with hyperventilation periods. It may rarely occur in intellectually normal children with behavioural disturbances. The diagnosis rests on a peculiar polygraphic sequence (Aicardi et al. 1988). Treatment with fenfluramine may be effective.

ANOXIC SEIZURES DUE TO RESPIRATORY OBSTRUCTION
These are infrequent in children, although accidental suffocation or strangulation does occur. Induction of anoxic seizures by an adult, usually the mother, is a relatively common form of the *Munchausen syndrome by proxy* or Meadow syndrome (Rosenberg 2003, Galvin et al. 2005). The diagnosis may be difficult, especially if the mother presses the baby's face into her breast. The constant presence of the mother at the onset of each episode is an essential clue, and a final diagnosis can be estabished by prolonged polygraphic recording (Stephenson et al. 2004) or by covert EEG–video monitoring, which, however, raises delicate ethical and legal problems (Bauer 2004).

SYNCOPES OF CARDIAC ORIGIN
Syncopes of cardiac origin are much rarer than reflex vasovagal or cardioinhibitory attacks. They represented only 6% of 108 syncopes studied by McHarg et al. (1997). It is important to recognize them because they may be due to dangerous conditions that may result in sudden death, so that preventive treatment and monitoring are essential. Cardiac disorders responsible for syncopes include valvular disorders such as aortic stenosis, which can produce syncopes on effort; postoperative conduction blocks; cardiomyopathies sometimes associated with myopathies; and intrinsic disturbances of cardiac rhythm such as Wolff–Parkinson–White syndrome, congenital atrioventricular block and the long Q-T syndromes. These syndromes are the expression of channelopathies involving specific sodium or potassium channels and include several distinct syndromes (long and short Q-T syndromes, Brugada syndrome, Ward–Romano syndrome, Jervell–Lange–Nielsen syndrome). Molecular genetic studies have shown that at least seven different long Q-T syndromes exist including: potassium channel mutations (LQT2) on chromosome 7q35–q36, sodium channel protein mutation on chromosome 3 (LQT3), ras-1 protein gene mutations on chromosome 11p (Towbin 1995, Sarkozy and Brugada 2005, Wolpert et al. 2005). They are genetically transmitted, which has an impact on diagnosis, counselling and treatment, and may be recessive or dominant (Avanzini et al. 2004). Associated features, e.g. deafness in the recessive Jervell–Lange–Nielsen syndrome (Chapter 18), may be present. All these syndromes can mimic epilepsy (Gordon 1994b, Pacia et al. 1994) and can result in sudden death (Goldenberg et al. 2005). Occurrence of episodes during sleep or exercise may be a hint to the correct diagnosis. Attacks can also be precipitated by emotion or stress. Such circumstances as well as a

family history of sudden death or 'epilepsy', or a personal history of chest pains, palpitations or a surgically repaired heart defect require full cardiac investigation. The corrected Q-Tc interval is prolonged in most cases, although occasional cases of cardiac syncope with a normal Q-T have been reported, so the ECG should be systematically recorded with the EEG in patients with unexplained loss of consciousness (Bricker et al. 1984). Prolonged ECG recording and effort test may be indicated in selected cases (Nousiainen et al. 1989), especially when a history of familial syncope or sudden death is present. In some cases, a pacemaker should be inserted as sudden death is possible.

Acute attacks of hyperpnoea and cyanosis are a common feature of congenital cyanotic cardiopathies. They may result in loss of consciousness and may be followed by hemiplegia of vascular origin (Chapter 22). Severe apnoea may also be a feature of the syndrome of alternating hemiplegia (Bourgeois et al. 1993).

EPISODES OF APNOEA OR BRADYCARDIA IN YOUNG INFANTS: NEAR-MISS SUDDEN INFANT DEATH SYNDROME (SIDS); APPARENT LIFE-THREATENING EVENTS

Study of the sudden infant death syndrome is beyond the scope of this book. However, some near-miss SIDS cases may be easily mistaken for epileptic events, the more so as they can be followed by neurological sequelae and episodes of status epilepticus (Constantinou et al. 1989). Indeed, the true sequence of events may be impossible to establish in some cases. Less severe episodes may manifest as briefer episodes of apnoea, with hypo- or hypertonia and a change of colour that may be wrongly interpreted as epileptic phenomena. Such events may occur in the first few days of life in apparently healthy babies (Grylack and Williams 1996).

Screening for infants at risk of sudden death has been extensively investigated. Most studies have found no precise correlation between polygraphic recordings and the later occurrence of sudden death (Reerink et al. 1995), so that indications for use of electronic monitors in the home remain tentative. In preterm infants, episodes of marked desaturation can occur without apnoea and remain undetectable by monitoring (Poets et al. 1995).

The awake apnoea syndrome consists of apnoeic–bradycardic episodes and may be causally related to the presence of gastro-oesophageal reflux (Pedley 1983, Spitzer et al. 1984, See et al. 1989, Page and Jeffery 2000) or to oesophageal spasm (Fontan et al. 1984). The attacks resemble syncope and are often preceded by restlessness and an apprehensive look and accompanied by opisthotonus, so the misdiagnosis of epilepsy is not rare. Such attacks may respond to the treatment of gastro-oesophageal reflux, although this is debated (Brand et al. 2005).

Other causes of apnoea in neonates and infants appear in Table 16.2.

ACUTE PSYCHIATRIC MANIFESTATIONS

Acute psychiatric manifestations represented the second most common cause of a wrong diagnosis of epilepsy in Jeavons'

experience (1983). In most of these cases the resemblance to epileptic seizures is only superficial, and such episodes as attacks of anxiety, acute phobic episodes, attacks of epigastric or laryngeal sensation of pressure, fugues and recurrent episodes of feelings of derealization often do not raise major diagnostic problems. However, panic attacks are sometimes mistaken for epilepsy (Genton et al. 1995). Hallucinations due to schizophrenia, or to schizophrenia-like states due to substance abuse (Chapter 12), and acute confusional episodes may be difficult to distinguish from some types of nonconvulsive status epilepticus. Recurrent episodes of abnormal paroxysmal behaviour may be due to intermittently manifesting metabolic diseases such as hyperammonaemia or hypoglycaemia, and metabolic screening is in order when such diagnoses are considered. *Munchausen syndrome by proxy* may also be regarded as a cause of psychogenic seizures. It can cause great diagnostic difficulties. The mothers, most often the offenders, may invent a story of seizures and, sometimes, tell it with great sophistication (Meadow 1984, 1991) or even teach the child that s/he has epilepsy, so that the child invents the episodes (Croft and Jervis 1989).

Attacks of rage may occur in adolescents and older children and are sometimes referred to as manifestations of the *episodic dyscontrol syndrome* (Elliott 1984). Such attacks may be a cause of physical aggression and may be associated with some obscuration of consciousness and postictal sleep. However, at times the attacks occur following only very slight provocations, and the aggression is clearly directed, which differs from what is seen in patients with complex partial seizures fighting against restraint.

PSEUDOSEIZURES (NON-EPILEPTIC SEIZUTES)
Pseudoepileptic seizures, also known as pseudoseizures, hysterical attacks, psychic or psychogenic seizures, can be very difficult to distinguish from true epileptic attacks (Holmes et al. 1980). They are frequent in adolescents and may occur in children as early as 4 years of age (Kramer et al. 1995). They can occur even during apparent sleep (Harden et al. 2003) and in children with neurodevelopmental impairment (Neill 1990). Pseudoseizures are commonly observed in children who also have epileptic seizures and are one important cause of apparent 'intractability' of epilepsy (Aicardi 1988). They may also occur in children who have never had epileptic attacks (Holmes et al. 1980, Lesser 1996).

Pseudoseizures can mimic any type of seizures, especially generalized ones, but unilateral or focal attacks may be seen and even EEG may not be sufficient for differential diagnosis from epileptic seizures as organic frontal seizures may not have an EEG expression (Chapter 15). Most pseudoseizures differ from true seizures by the nature of movements, which are not typical clonias but rather semipurposeful activity, by their violent and theatrical expression and by a nonstereotyped pattern. In one series of 21 children (Wyllie et al. 1990), 10 had episodes of unresponsiveness, generalized limb jerking and thrashing movements, and 6 had episodes of staring and unresponsiveness. Most children were responsive immediately after the paroxysm. The average age of 43 patients studied by Lancman et al. (1994b) was 12.4 years at onset of seizures and 15 years when the diagnosis

TABLE 16.2
TABLE 16.2
Main causes of apnoea in infants and children

Cause	References
Neonates and infants	
Apnoea related to acute neurological disturbances	
Acute hypoxic–ischaemic encephalopathy	Chapter 1
Spinal cord birth injury	Lee et al. (2004)
Neonatal and infantile seizures	Watanabe et al. (1982), Chapter 15
Apnoea related to chronic neurological disturbances	
CNS malformations	
Joubert syndrome	Chapter 2
Chiari II malformation	Chapter 2
Dandy–Walker syndrome	Chapters 2, 6
Peripheral malformations	
Vocal cord paralysis	Lee et al. (2004), Dinwiddie (2004)
Moebius syndrome	Sadarshan and Goldie (1985)
Pierre Robin syndrome	Buchenau et al. (2007)
Hyperekplexia	Nigro and Lim (1992), Rivera et al. (2006)
Neuromuscular diseases	
Congenital muscular dystrophies	Chapter 21
Congenital myopathies	
Spinal muscular atrophy	Chapter 19
Congenital central alveolar hypoventilation	This chapter
Metabolic diseases	Chapter 8
Hypoglycaemia	
Organic acidurias	
Nonketotic hyperglycinaemia	
Leigh syndrome and other mitochondrial diseases	Cummiskey et al. (1987), Grattan-Smith et al. (1990)
Gastrointestinal disturbances	
Gastro-oesophageal reflux[1], hiatus hernia	Molloy et al. (2005), Mousa et al. (2005)
Older children	
Rett syndrome	Hagberg et al. (1983)
Familial encephalopathy with permanent periodic breathing	Magaudda et al. (1987)
Neuromuscular disorders	
CNS diseases	Southall et al. (1990)
Epilepsy (status or isolated seizures)	Chapter 15
Mitochondrial encephalomyopathy with sleep apnoea	Tatsumi et al. (1988)
Obstructive sleep apnoea syndrome	This chapter
Obstructive apnoea due to hypertrophy of amygdalae	Nixon and Brouillette (2005)
Central apnoea of unknown cause	American Academy of Pediatrics Task Force on Infantile Apnea (1985)
Obesity (Pickwickian syndrome)	Mokhlesi et al. (2007)
Pulmonary diseases, especially bronchiolitis	Henderson (2005)
Common apnoeas of poorly understood mechanism	
Apnoea of prematurity[2]	Poets et al. (1995), Stokowski (2005)
Apparent life-threatening events (ALTE)[3]	Dewolfe (2005), Brand et al. (2005)

[1]Gastrointestinal reflux remains a deleted cause of apnoea.
[2]Exclusion diagnosis.
[3]Apnoea, pallor, cyanosis, impression of imminent death. About half the cases are due to known disorders (respiratory, digestive, neurological or cardiac); the remaining cases are idiopathic and may be related to the sudden infant death syndrome and to sudden unexpected death in epilepsy patients (SUDEP) (see Chapter 15).

was made. Twenty-one of them received antiepileptic agents, and the majority of episodes consisted of violent uncoordinated movements and generalized trembling, although a few patients had only staring seizures. The average duration of attacks was 5.6 minutes, although Bhatia and Sapra (2005) oberved that their patients tended to have long attacks lasting 10–35 minutes. Induction of seizures by suggestion (Lancman et al. 1994a) may be helpful. However, the personality of the parents and/or patient and the way they describe the attacks may give rise to serious difficulties. In addition some epileptic seizures, especially frontal ones, may easily suggest hysteria or simulation. Weinstock et al. (2003) reported on 5 children with 'hyperkinetic' attacks mimicking frontal lobe seizures, which are particularly difficult to identify. A nonparoxysmal EEG is an important argument but certainly does not exclude the diagnosis as movement artefacts may render the EEG uninterpretable and normal tracings occur occasionally in 'organic' frontal seizures, and close EEG–video observation of the patients and tests of provocation may be necessary to firmly establish the diagnosis (Wyllie et al. 1990). Conversely, recording of typical EEG discharges concomitant to clinical events excludes the diagnosis of pseudoseizures. Prolonged video recording can be especially useful in this regard (Chapter 15).

Pseudo-status epilepticus is relatively frequent in adult patients and can be seen also in children (Tuxhorn and Fischbach 2002). Recognition of such cases is essential as the diagnosis of epilepsy often results in prolonged and increasingly heavier drug therapy, which may have disastrous effects.

Pseudoseizures masquerading as *absences* have been observed in 18 children with hyperventilation syndrome by North et al. (1990). The EEG of these patients showed bursts of slow-wave activity without spikes, corresponding to apparently impaired awareness and responsiveness. A similar EEG change associated with altered responsiveness can be observed during hyperventilation in normal children (Epstein et al. 1994).

Once the diagnosis is established, previous drug treatment, if any, should be rapidly discontinued. Some form of psychiatric treatment seems beneficial, at least in the short term (Holmes et al. 1980). The short-term outcome was favourable in 16 of the 21 children in the series of Wyllie et al., but only 10 of 22 children followed-up for 40 months or more by Lancman et al. (1994b) were seizure-free at last visit. Gudmunsson et al. (2001) found that 14 of 17 children and adolescents with pseudoseizures were symptom-free after an average duration of treatment of 1.5 years and could resume school. A firm diagnosis is critical so that a shift away from antiepileptic medication and toward psychiatric therapy becomes possible.

THE HYPERVENTILATION SYNDROME

Hyperventilation syndrome is relatively common, especially in adolescent girls. The term implies that ventilatory effort is greater than necessitated by metabolic demands. Patients complain variably of chest pain, light-headedness and dyspnoea. Pseudo-absence spells and syncopes may suggest the diagnosis of epilepsy. The diagnosis rests on a high index of suspicion and on the presence of the typical symptoms. Rebreathing in a plastic or paper bag enables control of the symptoms of an impending attack and has both diagnostic and therapeutic value. Underlying family problems should be looked for, but the outlook is somewhat guarded as many children go on to hyperventilate and show chronic anxiety as adults (Herman et al. 1981, Oren et al. 1987).

SEIZURES OF TOXIC ORIGIN

Attacks of sudden loss of consciousness, often with convulsions or other neurological phenomena, should always raise the suspicion of toxicity (see Chapter 12). Predominantly motor manifestations may occur following use of an increasing number of drugs. Such seizures are often dystonic in nature, with recurrent episodes of stiffness, hyperextension of the head and opisthotonus. Oculogyric crises are frequent. Any recurrent attack with extrapyramidal manifestation must suggest the diagnosis of drug intoxication, even though any such possibility is denied by the parents or custodians. The drugs most commonly in cause are psychotropic drugs such as phenothiazines and butyrophenones

(Pranzatelli 1996) and metoclopramide (Leopold 1984), but a vast number of agents are being progressively added to the list (Elzinga-Huttenga et al. 2006) and a review of these is beyond the scope of this book. The important point is that any acute neurological or psychiatric manifestation in a child or an adolescent should immediately suggest such a possibility and makes a thorough investigation imperative, regardless of the denegations of parents or relatives. A familial susceptibility to drugs may exist. Consciousness is preserved in many cases and this does not rule out intoxication that can produce other neurological manifestations with intact vigilance. Urine examination for the commonly responsible drugs should be performed, and more specialized research can be required in case of doubt.

Most acute drug reactions are self-limited. Treatment with intravenous benztropine or diphenhydramine is useful for controlling rapidly severe dystonic–dyskinetic attacks, although some cases may be resistant to high doses (Leopold 1984).

Rare cases of attacks of endogenous toxic origin (e.g. mastocytoma) are on record (Krowchuk et al. 1994).

TETANY

Tetany is a manifestation of peripheral nerve hyperexcitability. The term is often used to designate convulsions due to hypocalcaemia in the newborn infant (Chapters 1, 15).

In older infants and children, tetany proper is characterized by episodes of tonic muscular spasms and paraesthesias affecting the distal territory of nerves, often precipitated by hyperventilation or ischaemia of the limbs. The clinical manifestations of classical tetany do not appear before 3 months of age. The so-called carpopedal spasm is the most striking manifestation. It appears abruptly and affects primarily the fingers, which are flexed at the proximal joint and extended at the distal joints, with the thumbs strongly adducted and opposed. The feet may be similarly involved. Consciousness is clear. Laryngospasm often occurs, simultaneously with carpopedal spasm or independently. The vocal cords are adducted so that inspiration becomes noisy, and complete interruption of respiration may rarely occur. Between spasms, signs of latent tetany may be present but the Chvostek sign is not characteristic as it occurs in some normal children. Nerve hyperexcitability is expressed electrophysiologically by repetitive EMG activity (multiplets) elicited by cuff-ischaemia of the arm, but is present also in 20–30% of normal individuals (Eisinger 1987). Tetany is usually due to hypocalcaemia and/or hypomagnesaemia but may also occur in normocalcaemic persons. In such cases, tetany appears to be the consequence of a decrease in the level of ionized calcium with a normal level of total calcium. Such a decrease in ionization of calcium can be due to alkalosis as a result of hyperventilation or of repeated vomiting as in pyloric stenosis. Vitamin D deficiency is now a rare cause of tetany. Postoperative hypoparathyroidism and pseudohypoparathyroidism are more frequently the cause (Wilson and Hall 2002). Hypomagnesaemia with secondary hypocalcaemia is more rarely a cause (Visudhipan et al. 2005). In patients with hypoparathyroidism and pseudohypoparathyroidism, headaches, extrapyramidal signs and calcification of the basal ganglia can be found. Patients with pseudohypoparathyroidism, in addition, are obese, below average height, with a moon-shaped facies and short metacarpals. Mental retardation, cataracts, enamel defect and decreased olfaction and auditory acuity are additional features (Ellie et al. 1989). In all types, epileptic seizures can occur at any age and are, in fact, more commonly observed than the muscle spasms of classical tetany.

The treatment of tetany consists of parenteral administration of calcium salts and vitamin D, and occasionally of magnesium salts.

BENIGN PAROXYSMAL VERTIGO AND PAROXYSMAL TORTICOLLIS OF INFANCY

PAROXYSMAL VERTIGO

This condition is characterized by recurrent attacks of vertigo that affect equally boys and girls between 1 and 5 years of age (Koenigsberger et al. 1970). The attacks are brief, lasting from one to several minutes, and come on suddenly without known precipitant. The child appears in distress, pale but conscious, and may stagger or fall during the attacks. Often, s/he will lie down on the floor, refusing to move. Nystagmus may be noted during attacks. The frequency of attacks is commonly one to a few per month. Many children have fewer than five attacks in total. Affected children appear otherwise normal, and in my experience all examinations are negative, although abnormalities in labyrinthine function were reported by Koenigsberger and colleagues. The outcome is consistently favourable. Attacks disappeared within 3 months to 8 years in all 19 cases studied by Lindskog et al. (1999). After a follow-up of 13–21 years, 4/19 had developed migainous headache; 7 had a family history of migraine. Most children cease having attacks by 5–6 years of age.

Benign paroxysmal positional vertigo, an entity well known in adults, may occur in children. Marcelli et al. (2006) observed 9 patients who had normal vestibular tests and responded to the classic Dix–Hallpike therapeutic manoeuvre.

BENIGN PAROXYSMAL TORTICOLLIS OF INFANCY

Benign paroxysmal torticollis of infancy (Cohen et al. 1993) is probably closely related to paroxysmal vertigo. The disorder appears before 1 year of age and sometimes from the early weeks of life. The attacks last commonly several hours and up to 2–3 days. They are marked by repeated vomiting, apparent discomfort and tilting of the head to one side, often with eye movements. The affected side may change with successive attacks. The head can be passively returned to the neutral position but the tilting recurs immediately. In some cases, there may be inclination of the trunk to the same side, sometimes with a degree of ipsilateral stiffness. Ataxia is common, especially in later attacks. If the child can walk, s/he is apt to veer towards the side to which the head is tilted. Although the clinical picture may be impressive, even suggesting a posterior fossa tumour, the abnormalities rapidly subside leaving a completely normal child free of any neurological

anomaly. The diagnosis is greatly helped by a history of previous similar episodes. If these are absent, neuroradiological assessment may be necessary. Familial occurrence has been reported (Giffin et al. 2002) and may be associated with a mutation in the *CACNA1* gene, again suggesting a relationship with migraine, which has been suggested for both paroxysmal vertigo and torticollis. A family history of migraine is useful for the diagnosis. In some patients, typical migraine will follow the torticollis as the child grows older (Deonna 1988). Other vertiginous episodes may occur in children and are caused by drug intoxication or by acute labyrinthitis of infectious origin (Chapter 18).

EPISODIC ATAXIAS

Benign vertigo of children may be related to recurrent ataxia, a familial condition with dominant (Vighetto et al. 1988) or possible X-linked (Livingstone et al. 1984) inheritance. Both vertigo and recurrent ataxia have been reported in the same patient (Tibbles et al. 1986). Attacks of episodic ataxia may last from a few hours to a few days. The origin of the ataxia (vestibular or cerebellar) is not clear but the condition belongs to the ionic channel disorders or 'channelopathies' (Gordon 1998, Graves and Hanna 2005, Kass 2005). At least two distinct forms are known, termed episodic ataxias types 1 and 2 (EA1 and 2). EA1 is characterized by brief episodes lasting seconds to minutes, with onset in early childhood and often induced by startle or exercise, and by the interictal presence of continuous myokymia (Brunt and Van Weerden 1990, Jen 2000). The disease maps to chromosome 12p13 and represents one type of potassium channel disease (KCN A1). EA2 is a calcium channel disorder linked to chromosome 19q13 at the same locus as familial hemiplegic migraine type 1 and SCA6 ataxia (Baloh et al. 1997, Jen et al. 2004), but the mutation is different (Greenberg 1997, Tonelli et al. 2006). It is often associated with nystagmus and may have quite variable manifestations; in some patients cerebellar signs are present, and in some families cases of fixed ataxia may coexist with cases of purely episodic disturbances.

Patients with episodic ataxia often respond to acetazolamide, which interrupts or prevents attacks. Sodium valproate may be a necessary adjunct to acetazolamide (Scoggan et al. 2006). An occasional patient will respond to the calcium-blocking agent flunarizine rather than acetazolamide (Boel and Casaer 1988). EA1 may respond to sulthiame (Brunt and Van Weerden 1990), acetazolamide or phenytoin (Griggs and Nutt 1995).

Autosomal dominant periodic cerebellovestibular ataxia with defective smooth pursuit movements may be genetically distinct from other autosomal dominant ataxias (Damji et al. 1996). Other familial ataxias variably accompanied by vertigo, defective smooth ocular pursuit and/or tinnitus and clinically and genetically distinct from EA1 and EA2 have been reported, and the term episodic ataxia type 3 has been proposed (Steckley et al. 2001). However, the nosology of these rare cases remains uncertain. Nonfamilial cases are on record (Verlooy and Velis 1985). Table 16.3 indicates the main causes of intermittent ataxia in childhood, and Table 16.4 lists the main types of genetically determined cerebellovestibular ataxia.

TABLE 16.3
Intermittent and recurrent ataxias in children*

Type	References
Vestibular	
Paroxysmal vertigo	Lindskog et al. (1999)
Perilymphatic fistula	Chapter 18
Endolymphatic hydrops	Idem
Vascular	
Basilar migraine	Lapkin and Golden (1978)
Transient ischaemic attacks	Chapter 14
Sickle cell disease	
Vasculitis	
Arterial dissection	
Emboli in posterior circulation	
Subclavian steal	Kurlan et al. (1984)
Metabolic	
Hypoglycaemia	Chapter 8
Electrolyte disturbances	Chapter 22
Hypoxia	Idem
Urea cycle disorders, esp. ornithine transcarbamylase deficiency	Chapter 8
Organic acidaemias including biotinidase and holocarboxylase deficiency	Idem
Propionic and methylmalonic acidaemias	Idem
Leucinosis (intermittent forms)	Idem
Leigh syndrome	Idem
Pyruvate dehydrogenase deficiency	Idem
Hartnup disease	Idem
Carnitine acyltransferase deficiency	Idem
Porphyrias	
Toxic	Chapter 12
Drug ingestion, especially antiepileptic, benzodiazepines	
Munchausen syndrome by proxy	
Demyelinating diseases	
Multiple sclerosis	Chapter 11
Tumours (fluctuations due to oedema)	Chapter 13
Epilepsy	
Epileptic pseudoataxia	Bennett et al. (1982)
Recurrent genetic ataxias	
Episodic ataxia type 1 (with continuous myokymias) (EA1)	Brunt and Van Weerden (1990)
Episodic ataxia type 2 (EA2)	Greenberg (1997), Griggs and Nutt (1995)
X-linked intermittent	Livingstone et al. (1984)
Dominant with vertigo[1]	Tibbles et al. (1986), Steckley et al. (2001)
Isolated periodic nystagmus	Valmaggia and Gottlob (2000)
Nystagmus and vertigo	Farris et al. (1986)

[1]Such cases have sometimes been referred to as episodic ataxia type 3 (EA3).

PAROXYSMAL DYSTONIA, DYSKINESIA AND CHOREOATHETOSIS

The paroxysmal dyskinesias are a complex group of conditions whose main feature is the occurrence of transient attacks of extrapyramidal movements but whose circumstances of occurrence and aetiology are diverse. Lance (1977) classified the primary paroxysmal dystonias into two subtypes: kinesigenic choreoathetosis and paroxysmal dystonic choreoathetosis. Additional types were later included in the classification proposed by Demirkiran and Jankovic (1995): intermediate cases induced by prolonged exercise, nonkinesigenic dyskinesias and hypnogenic dyskinesia. A majority of their 64 patients had acquired dyskinesia, and in contrast to most previous reports a family history was found in only 13 families.

PAROXYSMAL KINESIGENIC CHOREOATHETOSIS

This disorder is characterized by predominantly unilateral or bilateral attacks of dystonic movements or chorea that are precipitated by sudden movement (Bhatia 2001). Attacks usually last one to a few minutes and may occur up to 100 times daily. Some patients describe an aura of tightness or tingling in the affected segment. Consciousness is preserved, but the bizarre, often writhing and sometimes violent ballistic movements may result in falls. About three quarters of the cases are familial, with a dominant transmission. Other cases may represent new mutations or acquired disease. Gay and Ryan (1994) have reviewed the acquired causes of dyskinesia and reported a case induced by methylphenidate. Zorzi et al. (2003) reported that 5 of their 14 cases were due to acquired disorders such as cerebral palsy, stroke or inflammatory disease. Hart et al. (1995) reported a case of paroxysmal dystonia in a patient who also had episodes of hemiplegia, thus representing an intermediary form between dystonias and alternating hemiplegia. Episodes of paroxysmal ballismus precipitated by fever in children with dyskinetic cerebral palsy have been described by Harbord and Kobayashi (1991). In rare adult patients, paroxysmal choreoathetosis has been the presenting manifestation of diabetes mellitus (Haan et al. 1989). Paroxysmal dystonia has also been recorded in patients with cystinuria (Cavanagh et al. 1974) and with Hartnup disease (Darras et al. 1989).

Idiopathic paroxysmal kinesigenic dyskinesia in many cases responds favourably to anticonvulsant drugs, especially carbamazepine and phenytoin (Lance 1977, Bhatia 2001). The disorder does not affect lifespan but may be socially embarrassing. In some resistant cases, flunarizine has brought about control of the attacks (Lou 1989), but occasional cases are resistant to all known agents.

PAROXYSMAL DYSTONIC CHOREOATHETOSIS OF MOUNT AND REBACK

In this form, attacks are not precipitated by movement but rather by stress, coffee or alcohol (Lance 1977, Bressman et al. 1988). Attacks are usually much longer than in kinesigenic forms, lasting from 10 minutes to several hours, and occur less frequently. The condition is rare and appears to be inherited as a dominant mendelian trait. A gene (FPD1) mapping to chromosome 2q has been identified but there is also evidence for at least another gene in chromosome 1p (Hofele et al. 1997). Paroxysmal choreoathetosis generally does not respond to anticonvulsant agents, with the exception of the benzodiazepines, especially clonazepam and oxazepam. Acetazolamide has been used successfully in a patient who also had familial ataxia, and sublingual lorazepam may be effective.

TABLE 16.4
Genetically determined dominantly inherited vestibulocerebellar ataxias

Disorder	Gene locus	Clinical features	Remarks	References
Episodic ataxia type 1 (EA1)	12q13	Brief episodes of ataxia; permanent myokymias	K channel disorder, often sensitive to acetazolamide	Lubbers et al. (1995), Kullmann (2002)
Episodic ataxia type 2 (EA2)	19p13	Episodic ataxia with long episodes, tendency to become fixed; permanent nystagmus	Ca channel disorder often sensitive to acetazolamide	Kullmann (2002)
Periodic vestibulocerebellar ataxia (EA3)[1]	?	Autosomal dominant. Nystagmus; defective smooth pursuit; vertigo	Not linked to chromosome 19	Damji et al. (1996)
Episodic ataxia–vertigo and tinnitus (EA4)[1]	?	Autosomal dominant. Vestibular and auditory anomalies; defective smooth pursuit; vertigo	Not linked to EA1 or EA2 loci	Steckley et al. (2001)
Acute paroxysmal choreoathetosis/spasticity	1p	Predominant choreoathetosis; ataxia	K channel disorder	Auburger et al. (1996)

[1]Denominations EA3 and EA4 suggested by Steckley et al. (2001).

EXERCISE-INDUCED PAROXYSMAL DYSKINESIA

In this uncommon form (Lance 1977), dystonic/dyskinetic attacks are precipitated by prolonged exercise. The attacks usually supervene after 30–60 minutes of exercise and last 5–30 minutes. They may also respond to carbamazepine. Similar cases associated with epileptic seizures have been reported. Margari et al. (2000) described 6 patients with mostly generalized benign epilepsy and exercise-induced dyskinesia; Guerrini et al. (2002) observed 3 children with early-onset absence seizures before age 6 months who developed exercise-induced dyskinesia, and Zorzi et al. (2003) reported on nonkinesigenic paroxysmal dyskinesia among 14 children.

PAROXYSMAL CHOREOATHETOSIS AND INFANTILE BENIGN SEIZURES

Children with benign infantile seizures (Chapter 15) can develop, after a period of months to several years, paroxysmal dyskinetic attacks that usually are kinesigenic in type and respond to carbamazepine (Szepetowski et al. 1997). Dykinesia is not associated with seizure recurrences, and the outcome seems to be benign. This syndrome has been shown to be linked to several loci on chromosome 16 (Valente et al. 2000) but no gene has been identified. Interestingly, several studies of infantile convulsions, either isolated or followed by or associated with idiopathic epilepsy syndromes, including benign rolandic epilepsy (Guerrini 2002), have reported genetic mapping to the same chromosome, indicating the probable presence of a cluster of genes involved in neuronal excitability.

OTHER IDIOPATHIC PAROXYSMAL DYSKINESIAS

Cases of dystonias with more variability in expression and response to pharmacological agents have been reported (Bressman et al. 1988). Hemidystonia induced by prolonged exercise and cold has been reported by Wali (1992). A rare distinct type known as autosomal dominant paroxysmal choreoathetosis with spasticity (CSE) maps to chromosome 1p in the vicinity of a potassium gene channels cluster (Auburger et al. 1996). Symptomatic forms of paroxysmal dyskinesia do occur; Zorzi et al. (2003) observed 5 symptomatic cases in their series of 14 patients.

Paroxysmal kinesigenic dystonias should be distinguished from other types of attack especially when these are precipitated by sensory stimuli. These include cataplexy–narcolepsy, Nieman–Pick C disease, hyperekplexia and the Coffin–Lowry syndrome (Nelson and Hahn 2003, Stephenson et al. 2005).

Nocturnal paroxysmal dystonia is discussed on p. 686.

Paroxysmal dystonia of infancy was reported in 9 infants aged 1–5 months (Angelini et al. 1988). It consists of brief, frequently repeated episodes of opisthotonus and/or symmetrical or asymmetrical dystonia of the upper limbs. The frequency decreases with age, and the attacks disappear altogether between 8 and 22 months.

The *neck–tongue syndrome* (Orrell and Marsden 1993) consists of paroxysmal dystonia of the tongue upon rotation of the head.

BENIGN MYOCLONUS OF INFANCY

Benign myoclonus of infancy is different from benign neonatal sleep myoclonus (see below). The condition is described in Chapter 15 as it mimics infantile spasms, although without EEG abnormalities and with an excellent prognosis. Familial recurrence has been reported (Galletti et al. 1989).

EXCESSIVE STARTLE DISEASE

Excessive startle can be observed in many neurological diseases. Truly pathological disease on the other hand is uncommon but may be idiopathic or result from extensive CNS damage.

HYPEREKPLEXIA

Hyperekplexia or startle disease is characterized by a strikingly excessive startle elicited by auditory, visual and tactile sensory stimuli that fail to produce similar responses in normal persons.

There is little or no habituation of the startle reflexes. Tactile stimuli are particularly effective and slow to non-habituating to light touch, whereas proprioceptive stimuli are minimally or not effective in idiopathic forms (Shahar and Raviv 2004). Nose-tapping is especially effective (Shahar et al. 1991).

HEREDITARY HYPEREKPLEXIA

This disorder is caused by several mutations in the alpha 1 subunit of the inhibitory glycine receptor gene *GLRA1* on chromosome 5q33–q35 (Ryan et al. 1992, Shiang et al. 1995) and is mostly dominantly transmitted, although rare recessive forms are known to exist (Rees et al. 1994, Coto et al. 2005). More genetic heterogeneity is possible. Some cases are associated with compound heterozygosity for two different mutant alleles. Familial cases without mutation in the glycine receptor gene are known (Tijssen et al. 2002). The disease exists in two forms: a *major form* in which the startle response is not only quantitatively different from normal but also features momentary generalized stiffness with loss of postural control, producing unprotected falls 'en statue', and episodes of prolonged apnoea that can require resuscitation and even even be lethal, in response to minor stimuli such as touching the nose (Pascotto and Coppola 1992); and a *minor form* in which the excessive startle response is isolated. The latter form usually is not associated with detected mutations (Bakker et al. (2006). The attacks are different from epileptic seizures and the ictal EEG does not show paroxysmal activity, although spikes of uncertain significance have been described (Matsumoto et al. 1992). Intrauterine abnormal movements precipitated by noises occur in some cases (Vigevano et al. 1989).

In severe cases, infants also exhibit marked hypertonia from birth that disappears during sleep. Umbilical and inguinal hernias are frequently present and are probably the consequence of increased abdominal pressure due to permanent muscle contraction. At the time of spontaneous decrease of hypertonia, after the end of the first year of life, violent, often repetitive jerks of the limbs on falling asleep may appear (Andermann and Andermann 1988). The neonatal manifestations of the disease were initially reported as the *'stiff baby syndrome'* or *'congenital stiff-man syndrome'* (Sander et al. 1980) before the identity of the two conditions was recognized.

The two forms may coexist in the same family and may not be associated with known mutations (Tijssen et al. 2002).

SPORADIC CASES

Sporadic cases, which can be major or minor, have been described (Shahar and Raviv 2004). They may be more common than usually thought. Shahar and Raviv described 39 cases, 9 of which were of a major type with typical symptoms including severe apnoeic attacks. Interestingly, some have recently been shown to be due to mutations in the *GLAR2* gene that codes for another postsynaptic glycine receptor (Rees et al. 2006). According to Shahar and Raviv (2004), these infants do not respond to proprioceptive stimuli in contrast with brain-damaged infants.

Cases secondary to CNS disorders may be relatively common. Such cases are due to extensive brain lesions and are difficult to distinguish from excessive startle reflexes in infants with marked neurological signs and brisk reflexes. Acquired symptomatic causes of hyperekplexia and related excessive startle diseases have been extensively discussed by Brown et al. (1991).

Cases of late-onset hyperekplexia may occur and may respond to sodium valproate (Dooley and Andermann 1989). Other atypical cases include neonatal hyperekplexia followed by hypotonia and lethal status epilepticus (Lerman-Sagie et al. 2004).

OUTCOME AND TREATMENT

The outcome of hyperekplexia is not entirely benign, especially because of repeated falls and episodes of apnoea, and the possibility of death during a tonic paroxysm. In general, the symptoms tend to decrease with increasing age, and only the excessive startle persists.

Treatment with clonazepam or clobazam and valproic acid (Dooley and Andermann 1989) is usually effective but does not totally suppress the symptoms. Many patients respond well to benzodiazepines and may become completely normal after the age of 2 years. The attacks can be arrested by sudden flexion of the head and limbs that may be a life-saving manoeuvre (Vigevano et al. 1989).

JUMPING

Jumping has been known for a long time in various populations under picturesque names such as 'jumping Frenchmen of Maine', 'latah' or 'myriachit'. The exact nosological situation of these disorders remains uncertain (Saint-Hilaire et al. 1986).

STARTLE EPILEPSY

Startle epilepsy is discussed in Chapter 15.

OTHER PAROXYSMAL ABNORMAL MOVEMENTS

SHUDDERING ATTACKS

Shuddering attacks in infants (Pachatz et al. 2002) may be the same phenomenon as benign infant myoclonus. They have been observed as a premonitory symptom of the later development of essential tremor, although they may remain isolated (Holmes and Russman 1986).

SANDIFER SYNDROME

Sandifer syndrome is the name given to the contortions of the neck and associated abnormal postures observed in children with hiatus hernia (Mandel et al. 1989). The movements had previously been regarded as voluntary, and the mistaken diagnosis of dystonia is often considered. The movements primarily consist of sudden extension of the neck in an opisthotonic position, often with continuous twisting of the head from side to side. In some cases, extraordinary positions are assumed. Less spectacular manifestations may be more common and often go unrecognized (Werlin et al. 1980). Occurrence of attacks during the postprandial period can orient the diagnosis. The presence of hiatus hernia or even only of reflux (Garrotxateji et al. 1996) in association with such a dyskinesia allows the correct diagnosis to be made and appropriate therapy to be given. Medical treatment may not be sufficient and fundoplication is often necessary.

HEAD MOVEMENTS AND VISUAL ANOMALIES

A number of abnormal head postures or head movements can be a consequence of visual anomalies. The commonest is head tilt associated with paralysis of the oblique muscles. The head thrusts, characteristic of Cogan ocular motor apraxia, are not infrequently mistaken for myoclonic attacks or tics (Chapter 17). Some severely visually impaired patients seek to use rocking movements in an effort to improve their vision (Boyle et al. 2005)

Benign paroxysmal tonic upgaze of childhood is sometimes associated with forward flexion of the head. Ataxia and repeated falls have been reported (Ouvrier and Billson 1988, Deonna et al. 1990). The disorder is sometimes familial and may respond to L-dopa and be related to dopa-sensitive dystonia (Campistol et al. 1993) (Chapter 17).

DYSKINESIAS INDUCED BY TRANSIENT CEREBRAL ISCHAEMIA

Abnormal movements may be seen in patients with vascular disease and are well known in adults (Yanagihara et al. 1985). I have seen similar localized rhythmic movements in a child with thrombotic occlusion of the sylvian artery.

ABNORMAL MOVEMENTS IN NEONATES

Jitteriness in newborn infants is a common phenomenon (Parker et al. 1990, Shuper et al. 1991) without pathological significance and is mainly a differential diagnosis of neonatal convulsions (Chapter 15). Pathological myoclonus may also be observed in neonates with various disorders (Scher 1985).

RHYTHMIAS, MANNERISMS, GRATIFICATION PHENOMENA, MASTURBATION

Infants and young children often engage in repetitive rhythmic movements such as body-rocking or head-banging. Such movements may occur during the day, especially at the time of going to bed or when the child is bored. The movements generally disappear before 3 years of age. Nocturnal head bobbing or lateral movements occurring at night in a rhythmical manner are known as *jactatio capitis nocturna*. Jactatio capitis is a normal phenomenon that occurs in 3–15% of normal children in the first year of life. *Head-banging* is also a normal phenomenon in most cases that usually occurs at the time of going to bed and may last for long periods. Excessive head-banging may occur in normal children. Stereotypies also occur in older children and may present in very variable circumstances and can suggest epileptic events. In rare cases, stereotypies proved to be epileptic phenomena (Deonna et al. 2002).

Gratification phenomena (Brett 1997) are stereotyped movements that occur while the child appears withdrawn and from which s/he seems to derive great pleasure. The movements have a ritualistic quality and appear electively when the child is bored. Masturbation is commoner in girls in the younger age group. When bored or alone the child will adduct her thighs, stiffen, become flushed and perspire. Such episodes, which are associated with a blank stare, are often mistaken for epileptic seizures (Pranzatelli and Pedley 1991). They are completely benign and do not require any treatment.

MIGRAINE AND RELATED CONDITIONS

Migraine, chronic daily headache and tension-type headache are the most common headache-associated disorders in both children and adults. The term migraine designates a periodic disorder with symptom-free intervals, characterized by attacks of headache that have several (usually two or three) of the following features: throbbing nature, unilateral location, relief after sleep, presence of an aura, associated abdominal pain or nausea or vomiting, and a family history of similar condition (Prensky 1976, Barlow 1984, Deonna 1988).

The prevalence of migraine in childhood was 3.9% in the classic study of Bille (1962), using restrictive criteria. The incidence of migraine increases with increasing age from 2.7% at age 7, when there is a slight preponderance of boys, to 6.4% of boys and 14.8% of girls by age 14 years (Sillanpää 1983). An overall frequency of about 10% of children and adolescents is generally accepted.

AETIOLOGY AND PATHOPHYSIOLOGY

The aetiopathogenesis of migraine is imperfectly understood. Vascular changes clearly play an important role, and some forms of neurovascular instability of genetic origin must exist in migrainous patients. The frequency of a *positive family history* is very high. Prensky (1976) recorded an average incidence of 72%, and Barlow (1984) found a positive history in 89.7% of his patients. Stewart et al. (1997) in a population-based study found the risk of migraine to be 50% higher in patients with a family history than in controls. The mode of inheritance is uncertain, although a multifactorial mode seems likely. The syndrome is genetically heterogeneous, and some types (e.g. familial hemiplegic migraine) clearly follow a dominant pattern of inheritance (Stewart et al. 1997). It has been suggested that mutation of the *ATP1A2* gene, responsible for one form of hemiplegic migraine, may be a predisposing factor for a few cases of common migraine (Todt et al. 2005). It is possible that the same phenotype is the result of different genotypes, but a definitive answer must await the identification of suitable markers.

Most recent works have incriminated a primary neurogenic origin, rather than a primary vascular involvement. The mechanism of the attacks is at least partly understood. Migraine is now viewed as an inherited disorder with primary neuronal initiation of a cascade of neurochemical processes culminating in a spreading wave of cortical neuronal depolarization and regional oligaemia (Goadsby and Edvinsson 1993). Stimulation of the trigeminal ganglion results in the release of vasoactive substances including vasoactive intestinal peptide and substance P, which produce changes in cerebral blood flow and are responsible in some cases for the phenomenon of allodynia (change in the character of perception sensory stimuli, usually unpleasant). In classical migraine, a phase of hyperperfusion precedes the initial phase of neurological deficits and is followed by a period of oligaemia that begins posteriorly and moves anteriorly at a rate of 2mm per minute and appears to be responsible for the deficits. The pathophysiology of the aura is classically attributed to cortical ischaemia secondary to either vasospasm or arteriolar shunting (Lauritzen 1994, Woods et al. 1994). The pulsating headache is due to the pulsating and presumably dilated arteries associated with hyperaemia that follows the oligaemic phase. Associated shunting or vasoconstriction of the subcutaneous arterioles accounts for the frequently observable facial pallor, and in an occasional case segmental constrictions of the cerebral arteries have been documented by angiography. However, cerebral blood flow during the headache is highly variable (Olsen et al. 1987, Andersen et al. 1988). Increased flow cannot entirely account for the pain, and the mechanism of vasodilatation is not fully understood. In migraine without aura, the blood flow during attacks was not found to differ from postictal flow (Ferrari et al. 1995). A spreading inhibitory phenomenon, akin to *Leão spreading depression*, is thought to be responsible for the aura, but the origin of the inhibition remains unknown. There is still considerable controversy about the primary neurogenic or vascular mechanism of migraine.

CLINICAL FEATURES

The age at onset of migraine headaches can be very early in life. Holguin and Fenichel (1967) found that approximately 20% of patients had their first attack before 5 years of age. In many cases, attacks of headache have been preceded by recurrent abdominal pain and/or vomiting (see below) or by motion sickness, which is found in 45% of children with migraine, starting from age 2 years.

Classification of childhood migraine requires adaptation of the International Classification of Headache Disorders (ICHD-II) (Lipton et al. 2004) and has been extensively discussed (Hershey et al. 2005, Kienbacher et al. 2006) because atypical features, especially the frequency of bilateral headache and shorter duration of attacks, are common. Whatever the classification, two major forms of migraine with and without aura, otherwise known as classical and common migraine, are generally recognized.

The migraine headache is identical in both forms. A major feature of the pain is its throbbing character, and every effort should be made to recognize this feature without inducing the expected answer, by providing the child with several different words – if necessary supplemented by gestures – covering the main types of headache. Throbbing headache is present in 50–60% of cases of childhood migraine (Barlow 1984), and unilateral location is observed in 25–66% (for review, see Prensky 1976). The duration of headache in children is briefer than in adults, although in most cases it lasts for a few hours. Nausea and vomiting, photophobia and/or phonophobia, and pallor of the face and 'dark circles' under the eyes are frequent associated features.

The attacks may be precipitated by psychological factors, by certain foods, by physical exertion (Bille 1962), and by hormonal factors in adolescent girls. Such precipitating factors were present in 25% of the cases reported by Seshia et al. (1994).

Sleep is an effective manner of relieving migraine headache – this feature is of diagnostic value so should be asked about when taking the history – although many children resist sleep during the attack.

CLASSICAL MIGRAINE (MIGRAINE WITH AURA)

Classical migraine is defined as an idiopathic recurrent disorder manifesting with attacks of neurological symptoms unequivocally localizable to the cerebral cortex or brainstem, usually developing gradually over 5–20 minutes and lasting less than 60 minutes. The aura may be preceded by symptoms of irritability, pallor or undefinable premonitory feeling. Headache, nausea and/or photophobia normally follow the aura symptoms directly or after a free interval of less than an hour. The headache is generally contralateral to the sensory symptoms if it is lateralized at all, and usually lasts 4–72 hours although it may be completely absent (migraine aura without headache) (Lipton et al. 2004). The most common aura is one of sensory symptoms, mainly visual manifestations. Visual auras include photopsia, fortification spectra, negative scotomata that often consist of a cut-out of a portion of images with smooth, ragged or undulating edges but may also be hemianopic or quadrantic. Total blindness is rare (Bower et al. 1994). According to Panayiotopoulos (1994), elementary visual hallucinations in migraine are generally linear and black and white, which might help separate them from those in epilepsy. They may coexist with a scotoma or occur in isolation. More complex visual disturbances consist of illusions of micropsia, macropsia or distortion of objects and may not be described by young children for want of an appropriate vocabulary. Both the positive and the negative scotomata may be of either retinal or cortical origin. When only one eye is involved, a retinal origin (retinal migraine) is likely, whereas hemianopic scotomata are of cortical location.

An aura of light-headedness or vertigo is common, usually in combination with diplopia or blurred vision.

Other sensory auras include sensations of tingling or numbness that may involve both hands and the perioral area or be unilateral, distortions of body image usually associated with visual phenomena to produce the *'Alice in Wonderland syndrome'* (Golden 1979), and rarely auditory or olfactory symptoms (Fuller and Guiloff 1987), usually of an unpleasant character.

Hemiplegic and ophthalmoplegic migraine are currently classified as forms of classical migraine; they are described separately below, however, because of their special characteristics. They were previously known as complicated migraine.

In some children the aura may occur alone without subsequent headaches, nausea or abdominal pain (*acephalalgic migraine*). Such an occurrence is most frequently occasional but, in the rare patient, may be the only manifestation in a given epoch of the migraine (Barlow 1984, Shevell 1996).

COMMON MIGRAINE (MIGRAINE WITHOUT AURA)

Common migraine accounts for approximately 90% of all cases. Patients with common migraine have no aura before their headache attacks or have an aura only on rare occasions. In children the attacks are usually briefer than in older persons. They are associated with nausea and vomiting, photophobia and phonophobia.

The international criteria for common migraine include unilateral localization, and pain of a throbbing character that is moderate or severe and aggravated by physical activity. Such criteria, however, may not apply to children (Seshia et al. 1994), in whom bilateral headache and brief attacks of less than 2 hours are common.

HEMIPLEGIC AND OPHTHALMOPLEGIC MIGRAINE

Neurological signs that develop during the headache phase or persist for hours or days beyond the headache characterize complicated migraine. The term, not used in the International Classification, applies here to persistent visual manifestations such as scotoma or hemianopia but is mainly applied to hemiplegic and aphasic migraine, ophthalmoplegic migraine, confusional migraine and basilar artery migraine.

Some authors used the term synonymously with that of 'migraine accompagnée' to include cases with paraesthesiae, often unilateral and with a slow 'march' of several minutes duration, as well as cases with motor deficits, but it is used here only for cases with prolonged deficits.

The frequency of hemiplegic and ophthalmoplegic migraine is between 5% and 10% in series from referral centres, therefore lower in less biased series.

Hemiplegic migraine

Hemiplegic migraine most frequently occurs as a manifestation of the aura and remains confined to this stage of the attack. It is commonly associated with visual symptoms in the ipsilateral visual field and with ipsilateral sensory phenomena. Aphasia of a nonfluent type may also occur as an aura, often in association with other manifestations of left hemisphere affectation such as hemiparesis. In a second type of hemiplegic migraine, hemiparesis with or without aphasia appears after the aura or in its absence and persists for hours or even days. The hemiplegia may be dense and is often associated with confusion and agitation, thus suggesting a diagnosis of meningeal haemorrhage or other vascular accident. *Imaging* shows the absence of intracranial blood and in some cases a degree of swelling of the involved hemisphere. Prominent slow waves are present in EEG records and may persist up to several weeks. Angiography is better avoided because it may provoke vascular spasms in patients with migraine but has been normal when done. Remarkably, patients with this second type of hemiplegic migraine often have relatives affected with the same form of the disorder, and their recurrences tend to present in a similar manner. About half the familial cases have been mapped to chromosome 19q13 (Joutel et al. 1994) and were shown to result from mutations in the calcium channel gene *CACNA1A* (Ophoff et al. 1996). A second gene has been found on chromosome 1 (*ATP1A2*) (Riant et al. 2005). A third gene coding for the voltage-gated sodium channel SCN1A on chromosome 2q24 has been recently discovered (Dichgans et al. 2005). The same mutation in the *CACNA1* gene may have a widely variable clinical expression with classical migraine, hemiplegic migraine, migraine–coma or cerebellar ataxia in the same family (Wada et al. 2002).

Cases of transient hemiplegia during aura are not dominantly transmitted and represent a different condition. Some cases of familial hemiplegic migraine can be associated with marked MRI abnormalities of the white matter and have been found in families in which cerebral autosomal dominant arteriopathy with subcortical infarcts and leukoencephalopathy (CADASIL), also mapping to 19q, was present in other family members, suggesting a link between the two disorders. CADASIL is caused by mutations of the *NOTCH* gene (Chabriat et al. 1995, Hutchinson et al. 1995). This syndrome has not been decribed so far in children. The pattern of recurrence of attacks may change, however, sometimes after several years as in one of my patients who had attacks of hemiplegic migraine from 11 months of age and developed visual symptoms at age 10 years. In a number of cases, *chronic migraine* without paroxysmal episodes but with continuous headaches sets in.

Ophthalmoplegic migraine

Ophthalmoplegic migraine is characterized by the association of a recurrent IIIrd nerve palsy that develops during or following ipsilateral periorbital or temporal headache. The IVth and VIth nerves may be rarely affected. Permanent impairment of the IIIrd nerve may persist after repeated attacks. The syndrome is to be distinguished from other causes of IIIrd nerve palsy, from the painful ophthalmoplegia of Tolosa–Hunt (Chapter 17) and from congenital berry aneurysms. The onset may be as early as the first year of life. In young children, the headache may be absent or overlooked.

Gadolinium enhancement of the cisternal portion of the oculomotor nerve may be a useful sign (Wong and Wong 1997). The occurrence of *Raeder type II paratrigeminal syndrome* with oculosympathetic paresis as a migraine variant is on record (Shevell et al. 1993). Bilateral episodic mydriasis may be a migraine equivalent in childhood (Baziel et al. 1991).

CONFUSIONAL MIGRAINE

Confusional migraine is an uncommon type of migraine that often but not always follows a mild head trauma (Curtain et al. 2006). An acute confusional state is the presenting feature and headache is often insignificant. Confusion typically lasts for several hours and in some cases may progress to a stuporous state (Barlow 1984). Neurological signs are sometimes associated or alternate with confusion (Nezu et al. 1997). In a few patients, amnesia dominates the clinical picture so that the term transient global amnesia becomes appropriate (Sheth et al. 1995).

MIGRAINE–COMA

Rare cases of coma associated with features of migraine and with

TABLE 16.5
Main causes of persistent headache in childhood outside migraine

Cause	Characters of headache and possible associated symptoms or signs
Organic causes	
Brain tumours	Chronic, progressive, intermittent, often nocturnal, sometimes throbbing, mostly noncharacteristic. Vomiting, neurological signs
Vascular diseases	
Systemic infections	Acute, non-throbbing
Vascular malformations	Throbbing, fixed location. Seizures, neurological signs
Connective tissue diseases	Throbbing
Arterial hypertension	Acute, generalized, sometimes throbbing. Convulsions, transient visual disturbances
Congenital malformations and hydrocephalus	No characteristic quality. Large head and neurological signs
Infectious processes	
Paranasal sinusitis	Focal, acute or chronic, dull pain and pressure, location variable with sinus affected. Tenderness over sinus, nasal discharge
Intracranial suppuration and meningitis	Variable, often severe. Neurological and/or meningeal signs
Cervical osteoarthritis	Chronic, nonprogressive
Pseudotumour cerebri	Nondistinctive. Papilloedema, diplopia
Endocrine and metabolic causes, *e.g.* hypoglycaemia, recurrent metabolic disorders	Nondistinctive. Vomiting, lethargy
Cluster headaches	Characteristic periodicity, extreme pain usually not throbbing, facial pain in 30 per cent
Epileptic headache	Acute, non-throbbing, may be accompanied by vomiting; common in focal occipital epilepsy syndromes
Chronic daily headache	See text and Table 16.6
Post-traumatic headache	Pressure, aching, tightness. Anxiety or depression possible. No aura or visual or neurological symptoms
Psychogenic headache	Idem

frightening symptoms such as autonomic disturbances, apnoea sometimes of long duration, hypotension and cardiac irregularities have been reported (Fitzsimons and Wolfenden 1985, Curtain et al. 2006). In some of these, ataxia, nystagmus, myokymia and peduncular hallucinosis may be present (Zifkin et al. 1995) and cerebellar atrophy may be demonstrated (Elliott et al. 1996). Some cases can be extremely severe and life-threatening or even fatal (Kors et al. 2001). This may be due to cerebral oedema, which can also develop after mild head trauma without any migrainous symptom (Chapter 12).

BASILAR ARTERY MIGRAINE
Basilar artery migraine is an established 'complicated' form of migraine (Lapkin and Golden 1978). The main clinical features include variable associations of cranial nerve, cerebellar, cochleo-vestibular and corticobulbar signs and symptoms, together with visual disturbances attributable to the territory of the posterior cerebral arteries. This form is seen mainly in adolescent girls. Basilar migraine is one cause of intermittent ataxia (see Table 16.3). Visual symptoms are usually first in the sequence and consist of dimming of vision that may amount to almost total blindness. Consciousness may be impaired in some patients and true seizures have been observed. The EEG shows bilateral posterior slow waves, but intense epileptic activity has also been reported

so the syndrome may be difficult to distinguish from some forms of occipital epilepsy. Residual impairment is rare despite an often frightening symptomatology. However, multiple infarcts have been reported in some cases, even in childhood (Caplan 1991). This type of migraine may be related to amaurosis fugax, which is sometimes observed in adolescents and even in children (Appleton et al. 1988) and may occur as a post-traumatic phenomenon. The prognosis is excellent, and 13 patients followed for 10 years by Bower et al. (1994) remained symptom-free.

DIAGNOSIS OF MIGRAINE
The differential diagnosis of migraine (Table 16.5) includes a very large number of neurological, digestive, psychiatric and other conditions that cannot be discussed here. Only some difficult problems will be briefly considered.

Migraine and seizures coexist more often that would be expected by chance alone (Andermann and Lugaresi 1987). The relationship is a complex one: in some cases epilepsy may be the consequence of ischaemia during a severe migraine attack or the sequela thereof; in others it may be the result of a lesion such as an arteriovenous malformation (Barlow 1984). The occurrence of continuous spike–waves over the posterior part of the skull in association with both epileptic phenomena and migraine-like manifestation is of interest (Panayiotopoulos 1989). Usually the

EEG of patients with migraine is normal or shows focal or generalized slow waves, but focal spikes may be far more common than in control subjects (Kinast et al. 1982).

A further problem may be to differentiate postepileptic headache from migraine and sometimes to distinguish ictal manifestations of partial complex seizures, for example hallucinations or illusions, from those that occur in migraine (Seshia et al. 1985).

Syncopes may occur during a migraine attack in up to 1% of affected children. They may be particularly frequent in patients with basilar artery migraine.

Strokes can occur in adults during a migraine attack, especially during complicated attacks. The occurrence of strokes in children with migraine is certainly rare, if it exists at all (Rossi et al. 1990, Riikonen and Santavuori 1994, Nezu et al. 1997). The occurrence of strokes or stroke-like episodes in childhood migraine should arouse the suspicion of a mitochondrial encephalomyopathy (Chapter 8).

Mitochondrial disorders can present with migrainous features. Dvorkin et al. (1987) have reported on patients who presented in childhood or adolescence with severe migraine attacks, rapidly associated with epileptic seizures and episodes of epilepsia partialis continua. Most patients had a family history of migraine. CT usually showed hypodense lesions. Such cases are probably variants of the mitochondrial encephalopathy with stroke-like episodes and lactic acidosis (MELAS) syndrome and run an unfavourable course.

Cases of *migrainous headache with CSF pleocytosis* pose a nosologic more than a diagnostic problem. They often follow a common viral infection and present as classical migraine, often with hemiplegia. The CSF may contain up to several hundred cells, mostly lymphocytes. Imaging is normal and the course is favourable. The problems posed by such cases can be even more difficult in cases with only mild to moderate pleocytosis (Rossi et al. 1985, Caminero et al. 1998, Gomez-Aranda et al. 1997). Whether these cases are due to viral infections or represent a special, perhaps genetic, propensity to migrainous attacks in response to inflammation remains debated.

MIGRAINE EQUIVALENTS (ATYPICAL FORMS OF MIGRAINE AND/OR RELATED DISORDERS); THE 'PERIODIC SYNDROME', CYCLIC VOMITING AND ABDOMINAL MIGRAINE

In childhood, and especially in young children, paroxysmal episodes of disturbances of variable presentations have been considered as equivalents of migraine because of the frequency of familial antecedents and/or the later occurrence of migraine in the patients themselves. These include cyclic vomiting, recurrent abdominal pain and perhaps other periodic phenomena that have been described as the 'periodic syndrome', such as recurrent fever and paroxysmal limb pains. Al-Twajri and Shevell (2002) studied 108 such cases among 1106 migraineurs (9.8%). They recognized five types: paroxysmal torticollis in 11 children, benign paroxysmal vertigo in 41, abdominal migraine/cyclic vomiting in 20, and acute confusional migraine in 5. Girls were more commonly affected, except in confusional migraine. A family history of migraine was present in at least two thirds of children, and in some cases all, depending on the syndrome. Two forms may coexist, especially vomiting and abdominal syndrome.

CYCLIC VOMITING

Cyclic vomiting presents with repeated episodes of vomiting that may last hours or days and may lead to dehydration and ketosis. Abdominal discomfort is frequent. It is a common condition that may affect up to 10% of children (Wang et al. 2004). The onset is commonly in the third or fourth year of life. Two thirds of patients in one study (Al-Twajri and Shevell 2002) developed migraine headache in later childhood. Some authors think that the syndrome is inherited from the mother (Boles et al. 2005), and Wang et al. (2004) suggested that it might be associated with certain mitochondrial DNA sequences. The same syndrome has been sometimes attributed to epilepsy, which is certainly exceptional. Although a psychosomatic origin has been suggested in some of the cases, organic factors seem predominant. The main differential diagnoses are with intestinal malformation or hiatus hernia (Gordon 1994a), and with ketotic or nonketotic hypoglycaemia and other metabolic disorders with periodic manifestations such as disorders of the urea cycle or of oxidation of fatty acids (see Chapter 8). Treatment with erythromycin (Vanderhoof et al. 1995) and with barbiturates may be efficacious. With the latter, Gokhale et al. (1997) obtained disappearance of the attacks in 11 of 14 children treated.

RECURRENT ABDOMINAL PAIN

Recurrent abdominal pain is much more commonly a psychosomatic disorder than a migrainous manifestation (Hockaday 1987). The incidence of recurrent abdominal pain is between 0.7% and 1.7% of all children, and the condition seems unrelated to migraine (Mortimer et al. 1993). In addition, a large number of medical and surgical conditions are manifested in this manner, including brain or spinal tumours. Abdominal migraine is usually associated with vomiting, and the pain is usually periumbilical in location and crampy or more commonly aching in nature (Symon and Russell 1986).

Other manifestations sometimes attributed to migraine include recurrent fever, episodic hypothermia (Ruiz et al. 2003), paroxysmal leg pain (Guiloff and Fruns 1988, Mortimer et al. 1993) and paroxysmal chest pain (for review, see Barlow 1984). A curious familial syndrome of elicited repetitive blindness associated with migraine or epilepsy with a benign course was reported by Le Fort et al. (2004).

THE TREATMENT OF MIGRAINE

Migraine in its severe forms is a serious condition that results in many personal and familial problems and interferes with schooling and other activities. Therapy is therefore important but has limited efficacy, and it is thus essential to discuss extensively the aims and limits of therapy with the patient and family. Treatment of migraine is empirically based and, at best, only partially successful. Although a huge number of treatments have been and still are used, only a few have been studied in a systematic manner

(Lewis 2004, Damen et al. 2005). Important basic points include reassurance that the condition is benign, avoidance of stressful situations and general advice about lifestyle, including avoidance of established trigger factors. The problem of chronic migraine and the role of overuse of analgesics in its genesis have been extensively discussed in adults but seem to be less common or less well known in children (Mack 2006).

Treatment of individual attacks is sufficient for most patients who have relatively rare episodes. It should be given early at the beginning of headache or at the time of aura if it is present. The drugs that have a demonstrated although moderate efficacy include ibuprofen, acetaminophen, which may abort attacks in less than 2 hours (Hämäläinen et al. 1997a), and nasal-spray sumatriptan, which may be more effective but with more side effects (Hämäläinen et al. 1997b). Sumatriptan by injection has not been shown to be useful in children and is expensive. Some patients find analgesic mixtures of aspirin, phenacetin and barbiturates valuable. Repeated use of such therapies can favour the chronicity of headache and should therefore be strictly controlled. Early treatment of the attack, less than 1 hour after the initial symptoms, is thought to be important but may be difficult to use in practice. Ergot derivatives used to be regarded as the drugs of choice, in combination with antalgic drugs or in isolation. However, their efficacy was not confirmed in systematic studies (Damen et al. 2005). Moreover, they should not be used more than twice weekly and their use in children must be very parsimonious (Silberstein and Young 1995). Antiemetics are useful in children with repeated vomiting and should be given in combination with an analgesic. Metoclopramide has the additional advantage of speeding up gastric emptying, thus increasing the absorption of analgesics.

Continuous prophylactic treatment (Barlow 1984) is necessary only when repeated attacks occur and are considered troublesome enough by the child and family. A vast number of drugs have been used but very few have a demonstrated efficacy (for review, see Welch 1993). Propanolol (10–20 mg t.i.d. in children over 7–8 years of age) may be effective provided the treatment is given for a long enough period in a high enough dosage (Rosen 1983). Pizotifen was found effective by some authors but had no effect in a relatively large series. Clonidine appeared to be useful in a pilot study of 40 children but this good result was not confirmed in a double-blind study. Phenytoin and phenobarbitone had been regarded as drugs of choice by some investigators (Barlow 1984) but their side effects are troublesome. Methysergide should not be used in children because of the grave side effects of retroperitoneal or pulmonary fibrosis. Calcium channel blocking agents are vasodilators that prevent the entry of calcium into vascular smooth muscle thus preventing their contraction. Cyproheptadine has been used in children at a dose of 0.2–0.4 mg/kg/day, and nifedipine at a dose of 1 mg/kg/day (Barlow 1984). Flunarizine has been also employed in children at a daily dose of 5–7.5 mg. *Sumatriptan*, a selective agonist of serotonin (SHT1) receptors that selectively constricts cranial blood vessels, has been shown to be effective and well-tolerated (Visser et al. 1996, Pakalnis et al. 2003), but is expensive and is in fact reserved for acute use. There is not yet enough experience with other triptans in children. Among the new antiepileptic drugs, some seem to offer promise. These include valproic acid or valproate that is effective in some patients and well tolerated (Serdaroglu et al. 2002) and levetiracetam. Topiramate has been found to reduce significantly the frequency of attacks in placebo-controlled trials in adults (Brandes et al. 2004, Silberstein et al. 2004, Rapoport et al. 2006) and in children (Winner et al. 2005) and may reverse the chronic course in overtreated patients (Mei et al. 2006). Because of the cost and possible toxicity of the drug, indications are limited to severe invalidating cases and the efficacy is not yet definitely established (Silberstein et al. 2006).

Behavioural therapy has been shown to have a favourable effect (Baumann 2002).

Identification of provocative foods or drinks may be helpful but requires a thorough history-taking and may need several trials.

CLUSTER HEADACHES OR MIGRAINOUS NEURALGIA

Cluster headaches appear to be genetically distinct from migraine although they belong to the group of vascular headaches. The fundamental defect is likely to be different from that in migraine, an hypothesis supported by the finding of elevated plasma serotonin and whole blood histamine levels, which is not the case in migraine. The condition is rare in children and exceptional below 10 years of age (McNabb and Whitehouse 1999, Lampl 2002). The characteristic periodicity is a basic feature. The headache often occurs one or several times in a 24-hour period, during periods that last for several weeks but occur only once or twice a year or even at wider intervals. The headache is unilateral and usually centres about the eye. It is extremely severe but not throbbing and lasts less than 30 minutes in most cases. In approximately one third of patients pain is located in the lower face. Ipsilateral lachrymation and nasal congestion occur in about 50% of attacks. The finding of a Horner syndrome is uncommon in children. Several cases were initially considered as psychogenic because attention was focused on agitation and strange behaviour.

Drugs effective in migraine may be used for cluster headaches, but resistant cases are frequent. Indomethacin may be useful, as may steroids; ergotamine and ergovonine malleate have also been used.

DIFFERENTIAL DIAGNOSIS OF HEADACHES IN CHILDHOOD

Headache is an extremely common complaint in childhood. In most cases it is due to benign causes, including acute infectious disorders, visual difficulties and the like. Intracranial hypertension is a major cause of headache (Chapter 13) that, although rare, should always be kept in mind; it commonly follows lumbar puncture. The diagnosis may be difficult when headache lasts for days or even weeks (Kuntz et al. 1992). In some cases such as brain tumours or abscesses, headache has a serious significance,

TABLE 16.6
Types of persistent headache in 175 children*

Subtype	Frequency n (%)	Girls n (%)	Boys n (%)	Female:male ratio
Chronic migraine	94 (54)	69 (73)	25 (27)	2.8:1
New daily persistent headache	40 (23)	27	13	2.1:1
Chronic tension headache	35 (20)	27	8	3.4:1
Hemicrania continua	6 (3)	4	2	2.0:1
Total	175 (100)	127 (73)	48 (27)	2.6:1

*Modified from Mack (2004). Data from a specialized headache clinic.

and the problem is to separate the rare case of headache of severe organic cause from the mass of benign cephalalgias. A list of the main causes of subacute and chronic headache appears in Table 16.5. For all children, a detailed personal and family history, full neurological examination and measurement of blood pressure are in order. Imaging is not indicated for most cases, especially those of common migraine, and only a few basic laboratory investigations should be performed.

CHONIC DAILY HEADACHE IN CHILDREN

Chronic headache is frequent in children. It is usually benign. Abu-Arafeh and Macleod (2005) in a study of 815 cases found that in only 3 children it was due to serious intracranial pathology and in only 1 of these was the finding unexpected. The revised International Classification of Headache Disorders (Olesen and Steiner 2004) defines chronic daily headache as the presence of headache for at least 15 days in a 1-month period over a period of at least 3 months with no underlying pathology. It represents 30% of cases observed in headache specialty clinics. Onset is on average around 8–10 years of age but may be earlier. The pain is typically bilateral, pressing or tightening and mild to moderate in intensity. It is not associated with nausea, vomiting or transient neurological disturbances. This disorder can be divided into several subcategories (Mack 2004) (Table 16.6). However, many cases do not fulfil the International Headache Society criteria (Balottin et al. 2005). The most frequent type is chronic migraine succeeding to the usual paroxysmal type, which may result in part from uncontrolled overuse of antalgics. *Chronic tension-type headache* and *new daily headaches* are next in frequency. The onset is usually sudden and often follows an acute common illness. The long-term outcome is favourable but the condition may result in serious school and sleep problems (Wiendels et al. 2005). Psychogenic factors probably play a role that increases significantly in adolescent patients.

The *treatment* of chronic headache is difficult. A thorough discussion of the issue with the patient and family is essential. Common sources of anxiety and concern should be looked for. In some children and adolescents, moderate to severe depression may be a factor and such patients should be referred to a psychiatrist. In less severe cases, it is important to discuss frankly the patient's problem and to try to resolve the anxiety or conflict. Antidepressant drugs are only rarely indicated. In children younger than 7 years, migraine is by far the most common cause

of headache. Chu and Shinnar (1992) found that 75% of such children had migraine (72 of 78 had common migraine) and 12% had post-traumatic headache. None of their 104 patients had a sinister cause to their complaint.

OTHER HEADACHES

Headache may be due to drugs or toxins such as alcohol, which are increasingly used by adolescents in many parts of the world; marijuana, which is a peripheral vasodilator; caffeine withdrawal; and certain food additives such as monosodium glutamate, which is used in Chinese cooking and produces vasodilation. Sodium glutamate appears to be the cause of the 'Chinese restaurant syndrome', while nitrites may be responsible, in the USA, for 'hot dog headache'. Benign exertional headache occurs in adolescents following strenuous exercise. The diagnosis is easy as pain begins during or just following exercise and may last minutes to hours. The SUNCT syndrome (short-lasting unilateral neuralgiform headache attacks with conjunctival injection and tearing) is a syndrome of trigeminal autonomic cephalalgia rare in children (Sékhara et al. 2005).

ALTERNATING HEMIPLEGIA OF CHILDHOOD

Alternating hemiplegia was initially described as a variant of hemiplegic migraine. However, the condition is so different from classical migraine that it should be regarded as a specific disorder (Bourgeois et al. 1993). Its mechanism remains obscure. The disease certainly goes undiagnosed in many cases.

The onset of the disorder is almost always in the first year and usually in the first 6 months of life; a few late-onset cases are on record (Mikati et al. 2000).

Paroxysmal manifestations appear first, sometimes even in the neonatal period (Aicardi 2002). They consist of attacks of hemiplegia that are never isolated but variously combined with tonic attacks, ocular motor manifestations and autonomic phenomena. The clinical findings in 30 personal cases are listed in Table 16.7. Localized or generalized tonic and dystonic attacks and episodes of nystagmus often precede the hemiplegias by weeks to months.

The frequency of episodes is usually high, with attacks of hemiplegia occurring several times a month and lasting from a few minutes to several days. A characteristic feature in most cases

TABLE 16.7
Clinical findings in 30 cases of alternating hemiplegia of childhood

Sex: 17 girls, 13 boys

Age of onset of attacks: 3 days – 13 months

Onset with tonic attacks: 11

Paroxysmal features

Onset with tonic attacks: 14

Onset with bouts of hemiplegia: 5

Hemiplegic episodes: 30 (shifting bilateral involvement in 25)

Tonic attacks: 27 (unilateral in all cases; bilateral attacks in 9)

Paroxysmal nystagmus: 23 (unilateral in 17)

Paroxysmal strabismus: 11

Screaming, apparent pain: 28

Vasomotor disturbances: 23 (pallor, flushing, coldness, sometimes unilateral)

Disappearance with sleep: 30

Paroxysmal respiratory disturbances: 14 (dyspnoea cyanosis, may be life-threatening)

Nonparoxysmal features

Mental retardation (learning difficulties): 25

Neurological signs

    Choreoathetosis: 29

    Ataxia: 27

    Pyramidal tract signs: 9

---

is the occurrence of episodes in which the hemiplegia shifts from one side to the other, with a period of bilateral paralysis associated with mutism, difficulties in swallowing and drooling (Krägeloh and Aicardi 1980). Severe quadriplegic attacks with amimia, malaise and decreased consciousness are often observed (Fusco and Vigevano 1995). Frightening, possibly life-threatening episodes of apnoea occur in some patients. A very characteristic feature is the disappearance of all symptoms on falling asleep. In prolonged attacks, the child is normal on waking up but all symptoms return within 10–20 minutes. Parents often take advantage of this short period to feed the child.

A benign form has been reported by Andermann et al. (1994). In their two patients, the attacks occurred during sleep. A case associated with paroxysmal dystonia is on record (Kemp et al. 1995).

Nonparoxysmal manifestations are present in all patients after a course of a few months or years and run a progressive course. They include mental retardation of variable degree, choreoathetosis and dystonia, ataxia and sometimes pyramidal tract signs. All laboratory investigations and neuroradiological studies including MRI have been negative. Transient muscle mitochondrial abnormalities have been reported (Kemp et al. 1995) but are inconstant (Kyriakides and Drousiotou 1994). Single photon emission computed tomography (SPECT) has shown variable changes in perfusion, depending probably on the timing of examination (Andermann et al. 1995). Ictal EEGs show only a moderate slowing on the affected side.

The clinical picture of the classical form is so characteristic that there are few differential diagnoses. Initially, however, the occurrence of unilateral tonic seizures followed by hemiplegia makes the diagnosis of partial epileptic seizures difficult to avoid for physicians not familiar with the disease. In about half the patients,

true seizures may occur with or without temporal relationship to the hemiplegias. However, the phenotypic variability may be greater than previously thought (Saltik et al. 2004). In about half the patients, true seizures may occur with or without temporal relationship to the hemiplegias. The differential diagnosis is discussed by Andermann et al. (1995), and the main causes of paroxysmal hemiplegia are listed in Table 16.8.

The cases of cutis marmorata congenita with recurrent alternating hemiplegia described by Baxter et al. (1993) can closely simulate the disorder.

Dominant transmission has been reported in a family with affected members with typical but less severe symptoms and a later onset up to 3 years of age (Mikati et al. 1992), and two pairs of affected monozygotic twins and a few cases of apparently recessive transmission are also on record, but the vast majority of cases are sporadic.

The outcome is variable; some children may reach a normal or borderline intellectual level but most have moderate or severe mental retardation and almost all have a chronic movement disorder (Aicardi 2002).

The pathogenesis of the condition is unknown. Abnormalities of the blink reflex suggest involvement of the brainstem (Rinalduzzi et al. 2004). An ionic channel disorder appears probable. Two cases have been attributed to mutation in the second gene of familial hemiplegic migraine, *ATP1A2* (Bassi et al. 2004, Swoboda et al. 2004). However, no mutations in this gene were found by Kors et al. (2004) or in several unpublished cases. Given the difficulty of separating such cases from hemplegic migraine, this attribution remains uncertain.

Treatment with the calcium entry blocker flunarizine (Casaer et al. 1987, Silver and Andermann 1993, Andermann et al. 1995) reduces the frequency and duration of attacks in about half the cases. Other agents, including the NMDA receptor antagonist memantine, which has been found effective in a few patients (Korinthenberg 1996), and chloral hydrate or niaprazine, which if given at the onset of an attack may abort it (Veneselli and Biancheri 1997), are of uncertain efficacy. Recently, treatment with topiramate was found effective in a few children (Di Rosa et al. 2006, Jiang et al. 2006).

PAROXYSMAL DISTURBANCES OF CONSCIOUSNESS

The recurrence of variable degrees of disturbed consciousness from coma and stupor to lethargy and confusion is a common and difficult diagnostic problem. Most of the conditions that give rise to such problems are described in other chapters. Table 16.9 gives a list of responsible disorders to help diagnostic orientation. In most disorders, the diagnosis is suggested by a history of previous similar events and/or by a family history of similar cases. Metabolic disorders are particularly apt to present with recurrent disturbances of consciousness, often associated with vomiting and precipitated by infections and fasting. The possibility of drug toxicity should always be considered in such cases. A syndrome of idiopathic recurrent stupor (Tinuper et al. 1994, Lugaresi et

TABLE 16.8

TABLE 16.8
Main causes of recurrent hemiplegia in children

	Genetics*	References
Vascular diseases		
Thrombotic		
Homocystinuria	AR	Chapter 14
Dysproteinaemia	AR or AD	Idem
Fabry disease	AR	Chapter 8
Sickle cell disease	AD	Chapter 14
Fibromuscular dysplasia	AD, S	Idem
Hereditary polycythaemia	AD, AR	Idem
Protein C deficiency	AD	Idem
Resistance to activated protein C (factor Leyden)	AR	Idem
Factor XII deficiency	AR	Idem
Cutis marmorata congenita	S	Baxter et al. (1993)
Rendu–Osler–Weber disease	AD	Myles et al. (1970)
Embolic		
Mitral valve disease	S	Riela and Roach (1993)
Mitral valve prolapse	AD, S	Idem
Auricular myxoma	AD, AR?, S	Idem
Cardiomyopathies	AD, AR, S	Chapter 14
Conduction defects	S or AD	This chapter
Haemorrhagic diseases		
Coagulopathies	XR, AR	Chapter 14
Platelet disorders	XR, AD, AR	Idem
Arteriovenous malformations	S	Idem
Metabolic diseases		
MELAS	AR	Chapter 8
Kearn–Sayre syndrome	Usually S	Idem
Phosphoglycerol kinase deficiency (stroke-like episodes, sometimes myoglobinuria)	AR	DiMauro et al. (1982)
Carbohydrate-deficient glycoprotein syndrome[1]	AR	Jaeken and Carchon (1993)
Sulfite oxidase deficiency	AR	Chapter 8
Lactic acidosis	XR, AR, AD	Idem
Organic acidaemia (metabolic strokes)	AR	Idem
Pyruvate dehydrogenase deficiency		Silver et al. (1995)
Ammonia cycle disorders	AR, XR	Sperl et al. (1997)
Miscellaneous genetic diseases		
Hemiplegic migraine	AD	This chapter
Fibromuscular dysplasia	S	Chapter 14
Neurocutaneous diseases (tuberous sclerosis, neurofibromatosis)	AD	Chapter 3
Non-genetic diseases		
Demyelinating diseases		Riikonen and Donner (1987), Khan et al. (1995), Dale and Cross (1999)
Connective tissue diseases		Chapter 11
Alternating hemiplegia of childhood and variants[2]	S, rarely AD or AR?	Mikati et al. (1992), Aicardi (2002)

*AR = autosomal recessive, AD = autosomal dominant, S = sporadic, XR = X-linked recessive.
[1]Stroke-like episodes are on record but their pathological basis is not demonstrated.

al. 1998) in adolescents and young adults has been attributed to the accumulation of an endogenous ligand of benzodiazepine receptors, endozepine-4, and may respond to flumazenil, which blocks benzodiazepine receptors. This syndrome has also been reported in children (Soriani et al. 1997). The diagnosis demands exclusion of covert administration of exogenous benzodiazepines (Granot et al. 2004). However, a number of synthetic benzodiazepines are difficult to detect by conventional methods thus casting doubt on the very concept of endozepine stupor (Cortelli et al. 2005). Associated phenomena may include hypothermia in Shapiro syndrome (Sheth et al. 1994) or, rarely, hyperthermia in the so-called reverse Shapiro syndrome (Hirayama et al. 1994).

TABLE 16.9
Main causes of recurrent obtundation or coma

Disorder	References
Metabolic diseases	Chapters 8, 22
Hypoglycaemia	
Urea cycle disorders	
Mitochondrial disorders	
Organic acidurias	
Diabetes mellitus	
Fructose intolerance	
Glycogenosis type I	
Glutaric aciduria type 2	
Biotinidase deficiency	
Pyruvate dehydrogenase deficiency	
Fatty acid oxidation defects (recurrent Reye-like episodes)	
Addisonian crises	
Methylene-tetrahydrofolate reductase deficiency	Walk et al. (1994)
Epilepsy	
Nonconvulsive status epilepticus	Bennett et al. (1982)
Benign occipital epilepsy	Panayiotopoulos (1989)
Migraine	
Basilar artery migraine	Lapkin and Golden (1978)
Migraine–coma	Zifkin et al. (1995)
Hypertensive encephalopathy	Hauser et al. (1988)
Recurrent stroke-like episodes	Chapters 8, 14
MELAS, Kearns–Sayre and other mitochondrial diseases	
Carbohydrate-deficient glycoprotein syndromes	
Other vascular disorders	
Intoxication	Chapter 12
Pharmaceutical agents	
Organic solvents	
Street drugs	
Idiopathic recurrent stupor due to accumulation of endozepine	Tinuper et al. (1994), Lugaresi et al. (1998)
Associated with hypothermia and autonomic disturbances with or without agenesis of the corpus callosum (Shapiro syndrome)	Sheth et al. (1994)
Hypersomnias[1]	This chapter
Narcolepsy	
Idiopathic hypersomnia	
Kleine–Levin syndrome	

[1]Rarely is the disturbance of consciousness sufficient to suggest coma.

PAROXYSMAL DISORDERS OF SLEEP

The mechanisms and role of sleep are still mysterious. In children, sleep has different neurophysiological and clinical features from that in adults, and maturational changes with age in the development of clinical and EEG sleep stages have been extensively studied (review in Dan and Boyd 2006).

Childhood sleep disorders are one of the most prevalent complaints in paediatrics (Halbower and Marcus 2003); childhood obstructive sleep apnoea, for example, has a prevalence of 2%. Some of them, e.g. narcolepsy, are often not recognized and raise considerable diagnostic problems. However, most disturbances of sleep in children are transient and benign and require only counselling and reassurance. A few common and/or important disorders are discussed in this section.

NIGHT TERRORS AND NIGHTMARES

Night terrors usually occur between the ages of 18 months and 5 years (Guilleminault 1987a) and are associated with partial arousal from deep slow sleep (stages III–IV). They supervene mainly during the first hours of sleep. The child starts screaming and usually sits up, looking terrified. Although s/he appears to be awake, s/he does not recognize her/his parents and cannot be consoled. An episode lasts a few minutes, the child goes back to sleep and keeps no memory of the event. Night terrors often tend to occur every night for periods then disappear. They may persist to age 8 years in half the children and up to adolescence in one third (DiMario and Emery 1987).

Nightmares may produce a similar picture but take place during REM sleep.

Both night terrors and nightmares are benign conditions and require only reassurance.

SOMNAMBULISM (SLEEPWALKING)

Somnambulism is frequent in older children and adolescents. It is the consequence of incomplete arousal that permits some semi-purposeful activity without clear consciousness or memory of the event. The episodes are usually brief, and the activity in which the child engages is usually of simple type such as going to the bathroom. Somnambulism may be associated with somniloquy. It is characterized neurophysiologically by an incomplete arousal from slow sleep (Pedley 1983). Hereditary factors may play a role in its genesis.

Night terrors and sleepwalking occur together in more than half the cases and share the same genetic predisposition (DiMario and Emery 1986). They are grouped together under the term 'non-REM parasomnias'.

HYPNAGOGIC PHENOMENA

These are brief episodes of auditory or visual hallucinations or distortions of perception, especially auditory or proprioceptive, that occur in the transition between wakefulness and sleep, most commonly on going to sleep. They may be a part of the narcolepsy tetrad (see below) but much more commonly are a normal phenomenon.

RAPID EYE MOVEMENT (REM) SLEEP BEHAVIOUR DISORDER

Unconscious violent behaviour may arise from REM sleep in adolescents and adults. The syndrome is rare in childhood (Trajanovic et al. 2004).

ABNORMAL MOVEMENTS IN SLEEP

The *restless legs syndrome* can occur in children and adolescents (Kotagal and Silber 2004). It is characterized by an irresistible urge to move the limbs, usually accompanied by a peculiar discomfort in the lower limbs. It is a cause of difficulties in initiating or maintaining sleep and of daytime sleepiness. A similar family history is frequent. Walters et al. (1994) reported dominantly inherited cases in children with the typical features of urge to move, paraesthesiae, motor restlessness and periodic limb movements (nocturnal myoclonus). The syndrome may be associated with iron deficiency. Affected children may be misdiagnosed as hyperactive or irritable. The syndrome may be one cause of the so-called 'growing pains'.

Periodic movements of sleep may be associated with restless legs. They are more or less rhythmical and are sometimes recognized only by pain in the legs on awakening (Martinez and Guilleminault 2004). Association with ADHD, narcolepsy and other sleep disorders is frequent (Picchietti and Walters 1999). Treatment with the dopamine agonist pramipexol or with gabapentin or the benzodiazepines can be useful.

Other involuntary movements of sleep in children include include myoclonic jerks on falling asleep (Oswald 1959), nocturnal myoclonus that may be more or less rhythmical, jactatio capitis nocturna (see above), and the nocturnal jerks sometimes associated with hyperekplexia (see above).

Benign neonatal sleep myoclonus is a well-defined and easily diagnosed condition, even though it is often mistaken for epileptic seizures or even status epilepticus. Rhythmical jerks of the limbs may be generalized or localized and occur in brief or more prolonged bursts that can be repeated for hours. The trunk and face remain unaffected and the jerks immediately cease on awakening (Resnick et al. 1986, Di Capua et al. 1993). Induction of the myoclonus by shaking the crib is a useful diagnostic manoeuvre (Alfonso et al. 1995). The myoclonus usually disappears in a few weeks but can persist up to several months. Physiological myoclonus should be differentiated from pathological newborn myoclonus, which is not sleep-related, may involve the face and trunk, and is associated with EEG abnormalities (Scher 1985, Alfonso et al. 1993).

Nocturnal paroxysmal dystonia (Lugaresi et al. 1986) is characterized by sleep-related seizures with choreoathetoid, dystonic and ballistic movements occurring every night in adult patients. Similar cases occur occasionally in children. The symptomatology is similar to that of some frontal lobe seizures, and the disease often responds well to carbamazepine. Two subtypes are observed: short repeated attacks lasting only seconds to minutes, and long-lasting episodes. It is currently recognized as a form of frontal lobe epilepsy that may be familial (Chapter 15).

SLEEP APNOEA SYNDROMES
Several syndromes are characterized by the occurrence of abnormally frequent or prolonged episodes of apnoea during sleep (see Table 16.2). Normally, there is an irregular breathing pattern during REM sleep with frequent periods of apnoea lasting less than 10 seconds. Sleep apnoeas are a disabling problem because of their interference with sleep, which in some children is a contributory factor in growth impairment, school difficulties, and learning and behavioural problems (Nixon and Brouillette 2005). Episodes of apnoea that occur during sleep may be of three types (Guilleminault 1987b). *Obstructive apnoea* is the unsuccessful

maintenance of an airflow in spite of respiratory effort. *Central apnoea* is arrest of respiration because its fails to be initiated by the respiratory centres. *Mixed apnoea* combines both mechanisms.

OBSTRUCTIVE SLEEP APNOEA SYNDROME
This syndrome is defined by the occurrence of at least 30 apnoeic episodes lasting more than 10 seconds in a 7-hour sleep period (Guilleminault 1987b). Associated symptoms and signs may include daytime sleepiness, loud snoring, insomnia, enuresis, behavioural changes and declining school performance. Diagnosis depends on history, and in some cases bursts of increased activity and respiratory pauses during sleep wrongly suggest epilepsy. Polygraphic recording of the EEG, pneumogram and cardiogram are of great use, as is, especially, continuous recording of blood O_2 saturation (Gordon 1988). Severe complications may result, including cor pulmonale, failure to thrive and permanent neurological damage (Oren et al. 1987). Treatment by tonsillectomy and adenoidectomy or, in severe cases, by tracheostomy, or by alternative methods such as nasal continuous positive airway pressure (Guilleminault et al. 1986, Marcus et al. 1995, Nixon and Brouillette 2005) can produce spectacular improvement, but residual obstruction is not rare. Continous positive airway pressure may also be useful during daytime (Hoban 2005). Rare familial forms of sleep apnoea syndrome with additional features such as anosmia and colour blindness are on record (Manon-Espaillat et al. 1988). Symptomatic cases of obstructive sleep apnoea are not infrequent in patients with primary neurological conditions, especially abnormalities of the cervicomedullary junction (Chapter 2) or myotonic dystrophy (Chapter 19).

A *syndrome of increased airway resistance* appears to be more frequent than the obstructive sleep apnoea syndrome (Guilleminault et al. 1996). In such children, an increased respiratory effort is required to overcome the airway resistance, resulting in disturbed sleep with abnormal brief episodes of rapid shallow respiration, daytime sleepiness and fatigue, although polygraphic recording does not demonstrate obstructive apnoea, thus leading to sleep disturbances being erroneously ruled out. An increased frequency of night terrors and somnambulism may be observed.

CONGENITAL CENTRAL ALVEOLAR HYPOVENTILATION SYNDROME
Also known as 'Ondine's curse', this is a rare syndrome, considerably less frequent than obstructive sleep apnoea syndrome, characterized by the depression of central ventilatory drive during quiet sleep. This results in central apnoeas during sleep that are rapidly lethal if untreated. Trang et al. (2005) reported on 70 cases from France. They found an overall fatality rate of 38%, 43 patients surviving at a mean age of 9 years at the time of the study. Forty-nine of 50 who lived beyond 1 year of age received night-time ventilation. Additional problems may include swallowing difficulties. Abnormalities of the brainstem auditory evoked potentials have been found in congenital, idiopathic cases (Beckerman et al. 1986). A history of hydramnios is present in some cases (Alvord and Shaw 1989). Hirschsprung disease (Commare et al. 1993) is 10–20 times more common in children with

apnoea than in the general population and neural crest tumours can also be associated. Cases associated with ophthalmoplegia (Dooling and Richardson 1977) and glaucoma (Walsh and Montplaisir 1982) have been reported.

Most cases of Ondine's curse are genetically determined and result from a frameshift mutation causing an expansion of a polyalanine repeat in the *PHOX2B* gene (Amiel et al. 2003; Weese-Mayer et al. 2003, 2005; Trochet et al. 2005). The association of apnoea with Hirschsprung disease had previously been attributed to mutations of the *RET* (receptor tyrosine kinase) gene, which appears to be much rarer. An occasional case may be due to inflammatory or other disorders of the brainstem (Jensen et al. 1988, Miyazaki et al. 1991), and the disorder may be associated with neurocristopathies.

Rare cases may occur in later life as a result of neurological disease (Giangaspero et al. 1988, Jensen et al. 1988).

OTHER SYNDROMES FEATURING SLEEP APNOEA

The *Pickwickian syndrome* is a syndrome of hypoventilation with episodes of apnoea observed in some obese children. It is probably due, at least in part, to limitation of diaphragm movements by fat accumulation with resulting oxygen desaturation and hypercapnia. Daytime somnolence is a consequence of the disturbance of night sleep by apnoea.

Other neurological syndromes include, among their major features, apnoea or abnormal respiratory patterns. Rett syndrome (Chapter 9) is probably the most common syndrome associated with episodes of awake apnoea. Boltshauser et al. (1987) and Magaudda et al. (1987) have reviewed these syndromes, which include Joubert syndrome, Mohr syndrome and Dandy–Walker syndrome (Bordarier and Aicardi 1990). Magaudda et al. (1988) have described a syndrome of familial, fixed, congenital encephalopathy with undifferentiated sleep–waking EEG cycle, excessive startles and continuous periodic breathing.

Episodes of 'microsleep' occur especially in patients with nocturnal insomnia (Tassinari 1976), can be mistaken for epileptic absences and may have the same unpleasant or dangerous consequences for the patients.

SYNDROMES OF HYPERSOMNIA

NARCOLEPSY–CATAPLEXY

Narcolepsy consists of attacks of irrepressible sleep occurring during daytime, most often during monotonous activity. In most patients, the attacks, which last usually 10–20 minutes, appear on a background of more or less continuous sleepiness. Hypersomnia in narcolepsy is usually associated with one or more of the other elements of the tetrad of symptoms – cataplexy, hypnagogic hallucinations and sleep paralysis – but these do not necessarily occur together. *Cataplexy* is a sudden loss of muscle tone, precipitated by laughter or excitement. It results in the patient falling to the ground without losing consciousness. It should be distinguished from epilepsy (Macleod et al. 2005), hyperekplexia, Niemann–Pick C disease, and sudden falls that occur in patients with the Coffin–Lowry syndrome. The full tetrad occurs in only 10% of adult patients. Many children present with behaviour

problems or learning difficulties, both consequences of sleepiness and efforts to stay awake (Winter et al. 1996). Narcolepsy is said to be unusual in children, and only short paediatric series are on record (Young et al. 1988), but this is probably the result of the disease not being thought of before adolescence or adulthood. In fact, many adults with narcolepsy retrospectively admit to having had the condition since childhood, and about 80% of cases have their onset before 20 years of age and up to 30% before age 15. The earliest recorded onset was in a 2-year-old child (Winter et al. 1996). From a neurophysiological point of view, narcolepsy is characterized by a short latency (less than 10 minutes) from sleep onset to the stage of rapid eye movements (REM sleep). A *multiple sleep latency test* records the time to going to sleep; a positive test is confirmatory rather than conclusive. A total REM latency period of less than 7 minutes or the occurrence of two sleep-onset REM periods is found in 83% of patients (Moscovich et al. 1993). However, not every episode of sleep need be associated with early-onset REM, which occurs in less than half the episodes (Aldrich 1990). The diagnosis is best assured when a history of cataplexy is present.

Recent studies have demonstrated that most cases of narcolepsy are associated with deficiency of hypocretin (orexin) as shown by the low or absent concentration in CSF. Hypocretin is a hormone produced by neurons in the posterior lateral hypothalamic nuclei that plays an important role in sleep and also in appetite and behaviour (Baumann and Bassetti 2005). Interestingly, deficiency of hypocretin is found in over 90% of cases that feature cataplexia but much less frequently in isolated narcolepsy and in familial forms (Dauvilliers et al. 2003), suggesting heterogeneity of the disease. Several loci have been mapped on chromosome 17q21 (Mignot et al. 2001) and on chromosomes 4p and 21q. The gene(s) for narcolepsy may act through an autoimmune mechanism resulting in loss of orexin/hypocretin neurons (Dauvilliers et al. 2007). The relationships of the gene(s) with the HLA system are indicated by the frequency of the HLA-DR2 group. However, there is evidence that non-HLA genes also confer susceptibility to the disorder.

Ninety-eight per cent of the cases of narcolepsy–cataplexy occur in patients who belong to the HLA-DR2 or DQw1 groups (Kramer et al. 1987), although rare genuine cases exist that do not belong to these HLA groups (Confavreux et al. 1988). This relationship is present only in idiopathic cases; it does not hold for the cases of narcolepsy due to acquired brain injury (Aldrich and Naylor 1989) that can rarely be observed with hypothalamic or with pontomedullary (D'Cruz et al. 1994) lesions. Such lesions most commonly induce coma or permanent hypersomnia or sleepiness. Narcolepsy may be genetically related to some instances of idiopathic hypersomnia, in which the incidence of HLA-DR2 may be as high as 60% (Parkes and Lock 1989).

The typical tetrad of narcolepsy–cataplexy is rarely complete. Narcolepsy proper refers to the brief attacks of sleep that occur 3–5 times daily on average. Half the patients are easy to awaken during an attack and most feel refreshed afterwards. It occurs by definition in all patients and is usually the sole manifestation before adolescence.

Hypnagogic hallucinations (see p. 685) and *sleep paralysis* are uncommon. The latter consists of generalized hypotonia with inability to move during the transition between sleep and wakefulness. Partial paralysis with inability to move any one body part is more common. Nocturnal insomnia is also a frequent complaint of narcoleptic patients. In young children, day naps are often long (20–120 minutes) and unrefreshing, and the response to stimulants is poor (Kotagal et al. 1990).

Episodes of amnesic automatism simulating epilepsy occur in 8% of patients (Aldrich 1990, Schenck and Mahowald 1992).

Sleep paralysis, cataplexy and hypnagogic hallucinations appear to reflect the fact that the motor manifestations of REM sleep, whose immediate or rapid onset after falling asleep characterizes narcolepsy, may also occur in slight chronological dissociation from the behavioural component of sleep in narcoleptic individuals.

The course of narcolepsy is lifelong and often psychologically distressing. A good regimen of sleep is an essential component of therapy. This includes a regular schedule of night sleep, the avoidance of long naps, and the provision of short periods of day rest. Methylphenidate and the amphetamines may help some patients but their action is often transitory. Imipramine, 50 mg t.i.d., has a beneficial effect on cataplexy. Treatment of narcolepsy with modafinil (Bastuji and Jouvet 1988) or selegiline (Hublin et al. 1994) is effective to alleviate the symptoms. Tyrosine seems to produce a subjective improvement in both adults and children (Winter et al. 1996), perhaps by increasing central catecholamine release. Sodium oxylate seems promising for the treatment of cataplexy (Mamelak et al. 2001, Xyrem International Study Group 2005). Making the correct diagnosis, which is often missed (Stores 2006), and simple reassurance that the disorder is not a psychiatric one are of great importance. Isolated cataplexy has been reported with pontomedullary lesions (D'Cruz et al. 1994) in patients with Coffin–Lowry syndrome (Stephenson et al. 2005), and in patients with Niemann–Pick C disease and with Norrie syndrome (Chapter 17), in which it may account for the atonic attacks previously reported (Vossler et al. 1996).

OTHER SYNDROMES WITH HYPERSOMNIA

Hypersomnia is encountered in patients with nocturnal insomnia, especially in children with the obstructive sleep apnoea syndrome or the increased airway resistance syndrome, which are probably the most common causes of diurnal hypersomnia.

Depression and neurotic states are a frequent cause of hypersomnia in adolescent patients.

Occasional cases of recurrent hypersomnia are caused by lesions of the third ventricle or brainstem such as tumours or sequelae of encephalitis, trauma or vascular accidents (Plazzi et al. 1996, Autret et al. 2001).

Kleine–Levin syndrome

The syndrome of Kleine–Levin has been described in Chapter 4, and only the pathogenesis and the required investigations for affected patients are discussed here.

Hypothalamic dysfunction may account for the symptomatology because: (a) the appetite and sleep symptoms implicate hypothalamic systems; (b) the syndrome occurs mostly in the teenage period; (c) it affects mostly boys and its episodic nature could be seen as a counterpart to variable behaviour in connection with onset of menarche in girls; and (d) some EEG findings are compatible with hypothalamic dysfunction.

The work-up should include a neuropsychiatric assessment. If the history and symptoms are typical there is no need for further work-up, but in case of doubt, neurological and laboratory tests to exclude other neurological disorders and metabolic problems may be essential. A urine and/or blood screen for narcotics and other drugs might also be appropriate in some cases. The EEG sometimes shows mild to moderate increase of low-frequency activity, and there may be subtle signs of damage to the CSF blood–brain barrier.

Treatment of the syndrome is detailed in Chapter 4.

INSOMNIA

Many young children have periods when they have difficulty going to sleep. This is a physiological event that should be dealt with gently by parents.

The phenomenon occurs less commonly in school-age children, in whom it is often related to anxiety, especially based on school problems or emotional difficulties. Difficulties in getting to sleep are also common in hyperkinetic children (Chapter 26) and in children with learning difficulties (Ferber 1987).

Certain drugs such as phenobarbitone are an often unrecognized cause of sleep disturbances in epileptic toddlers or children. Sometimes, a true depressive state is responsible for insomnia.

In a significant proportion of cases no cause is found, and the prognosis is variable, as some cases persist into adolescence and adulthood.

In many children with neurodevelopmental disabilities and in blind children, the circadian rhythms are considerably disturbed and this often produces severe family life disruption. Melatonin may be a potent treatment of such cases (Jan and Freeman 2004, Phillips and Appleton 2004).

In most cases no drug therapy is indicated. In rare patients the use of hypnotics such as nitrazepam or chloral hydrate may be considered, especially when severe daily fatigue results from insomnia.

Nocturnal awakening in young children, followed by resumption of sleep in the small hours of the morning is a fairly common and benign behaviour that requires no more than reassurance. Seizures are a rare cause of insomnia responsible for excessive daytime somnolence. In some cases, the seizures are limited to awakening associated with paroxysmal EEG bursts (Peled and Lavie 1986).

REFERENCES

Abu-Arafeh I, Macleod S (2005) Serious neurologic disorders in children with chronic headache. *Arch Dis Child* 90: 937–40.
Aicardi J (1988) Clinical approach to the management of intractable epilepsy. *Dev Med Child Neurol* 30: 429–40.
Aicardi J (2002) Alternating hemiplegia of childhood. In: Guerrini R, Aicardi J, Andermann F, Hallett M, eds. *Epilepsy and Movement Disorders*. Cambridge: Cambridge University Press, pp. 379–92.

Aicardi J (2003) Diagnosis and differential diagnosis. In: Arzimanoglou A, Guerrini R, Aicardi J, eds. *Epilepsy in Children, 3rd edn*. Philadelphia: Lippincott, Williams & Wilkins, pp. 325–41.

Aicardi J, Gastaut H, Mises J (1988) Syncopal attacks compulsively self-induced by Valsalva's maneuver associated with typical absence seizures: a case report. *Arch Neurol* 45: 923–5.

Aldrich MS (1990) Narcolepsy. *N Engl J Med* 323: 389–94.

Aldrich MS, Naylor MW (1989) Narcolepsy associated with lesions of the diencephalon. *Neurology* 39: 1505–8.

Alfonso I, Papazian O, Rodriguez JA, Jeffries H (1993) Benign neonatal sleep myoclonus. *Int Pediatr* 8: 250–2.

Alfonso I, Papazian O, Aicardi J, Jeffries HE (1995) A simple maneuver to provoke benign neonatal sleep myoclonus. *Pediatrics* 96: 1161–3.

Al-Twajri WA, Shevell MI (2002) Pediatric migraine equivalents: occurrence and clinical features in practice. *Pediatr Neurol* 26: 365–8.

Alvord EC, Shaw CM (1989) Congenital difficulties with swallowing and breathing associated with maternal polyhydramnios: neurocristopathy or medullary infarction? *J Child Neurol* 4: 299–306.

American Academy of Pediatrics Task Force on Infantile Apnea (1985) Prolonged infantile apnea: 1985. *Pediatrics* 76: 129–31.

Amiel J, Laudier B, Attie-Bitach T, et al. (2003) Polyalanine expansion and frameshift mutations of the paired-like homeobox gene PHOX2B in congenital central hypoventilation syndrome. *Nat Genet* 33: 459–61.

Andermann E, Andermann F, Silver K, et al. (1994) Benign familial nocturnal alternating hemiplegia of childhood. *Neurology* 44: 1812–4.

Andermann F, Andermann E (1988) Startle disorders of man: hyperekplexia, jumping and startle epilepsy. *Brain Dev* 10: 213–22.

Andermann F, Lugaresi E, eds. (1987) *Migraine and Epilepsy*. London: Butterworths.

Andermann F, Aicardi J, Vigevano F, eds. (1995) *Alternating Hemiplegia of Childhood*. New York: Raven Press.

Andersen AR, Friberg L, Olsen TS, Olesen J (1988) Delayed hyperemia following hypoperfusion in classic migraine. Single photon emission computed tomographic demonstration. *Arch Neurol* 45: 154–9.

Angelini L, Rumi V, Lamperti E, Nardocci N 1988) Transient paroxysmal dystonia in infancy. *Neuropediatrics* 19: 171–4.

Appleton R, Farrell K, Buncic JR, Hill A (1988) Amaurosis fugax in teenagers: a migraine variant. *Am J Dis Child* 142: 331–3.

Auburger G, Ratzlaff T, Lunkes A, et al. (1996) A gene for autosomal dominant paroxysmal choreoathetosis/spasticity (CSE) maps to the vicinity of a potassium channel gene cluster on chromosome 1p, probably within 2 cM, between D1S443 and D1S197. *Genomics* 31: 90–4.

Auduy B (1988) [Acute cardiorespiratory failure after niaprazine absorption.] *Arch Fr Pediatr* 45: 439 (letter) (French).

Autret A, Lucas B, Mondon K, et al. (2001) Sleep and brain lesions: a critical review of the literature and additional new cases. *Neurophysiol Clin* 31: 356–75.

Avanzini G, Franceschetti S, Avoni P, Liguori R (2004) Molecular biology of channelopathies: impact on diagnosis and treatment. *Expert Rev Neurother* 4: 519–39.

Bakker MJ, van Dijk JG, van der Maagdenberg AM, Tijssen MA (2006) Startle syndrome. *Lancet Neurol* 5: 513–24.

Baloh RW, Yue Q, Furman JM, Nelson SF (1997) Familial episodic ataxia: clinical heterogeneity in four families linked to chromosome 19p. *Ann Neurol* 41: 8–16.

Balottin U, Termine C, Nicoli F, et al. (2005) Idiopathic headache in children under 6 years of age: a follow-up study. *Headache* 45: 705–15.

Barlow CF (1984) *Headaches and Migraine in Childhood. Clinics in Developmental Medicine no. 91*. London: Spastics International Medical Publications.

Bassi MT, Bresolin N, Tonelli A, et al. (2004) A novel mutation in the ATP1A2 gene causes alternating hemiplegia of childhood. *J Med Genet* 41: 621–8.

Bastuji H, Jouvet M (1988) Successful treatment of idiopathic hypersomnia and narcolepsy with modafinil. *Prog Neuropsychopharmacol Biol Psychiatry* 12: 695–700.

Battaglia A, Guerrini R, Gastaut H (1989) Epileptic seizures induced by syncopal attacks. *J Epilepsy* 2: 137–46.

Bauer KA (2004) Covert videosurveillance of parents suspected of child abuse: the British experience and alternative approaches. *Theor Med Bioeth* 25: 311–27.

Baumann CF, Bassetti CL (2005) Hypocretins (orexins) and sleep–wake disorders. *Lancet Neurol* 4: 673–82.

Baumann RJ (2002) Behavioral treatment of migraine in children and adolescents. *Paediatr Drugs* 4: 555–61.

Baxter P, Gardner-Medwin D, Green SH, Moss C (1993) Congenital livedo reticularis and recurrent stroke-like episodes. *Dev Med Child Neurol* 35: 917–21.

Baziel GM, Van Engelen MD, Willy O, et al. (1991) Bilateral episodic mydriasis as a migraine equivalent in childhood: a case report. *Headache* 31: 375–7.

Beckerman R, Meltzer J, Sola A, et al. (1986) Brain-stem auditory response in Ondine's syndrome. *Arch Neurol* 43: 698–701.

Bennett HS, Selman JE, Rapin I, Rose A (1982) Nonconvulsive epileptiform activity appearing as ataxia. *Am J Dis Child* 136: 30–2.

Bhatia KP (2001) Familial (idiopathic) paroxysmal dyskinesias: an update. *Semin Neurol* 21: 69–74.

Bhatia MS, Sapra S (2005) Pseudoseuzures in children: a profile of 50 cases. *Clin Pediatr* 44: 617–21.

Bille B (1962) Migraine in school children. A study of the incidence and short-term prognosis, and a clinical, psychological and electroencephalographic comparison between children with migraine and matched controls. *Acta Paed Suppl* 136: 1–151.

Bodiou C, Bavoux F (1988) [Niaprazine and side effects in pediatrics. Cooperative evaluation of French centers of pharmacovigilance.] *Therapie* 43: 307–11 (French).

Boel P, Casaer P (1988) Familial periodic ataxia responsive to flunarizine. *Neuropediatrics* 19: 218–20.

Boles RG, Adams K, Li BV (2005) Maternal inheritance in cyclic vomiting syndrome. *Am J Med Genet A* 133: 71–9.

Boltshauser E, Lange B, Dumermuth G (1987) Differential diagnosis of syndromes with abnormal respiration (tachypnea–apnea). *Brain Dev* 9: 462–5.

Bordarier C, Aicardi J (1990) Dandy–Walker syndrome and agenesis of the cerebellar vermis: diagnostic problems and genetic counselling. *Dev Med Child Neurol* 32: 285–94.

Bourgeois M, Aicardi J, Goutières F (1993) Alternating hemiplegia of childhood. *J Pediatr* 122: 673–9.

Bower S, Dennis M, Warlow C, et al. (1994) Long term prognosis of transient lone bilateral blindness in adolescents and young adults. *J Neurol Neurosurg Psychiatry* 57: 734–6.

Boyle NJ, Jones DH, Hamilton R, et al. (2005) Blindsight in children: does it exist and can it be used to help the child? Observations on a case series. *Dev Med Child Neurol* 47: 699–702.

Brand DA, Altman RL, Purtill K, Edwards KS (2005) Yield of diagnostic testing in infants who have had apparent life-threatening events. *Pediatrics* 115: 885–93.

Brandes JL, Saper JA, Diamond M, et al. (2004) Topiramate for migraine prevention: a randomized controlled trial. *JAMA* 291: 965–73.

Breningstall GN (1996) Breath-holding spells. *Pediatr Neurol* 14: 91–7.

Bressman SB, Fahn S, Burke RE (1988) Paroxysmal non-kinesigenic dystonia. *Adv Neurol* 50: 403–13.

Brett EM, ed. (1997) *Paediatric Neurology, 3rd edn*. Edinburgh: Churchill Livingstone.

Bricker JT, Garson A, Gillette PC (1984) A family history of seizures associated with sudden cardiac deaths. *Am J Dis Child* 138: 866–8.

Brown P, Rothwell JC, Thompson PD, et al. (1991) The hyperekplexias and their relationship to the normal startle reflex. *Brain* 114: 1903–28.

Brunt ERP, Van Weerden TW (1990) Familial paroxysmal kinesigenic ataxia and continuous myokymia. *Brain* 113: 1361–82.

Buchenau W, Urschitz MS, Sautermeister J, et al. (2007) A randomized clinical trial of a new orthodontic appliance to improve upper airway obstruction in infants with Pierre Robin sequence. *J Pediatr* 151: 145–9.

Camfield PR, Camfield CS (1990) Syncope in childhood: a case control clinical study of the familial tendency to faint. *Can J Neurol Sci* 17: 306–8.

Caminero AB, Pareja JA, Arpa J, et al. (1998) Migrainous syndrome with CSF pleocytosis. SPECT findings. *Headache* 37: 511–5.

Campistol J, Prats JM, Garaizar C (1993) Benign paroxysmal tonic upgaze of childhood with ataxia. A neuro-ophthalmological syndrome of familial origin? *Dev Med Child Neurol* 35: 436–9.

Caplan LR (1991) Migraine and vertebrobasilar ischemia. *Neurology* 41: 55–61.

Casaer P, Aicardi J, Curatolo P, et al. (1987) Flunarizine in alternating hemiplegia in childhood. An international study in 12 children. *Neuropediatrics* 18: 191–5.

Cavanagh NDC, Bicknell J, Howard E (1974) Cystinuria with mental retardation and paroxysmal dyskinesia in two brothers. *Arch Dis Child* 49: 662–4.

Chabriat H, Tournier-Lasserve E, Vahedi K, et al. (1995) Autosomal dominant migraine with MRI white-matter abnormalities mapping to the CADASIL locus. *Neurology* 45: 1086–91.

Chu ML, Shinnar S (1992) Headaches in children younger than 7 years of age. *Arch Neurol* 49: 79–82.

Cohen HA, Nussinovitch M, Ashkenasi A, et al. (1993) Benign paroxysmal torticollis in infancy. *Pediatr Neurol* 9: 488–90.

Commare MC, François B, Estournet B, Barois A (1993) Ondine's curse: a discussion of five cases. *Neuropediatrics* 24: 313–8.

Confavreux C, Gebuhrer L, Betuel H, et al. (1988) [HLA and narcolepsy. Apropos of 28 cases including 2 negative HLA-DR2.] *Rev Neurol* 144: 327–31 (French).

Constatinou JF, Gillis J, Ouvrier RA, Rahilly PM (1989) Hypoxic–ischaemic encephalopathy after near-miss sudden death syndrome. *Arch Dis Child* 64: 743–8.

Cooper CJ, Ridker P, Shea J, Creager MA (1994) Familial occurrence of neuro-cardiogenic syncope. *N Engl J Med* 331: 205 (letter).

Cortelli P, Avallone R, Baraldi M, et al. (2005) Endozepines in recurrent stupor. *Sleep Med Rev* 9: 477–87.

Coto E, Armenta D, Espinosa R, et al. (2005) Recessive hyperekplexia due to a new mutation (R100H) in the GLRA1 gene. *Mov Disord* 20: 1626–9.

Croft RD, Jervis M (1989) Munchausen's syndrome in a 4 year old. *Arch Dis Child* 64: 740–1.

Cummiskey J, Guilleminault C, Davis R, et al. (1987) Automatic respiratory failure, sleep studies and Leigh's disease (case report). *Neurology* 37: 1876–8.

Curtain RP, Smith RL, Ovcaric M, Griffiths LR (2006) Minor head trauma-induced sporadic hemiplegic migraine coma. *Pediatr Neurol* 34: 329–32.

Dale RC, Cross JH (1999) Ictal hemiparesis. *Dev Med Child Neurol* 41: 344–7.

Damen L, Bruijn JK, Verhagen AP (2005) Symptomatic treatment of migraine in children: a systematic review of medication trials. *Pediatrics* 116: 295–302.

Damji KF, Allingham RR, Pollock SC, et al. (1996) Periodic vestibulocerebellar ataxia, an autosomal dominant ataxia with defective smooth pursuit, is genetically distinct from other autosomal dominant ataxias. *Arch Neurol* 53: 338–44.

Dan B, Boyd SG (2006) A neurophysiological perspective on sleep and its maturation. *Dev Med Child Neurol* 48: 773–9.

Daniels SR, Bates SR, Kaplan S (1987) EEG monitoring during paroxysmal hyperpnea of tetralogy of Fallot: an epileptic or hypoxic phenomenon? *J Child Neurol* 2: 98–100.

Darras BT, Ampola MG, Dietz WH, Gilmore HE (1989) Intermittent dystonia in Hartnup disease. *Pediatr Neurol* 5: 118–20.

Dauvilliers Y, Baumann CR, Carlander B, et al. (2003) CSF hypocretin-1 levels in narcolepsy, Kleine–Levin syndrome and other hypersomnias and neurological conditions. *J Neurol Neurosurg Psychiatry* 74: 1667–73.

Dauvilliers Y, Arnulf I, Mignot E (2007) Narcolepsy with cataplexy. *Lancet* 369: 499–511.

D'Cruz OF, Vaughn BV, Gold SH, Greenwood RS (1994) Symptomatic cataplexy in pontomedullary lesions. *Neurology* 44: 2189–91.

Demirkiran M, Jankovic J (1995) Paroxysmal dyskinesias: clinical features and classification. *Ann Neurol* 38: 571–9.

Deonna T (1988) Paroxysmal disorder which may be migraine or may be confused with it. In: Hockaday J, ed. *Migraine in Childhood*. London: Butterworths, pp. 75–87.

Deonna T, Roulet E, Meyer HU (1990) Benign paroxysmal tonic upgaze of childhood—a new syndrome. *Neuropediatrics* 21: 213–4.

Deonna T, Fohlen M, Jalin J, et al. (2002) Epileptic stereotypies in children? In: Guerrini R, Aicardi J, Andermann F, Hallett M, eds. *Epilepsy and Movement Disorders*. Cambridge: Cambridge University Press, pp. 319–32.

Desai P, Talwar D (1992) Nonepileptic events in normal and neurologically handicapped children: a video–EEG study. *Pediatr Neurol* 8: 127–9.

Dewolfe CC (2005) Apparent life-threatening events: a review. *Pediatr Clin North Am* 52: 1127–46.

Di Capua M, Fusco L, Ricci S, Vigevano F (1993) Benign neonatal sleep myoclonus: clinical features and video–polygraphic recordings. *Mov Disord* 8: 191–4.

Dichgans M, Freilinger T, Eckstein G, et al. (2005) Mutation in the neuronal voltage-gated sodium channel SCN1A in a familial hemiplegic migraine. *Lancet* 366: 371–7.

DiMario FJ, Burleson JA (1993) Autonomic nervous system function in severe breath-holding spells. *Pediatr Neurol* 9: 268–74.

DiMario FJ, Emery ES (1987) The natural history of night terrors. *Clin Pediatr* 26: 505–11.

DiMauro S, Miranda AF, Olarte M, (1982) Muscle phosphoglycerate mutase deficiency. *Neurology* 32: 584–91.

Dinwiddie R (2004) Congenital upper airway obstruction. *Paediatr Respir Rev* 5: 17-24.

Di Rosa G, Spanò M, Pustorini G, et al. (2006) Alternating hemiplegia of childhood successfully treated with topiramate: 18 months of follow-up. *Neurology* 66: 146.

Dooley JM, Andermann F (1989) Startle disease or hyperekplexia: adolescent onset and response to valproate. *Pediatr Neurol* 5: 126–7.

Dooling EC, Richardson EP (1977) Ophthalmoplegia and Ondine's curse. *Arch Ophthalmol* 95: 1790–3.

Dvorkin GS, Andermann F, Carpenter S, et al. (1987) Classical migraine, intractable epilepsy and multiple strokes: a syndrome related to mitochondrial encephalomyopathy. In: Andermann F, Lugaresi E, eds. *Migraine and Epilepsy*. London: Butterworths, pp. 203–32.

Eisinger J (1987) Repetitive electromyographic activity, spasmorhythmia and spasmophilia. *Magnesium* 6: 65–73.

Ellie E, Julien J, Ferrer X, et al. (1989) Extensive cerebral calcification and retinal changes in pseudohypoparathyroidism. *J Neurol* 236: 432–4.

Elliott FA (1984) The episodic dyscontrol syndrome and aggression. *Neurol Clin* 2: 113–25.

Elliott MA, Peroutka SJ, Welch S, May EF (1996) Familial hemiplegic migraine, nystagmus, and cerebellar atrophy. *Ann Neurol* 39: 100–6.

Elzinga-Huttenga J, Heckster Y, Bilj A, Rotteveel J (2006) Movement disorders induced by gastrointestinal drugs: two pediatric cases. *Neuropediatrics* 37: 102–6.

Epstein MA, Duchowny M, Jayakar P, et al. (1994) Altered responsiveness during hyperventilation-induced EEG slowing: a non-epileptic phenomenon in normal children. *Epilepsia* 35: 1204–7.

Farris BK, Smith JL, Ayyar R (1986) Neuro-ophthalmologic findings in vestibulocerebellar ataxia. *Arch Neurol* 43: 1050–3.

Ferber R (1987) The sleepless child. In: Guilleminault C, ed. *Sleep and its Disorders in Children*. New York: Raven Press, pp. 141–63.

Ferrari MD, Haan J, Blokland JA, et al. (1995) Cerebral blood flow during migraine attacks without aura and effect of sumatriptan. *Arch Neurol* 52: 135–9.

Fitzsimons RB, Wolfenden WH (1985) Migraine coma. Meningitic migraine with cerebral oedema associated with a new form of autosomal dominant cerebellar ataxia. *Brain* 108: 555–77.

Fontan JP, Heldt GP, Heyman MB, et al. (1984) Esophageal spasm associated with apnea and bradycardia in an infant. *Pediatrics* 73: 52–5.

Fuller GN, Guiloff RJ (1987) Migrainous olfactory hallucinations. *J Neurol Neurosurg Psychiatry* 50: 1688–90.

Fusco L, Vigevano F (1995) Alternating hemiplegia of childhood: clinical findings during attacks. In: Andermann F, Aicardi J, Vigevano F, eds. *Alternating Hemiplegia of Childhood*. New York: Raven Press, pp. 29–41.

Galletti F, Brinciotti M, Emanuelli O (1989) Familial occurrence of benign myoclonus of early infancy. *Epilepsia* 30: 579–81.

Galvin HK, Newton AW, Vandeven AM (2005) Update on Munchausen syndrome by proxy. *Curr Opin Peediatr* 17: 252–7.

Garrotxategi P, Reguilon ML, Arana J, et al. (1996) Gastroesophageal reflux in association with the Sandifer syndrome. *Eur J Pediatr Surg* 5: 203–5.

Gastaut H (1974) Syncopes: generalised anoxic seizures. In: Vinken PJ, Bruyn GW, eds. *Handbook of Clinical Neurology, vol. 15. The Epilepsies*. Amsterdam: North Holland, pp. 815–35.

Gastaut H (1980) [A little known neurological syndrome in a mentally retarded child: compulsive syncope self-induced by Valsalva manoeuvre.] *Bull Acad Natl Med* 164: 713–7 (French).

Gastaut H, Zifkin B, Rufo M (1987) Compulsive respiratory stereotypies in children with autistic features: polygraphic recording and treatment with fenfluramine. *J Autism Dev Disord* 17: 391–406.

Gay CT, Ryan SG (1994) Paroxysmal kinesigenic dystonia after methylphenidate administration. *J Child Neurol* 9: 45–6.

Genton P, Bartolomei F, Guerrini R (1995) Panic attacks mistaken for relapse of epilepsy. *Epilepsia* 36: 48–51.

Giangaspero F, Schiavina M, Sturani C, et al. (1988) Failure of automatic control of ventilation (Ondine's curse) associated with viral encephalitis of the brain stem: a clinicopathologic study of one case. *Clin Neuropathol* 7: 234–7.

Giffin NJ, Benton S, Goadsby PJ (2002) Benign paroxysmal torticollis of infancy: four new cases with linkage to the CACNA1 mutation. *Dev Med Child Neurol* 44: 490–3.

Goadsby PJ, Edvinsson L (1993) The trigeminovascular system and migraine: studies characterizing cerebrovascular and neuropeptide changes seen in humans and cats. *Ann Neurol* **33**: 48–56.

Gokhale R, Huttenlocher PR, Brady L, Kirschner BS (1997) Use of barbiturates in the treatment of cyclic vomiting during childhood. *J Pediatr Gastroenterol Nutr* **25**: 64–7; erratum 559.

Golden GS (1979) The Alice in Wonderland syndrome in juvenile migraine. *Pediatrics* **63**: 517–9.

Goldenberg I, Moss AJ, Zareba W (2005) Sudden cardiac death without structural heart disease: update of the long QT and Brugada syndromes. *Curr Cardiol Rep* **7**: 349–56.

Gomez-Aranda F, Canadellas F, Martin-Masso JF, et al. (1997) Pseudomigraine with temporary neurological symptoms and lymphocytic pleocytosis: a report of 50 cases. *Brain* **120**: 1105–13.

Gordon N (1987) Breath-holding spells. *Dev Med Child Neurol* **29**: 811–4.

Gordon N (1988) Nasal obstruction in childhood: the obstructive sleep apnoea syndrome. *Dev Med Child Neurol* **30**: 261–5.

Gordon N (1994a) Recurrent vomiting in childhood, especially of neurological origin. *Dev Med Child Neurol* **36**: 463–7.

Gordon N (1994b) The long Q-T syndromes. *Brain Dev* **16**: 153–5.

Gordon N (1998) Episodic ataxia and channelopathies. *Brain Dev* **20**: 9–13.

Granot R, Berkovic S, Patterson R, et al. (2004) Endozepine stupor: disease or deception? A critical review. *Sleep* **27**: 1597–9.

Grattan-Smith PJ, Shield LK, Hopkins IJ, Collins KJ (1990) Acute respiratory failure precipitated by general anaesthesia in Leigh syndrome. *J Child Neurol* **5**: 137–41.

Graves TD, Hanna MG (2005) Neurological channelopathies. *Postgrad Med J* **81**: 20–31.

Greenberg DA (1997) Calcium channels in neurological disease. *Ann Neurol* **42**: 275–82.

Griggs RC, Nutt JG (1995) Episodic ataxias as channelopathies. *Ann Neurol* **37**: 285–7.

Grylack LJ, Williams AD (1996) Apparent life-threatening events in presumed healthy neonates during the first three days of life. *Pediatrics* **97**: 349–51.

Gudmunsson O, Prendergast M, Foreman D, Cowley S (2001) Outcome of pseudoseizures in children and adolescents: a 6-year symptom survival analysis. *Dev Med Child Neurol* **43**: 547–51.

Guerrini R, Sanchez-Carpintero R, Deonna T, et al. (2002) Early-onset absence epilepsy and paroxysmal dyskinesia. *Epilepsia* **43**: 1224–9.

Guilleminault C (1987a) Disorders of arousal in children: somnambulism and night terrors. In: Guilleminault C, ed. *Sleep and its Disorders in Children*. New York: Raven Press, pp. 243–52.

Guilleminault C (1987b) Sleep apnea in the full-term infant. In: Guilleminault C, ed. *Sleep and its Disorders in Children*. New York: Raven Press, pp. 195–211.

Guilleminault C, Nino-Murcia G, Heldt G, et al. (1986) Alternative treatment to tracheostomy in obstructive sleep apnea syndrome: nasal continuous positive airway pressure in young children. *Pediatrics* **78**: 797–802.

Guilleminault C, Pelayo R, Leger D, et al. (1996) Recognition of sleep-disordered breathing in children. *Pediatrics* **98**: 871–82.

Guiloff RJ, Fruns M (1988) Limb pain in migraine and cluster headache. *J Neurol Neurosurg Psychiatry* **51**: 1022–31.

Haan J, Kremer HPH, Padberg GWAM (1989) Paroxysmal choreoathetosis as presenting symptom of diabetes mellitus. *J Neurol Neurosurg Psychiatry* **52**: 133 (letter).

Hagberg B, Aicardi J, Dias K, Ramos O (1983) A progressive syndrome of autism, dementia, ataxia and loss of purposeful use of hands in girls: Rett syndrome: report of 35 cases. *Ann Neurol* **14**: 471–9.

Halbower AC, Marcus CL (2003) Sleep disorders in children. *Curr Opin Pulm Med* **9**: 471–6.

Hämäläinen ML, Hoppu K, Santavuori P (1997a) Sumatriptan for migraine attacks in children: a randomized placebo-controlled study. Do children with migraine respond to oral sumatriptan differently from adults? *Neurology* **48**: 1100–3.

Hämäläinen ML, Hoppu K, Valkeila E, Santavuori P (1997b) Ibuprofen or acetaminophen for the acute treatment of migraine in children: a double-blind, randomized, placebo-controlled, crossover study. *Neurology* **48**: 103–7.

Harbord MG, Kobayashi JS (1991) Fever producing ballismus in patients with choreoathetosis. *J Child Neurol* **6**: 49–52.

Harden CL, Burgut FT, Kanner AM (2003) The diagnostic significance of video–EEG monitoring findings on pseudoseizure patients differs between neurologists and psychiatrists. *Epilepsia* **44**: 453–6.

Hart YM, Tampieri D, Andermann E, et al. (1995) Alternating paroxysmal dystonia and hemiplegia in childhood as a symptom of basal ganglia disease. *J Neurol Neurosurg Psychiatry* **59**: 453–4 (letter).

Hauser RA, Lacey M, Knight MR (1988) Hypertensive encephalopathy. Magnetic resonance imaging demonstration of reversible cortical and white matter lesions. *Arch Neurol* **45**: 1078–83.

Henderson J (2005) Respiratory support of infants with bronchiolitis related apnoea: is there a role for negative pressure? *Arch Dis Child* **90**: 224–5.

Herman SP, Stickler GB, Lucas AR (1981) Hyperventilation syndrome in children and adolescents. Long-term follow-up. *Pediatrics* **67**: 183–7.

Hershey AD, Winner P, Kabbouche MA, et al. (2005) Use of ICHD-II criteria in the diagnosis of pediatric migraine. *Headache* **45**: 1288–97.

Hirayama K, Hoshino Y, Kamashiro H, Yamamoto T (1994) Reverse Shapiro's syndrome. A case of agenesis of the corpus callosum associated with periodic hyperthermia. *Arch Neurol* **51**: 494–6.

Hoban TF (2005) Obstructive sleep apnea in children. *Curr Treat Options Neurol* **7**: 353-361.

Hockaday JM (1987) Migraine and its equivalents in childhood. *Dev Med Child Neurol* **29**: 265–70.

Hofele JM, Benecke R, Auburger G (1997) Gene locus FPD1 of the dystonic Mount–Reback type of autosomal dominant paroxysmal choreoathetosis. *Neurology* **49**: 1252–7.

Holguin J, Fenichel G (1967) Migraine. *J Pediatr* **70**: 290–7.

Holmes GL, Russman BS (1986) Shuddering attacks. *Am J Dis Child* **140**: 72–4.

Holmes GL, Sackellares JC, McKiernan J, et al. (1980) Evaluation of childhood pseudoseizures using EEG telemetry and video tape monitoring. *J Pediatr* **97**: 554–8.

Horrocks IA, Nechay A, Stephenson JB, Zuberi SM (2005) Anoxic–epileptic seizures: observational study of epileptic seizures induced by syncope. *Arch Dis Child* **90**: 1283–7.

Hublin C, Partinen M, Heinonen EH, et al. (1994) Selegiline in the treatment of narcolepsy. *Neurology* **44**: 2095–101.

Hutchinson W, O'Riordan J, Javed M, et al. (1995) Familial hemiplegic migraine and autosomal dominant arteriopathy with leukoencephalopathy (CADASIL). *Ann Neurol* **38**: 817–24.

Jaeken J, Carchon H (1993) The carbohydrate-deficient glycoprotein syndromes: an overview. *J Inherit Metab Dis* **16**: 813–20.

Jan JE, Freeman RD (2004) Melatonin therapy for circadian rhythm sleep disorders in children with multiple disabilities: what have we learned in the last decade? *Dev Med Child Neurol* **46**: 776–82.

Jeavons PM (1983) Non-epileptic attacks in childhood. In: Rose FC, ed. *Research Progress in Epilepsy*. London: Pitman, pp. 224–30.

Jen J (2000) Familial episodic ataxias and related channel disorders. *Curr Treat Options Neurol* **2**: 429–31.

Jen J, Kim GW, Baloh RW (2004) Clinical spectrum of episodic ataxia type 2. *Neurology* **62**: 17–22.

Jensen TH, Hansen PB, Brodersen P (1988) Ondine's curse in Listeria monocytogenes brain stem encephalitis. *Acta Neurol Scand* **77**: 505–6.

Jiang WJ, Chi ZF, Ma L, et al. (2006) Topiramate: a new agent for patients with alternating hemiplegia of childhood. *Neuropediatrics* **37**: 229–33.

Joutel A, Ducros A, Vahedi K, et al. (1994) Genetic heterogeneity of familial hemiplegic migraine. *Am J Hum Genet* **55**: 1166–72.

Kass RS (2005) The channelopathies: novel insights into molecular and genetic mechanisms of human disease. *J Clin Invest* **115**: 1986–9.

Kemp GJ, Taylor DJ, Barnes PRJ, et al. (1995) Skeletal muscle mitochondrial dysfunction in alternating hemiplegia of childhood. *Ann Neurol* **38**: 681–4.

Khan S, Yakub BA, Poser CM, et al. (1995) Multiphasic disseminated encephalomyelitis presenting as alternating hemiplegia. *J Neurol Neurosurg Psychiatry* **58**: 467–70.

Kienbacher C, Wober C, Zesch H, et al. (2006) Clinical features, classification and prognosis of migraine and tension-type headache in children and adolescent: a long-term follow-up study. *Cephalalgia* **26**: 820–30.

Kinast M, Lenders H, Rothner AD, Erenberg G (1982) Benign focal epileptiform discharges in childhood migraine. *Neurology* **32**: 1309–11.

Koenigsberger MR, Chutorian AM, Gold AP, Schvey MS (1970) Benign paroxysmal vertigo of childhood. *Neurology* **20**: 1108–13.

Korinthenberg R (1996) Is infantile alternating hemiplegia mediated by glutamate toxicity and can it be treated with memantine? *Neuropediatrics* **27**: 277–8.

Kors EE, Terwindt GM, Vermeulen FM, et al. (2001) Delayed central edema and fatal coma after minor head trauma. *Ann Neurol* **49**: 753–60.

Kors EE, Vanmolkot KR, Haan J, et al. (2004) Alternating hemiplegia of childhood: no mutations in the second familial hemiplegic migraine gene ATP1A2. *Neuropediatrics* **35**: 293–4.

Kotagal S, Silber MH (2004) Childhood-onset restless legs syndrome. *Ann Neurol* **56**: 803–7.

Kotagal S, Hartse K, Walsh JK (1990) Characteristics of narcolepsy in pre-teenaged children. *Pediatrics* **85**: 205–9.

Krägeloh I, Aicardi J (1980) Alternating hemiplegia in infants: report of five cases. *Dev Med Child Neurol* **22**: 784–91.

Kramer RE, Dinner DS, Braun WE, et al. (1987) HLA-DR2 and narcolepsy. *Arch Neurol* **44**: 853–5.

Kramer U, Carmant L, Riviello JJ, et al. (1995) Psychogenic seizures: videotelemetry observations in 27 patients. *Pediatr Neurol* **12**: 39–41.

Krowchuk DP, Williford PM, Jorizzo JL, Kandt RS (1994) Solitary masto-cytoma producing symptoms mimicking those of a seizure disorder. *J Child Neurol* **9**: 451–3.

Kullmann DM (2002) The neuronal channelopathies. *Brain* **125**: 1177–95.

Kuntz KM, Kokmen E, Stevens JC, et al. (1992) Post-lumbar puncture headaches: experience in 501 consecutive procedures. *Neurology* **42**: 1884–7.

Kurlan R, Krall RL, Deweese JA (1984) Vertebrobasilar ischemia after total repair of tetralogy of Fallot: significance of subclavian steal created by Blalock–Taussig anastomosis. Vertebrobasilar ischemia after the correction of tetralogy of Fallot. *Stroke* **15**: 359–62.

Kyriakides T, Drousiotou A (1994) No structural or biochemical evidence for mitochondrial cytopathy in a case of alternating hemiplegia of childhood. *Ann Neurol* **36**: 805–6 (letter).

Lampl C (2002) Childhood-onset cluster headache. *Pediatr Neurol* **27**: 138–40.

Lance JW (1977) Familial paroxysmal dystonic choreoathetosis and its differentiation from related syndromes. *Ann Neurol* **2**: 285–93.

Lancman ME, Asconapé JJ, Craven WJ, et al. (1994a) Predictive value of induction of psychogenic seizures by suggestion. *Ann Neurol* **35**: 359–61.

Lancman ME, Asconapé JJ, Graves S, Gibson PA (1994b) Psychogenic seizures in children: long-term analysis of 43 cases. *J Child Neurol* **9**: 404–7.

Lapkin M, Golden G (1978) Basilar artery migraine. A review of 30 cases. *Am J Dis Child* **132**: 278–81.

Lauritzen M (1994) Pathophysiology of the migraine aura. The spreading depression theory. *Brain* **117**: 199–210.

Lee CC, Su BH, Lin HC, et al. (2004) Outcome of vocal cord paralysis in infants. *Acta Paediatr Taiwan* **44**: 278–81.

Le Fort D, Safran AB, Picard F, et al. (2004) Elicited repetitive daily blindness: a new familial disorder relating to migraine and epilepsy. *Neurology* **63**: 348–50.

Lempert T, Bauer M, Schmidt D (1994) Syncope: a videometric analysis of 56 episodes of transient cerebral hypoxia. *Ann Neurol* **36**: 233–7.

Leopold NA (1984) Prolonged metoclopramide-induced dyskinetic reaction. *Neurology* **34**: 238–9.

Lerman-Sagie T, Watemberg N, Vinkler C, et al. (2004) Familial hyperekplexia and refractory status epilepticus: a new autosomal recessive syndrome. *J Child Neurol* **19**: 522–5.

Lesser RP (1996) Psychogenic seizures. *Neurology* **46**: 1499–507.

Lewis DW, Frank CM (1993) Hair-grooming syncope seizures. *Pediatrics* **91**: 836–8.

Lewis DW (2004) Toward a definition of childhood migraine. *Curr Opin Pediatr* **16**: 628–36.

Lindskog U, Olkvist L, Noaksson L, Wallquist J (1999) Benign paroxysmal vertigo in childhood: a long-term follow-up study. *Headache* **19**: 33–7.

Lipton RB, Bigal ME, Steiner TJ, et al. (2004) Classification of primary headache. *Neurology* **63**: 427–35.

Livingstone IR, Gardner-Medwin D, Pennington RJT (1984) Familial intermittent ataxia with possible X-linked inheritance. *J Neurol Sci* **64**: 89–97.

Lombroso CT, Lerman P (1967) Breath-holding spells (cyanotic and pallid infantile syncope). *Pediatrics* **39**: 563–81.

Lou HC (1989) Flunarizine in paroxysmal choreoathetosis. *Neuropediatrics* **20**: 112 (letter).

Lubbers WJ, Brunt ERP, Scheffer H, et al. (1995) Hereditary myokymia and paroxysmal ataxia linked to chromosome 12 is responsive to acetazolamide. *J Neurol Neurosurg Psychiatry* **59**: 400–5.

Lugaresi E, Cirignotta F, Montagna P (1986) Nocturnal paroxysmal dystonia. *J Neurol Neurosurg Psychiatry* **49**: 375–80.

Lugaresi E, Montagna P, Tinuper P, et al. (1998) Endozepine stupor. Recurring stupor linked to endozepine-4 accumulation. *Brain* **121**: 127–33.

Mack KJ (2004) What incites new daily persistent headache in children? *Pediatr Neurol* **31**: 122–5.

Mack KJ (2006) Episodic and chronic migraine in children. *Semin Neurol* **26**: 223–31.

Macleod S, Ferrie C, Zuberi SM (2005) Symptoms of narcolepsy in children misinterpreted as epilepsy. *Epil Disord* **7**: 13–7.

Magaudda A, Tassinari CA, Bureau M, et al. (1987) Awake apnea syndromes: differential diagnosis with epileptic seizures and correlation with Rett syndrome: report of 28 cases. In: Wolf P, Dam M, Janz D, Dreifuss FE, eds. *Advances in Epileptology, vol. 46.* New York: Raven Press, pp. 245–50.

Magaudda A, Genton P, Bureau M, et al. (1988) Familial encephalopathy wth permanent periodic breathing: 4 cases in 2 unrelated families. *Brain Dev* **10**: 110–9.

Mamelak M, Kesler A, Vainstein G, et al. (2001) A pilot study of the effects of of sodium oxylate on sleep architecture and daytime alertness in narcolepsy. *Sleep* **27**: 1327–34.

Mandel H, Tirosh E, Berant M (1989) Sandifer syndrome reconsidered. *Acta Paed Scand* **78**: 797–9.

Manon-Espaillat R, Gothe B, Adams N, et al. (1988) Familial "sleep apnea plus" syndrome: report of a family. *Neurology* **38**: 190–3.

Marcelli V, Piazza F, Pisani F, Marciano E (2006) Neuro-otological features of benign paroxysmal vertigo and benign positional paroxysmal vertigo in children: follow-up study. *Brain Dev* **28**: 80–4.

Marcus CL, Davidson Ward SL, Mallory GB, et al. (1995) Use of nasal continuous positive airway pressure as treatment of childhood obstructive sleep apnea. *J Pediatrics* **127**: 88–94.

Margari L, Perniola T, Illiceto G, et al. (2000) Familial paroxysmal exercise-induced dyskinesia and benign epilepsy: a clinical and neurophysiological study of an uncommon disorder. *Neurol Sci* **21**: 165–72.

Martinez S, Guilleminault C (2004) Periodic leg movements in prepubertal children with sleep disturbance. *Dev Med Child Neurol* **46**: 765–70.

Matsumoto J, Fuhr P, Nigro M, Hallett M (1992) Physiological abnormalities in hereditary hyperekplexia. *Ann Neurol* **32**: 41–50.

McHarg ML, Shinnar S, Rascoff H, Walsh CA (1997) Syncope in childhood. *Pediatr Cardiol* **18**: 367–71.

McNabb S, Whitehouse W (1999) Cluster headache in children. *Arch Dis Child* **81**: 511–2.

Meadow R (1984) Fictitious epilepsy. *Lancet* **2**: 25–8.

Meadow R (1991) Neurological and developmental variants of Munchausen syndrome by proxy. *Dev Med Child Neurol* **33**: 270–2.

Mei D, Ferraro D, Zelano G, et al. (2006) Topiramate and triptans revert chronic migraine with medication overuse to episodic migraine. *Clin Neuropharmacol* **29**: 269–75.

Metrick ME, Ritter FJ, Gates JR, et al. (1991) Nonepileptic events in childhood. *Epilepsia* **32**: 322–8.

Mignot E, Lin L, Rogers W, et al. (2001) Complex HLA-DR and -DQ interactions confer risk of narcolepsy–cataplexy in three ethnic groups. *Am J Hum Genet* **68**: 686–99.

Mikati MA, Maguire H, Barlow CF, et al. (1992) A syndrome of autosomal dominant alternating hemiplegia: clinical presentation mimicking intractable epilepsy; chromosomal studies; and physiologic investigations. *Neurology* **42**: 2251–7.

Mikati MA, Kramer U, Zupanc ML, Shanahan RJ (2000) Alternating hemiplegia of childhood: clinical manifestations and long-term outcome. *Pediatr Neurol* **23**: 134–41.

Miyazaki M, Hashimoto T, Sakumura N, et al. (1991) Central sleep apnea and arterial compression of the medulla. *Ann Neurol* **29**: 564–5.

Mokhlesi B, Tulaimat A, Faibussowitsch I, et al. (2007) Obesity hypoventilation syndrome: prevalence and predictors in patients with obstructive sleep apnea. *Sleep Breath* **11**: 117–24.

Molloy EJ, Di Fiore JM, Martin RJ (2005) Does gastroesophageal reflux cause apnea in preterm infants? *Biol Neonat* **87**: 254–61.

Mortimer MJ, Kay J, Jaron A (1993) Clinical epidemiology of childhood abdominal migraine in an urban general practice. *Dev Med Child Neurol* **35**: 243–8.

Moscovitch A, Partinen M, Guilleminault C (1993) The positive diagnosis of narcolepsy and narcolepsy's borderland. *Neurology* **43**: 55–60.

Mousa H, Woodey JM, Metheney M, Hayes J (2005) Testing the association between gastroesophageal reflux and apnea in infants. *J Pediatr Gastoenterol Nutr* **41**: 169–77.

Myles ST, Needham CW, LeBlanc FE (1970) Alternating hemiparesis associated with hereditary hemorrhagic telangiectasia. *Can Med Assoc J* **103**: 509–511.

Neill JC (1990) Pseudoseizures in impaired children. *Neurology* **40**: 1146 (letter).

Nelson GB, Hahn JS (2003) Stimulus-induced drop episodes in Coffin–Lowry syndrome. *Pediatrics* **111**: e197–202.

Nezu A, Kimura S, Ohtsuki N, et al. (1997) Acute confusional migraine and migrainous infarction in childhood. *Brain Dev* **19**: 148–51.

Nigro MA, Lim HC (1992) Hyperekplexia and sudden neonatal death. *Pediatr Neurol* **8**: 221–5.

Nixon GM, Brouillette RT (2005) Sleep. 8: Paediatric obstructive sleep apnoea. *Thorax* **60**: 511–6.

North KN, Ouvrier RA, Nugent M (1990) Pseudoseizures caused by hyperventilation resembling absence epilepsy. *J Child Neurol* **5**: 288–94.

Nousiainen U, Mervaala E, Uusitupa M, et al. (1989) Cardiac arrhythmias in the differential diagnosis of epilepsy. *J Neurol* **236**: 93–6.

Olesen J, Steiner TJ (2004) The International Classification of Headache Disorders, 2nd edn (ICDH-II). *J Neurol Neurosurg Psychiatry* **75**: 808–11.

Olsen TS, Friberg L, Lassen NA (1987) Ischemia may be the primary cause of the neurologic deficits in classic migraine. *Arch Neurol* **44**: 156–61.

Ophoff RA, Terwindt GM, Vergouwe MN, et al. (1996) Familial hemiplegic migraine and episodic ataxia type-2 are caused by mutations in the Ca2+ channel gene CACNL1A4. *Cell* **87**: 543–52.

Oppenheimer SM, Cechetto DF, Hachinski VC (1990) Cerebrogenic cardiac arrhythmias: cerebral electrocardiographic influences and their role in sudden death. *Arch Neurol* **47**: 513–9.

Oren J, Kelly DH, Shannon DC (1987) Long-term follow-up of children with congenital central hypoventilation syndrome. *Pediatrics* **80**: 375–80.

Orrell RW, Marsden CD (1993) The neck–tongue syndrome. *J Neurol Neurosurg Psychiatry* **57**: 348–52.

Oswald I (1959) Sudden bodily jerks on falling asleep. *Brain* **82**: 92–103.

Ouvrier RA, Billson F (1988) Benign paroxysmal tonic upgaze of childhood. *J Child Neurol* **3**: 177–80.

Pachatz C, Fusco L, Vigevano F (2002) Shuddering and benign myoclonus of early infancy. In: Guerrini R, Aicardi J, Andermann F, Hallett M, eds. *Epilepsy and Movement Disorders*. Cambridge: Cambridge University Press, pp. 343–51.

Pacia SV, Devinsky O, Luciano DJ, Vazquez B (1994) The prolonged QT syndrome presenting as epilepsy: a report of two cases and literature review. *Neurology* **44**: 1408–10.

Page M, Jeffery H (2000) The role of gastro-oesophageal reflux in the etiology of SIDS. *Early Hum Dev* **59**: 127–49.

Pakalnis A, Kring D, Paolicchi J (2003) Parental satisfaction with sumatriptan nasal spray in childhood migraine. *J Child Neurol* **18**: 772–5.

Panayiotopoulos C (1989) Benign nocturnal childhood occipital epilepsy: a new syndrome with nocturnal seizures, tonic deviation of the eyes, and vomiting. *J Child Neurol* **4**: 43–8.

Panayiotopoulos C (1994) Elementary visual hallucinations in migraine and epilepsy. *J Neurol Neurosurg Psychiatry* **57**: 1371–4.

Parker S, Zuckerman B, Bauchner H, et al. (1990) Jitteriness in full-term neonates: prevalence and correlates. *Pediatrics* **85**: 17–23.

Parkes JD, Lock CB (1989) Genetic factors in sleep disorders. *J Neurol Neurosurg Psychiatry* **52** Suppl: 101–8.

Pascotto A, Coppola G (1992) Neonatal hyperekplexia: a case report. *Epilepsia* **33**: 817–20.

Patel H, Garg BP, Markand ON (1994) Bathing epilepsy: video/EEG recording and literature review. *J Epilepsy* **7**: 290–4.

Pedley TA (1983) Differential diagnosis of episodic symptoms. *Epilepsia* **24** Suppl 1: S31–44.

Peled R, Lavie P (1986) Paroxysmal awakenings from sleep associated with excessive daytime somnolence: a form of nocturnal epilepsy. *Neurology* **36**: 95–8.

Pelekanos JT, Dooley JM, Camfield PR, Finley J (1990) Stretch syncope in adolescence. *Neurology* **40**: 705–7.

Picchietti DL, Walters AS (1999) Moderate to severe limb movement disorder in childhood and adolescence. *Sleep* **22**: 297–300.

Phillips L, Appleton RE (2004) Systematic review of melatonin treatment in children with neurodevelopmental disabilities and sleep impairment. *Dev Med Child Neurol* **46**: 771–5.

Plazzi G, Montagna G, Provini F, et al. (1996) Pontine lesions in idiopathic narcolepsy. *Neurology* **46**: 1250–4.

Poets CF, Stebbens VA, Richard D, Southall DP (1995) Prolonged episodes of hypoxemia in preterm infants undetectable by cardiorespiratory monitors. *Pediatrics* **95**: 860–3.

Pranzatelli MR (1996) Antidyskinetic drug therapy for pediatric movement disorders. *J Child Neurol* **11**: 355–9.

Pranzatelli M, Pedley TA (1991) Differential diagnosis in children. In: Dam M, Gram L, eds. *Comprehensive Epileptology*. New York: Raven Press, pp. 423–47.

Prensky AL (1976) Migraine and migrainous variants in pediatric patients. *Pediatr Clin North Am* **23**: 461–71.

Rapoport A, Maushop A, Diener H, et al. (2006) Long-term migraine prevention with topiramate: open-label extension of pivotal trials. *Headache* **46**: 1151–60.

Reerink JD, Peters ACB, Verloove-Vanhorick SP, et al. (1995) Paroxysmal phenomena in the first two years of life. *Dev Med Child Neurol* **37**: 1094–100.

Rees MI, Andrew M, Jawad S, et al. (1994) Evidence for recessive as well as dominant forms of startle disease (hyperekplexia) caused by mutations in the alpha-subunit of the inhibitory glycine receptor. *Hum Mol Genet* **3**: 2175–9.

Rees MI, Harvey K, Pearce BR, et al. (2006) Mutations in the gene encoding GlyT2 (SLC6A5) define a presynaptic component of human startle disease. *Nat Genet* **38**: 801–6.

Resnick TJ, Moshé SL, Perotta L, Chambers HJ (1986) Benign neonatal sleep myoclonus: relationship to sleep states. *Arch Neurol* **43**: 266–8.

Riant F, De Fusco M, Aridon P, et al. (2005) ATP1A2 mutation in 11 families with familial hemiplegic migraine. *Hum Mutat* **26**: 281.

Riela AR, Roach ES (1993) Etiology of stroke in children. *J Child Neurol* **8**: 201–20.

Riikonen R, Donner M (1987) Chronic relapsing course of encephalomyeloradiculopathy in a 6-year-old boy. *Neuropediatrics* **18**: 235–8.

Riikonen R, Santuavori P (1994) Hereditary and acquired risk factors for childhood stroke. *Neuropediatrics* **25**: 227–33.

Rinalduzzi S, Valeriani M, Vigevano F (2004) Brainstem dysfunction in alternating hemiplegia of childhood: a neurophysiological study. *Cephalalgia* **26**: 511–9.

Rivera S, Villega F, de Saint-Martin A, et al. (2006) Congenital hyperekplexia: five sporadic cases. *Eur J Pediatr* **165**: 104–7.

Rosen JA (1983) Observations on the efficacy of propanolol for the prophylaxis of migraine. *Ann Neurol* **13**: 92–3.

Rosenberg DA (2003) Munchausen syndrome by proxy: medical diagnostic criteria. *Child Abuse Negl* **27**: 421–30.

Rossi LN, Vassella F, Bajc O, et al. (1985) Benign migraine-like syndrome with CSF pleocytosis in children. *Dev Med Child Neurol* **27**: 192–8.

Rossi LN, Penzien JM, Deonna T, et al. (1990) Does migraine-related stroke occur in childhood? *Dev Med Child Neurol* **32**: 1016–21.

Ruiz C, Gener B, Garaizar C, Prats JM (2003) Episodic spontaneous hypothermia: a periodic childhood syndrome. *Pediatr Neurol* **28**: 304–6.

Ryan SG, Sherman SL, Terry JC, et al. (1992) Startle disease, or hyperekplexia: response to clonazepam and assignment of the gene (STHE) to chromosome 5q by linkage analysis. *Ann Neurol* **31**: 663–8.

Sadarshan A, Goldie WD (1985) The spectrum of congenital facial diplegia (Moebius syndrome). *Pediatr Neurol* **1**: 181-4.

Saint-Hilaire MH, Saint-Hilaire JM, Granger L (1986) Jumping Frenchmen of Maine. *Neurology* **36**: 1269–71.

Saltik S, Cokar O, Uslu T, et al. (2004) Alternating hemiplegia of childhood: presentation of two cases regarding the extent of variability. *Epileptic Disord* **6**: 45–8.

Sander JE, Layzer RB, Goldsobel AB (1980) Congenital stiff-man syndrome. *Ann Neurol* **8**: 195–7.

Sarkozy A, Brugada P (2005) Sudden cardiac death and inherited arrhythmia syndromes. *J Cardiovasc Electrophysiol* **16** Suppl 1: S8–20.

Schenck CH, Mahowald MW (1992) Motor dyscontrol in narcolepsy: rapid eye movement (REM) sleep without atonia and REM sleep behavior disorder. *Ann Neurol* **32**: 3–10.

Scher MS (1985) Pathologic myoclonus of the newborn: electrographic and clinical correlations. *Pediatr Neurol* **1**: 324–8.

Scoggan KA, Friedman JH, Bulman DE (2006) CACNA1A mutation in a EA-2 patient responsive to acetazolamide and valproic acid. *Can J Neurol Sci* **33**: 68–72.

See CC, Newman LJ, Berezin S, et al. (1989) Gastroesophageal reflux-induced hypoxemia in infants with apparent life-threatening events. *Am J Dis Child* **143**: 951–4.

Sékhara T, Pelc K, Mewasingh LD, et al. (2005) Pediatric SUNCT syndrome. *Pediatr Neurol* **33**: 206–7.

Serdaroglu G, Erhan E, Tejgul H, et al. (2002) Sodium valproate prophylaxis in childhood migraine. *Headache* **42**: 819–22.

Seshia SS, Reggin JD, Stanwick RS (1985) Migraine and complex seizures in children. *Epilepsia* **26**: 232–6.

Seshia SS, Wolstein JR, Adams C, et al. (1994) International Headache Society criteria and childhood headache. *Dev Med Child Neurol* **36**: 419–28.

Shahar E, Raviv R (2004) Sporadic major hyperekplexia in neonates and infants: clinical manifestations and outcome. *Pediatr Neurol* **31**: 30–4.

Shahar E, Brand N, Uziel Y, Barak Y (1991) Nose tapping test inducing a generalized flexor spasm: a hallmark of hyperekplexia. *Acta Paediatr Scand* **80**: 1073–7.

Sheth RD, Barron TF, Hartlage PL (1994) Episodic spontaneous hypothermia with hyperhydrosis: implications for pathogenesis. *Pediatr Neurol* **10**: 58–60.

Sheth RD, Riggs JE, Bodensteiner JB (1995) Acute confusional migraine: variant of transient global amnesia. *Pediatr Neurol* **12**: 129–31.

Shevell MI (1996) Acephalalgic migraines of childhood. *Pediatr Neurol* **14**: 211–5.

Shevell MI, Silver K, Watters GV, Rosenblatt B (1993) Transient oculosympathetic paresis (group II Raeder paratrigeminal neuralgia) of childhood: migraine variant. *Pediatr Neurol* **9**: 289–92.

Shiang R, Ryan SG, Zhu YZ, et al. (1995) Mutational analysis of familial and sporadic hyperekplexia. *Ann Neurol* **38**: 85–91.

Shuper A, Zalzberg J, Weitz R, Mimouni M (1991) Jitteriness beyond the neonatal period: a benign pattern of movement in infancy. *J Child Neurol* **6**: 243–5.

Silberstein SD, Young WB, for the Working Panel of the Headache and Facial Pain Section of the American Academy of Neurology (1995) Safety and efficacy of ergotamine tartrate and dihydroergotamine in the treatment of migraine and status migrainosus. *Neurology* **45**: 577–84.

Silberstein SD, Neto W, Scmitt J, et al. (2004) Topiramate in migraine prevention. *Arch Neurol* **61**: 490–5.

Silberstein SD, Hulihan J, Karim MR, et al. (2006) Efficacy and tolerability of topiramate 200 mg/d in the prevention of migraine with/without aura in adults: randomized, placebo-controlled, double-blind, 2-week pilot study. *Clin Ther* **28**: 1002–11.

Sillanpää M (1983) Changes in the prevalence of migraine and other headache during the first seven school years. *Headache* **23**: 15–9.

Silver K, Andermann F (1993) Alternating hemiplegia of childhood: a study of 10 patients and results of flunarizine treatment. *Neurology* **43**: 36–41.

Silver K, Scriver C, Arnold DL, et al. (1995) Alternating hemiplegia of childhood associated with mitochondrial disease—a deficiency of pyruvate dehydrogenase. In: Andermann F, Aicardi J, Vigevano F, eds. *Alternating Hemiplegia of Childhood*. New York: Raven Press, pp. 165–71.

Soriani S, Carrozzi M, De Carlo L, et al. (1997) Endozepine stupor in children. *Cephalalgia* **17**: 658–61.

Southall DP, Talbert DG, Johnson P, et al. (1985) Prolonged expiratory apnoea: a disorder resulting in episodes of severe arterial hypoxaemia in infants and young children. *Lancet* **2**: 571–7.

Southall DP, Lewis GM, Buchanan R, Weller RO (1987) Prolonged expiratory apnoea (cyanotic 'breath-holding') in association with a medullary tumour. *Dev Med Child Neurol* **29**: 789–93.

Southall DP, Samuels MP, Talbert DG (1990) Recurrent cyanotic episodes with severe arterial hypoxaemia and intrapulmonary shunting: a mechanism for sudden death. *Arch Dis Child* **65**: 953–61.

Sperl W, Felber S, Skladal D, Wermuth B (1997) Metabolic stroke in carbamyl phosphate synthetase deficiency. *Neuropediatrics* **28**: 229–34.

Spitzer AR, Boyle JT, Tuchman DN, Fox WW (1984) Awake apnea associated with gastroesophageal reflux: a specific clinical syndrome. *J Pediatr* **104**: 200–5.

Steckley JE, Ebers GS, Cadez MZ, McLachlan RS (2001) An autosomal dominant dsisorder with episodic ataxia, vertigo and tinnitus. *Neurology* **57**: 1499–502.

Stephenson JBP (1980) Reflex anoxic seizures and ocular compression. *Dev Med Child Neurol* **22**: 380–6.

Stephenson JBP (1990) *Fits and Faints. Clinics in Developmental Medicine no. 109*. London: Mac Keith Press.

Stephenson J, Breningstall G, Steer C, et al. (2004) Anoxic–epileptic seizures: home video recording of epileptic seizures induced by syncope. *Epileptic Disord* **6**: 14–9.

Stephenson JBP, Hoffmann MC, Russell AJ, et al. (2005) The movement disorders of Coffin–Lowry syndrome. *Brain Dev* **27**: 108–13.

Stewart WF, Staffa J, Lipton RB, Ottman R (1997) Familial risk of migraine: a population-based study. *Ann Neurol* **41**: 166–72.

Stokowski LA (2005) A primer on apnea of prematurity. *Adv Neonat Care* **5**: 155–70.

Stores G (2006) The protean manifestations of childhood narcolepsy and their misinterpretation. *Dev Med Child Neurol* **48**: 307–10.

Swoboda KJ, Kanavakis E, Xaidara A, et al. (2004) Alternating hemiplegia of childhood or familial hemiplegic migraine? *Ann Neurol* **55**: 884–7.

Symon DNK, Russell G (1986) Abdominal migraine: a childhood syndrome defined. *Cephalalgia* **6**: 223–8.

Szepetowski P, Rochette J, Berquin P, et al. (1997) Familial infantile convulsions and paroxysmal choreoathetosis: a new neurological syndrome linked to the pericentromeric region of human chromosome 16. *Am J Hum Genet* **61**: 889–98.

Tassinari CA (1976) [Nosology and boundaries of syndromes with periodic respiration during sleep (Pickwickian syndrome, Ondine's syndrome, obstruction of the superior airway, microsleep syndrome, insomnia, and narcolepsy).] *Rev Electroencephalogr Neurophysiol Clin* **6**: 53–61 (French).

Tatsumi C, Takahashi M, Yorifuji S, et al. (1988) Mitochondrial encephalomyopathy with sleep apnea. *Eur Neurol* **28**: 64–9.

Tibbles JAR, Camfield PR, Cron CC Farrell K (1986) Dominant recurrent ataxia and vertigo of childhood. *Pediatr Neurol* **2**: 35–8.

Tijssen MA, Vergouwe MN, van Dijk JG, et al. (2002) Major and minor forms of hereditary hyperekplexia. *Mov Disord* **17**: 826–30.

Tinuper P, Montagna P, Plazzi G, et al. (1994) Idiopathic recurring stupor. *Neurology* **44**: 621–5.

Todt U, Dichgans M, Jurkat-Rott K, et al. (2005) Rare missense variants in ATP1A2 in families with clustering of common forms of migraine. *Hum Mutat* **26**: 315–21.

Tonelli A, D'Angelo MG, Salati R, et al. (2006) Early onset, non fluctuating spinocerebellar ataxia and a novel mutation in CACNA1A gene. *J Neurol Sci* **241**: 13–7.

Towbin JA (1995) New revelations about the long-QT syndrome. *N Engl J Med* **333**: 384–5.

Trajanovic NN, Voloh I, Shapiro CM, Sander P (2004) REM sleep behavior disorder in a child with Tourette syndrome. *Can J Neurol Sci* **31**: 572–5.

Trang H, Dehan M, Beaufils F, et al. (2005) The French Congenital Central Hypoventilation Syndrome Registry: general data, phenotype, and genotype. *Chest* **127**: 72–9.

Trochet D, O'Brien LM, Gozal D, et al. (2005) PHOX2B genotype allows for prediction of tumor risk in congenital central hypoventilation syndrome. *Am J Hum Genet* **76**: 421–6.

Tuxhorn IE, Fischbach HS (2002) Pseudo status epilepticus in children. *Pediatr Neurol* **27**: 407–9.

Valente EM, Spacey SD, Walli GM, et al. (2000) A second paroxysmal kinesigenic choreoathetosis locus (FKD2) mapping on 16q13–q22.1 indicates a family of genes which give rise to paroxysmal disorders on chromosome 16. *Brain* **123**: 2040–5.

Valmaggia G, Gottlob I (2000) Periodic alternating nystagmus in two children with a similar, unusual phenotype. *Pediatr Neurol* **23**: 432–5.

Vanderhoof JA, Young R, Kaufmann SS, Ernst L (1995) Treatment of cyclic vomiting in childhood with erythromycin. *J Pediatr Gastroenterol Nutr* **21** Suppl 1: S60–2.

Veneselli E, Biancheri R (1997) Alternating hemiplegia of childhood: treatment of attacks with chloral hydrate and niaprazine. *Eur J Pediatr* **156**: 157–8 (letter).

Verlooy P, Velis DN (1985) Non-familial periodic ataxia responding to acetazolamide. *Clin Neurol Neurosurg* **87**: 35–7.

Vigevano F, Di Capua M, Dalla Bernardina B (1989) Startle disease: an avoidable cause of sudden infant death. *Lancet* **1**: 216 (letter).

Vighetto A, Froment JC, Trillet M, Aimard J (1988) Magnetic resonance imaging in familial paroxysmal ataxia. *Arch Neurol* **45**: 547–9.

Visudhiphan P, Visudtibhan A, Chiemchanya S, Khongkhatithum C (2005) Neonatal seizures and familial hypomagnesemia with secondary hypocalcemia. *Pediatr Neurol* **33**: 202–5.

Visser WH, de Vriend RH, Jaspers NMWH, Ferrari MD (1996) Sumatriptan in clinical practice: a 2-year review of 453 migraine patients. *Neurology* **47**: 46–51.

Vossler DG, Wyler AR, Wilkus RJ, et al. (1996) Cataplexy and monoamine oxidase deficiency in Norrie disease. *Neurology* **46**: 1258–61.

Wada T, Kobayashi N, Takahashi Y, et al. (2002) Wide variability in a family with CACNA1A T666m mutation: hemiplegic migraine, coma, and progressive ataxia. *Pediatr Neurol* **26**: 47–50.

Wali GM (1992) Paroxysmal hemidystonia induced by prolonged exercise and cold. *J Neurol Neurosurg Psychiatry* **55**: 236–7 (letter).

Walk D, Kang SS, Horwitz A (1994) Intermittent encephalopathy, reversible nerve conduction slowing, and MRI evidence of cerebral white matter disease in methylenetetrahydrofolate reductase deficiency. *Neurology* **44**: 344–7.

Walsh JF, Montplaisir J (1982) Familial glaucoma and sleep apnea: a new syndrome. *Thorax* **37**: 845–9.

Walters AS, Picchietti DL, Ehrenberg BL, Wagner ML (1994) Restless legs syndrome in childhood and adolescence. *Pediatr Neurol* **11**: 241–5.

Wang Q, Ito M, Adams K, Li BU, et al. (2004) Mitochondrial DNA control region sequence variation in migraine headache and cyclic vomiting syndrome. *Am J Med Genet A* **131**: 50–8.

Watanabe K, Hara K, Miyazaki S, et al. (1982) Apneic seizures in the newborn. *Am J Dis Child* **136**: 980–4.

Weese-Mayer DE, Berry-Kravis EM, Zhou L, et al. (2003) Idiopathic congenital hypoventilation syndrome: analysis of genes pertinent to early autonomic nervous system embryologic development and identification of mutations in PHOX2b. *Am J Med Genet A* **123**: 267–78.

Weese-Mayer DE, Berry-Kravis EM, Marazita ML (2005) In pursuit (and discovery) of genetic basis for congenital central hypoventilation syndrome. *Respir Physiol Neurobiol* **149**: 73–82.

Weinstock A, Giglio P, Kerr SL, et al. (2003) Hyperkinetic seizures in children. *J Child Neurol* **18**: 517–24.

Welch KM (1993) Drug therapy of migraine. *N Engl J Med* **329**: 1476–83.

Werlin SL, D'Souza BJ, Hogan WJH, et al. (1980) Sandifer syndrome: an unappreciated clinical entity. *Dev Med Child Neurol* **22**: 374–8.

Wiendels NJ, van der Geest MC, Neven AK, et al. (2005) Chronic daily headache in children and adolescents. *Headache* **45**: 678–83.

Wilson LC, Hall CM (2002) Albright's hereditary osteodystrophy and pseudohypoparathyroidism. *Semin Musculoskelet Radiol* **6**: 273–83.

Wilson D, Moore P, Finucane AK, Skinner JR (2005) Pacing in the management of severe pallid breath-holding atacks. *J Pediatr Child Health* **41**: 228–30.

Winner P, Pearlman EM, Linder SL, et al. (2005). Topiramate for migraine prevention in children: a randomized, double-blind, placebo-controlled trial. *Headache* **45**: 1304–12.

Winter E, Prendergast M, Green A (1996) Narcolepsy in a 2-year-old boy. *Dev Med Child Neurol* **38**: 356–9.

Wolpert C, Schimpf R, Veltmann C, et al. (2005) Clinical characteristics and treatment of short QT syndrome. *Expert Rev Cardiovasc Ther* **3**: 611–7.

Wong V, Wong WC (1997) Enhancement of oculomotor nerve: a diagnostic criterion for ophthalmoplegic migraine? *Pediatr Neurol* **17**: 70–3.

Woods RP, Iacoboni M, Mazziotta JC (1994) Brief report: bilateral spreading cerebral hypoperfusion during spontaneous migraine headache. *N Engl J Med* **331**: 1689–92.

Woody RC, Kiel EA (1986) Swallowing syncope in a child. *Pediatrics* **78**: 507–9.

Wyllie E, Friedman D, Rothner D, et al. (1990) Psychogenic seizures in children and adolescents: outcome after diagnosis by ictal video and electroencephalographic recording. *Pediatrics* **85**: 480–4.

Xyrem International Study Group (2005) Further evidence supporting the use of sodium oxylate for treatment of cataplexy: a double-blind placebo-controlled study in 228 patients. *Sleep Med* **6**: 415–21.

Yanagihara T, Piepgras DG, Klass DW (1985) Repetitive involuntary movement associated with episodic cerebral ischemia. *Ann Neurol* **18**: 244–50.

Young D, Zorick F, Wittig R, et al. (1988) Narcolepsy in a pediatric population. *Am J Dis Child* **142**: 210–3.

Zifkin BG, Arnold DL, Andermann F, Andermann E (1995) Familial hemiplegic migraine with altered consciousness followed by peduncular hallucinosis: migraine coma as a disorder of brain energy metabolism and possible relevance to alternating hemiplegia of childhood. In: Andermann F, Aicardi J, Vigevano F, eds. *Alternating Hemiplegia of Childhood*. New York: Raven Press, pp. 179–87.

Zorzi G, Conti C, Erba A, et al. (2003) Paroxysmal dyskinesias in children. *Pediatr Neurol* **28**: 168–72.

PART VIII

DISORDERS OF THE OCULAR, VISUAL, AUDITORY AND VESTIBULAR SYSTEMS

Disorders of the visual, visuomotor, auditory and vestibular systems are of considerable importance in neurology in general and especially in child neurology. The information collected through these major sensory channels plays a decisive role in the development and function of the CNS, and their main dys-functions justify a separate study. Many of these disorders have been described elsewhere in this book, but a number of relatively common conditions do not fit into any of the preceding chapters and warrant a description of their own because of their frequency or therapeutic or diagnostic importance.

17

DISORDERS OF OCULAR MOTOR AND VISUAL FUNCTIONS

Jean Aicardi and Carey Matsuba

The visual system plays a primary role in the exploration and analysis of the external world. Proper functioning of this system requires the integrity of an extremely complex neuronal network that is easily disturbed by a vast number of CNS disorders. Such disturbances include defects of ocular motility that result not only from peripheral nerve involvement, but also from affectation of the highly complex systems that maintain binocular vision, stability of gaze and other mechanisms necessary for the adequate collection and interpretation of visual information. Transmission of visual information received by the retina to the occipital cortex and processing of this information can also be impeded or disturbed by the many pathological processes that, in turn, may influence the ocular motor system. Clinical and electrophysiological analysis of visual system disorders is a sensitive means of exploring CNS function and the abnormalities of ocular movements and visual perception. It constitutes an essential part of the neurological examination.

DISORDERS OF OCULAR MOTOR FUNCTION

INVOLVEMENT OF PERIPHERAL OCULAR MOTOR NERVES OR THEIR NUCLEI (Leigh and Zee 2006)

The movements of the eyeballs are controlled by the IIIrd, IVth and VIth cranial nerves through the muscles that they innervate. Paralysis of one or several of these muscles results in ophthalmoplegia, which may be acquired or congenital and occur isolated or in combination. Such paralysis should be distinguished from nonparalytic strabismus, which is a very common condition affecting 3–4% of all children and whose study is beyond the scope of this book (see Taylor and Hoyt 2005).

ACQUIRED OPHTHALMOPLEGIA

Ophthalmoplegia can be due to a large number of causes, most of which have been described in the previous chapters.

Acquired IIIrd nerve palsies

Acquired IIIrd nerve palsies are common. The most frequent causes (Table 17.1) are closed head trauma, infections, tumours, and vascular causes including migraines (Ing et al. 1992). Typically, the IIIrd nerve is damaged through its course, as nuclear and fascicular IIIrd nerve palsies are rare. If a nuclear IIIrd nerve palsy is present, bilateral signs are likely, whereas fascicular palsies tend to be unilateral. The age of onset and the underlying cause are determining factors in the prognosis of the disease.

The most common cause of an acquired IIIrd nerve palsy is trauma. Traumatic palsies result from haemorrhage or oedema into the nerves or muscles or from avulsion or lacerations of these structures (Miller 1985). Third nerve palsies often clear spontaneously, but infrequently they persist or show evidence of aberrant regeneration, the first signs of which may appear by 4–6 weeks following the causal lesion or infection (Walsh and Hoyt 1969, Miller 1985). The diagnosis of traumatic palsy may be difficult, particularly when the trauma has been minimal or not reported, or when the paralysis is delayed, or when there are complications such as secondary orbital oedema, secondary increased intracranial pressure, infections, or vascular disorders such as carotid–cavernous fistulae (Marmor et al. 1982). In such cases, neuroimaging investigation is indicated because trauma may be the only precipitating factor of paralysis of a nerve already compromised by a chronic (compressive) lesion.

Infection is the next most common cause, especially meningitis (Miller 1985), encephalitis and abscesses. Partial palsy may be due to frontal sinusitis (Coker and Ros 1996). Tumours may present as an isolated IIIrd nerve palsy, especially craniopharyngiomas. With brainstem tumours other neurological signs become rapidly obvious. Acute painful unilateral IIIrd nerve palsy may represent an ophthalmoplegic migraine. Typically, there is a history of migraine. Generally, symptoms start in the first decade and resolve over a period of weeks. Steroids may reduce the length of symptoms. Relapses can occur.

Acquired IVth nerve palsies

Acquired IVth nerve palsies are mainly of traumatic origin (Keane 1993). Avulsion of the superior oblique pulley may explain the relative frequency of paralysis of this muscle (von Noorden et al. 1986). The nerve can also be injured by inflammation or compression in its long course (Sydnor et al. 1982). Rare causes such as infection, tumours and raised intracranial pressure have been documented. Nuclear and fascicular IVth nerve palsies typically result from posterior fossa tumours. Fourth nerve paralysis is typically unilateral in more than 60% of cases and resolves in two

TABLE 17.1
Causes and clinical features of acquired ocular motor nerve paralysis

Site of lesion	Clinical features	Main causes
Oculomotor nuclei	Bilateral involvement frequent, often associated with gaze palsies. Internal ophthalmoplegia indicates midline lesion. Symmetrical ptosis may exist in isolation	Brainstem tumours and other tumours (pineal region, diencephalon). Infections and inflammation, e.g. brainstem encephalitis, multiple sclerosis. Vascular disease and vascular malformations. Degenerative diseases (Wernicke, Leigh)
Fascicular portion (between nuclei and emergence from peduncle)	Similar to nuclear involvement but rarely bilateral	Brainstem intrinsic disease
Interpeduncular fossa	May be associated with involvement of pyramidal tract. Pupillary dilatation and accomodative paralysis present	Basilar meningitis. Aneurysms of rostral basilar artery (rare). Dermoid cysts
At or near entrance into dura	Pupillary involvement prominent especially with herniation	Frontal trauma. Aneurysms. Transtentorial herniation from expanding supratentorial masses or haematomas
In cavernous sinus	Associated involvement of other nerves (V, VI, IV, oculosympathetic)	Sinus thrombosis. Aneurysms. Carotid–cavernous fistulas. Pituitary adenomas. Chordomas and other basilar tumours
Orbital apex and/or superior orbital fissure	Involvement may be partial as the nerve divides into two branches. Pupillary involvement only with affectation of lower trunk	Tolosa–Hunt syndrome. Orbital pseudotumour. Orbital cellulitis. Orbital tumours
Diffuse, undetermined or variable	Variable. Associated paralyses in some cases	Ophthalmoplegic migraine. Sarcoidosis, Whipple disease, some toxic causes such as drugs (e.g. anticonvulsants, aspirin). Miller Fisher syndrome and related cranial polyneuropathies, postviral palsies. Diabetes mellitus (exceptional)

thirds (Sydnor et al. 1982). Fourth nerve palsies often clear spontaneously after several months, but infrequently they persist or show evidence of aberrant regeneration, the first signs of which may appear by 4–6 weeks following the causal lesion or infection (Walsh and Hoyt 1969, Miller 1985).

Acquired VIth nerve palsies

As with the other oculomotor cranial nerves, the most common cause of VIth nerve palsy in infants is trauma. Other pathologies including tumour, infection and increased intracranial pressure may also lead to paresis (Table 17.2). Paralysis of the VIth nerve is sometimes observed in newborn infants, probably as a result of birth trauma (de Grauw et al. 1983), and usually disappears spontaneously in a few weeks. Tumours are the most common cause in older children, and the nerve is especially sensitive to any cause of high intracranial pressure including pseudotumour cerebri. Meningitis and postnatal trauma can also produce lateral rectus paralysis (Afifi and Menezes 1992). Acquired paralysis of the VIth nerve may be difficult to distinguish from the sudden appearance of a squint due to a decompensation of refractive error or other visual disturbance, often at the time of an acute infectious disorder (Watson and Fielder 1987).

Postinfectious VIth nerve palsy secondary to a viral infection may be diagnosed on the basis of history, although the diagnosis is often made without definitive proof. The onset is sudden and the involvement is generally unilateral. The child complains of diplopia, and the paralytic strabismus is observed. Full motility is restored within 6–12 months. A recurrent form has been reported (Afifi et al. 1990, Cohen et al. 1993).

Involvement of the VIth nerve may be a part of the *Gradenigo syndrome*, which commonly occurred as a complication of mastoiditis when the infection reached the apex of the petrous, though such cases are now exceptional. Due to the proximity of the cavum trigeminale, the Vth nerve is also affected with pain in the face and eye, and the facial nerve may be involved in its petrous canal. Rarely, Gradenigo syndrome can be a consequence of T-cell lymphoma (Norwood and Haller 1990). The syndrome is now more commonly seen with orbital or retro-orbital disease (Taylor 1997).

Combined ophthalmoplegias

On occasion, ophthalmoplegia may involve a combination of nerves. An example is the Miller Fisher syndrome. Miller Fisher syndrome, a variant of Guillain–Barré syndrome, results in ophthalmoparesis of one or a combination of the IIIrd, IVth and VIth cranial nerves with pupil involvement. It is associated with the presence of serum anti-GQ1b IgG antibodies. The involvement appears to be primarily in the periphery, although some oculocephalic manoeuvres may suggest a supranuclear component. Typically, function slowly recovers spontaneously or following

TABLE 17.2
Causes and clinical features of paralysis of the abducens and trochlear nerves

Site of lesion	Clinical features	Causes
Nucleus of IVth nerve	Difficult to determine and to differentiate from IIIrd nerve nuclei involvement and from supranuclear lesions	Brainstem tumours. Inflammatory or demyelinating disease. Vascular obstruction and malformations
Peripheral IVth nerve	Difficult to make a topical diagnosis. Head tilt toward the opposite shoulder	Head trauma
Nucleus of VIth nerve	Conjugate gaze palsy to the ipsilateral side. Does not produce isolated lateral rectus palsy	Same as IVth nerve nucleus involvement
Subarachnoid segment of VIth nerve	Isolated lateral rectus palsy	Aneurysm of basilar artery or its branches. Space-occupying supratentorial lesion (downward movement of neuraxis). Arnold–Chiari malformation. Meningitis and infiltration of the basal meninges
Extradural VIth nerve	Gradenigo syndrome. Involvement of VIIth nerve and gasserian ganglion: pain in the face, reduced corneal sensitivity	Mastoiditis. Rarely bone tumours
Inferior petrosal sinus	May be similar to Gradenigo syndrome	Mastoiditis. Dural arteriovenous malformations of posterior fossa. Fracture of temporal bone. Primitive trigeminal artery
Cavernous sinus and/or superior orbital fissure	Associated involvement of other cranial nerves	Aneurysm, carotid cavernous fistulae, tumours, thrombosis of cavernous sinus
Sphenopalatine fossa	Loss of tearing due to involvement of 2nd division of Vth nerve	Tumours of skull base
Orbit	Indistinguishable from myogenic involvement except by EMG	Tumours, inflammatory lesions
Diffuse, undetermined or variable	Isolated VIth nerve palsy	Postinfectious paralysis, diabetes (rare), migraine (rare), cranial polyneuropathy and Miller Fisher syndrome

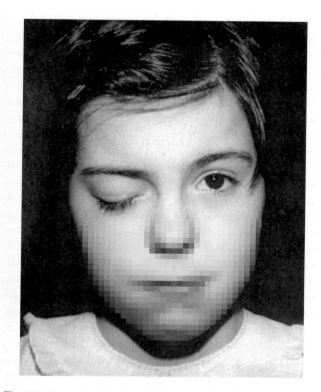

Fig. 17.1. Acquired ophthalmoplegia in 8-year-old girl with Tolosa–Hunt syndrome.

treatment with plasmaphoresis. An association has been observed following *Camplyobacter jejuni* infection, which is thought to induce antiganglioside antibodies (Ang 2001).

Another example of a combined ophthalmoplegia is the *Tolosa–Hunt syndrome* (Fig. 17.1). Tolosa–Hunt syndrome is characterized by a dull, persistent pain around the affected eye, ophthalmoplegia and, sometimes, involvement of the optic nerve, the first and/or second branches of the trigeminal nerves and the sympathetic innervation of the affected eye (Goto et al. 1989, Gordon 1994). The IIIrd nerve is usually involved first and more severely than others, but all three ocular motor nerves may be affected. The diagnosis requires exclusion of other known causes of painful ophthalmoplegia such as infection, neoplasm or lymphoma (Spector and Fiandaca 1986). CT may show a high-density area in the orbit, and orbital phlebography may show occlusion of the superior ophthalmic vein (Goadsby and Lance 1989). Subtle MRI abnormalities such as thickening of the external wall of the cavernous sinus are being increasing recognized (Ganesan et al. 1996), and detailed imaging of the cavernous sinus is now essential in the investigation of apparently isolated, even painless, cranial nerve palsies. The course usually extends over weeks or, rarely, months. Corticosteroid administration is valuable in the treatment and frequently has a dramatic effect. The condition is related to orbital pseudotumour (Grossniklaus et al. 1985, Rohr and Gauthier 1988), which may be either acute or chronic.

701

This so-called sclerosing orbital pseudotumour (Abramovitz et al. 1983) does not respond to steroids. Pseudotumour is rarely seen in children and is usually associated with displacement of the globe downward and outward, as well as with oedema and inflammation of the eyelids, both signs that are not present with Tolosa–Hunt syndrome. Pseudotumours may be difficult to differentiate from lymphomas and other tumours (Flanders et al. 1989).

Acute rectus muscle palsy as a result of orbital myositis (Pollard 1996) is also closely related to orbital pseudotumour and Tolosa–Hunt syndrome. CT or MRI shows swelling of the affected muscle, usually the lateral rectus but occasionally the medial or superior rectus. Muscle involvement has also been observed in Graves ophthalmopathy in infants and adolescents (Uretsky et al. 1980).

The painful ophthalmoplegia of Tolosa–Hunt syndrome may be difficult to distinguish from ophthalmolplegic migraine, although involvement of the Vth nerve, increased erythrocyte sedimentation rate and a long duration of pain favour the former diagnosis (Kandt and Goldstein 1985). Enlargement of the optic nerve sheath and of the extraocular muscles is also an argument in favour of Tolosa–Hunt syndrome. Treatment with prednisone (1–1.5 mg/day) produces disappearance of pain and of ophthalmoplegia, the latter after several days or weeks. Recurrences may occur on discontinuation of treatment or in spite of it. Involvement of the facial nerve is not rare (Swerdlow 1980). Some authors suggest that the Tolosa–Hunt syndrome may be a form of recurrent cranial nerve neuropathy because of the relative frequency of recurrences that may affect the contralateral side and the involvement of different cranial nerves (Barontini et al. 1987).

Cavernous sinus thrombosis may resemble the Tolosa–Hunt syndrome when it produces unilateral (and sometimes bilateral) ophthalmolplegia. However, fever and septic signs are usually marked and there is proptosis and orbital congestion. Vigorous antibiotic treatment is urgently indicated before meningeal involvement sets in (Harbour et al. 1984).

CONGENITAL OPHTHALMOPLEGIA
Congenital ophthalmolplegia and ptosis are often not recognized until relatively late or are discounted as representing 'physiological' or pathological strabismus. For this reason, the diagnosis of congenital ophthalmolplegia should not be excluded on the basis of the child having no ophthalmoplegia at birth by history. Photographs can be extremely useful.

Congenital IIIrd nerve palsy
This condition is relatively uncommon. In the vast majority, it is unilateral. All bilateral congenital IIIrd nerve palsies are associated with additional neurological signs due to anomalous brain development or prenatal damage (Flanders et al. 1989). Anomalies in brain development, intrauterine injury (vascular, teratogenic or infectious) and perinatal damage are possible causes.

Congenital IIIrd nerve palsy presents with ptosis, exotropia and hypotropia of the involved eye. The paralysis is generally unilateral and complete, although the pupil may be of normal size or even small because of aberrant regeneration. This is exotropia

and usually amblyopia of the affected eye. In most cases, evidence of aberrant regeneration is present in the form of lid retraction and/or papillary constriction on attempted adduction (Prats et al. 1993). Cyclic phenomena, with spasm of adduction, papillary constriction and lid elevation alternating with adductor paresis, ptosis and papillary constriction may occur. Surgical management of the strabismus involves resection of the medial rectus, but is of purely cosmetic value.

Congenital IVth nerve palsy
Congenital trochlear nerve paralysis is the commonest of congenital ocular motor palsies. There is usually no associated neurological or developmental anomaly, but occasionally trauma has been associated (Reynolds et al. 1984). Almost all cases are unilateral (Von Noorden et al. 1986). The presenting complaint is frequently a head tilt away from the paralysed side or even scoliosis. When the head is tilted to the paralytic side, hypertropia becomes evident. Surgical therapy is important to avoid torticollis and scolisosis. Congenital IVth nerve palsy has been reported with occult cranium bifidum (Bale et al. 1988) and as a familial occurrence (Astle and Rosenbaum 1985).

Congenital VIth nerve palsy
Abducens nerve palsy is rarely seen in healthy neonates, suspected to be a result of focal damage to the peripheral nerve. Often when present it may go unrecognized. Congenital VIth nerve palsies can be unilateral or bilateral and, in the latter case, is easily confused with non-paralytic strabismus. It may be a part of the Moebius syndrome (Chapter 19). The prognosis is typically good, with many children developing binocular vision.

Duane retraction syndrome
Duane retraction syndrome is characterized by a palsy of the lateral rectus, limitation of adduction, and narrowing of the palpebral fissure because of globe retraction on attempted adduction. The syndrome is more often unilateral than bilateral and has been attributed to fibrosis of the lateral rectus, but its pathogenesis is more complex and neural in origin (Huber 1974, Miller 1985, Taylor 1997). Retraction on adduction is due to co-contraction in the superior and inferior as well as the lateral rectus, indicating absence of the VIth nerve, the IIIrd nerve supplying all the extraocular muscles in an abnormal manner. Interestingly, a majority of children with Duane syndrome are able to maintain binocular vision by turning their head toward the side of the lesion. Abnormalities of the brainstem auditory evoked potentials have also been found (Jay and Hoyt 1980). There has been more evidence to suggest that Duane syndrome is caused by a neurogenic brainstem ocular motor dysfunction. Duane syndrome is often associated with additional brainstem anomalies. More complex forms associated with Marcus Gunn phenomenon (Isenberg and Blechman 1983) (see below) or with the 'crocodile tears' phenomenon (Biedner et al. 1979) are on record, indicating that the tendency to abnormal synkinesis may be widespread. Crocodile tears are thought to be due to a discrete lesion in the vicinity of the abducens nucleus with innervation of both the lateral rectus and

TABLE 17.3
Types and causes of gaze palsies in children

Vertical gaze palsy
Tumours (of pineal region and brainstem)
Sylvian aqueduct syndrome in hydrocephalus, especially aqueductal stenosis
Niemann–Pick C disease (DAF syndrome)[1]
Gaucher disease
Miller Fisher syndrome
Abetalipoproteinaemia (vitamin E deficiency)
Vitamin B_{12} deficiency
Congenital vertical ocular motor apraxia

Horizontal gaze palsy
Frontal lobe destructive lesions (area 8)
Brainstem (pontine) tumours
Central pontine myelinolysis
Familial congenital gaze palsy

Internuclear ophthalmoplegia
Brainstem tumours
Brainstem vascular lesions
Multiple sclerosis
Toxic causes

Convergence palsy
Trauma (may be minor)
Tumour of pineal region

Ocular motor apraxia (paresis or slowing of saccadic eye movements)
Cogan disease (congenital ocular motor apraxia)
Ataxia–telangiectasia
Ataxia–ocular motor apraxia (Chapter 9)
Gaucher disease
Spinocerebellar degenerations

[1]DAF syndrome: downward gaze palsy, ataxia and foam cells.

the salivary gland by ocular motor fibres. Several different phenotypes have been described, involving a number of different chromosome mutations. In some cases, it may be transmitted as an autosomal dominant condition.

Fibrosis of extraocular muscles (congenital familial external ophthalmoplegia)

This disorder is characterized by the local (Prakash et al. 1985) or diffuse (Hiatt and Halle 1983) replacement of muscle fibres by fibrous connective tissue. Most cases are dominantly inherited. The only manifestation is restricted ocular motility in the fields of affected muscles. Ptosis is generally present. Diagnosis can be made through the biopsy of the fibrotic muscles. The classical type, linked to chromosome 12, was shown by Engle et al. (1997) to be associated with absence of the nucleus and nerve fibres normally forming the upper part of the IIIrd nerve complex. Since then, several phenotypes of congenital fibrosis have been described (Engle et al. 1994, 2002; Yazdani and Traboulsi 2004).

Brown syndrome

Brown syndrome is caused by shortening of the superior oblique muscle or tendon (Walsh and Hoyt 1969) and is closely related to fibrosis of extraocular muscles. Passive elevation of the globe in adduction is restricted, as is voluntary elevation. Acquired cases may occur as a result of rheumatoid arthritis (Wang et al.

1984) or trauma. Surgical treatment can produce cosmetic benefit in cases of muscle fibrosis.

Congenital ptosis

Congenital ptosis is a common condition caused by absence or fibrosis of the levator palpebrae. Familial cases may occur although the condition is usually sporadic (Walsh and Hoyt 1969). Seventy per cent of cases are unilateral, and in rare cases, ptosis is associated with extraocular muscle involvement. Some patients demonstrate a synkinesis between the movements of the jaw and those of the upper lid such that lowering the jaw or moving it sideways produces elevation of the lid which is especially striking in infants when sucking, the so-called jaw-winking or *Marcus Gunn phenomenon* (Pratt et al. 1984). An inverted Marcus Gunn phenomenon in which there is drooping of the lid on opening of the mouth has been reported as a congenital (Lubkin 1978) or acquired (Rana and Wadia 1985) phenomenon. The mechanism of this phenomenon may be aberrant regeneration, but a central mechanism is possible and has also been proposed for other synkineses (McLeod and Glaser 1974).

Congenital ptosis should be distinguished from acquired ptosis, and especially from myasthenia gravis. Corrective surgery is indicated in severe cases for cosmetic reasons or when vision is impaired by the drooping lid.

GAZE PALSIES

Gaze palsies are due to involvement of the supranuclear pathways that control the orientation of the head and eyes (Daroff and Troost 1978). Such control is integrated at several levels including the vestibular nuclei, other brainstem structures, the basal nuclei and the cerebral cortex (Pierrot-Deseilligny et al. 1997). The diagnosis of supranuclear ocular palsies rests on the characteristics of abnormal head movements and on the demonstration that the eyes can move normally in response to the doll's head manoeuvre, caloric testing and Bell's phenomenon. The main causes of gaze palsies are listed in Table 17.3 and only some of the manifestations and causes will be discussed here.

Horizontal gaze palsies

Horizontal gaze palsy may occur sporadically or as part of an hereditary condition. It can be due to a cortical lesion in the contralateral frontal lobe (area 8), in the anterior occipital lobe or in the ipsilateral para-abducens pontine nucleus. It is not uncommonly associated with other neurological anomalies, including hemiplegia, or with more complex disturbances such as hemineglect or hemianopia. In addition, some systemic features can also be found including musculoskeletal anomalies such as kyphoscoliosis (Steffen et al. 1998) and ear dysplasia.

Subcortical (pontine) lesions are a common manifestation of brainstem glioma, less commonly of vascular malformations or destructive lesions. They may be a sign of central pontine myelinolysis (Chapter 21). Pontine gaze palsy can be difficult to distinguish from Moebius syndrome or other causes of bilateral VIth nerve palsy. Familial congenital gaze palsy has been reported (Vetterli and Henn 1981, Jen et al. 2002).

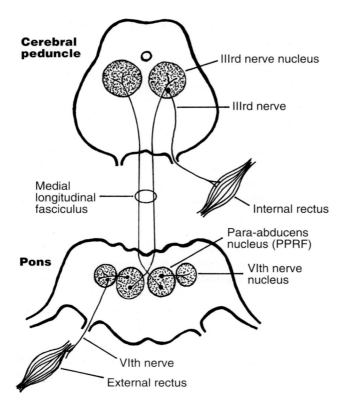

Cerebral peduncle

IIIrd nerve nucleus

IIIrd nerve

Medial longitudinal fasciculus

Internal rectus

Para-abducens nucleus (PPRF)

Pons

VIth nerve nucleus

VIth nerve

External rectus

Fig. 17.2. Internuclear ophthalmoplegia. On attempted gaze to either side, there is no contraction of the internal rectus, due to involvement of the medial longitudinal fasciculus which prevents transmission of influx from the pontine centre for lateral gaze (para-abducens nucleus in the paramedian pontine reticular formation: PPRF) to the contralateral IIIrd nerve nucleus, resulting in disconjugate lateral gaze. In unilateral lesions of the medial longitudinal fasciculus, the internuclear ophthalmoplegia is also unilateral. There is usually associated nystagmus of the abducting eye.

Vertical gaze palsies

Paralysis of vertical gaze, especially upward gaze, may be difficult to distinguish from a simple difficulty in looking upwards, which is frequent in patients with mild disturbances of consciousness and even in fatigued patients. Transient disturbances in supranuclear vertical gaze occur in up to 2% of healthy neonates with downward deviation of gaze (Hoyt et al. 1980). They can be associated with upbeat nystagmus (Goldblum and Effron 1994). Yokochi (1991) reported episodes of downward gaze deviation in 13 neurologically impaired preterm or term infants with a history of perinatal asphyxia. These episodes lasted several seconds each during wakefulness. All patients had imaging evidence of periventricular leukomalacia, involving predominantly the optic radiations, and half of them had mental retardation or cerebral palsy at 5 years of age. However, similar episodes with a benign course have also been reported (Kleiman et al. 1994).

Paroxysmal tonic upgaze

Ouvrier and Billson (1988) reported a syndrome, which they termed *benign paroxysmal tonic upgaze of childhood*, characterized by episodes of sustained tonic conjugate upward deviation of the eyes, lasting from 30 minutes to several hours, with compensatory forward bending of the head. On attempted downward gaze, downbeating ocular saccades would occur. Symptoms were fluctuating, increased by fatigue and intercurrent illnesses and relieved by sleep. The onset was between 6 and 24 months of age. Affected children had no other difficulty except mild ataxia. All symptoms spontaneously disappeared in a few weeks or months. Similar cases have been reported by Deonna et al. (1990) and by Guerrini et al. (1998), who also mentioned the occurrence of occasional atonic falls. Very similar symptoms but with an earlier onset in the first month of life have also been described (Ahn et al. 1989).

Familial cases of this syndrome have been reported, and the episodes of downward gaze can be abolished by low-dose L-dopa treatment, suggesting a possible link to dopa-sensitive dystonia (Campistol et al. 1993). Association with psychomotor retardation has been rarely reported (Sugie et al. 1995). However, recent work (Hertle et al. 1998) indicates a less favourable outcome with respect to both cognition and fine motor control.

Paralysis of vertical gaze that has been described in intoxication with anticonvulsants, antidepressants and other drugs may be explained in part by the disturbance of consciousness, but this does not apply to all cases and true ophthalmoplegia has been repeatedly observed.

The most important cause of vertical gaze palsy is represented by tumours in the pineal region. The sylvian aqueduct syndrome can also be seen in patients with hydrocephalus due to aqueductal stenosis. The syndrome features associated eyelid retraction, mydriasis with dilated pupils with better contraction to near objects than to light (light–near dissociation), skew deviation of the eyes, and sometimes convergent–retraction nystagmus (nystagmus retractorius) and disturbances in horizontal gaze. The pretectal syndrome has been reviewed in detail by Keane (1990). Disorders of the basal ganglia such as Huntington disease are frequently associated with vertical supranuclear gaze palsies. Vertical downward gaze palsy is also a feature of Niemann–Pick and Gaucher diseases. In the latter case, paralysis of horizontal gaze is frequently associated (Grosse-Tsur et al. 1989) and may be isolated (Patterson et al. 1993).

Keane and Finstead (1982) have reported that isolated upward gaze palsy may be the initial manifestation of the Miller Fisher syndrome, and Sandyk (1984) has described the same phenomenon in vitamin B_{12} deficiency.

Internuclear ophthalmoplegia

Internuclear ophthalmoplegia is characteristic of the involvement of the medial longitudinal fasciculus that connects the abducens nucleus on one side and the opposite ocular motor nucleus to permit conjugate lateral gaze (Fig. 17.2). When these nuclei are disconnected, attempted lateral movements produce abduction of the eye ipsilateral to the fasciculus lesion and absence of the normal adduction of the contralateral eye. The phenomenon may be uni- or bilateral and is mainly due to multiple sclerosis, although, in children, brainstem tumours and head trauma (Mueller et al. 1993) may be a more frequent cause. Other causes such as metabolic, immunological and inflammatory processes have been associated. In mild cases, contraction of the medial lateral rectus may be present but slower than that of the lateral rectus. Nystagmus of the abducting eye is usually present. The 'one-and-a-half syndrome' is a variant characterized by complete lateral gaze palsy to one side ('one') with contralateral paralysis of the adduction ('and-a-half'). It is caused by a lesion involving the parapontine reticular formation and the longitudinal fasciculus on the same side (Pierrot-Deseilligny et al. 1981, Wall and Wray 1983).

Convergence palsy

Convergence palsy is an inability to adduct both eyes in the absence of medial rectus paralysis. The commonest cause is probably closed head injury (Krohel et al. 1986). Convergence palsy may be encountered even following minor head trauma. It is necessary before accepting the diagnosis of convergence palsy to rule out the presence of a tumour of the quadrigeminal plate or neighbouring structures. Treatment of post-traumatic convergence palsy consists of convergence exercises and/or wearing prisms.

OCULAR MOTOR APRAXIA

Ocular motor apraxia is characterized by abnormal movements of the head and eyes when changes in gaze are being attempted. In its complete form, initiation of a saccade may take up to one second, and the movement is slow and hypometric so that several successive hypometric saccades may be necessary to bring the eyes to the desired position. In fact, refixation is commonly performed by head turning rather than by eye deviation. During head rotation, there may be deviation of the eyes in the opposite direction (contraversion), with secondary realignment of the eyes and head when the new objective has been reached (Zee et al. 1977). The anomaly is limited to horizontal saccades, whilst vestibular reflex movements, pursuit (slow) movements and vertical saccades are normal.

Most cases are idiopathic. A few cases have been associated with chromosomal abnormalities (Martin Carballo et al. 1993) or with immune deficiency (Narbona et al. 1980). Shawkat et al. (1995) reported that 38 of 62 scans in such children were abnormal, showing delayed myelination, agenesis of the corpus callosum and cerebellar vermian abnormalities, and suggested that lesional causes of delayed saccades may be more common than previously thought. Rare cases of vertical ocular motor apraxia are on record (Hughes et al. 1985, Ebner et al. 1990). The patient of Ebner et al. had a bilateral lesion at the mesencephalic–diencephalic junction demonstrated by CT.

Ocular motor apraxia should be distinguished from abnormal eye movements observed in children with very low visual acuity who tend to use head movements rather than saccades for looking at targets (Jan et al. 1986) and in children with severe strabismus and low acuity. A syndrome of saccade palsy associated with retinal dystrophy reported by Moore and Taylor (1984) may be simply due to the low visual acuity of affected children.

Ocular motor apraxia is observed as a specific congenital disease known as Cogan disease and in various CNS disorders, including perinatal conditions like cerebral palsy, congenital malformations, neurodegenerative conditions (Le Ber et al. 2003, 2004), infections and tumours.

Cogan disease or congenital ocular motor apraxia is generally recognized after 6–12 months of age because of the occurrence of head thrusts that may be mistaken for tics or even epileptic seizures. Vertical saccades are normal, and mental development is usually preserved. However, many children have clumsiness, difficulties with equilibrium and learning problems. The disease is genetically determined in rare cases, probably transmitted as a recessive trait the expression of which may be very mild, limited for instance to slowness or absence of optokinetic nystagmus. The prognosis is generally favourable with a tendency towards improvement (Zee et al. 1977). In addition, older patients tend to use more unobtrusive manoeuvres than head thrusts such as forced blinking for refixation. However, learning problems and clumsiness may be a very significant associated disability (Rappaport et al. 1987, Marr et al. 2005).

Abnormal eye movements reminiscent of those of Cogan disease may be seen in association with callosal agenesis or vermian aplasia (Bordarier and Aicardi 1990, Leão and Ribeiro-Silva 1995, Kondo et al. 2007). Slowness of saccades has also been reported with Friedreich disease (Kirkham et al. 1979) and other rare spinocerebellar degenerations (Wadia and Swami 1971) including a syndrome of ataxia–ocular motor apraxia (Aicardi et al. 1988; Chapter 8). Abnormal movements are also observed in children with albinism (Collewijn et al. 1985).

NYSTAGMUS

Nystagmus is an involuntary, rhythmical, conjugate oscillatory movement of the eyes (Dell'Osso 1984, Hoyt 1987, Troost 1989) that may occur in any plane. It is due to dysfunction of the complex mechanisms that maintain ocular fixation. The clinical description of nystagmus is usually based on the direction of the fast component and is termed horizontal, vertical or rotary, or any combination of these. The nystagmus may be conjugate or dysconjugate. A long recognized distinction is between jerk nystagmus, in which there is a slow initiating component followed by a fast corrective component, and pendular nystagmus in which the oscillations are of equal speed. However, the distinction between pendular and jerk oscillations may be difficult and even meaningless as the form of eye movements may change with gaze or other factors. In pendular nystagmus, the oscillations are slow in each direction, at least in the primary position of gaze, but may change to jerk nystagmus on lateral gaze. The most common form of jerk nystagmus is gaze-evoked nystagmus due to a deficit in the mechanisms responsible for holding the eyes in an eccentric position, whose seat is in the posterior fossa. The intensity of jerk nystagmus increases in the horizontal plane when gaze is in the direction of the fast phase (Alexander's law).

There are many types of nystagmus. Pendular nystagmus may be congenital or acquired. Acquired causes may be due to neurological diseases of the brainstem or cerebellum.

Common jerk nystagmus includes vestibular and gaze-evoked nystagmus. Vestibular nystagmus is also a common type of jerk nystagmus and may result from involvement of the vestibular end organ or central pathways and nuclei (Daroff et al. 1978). Central causes are usually uniplanar in contrast to

TABLE 17.4
Various types of nystagmus

Type	Origin	References
Pendular	Congenital; rarely acquired loss of vision	Troost (1989)
	Acquired neurological diseases of brainstem/cerebellum or diffuse degenerations	Harris (1997)
Latent (seen only with monocular vision)	Congenital	Dell'Osso et al. (1979)
Acquired horizontal jerk nystagmus		
Vestibular	Peripheral end-organ (horizontal rotary); central (pure vertical or horizontal)	Troost (1981)
Gaze-evoked/gaze-paretic	Posterior fossa structures; if vertical: brainstem+ cerebellum	Spector and Troost (1981)
Rotary	Vestibular central; medullary lesions; congenital	Troost (1989)
Upbeat	Congenital; acquired brainstem disease; Wernicke encephalopathy	Daroff and Troost (1973)
Downbeat	Chiari I malformation; other lesions of cervicomedullary junction	Pedersen et al. (1980), Baloh and Spooner (1981), Halmagyi et al. (1983)
See-saw (binocular pendular torsional oscillations with superimposed vertical vector moving the eyes in opposite directions)	Lesions of chiasma + floor of 3rd ventricle	Dell'Osso et al. (1974), Daroff et al. (1978)
Retractorius	Quadrigeminal plate; pineal tumours	Walsh and Hoyt (1969)
Periodic alternating (beating successively in one then the opposite direction)	Similar to downbeat nystagmus	Baloh et al. (1976)
Dissociated (major asymmetry between eyes)	Posterior fossa lesions	Cogan (1963)
Voluntary nystagmus	May be a manifestation of hysteria	Walsh and Hoyt (1969)

peripheral causes, which are commonly torsional or multiplanar. Visual fixation typically inhibits peripheral vestibular nystagmus, but not central vestibular nystagmus. In gaze-evoked nystagmus, the jerk nystagmus occurs in the direction of eccentric gaze. Posterior fossa structural diseases are commonly implicated. Also, drugs, particularly anticonvulsants, are known to lead to the phenomenon.

In periodic alternating nystagmus, the null point shifts position in a cyclic pattern. Periodic alternating nystagmus is typically congenital and benign, but it has been associated with neurodegenerative conditions like ataxia–telangiectasia, and vestibulocerebellar lesions (Shallo-Hoffman and Riordan-Eva 2001). In some cases, periodic alternating nystagmus may respond to oral baclofen. Other less common types of nystagmus are summarized in Table 17.4.

Latent nystagmus occurs when a single eye is covered. It may be 'manifest–latent' in children with strabismus who are actually viewing with a single eye at a time, even though both eyes are open.

The differential diagnosis of nystagmus includes many ophthalmological and neurological conditions. Nystagmus should be differentiated from the roving movements of blind children with pregeniculate lesions. Such movements are indicative of extremely poor vision or complete blindness and may be replaced by nystagmus when some useful vision develops in infants a few months of age (Jan et al. 1986, Kompf and Piper 1987).

The differential diagnosis of nystagmus has been reviewed by Gresty et al. (1984).

Acquired nystagmus
Acquired nystagmus is usually of the jerk type with a horizontal or horizontal–rotary form. The main causes of acquired nystagmus are indicated in Table 17.4. It is important to keep in mind that drug toxicity is a common cause of jerk nystagmus of horizontal or vertical types, and that certain forms of nystagmus, e.g. see-saw nystagmus and downbeat nystagmus (Hanegan et al. 1983), are electively caused by certain conditions such as chiasmatic lesions or the Chiari I malformation.

Monocular vertical oscillations may also occur in amblyopic patients, the so-called Hermann–Bielschowsky phenomenon (Smith et al. 1982). Many other types of ocular oscillations are recognized. Some of them are listed in Table 17.5, together with their probable or possible anatomical origin and causes.

TABLE 17.5
Some ocular movements related to or mimicking nystagmus

Type of movement	Clinical features (and common causes)	Reference
Square-wave jerks	Barely visible jerks on steady fixation or smooth pursuit (1–5° saccades) away from fixation point, followed after 200 ms interval by refixation. Only larger jerks clinically visible. (Most common abnormality with cerebellar disease)	Daroff et al. (1978)
Ocular dysmetria	Undershooting followed by brief small-amplitude saccadic oscillations or overshooting followed by single or several corrective saccades on refixation. (Cerebellar disease)	Daroff et al. (1978)
Ocular flutter and macrosaccadic oscillations	Brief binocular, purely horizontal oscillations occurring spontaneously during straight-ahead fixation. Crescendo amplitude; no intersaccadic latency; whole burst lasts 1–2 secs. (Cerebellar disease)	Cogan (1954)
Opsoclonus	Very fast saccadic eye movements in all directions occurring in sudden bursts. (Neuroblastoma, opsomyoclonic syndrome, diffuse cerebellar disease)	Cogan (1954)
Ocular bobbing	Fast downward movement of both eyes followed by slow drift back to mid-position. (Severe brainstem dysfunction, comatose patients)	Mehler (1988)
Ocular dipping	Slow downward and fast upward movement and spontaneous roving horizontal movements. (Same as bobbing)	Ropper (1981)
Superior oblique myokymia	Small-amplitude torsional monocular movement with oscillopsia. (Nonpathological phenomenon. Benign like palpebral myokymia)	Hoyt and Keane (1970)

Congenital nystagmus

Congenital nystagmus is usually recognized shortly after birth but may be of the latent type and not detected until visual acuity testing. It may be delayed up to several months of age, especially when sensory in type. It persists throughout life and may be ignored by the patient. There is no widely accepted classification of nystagmus. Often, congenital nystagmus may be categorized into congenital idiopathic nystagmus, sensory defect nystagmus and neurological nystagmus.

There are numerous causes of congenital nystagmus. It may be genetically determined, and can be transmitted as an autosomal recessive, autosomal dominant or X-linked character (Dell'Osso et al. 1974).

Congenital nystagmus usually oscillates in a constant direction; up to 40 wave forms have been described, most of which are specific for congenital nystagmus but require specialized recordings for their recognition. Such recordings are difficult to calibrate in children (Baker et al. 1995) and careful clinical examination is essential.

Clinically, congenital nystagmus remains horizontal during vertical gaze rather than converting to gaze-evoked vertical nystagmus (Troost 1989). Head nodding or shaking is present in 6.6–8.0% of children with congenital nystagmus, regardless of the type (idiopathic or sensory) and mode of inheritance (Jan et al. 1990). It may be a means of improving foveation time and, therefore, visual acuity. A reduction in visual acuity is seen in about half of the children (Dell'Osso et al. 1974, Troost 1989, Jan et al. 1990), but in the presence of 'sensory' nystagmus, low visual acuity is commonly seen (Jan et al. 1986, 1990).

Congenital nystagmus is commonly associated with strabismus and other ocular abnormalities (Hertle and Dell'Osso 1999, Abadi and Bjerre 2002). Additional features of congenital nystagmus are shown in Table 17.6. A unique feature of congenital nystagmus is the so-called inverted optokinetic nystagmus: the fast components are in the direction of rotation of the drum instead of the opposite, which is normal (Halmagyi et al. 1980).

In patients with albinism, nystagmus is commonly seen. Often, jerk nystagmus may reverse direction. Interestingly, children with albinism have an excess proportion of nondecussated retinofugal fibres so that only the innermost parts of the nasal fields have a crossed cortical projection. This anomaly can be detected by study of the visual evoked potentials and, in some cases, by MRI demonstration of a sagittally split chiasma (Apkarian et al. 1995).

Ocular oscillations different from nystagmus (Table 17.5)

There are a number of ocular movements that may mimic nystagmus. Square wave jerks represent an abnormal eye movement. They consist of a conjugate displacement of the eyes up to 5 degrees from fixation, followed by a refixation saccade. They are often barely visible because of small amplitude. Although square wave jerks can be seen in normal patients, they have been associated with cerebellar disease, progressive supranuclear palsy and multiple sclerosis (Dell'Osso et al. 1975).

Opsoclonus is characterized by chaotic, rapid oscillations in all planes of gaze. Opsoclonus is exceptionally observed in newborn infants (Hoyt 1977). It may also be seen in some viral infections and in association with neuroblastoma (Chapter 10).

TABLE 17.6
Main features of congenital nystagmus*

Binocular
Similar amplitude in both eyes
Uniplanar, usually horizontal (may be vertical, rotary)
Increased by attempts at fixation
Inversion of the optokinetic reflex[1]
Associated head oscillations (in some types)
Abolished in sleep
Distinctive waveforms (require special recording systems)

*Adapted from Troost (1989).
[1]See Halmagyi et al. (1980) for details.

In children with neural crest tumours or brainstem encephalitis, opsoclonus is accompanied by diffuse or focal myoclonus.

Ocular flutter and ocular hypermetria may be seen in patients with inflammatory or other disorders of the cerebellum (Cogan 1954).

Spasmus nutans

Spasmus nutans consists of a triad of nystagmus (high frequency, small amplitude, dysconjugate oscillations), head shaking and head tilt (torticollis). Symptoms appear usually toward the end of the first year of life or during the second year. All three components need not be present at the same time, and head tilt and nodding movements may be transitory or be absent altogether. The nystagmus is constant. It may be binocular but is often predominantly or exclusively monocular. Vision is typically normal. The head shaking is horizontal, vertical or gyral, with a rate of 60–120 per minute, while the rate of eye oscillations is around 300 per minute. The nystagmus and head shaking occur in bursts lasting 5–30 seconds in association with fixation. Although infrequent, spasmus nutans is the commonest cause of unilateral nystagmus in infants (Weissman et al. 1987) and should be included in the diagnosis of all cases of unilateral nystagmus (Farmer and Hoyt 1984). The cause of the disorder is unknown and the course is benign with resolution in a few months to 2 years. However, cases of 'sinister' spasmus nutans due to optic gliomas are on record (Albright et al. 1984, King et al. 1986), so that imaging is indicated in all cases, even when the typical picture is present. Retinal disease can also be a cause (Lambert and Newman 1993), and spasmus nutans has been reported in association with unilateral poor vision due to anterior pathway lesions.

DISORDERS LEADING TO VISUAL IMPAIRMENT

THE ASSESSMENT OF VISION

Conditions that lead to a reduction in visual acuity or visual field are not uncommon. Often, these conditions are associated with systemic disorders. Therefore, careful history taking and examination are needed. A full ophthalmological assessment includes fundoscopic examination, evaluation of visual acuity and visual fields testing. Such examinations are difficult in infants and young children (Hoyt et al. 1982). Assessment should include

identification of reflex responses, such as papillary light reflex, which are reliably present after 31 weeks gestation. A blink response to light develops at approximately the same period (dazzle reflex), but the blink response to threat is unreliable and late in appearance. Fixation and following are present from very early in life. Infants turn their head towards a diffuse light from a few days of age. The human face, at a distance of approximately 30 cm, is the best target for fixation. Following in the vertical plane is particularly useful as vertical eye movements are not normally random movements and are therefore more reliable than horizontal ones. Nystagmus induced by rotation about the body axis is present in normal term babies, but is inhibited within a few seconds by visual fixation, whereas in blind children it may persist for 15 seconds.

Standard visual acuity charts should be used to measure visual acuity. However, this is not practical in nonverbal children. In these cases, the preferential looking technique offers an estimate of visual acuity (McDonald et al. 1985, Atkinson and van Hof-van Duin 1993); in the absence of standardized tests, functional measures can also be used. On occasion, these children may be considered to be blind, if there is obviously no vision or if they notice large objects only a few feet away (Jan et al. 1977). Similarly, standard visual field testing, such as Goldmann perimetry, can be performed. In young children, visual field is commonly tested by confrontational methods.

On occasion, additional testing is helpful in the evaluation of the visual pathways. The visual evoked response to flashes is an excellent technique to demonstrate the integrity of the visual pathways without patient cooperation (Baker et al. 1995). A positive cortical wave with a peak latency of 300 ms is first demonstrable at 30 weeks gestation. The latency then declines by about 10 ms each week through the last 10 weeks of gestation (Taylor et al. 1987, Leaf et al. 1995). By about 3 months of age, the morphology and latency of the visual evoked responses are relatively mature, but interpretation of the response at earlier periods remains difficult. Further visual evoked procedures, such as pattern, shifting orientation and sweep, are being used, which can be used to provide greater information regarding the visual axis. Additional vision tests, such as electroretinography, can be used to assist in the diagnosis of many retinal diseases.

For central causes of vision loss, neuroimaging techniques may be useful in the assessment of children with visual difficulties (Flodmark et al. 1990) as they can detect associated cerebral malformations such as absence of the septum pellucidum or agenesis of the corpus callosum. Further, imaging may also be useful in demonstrating lesions of the optic radiations, especially dilatation of the occipital horns and periventricular leukomalacia (Van Nieuwenhuizen and Willemse 1988, Scher et al. 1989).

The assessment of the child helps not only identify a diagnosis, but can also be used to initiate childhood developmental support for children who have a vision loss. Vision loss is variably defined. The definition of legal blindness in Canada and the USA specifies that distance visual acuity should be no more than 20/200 in the better eye with correction, or that the widest diameter of vision should subtend an angle of no more than 20°.

In the UK, an acuity of 3/60 or less in the better eye is legally required. Such definitions may not applicable to younger children, as visual acuity measures are not always accurate in some clinical settings. In addition, visual acuity and visual functions develop over time. Therefore, younger children whose visual acuity is suboptimal by adult standards may not have a visual impairment compared with same-aged children.

Amblyopia is clinically defined as a significant reduction in visual acuity, despite appropriate correction of a refractive error (Friendly 1987). It is the most common cause of unilateral vision loss. Typically, the examination reveals factors that lead to amblyopia, such as anisometropia, strabismus, monocular form deprivation or a combination of these. Unlike many causes of vision loss, amblyopia can be treated, leading to improvement in visual acuity.

FEATURES OF EARLY-ONSET BILATERAL VISION LOSS

Congenital blindness is usually easily detected, except in young infants with severe deficit of cognitive and relational functions in whom the distinction between blindness and indifference to surroundings may be difficult to establish.

Visual acuity loss associated with lesions of pregeniculate optic pathways is most common. In children with involvement of eye media and/or retina, eye-pressing with thumb and fingers is common (Jan et al. 1983). The mechanism of this digito-ocular phenomenon may be related to the production of phosphenes and other visual sensations by mechanical pressure. The presence of intense eye-pressing should suggest the possibility of retinal disease. It is especially common in blind children with mental retardation.

Visual impairment due to optic atrophy and other pregeniculate lesions is often accompanied by abnormal eye movements that may be of a 'searching' or roving type, in cases of total blindness, or of congenital nystagmus type when some useful vision is preserved or recovery takes place following an early period of complete visual impairment (Jan et al. 1986). More central causes of visual impairment are not always associated with these roving eye movements (Whiting et al. 1985); however, oculomotor apraxias and dyskinetic eye movements may be seen in these cases (Matsuba and Jan 2006).

In addition to visual dysfunction, blindness may be responsible for some neurological manifestations such as hypotonia and delayed motor development (Jan and Scott 1974). However, gross retardation is never explained by visual disturbances. Sonksen (1993) followed 600 children with severe visual impairment and carefully assessed the development of their language and social skills. She emphasized the importance of early diagnosis and management to compensate for the increased vulnerability of these children. Visual impairment can also be responsible for EEG abnormalities, particularly the occurrence of occipital spikes that may result from deafferentation of the occipital cortex (Jan and Wong 1988). Such spikes are not indicative of epilepsy, if no clinical seizures are present, and do not require treatment.

Congenital blindness may be difficult to distinguish from *delayed visual maturation* (Tresidder et al. 1990, Fielder and Mayer 1991). This condition is defined as reduced or absent visual responsiveness with normal ophthalmological examination present from birth but with subsequent improvement at several months of age. The diagnosis is made retrospectively and by exclusion of the visual system for other disease. It is essential that the vision should improve with time, but may not be normal, as delayed visual maturation is often associated with ocular and systemic diseases.

There have been several classifications for delayed visual maturation. Uemura et al. (1981) have used a three-type classification where type I comprises patients with delayed visual maturation with no other anomalies; type II, patients with delayed visual maturation with systemic disease such as a seizure disorder or cognitive impairment; and type III, patients with delayed visual maturation with additional ocular visual abnormality. Similarly, Fielder and Mayer (1991) distinguished four types: type I in which there is no ocular or CNS defect; type II where neurological abnormalities are associated; type III in children with albinism and infantile nystagmus: and type IV, in which severe structural eye abnormalities are present.

Clinically, a 'roving' nystagmus may be present in some infants when visual recovery begins. Transient strabismus is frequent. Fundoscopic examination is normal but the infantile optic disc is paler than that of older children, and the fundus and macula may be somewhat mottled so that an erroneous diagnosis of optic atrophy or retinopathy may be entertained. Delayed maturation of the visual evoked response may be found with abnormal shape, including absence of negative deflections following the first potential (Mellor and Fielder 1980) and increased latency of the evoked response. The electroretinogram (ERG) is typically normal. Recovery occurs after the age of 4–6 months, although it is dependent upon the type. Children with systemic conditions have a worse prognosis. Nystagmus and low acuity may persist in some infants. The cause of this condition is unknown.

CAUSES OF VISUAL IMPAIRMENT

There are vast numbers of CNS, optic nerve, retinal and ocular structure disorders that lead to dysfunction in the visual pathways. Often, these problems are associated with a number of systemic and neurological diseases. The following paragraphs discuss some common conditions that result in a loss of visual field of visual acuity. The main causes of blindness in childhood are listed in Table 17.7.

CORTICAL VISUAL IMPAIRMENT

In adults, the term cortical blindness describes often complete vision loss due to bilateral damage to the occipital cortex. However, children who present with damage to the occipital cortex present differently than adults. Because these children often have partial vision loss, the term cortical visual impairment was introduced (Jan et al. 1987). In the mid 1980s, this form of visual impairment was being increasingly identified (Whiting et al. 1985, Roland et al. 1986). The term cortical visual impairment applies to a bilateral reduction in visual acuity due to damage of the

TABLE 17.7

Main causes of blindness or severe visual impairment in childhood

Diseases of the anterior visual pathway[1]
Corneal anomalies (scars or metabolic disorders)
Congenital cataracts (hereditary, prenatal infections, metabolic diseases, unknown causes)
Retinopathy of prematurity
Retinitis pigmentosa (several types)
Infectious retinal disease (*e.g.* toxoplasmosis, rubella)
Leber congenital amaurosis
Metabolic and heredodegenerative retinal diseases
Optic nerve hypoplasia
Leber hereditary optic neuropathy
Acquired optic atrophy (see Table 17.8)

Diseases of the posterior visual pathway*
Congenital occipital malformations
Periventricular leukomalacia (due to preterm birth, pre- or postnatal hypoxic–ischaemic events)
Occipital infarcts (thrombosis or compression of posterior cerebral arteries)
Diffuse circulatory failure (vascular collapse, heart failure, status epilepticus, malaria)
Raised intracranial pressure (especially shunt failure)
Heredodegenerative diseases

[1]Many causes can involve both anterior and posterior pathways.

occipital cortex, in particular the calcarine cortex. In some children, central vision loss may primarily result from deep subcortical white matter insults such as periventricular leukomalacia. As a result, the term cerebral visual impairment is commonly used, as it is more inclusive.

The early diagnosis of cortical visual impairment remains essentially clinical. Children may undergo multiple investigations, but the results must be interpreted with caution. Visual evoked responses may be deceptive, as they may be normal despite profound visual loss (Taylor and McCulloch 1991, Wong 1991). An extinguished ERG can be helpful, but may be absent in blindness not due to involvement of the retinal sensory epithelium. Study of the optokinetic nystagmus may be helpful for the diagnosis of malingering if special equipment is available, but in most cases clinical assessment is the best option.

Cortical/cerebral visual impairment (CVI) is now the most common cause of visual acuity loss in young children in developed countries. Traditionally, CVI has been defined as a reduction in visual acuity and/or visual field. However, CVI has also been used to describe eye movement abnormalities and poor visual attention (Weiss et al. 2001). In the presence of acuity loss, it is associated with significant comorbidities including cognitive and motor impairments. Typical causes include perinatal hypoxic–ischaemia, especially in preterm infants with periventricular leukomalacia (Lanzi et al. 1998, Ng et al. 1989), infections, hydrocephalus, trauma and structural brain anomalies. Rarer aetiologies include hypoglycaemia, seizures, and inflammatory and neurodegenerative conditions. Fortunately, unlike in adults, children with vision loss due to occipital cortex injury often have improvement in their visual acuity over time (Roland et al. 1986).

The underlying neurological structural abnormality varies, often dependent upon the onset of the injury, preterm versus term, as well as the type of injury. In preterm children, the most common site of injury is to the periventricular white matter. Often, white matter disease can be divided into hypoperfusion and haemorrhagic. In addition, profound hypotensive injuries in preterm children may lead to deep grey matter and brainstem injuries. In term children, watershed areas are affected, more likely occurring in the frontal and parietal–occipital regions.

Acquired CVI is frequent in children. Often, some degree of vision is usually preserved. Many children present with puzzling visual behaviour and can be shown to have field and/or agnosic deficits, including difficulties with recognition, orientation and depth, movement and simultaneous perception (Jan et al. 1987, Jan 1993). CVI may be transient or lasting. Transient CVI is frequent following head trauma (Eldridge and Punt 1988), and may be a manifestation of epilepsy, migraine or other acute conditions (Barnet et al. 1970) such as hypoglycaemia (Garty et al. 1987).

Lasting acquired CVI can be a complication of infections, especially purulent meningitis or herpes encephalitis; of acute hypoxia following vascular collapse; of acute dehydration; of status epilepticus; of pernicious attacks of malaria; and of severe head trauma. It may also result from shunt dysfunction in hydrocephalus (Arroyo et al. 1985, Connolly et al. 1991) as a result of infarction in the territory of both posterior cerebral arteries due to their compression while crossing the tentorial edge. Extensive cortical malformations are a less frequent cause (Jan 1993).

Although there may be complete loss of vision lasting weeks or months, most patients recover some degree of vision, even though permanent field defects and low acuity almost always persist (Lambert et al. 1987, Matsuba and Jan 2006). The clinical features of CVI often make its recognition difficult, especially in children with cognitive and/or behavioural manifestations. It is occasionally difficult to distinguish CVI from optic ataxia or dyskinetic eye movements, where major disturbances in reaching for objects easily suggest blindness (Perenin and Vighetto 1988, Jan et al. 2001).

Ventral and dorsal visual pathways
Vision influences many areas of childhood development. In the neonatal period, infants develop visual attention. Once visual attention is developed, the infant will begin to reach to interact with near objects. Subsequently, vision encourages children to explore more distant objects through visuomotor skills. The complex visual and environmental interaction is influenced by multiple comprehensive visual modules. These modules are separated into two main cortical pathways, the dorsal and ventral streams (Milner and Goodale 1995). The ventral stream links the occipital and temporal lobes. Its connections have been associated with recognition of geometric forms, route finding and visual memory. The dorsal stream runs between the occipital and parietal lobes, subserving the ability to process the whole visual scene. It is mostly concerned with perception of movement and visuomotor performance.

Interference with these pathways does not necessarily include a reduction in visual acuity or field but can have functional consequences (Goodale and Westwood 2004). It is thought that

for a cochlear implant should be screened for metabolic conditions, especially those children with an affected sibling, those from a consanguineous marriage, and those in whom there is a family history of profound hearing impairment, particularly if associated with developmental delay or dysmorphic features. Metabolic screening should include blood gases, mucopolysaccharides and oligosaccharides, amino acids, very long chain fatty acids, blood lactate, urine sugar reducing substances and phytanic acid.

The purpose of investigation incorporates establishing the cause of the hearing loss, gathering information that is relevant to the hearing loss management, investigating for coexisting medical problems, establishing a prognosis for the child and the family, and in addition informing epidemiology and thus planning for effective hearing loss prevention and surveillance programmes and assessing how best to meet the needs of managing children with a hearing loss.

AUDIOLOGICAL ASSESSMENT

A wide range of behavioural tests of hearing for typically developing infants aged over 6 months is available, which can be adapted for delayed development provided the child has sufficient development to cope with the strictures of the testing situation. Behavioural tests of hearing when conducted with precision complement the role of electrophysiological techniques. Behavioural testing includes the distraction test, visual reinforcement audiometry, the performance test for which a child is conditioned to perform a simple action in response to a sound stimulus, and pure tone audiometry. In addition, there are a range of tests of auditory discrimination of speech (Hickson 2002).

Objective physiological measures are more appropriate to detect hearing impairment in newborns and very young infants and for children who are unable to cooperate with behavioural testing. These techniques include otoacoustic emission (OAE) testing (either transient-evoked or distortion-product) and auditory brainstem responses (ABRs). These technologies comprise noninvasive recordings of physiological activity that underlie normal auditory function. The two measures are highly correlated with a degree of peripheral hearing sensitivity.

OAEs are sensitive to outer hair cell dysfunction and testing can detect sensory hearing loss. The recordings are reliable in neonates in response to stimuli and a frequency range above 1500 Hz. Because OAEs are also sensitive to outer ear canal obstruction and middle ear effusion, a positive test result can occur in the presence of normal cochlear function but temporary conductive dysfunction. As OAE responses are generated within the cochlear by the outer hair cells the technique does not detect VIIIth nerve or auditory brainstem pathway dysfunction. Therefore OAE testing may not detect infants with auditory neuropathy or neural conduction disorders without concomitant sensory outer hair cell dysfunction.

In contrast, the ABR reflects activity of the cochlear, auditory nerve and auditory brainstem pathways. The click-evoked ABR is highly correlated with hearing sensitivity in the frequency range 1000–8000 Hz. Because the ABR is sensitive to auditory nerve and brainstem dysfunction, ABR screening can lead to a positive result in the absence of peripheral (i.e. middle ear or cochlear) hearing loss but in the presence of auditory neuropathy or neural conduction disorders in newborns.

An audiological test battery to assess the integrity of the auditory system should include OAEs, a measure of middle ear function, acoustic reflex thresholds, observation of the infant's behavioural response to sound, and parental reports of emerging communication and auditory behaviours. There should be appropriate measures of middle ear function including reflectance tympanometry using appropriate frequency probe stimuli, bone conduction ABR or pneumatic otoscopy (Joint Committee on Infant Hearing 2000).

NEONATAL HEARING SCREENING

Many countries have adopted universal newborn screening programmes. Whilst there is consensus from a number of influential advisory bodies (Joint Committee on Infant Hearing 2000), the long-term affectiveness of these programmes has not been established (Puig et al. 2005). However, studies of language ability after early detection of permanent childhood hearing impairment through neonatal screening has confirmed improved receptive language scores (Kennedy et al. 2006). The advocates of neonatal hearing screening propose that all infants should have access to hearing screening using a physiological measure and that infants with confirmed permanent hearing loss should receive appropriate services before the age of 6 months. The target for universal neonatal hearing screening programmes is a permanent bilateral or unilateral sensory or conductive hearing loss averaging 30–40 dB or more in the frequency region important for speech recognition at 500–4000 Hz. Infants who pass a newborn hearing screen but who have risk indicators for other auditory disorders or speech and language delay should receive ongoing audiological and medical surveillance. All programmes must be in a position to take forward the care of an infant who has been identified as having a hearing loss through a neonatal newborn hearing screening programme. The doctor involved must have an appropriate level of competence and would therefore usually be an audiological physician or a community doctor in audiology, or a paediatrician or otolaryngologist with an appropriate level of training.

AETIOLOGY OF SENSORINEURAL HEARING IMPAIRMENT

GENETIC CAUSES

This is a rapidly advancing field, traditionally categorized into syndromic (30%) and non-syndromic (70%) causes (Friedman and Griffith 2003, Nance 2003). While it is still helpful to make this distinction initially clinically, it is important to appreciate that some syndromic conditions may simply appear non-syndromic because the wider manifestations of the disorder have not been recognized, e.g. prolonged QT intervals in Jervell–Lange-Neilson syndrome, thyroid dysfunction in Pendred syndrome, and retinitis pigmentosa in Usher syndrome. At a molecular level, the distinction can also be confusing. Whilst 50% of non-syndromic sensorineural hearing loss arises from mutations in *connexin-26*, other connexin genes can have associated abnormalities, e.g. dermatological abnormalities with *connexin-30* and *connexin-31*, palmo-plantar hyperkeratosis with a dominant *G59A* allele, mutilating keratoderma associated with the *D66H* allele, and neurological abnormalities with *connexin-32* seen in X-linked Charcot–Marie–Tooth disease. Around 33 recessive, 41 dominant and five X-linked loci have been mapped for non-syndromic genetic deafness. Despite the very large number of loci that have been identified, most cases of genetic deafness are caused by these mutations that involve a single gene from the connexins (Denoyelle et al. 1999).

The connexins are a family of genes that code for the subunits of gap junction proteins. Gap junctions form when the hexameric hemi-connexins on the surface of two adjacent cells join to form a complete gap junction. The resulting channels permit the flow of ions and small molecules between the cells. The GJB2 gene at the locus 13q12–13 is one of the more commonly clinically available genetic tests for non-syndromic deafness, the others being for *SLC26A4* and *WFS1* (Smith 2004). These genes make a substantial contribution to the total genetic deafness mutation load and they are relatively easy to screen for. *GJB2* at the DFNB1 locus results in autosomal recessive non-syndromic deafness. *GJB2* encodes the transmembrane protein called connexin-26, which oligomerizes with five other connexins to form a connexon that is the constituent component of gap junctions. The severity of hearing loss in *connexin-26* gene mutations is extremely variable and cannot be predicted even within families, although it has been shown to be non-progressive in most cases on follow-up into young adult life (Denoyelle et al. 1999). The *DFNB1* gene responsible for this recessive, non-syndromic sensorineural hearing loss causes approximately 15% of all infant hearing losses. It is important to consider testing for this common mutation as this will detect 95% of instances in caucasian families who are not consanguineous. If the test is positive, then there is no further requirement for CT, perchlorate washout or investigations for retinitis pigmentosa (Joint Committee on Infant Hearing 2000).

DFNA36 mutation hearing loss is a condition of early onset and rapid progression of dominant non-syndromic deafness (Makishima et al. 2004).

Mutations of several genes that encode for a variety of different myocins, psychoskeletal motor proteins that create tension or facilitate the movement of cell components along actin filaments, are associated with hearing loss: *MYO6*, *MYO7A*, *MYO15A*, *MYO1A* and *MYO3A* (Ben-Yosef and Friedman 2003).

The *A1555G* mitochondrial mutation infers susceptibility to normal doses of aminoglycosides, an example of a situation in which genetic vulnerability combined with environmental risk factors results in sensorineural hearing loss.

GENETIC SYNDROMES

Again, progress in this area is very fast and there are an increasing number of conditions in which molecular analysis can confirm diagnosis: Waardenburg syndromes types I–IV, Treacher Collins syndrome, Alport syndrome, branchio-otorenal syndrome, Usher syndrome, Jervell–Lange-Neilsen syndrome, Pendred syndrome, Charcot–Marie–Tooth disease, and craniosynostosis–deafness. The three syndromes of Jervell–Lange-Neilsen, Pendred and Usher may all initially appear to be non-syndromic until the involvement of other organs is recognized.

Prolonged QT syndrome/Jervell–Lange-Nielsen syndrome
Mutations in the various potassium channel genes may result in the long QT syndrome, and when this is associated with congenital sensorineural deafness it is known as the Jervell–Lange-Nielsen syndrome (JLNS) (Neyroud et al. 1997). The prevalence is 0.21% in children with congenital deafness (Ocal et al. 1997) (Chapter 16). Prolongation of the QT interval is seen on the EEG and reflects a defective cardiac repolarization that can lead to recurrent attacks of syncope, ventricular arrythmia and sudden death. Syncopal attacks can be precipitated by fright. The long QT syndrome is defined on the basis of a QTc (corrected QT) interval >470 ms in asymptomatic individuals. The *KVLQT1* gene that causes JLNS also causes Ward–Romano syndrome, in which there is no hearing loss. *KVLQT1* maps to chromosome 11p15.5 (JLNS1 locus); a recessive mutation involving another potassium channel gene, *KCNE1*, at the JLNS2 locus on chromosome 21q22.1 may produce an identical phenotype that affects the active potassium transport system in the hair cells of the cochlear. Another potassium channel gene, *KCNQ4*, which is limited to the outer hair cells, has mutations that cause a relatively common dominant form of progressive hearing loss that typically begins in the first two decades of life, firstly involving the high frequencies and then progressing within a decade to profound deafness.

All hearing-impaired children should have an ECG, and if it is marginal or abnormal they should be referred to a cardiologist for further investigation as they may require further monitoring with ECG and exercise testing to establish whether there is a prolonged QT interval. This is associated with a high risk of syncope and sudden death during the first year of life or later and there is also a vestibular areflexia.

Pendred syndrome
Pendred syndrome, which arises from mutations in *SLC26A4*, is the most common cause of syndromic deafness, accounting for more than 5% of all autosomal recessive hearing loss cases. It is characterized by bilateral sensorineural hearing loss associated with goitre with or without hypothyroidism (Reardon et al. 1997). There appears to be a relationship between the severity of the hearing impairment and the degree of hypothyroidism. The deafness is congenital and associated with temporal bone abnormalities that range from isolated enlargement of the vestibular aqueduct to Mondini dysplasia, which is a more complex malformation that also includes cochlear hypoplasia (Napiontek et al. 2004). The hearing loss is usually profound but can be variable in onset, rapidly progressing and unilateral. The goitre generally

develops after the age of 10 years, and the thyroid dysfunction is variable. The sensorineural deafness is occasionally associated with disturbed vestibular function.

Usher syndrome

Usher syndrome affects 2–4% of all cases with profound deafness and 50% of the deaf–blind population. Usher syndrome type I is characterized by vestibular dysfunction, profound congenital hearing loss and early onset of retinitis pigmentosa. The progressive degeneration of the retina results in loss of night vision and restriction of visual fields leading to blindness. Type I is distinguished from type II by this early onset of retinitis pigmentosa. Type II also has a generally less severe hearing loss and normal vestibular function. Usher syndrome type III is characterized by a progressive postlingual hearing loss and varying severity of retinitis pigmentosa, without a vestibular component. Usher syndrome is phenotypically and genotypically complex with, for example, USH1 loci mapping to 10q21–22 and 11q13.5 (Ben-Yosef and Friedman 2003).

Alport syndrome

In this condition, the hearing loss may not present until the age of 8–10 years, and 50% of those affected have progressive bilateral hearing loss that involves high frequencies initially. There is a progressive nephritis. The incidence is 1 in 10,000 births, and X-linked, autosomal recessive and autosomal dominant varieties occur. Haematuria is seen in the first decade of life, and diagnosis is based on this plus a family history of haematuria or renal failure, characteristic renal biopsy findings, sensorineural hearing loss, and ophthalmic signs of anterior lenticonus or macular flecks. Ocular findings might also include congenital cataracts and spherophakia. The disease results from mutations involving one or other of three tissue-specific polypeptide subunits of collagen that are encoded by the COL4A3, COL4A4 and COL4A5 genes. The COL4A5 gene is located at Xq22, while the genes coding for 3 and 4 collagens are next to each other on 2q35.

Alström syndrome

Alström syndrome is a recessively inherited genetic disorder caused by mutation of the ALMS1 gene (Hearn et al. 2002) and characterized by congenital retinal dystrophy that leads to blindness, sensorineural hearing impairment, childhood obesity, insulin-resistant type 2 diabetes mellitus, and hypertriglyceridaemia that can precipitate pancreatitis and pulmonary symptoms (Michaud et al. 1996). Among 182 cases studied by Marshall et al. (2005), 20% showed neurological symptoms, including clonic tic and absence seizures, while developmental motor or language delays were observed in almost 50%. There were fibrotic infiltrations of multiple organs including kidney, heart, liver, lung, bladder, gonads and pancreas.

Waardenburg syndrome

Waardenburg syndrome affects 1–2% of individuals with profound hearing loss, which can be bilateral or unilateral and is associated with defects in tissues and structures derived from neural crest cells (Liu et al. 1995). Pigmentary abnormalities include brilliant blue eyes, complete or segmental heterochromia, and patches of cutaneous hyper- or hypopigmentation. There is lateral displacement of the inner canthi of the eyes, a pinched appearance of the nose and synophrys. Gastrointestinal symptoms can occur, and there may be a history of Hirschprung disease. There is an increased incidence of neural tube defects and limb defects. There are at least eight loci that contribute to the phenotype. Waardenburg syndrome type I can result from more than 50 different mutations involving the PAX3 gene on 2q35. Waardenburg type IIA results from mutations at the MITF locus on 3q12 and this condition has less frequent eyelid anomalies and a higher degree of deafness and heterochromia. Some Waardenburg type IIA patients have albinism, with or without freckling, and this is known as the Tietz syndrome. A number of other loci have been described such as those in Waardenburg type III, a condition that features various limb defects. The mechanism here appears to be that the cochlear neural crest cells that contribute to the intermediate layer of the stria vascularis are affected and are likely to be the cause of the deafness as the stria cannot maintain the critical endocochlear potential that is required for the hair cells to function normally.

Brown–Vialetto–Van Laere syndrome

This is a rare disease of unknown origin that is considered to be part of a group of motor neuron diseases with pontobulbar palsy and deafness. The bilateral sensorineural deafness can be accompanied by a variety of cranial nerve disorders that usually involve the motor components of the lower cranial nerves but might also involve spinal motor nerves and upper motor neurons. There are both familial and sporadic cases. Some neurophysiological studies show evidence of nerve damage with subsequent improvement, which raises the possibility that the disorder is due to primary nerve damage rather than motor neuron disorder (Degrandis 2005, Prabhu 2005).

Wolfram syndrome

Wolfram syndrome is an autosomal recessive disease characterized by diabetes insipidus, diabetes mellitus, optic atrophy and deafness, which arises from mutations of WFS1. There is high-frequency hearing loss, and the condition can also involve peripheral neuropathy with urinary tract atony and psychiatric illness. A dominant low-frequency sensorineural hearing loss can also be caused by mutations in WFS1 (Lesperance 2003). As routine newborn hearing screening will not typically identify hearing loss affecting frequencies below 2000 Hz, children at risk of deafness in Wolfram syndrome need to be specifically monitored.

Congenital fixation of the stapes footplate with perilymphatic gusher

This is an X-linked syndrome featuring mixed or sensorineural deafness, the conductive component of which involves congenital fixation of the stapes footplate. If attempts are made to mobilize this, there is a profuse flow of endolymphatic fluid. CT shows dilatation of the internal auditory meatus with an abnormal communication between the subarachnoid space and the cochlear endolymph. Carrier females may have a mild hearing loss and a less severe abnormality of the inner ear. The locus maps to Xq21.1; in many families the mutation has been shown to be a deletion, and it can sometimes involve nearby genes for mental retardation and choroideraemia.

Syndromic hearing loss associated with dermatological disorders
There are at least five dermatological disorders that are associated with syndromic hearing loss; these also involve a wide variety and severity of organ involvement. An example is the Bart–Pumphrey syndrome, which is an autosomal dominant disorder characterized by sensorineural hearing loss, palmoplanter keratoderma, knuckle pads and leukonychia (Richard et al. 2004).

Dominant optic atrophy, sensorineural hearing loss, ptosis and ophthalmoplegia
This syndrome is caused by a missense mutation in *OPA1* (Payne et al. 2004). *OPA1* is a nuclear gene but the gene product localizes to mitochondria, suggesting that mitochondrial dysfunction might be the common pathway to many forms of syndromic and non-syndromic optic atrophy, hearing loss and external ophthalmoplegia.

Craniofacial abnormality syndromes
A large number of syndromic conditions with craniofacial abnormalities are associated with deafness, some of which have delineation of the underlying molecular basis of the hearing impairment. An example is branchio-otorenal syndrome, associated with mutations in *EYA1* and *EYA4* genes affecting transcription factors. This syndrome may have associated Mondini-type cochlear hypoplasia with hypoplastic and displaced ossicles. Renal ultrasound may demonstrate agenesis or hypoplasia or dysplasia of the kidneys.

Children with profound or progressive hearing loss and craniofacial abnormalities are more likely to have abnormal CT findings. Dilated vestibular aqueduct correlates with the presence of progressive hearing impairment. CT of the petrous temporal bones has been found to be abnormal in 6.8–12.8% of bilateral sensorineural hearing loss and in up to 30% of cochlear implant candidates. Mondini-type dysplasia is the presence of a cochlear with a normal basal turn and a distal sac. Semicircular canals are absent or dysplastic in the CHARGE association (colobomata, heart defect, atresia of the choanae, retarded growth/development, genital hypoplasia, and ear anomalies or deafness) and in the Vater–Rapadilino syndrome (Vater is the association of vertebral defects, anal atresia/stenosis, tracheo-oesophageal fistula, radial defects and renal anomalies, while Rapadilino includes radial defects, absent/hypoplastic patellae, high cleft palate, diarrhoea and dislocated joints, little size, a long slender nose and normal intelligence with hearing loss also a feature) (Bamiou et al. 2000a).

Sensorineural hearing loss with chromosomal abnormalities
Chromosomal abnormalities occur in around 5% of children with sensorineural hearing loss. Hultcrantz (2003) reported that 61% of females with Turner syndrome suffered from otitis media and sensorineural dip in hearing; in some cases this was observed as early as 6 years of age and progressed over time.

6q minus syndrome can be accompanied by a bilateral severe sensory hearing loss. This rare disorder, due to a monosomy or trisomy of 6q results in mental retardation, microcephaly, asymmetrical face, broad nasal bridge, hypertelorism, epicanthus, strabismus, high arched palate, ventricular septum defect and seizures. Tetraplegia and diaphragmatic hernia have also been described (Schuster et al. 2003).

HEARING LOSS WITH NEUROLOGICAL DISEASE
An inherited disorder of white matter with ataxia, leukodystrophy and sensorineural hearing loss progressing to complete deafness by the age of 12 years was reported by Leuzzi et al. (2000). Familial cerebellar ataxia with hypergonadotropic hypogonadism and sensorineural deafness has been described, but generally with the hearing loss developing in adult life (Storey 2001, Georgopoulos et al. 2004).

Children with *autism* have an increased rate of audiological problems, with one group describing profound bilateral hearing loss in 3.5% of cases (Rosenhall et al. 1999). Discomfort with sound was common, affecting 18% of cases; serous otitis media occurred in 23.5%, with an associated conductive hearing loss in 18.3%.

Prevalence of sensorineural hearing loss of 17.3% has been described in Rett syndrome and was increased in the older participants and in those who had had seizures requiring the use of anticonvulsants in the study by Pillion et al. (2003).

Sensorineural hearing loss may be associated with neurodegenerative disorders such as Hunter syndrome, and with sensorimotor neuropathy in Friedreich ataxia and Charcot–Marie–Tooth syndrome.

Refsum Disease
Refsum disease is characterized by retinitis pigmentosa, anosmia, chronic sensorimotor neuropathy and ataxia. Hearing loss is common, so those patients who report hearing difficulties should have a full audiometric investigation (Bamiou et al. 2003). There is a range of hearing loss types in the condition, varying from mild, predominantly high frequency, to moderate, as well as some evidence to suggest that there may be subtle auditory nerve involvement. Oysu et al. (2001) described the absence of auditory brainstem responses but the presence of otoacoustic emissions in a case of Refsum disease with hearing loss. This suggests that the hearing loss might be secondary to auditory neuropathy, with the hearing abnormality determined from the post-outer hair cells level. There may therefore be limited benefits and a risk of noise-induced damage to outer hair cells with the use of hearing aids so the latter should be carefully considered and otoacoustic emission measurements undertaken for individuals with Refsum disease.

Mitochondriopathies
Cosegregation of the mitochondrial DNA A1555G and G4309A

mutations has been described that results in deafness and mitochondrial myopathy. Symptoms included progressive external ophthalmoplegia, exercise intolerance and deafness after aminoglycoside exposure (Campos et al. 2002). Mitochondrial cytopathies can present with a variety of symptoms but occasionally sensorineural hearing loss is the first manifestation, and some patients have been described who have responded well to cochlear implantation.

Sensorineural hearing loss is a common symptom in patients with myoclonic epilepsy associated with ragged-red fibres (MERRF). In this situation pure-tone threshold audiometry can show bilateral sloping type sensorineural hearing loss and the primary lesion appears to be in the cochlear, although there may be some involvement with retrocochlear structures (Tsutsumi et al. 2001).

There is a high incidence (42%) of sensorineural hearing loss in children with mitochondrial encephalopathies including Kearns–Sayre syndrome, Friedreich ataxia and MELAS (mitochondrial encephalopathy, lactic acidosis and stroke-like episodes). The hearing impairment is progressive but does not have a prognostic value for understanding the progression of the underlying disorder. Findings suggest that there may be cochlear and retrocochlear involvement (Zwirner and Wilichowski 2001). Histopathology in MELAS has shown that there is severe degeneration of the stria vascularis and degenerative change of spiral ganglion cells that causes the sensorineural hearing loss (Karkos et al. 2005).

BIOPTERIN DEFICIENCY (Chapter 8)
Three quarters of affected infants will develop a hearing loss that may be profound and that persists even after treatment is instigated (Wolf et al. 2002). Hearing loss can be completely prevented by presymptomatic diagnosis and the administration of supplemental biotin.

THE MOLECULAR BASIS FOR HEARING IMPAIRMENT

Mutations that affect transcription factors, intracellular proteins, transmembrane proteins, extracellular proteins and energy production can all result in hearing impairment (see Nance 2003 for a full review).

Mutations affecting transcription factors can result in severe forms of deafness. Defects in the PAX3, MITF and SOX10 genes cause forms of Waardenburg syndrome. Mutations that involve the POU4F3 and POU3F4 genes result in a dominant form of progressive hearing loss and the X-linked syndrome of congenital fixation of the stapes footplate. Branchio-oto-renal syndrome results from mutations involving the EYA1 and EYA4 genes.

Mutations that affect intracellular proteins can give rise to atypical myosins; different mutations in MYO7A can cause either dominant or recessive Usher syndrome; mutations involving MYO6 and MYH9 lead to progressive forms of dominant hearing loss; and MYO15 defects produce a profound congenital form of recessive hearing loss.

Mutations that give rise to abnormal structural proteins, such as those caused by defects in DIAPH1 and STRC, result in a progressive dominantly inherited hearing loss. The two genes are highly expressed in the hair cells where they promote actin polymerization and the production of stereocilin, which is a component of microvilla proteins. Mutations involving the TCOF1 gene on 5q31 cause Treacher Collins syndrome.

Mutations that affect transmembrane proteins can result in channelopathies, and these mutations involve at least three members of the connexin family of gap junction proteins: CX26, CX30 and CX43. Two potassium channel genes, KBLQT1 and KCNE1, maintain normal homeostasis of the cochlear endolymph, and defects in these genes cause two forms of the recessive Jervell–Lange-Nielsen syndrome. Defect in SLC26A4, which codes for a membrane-bound protein that is involved in ion transport, is the cause of Pendred syndrome.

CDH23 on 10q21 is a member of a calcium-dependent family of genes, the cadherins, that mediate cell adhesion, and abnormalities of this gene are known to result in deafness.

Mutations that involve the three collagen genes, COL2A1, COL1A2 and COL11A1, result in disturbance of extracellular protein and are the cause of three recognized forms of Stickler syndrome, while mutations involving COL4A5, COL4A3 and COL4A4 result in the autosomal and sex-linked forms of Alport syndrome.

Finally, hearing loss can result from abnormalities in energy production. As nuclear and cytoplasmic genes are active in the mitochondria at the site of oxidative phosphorylation, hearing loss can be part of a large number of complex neurological syndromes that involve deletions in the mitochondrial DNA or point mutations that involve mitochondrial t-RNAs. There is also the deafness/dystonia peptide, which is the product of a gene on Xq22 that produces deafness, blindness, retardation and dystonia in the Tranebjaerg syndrome.

CONGENITAL INFECTION

RUBELLA
Hearing impairment may be an isolated sequela of congenital infection with rubella, but rubella infection is currently very rare in the UK and the National Congenital Rubella Surveillance Programme reported that the incidence of congenital rubella births had fallen to an average of 4 per year over the period 1991–1995 (Miller et al. 1997). Even following a resurgence of infection in the community, only 12 congenital rubella births were reported in 1996 (Tookey and Peckham 1999). However, it is important to remember that the uptake of vaccine varies across countries and this can result in cohorts of susceptible women (Crowcroft and Pebody 2004).

CYTOMEGALOVIRUS (Chapter 10)
Twenty to 30 per cent of all deafness cases may be caused by cytomegalovirus (CMV), and congenital CMV infection results in sensorineural hearing loss in around one fifth of affected children (Barbi et al. 2003). Hearing loss may be progressive or fluctuating, and infants will need to be kept under review. However, ganciclovir therapy (Kimberlin et al. 2003) begun in the neonatal period in

symptomatically infected infants with CMV infection involving the central nervous system may prevent hearing deterioration at 6 months or even over 1 year. However, neutropenia is common during therapy affecting almost two thirds of treated infants.

TOXOPLASMOSIS
Congenital toxoplasmosis may cause hearing loss (Chapter 10).

SYPHILIS
Syphilis can also cause hearing loss in the secondary or tertiary phase, and a positive FTA-ABS test assists in diagnosis.

PERINATAL CAUSES OF SENSORINEURAL HEARING LOSS

The prevalence of significant sensorineural hearing impairment in children with birthweight <1500 g is around 51 per 10,000, compared to an overall rate of 5.3, thus almost 10 times the background level (Van Naarden and Decoufle 1999). All infants who experience an illness or condition that requires admission of 48 hours or greater to a neonatal intensive care unit should be considered as being at risk for sensorineural hearing loss (Joint Committee on Infant Hearing 2000). This risk is increased in the presence of intrauterine infections such as CMV, herpes simplex, toxoplasmosis or rubella, findings of stigmata or other features associated with a syndrome known to include a sensorineural and/or conductive hearing loss, a family history of permanent childhood sensorineural hearing loss, and craniofacial anomalies including those with morphological abnormalities of the pinnae and ear canal. Neonatal indicators include in particular hyperbilirubinaemia at a serum level requiring exchange transfusion, persistent pulmonary hypertension of the newborn that required mechanical ventilation, and conditions that have required the use of extracorporeal membrane oxygenation. Even short-term episodes of hyperbilirubinaemia can result in temporary and permanent evoked potential abnormalities including auditory brainstem threshold changes and prolonged auditory brainstem response wave (I–V) latencies, which suggests that both peripheral and central nervous systems are vulnerable to bilirubin insult. High sound pressure levels above 90 dB can cause damage to the inner ear and result in permanent hearing loss, and babies born to mothers exposed to noisy surroundings such as incubator noise and recreational activities such as fireworks may be at greater risk (Chang and Merzenich 2003).

POSTNATAL ACQUIRED HEARING IMPAIRMENT

MENINGITIS AND CENTRAL NERVOUS SYSTEM INFECTION
Meningitis is the most frequent cause of acquired sensorineural hearing loss in childhood. The risk of this sequela is increased with the development of hydrocephalus and/or if the child is aged below 1 month or over 5 years and the CSF glucose concentration is less than 2.2 mmol/L. Additional risk factors that increase the likelihood of a hearing loss following non-haemophilus bacterial meningitis include duration of symptoms before admission of over 2 days, absence of petechiae, cerebrospinal fluid glucose level <0.6 mmol/L, a *Streptococcus pneumoniae* infection and ataxia (Koomen et al. 2003). Most commonly there is either a completely flat audiogram or a predominantly high-frequency hearing loss. Brainstem auditory evoked potentials (BAEPs) from 101 children with bacterial or aseptic meningitis showed a frequency of BAEP impairment of 35% among those with bacterial meningitis, with 31% experiencing hearing loss on discharge, compared with rates of 21% and 14% respectively for aseptic meningitis. Most of the BAEP impairment in the bacterial meningitis cases was associated with Haemophilus influenzae infection. Follow-up in this situation with BAEPs is necessary for those children with initially abnormal findings as a small number return to normal and some deteriorate further (Bao and Wong 1998).

Since the introduction of the *H. influenzae* type B vaccine, *S. pneumoniae* has emerged as a dominant causative organism of bacterial meningitis in children, and 14% of 79 children with confirmed bacterial meningitis in one clinical series experienced permanent sensorineural hearing loss after confirmed bacterial meningitis (Wellman et al. 2003). Routine inpatient audiological screening of postmeningitic children has been advocated in order to avoid compliance problems with outpatient audiological assessment. High-frequency hearing loss has been described following Epstein–Barr virus infection, and sensorineural hearing loss is an important complication of mumps with mumps meningoencephalitis increasing this risk (Kanra et al. 2002).

OTOTOXICITY: DRUG-INDUCED HEARING LOSS
A wide range of drugs are associated with autotoxicity, including antimalarial drugs such as quinine and chloroquine, nonsteroidal anti-inflammatories including salicylate and indomethacin, loop diuretics including furosemide, chelating agents such as deferoxamine, and antibiotics including the aminoglycosides and other antimicrobials agents: chloramphenicol, colistin, erythromycin, minocycline, polymyxin B and vancomycin; these are reviewed by Schacht (2006).

Aminoglycoside ototoxicity occurs sporadically but also within families in association with a mitochondrial DNA (mtDNA) 155A to G point mutation in the 12S ribosomal RNA gene. Transmission of the same predisposing mutation can render individuals susceptible to sensorineural hearing loss following treatment with streptomycin (Fischel-Ghodsian et al. 1997, Gardner et al. 1997). Aminoglycosides can affect the vestibular system or result in destruction of hair cells in the organ of Cortey, depending on the type of aminoglycoside.

Ototoxicity to the cochlear or vestibular system can also follow the application of ototopic antibiotic ear drops (Matz 2004).

HEARING IMPAIRMENT ASSOCIATED WITH HAEMATOLOGICAL AND IMMUNOLOGICAL DISORDERS
The prevalence of sensorineural hearing loss is raised in sickle cell disease (Mgbor and Emodi 2004).

TABLE 18.1
Conductive hearing loss associated with skeletal dysplasias

Condition	Inheritance	References
Melnick–Needles syndrome	AD	Robertson et al. (1997)
Oto-palato-digital syndrome type II	XL	Zaytoun et al. (2002)
Autosomal dominant skeletal dysplasia with congenital stapes ankylosis	AD	Hilhorst-Hofstee et al. (1997), Brown et al. (2003)
Cerebrocostomandibular syndrome	AD	van den Ende et al. (1998)
Teunissen–Cremers syndrome	AD	Weekamp et al. (2005)
Van Buchem disease	AD	Vanhoenacker et al. (2003)
Cleidocranial dysplasia	AD	Visosky et al. (2003), Suba et al. (2005)
Dyschrondrosteosis	AD	De Leenher et al. (2003)
Osteogenesis imperfecta	Various (7 different types)	Imani et al. (2003)

AD = autosomal dominant; XL = X-linked.

High-frequency hearing loss and middle ear conductive loss have been described in leukaemia and thalassaemia. The thiamin-responsive megaloblastic anaemia also known as Rogers syndrome is an early-onset autosomal recessive disorder defined by the occurrence of megaloblastic anaemia, diabetes mellitus and sensorineural deafness (Neufeld et al. 1997).

There are reports of a possible autoimmune-related sensorineural hearing loss, and examination of erythrocyte sedimentation rate and immunoglobulins with their subclasses, complement studies and autoantibodies may be informative (Bamiou et al. 2000a).

OTOTOXICITY FROM ANTINEOPLASTIC CHEMOTHERAPY AND RADIOTHERAPY

Children treated for megaloblastoma, osteosarcoma and neuroblastoma have a greater incidence and severity of hearing loss as a sequela of treatment. Bilateral decreases in hearing were seen in 61% of 67 patients studied by Knight et al. (2005), and their median time to hearing loss was 135 days. Platinum compounds cysplatin and carboplatin are essential components in the chemotherapeutic treatment of a variety of paediatric malignancies. However, platinum agents have adverse effects including ototoxicity and associated permanent hearing loss. This is manifested as bilateral high-frequency sensorineural hearing loss, and with continued administration and cumulative dose, the hearing loss tends to increase in severity and progressively spreads to affect hearing at lower frequencies. Hearing loss can also progress after the completion of treatment and this has been reported in 15–20% of patients. Prior or concurrent craniospinal radiation enhances the ototoxicity of cysplatin. Young age at the time of treatment also increases a child's risk for ototoxicity (Knight et al. 2005). In addition to these agents, aminoglycosides and irradiation can adversely affect high-frequency hearing. A progressive hearing loss can occur after stereotactic radiation treatment in the management of posterior fossa tumours (Jackson et al. 2000).

NEUROFIBROMATOSIS

Neurofibromatosis type 2 can give rise to a vestibular schwan-noma that commonly presents with deafness and is sometimes associated with tinnitus, a facial nerve paralysis or headache. Vestibular schwannomas may be bilateral, and a few selected patients may benefit from auditory brainstem implants. Hearing loss can also occur in neurofibromatosis type 1 (Samii et al. 1997, Cunningham et al. 2005).

POST-TRAUMATIC HEARING LOSS

Falls and blows to the head that result in temporal bone fracture can result in hearing loss in over 80% of cases. Post-traumatic hearing loss may be related to a post-traumatic perilymphatic fistula, while minor head trauma may be associated with a progressive sensorineural hearing loss in the presence of a dilated vestibular aqueduct.

CONDUCTIVE HEARING LOSS

OTITIS MEDIA WITH EFFUSION

Otitis media with effusion (OME) affects 10–30% of 1- to 3-year-olds, and by the age of 4 years the cumulative incidence is 80%. By definition, OME involves a middle ear effusion without signs or symptoms of an acute infection and it is a sequel to acute otitis media. It can result in a conductive hearing loss of around 25–30 dB. Children with positive single tests need to begin a period of observation, as it seems that only long-term OME requires treatment (Butler and MacMillan 2001). Therapies offered for OME include decongestants, mucolytics, steroids, antihistamines and antibiotics, and myringotomy as the surgical treatment. A Cochrane review of treatment efficacy for children who were otherwise typically developing showed that the benefits of grommets was small. There is also a risk of tympanosclerosis from surgical procedures (Lous et al. 2005). A large trial (Paradise et al. 2005) followed children prospectively from the age of 2 months and then assigned those who had persistent middle ear effusion before the age of 3 years on a random basis to the insertion of tympanostomy tubes. There was no significant difference at the age of 6 years in the outcome measures of intelligence, language skills, central auditory processing, behaviour and emotion.

Measures of intellectual and language ability at the age of 6 are strongly predictive of later academic performance, so the authors concluded that it was unlikely that these children would develop later developmental difficulties. Lous et al. (2005), however, stressed that clinicians need to make decisions regarding treatment for children who have speech and language delays, behavioural and learning problems or defined clinical syndromes on an individual basis because such children have been excluded from the primary studies looking at the effectiveness of treatment of OME.

CONDUCTIVE LOSS FROM ISOLATED ANOMALIES OF THE STRUCTURE OF THE EAR

There is an autosomal dominant inheritance of round window atresia (Linder et al. 2003) and familial lateral semicircular canal malformation with external and middle ear abnormality (Matsunaga and Hirota 2003). There is also a dominant hereditary conductive hearing loss due to an ossified stapedius tendon.

There are a number of genetic causes of conductive hearing loss such as Mondini defect, which is a congenital malformation of the inner ear that is commonly associated with a sensorineural hearing impairment and also in some cases with CSF otorrhea or rhinorrhea and recurrent meningitis. Ossicular chain aplasias are described.

Apert syndrome is associated with craniosynostosis, midfacial malformations, and syndactyly of the hands and feet; it accounts for 4.5% of all cases of craniosynostosis. Congenital hearing impairment affects 3–6% of cases. Otitis media with effusion is the most common abnormality, and there is also an increased incidence of congenital ossicular abnormalities with ossicular chain fixation and congenital conductive hearing loss (Rajenderkumar et al. 2005a,b).

CONDUCTIVE HEARING LOSS ASSOCIATED WITH SKELETAL DYSPLASIAS

Many different forms of skeletal dysplasia have a conductive hearing loss component (Hilhorst-Hofstee et al. 1997, van den Ende et al. 1998, Brown et al. 2003, De Leenheer et al. 2003, Imani et al. 2003, Vanhoenacker et al. 2003, Visosky et al. 2003, Daneshi et al. 2005, Weekamp et al. 2005). Associated features are variable. The reader is referred to references in Table 18.1 for details.

Although these conditions are rare, it is important to appreciate that the diagnosis may be missed in females who have very mild craniofacial anomalies and whose deafness may be mistakenly attributed to an isolated ossicular deformity (Robertson 1997).

FANCONI ANAEMIA

Many morphological anomalies affecting the structures of the ear, head and neck are reported in Fanconi anaemia, although they are present in only a minority of patients. Conductive hearing loss, external auditory canal stenosis and auricular malformation have been described (Santos et al. 2002).

AUDITORY NEUROPATHY

The term auditory neuropathy describes functional disturbance or pathological change in the peripheral nervous system, although in this situation the exact site of a lesion is not known. Auditory neuropathy is a sensorineural disorder characterized by absent or abnormal auditory evoked potentials and normal cochlear outer hair cell function. In auditory neuropathy children show repeatable cochlear microphonic potentials in the absence of click-evoked auditory brainstem responses. Whilst the audiometric findings for some children with auditory neuropathy vary significantly, thresholds on behavioural testing range from normal to profound levels. Speech discrimination skills are also very variable, and in one series (Rance et al. 1999) half of the subjects showed little understanding or even awareness of speech inputs in both unaided and aided conditions. However, some children who scored at significantly impaired levels on a speech discrimination task did benefit from the provision of amplification. Auditory neuropathy can follow a compromised neonatal course, particularly in the presence of neonatal hyperbilirubinaemia, and it can also be seen in children who have a family history of childhood hearing loss (Joint Committee on Infant Hearing 2000). Auditory neuropathy can be associated with a loss of myelin. The pathophysiological changes in neural conduction properties associated with demyelination are likely to have a profound effect on auditory evoked responses as they are dependent on relatively precise synchronous response of a population of auditory nerve fibres to a transient acoustic stimulus. Auditory neuropathy has been described in Charcot–Marie–Tooth disease type 1 and in adrenoleukodystrophy.

MANAGEMENT OF SENSORINEURAL HEARING IMPAIRMENT

Permanent childhood hearing impairment can have a devastating impact on communication skills, educational attainments and quality of life, with resultant high cost to society. Outcomes are improved for children with congenital impairments if they are diagnosed and intervention commences by 6 months of age (Fortnum et al. 2001, Kennedy et al. 2006). Families should expect choice and confidentiality and communication in their native language. This communication should include: information about childhood hearing loss, the prevalence and effects of early hearing loss, the potential benefits and risks of screening and evaluation procedures, and prognosis and intervention. Hearing aid fitting may be indicated to give the child access to amplified speech. Cochlear implantation for profoundly deaf children continues to be offered at an earlier age of identification. Health, social services and education agencies all need to be associated with the child's early intervention.

The views and interests of individuals who are affected with deafness must be considered when developing policies regarding the appropriate use of genetic testing and counselling for families who carry the genes associated with hearing loss. The Joint Committee on Infant Hearing (2000) suggested benchmarks and quality indicators of service with comprehensive coordinated services between the infant's home, family, related professionals with expertise in hearing loss, and state and global agencies who are responsible for provision of services to children with hearing loss. Infants referred from universal neonatal hearing screening should have audiological and medical evaluations before the age of 3 months. Infants who are at risk of progressive or delayed-onset sensorineural hearing loss or conductive hearing loss should have audiological monitoring every 6 months until the age of 3 years. Early intervention services need to be designed to meet the individualized needs of the infant and family and to address the child's acquisition of communication with competent social skills, emotional well-being and positive self-esteem. Communication support planning needs to consider both a visual language and other sign systems as well as auditory oral communication.

HEARING AIDS

The successful rehabilitation of the deaf child employing hearing aids depends on careful assessment of hearing in all frequencies, individualized hearing aid prescription, and attentive follow-up and educational support. The primary aim is to make speech accessible for the child, and if insufficient care is taken in matching the aid to the child's needs, the aid will be rejected. Hearing aid technology advances rapidly but it cannot as yet completely compensate for the damaged human ear. This is because the mammalian cochlear outer hair cell system is a biologically active process that amplifies in a highly frequency-selective manner and with nearly instantaneous response (Dallos 1992). There are two reasons why an impaired ear cannot have its narrow tuning restored by a hearing aid: (i) because the outer hair cell system responsible for the tuning is compromised, and (ii) because hearing aids must amplify gain to input signals and therefore stimulate the cochlear at moderate and high levels where tuning is no longer narrow, even in a normal ear. This means that even the narrower span compression system will still produce broader than normal excitation in an impaired ear.

Hearing aids are either analogue or digital (Mueller 2000, Trine and Van Tasell 2002), depending on the technology used to process sound. They can come as a behind the ear hearing aid, an in the ear or in the canal aid, or a body-worn hearing aid. There are also bone conduction hearing aids for people with conductive hearing loss or people who cannot wear a conventional hearing aid, where the sound is delivered through the skull by vibration. An analogue hearing aid has a microphone that picks up sound and converts it into small electrical signals that vary according to the pattern of the sound; the signals are then amplified by transistors and fed to the earphone on the hearing aid so that they can be heard. Most of the more satisfactory analogue hearing aids compress the sound using automatic gain control. This amplifies quiet sounds until they are loud enough to be heard but gives less amplification to sounds that are already loud so that the child is protected against uncomfortably loud sound levels. In contrast, digital aids take the signal from the microphone and convert it into numerical data that can be manipulated by a computer in the hearing aid. This makes it possible to tailor and process sounds very precisely in ways that are not possible with analogue aids. Digital aids can be very finely adjusted to suit individual needs. They may have acoustic feedback suppression or feedback cancellation which helps reduce whistling noises.

INDUCTION LOOP AND INFRARED SYSTEMS

The loop system helps deaf people who use a hearing aid or loop listener to hear sound more clearly by reducing or cutting out background noise. Anyone sitting in an area of loop can pick up the sound if they switch their hearing aid or loop listening aid to the T setting. Electrical equipment and wiring can cause interference. As an alternative, an infrared system can be fitted; infrared receivers are not usually prone to interference, unless they are in direct sunlight.

RADIO MICROPHONE SYSTEMS

These systems are designed for use in classrooms or similar settings and they can help deaf learners hear the teacher or lecturer from a distance. Learners will need to be wearing hearing aids to benefit from them, and some systems also work with cochlear implants. The lecturer wears a clip-on microphone and the deaf learner wears the receiver.

SOUNDFIELD SYSTEMS

A soundfield system amplifies the teacher's voice at a low level and distributes it around the room from speakers mounted above head height. Deaf learners seated anywhere in the room will be able to hear equally well.

COCHLEAR IMPLANTATION

In cochlear implantation the sensory organ of the ear is replaced by an implantable electronic prosthesis. This cochlear implant stimulates the auditory nerve by electrical pulses and thus generates the sensation of hearing along the auditory pathway. In cochlear implants, the electrical signal provided by the device bypasses the portion of the auditory pathway linked to internal hair cells and the synapse to the auditory nerve fibre and stimulates the spiral ganglion cells directly. Cochlear implants in prelingually deaf children permit improved development of speech reception, language acquisition and reading comprehension (Rubinstein 2002, Francis and Niparko 2003, Ramsden 2004).

Cochlear implantation is a valuable intervention for the acquisition of speech perception and verbal language for children with severe to profound hearing impairment (Ramsden 2004, Francis and Niparko 2003). Early identification of the hearing loss, early hearing aid use, and language intervention and cochlear implantation by 2 years of age are positive predictors for language acquisition, which can even approach the levels of normal hearing children. Although implantation of children under the age of 2 years is potentially associated with higher surgical and anaesthesia risk, many results have been very positive (Rubinstein 2002). A late age of implantation does not preclude beneficial development of vocabulary (El-Hakim et al. 2001). Variations in the temporal bone anatomy in some patients such as those with CHARGE association can give increased technical challenges and an increased risk to the facial nerve during cochlear implantation. Cochlear implantation in children with inner ear malformations can give rise to complications such as CSF leak but can be a successful method of rehabilitation (Woolley et al. 1998). Children who have their hearing loss identified by the age of 6 months have been demonstrated to have significantly better language scores than children identified after this period (Yoshinaga-Itano et al. 1998).

PROGNOSIS

Studies from animal models and infant language acquisition suggest that early intervention with aiding is the aspiration in hearing impairment. However the literature also suggests that there are other important factors that influence prognosis. A report from a geographic cohort of intellectually normal children who had undergone neonatal screening for high risk infants revealed outcomes that were strongly related to the severity of the hearing impairment and not to the age of diagnosis. The non-verbal IQ also had an impact on prognosis in this report (Wake et al. 2005).

It is important to consider that up to 40% of children with a confirmed hearing loss have developmental delays or other disabilities. These need to be taken into account in the evaluation of a child who is failing to show the development of speech production that might be otherwise expected after successful aiding. Speech perception abilities of cochlear implant users and hearing aid users suggest that the performance of an average implant user is similar to that of a hearing aid user with a hearing loss of 70–90 dB. Cochlear implantation in infants between the ages of 6 and 18 months can give a good outcome, with prelexical babbling correlating significantly with the age of implantation (Schauwers et al. 2004). Speech and language proficiency is greater for children who had exhibited normal hearing for even a short period after birth and who received their cochlear implant shortly after losing their hearing (Geers 2004). Improvements in speech can continue over many years. Six years after cochlear implantation, a child's speech acquisition process is incomplete and there is no evidence of a plateau in performance, with the mean number of intelligible words per utterance increasing from 0.15 to 4.2. In children exposed to aural/oral communication rehabilitation, the age at implantation is an important variable affecting the level of speech production achieved by prelinguistically deaf cochlear implant users. The percentage of intelligible syllables shows a dramatic improvement in intelligibility in the first three years after implantation (Blamey et al. 2001).

CENTRAL AUDITORY PROCESSING DISORDERS

Central auditory processing disorder (CAPD) is an inability or impaired ability to attend, to discriminate, recognize, remember or comprehend information presented through the auditory channels even though the child has normal intelligence and hearing sensitivity (Keith and Pensak 1991). Functionally, the child shows a range of difficulties with: the localization of sound; binaural synthesis, in that stimuli presented simultaneously or alternately to opposite ears are incompletely perceived; and figure ground difficulties in which a primary signal or message is difficult for the child to perceive in the presence of competing sounds. In addition there are problems with binaural separation, memory for auditory stimuli, forming words out of separately articulated phonemes, discriminating two acoustic stimuli, perceiving whole words or messages when parts are omitted, showing listening attention over a reasonable period of time, associating correspondence between a non-linguistic source and its sound, and establishing a correspondence between the linguistic sound and the meaning.

Children with central auditory processing disorders show behavioural symptoms with: inconsistent responses to auditory stimuli; requesting that information be repeated; poor auditory attention; difficulty listening if there is background noise; easy distractability; problems with phonics and discrimination of speech sounds; poor auditory memory; and poor development of spoken and written language skills (Gordon and Ward 1995).

CAPDs would arise from situations in which information from the cochlear nucleus in the brainstem is affected in relaying to the auditory cortex or subsequently when handled by the cortical and subcortical auditory areas in order that audition can be fully appreciated and interpreted. Two main areas of controversy in the concept of CAPDs relate to how best to assess the symptomatology and avoid misinterpretation when, for instance, the primary reason for the child's presentation lies with an intellectual or attentional deficit, and how best to objectively measure the degree of processing dysfunction. Also, children may have a common aetiology such as hypoxic damage that has resulted in impairment to the auditory nuclei, brainstem and cerebral cortex and may be associated with a more peripheral sensorineural hearing loss. A number of acquired conditions that may result in CAPD have been described, including tumours of the auditory areas, meningitis, Lyme disease, head trauma, cerebral vascular accidents, heavy metal exposure, adrenoleukodystrophy, epilepsy and Landau–Kleffner syndrome (Bamiou et al. 2001).

CAPDs can also give rise to difficulties in modulating sound. Abnormal responses to sound can result in hyperacusis, which is a lowered hearing threshold; odynacusis, which is a lowered pain threshold for loud sounds; and auditory allodynia, which is a substantial aversion to or fear of certain sounds that are not normally found aversive. Some children also show auditory fascinations where there is a substantial attraction to or fascination with certain sounds.

Odynacusis is found in the majority of people with Williams syndrome. When pain is due to outer hair cell damage, it is termed 'recruitment'. People with Williams syndrome have a heightened non-habituating fear of certain sound classes. Typical populations will experience aversion to loud or startling sounds, or sounds that have an association with danger, such as sirens and babies crying or people screaming, but the response to sounds by people with Williams syndrome can be atypical in the magnitude of the reaction and in the types of sounds that the individual finds

19
DISEASES OF THE MOTOR NEURON

Since the almost complete disappearance of acute anterior poliomyelitis in industrialized countries, chronic degenerative diseases now account for most cases of anterior horn cell disease. In some developing countries, however, acute poliomyelitis remains a cause of involvement of the motor neurons of the spinal cord.

SPINAL MUSCULAR ATROPHY (SMA)

The spinal muscular atrophies constitute a heterogeneous group of disorders characterized by progressive degeneration of the anterior horn cells in the spinal cord and often of cells of the motor nuclei in the brainstem. Collectively, they represent the commonest degenerative disorder of the CNS and the second most frequent lethal genetic disorder of childhood after mucoviscidosis. Most are genetic diseases, with various modes of inheritance. Onset may be at any age from early infancy, or even the prenatal period, to adulthood. The mechanisms responsible for neuronal degeneration and death are still incompletely understood.

Involvement of the motor neurons may be diffuse or restricted to certain muscle groups. Most commonly, muscular weakness and wasting involve the proximal part of the limbs, but distal, scapulohumeral, facioscapulohumeral and segmental forms are known, and both the topography of involvement and mode of inheritance are important for the diagnosis.

Recently, considerable evidence that these disorders can also affect axons and a number of neurons outside the anterior horn cells has been presented.

CLASSIFICATION OF THE SMAs (Table 19.1)
Classification is difficult and several systems have been proposed, none of which is entirely satisfactory. Agreement has been reached regarding classification of the most common forms into three types. Type I, or Werdnig–Hoffmann disease, designates the easily recognizable early-onset acute form. The chronic forms are divided into type II, in which onset is later in the first year and the topography of weakness is diffuse with resulting deformities and severe disability, and the milder type III, also known as Kugelberg, Kugelberg–Welander or Wohlfart–Kugelberg disease, which has a later onset and mostly proximal involvement (Pearn 1980, Emery 1994). Dubowitz (1999) proposed the addition of a very severe form of prenatal onset (type 0) resulting in intra-uterine death or brief survival only with immediate need for respiratory support. There is in fact evidence that the SMAs may form a phenotypic continuum with intermediates between all the three classical types (Iannaccone 1998, Dubowitz 1999). This classification has supplanted previous schemes. The classical SMAs fulfil the following criteria (Munsat and Davies 1992): symmetrical muscle weakness of trunk and limbs more marked proximally than distally and predominating in the lower limbs; presence of tongue fasciculations and/or of tremor of the fingers, the latter also known as minipolymyoclonus, which is characteristic of anterior horn cell disease; EMG and biopsy demonstrating typical neurogenic abnormalities. Conversely, criteria of exclusion are: sensory involvement, evidence of CNS dysfunction, extensive arthrogryposis, elevation of creatine kinase to more than 10 times the maximum normal level, and reduction of nerve conduction velocity by more than 70%. However, some of these criteria need to be qualified in view of recent findings of more diffuse involvement. The three classical types have been shown to be allelic and linked to chromosome 5q13 markers (Brzustowicz et al. 1990; Melki et al. 1990a,b), and a gene at this locus, the *SMN* (survival motor neurons) gene, encoding a hitherto unknown protein of 294 amino acids, has been identified (Melki et al. 1994, Lefebvre et al. 1995). Deletion of exon 7 of this gene is found in 85–95% of all types of SMA (Rodrigues et al. 1996). Homozygous deletion of the *SMN* gene was found in 93% and interruption of the gene in 5.6% of patients with severe SMA. In general, severe forms are associated with large deletions that also remove adjacent genes (especially the *DNAI* gene), but deletion of exon 7 is sufficient to result in severe forms. In rare cases, the gene is neither lacking nor truncated, but a point mutation is present in exon 7, supporting the view that the *SMN* gene – and especially exon 7 – is responsible for the SMA phenotype. However, the *SMN* gene is present in two copies (telomeric or *SMN1* and centromeric or *SMN2*), and *SMN2* is able to code for some protective protein and may have a compensatory role and could rescue function of *SMN1*, even though this rescue may not be sufficient in most cases. As a result the number of copies of the *SMN2* gene can influence the severity of the clinical picture. Rare cases of normal carriers with homologous deletion of the *SMN1* gene have been identified (Cobben et al. 1995, Prior et al. 2004). In some such cases, a compensatory role of the *SMN2* gene has been considered, so some uncertainties persist even though the role of the *SMN1* gene is clearly essential. Some investigators (DiDonato et al. 1997) have proposed that conversion (i.e. exchange of DNA sequences between central and telomeric SMN genes so that the telomeric locus now possesses nucleotides normally associated with the centromeric locus,

TABLE 19.1
Classification of the main types of spinal muscular atrophy (SMA) in children

Type	Principal synonyms	Inheritance	Gene	Locus
SMA type I	Werdnig–Hoffmann disease; acute infantile SMA	AR	SMN1[1]	5q13
Chronic SMA				
Type II	Arrested Werdnig–Hoffmann disease; chronic generalized SMA	AR	SMN1[1]	5q13
Type III	Kugelberg disease; Kugelberg–Welander disease; Wohlfart–Kugelberg–Welander disease	AR	SMN1[1]	5q13
Spinal muscular atrophy with respiratory distress (SMARD1)	Severe infantile axonal neuropathy with respiratory failure (SIANRF)	AR	IGHMBP2[2]	11q13–q21
Severe forms of SMA				
Congenital SMA	Type 0 SMA	AR	SMN2[2]	?
SMA with pontocerebellar hypoplasia	Amyotrophic cerebellar hypoplasia; pontocerebellar hypoplasia type 1	AR	?	?
SMA with arthrogryposis and multiple bone fractures	—	AR	?	?
Benign familial SMA with hypertrophy of the calves	—	AD; XL?	?	?
Distal SMAs (several types)	Progressive SMA (Charcot–Marie type)	AD or AR	?	12q24?
Scapulohumeral and facioscapulohumeral SMA	Neurogenic facioscapulohumeral and scapulohumeral syndromes	AD, AR, XL?	?	?
Complex patterns of SMA	Madras type of SMA	?	?	?
Bulbopontine and bulbar types of neurogenic atrophy[3]				
Type 1	Brown–Vialetto–Van Laere syndrome	AR?[4]	?	?
Type 2	Fazio–Londe disease	AD, AR, XL	?	?

AR = autosomal recessive; AD = autosomal dominant; XL = X-linked.
[1]See text for genetic details.
[2]Probable.
[3]Spinal involvement is frequent but not constant.
[4]Dominant transmission in rare families.

which is unable to code for exon 7 but can code for exon 8) is frequently the cause of types II and III SMA. Such conversion, indistinguishable from deletion of exon 7 with usual techniques, has been thought to be commonly associated with chronic, relatively benign SMAs, while true deletion of exon 7 causes type I. However, it seems that deletion rather than conversion is implied in many cases, and multiple copies of the SMN2 gene are not consistently able to rescue most cases of deletion of SMN1 (Diep Tran et al. 2001, Harada et al. 2002).

Not all cases of SMA are associated with deletion of the SMN genes. Some less common forms of SMA are not linked to this gene or to chromosome 5. These include the SMARD1 syndrome with severe diaphragmatic paralysis (see below), cases of pontocerebellar atrophy with SMA (Chapter 9), some of the cases of SMA associated with arthrogryposis and congenital fractures, and rare cases of SMA with myoclonic epilepsy (Haliloglu et al. 2002, Striano et al. 2004). However, some cases with associated congenital heart disease and some cases with arthrogryposis and congenital fractures show the same deletion of exon 7 as the classical type (Bürglen et al. 1996, Melki and Munnich 1996, Garcia-Cabezas et al. 2004).

ACUTE INFANTILE SPINAL MUSCULAR ATROPHY, WERDNIG–HOFFMANN DISEASE, SMA TYPE I

The incidence of SMA type I is 1 per 20,000 live births, and the gene carrier frequency is 1 in 60–80 (Pearn 1980). It is associated with a deletion of exon 7 of the SMN gene in over 95% of cases. A deletion in the NAIP (neuronal apoptosis inhibitory protein) gene is also found in 50–60% of cases of SMA type I (Rodrigues et al. 1996), and large deletions of the 5q13 region seem to be correlated with the severe type of SMA (Spiegel et al. 1996). However, 27% of SMA type I cases have only a deletion of the SMN gene. Deletions in exon 3 have been found in some patients without exon 7 deletion (Cobben et al. 1995), resulting in a frameshift and a premature stop codon.

PATHOLOGY
Pathologically there is conspicuous loss of anterior horn cells. Residual motor neurons are in the process of degenerating with chromatolysis and eventual phagocytosis by satellite cells. Neurons in the cervical cord may be strikingly preserved (Kuzuhara and Chou 1981). Glial bundles have been observed in the anterior roots (Chou and Nonaka 1978) and in the posterior roots,

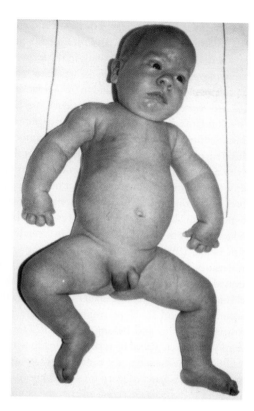

Fig. 19.1. Werdnig–Hoffmann disease (spinal muscular atrophy type I). Note narrow chest due to paralysis of intercostal mucles, flexion position of fingers, retrognathism and alert look.

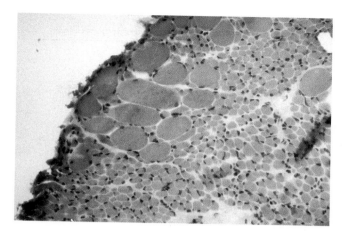

Fig. 19.2. Werdnig–Hoffmann disease. Muscle biopsy specimen showing fascicular atrophy typical of anterior horn cell involvement. Note that atrophic fibres keep a rounded contour that is unusual in spinal muscular atrophy of later onset, in which angular atrophic fibres are the rule. (Courtesy Dr MC Routon, Hôpital Saint Vincent de Paul, Paris.)

which are also shrunken. The significance of this finding remains obscure. Evidence of peripheral nerve involvement with loss of large myelinated axons (Chien and Nonaka 1989) is consistent with wallerian degeneration rather than indicating a dying-back process. However, more extensive sensory involvement is present in some cases (Anagnostou et al. 2005), and sensory neuropathy has been shown by systematic study of sural nerve biopsy and decreased sensory conduction velocity in 6 of 7 cases of type I SMA confirmed by molecular studies but not in types II and III (Rudnik-Schöneborn et al. 2003b). Supraspinal lesions are regularly present in the motor nuclei of the brainstem, notably in the hypoglossal nucleus, nucleus ambiguus and facial nucleus. Thalamic involvement is also a common feature. Such lesions may be responsible for alteration of sensory evoked potentials including somatic and visual potentials reported by Cheliout-Héraut et al. (2003).

CLINICAL FEATURES
The clinical manifestations of the disease are characteristic, permitting an almost immediate diagnosis except at the very onset. In about 30% of cases, the disorder has a prenatal onset and the infant is born with proximal weakness of the limbs and areflexia. The weakness spreads rapidly and, within a few weeks, there is marked quadriplegia with some preservation of distal movements, especially in the upper limbs. The paralysis is symmetrical and also involves axial muscles especially of the neck.

Paralysis of the intercostal muscle is a key feature of the condition. It produces a characteristic deformity of the thorax that is flattened laterally and remains immobile or paradoxically decreases in circumference during inspiratory movements, whereas the abdomen bulges, in a see-saw movement. Respiratory motions are performed almost exclusively by the diaphragm, which is spared until the late stages of the disease. Retrognathism, sometimes associated with fasciculations of the chin muscles, is constant and, together with preserved eye movements and vivid look, completes the characteristic appearance of the patients (Fig. 19.1).

Deep tendon reflexes are abolished. Tongue fasciculations are often present but may be difficult to distinguish from the frequent tremulous tongue movements of normal infants. There is no sensory loss, no pyramidal tract signs and no sphincter disturbances. Intelligence is preserved and the infants are usually described as very attractive.

The disorder in most cases is rapidly progressive, especially in prenatal forms and in acute cases of early onset. Death occurs within the first 18 months of life in 80% of cases and results from respiratory insufficiency, often precipitated and aggravated by intercurrent respiratory infections. Many infants have swallowing difficulties necessitating tube feeding. Patients with disease of neonatal onset often die before 3 months of age. Several reports (Russman et al. 1992, Iannacone et al. 1993) indicate a less gloomy outlook with much higher survival rates and better function, and Chung and Wong (2004) also found a significant improvement in outcome among Chinese children. However, some degree of selection of cases was not excluded and the prognosis of acute infantile SMA remains quite poor.

Type 0 SMA (Dubowitz 1999) designates the most extreme degree of the disease with prenatal onset resulting in death or inability to establish and sustain respiration from birth. This form requires immediate mechanical respiratory assistance, and attention to the major swallowing difficulties. Similar cases have

TABLE 19.2
Main causes of hypotonia in infants and young children[*]

Hypotonia with paralysis
  Spinal muscular atrophies
    Werdnig–Hoffmann disease (type I)
    Chronic spinal muscular atrophies (types II and III)
    Spinal muscular atrophy with respiratory distress (SMARD 1)
    Other rare forms
      With arthrogryposis
      With multiple bone fractures
      With pontocerebellar hypoplasia
  Congenital muscular dystrophies (Chapters 8, 21)
  Congenital myotonic dystrophy
  Congenital structural myopathies (Chapters 8, 21)
  Congenital and neonatal myasthenia (may last up to 1 year)
  Congenital neuropathies (Chapter 20)
  Disorders with combined CNS and PNS involvement
    Congenital disorder of glycosylation type I (Chapter 8)[1]
    Neuroaxonal dystrophy
    Mitochondrial diseases
    Peroxisomal diseases (Zellweger syndrome and neonatal adrenoleukodystrophy)
    Sensory neuropathy with spastic paraplegia (Cavanagh et al. 1979)
    Lowe syndrome (Charnas et al. 1988)

Hypotonia without paralysis
  CNS disorders
    Hypotonic cerebral palsy, especially the early stages of dystonic and ataxic cerebral palsy
    Metabolic disorders
      Aminoaciduria, organic acidurias, lactic acidosis, mitochondrial diseases, Leigh syndrome
      Lowe syndrome
      Degenerative diseases, e.g. leukodystrophies
      Glycogen storage disorders
    Chromosomal disorders
      Down syndrome
      Prader–Willi syndrome
    Nutritional and endocrine disorders
      Rickets, hypothyroidism, renal tubular acidosis
      Malnutrition, kwashiorkor
    Connective tissue disorders
      Ehlers–Danlos syndrome
      Congenital laxity of ligaments (arthrochalasis multiplex congenita)
      Osteogenesis imperfecta
      Mucopolysaccharidosis
    Benign congenital
      Dissociated motor development (hypotonia and delayed walking contrasting with fine motor development – Hagberg and Lundberg 1969), with or without 'shuffling'
      Benign idiopathic[2]

[*]Partially adapted from Dubowitz (1995).
[1]Cases with and without paralysis can occur.
[2]The existence of such cases is not proven.

been reported by MacLeod et al. (1999). Even within this form, variable degrees of severity can obtain, thus supporting the concept of a continuum of severity.

DIAGNOSIS
The diagnosis of SMA I can be confirmed by EMG examination, which shows neurogenic tracings with a reduced pattern of ac-

tivity during maximal effort, increased duration and amplitude of individual motor unit potentials, and increased incidence of polyphasic potentials. Spontaneous activity, in the form of rhythmical firing of motor units, is present in 69% of cases, and fibrillation and positive sharp waves are found in 35% (Hausmanowa-Petrusewicz and Karwanska 1986), but fasciculations are rarely visible in small infants. Large potentials are due to increased size of regenerating motor units adopted by remaining anterior horn cell neurons. Polyphasic potentials are common and probably result from the presence in muscles of numerous groups of small fibres without any sign of reinnervation and of the less tightly packed fibres within the motor unit. Motor nerve conduction velocities are normal or slightly slowed in most patients, but more marked reduction may be observed, especially in severely affected patients (Imai et al. 1990).

Serum creatine kinase is usually normal, although it may be mildly elevated in infants with a rapidly progressive form.

Muscle biopsy shows fascicles of small rounded fibres that belong to both types I and II. Hypertrophic fibres are scattered among atrophic fascicles and belong to type I. The normal checkerboard pattern is replaced by type grouping in which large numbers of fibres of the same type are contiguously arranged (Fig. 19.2). Muscle biopsy is *not* necessary for the diagnosis of SMA when clinical and EMG data are characteristic, and confirmation is best provided by genetic testing. Indeed, biopsy may be difficult to interpret in early cases or due to sampling problems, at a time when clinical and EMG diagnosis does not raise any difficulty when interpreted in the light of clinical evidence.

Diagnostic tests based on DNA analysis now replace previous diagnostic techniques. They are also effective for prenatal diagnosis (Stewart et al. 1998, Milunsky and Cheney 1999) and have a high level of reliability provided maternal DNA contamination is avoided. Jedrzejowska et al. (2005) were able to make the diagnosis in 263 of 266 cases (96.6%) tested using detection of exon 7 by standard PCR and a quantitative real-time PCR for more complex cases. Reliable preimplantation diagnosis is now possible (Malcov et al. 2004, Burlet et al. 2005).

The *differential diagnosis* of SMA type I is usually easy even though there are many causes of hypotonia in infancy (Table 19.2). *Congenital myopathies and congenital muscular dystrophies* may present in a similar manner with absent tendon reflexes. *Respiratory involvement* is different in such cases, with anteroposterior flattening of the chest as opposed to lateral compression in SMA. Facial affectation is usually present, and a neurogenic EMG pattern is not observed. Creatine kinase levels are raised. *Myasthenia gravis* should always be considered because it is a treatable condition but the clinical picture is different with predominant facial and ocular involvement in most cases. *Transection of the spinal cord* and congenital spinal tumours occasionally produce superficially similar features, especially with regard to respiratory muscle involvement and thoracic deformity. Systematic exploration of sensation in the lower part of the body and search for minor pyramidal tract signs are therefore important. *Infantile type 2 glycogenosis (Pompe disease)*, which produces a similar extensive muscle involvement, is invariably associated with cardiac affectation and often with CNS signs. Rare cases of *congenital or early neuropathy* are on record (Korinthenberg et al. 1997). Such patients have marked reduction of nerve conduction velocity and may have evidence of sensory impairment. The CSF may contain excess protein (Chapter 20). A rare mitochondrial disease with *cytochrome c deficiency* produces severe hypotonia with respiratory failure in the neonatal period. Renal tubular symptoms and CNS anomalies may be associated (DiMauro et al. 1985). An exceptional form of this disease is due to transient deficiency of cytochrome c and recovers with delayed maturation of the enzyme (Zeviani et al. 1987). Exceptional cases of type IV glycogenosis can also produce a similar picture (Tay et al. 2004).

MANAGEMENT

No effective treatment is yet available. Vigorous treatment of respiratory infections is indicated. Mechanical ventilation promotes expansion and growth of the lungs and can prolong survival of affected infants and alleviate parents' distress, but the intensity of therapy and especially the indications for long-term mechanical ventilation are extremely difficult to determine from a humane as well as from an ethical point of view (Gilgoff et al. 1989, Gordon 1991).

ATYPICAL FORMS AND THE LIMITS OF WERDNIG–HOFFMANN DISEASE

Spinal muscular atrophy with respiratory distress type 1 (SMARD1)

SMARD1 spinal muscular atrophy with paralysis of the diaphragm of early onset was initially regarded as an atypical form of SMA (McWilliam et al. 1985) in spite of the usual preservation of diaphragmatic function in the SMAs. In fact, it is due to a different genetic abnormality with mutations in the gene of the immunoglobulin μ binding protein 2 (*IGHMBP2*) on chromosome 11q13–q21. Several different mutations have been described, indicating allelic heterogeneity (Maystadt et al. 2004). The disease is inherited as an autosomal recessive condition and represents approximately 1% of early-onset SMA cases. It is clinically heterogeneous, with variable course. In most cases (Viollet et al. 2002, Grohmann et al. 2003, Pitt et al. 2003, Rudnik-Schöneborn et al. 2004) the clinical onset is within the first months of life, starting with generalized hypotonia, weak cry, stridor and foot deformities. Intrauterine growth retardation indicates abnormal prenatal development in three quarters of infants, and preterm birth occurs in over one third of gestations. Diaphragmatic palsy is usually apparent by 6 months to 1 year of age, often requiring permanent ventilation. Progressive distal muscular atrophy and joint contractures become rapidly apparent. Hand drops and fatty pads on the fingers are suggestive. Facial weakness is not a feature. Evidence of peripheral sensory and autonomic nerve involvement is often present, and the condition is also considered by some as a type of peripheral neuropathy (Pitt et al. 2003, Duval-Beaupere et al. 1994, Diers et al. 2005). Voiding dysfunction may occur, and evidence of autonomic dysfunction can be found with cardiac arrhythmia, hypertension and excessive sweating in some children. Decrease in conduction

velocity and EMG evidence of denervation are present in the majority of children. Progression of the disease is slow but respiratory distress is threatening and bulbar weakness may develop in some cases (Rudnik-Schöneborn et al. 2004). Prenatal diagnosis is possible (Grohmann et al. 2003, Sangiuolo et al. 2004).

However, the age of onset and severity may be variable even within the same family, with some patients having normal muscle strength until adult age and normal diaphragm function into adulthood (Viollet et al. 2002).

Amyotrophic pontocerebellar hypoplasia

A severe form of congenital SMA has been observed in a few families in association with pontocerebellar hypoplasia (see also Chapter 9). Such patients also have severe developmental delay, anterior horn cell involvement, evidence of peripheral nerve affectation with markedly slowed motor conduction velocities (Goutières et al. 1977, Kamoshita et al. 1990) and severe developmental delay. This condition features evidence of both spinocerebellar degeneration and malformation of the vermis and anterior lobe of the cerebellum, with severe hypoplasia also affecting the brainstem, and has also been termed infantile neuronal degeneration (Steinman et al. 1980), Norman disease (Kamoshita et al. 1990) and *pontocerebellar hypoplasia type 1* (Barth 1993). The disease features extensive contractures and is often rapidly lethal. However, some patients can present with milder symptoms and can survive to several years (Muntoni et al. 1999, Rudnik-Schöneborn et al. 2003a). The disorder is not linked to chromosome 5.

SMA with arthrogryposis and multiple bone fractures

This is an often rapidly lethal disorder (Van Toorn et al. 2002, Felderhoff-Mueser et al. 2002) and, like the previous two disorders, it is not related to a deletion in the SMN gene in all cases (Rudnik-Schöneborn et al. 1996), although Bürglen et al. (1996) demonstrated deletion of exon 7 in six of 12 infants with SMA with arthrogryposis, and Garcia-Cabezas et al. (2004) reported on a child with fractures and deletion of the *SMN1* gene.

SMA initially limited to, or clearly predominating in the cervical muscles (Fig. 19.3)

Some cases of progressive SMA involving initially and predominantly the cervical muscles may be distinct from classical Werdnig–Hoffmann disease (Goutières et al. 1991). Affected children may be able to walk. Secondary diffusion occurs in a descending manner with intercostal muscle paralysis eventually leading to respiratory failure and death. No DNA study was available in these cases.

Progressive SMA with ophthalmoplegia and pyramidal symptoms

This association has been observed in two siblings (Hamano et al. 1994). Similar cases with involvement of motor and sensory nerves and a rapidly lethal course have been shown to be associated with large deletions involving the *SMN* gene and several flanking markers (Korinthenberg et al. 1997).

Such atypical forms have bred true in several families, indicating that SMA is not a homogeneous group.

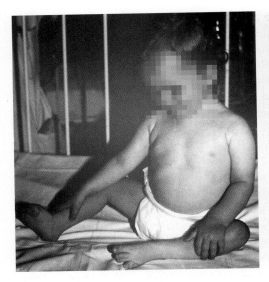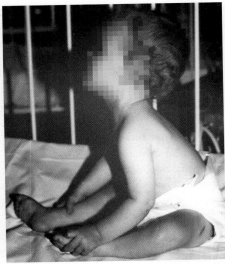

Fig. 19.3. Spinal muscular atrophy with cervical predominance. *(Left)* Head in forward flexion, the patient being unable to keep it erect. *(Right)* After being pulled back, the head cannot be put back to the forward position. (14-month-old girl with complete paralysis of both anterior and posterior cervical muscles with preservation of normal strength in lower limbs but some weakness and wasting of upper limbs.)

Acute-onset forms

Acute-onset forms following intercurrent infections have been reported (Robb et al. 1991).

CHRONIC SMA TYPE II, ARRESTED WERDNIG–HOFFMANN DISEASE

Type II SMA is also inherited as an autosomal recessive character in at least 90% of cases. According to the English SMA Study, the gene carrier frequency is 1 in 76–111 for the chronic forms (Pearn 1978, 1980). The different expression of the acute and chronic forms in which a similar DNA abnormality is present is as yet not understood. However, deletion of the *NAIP* gene has been found only exceptionally in SMA types II and III, and large-scale deletions of the 5q13 region are suggestive of Werdnig–Hoffmann disease (Burlet et al. 1996, Wang et al. 1997). The number of copies of the *SMN2* gene probably plays a role by coding for some active protein but cannot account for all the differences (Diep Tran et al. 2001, Harada et al. 2002, Prior et al. 2004). The pathology is similar to that of type 1 although less severe. In addition, the expression of neurofilaments is normal, contrary to what is observed in type I SMA (Araki et al. 2003).

Type II SMA has its onset after 3 months of age, although the exact date of the first manifestations is difficult to determine (Zerres et al. 1995, 1997) and may overlap with that of the acute form. Rare cases of occurrence of both type I and type II cases in the same pedigree are on record, but, much more frequently, this is only apparent and results from slow course of a few type I cases. The onset is generally insidious, the infant initially developing normally and attaining the first motor milestones up to the sitting position. Acquisition of standing posture is not acquired and even the sitting position is often abnormal with excessive curvature of the back. In some cases, onset is earlier with failure to reach more than head control. Conversely, in a few patients there is fairly rapid onset of weakness in the legs with loss of previous mobility. Eventually, weakness and atrophy are widespread, although some predominance in muscles of the pelvic girdle may persist.

The *course* is initially one of slowly progressive weakness and wasting. Stabilization is common after 1–2 years although there is no improvement, and late resumption of progression is rare. Deep tendon reflexes are abolished, except occasionally the distal reflexes. Fasciculations are often visible, and minipolymyoclonus is common. Swallowing usually remains normal. Involvement of intercostal muscles is present in about half the cases and, in such instances, develops before the age of 3 years. During childhood, contractures tend to develop and major deformities are extremely common (Fig. 19.4). These include hip dislocation and kyphoscoliosis that favours the development of respiratory complications (Merlini et al. 1989). Such complications may in turn precipitate neurological decompensation. Even with the best prevention of orthopaedic deformities, ambulation is never achieved when onset is before 2 years. Most patients survive to adult age. In the large series of Zerres et al. (1997) survival rates were 98.5 % at 5 years and 28.5% at 25 years of age. Mean age at death was 30 years in the study by Pearn et al. (1978), but longer survival is now more frequent not only in the intermediate types but also in classical forms.

The *pathological and EMG features* are similar to those of type I SMA. However, electrical fasciculation is often observed and pseudomyotonic discharges may be seen (Hausmanowa-Petrusewicz and Karwanska 1986). Motor nerve conduction velocities are mildly decreased, especially in the distal portions of nerves (Imai et al. 1990).

The *management* of patients with type II SMA poses numerous problems. Physiotherapy, prevention of deformities and attempts at verticalization are of utmost importance. Physiotherapy aims at maintaining articular motility and preventing muscle retractions and consequent deformities. Light orthoses can be used early for the same purpose. Prevention of scoliosis is especially important (Barois et al. 1989), whether by orthopaedic or surgical intervention.

Assisted non-invasive night-time ventilation by facial mask or buccal canula may be necessary for patients with intercostal muscle involvement. It should be started early enough to promote pulmonary growth and to maintain elasticity of the thorax (Duval-Baupère et al. 1985). According to Mellies et al. (2004), disordered sleep breathing is common but often unrecognized, and ventilatory assistance improves sleep and quality of life. Long-term mechanical ventilation raises a number of ethical and practical problems (Gilgoff et al. 1989).

Cognition is normal in the chronic forms of SMA. Language development was reported to be precocious in type II cases (Bénomy and Bénomy 2005). Spatial cognition was also found normal (Rivière and Lécuyer 2002). Integration of affected children into normal schools can be realized through the use of specially adapted school material and electric wheelchairs. Orientation of these normally intelligent patients toward activities that they will be able to perform, such as mathematics and writing, is a most essential part of overall management. Active psychological support of the patients and families should be provided.

CHRONIC SMA TYPE III (KUGELBERG DISEASE, KUGELBERG–WELANDER DISEASE, PSEUDOMYOPATHIC SMA, WOHLFART–KUGELBERG–WELANDER DISEASE)

This form is also transmitted as an autosomal recessive trait, although sporadic cases are not uncommon. It is also associated, in most cases, with a deletion in the *SMN1* gene. The onset of the disease may be at any age between infancy and early childhood and is extremely insidious. Two subtypes are often recognized: patients with subtype IIIa walk before age 3 years, those with IIIb after this age, and this difference may have a bearing on the prognosis (Rudnik-Schöneborn et al. 2001).

The parents may first notice the small volume of the child's thigh muscles or that s/he has difficulty rising from the floor. Weakness and amyotrophy clearly predominate on the proximal segment of the lower limbs and may involve electively the quadriceps. Examination shows a positive Gowers manoeuvre, wasting of proximal muscles and absent knee jerks with preservation of ankle jerks and of reflexes of the upper limbs. The picture thus bears a close clinical resemblance to the muscular dystrophies with a waddling gait. Calf hypertrophy may be present in some patients, completing the resemblance to Duchenne dystrophy (Bouwsma and Van Wijngaarden 1980). The disease progresses very slowly towards the distal lower limbs and/or the proximal upper limbs. Pes cavus is frequent. Many patients show a coarse *tremor of the hands* (Dawood and Moosa 1983) that is probably related to imperfect synchronization of a diminished number of

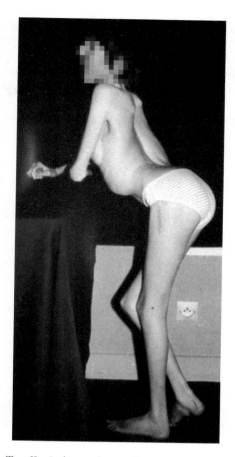

Fig. 19.4. Type II spinal muscular atrophy. Diffuse amyotrophy of limbs and marked kyphoscoliosis in 14-year-old girl. (Courtesy Dr J-P Padovani, Hôpital des Enfants Malades, Paris.)

large motor units resulting from collateral reinnervation of fibres by remaining neurons. The ECG shows tremulousness of the baseline, presumably reflecting the same muscular tremor. Most affected individuals can continue to lead normal lives into adulthood (Zerres et al. 1995, 1997) but some cases run a faster course; orthopaedic complications can produce severe functional limitations which should be avoided by appropriate physiotherapy and/or orthopaedic management. Proper counselling with insistence upon acquisition of skills likely to be maintained over long periods is of utmost importance. In rare cases, congenital (Oka et al. 1995) or progressive (Alberfeld and Namba 1969) ophthalmoplegia is associated.

Distinguishing type III SMA from muscular dystrophy may be difficult as the clinical picture may be suggestive and the creatine kinase level may be moderately elevated. Muscle biopsy is sometimes difficult to interpret, as 'myopathic' changes such as split or necrotic fibres, central nuclei and some increase in fibrous and fatty tissue may be observed. EMG is the best examination and is sufficient for the diagnosis in this writer's experience. In addition to myogenic diseases, differential diagnosis also includes rare diseases such as 'adult-type' gangliosidosis that may present with isolated anterior horn cell involvement (Navon et al. 1995) and exceptional cases of intramedullary tumours presenting as isolated SMA (Aysun et al. 1993).

The *management* of type III SMA is based on physiotherapy and prevention of contractures and retractions. In both types II and III, several trials of drugs that can provoke changes in the reading of DNA have been made. These include gabapentin (Miller et al. 2001, Merlini et al. 2003), riluzole (Russman et al. 2003), phenylbutyrate (Mercuri et al. 2004a). Despite some positive results, none has reached practical use. Gene therapy is being studied (DiDonato et al. 2003).

DIAGNOSIS BY MOLECULAR GENETICS OF THE RECESSIVE PROXIMAL SMAS

Diagnosis of the three classical types of SMA by molecular genetics is possible, mostly by demonstration of homozygous deletion of exon 7 in the *SMN1* gene (Melki et al. 1994). However, a deletion is not present in a variable but small proportion of patients with SMA; rare persons with homozygous deletion may be phenotypically unaffected; and the relationship of the *SMN* genes to SMA has not yet been fully determined.

Approximately 10% of SMA cases (e.g. SMARD1, SMA with olivopontocerebellar atrophy) are not associated with a deletion or linked to chromosome 5 (Novelli et al. 1995, Rudnick-Schöneborn et al. 1995). Conversely, a number of cases in which one or several of the accepted exclusion criteria (Munsat and Davies 1992) are present may show a typical deletion, including cases with CNS dysfunction, arthrogryposis or associated malformations (Rudnik-Schöneborn et al. 1996).

DNA analysis makes prenatal diagnosis of most types of classical SMA possible and reliable (Cobben et al. 1993, Wirth et al. 1995). A DNA test using polymerase chain reaction is available (Van der Steege et al. 1995). The basis of this test is demonstration of homozygous deletion of exon 7 of the *SMN* gene. It is relatively easy to perform but may be negative in around 2% of affected children who harbour a different DNA defect (Raymond 1997).

OTHER TYPES OF SMA

DOMINANT DIFFUSE (OR PROXIMAL) FORMS OF CHRONIC SMA

Dominant forms of chronic SMA are uncommon in childhood (Emery et al. 1976a,b; Pearn et al. 1978; Boylan and Cornblath 1992). These forms usually have a slowly progressive course. They represent less than 2% of childhood cases but up to 30% of adult cases (Pearn 1978) and are also known in adults as *type IV SMA*. There may be two distinct genes: early-onset forms begin between birth and 8 years of age and do not have a marked selectivity for proximal muscles; late-onset forms are seen in young adults and have a marked proximal selectivity. A few families with early-onset SMA affecting predominantly the lower limbs with feet deformity and severe interference with ambulation have been recently reported (Merçuri et al. 2004b). Clinically similar cases have been shown to map to chromosome 12q23–q24 (van der Vleuten et al. 1998). Some other cases of chronic SMA may represent non-genetic phenocopies or new dominant mutations (Pearn 1980).

SEX-LINKED SMA

Rare cases of sex-linked SMA are on record in adults (Paulson et al. 1980) and in children (Skre et al. 1978). In the kindred reported by Skre et al., some patients had a pattern of diffuse involvement and others a scapuloperoneal pattern. These X-linked forms may be different from the proximal form of adult proximal neuronopathy, or *Kennedy disease* (Guidetti et al. 1986), which features bulbar muscle involvement, gynaecomastia and frequent asymmetry of involvement in addition to proximal SMA. The gene is located on the proximal long arm of chromosome X and includes a CAG repeat whose expansion is associated with the clinical disease. The gene codes for cell surface androgen receptor (Doyu et al. 1992).

DISTAL SMA

This form presents with features similar to those of the peroneal muscle atrophies. In the large series of Harding and Thomas (1980) it accounted for 13% of 262 cases. At least seven genes have been implicated (Dierick et al. 2008) but there is no linkage to chromosome 5. Dominant inheritance was predominant, but recessive forms are also known (Harding and Thomas 1980) and sporadic cases are frequent. There is a marked excess of males especially in mild forms, suggesting an X-linked inheritance in some families. The disease is difficult to distinguish from the neural peroneal atrophies, especially as these may not show any sign of sensory impairment at onset. Criteria for diagnosis should therefore include: (1) distal muscular atrophy usually predominant in the lower limbs; (2) absence of sensory anomalies; (3) concordant EMG and pathological evidence of anterior horn cell affectation; and (4) a period of at least 18 months free of sensory signs (Harding and Thomas 1980). Pes cavus, often severe, is a common presenting sign. Ankle jerks and upper-limb tendon reflexes are often preserved in contrast to what is seen in Charcot–Marie–Tooth disease. Age of onset varies from infancy to middle life and may differ within the same kindred (Boylan et al. 1995). Cases mapping to chromosome 12q24 are on record (De Angelis et al. 2002). The course is usually slow but progressive, patients needing calipers or other walking aids by 25–30 years of age, although many are only moderately disabled in adulthood. In rare forms, the upper extremities are affected first and predominantly, with a slow course (Timmerman et al. 1996, Hedge et al. 2001). These forms seem to be dominantly inherited or sporadic. An association with *optico-acoustic atrophy* has been reported (Chalmers and Mitchell 1987). A previously described association of distal SMA with vocal cord paralysis (Boltshauser et al. 1989) has been shown to be due to a neuropathy rather than to anterior horn cell disease. Bertini et al. (1989) reported the association of a distal SMA with diaphragmatic paralysis.

SCAPULOPERONEAL SMA

The scapuloperoneal syndrome, characterized by wasting and weakness in the shoulder girdle and anterior muscles of the leg, can be due to myopathic, neural or anterior horn cell involvement. The latter type is the most common (Mercelis et al. 1980). It is usually inherited as an autosomal dominant trait but recessive inheritance and X-linked transmission (Thomas et al. 1972) may occur. A linkage to chromosome 12q24–31 was found in one kindred (Isozumi et al. 1996). Some investigators (e.g. Dubowitz 1995) have expressed doubts about the reality of SMA as a cause of scapuloperoneal syndrome.

Facioscapuloperoneal SMA is a rare type that simulates the more common facioscapulohumeral muscular dystrophy. The genetic transmission is autosomal dominant. Onset is by facial diplegia with progressive downward extension of weakness (Furukawa and Toyokura 1976). In one child, optic atrophy and sensory and autonomic disturbances were associated (Schmitt et al. 1994).

Benign Familial SMA with Hypertrophy of the Calves

Hypertrophy of the calves may be relatively common in chronic SMAs (Bertorini and Igarashi 1985). Bouwsma and Van Wijngaarten (1980) found it in 29 of 100 patients. All were males, suggesting that an X-linked factor might be at play. D'Alessandro et al. (1982) described a dominant form in a father and son.

UNCONVENTIONAL PATTERNS OF SMA
Monomelic or Asymmetrical SMA
A monomelic or clearly asymmetrical form of progressive SMA has been reported, originally from Japan where the condition seems to be prevalent (Hirayama et al. 1987), and subsequently also in other countries (Tandan et al. 1990, Liu and Specht 1993, Restuccia et al. 2003). The disease predominantly affects males, and clinical features of the condition include a juvenile onset, between 15 and 25 years, of an insidiously progressive muscular atrophy not precipitated by any infection or trauma. The atrophy does not involve the brachioradialis muscle and is associated with weakness exaggerated by cold (cold paresis) and with fine irregular tremor. Both sides may be involved, almost always in a very asymmetrical manner. Denervation changes are shown by EMG and muscle biopsy, and are often bilateral (Misra et al. 2005) even when clinical involvement appears to be unilateral. There is no sensory impairment, and conduction velocities are normal. The disorder is usually sporadic but a few familial cases are known (Tandan et al. 1990). Pathological lesions (Hirayama et al. 1987) include shrinkage and necrosis of large and small motor nerve cells. Several recent studies point to the probability of a cervical myelopathy associated with venous dilatation associated with neck flexion of traumatic origin (Hirayama and Tokumaru 2000, Restuccia et al. 2003, Baba et al. 2004).

Complex Patterns of SMA
Juvenile motor neuron disease is common in southern India. The best-defined type is known as Madras type. The disease is usually sporadic; it predominates in males and its onset is during the second decade of life. The upper limbs are initially and preferentially affected, although the lower limbs eventually become involved. Sensorineural deafness is present in one third of the patients, and bulbar involvement is is found in about 40% of cases (Gourie-Devi and Suresh 1988). The disease is slowly pro-

gressive and not uncommonly becomes arrested. A variant with optic atrophy and cerebellar involvement has been described (Gourie-Devi and Nalini 2003).

BULBAR AND BULBOPONTINE TYPES OF NEUROGENIC MUSCULAR ATROPHY; CHILDHOOD AND JUVENILE PROGRESSIVE BULBAR PALSY; BULBAR HEREDITARY NEUROPATHY TYPE 2 (BHN2)
Progressive bulbar palsy is a form of motor neuron disease with predominant involvement of bulbar muscles, although muscles innervated by pontine, spinal and, occasionally, midbrain motor neurons may also be involved.

Only those cases with 'pure' involvement of brainstem nuclei are considered here. Some cases that feature both bulbar paralysis and extensive involvement of limb and trunk muscles are difficult to differentiate from the SMAs. Cases with definite involvement of the long tracts, especially the corticospinal tracts, can be regarded as a form of lateral amyotrophic sclerosis and are studied later in this chapter. The mere presence of some pyramidal tract signs may not be sufficient for exclusion from the syndrome.

The eponym *Fazio–Londe disease* is often applied to the childhood form. Age of onset may be variable within the same kindred (Albers et al. 1983). Typically the disease begins between 2 and 12 years by nasal speech, stridor and often repeated respiratory infections. Dysphagia, facial diplegia and sometimes oculomotor paralyses progressively develop and may lead to death in around 18 months to 10 years (Della Giustina et al. 1979, Beauvais et al. 1988). Involvement of the spinal musculature is variable. McShane et al. (1992) reported five cases and distinguished three different forms: a dominant type is exceptional; recessive forms can present with early onset before 2 years of age, stridor and respiratory difficulties resulting from vocal cord paralysis, and involvement of the lower cranial pairs, the facial nerve and, sometimes, the oculomotor nuclei, and are often lethal in 2–3 years. A more benign and protracted form features dysarthria, dysphagia and facial weakness rather than respiratory symptoms and may be seen even in adults. There is a strong concordance of each pattern within the same family. Pathologically, there is marked degeneration of the cranial motor nuclei with variable involvement of motor neurons in the spinal cord.

Cases of childhood and juvenile progressive bulbar palsy usually have dominant or recessive inheritance (Beauvais et al. 1988), or rarely are X-linked (Boz et al. 2002). Recessively inherited forms are not necessarily severe (Beauvais et al. 1988). This disorder should be differentiated from other lesions of the brainstem such as myasthenia gravis, tumours or encephalitis, from Miller Fisher syndrome, and from the rare cases of congenital oculobulbar palsy (Jennekens et al. 1992) that may be related to congenital myasthenia.

Brown–Vialetto–Van Laere Syndrome (Bulbar Hereditary Neuropathy Type 1)
Juvenile-onset bulbospinal muscular atrophy also occurs in asso-

ciation with deafness (Brown–Vialetto–Van Laere syndrome). In this rare, probably autosomal recessive syndrome, bilateral neural deafness first appears in late childhood or adolescence. Vestibular areflexia is associated. Subsequently, involvement of several cranial nerves appears, causing facial diplegia, dysarthria and dysphagia. Infantile onset with secondary development of deafness has been reported (Voudris et al. 2002). Optic atrophy is occasionally observed as well as mild cerebellar and pyramidal signs (Brucher et al. 1981). The course of the disease is slow and some patients may survive to their fourth decade, but respiratory insufficiency and swallowing difficulties eventually develop and lead to death (Gallai et al. 1981, Summers et al. 1987). Degenerative lesions of the first and second neurons of the auditory and vestibular pathways are evident along with gliosis of the vestibular and cochlear nuclei and superior olives. The condition is apparently inherited as an autosomal recessive trait.

ASSOCIATED OR COMPLICATED SMAs
SMA occurs in association with involvement of CNS structures in several rare multisystem disorders, the most important being amyotrophic lateral sclerosis (ALS), which is mostly a sporadic disease of adults and clinically is characterized by the association of lower motor involvement with pyramidal tract signs. About 10% of cases are genetically determined, caused by at least eight different mutations. ALS occurs rarely in young individuals (juvenile ALS), and several mutations and clinical pictures have been described.

Juvenile Amyotrophic Lateral Sclerosis
The clinical presentation of juvenile ALS is variable. Most cases seem to belong to ALS2, and present as a chronic condition with upper-limb amyotrophy and sometimes also bulbar amyotrophy, with bilateral pyramidal tract signs, and closely resemble adult amyotrophic lateral sclerosis but with a relatively benign, slow course and a familial (autosomal recessive) origin. True cases of ALS are difficult to separate from other conditions with chronic amyotrophy and some forms of familial spastic paraplegia. The patients reported from Tunisia by Ben Hamida et al. (1990) belonged to three subgroups. The largest group consisted of clinically typical cases and these were later shown by Hentati et al. (1994) to be linked to mutation of a gene on chromosome 2q33, coding for the protein alsin. The other two groups included cases of spastic paraplegia associated with peroneal atrophy or with spastic and pseudobulbar syndrome and are regarded as a form of hereditary spastic paraplegia, one of which is associated with a mutation in the alsin gene (Gros-Louis et al. 2003) (Chapter 9).

Infantile-onset ascending hereditary spastic paralysis (IAHSP) (Eymard-Pierre et al. 2002) is clinically distinct from ALS but is also due to mutation in the alsin gene. Lesca et al. (2003) reported on 16 cases of IAHSP in 11 families from Europe and North Africa. These were characterized by an onset in the first 2 years of life of a spastic paraplegia ascending to involve the upper limbs at the end of the first decade, then slowly progressing during the second decade, to result in tetraplegia, anarthria, dys-

phagia and slow eye movements. Intellect remained normal and the patients had a prolonged survival. There was no evidence of lower motor neuron affectation. Imaging showed bilateral hypersignal in the posterior arm of the internal capsule and some degree of cortical atrophy in the oldest patients. A mutation of the alsin gene was found in four of 10 families studied, but was excluded in another case. The syndrome is thus genetically heterogeneous. Despite the presence of an alsin mutation it is clearly different from ALS but its nosological situation remains unclear (Eymard-Pierre et al. 2006).

The other types of early-onset ALS are very rare. ALS 4 resembles purely motor neuropathy with some pyramidal components and no bulbar signs and is linked to 9q34 (De Jonghe et al. 2002). ALS 5 is linked to chromosome 15q15.1–15q21.1 (Hentati et al. 1994) with clinical features of adult ALS but a more benign course.

A familial degenerative disease of the anterior horn cells and pyramidal tracts, often in association with parkinsonism, dementia and a lethal course is still seen among the Chamorro people on the island of Guam although its frequency has dramatically declined. The cause remains enigmatic (Galasko et al. 2002).

SMA may also occur in association with involvement of the posterior columns of the spinal cord (Engel et al. 1959), and more complex cases including pyramidal, spinocerebellar and thalamic involvement are known (Grunnet and Donaldson 1985).

Primary Lateral Sclerosis
This condition is exceptional in children (Grunnett et al. 1989). It presents with progressive spastic and bulbar syndrome (Lerman-Sagie et al. 1996). Familial cases associated with a pseudobulbar syndrome and gaze paresis have been reported by Gascon et al. (1995). A mutation in the alsin gene on chromosome 2q33 has been found in some cases (Yang et al. 2001).

Agenesis of the Corpus Callosum with Neuronopathy (Andermann Syndrome)
A syndrome featuring agenesis of the corpus callosum, anterior horn cell disease, a mixed sensory and motor neuropathy, and facial dysmorphism occurs in Quebec and is inherited as an autosomal recessive trait (Larbrisseau et al. 1984, Hauser et al. 1993). The gene has been identified (Howard et al. 2002). Mild mental retardation is also a feature. The course is slowly progressive but lifespan seems to be normal (Chapters 2 and 20).

Other Complicated SMAs
The adult form of hexosaminidase A deficiency can occur in childhood. It regularly features anterior horn cell involvement with a slowly progressive course, beginning in half the cases before age 10 years. Associated dystonia and pyramidal tract signs are frequent (Specola et al. 1990) but pure affectation of the anterior horn cells is occasionally seen (Johnson et al. 1982).

SMA with Retinitis Pigmentosa
Rare cases of familial progressive atrophy of the arms, shoulders, neck and chest with loss of tendon reflexes and associated deaf-

TABLE 19.3
Disorders with associated peripheral and CNS involvement

Disease	References
With predominant involvement of spinal cord, especially anterior horn cells	
Infantile neuroaxonal dystrophy	Chapter 9
Hexosaminidase A deficiency	Chapter 8
Neuronal inclusion disease	Chapter 9
Amyotrophic cerebellar hypoplasia (pontocerebellar hypoplasia with anterior horn cell disease, Norman disease)	Chapters 9, 20
Andermann syndrome (callosal agenesis and neuronopathy)[1]	
Viral infections (poliomyelitis with brain involvement, West Nile encephalitis, tick-borne meningoencephalitis)	This chapter
Triose-phosphate isomerase deficiency	Poll-Thé et al. (1985)
Rett syndrome	
With predominant involvement of nerves	
Leukodystrophies	Chapters 8, 9
Metachromatic	
Krabbe	
Cockayne	
Pelizaeus–Merzbacher (some cases)	Chapter 9
Spinocerebellar degenerations	Chapter 9
Friedreich ataxia	
Troyer syndrome	
IOSCA (infantile-onset spinocerebellar ataxia)	
Charlevoix–Saguenay ataxia)	
Machado–Joseph disease (SCA3)	
Behr syndrome	
Spastic paraplegia with neuropathy	
Metabolic and degenerative diseases	
Adrenomyeloneuropathy	Chapter 8
Bassen–Korzweig disease (abetalipoproteinaemia)	Chapters 8, 9
Vitamin E malabsorption	Chapters 8, 20
Giant axonal neuropathy	Chapter 20
Refsum disease	Chapters 8, 20
Leigh disease	Jacobs et al. (1990)
Mitochondrial cytopathy, especially MELAS, Leigh/NARP, MNGIE[2]	Chapter 8
Glycosylation defects (esp. type 1)	Chapter 8
Cerebrotendinous xanthomatosis	Chapter 8
Sialosidosis 1	Steinman et al. (1980)
Lowe syndrome	Kawano et al. (1998)
Ataxia–telangectasia	Kwast and Ignatowicz (1990)
Malnutrition, folate deficiency	Chopra and Sharma (1992)
Short- and long-chain hydroxy acid deficiency (SCHAD, LCHAD)	Dionisi Vici et al. (1991), Tein et al. (1995)
Malignant diseases (leukaemia, lymphoma)	Chapter 13
Inflammatory diseases	
Inflammatory neuropathy with CNS involvement	Uncini et al. (1999)
Collagen disorders (e.g. lupus erythematosus)	Chapter 11
Dysimmune disorders	
Chediak–Higashi disease	Van Hale (1987), Barrat et al. (1988)
Lymphohistiocytosis	Boutin et al. (1988)
Toxic disorders	Chapters 12, 20

[1]Several mechanisms probably involved.
[2]NARP = neurogenic muscle weakness, ataxia, retinitis pigmentosa; MNGIE = mitochondrial neurogastrointestinal encephalomyopathy.

ness, typical bone corpuscle retinopathy and mental retardation have been described (Walsh and Hoyt 1969). A spastic component was probably present. The association of retinitis pigmentosa and muscle weakness is more commonly due to mitochondrial disease, and the weakness is then usually of myogenic origin (Chapter 8). Several other conditions featuring both peripheral and CNS involvement are listed in Table 19.3. In this table, disorders involving the axons rather than the anterior horn are also indicated, as the clinical problems they pose are very similar to those posed by anterior horn involvement.

ACQUIRED MOTOR NEURON DISEASES

Acquired motor neuron diseases are mainly of viral origin; the role of toxic, vascular or other environmental factors in the aetiology of amyotrophic lateral sclerosis and other related syndromes has been discussed by Wicklund (2005).

Most acquired viral diseases of the anterior horn cells run an acute course. They are mainly represented by *acute anterior poliomyelitis* and similar diseases due to enteroviruses other than the polioviruses.

Acute poliomyelitis is by far the commonest cause of acquired anterior horn cell disease. It unfortunately remains prevalent in some developing countries. In industrialized countries, only rare cases occur in unvaccinated children. Occasional cases of paralytic poliomyelitis due to attenuated live vaccine virus have been reported in recipients of the vaccine or in contacts, mainly in children with immunodeficiency. Poliomyelitis has been discussed in Chapter 10. Poliomyelitis-like diseases due to other enteroviruses including members of the Coxsackie and echo virus groups have been reported.

West Nile encephalomyelitis, a tick-borne flavivirus infection, has been responsible for epidemics of meningoencephalitis in several US states. It can also give rise to a poliomyelitis-like disease, with initial fever and meningeal signs with CSF pleocytosis, followed within a few days by focal asymmetical flaccid paralysis that may be more or less extensive (Jeha et al. 2003). The electrophysiological features are indistinguishable from those of paralytic poliomyelitis (Al-Shekhlee and Katirji 2004), and MRI can show high-density T_2 images in the anterior horn cell (Jeha et al. 2003). A similar disease might also result from infection by the flavivirus of Japanese encephalitis (Arya 1998). With the development of air travel, similar cases are likely to be observed in Europe. Rare cases of polio-like disease due to the virus of European tick-borne encephalitis have been reported (Aendekerk et al. 1996).

Hopkins syndrome, which consists of acute poliomyelitis-like paralysis following an attack of asthma, may be of viral origin (Arita et al. 1995).

REFERENCES

Aendekerk RP, Schrivers AN, Koehler PJ (1996) Tick-borne encephalitis complicated by a poliomyelitis-like syndrome following a holiday in central Europe. *Clin Neurol Neurosurg* 98: 262–4.
Alberfeld DC, Namba T (1969) Progressive ophthalmoplegia in Kugelberg–Welander disease. Report of a case. *Arch Neurol* 20: 253–6.

Al-Shekhlee A, Katirji B (2004) Electrodiagnostic features of acute paralytic poliomyelitis associated with West Nile virus infection. *Mucle Nerve* 29: 376–80.

Albers JW, Zimnowodzki S, Lowrey CM, Miller B (1983) Juvenile progressive bulbar palsy. Clinical and electrodiagnostic findings. *Arch Neurol* 40: 351–3.

Anagnostou E, Miller SP, Guiot MC, et al. (2005) Type I spinal muscular atrophy can mimic sensory–motor axonal neuropathy. *J Child Neurol* 20: 147–50.

Araki S, Hayashi M, Tamagawa K, et al. (2003) Neuropathological analysis in spinal muscular atrophy type II. *Acta Neuropathol* 106: 441–8.

Arita J, Nakae Y, Matsushima H, Maekawa K (1995) Hopkins syndrome: T2-weighted high intensity of anterior horn on spinal imaging. *Pediatr Neurol* 13: 263–5.

Arya SC (1998) Japanese encephalitis virus and poliomyelitis-like syndrome. *Lancet* 351: 1094–7.

Aysun S, Cinbis M, Özcan OE (1993) Intramedullary astrocytoma presenting as spinal muscular atrophy. *J Child Neurol* 8: 354–6.

Baba Y, Nakajima M, Utsunomiya H, et al. (2004) Magnetic resonance imaging of thoracic and epidural venous dilatation in Hirayama disease. *Neurology* 62: 1426–8.

Barois A, Estournet B, Duval-Beaupère G, et al. (1989) [Infantile spinal muscular atrophy.] *Rev Neurol* 145: 299–304 (French).

Barrat FJ, Auloge L, Postural F, et al. (1996) Genetic and physical mapping of the Chediak–Higashi syndrome on chromosome 1q42–43. *Am J Hum Genet* 59: 625–32.

Barth PG (1993) Pontocerebellar hypoplasias. An overview of a group of inherited neurodegenerative disorders with fetal onset. *Brain Dev* 15: 411–22.

Beauvais P, Roubergue A, Billette de Villemeur T, Richardet JM (1988) [Progressive bulbopontine paralysis in children.] *Arch Fr Pediatr* 45: 653–5 (French).

Ben Hamida M, Hentati F, Ben Hamida C (1990) Hereditary motor system diseases (chronic juvenile amyotrophic lateral sclerosis)—conditions combining a bilateral pyramidal syndrome with limb and bulbar amyotrophy. *Brain* 113: 347–63.

Bénomy C, Bénomy H (2005) Precocity of language and type II spinal muscular atrophy in 3–4-year-old children: a study of 12 cases. *Eur J Paediatr Neurol* 9: 71–6.

Bertini E, Gadisseux JL, Palmieri G, et al. (1989) Distal infantile spinal muscular atrophy associated with paralysis of the diaphragm: a variant of infantile spinal muscular atrophy. *Am J Med Genet* 33: 328–35.

Bertorini TE, Igarashi M (1985) Postpoliomyelitis muscle pseudohypertrophy. *Muscle Nerve* 8: 644–9.

Boltshauser E, Lang W, Spillmann T, Hof E (1989) Hereditary distal muscular atrophy with vocal cord paralysis and sensorineural hearing loss: a dominant form of spinal muscular atrophy? *J Med Genet* 26: 105–8.

Boutin B, Routon MC, Rocchiccioli F, et al. (1988) Peripheral neuropathy associated with erythrophagocytic lymphohistiocytosis. *J Neurol Neurosurg Psychiatry* 51: 291–4.

Bouwsma G, Van Wijngaarden GK (1980) Spinal muscular atrophy and hypertrophy of the calves. *J Neurol Sci* 44: 275–9.

Boylan KB, Cornblath DR (1992) Werdnig–Hoffmann disease and chronic distal spinal muscular atrophy with apparent autosomal dominant inheritance. *Ann Neurol* 32: 404–7.

Boylan KB, Cornblath DR, Glass JD, et al. (1995) Autosomal dominant distal spinal muscular atrophy in four generations. *Neurology* 45: 699–704.

Boz C, Sahin N, Kalay E, et al. (2002) X-linked spinal and bulbar muscular atrophy without proximal atrophy. *Clin Neurol Neurosurg* 105: 14–8.

Brucher JM, Dom R, Lombaert A, Carton H (1981) Progressive pontobulbar palsy with deafness: clinical and pathological study of two cases. *Arch Neurol* 38: 186–90.

Brzustowicz LM, Lehner T, Castilla LA, et al. (1990) Genetic mapping of childhood-onset spinal muscular atrophy to chromosome 5q11.2–13.3. *Nature* 344: 540–1.

Bürglen L, Amiel J, Viollet L, et al. (1996) Survival motor neuron deletion in the arthrogryposis multiplex congenita–spinal muscular atrophy association. *J Clin Invest* 98: 1130–2.

Burlet P, Bürglen L, Clermont O, et al. (1996) Large scale deletions of the 5q13 region are specific to Werdnig–Hoffmann disease. *J Med Genet* 33: 281–3.

Burlet, P, Frydman N, Gigarel N, et al. (2005) Improved single-cell protocol for preimplantation genetic diagnosis of spinal muscular atrophy. *Fertil Steril* 84: 734–9.

Cavanagh NPC, Eames RA, Galvin RJ, et al. (1979) Hereditary sensory neuropathy with spastic paraplegia. *Brain*: 102: 79–94.

Chaliout-Héraut F, Barois A, Urtizberea A, et al. (2003) Evoked potentials in spinal muscular atrophy. *J Child Neurol* 18: 383–90.

Chalmers N, Mitchell JD (1987) Optico-acoustic atrophy in distal spinal muscular atrophy. *J Neurol Neurosurg Psychiatry* 50: 238–9.

Charnas L, Bernar J, Pezeshkpour GH, et al. (1988) MRI findings and peripheral neuropathy in Lowe's syndrome. *Neuropediatrics* 19: 7–9.

Chien YY, Nonaka I (1989) Peripheral nerve involvement in Werdnig–Hoffmann disease. *Brain Dev* 11: 221–9.

Chopra JS, Sharma A (1992) Protein energy malnutrition and the nervous system. *J Neurol Sci* 110: 8–20.

Chou SM, Nonaka I (1978) Werdnig–Hoffmann disease: proposal of a pathogenetic mechanism. *Acta Neuropathol* 41: 45–54.

Chung BH, Wong VC (2004) Spinal muscular atrophy: survival patterns and functional status. *Pediatrics* 114: e548–53.

Cobben JM, de Visser M, Scheffer H, et al. (1993) Confirmation of clinical diagnosis in requests for prenatal prediction of SMA type 1. *J Neurol Neurosurg Psychiatry* 56: 319–21.

Cobben JM, van der Steege G, Grootscholten P, et al. (1995) Deletions of the survival motor neuron gene in unaffected siblings of patients with spinal muscular atrophy. *Am J Hum Genet* 57: 805–8.

D'Alessandro R, Montagna P, Govoni E, Pazzaglia P (1982) Benign familial spinal muscular atrophy with hypertrophy of the calves. *Arch Neurol* 39: 657–60.

Dawood AA, Moosa A (1983) Hand and ECG tremor in spinal muscular atrophy. *Arch Dis Child* 58: 376–8.

De Angelis MV, Gatta V, Stuppia L, et al. (2002) Autosomal dominant distal spinal muscular atrophy: an Italian family not linked to 12q24 and 7p14. *Neuromuscul Disord* 12: 26–30.

De Jonghe P, Auer-Grumbach M, Irobi J, et al. (2002) Autosomal dominant juvenile amyotrophic lateral sclerosis and distal hereditary motor neuronopathy with pyramidal tract signs: synonyms for the same disorder? *Brain* 125: 1320–5.

Della Giustina E, Ferrière G, Evrard P, Lyon G (1979) Progressive bulbar paralysis in childhood (Londe syndrome). A clinicopathological report. *Acta Paediatr Belg* 32: 129–33.

DiDonato CJ, Ingraham SE, Mendell JR, et al. (1997) Deletion and conversion in spinal muscular atrophy patients: is there a relationship with severity? *Ann Neurol* 41: 230–7.

DiDonato CJ, Parkes RJ, Kothary R (2003) Development of a gene therapy strategy for the restoration of survival motor neuron protein expression: implications for spinal muscular atrophy therapy. *Hum Gene Ther* 14: 179–88.

Diep Tran T, Kroepfl T, Saito M, et al. (2001) The gene–copy ratio of SMN1/SMN2 in Japanese carriers with type I spinal muscular atrophy. *Brain Dev* 23: 321–6.

Dierick I, Baets J, Irobu J, et al. (2008) Relative contribution of mutations in genes for autosomal dominant distal hereditary motor neuropathies: a genotype-phenotype correlation study. *Brain* 131: 1217–27.

Diers A, Kaczinski A, Grohmann K, et al. (2005) The ultrastructure of peripheral nerve, motor end-plate and skeletal muscle in patients suffering from chronic spinal muscular atrophy with respiratory distress type 1 (SMARD1). *Acta Neuropathol* 110: 289–97.

DiMauro S, Bonilla E, Zeviani M, et al. (1985) Mitochondrial myopathies. *Ann Neurol* 17: 521–38.

Dionisi Vici C, Burlina AB, Bertini E, et al. (1991) Progressive neuropathy and recurrent myoglobinuria in a child with long-chain 3-hydroxy-acyl-coenzyme A dehydrogenase deficiency. *J Pediatr* 118: 744–6.

Doyu M, Sobue G, Mukai E, et al. (1992) Severity of X-linked recessive bulbospinal neuronopathy correlates with size of the tandem CAG repeat in androgen receptor gene. *Ann Neurol* 32: 707–10.

Dubowitz V (1995) *Muscle Disorders in Children, 2nd edn.* Philadelphia: WB Saunders.

Dubowitz V (1999) Very severe spinal muscular atrophy (SMA type 0): an expanding clinical phenotype. *Eur J Paediatr Neurol* 3: 49–51.

Duval-Baupère G, Barois A, Quinet I, Estournet B (1985) [Thoracic, spinal and respiratory problems in children with prolonged infantile spinal amyotrophy.] *Arch Fr Pediatr* 42: 625–34 (French).

Duval-Baupère G, Litchy WJ, Minnerath S, et al. (1994) Hereditary motor and sensory neuropathy with diaphragm and vocal cord paresis. *Ann Neurol* 35: 608–15.

Emery AEH, ed. (1994) *Diagnostic Criteria for Neuromuscular Disorders, 2nd edn.* Baarn, The Netherlands: European Neuromuscular Centre.

Emery AEH, Davie AM, Holloway S, Skinner R (1976a) International collaborative study of the spinal muscular atrophies. Part 2. Analysis of genetic data. *J Neurol Sci* 30: 375–84.

Emery AEH, Hausmanowa-Petrusewicz I, Davie AM, et al. (1976b) International collaborative study of the spinal muscular atrophies. Part 1. Analysis of clinical and laboratory data. *J Neurol Sci* 29: 83–94.

Engel K, Kurland LT, Klatzo I (1959) An inherited disease similar to amyotrophic lateral sclerosis with a pattern of posterior column involvement: an intermediate form? *Brain* 82: 203–20.

Eymard-Pierre E, Lesca G, Dollet S, et al. (2002) Infantile onset ascending hereditary spastic paralysis is associated with mutations in the alsin gene. *Am J Hum Genet* 71: 518–27.

Eymard-Pierre E, Yamanaka K, Haeussler M, et al. (2006) Novel missense mutation in ALS2 gene results in infantile ascending hereditary spastic paralysis. *Ann Neurol* 59: 976–80.

Felderhoff-Mueser U, Grohmann K, Harder A, et al. (2002) Severe spinal muscular atrophy variant associated with congenital bone fractures. *J Child Neurol* 17: 718–21.

Furukawa T, Toyokura Y (1976) Chronic spinal muscular atrophy of facioscapulohumeral type. *J Med Genet* 13: 285–9.

Galan E, Kousseff BG (1995) Peripheral neuropathy in Ehlers–Danlos syndrome. *Pediatr Neurol* 12: 242–5.

Galasko D, Salmon DP, Craig UK, et al. (2002) Clinical features and changing pattern of neurodegenerative disorders on Guam, 1997–2000. *Neurology* 58: 90–97; comment 59: 1121; author reply 1121.

Gallai V, Hockaday JM, Hughes JT, et al. (1981) Ponto-bulbar palsy with deafness (Brown–Vialetto–Van Laere syndrome): a report of three cases. *J Neurol Sci* 50: 259–75.

Garcia-Cabezas MA, Garcia-Alix A, Martin Y, et al. (2004) Neonatal spinal muscular atrophy with multiple contractures, bone fractures, respiratory insufficiency and 5q13 deletion. *Acta Neuropathol* 107: 475–8.

Garg A (2004) Medical progress: Acquired and inherited lipodystrophies. *N Engl J Med* 350: 1220–34.

Gascon GG, Chavis P, Yaghmour A, et al. (1995) Familial childhood primary lateral sclerosis with associated gaze paresis. *Neuropediatrics* 26: 313–9.

Gilgoff IS, Kahlstrom E, McLaughlin E, Keens TG (1989) Long-term ventilatory support in spinal muscular atrophy. *J Pediatr* 115: 904–9.

Gordon N (1991) The spinal muscular atrophies. *Dev Med Child Neurol* 33: 934–8.

Gourie-Devi M, Nalini A (2003) Madras motor neuron disease variant, clinical features of seven patients. *J Neurol Sci* 209: 13–17

Gourie-Devi M, Suresh TG (1988) Madras pattern of motor neuron disease in South India. *J Neurol Neurosurg Psychiatry* 51: 773–7.

Goutières F, Aicardi J, Farkas A (1977) Anterior horn cell disease associated with ponto-cerebellar hypoplasia in infants. *J Neurol Neurosurg Psychiatry* 40: 370–8.

Goutières F, Bogicevic D, Aicardi J (1991) A predominantly cervical form of spinal muscular atrophy. *J Neurol Neurosurg Psychiatry* 54: 223–5.

Grohmann K, Varon R, Stolz P, et al. (2003) Infantile spinal muscular atrophy with respiratory distress type 1 (SMARD1). *Ann Neurol* 54: 19–24.

Gros-Louis F, Meijer IA, Hand CK, et al. (2003) An ASL2 gene mutation causes hereditary spastic paraplegia in a Pakistani kindred. *Ann Neurol* 53: 145–6.

Grunnet ML, Donaldson JO (1985) Juvenile multisystem degeneration with motor neuron involvement and eosinophilic intracytoplasmic inclusions. *Arch Neurol* 42: 1114–6.

Grunnet ML, Leicher C, Zimmerman A, et al. (1989) Primary lateral sclerosis in a child. *Neurology* 39: 1530–2.

Guidetti D, Motti L, Marcello N, et al. (1986) Kennedy disease in an Italian kindred. *Eur Neurol* 25: 188–96.

Hagberg B, Lundberg K (1969) Dissociated motor development simulating cerebral palsy. *Neuropadiatrie* 1: 187–99.

Haliloglu G, Chattopadhyay A, Skoradis L, et al. (2002) Spinal muscular atrophy with progressive myoclonic epilepsy: report of new cases and review of the literature. *Neuropediatrics* 33: 314–9.

Hamano K, Tsukamoto H, Yazawa T, et al. (1994) Infantile progressive spinal muscular atrophy with ophthalmoplegia and pyramidal symptoms. *Pediatr Neurol* 10: 320–4.

Harada Y, Sutomo R, Sadewa AH, et al. (2002) Correlation between SMN2 copy number and clinical phenotype of spinal muscular atrophy: three SMN2 copies fail to rescue some patients from the disease severity. *J Neurol* 249: 1211–9.

Harding AE, Thomas PK (1980) Hereditary distal spinal muscular atrophy. A report of 34 cases and a review of the literature. *J Neurol Sci* 45: 337–48.

Hauser E, Bittner R, Liegl C, et al. (1993) Occurrence of Andermann syndrome out of French Canada—agenesis of the corpus callosum with neuronopathy. *Neuropediatrics* 24: 107–10.

Hausmanowa-Petrusewicz I, Karwanska A (1986) Electromyographic findings in different forms of infantile and juvenile proximal spinal muscular atrophy. *Muscle Nerve* 9: 37–46.

Hedge MR, Chong B, Stevenson C, et al. (2001) Clinical and genetic analysis of four patients with distal upper limb spinal muscular atrophy. *Indian J Med Res* 114: 141–7.

Hentati A, Bejaoui K, Pericak-Vance MA, et al. (1994) Linkage of recessive familial amyotrophic lateral sclerosis to chromosome 2q33–q35. *Nat Genet* 7: 425–8.

Hirayama K, Tokumaru Y (2000) Cervical dural sac and spinal cord in juvenile muscular atrophy of distal extremities. *Neurology* 54: 1922–6.

Hirayama K, Tomonaga M, Kitano K, et al. (1987) Focal cervical poliopathy causing juvenile muscular atrophy of distal upper extremity: a pathological study. *J Neurol Neurosurg Psychiatry* 50: 285–90.

Howard HC, Dube MP, Prevost C, et al. (2002) Fine mapping the candidate region for peripheral neuropathy with or without agenesis of the corpus callosum in the French Canadian population. *Eur J Hum Genet* 10: 406–12.

Iannaccone ST (1998) Spinal muscular atrophy. *Semin Neurol* 18: 19–26.

Iannaccone ST, Browne RH, Samaha FJ, Buncher CR (1993) Prospective study of spinal muscular atrophy before age 6 years. DCN/SMA group. *Pediatr Neurol* 9: 187–93.

Imai T, Minami R, Nagaoka M, et al. (1990) Proximal and distal motor nerve conduction velocities in Werdnig–Hoffmann disease. *Pediatr Neurol* 6: 82–6.

Isozumi K, DeLong R, Kaplan S, et al. (1996) Linkage of scapuloperoneal spinal muscular atrophy to chromosome 12q24–31. *Hum Mol Genet* 5: 1377–82.

Jacobs JM, Harding BN, Lake BD, et al. (1990) Peripheral neuropathy in Leigh's disease. *Brain* 113: 447–62.

Jacome DE (1999) Epilepsy in Ehlers–Danlos syndrome. Epilepsia 40: 467–73.

Jedrzejowska M, Wiszniewski W, Zimowski J, et al. (2005) Application of a rapid non-invasive technique in the molecular diagnosis of spinal muscular atrophy (SMA). *Neurol Neurochir Pol* 39: 89–94.

Jeha LE, Sila CA, Lederman RJ, et al. (2003) West Nile virus infection: a new acute paralytic illness. *Neurology* 61: 55–9.

Jennekens FGI, Veldman H, Vroegindeweij-Claessens LJHM, et al. (1992) Congenital oculo-bulbar palsy. *J Neurol Neurosurg Psychiatry* 55: 404–6.

Johnson WG, Wigger HJ, Karp HR, et al. (1982) Juvenile spinal muscular atrophy: a new hexosaminidase deficiency phenotype. *Ann Neurol* 11: 11–6.

Kamoshita S, Takei Y, Miyao M, et al. (1990) Pontocerebellar hypoplasia associated with infantile motor neuron disease (Norman's disease). *Pediatr Pathol* 10: 133–42.

Kawano T, Indo Y, Nakazato H, et al. (1998) Oculocerebrorenal syndrome of Lowe: three mutations in the OCRL1 gene derived from three different phenotypes. *Am J Med Genet* 77: 348–55.

Korinthenberg R, Sauer M, Ketelsen UP, et al. (1997) Congenital axonal neuropathy caused by deletions in the spinal muscular atrophy region. *Ann Neurol* 42: 364–8.

Kuzuhara S, Chou SM (1981) Preservation of the phrenic motoneurons in Werdnig–Hoffmann disease. *Ann Neurol* 9: 506–10.

Kwast O, Ignatowicz R (1990) Progressive peripheral neuron degeneration in ataxia–telangiectasia: an electrophysiological study in children. *Dev Med Child Neurol* 32: 800–7.

Larbrisseau A, Vanasse M, Brochu P, Jasmin J (1984) The Andermann syndrome: agenesis of the corpus callosum associated with mental retardation and progressive sensorimotor neuropathy. *Can J Neurol Sci* 11: 257–61.

Lefebvre S, Bürglen L, Reboullet S, et al. (1995) Identification and characterization of a spinal muscular atrophy-determining gene. *Cell* 80: 155–65.

Lerman-Sagie T, Filiaso J, Smith DW, Korson M (1996) Infantile onset of hereditary ascending spastic paralysis with bulbar involvement. *J Child Neurol* 11: 54–7.

Lesca G, Eymard-Pierre E, Santorelli FM, et al. (2003) Infantile ascending hereditary spastic paralysis (IAHSP): clinical features in 11 families. *Neurology* 60: 674–82.

Liu GT, Specht LA (1993) Progressive juvenile segmental spinal muscular atrophy. *Pediatr Neurol* 9: 54–6.

MacLeod MJ, Taylor JE, Lunt PW, et al. (1999) Prenatal onset spinal muscular atrophy. *Eur J Paediatr Neurol* **3**: 65–72.

Malcov M, Schwartz T, Mei-Raz N, et al. (2004) Mutiplex nested PCR for preimplantation genetic diagnosis of spinal muscular atrophy. *Fetal Diagn Ther* **19**: 199–206.

Maystadt I, Zarhrate M, Landrieu P, et al. (2004) Allelic heterogeneity of SMARD1 at the IGHMBP2 locus. *Hum Mutat* **23**: 525–6.

McShane MA, Boyd S, Harding B, et al. (1992) Progressive bulbar paralysis of childhood. A reappraisal of Fazio–Londe disease. *Brain* **115**: 1889–900.

McWilliam RC, Gardner-Medwin D, Doyle D, Stephenson JBP (1985) Diaphragmatic paralysis due to spinal cord atrophy. *Arch Dis Child* **60**: 145–9.

Melki J, Munnich A (1996) Molecular genetics of spinal muscular atrophy. In: Arzimanoglou A, Goutières F, eds. *Trends in Child Neurology*. Paris: John Libbey, pp. 137–41.

Melki J, Abdelhak S, Sheth MF, et al. (1990a) The gene responsible for chronic proximal spinal muscular atrophies of childhood maps to chromosome 5q. *Nature* **344**: 767–8.

Melki J, Sheth P, Abdelhak S, et al. (1990b) Mapping of acute (type I) spinal muscular atrophy to chromosome 5q12–q14. *Lancet* **336**: 271–3.

Melki J, Lefebvre S, Bürglen P, et al. (1994) De novo and inherited deletions of the 5q13 region in spinal muscular atrophies. *Science* **264**: 1474–7.

Mellies U, Dehna-Schwake C, Fehling F, Voit T (2004) Sleep disordered breathing in spinal muscular atrophy. *Neuromusc Disord* **14**: 797–803.

Mercelis R, Demeester J, Martin JJ (1980) Neurogenic scapuloperoneal syndrome in childhood. *J Neurol Neurosurg Psychiatry* **43**: 888–96.

Mercuri E, Bertini E, Messina S, et al. (2004a) Pilot trial of phenylbutyrate in neuromuscular diseases. *Neuromusc Disord* **14**: 130–5.

Mercuri E, Messina S, Kinali M, et al. (2004b) Congenital form of spinal muscular atrophy predominantly affecting the lower limbs: a clinical and muscle MRI study. *Neuromusc Disord* **14**: 125–9.

Merlini L, Granata C, Bonfiglioli S, et al. (1989) Scoliosis in spinal muscular atrophy: natural history and management. *Dev Med Child Neurol* **31**: 501–8.

Merlini, L, Solari A, Vita G et al. (2003) Role of gabapentin in spinal muscular atrophy: results of a multicenter, randomized Italian study. *J Child Neurol* **18**: 537–541

Miller RG, Moore DH, Dronsky V, et al. (2001) A placebo-controlled trial of gabapentin in spinal muscular atrophy. *J Neurol Sci* **191**: 127–31.

Milunsky JM, Cheney SM (1999) Prenatal diagnosis of spinal muscular atrophy by direct molecular analysis. *Genet Test* **3**: 255–8.

Misra UK, Kalita L Mishra VN, et al. (2005) A clinical, magnetic resonance imaging, and survival motor neuron gene deletion study of Hirayama disease. *Arch Neurol* **62**: 120–3.

Munsat TL, Davies KE (1992) International SMA consortium meeting (26–28 June 1992, Bonn, Germany). *Neuromusc Disord* **2**: 423–8.

Muntoni F, Goodwin FG, Sewry C, et al. (1999) Clinical spectrum and diagnostic difficulties of infantile pontocerebellar hypoplasia type 1. *Neuropediatrics* **30**: 243–8.

Navon R, Khosravi R, Korczyn T, et al. (1995) A new mutation in the HEXA gene associated with a spinal muscular atrophy phenotype. *Neurology* **45**: 539–43.

Novelli G, Capon F, Tamisari L, et al. (1995) Neonatal spinal muscular atrophy with diaphragmatic paralysis is unlinked to 5q11.2–q13. *J Med Genet* **32**: 216–9.

Oka A, Matsushita Y, Sakakihara Y, et al. (1995) Spinal muscular atrophy with oculomotor palsy, epilepsy, and cerebellar hypoperfusion. *Pediatr Neurol* **12**: 365–9.

Paulson GW, Liss L, Sweeney PJ (1980) Late-onset spinal muscle atrophy. A sex-linked variant of Kugelberg–Welander. *Acta Neurol Scand* **61**: 49–55.

Pearn J (1978) Incidence, prevalence and gene-frequency studies of chronic childhood spinal muscular atrophy. *J Med Genet* **15**: 409–13.

Pearn J (1980) Classification of spinal muscular atrophies. *Lancet* **1**: 919–22.

Pearn J, Gardner-Medwin D, Wilson J (1978) A clinical study of chronic childhood muscular atrophy. A review of 141 cases. *J Neurol Sci* **38**: 23–37.

Pitt M, Houlden J, Jacobs Q, et al. (2003) Severe infantile neuropathy with diaphragmatic weakness and its relationship to SMARD1. *Brain* **126**: 2682–92.

Poll-Thé BT, Aicardi J, Girot R, Rosa R (1985) Neurological findings in triosephosphate isomerase deficiency. *Ann Neurol* **17**: 439–43.

Prior TW, Swoboda KJ, Scott HD, Hejmanowski AQ (2004) Homozygous SMN1 deletion in affected family members and modification of the phenotype by SMN2. *Am J Med Genet A* **130**: 307–10.

Raymond FL (1997) Spinal muscular atrophy of childhood: genetics. *Dev Med Child Neurol* **39**: 419–20.

Restuccia D, Rubino M, Valeriani M (2003) Cervical cord dysfunction during neck flexion in Hirayama's disease. *Neurology* **60**: 1980–83.

Rivière J, Lécuyer R (2002) Spatial cognition in young children with spinal muscular atrophy. *Dev Neuropsychol* **21**: 273–83.

Robb SA, McShane MA, Wilson J, Payan J (1991) Acute onset spinal muscular atrophy in siblings. *Neuropediatrics* **22**: 45–6.

Rodrigues NR, Owen N, Talbot K, et al. (1996) Gene deletions in spinal muscular atrophy. *J Med Genet* **33**: 93–6.

Rudnik-Schöneborn S, Wirth B, Röhrig D, et al. (1995) Exclusion of the gene locus for spinal muscular atrophy on chromosome 5q in a family with infantile olivopontocerebellar atrophy (OPCA) and anterior horn cell degeneration. *Neuromusc Dis* **5**: 19–23.

Rudnik-Schöneborn S, Forkert R, Hahnen E, et al. (1996) Clinical spectrum and diagnostic criteria of infantile spinal muscular atrophy: further delineation on the basis of SMN gene deletion findings. *Neuropediatrics* **27**: 8–15.

Rudnik-Schöneborn S, Hausmanowa-Petrusewicz I, Borkowska J, Zerres J (2001) The predictive value of achieved motor milestones assessed in 441 patients with infantile spinal muscular atrophy types II and III. *Eur Neurol* **45**: 174–81.

Rudnik-Schöneborn S, Goebel HH, Schlote W, et al. (2003a) Classical infantile spinal muscular atrophy with SMN deficiency causes sensory neuronopathy. *Neurology* **60**: 983–7.

Rudnik-Schöneborn S, Sztriha L, Aithala GR, et al. (2003b) Extended phenotype of pontocerebellar hypoplasia with infantile spinal muscular atrophy. *Am J Med Genet A* **117**: 10–7.

Rudnik-Schöneborn S, Stolz P, Varon R, et al. (2004) Long-term observations of patients with infantile spinal muscular atrophy with respiratory distress type 1 (SMARD1). *Neuropediatrics* **35**: 174–82.

Russman BS, Iannacone ST, Buncher CR, et al. (1992) Spinal muscular atrophy: new thoughts on the pathogenesis and classification schema. *J Child Neurol* **7**: 347–53.

Russman BS, Iannaccone ST, Samaha FJ (2003) A phase I trial of riluzole in spinal muscular atrophy. *Arch Neurol* **60**: 1601–3.

Sangiuolo F, Filareto A, Giardina E, et al. (2004) Prenatal diagnosis of spinal muscular atrophy with respiratory distress (SMARD1) in a twin pregnancy. *Prenat Diagn* **24**: 839–41.

Schmitt HP, Härle M, Koelfen W, Nissen KH (1994) Childhood progressive spinal muscular atrophy with facioscapulo-humeral predominance, sensory and autonomic involvement and optic atrophy. *Brain Dev* **16**: 386–92.

Skre H, Mellgren SI, Bergsholm P, Slagsvold JE (1978) Unusual type of neural muscular atrophy with a possible X-chromosomal inheritance pattern. *Acta Neuropathol Scand* **58**: 249–60.

Specola N, Vanier M, Goutières F, et al. (1990) The juvenile and chronic forms of GM2 gangliosidosis. Clinical and enzymatic heterogeneity. *Neurology* **40**: 145–50.

Spiegel R, Hagmann A, Boltshauser E, Moser H (1996) [Molecular genetic diagnosis and deletion analysis in type I–III spinal muscular atrophy.] *Schweiz Med Wochenschr* **126**: 907–14 (German).

Steinman GS, Rorke LB, Brown MJ (1980) Infantile neuronal degeneration masquerading as Werdnig–Hoffmann disease. *Ann Neurol* **8**: 317–24.

Stewart H, Wallace A, McGaughran J, et al. (1998) Molecular diagnosis of spinal muscular atrophy. *Arch Dis Child* **78**: 531–5.

Striano P, Boccella P, Sarappa C, Striano S (2004) Spinal muscular atrophy and progressive myoclonic epilepsy: one case report and characteristics of the epileptic syndrome. *Seizure* **13**: 582–6.

Summers BA, Swash M, Schwartz MS, Ingram DA (1987) Juvenile-onset bulbospinal muscular atrophy with deafness: Vialetto–Van Laere syndrome or Madras-type motor neuron disease? *J Neurol* **234**: 440–2.

Tandan R, Sharma KR, Bradley WG, et al. (1990) Chronic segmental spinal muscular atrophy of upper extremities in identical twins. *Neurology* **40**: 236–9.

Tay SK, Akman HO, Chang WK, et al. (2004) Fatal infantile neuromuscular presentation of glycogen storage disease type IV. *Neuromusc Disord* **14**: 253–60.

Tein I, Donner EJ, Hale DE, Murphy EG (1995) Clinical and neurophysiologic response of myopathy and neuropathy in long-chain L-3-hydroxyacyl-CoA dehydrogenase deficiency to oral prednisone. *Pediatr Neurol* **12**: 68–76.

Thomas PK, Calne DB, Elliott CF (1972) X-linked scapuloperoneal syndrome. *J Neurol Neurosurg Psychiatry* **35**: 208–15.

Timmerman V, De Jonghe P, Simokovic S, et al. (1996) Distal hereditary motor neuropathy type II (distal HMN II): mapping of a locus to chromosome 12q24. *Hum Mol Genet* **5**: 1065–9.

Uncini A, Di Muzio A, De Angelis MV, et al. (1999) Minimal and asymptomatic chronic inflammatory demyelinating polyneuropathy. *Clin Neurophysiol* **110**: 694–8.

Van der Steege G, Grootscholten PM, Van der Vlies P, et al. (1995) PCR-based DNA test to confirm clinical diagnosis of autosomal recessive spinal muscular atrophy. *Lancet* **345**: 985–6 (letter).

van der Vleuten AJ, van Ravenswaaij-Arts CM, Frijns CJ, et al. (1998) Localisation of the gene for a dominant congenital spinal muscular atrophy predominantly affecting the lower limbs to chromosome 12q23–q24. *Eur J Hum Genet* **6**: 376–82.

Van Hale P (1987) Chediak–Higashi syndrome. In: Gomez MR, ed. *Neurocutaneous Diseases: a Practical Approach.* London: Butterworths, pp. 209–13.

Van Toorn R, Davies J, Wilmshurst JM (2002) Spinal muscular atrophy with congenital fractures: post-mortem analysis. *J Child Neurol* **17**: 721–3.

Viollet L, Barois A, Rebeiz G, et al. (2002) Mapping of autosomal recessive chronic distal muscular atrophy to chromosome 11q13. *Ann Neurol* **51**: 585–92.

Voudris KA, Skardoutsou A, Vagiakou FA (2002) Infantile progressive bulbar palsy with deafness. *Brain Dev* **24**: 732–5.

Walsh FB, Hoyt WF (1969) *Clinical Neuro-ophthalmology, 3rd edn.* Baltimore: Williams & Wilkins.

Wang CH, Carter JA, Das K, et al. (1997) Extensive DNA deletion associated with severe disease alleles on spinal muscular atrophy homologues. *Ann Neurol* **42**: 41–9.

Wicklund MP (2005) Amyotrophic lateral sclerosis: possible role of environmental influences. *Neurol Clin* **23**: 461–84.

Wirth B, Rudnick-Schöneborn S, Hahnen E, et al. (1995) Prenatal prediction in families with autosomal recessive proximal spinal muscular atrophy (5q11.2–q13.3): molecular genetics and clinical experience in 109 cases. *Prenat Diagn* **15**: 407–17.

Yang Y, Hentati A, Deng HX, et al. (2001) The gene encoding alsin, a protein with three guanine nucleotide exchange factor domains, is mutated in a form of recessive amyotrophic lateral sclerosis. *Nat Genet* **29**: 160–5.

Yokochi K, Oda M, Satoh J, Morimatsu Y (1989) An autopsy case of atypical infantile motor neuron disease with hyaline intraneuronal inclusions. *Arch Neurol* **46**: 103–7.

Zerres K, Rudnik-Schöneborn S (1995) Natural history of proximal spinal muscular atrophy. Clinical analysis of 445 patients with suggestions for a modification of existing classification. *Arch Neurol* **52**: 518–23.

Zerres K, Rudnik-Schöneborn S, Forrest E, et al. (1997) A collaborative study on the natural history of childhood and juvenile onset proximal spinal muscular atrophy (types II and III SMA): 569 patients. *J Neurol Sci* **146**: 67–72.

Zeviani M, Peterson P, Servidei E, et al. (1987) Benign reversible muscle cytochrome c oxidase deficiency: a second case. *Neurology* **37**: 64–7.

20
DISORDERS OF THE PERIPHERAL NERVES

Robert Ouvrier and Jean Aicardi

This chapter considers only those disorders in which the primary pathological process affects the axons of motor or sensory cells or both, or their myelin sheath and associated Schwann cells. Diseases in which axonal damage results in primary lesions of the neuronal perikarya have been described in Chapter 19.

Hereditary neuropathies may be purely sensory in type. More often they involve both sensory and motor fibres. Nerve fibre function can be disturbed in several manners (Fig. 20.1). Wallerian degeneration occurs when an axon is separated from the cell perikaryon or when the cell dies. Axonal neuropathies are characterized primarily by involvement of the axon and may be the result of toxins, genetic disease, vascular disturbances and so on. In many cases, axonal neuropathies begin and remain more severe distally than proximally, perhaps because the enormous length of axons makes the metabolic needs of their most distal parts difficult to meet. This may also be due to disturbances in the axonal transport systems. In axonal neuropathies, nerve conduction velocities are normal or only slightly slowed despite evidence of denervation. Characteristically, the amplitude of sensory and compound muscle action potentials is reduced. Diseases of the Schwann cell and the myelin sheath are also due to multiple (genetic or acquired) causes, especially inflammatory diseases. The lesions are diffuse or segmental, limited to the length of nerve depending on one Schwann cell (internode). Such a process may produce a conduction block in some fibres in whole nerves or a slowing of nerve conduction velocities, either focal or generalized. Slowing may be diffuse and uniform as in some metabolic and hereditary neuropathies (Miller et al. 1985). Conduction block and temporal dispersion are indicative of multifocal segmental demyelination. Conduction block is defined at the cellular level as failure of an action potential to propagate throughout the length of an axon. When many individual axons are blocked, especially at a localized site, both the amplitude and the area under the curve of the evoked muscle action potential are reduced when proximal stimulation is compared to distal stimulation (beyond the region of conduction block) of the motor nerve. With pure temporal dispersion, increased duration occurs together with reduced amplitude but the area under the curve is preserved. Demyelination and axonal disease are not independent processes, but the exact nature of their relationship remains unclear.

HEREDITARY MOTOR AND SENSORY NEUROPATHIES (HMSNs)

The HMSNs are the most common degenerative disorders of the peripheral nervous system, accounting for approximately 40% of childhood chronic neuropathies (Ouvrier 1992). Degeneration of myelin sheaths and/or axons produces a predominantly distal paralytic amyotrophy involving preferentially the lower limbs and associated with areflexia. Sensory disturbances are overshadowed by motor involvement.

The current classification of the HMSNs remains based in part on their pathology (axonal or demyelinating), their electro-clinical manifestations, especially the motor and sensory conduction velocities, and their mode of inheritance. Progress in molecular genetics is rapidly changing the criteria for classification. Many of the HMSNs result in the clinical picture referred to as Charcot–Marie–Tooth (CMT) disease. In the recent past, neurologists have tended to use the term HMSN whereas geneticists prefer CMT. HMSN type I is synonymous with CMT 1 but there are some discrepancies in the nomenclature especially in regard to the rarer forms. For example, CMT 4 is classified as a demyelinating form of autosomal recessive HMSN, whereas HMSN type IV originally referred to Refsum disease. The CMT nomenclature will be used predominantly in this chapter. A composite classification is given in Table 20.1.

CMT 1 / HMSN I
CMT 1 is characterized pathologically by extensive segmental demyelination and remyelination with the development of 'onion bulbs' around nerve fibres, by slow motor and sensory nerve conduction velocities and by a dominant inheritance. However, both autosomal recessive (Harding and Thomas 1980a, Gabreëls-Festen et al. 1992) and X-linked forms have been reported (Hahn et al. 1990, Ionasescu et al. 1991). The prevalence of HMSN I is 3.8 per 100,000 population, accounting for about 50% of paediatric cases of hereditary neuropathies. Although the penetrance of the disease is high (83%), there is significant variability in clinical and pathological expression (Harding and Thomas 1980b). In some cases, the clinical and even nerve biopsy findings can be minimal, particularly in young children. Nevertheless, children affected by CMT 1A almost always show some

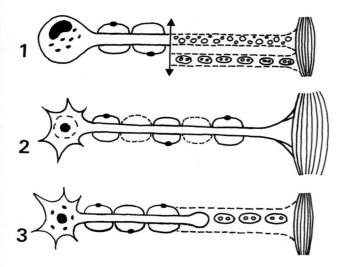

Fig. 20.1. Different types of peripheral nerve involvement.

1. Wallerian degeneration. Following interruption of axon, there is chromatolysis of the cell body. In distal axon, myelin initially disintegrates (upper part of schema). Later, Schwann cells divide and line up inside basement membrane to regenerate an axon (lower part of schema). Axonal sprouting is also observed. Nerve conduction is normal in proximal axon and absent distally. Muscle atrophy is present.

2. Segmental demyelination. Patchy damage to Schwann cells with secondary paranodal, axonal degeneration. Secondary remyelination generates short internodes with thin myelin sheath. Repeated episodes of demyelination and remyelination may produce 'onion bulb' formations. Conduction block or slowing of conduction in demyelinated segments. Increased mechanical irritability.

3. 'Dying back' neuropathy. Degeneration begins in terminal axon. Secondary demyelination often occurs. Conduction is normal proximally and absent distally in affected fibres. Preferential involvement of large fibres explains the mild/moderate reduction in nerve conduction velocity, as the measured velocity is that of small fibres.

manifestations by the age of 3 years. Mild and even asymptomatic cases occur (Thomas et al. 1997), and systematic examination of parents and relatives therefore improves the diagnostic yield in propositi. Most de novo duplications are of paternal origin (Palau et al. 1993, Harding 1995).

CMT 1 is genetically heterogeneous but more than 80% of childhood cases are linked to chromosome 17 (CMT 1A). The defect in such cases is usually a submicroscopic duplication, approximately 1.5 megabases in length, within band 17p11.2 (Raeymaekers et al. 1991). The duplication includes the gene encoding peripheral myelin protein 22 (PMP22) (Patel et al. 1992) so that the gene is present in three copies. In a few cases without duplication, a point mutation of the *PMP22* gene has been found (Roa et al. 1993), thus indicating that this gene is the disease gene in CMT 1. The duplication is thought to result from unequal crossing-over during meiosis. Deletions of the same region result in hereditary neuropathy with liability to pressure palsies (HNPP), which is described later (pp. 766–7). Cases of CMT 1A due to trisomy 17 have also been recorded. The mechanism by which overexpression of PMP22 (whether produced by having three copies of the *PMP22* gene or by a gain of function mutation) produces the clinical manifestations is not understood.

Mouse and rat models that overexpress PMP22 develop phenotypic features consistent with CMT 1, and the severity of demyelination is proportional to the level of PMP22 expression. PMP22 comprises only 2–5% of peripheral nervous system myelin. Impaired cellular trafficking appears to be a possible mechanism in several PMP22-related neuropathies (Lupski and Chance 2005).

In a few families, the disease is caused by mutations of the *MPZ (myelin P0)* gene (CMT 1B) which maps to chromosome 1q21–q23 (Warner et al. 1996). Mutations of both the *PMP22* and *MPZ* genes cause a variety of clinical pictures, ranging from congenital hypomyelination, through the Déjerine–Sottas phenotype to a CMT 1 phenotype or even, in the case of *MPZ*, to an axonal degenerative CMT syndrome (CMT 2), depending on the location and severity of the mutation (Warner et al. 1996). In our experience of paediatric cases, the clinical features of cases caused by point mutations are more severe than typical duplication-linked CMT 1A cases. The histopathological findings of CMT 1B are similar to those of CMT 1A but uncompacted myelin may be seen in a significant number of fibres and focal folding of myelin (tomacula) can also be prominent. MPZ constitutes about 50% of myelin protein and is important for the process of myelin adhesion (Shy 2005).

Some cases do not map to either of these loci. In some dominantly transmitted cases referred to as CMT 1C, mutations of *LITAF/SIMPLE*, a gene that may be involved in aberrant protein degradation, have been found (Street et al. 2003).

Confusingly, CMT 1D refers to CMT 1 caused by *heterozygous mutations* of the zinc finger transcription regulator *EGR2* (also known as *Krox 20*) which induces a transcription factor of many genes critical for the formation and maintenance of myelin (Warner et al. 1999). *Homozygous EGR2 mutations* cause a more severe autosomal recessive hypo- and de-myelinating neuropathy CMT 4E (see below).

X-LINKED CMT (CMT X)
In approximately 10% of cases, the disorder is linked to the X chromosome, where at least three different loci have been found (Ionasescu et al. 1991, 1992). The most frequent (X-linked dominant) form lies on the long arm at Xq13.1. Numerous mutations at this locus are known to involve the gene for connexin 32 (Bergoffen et al. 1993), a membrane-spanning gap junction protein localized adjacent to the nodes of Ranvier and the Schmidt–Lanterman incisures. Pedigrees show the expected absence of male-to-male transmission. Males are usually much more obviously affected than females but generally clinical involvement is less severe in the first decade than in those with CMT 1. On the other hand, the eventual degree of disability is greater in mature males with CMT X than in CMT 1. Occasional affected children may present with isolated deafness (Stojkovic et al. 1999) and some have had transient CNS symptomatology associated with white matter lesions (Haneman et al. 2003). The neurophysiological features of the X-linked type in males may resemble those of CMT 1, but average nerve conduction velocity (NCV) is about 10 m/s faster in CMT X males (mean peroneal

TABLE 20.1

Sub-classification of the Charcot–Marie–Tooth syndrome

Disorder (OMIM number)	Inheritance*	Chromosomal locus	Pathological mechanism	Histopathological/ neurophysiological features	Comments
CMT 1A (118220)	AD	1.5Mb duplication at 17p11.2–12	DNA duplication, PMP 22 protein	Sheath hypertrophy, onion bulb formation	Distal weakness, mild functional impairment, slowing of nerve conduction velocities (NCVs)
CMT 1B (118200)	AD	1q21–23	Duffy linked, myelin protein P_0 mutation	Similar to CMT 1A or more severe	Similar to CMT 1A or more severe (see CMT 3)
CMT1C (601098)	AD	16p13	LITAF/SIMPLE missense		
CMT 1D (607678)	AD	10q21.1–q22.1	EGR2/KROX20 mutations (heterozygous)		Autosomal recessive forms are labelled CMT 4E
CMT 1E (118300)	AD	17p11.2	PMP22 mutation		Associated with sensorineural deafness
CMT 1F (607734)	AD	8p21	NEFL mutation		Early-onset severe cases with slow NCVs. See CMT 2E for axonal phenotype
CMT 1	AR	Unknown. AR CMT 1 cases with known mutations are labelled CMT 4		Fewer classic onion bulbs, basal lamina bulbs more frequent. Tomacula present	Early onset, similar to CMT 1A but more severe
CMT X1 (302800)	XD	Xq13.1	Connexin 32 (gap junction protein GJB1) mutation	Demyelination and axonal degeneration. Minimal hypertrophy. Motor nerve conduction velocities (NCVs) lower than normal but faster than in CMT 1A	Absence of male-male transmission. Females mildly affected. Males more severely affected than in CMT 1A
CMT X2 (302801)	XR	Xp22.2	Unknown		Rare infantile onset ± intellectual disability. Females very mildly affected ± Spasticity
CMT X3 (302802)	XR	Xq26	Unknown		
CMT 2A (118210)	AD	1p36.2	Kinesin family 1B (KIF1B) mutation in one family	Axonal degeneration	CMT 2 cases have normal or near-normal NCVs with decreased compound muscle action potential (CMAP)
CMT 2A (608507)		1p36.2	Mutations of mitofusin 2 in others	Early- and late-onset cases	
CMT 2B (600882)	AD	3q21	RAB7 missense	Large and small fibre loss	Frequent foot ulcers and other sensory features
CMT 2B1 (605588)	AR	1q21.2–3	LMNA missense	Severe fibre loss	Described in a small Moroccan pedigree
CMT 2B2 (605589)	AR	19q13.3	Unknown		Described in a small inbred Costa Rican pedigree
CMT 2C (606071)	AD	12q23–24	Unknown		Severe, including respiratory failure and vocal cord weakness
CMT 2D (601472)	AD	7p15	GARS mutation		Clinically similar to CMT 2A, distal SMA
CMT 2E (607684)	AD	8p21	NEFL mutation		Demyelinating phenotypes are labelled CMT 1F
CMT 2F (606595)	AD	7q11–q21	HSPB1/HSP27 mutation		Small heat-shock protein B1
CMT 2G (608591)	AD	12q12–q13.3	Unknown		
CMT 2G (607706)	AR	8q13–q21.1	GDAP1 missense		3 kindreds, severe with vocal weakness
CMT 2H (607731)	AR	8q21.3	Unknown		Pyramidal features; described in a Tunisian kindred
CMT 2I (607677)	AD	1q22	MPZ (P_0) mutation		Late onset
CMT 2J (607736)	AR	1q22	MPZ (P_0) mutation		Sensory and pupillary abnormalities

→

Type	Inheritance	Locus	Gene/mutation	Pathology	Clinical features
CMT 2K (607831)	AR	8q13–q21.1	*GDAP1* missense		Most cases due to GDAP1 mutations are labelled CMT 4A
CMT 2L (608673)	AD	12q24	*HSPB8*		
CMT 3¹ (145900) (Déjerine–Sottas syndrome)	AR/AD	19q13.1, 17p11.2, 1q22 (a number of specific allelic variants have been reported)	Periaxin (*PRX*), *PMP22*, *MPZ* (P_0), *EGR2* mutations	Hypomyelination, basal lamina onion bulb formation. Motor NCVs <10 m/s	Clinically severe, infantile onset, global delay, cranial and spinal nerve involvement (shares common features with severe CMT 1A, especially in the tetrasomic homozygous variants)
CMT 4A (214400)	AR	8q13–q21.1	*GDAP1* mutation	Demyelination or axonal degeneration	Early and severe onset, complete distal (to elbows and knees) paralysis by teens. Often non-ambulatory
CMT 4B1 (601382)	AR	11q22	*MTMR2* mutation	Congenital hypomyelination, excessive myelin outfolding, onion bulbs, slow NCVs	Clinically mild to severe, early distal weakness and pes cavus. Cranial nerve signs. Confined to small pedigrees
CMT 4B2 (604563)	AR	11p15	*SBF2* mutation	As above (similar to CMT 4B1 and 4H)	Often associated with glaucoma
CMT 4C (601596)	AR	5q32	*KIAA1985* mutation		
CMT 4D (601455) Lom type	AR	8q24.3	*NDRG1* mutation		Closed gypsy pedigree, associated with deafness
CMT 4E (605253)	AR	10q21–22.1	*EGR2* (Krox20 mouse homolog) mutation		AD cases are labelled CMT 1D
CMT 4F (145900)	AR	19q13	Periaxin (*PRX*)		See CMT 3
CMT 4H (609311)	AR	12p11.21–q13.11	*Frabin/FGD4*	Demyelination. Myelin outfolding	Similar to CMT 4B
CMT 5 (600631)	AD	Not known. Linkages excluded at chromosomes 1, 3, 7, 10, 17	Unknown	Axonal degeneration	Pyramidal features, marked leg cramps, and often late onset
CMT intermediate A (608340)	AR	8q13–q21.1	*GDAP1* mutation	Intermediate NCVs	Turkish families, mixed axonal and demyelinating features. Fairly mild
CMT intermediate B (606482)	AD	19p13.2–p12	Dynamin 2 mutations		Intermediate NCVs. Occasional neutropenia
CMT intermediate C (608323)	AD	1p35	Unknown		2 unrelated families
CMT intermediate D (607791)	AD	1q22–q23	*MPZ* (P_0) mutation		
Hereditary neuropathy with liability to pressure palsies (HNPP) (162500)		1.5Mb deletion at 17p11.2–12	DNA deletion (or missense mutation) affecting PMP 22 protein synthesis	Presence of tomaculous changes on biopsy with uncompacted myelin. Mild slowing of motor NCVs, but conduction block may be present	Acute-onset focal weakness and sensory loss following nerve trauma. Often the functional deficit is temporary, returning to baseline levels over time. May be episodic
Roussy–Lévy syndrome (180800)		500Kb partial duplication at 17p11.2 and 1q22–q23	*PMP22* or *MPZ* (P_0) mutation		Similar features to CMT 1A but with associated gait ataxia and tremor. In later life may suffer neuropathic foot ulcers

*AD = autosomal dominant; AR = autosomal recessive; XD = X-linked dominant; XR = X-linked recessive.

¹The term CMT 3 should be reserved for hereditary neuropathies in which hypomyelination is the dominant feature. This would include hypomyelinating neuropathy, Déjerine–Sottas disease and congenital amyelinating neuropathy.

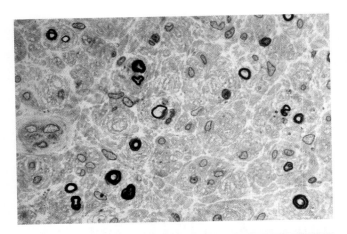

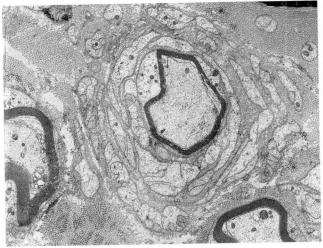

Fig. 20.2. Hereditary motor and sensory neuropathy type I. *(Top)* Prolifera-tion of Schwann cells with 'onion bulb' formations. Note also the small number of myelinated fibres. *(Bottom)* 'Onion bulb' formation as seen with electron microscope. The axon is thinly myelinated in comparison with two normal axons. (Courtesy Dr MC Routon, Hôpital Saint Vincent de Paul, Paris.)

greatest loss among those of large calibre. The distribution of fibre diameters is thus unimodal. Unmyelinated fibres are not affected. Proliferation of the sheath of Schwann produces the classical 'onion bulb' formations (Fig. 20.2) that can be shown by electron microscopy to contain only Schwann cells and their processes. Nerve-fibre teasing shows numerous images of segmental and paranodal demyelination and remyelination, predominating on the distal part of nerves. Pathological lesions, in particular onion bulbs, are nonspecific and indicate only the succession of demyelinating and remyelinating episodes that can also be observed in many other neuropathies. When marked, the process leads to hypertrophy of nerve roots and plexi. Degenerative changes in muscle are secondary to neural damage. The mechanism of the malady is still not fully understood. Nukuda and Dyck (1984) suggested that demyelination/remyelination might be secondary to alterations of the axons but the subsequent discovery of myelin protein mutations argues strongly for a primary Schwann cell defect (Lupski and Chance 2005).

In CMT X, the pathological lesions vary from predominant chronic de- and remyelination to, more commonly, a mixture of demyelination and axonal degeneration with moderate loss of myelinated fibres (Sander et al. 1997).

CLINICAL MANIFESTATIONS

Onset of CMT 1A is usually within the first decade, although cases of later onset are known. A very early onset during the neonatal period or the first year is not as rare as once thought (Ouvrier et al. 1987). Foot deformity or gait disturbances are the usual presenting manifestations. Pes cavus is typical and is often associated with hammer toes. Pes cavus has been attributed to imbalance between the long flexors and invertors of the ankle but involvement of the intrinsic muscles of the feet may be more important (Gallardo et al. 2006). Some children present with pes planus and marked valgus deviation of the feet. Pes planus was more common than pes cavus in a series of 17 children diagnosed early because of a positive family history; seven had areflexia and the ankle jerk was absent in only 3 of them (Feasby et al. 1992). Gait disturbances include poor stability or stepping gait, difficulties running and frequent falls. Such symptoms develop insidiously so that most patients are seen only after several years. The contrast between marked neurological signs and good preservation of function is then striking.

Examination reveals fairly symmetrical atrophy of the peroneal muscles (hence the term peroneal amyotrophy classically applied to CMT), later involving the calves and eventually the lower third of the thigh (Fig. 20.3). In the upper extremity, atrophy of the small muscles of the hand may occur, although weakness of the intrinsic muscles of the hands is quite often demonstrable. Asymmetrical and even unilateral involvement has been rarely reported (Ouvrier 1992). In many cases, muscle bulk may remain normal for prolonged periods, and in Aicardi's experience approximately half of affected children and adolescents do not have any wasting. Hypertrophy of the calves occurs in some families (Uncini et al. 1994).

Deep tendon reflexes, especially the ankle jerks, are often lost

NCV 31 m/s) than in CMT 1 males (mean peroneal NCV 22 m/s) (Nicholson and Nash 1993), whereas in females they are more axonal in type. It seems likely that most 'intermediate' types of CMT with mildly slowed conduction velocities are X-linked. There are other entities, e.g. *dynamin* mutations, which characteristically cause an intermediate form of CMT 1, sometimes associated with neutropenia (Züchner et al. 2005). A rare X-linked recessive axonal form maps to Xp22.2, and another axonal form with associated deafness and mental retardation maps to Xq24–q26 (Priest et al. 1995, Ouvrier et al. 2007).

PATHOLOGY

The pathology of CMT 1 has been studied mainly by muscle and nerve biopsy. Only a few post-mortem examinations have been reported: these cases showed degeneration of the posterior columns, some loss of anterior horn cells, and degeneration of the anterior and posterior spinal roots (De Recondo 1975). There is a reduction in the numbers of myelinated fibres, with the

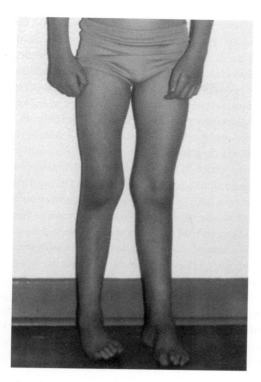

Fig. 20.3. Hereditary motor and sensory neuropathy type I in an 8-year-old girl. Note wasting of lower limbs below the lower third of thigh and deformed feet.

inflammatory polyneuropathy but a coincidence of two different nerve disorders seems unlikely. In practice a trial of steroids is indicated in cases with sudden deterioration.

DIAGNOSIS

The diagnosis of CMT 1 is easy in typical forms. The presence of sensory deficit is important to distinguish the condition from distal forms of myopathy or spinal amyotrophy. Slowing of motor and sensory nerve conduction velocities to less than 60% of the lower limit of normal values and increased distal latencies separate CMT 1 from CMT 2. There is no correlation between slowing of conduction velocities and clinical severity. Nerve conduction abnormalities appear early and are present in most CMT 1A cases by 3 years of age (Ouvrier 1992) or even earlier (Berciano et al. 1989), although they are sometimes inconclusive (Ryan and Jones 2004). Prolongation of distal latencies may precede slowing of nerve conduction (Garcia et al. 1998). Conduction velocities are usually abnormal in one of the parents, whether or not clinically affected. Neurogenic EMG changes are usually mild to moderate.

Nerve biopsy is not specific and is not necessary for diagnosis, especially when there is a clear family history of the disease. Testing of DNA for the presence of the chromosome 17p11.2 duplication detects most cases. When negative, more intensive analysis of the *PMP22*, *MPZ* or *LITAF* genes may be pursued. The main indication for biopsy would be differentiation from chronic inflammatory neuropathy. In such cases, nerve biopsy and/or a trial of steroid treatment may be warranted. Prenatal diagnosis is possible in principle, but the presence of a duplication or point mutation does not enable one to predict the severity of the disorder. Approximately 20% of affected individuals have a significant disability but a similar proportion remain asymptomatic.

Cases of CMT 1 are not uncommonly associated with tremor of the upper limbs and sometimes with some degree of clumsiness. Such cases are identical with the *Roussy–Levy syndrome* and do not deserve individualization. The family in the first reported case was shown to have a mutation of the *MPZ* gene (Plante-Bordeneuve et al. 1999) but a similar picture can be caused by *PMP22* gene mutations (Thomas et al. 1997). HMSN I is clearly different clinically and genetically from Friedreich ataxia with which it is all too often confused but whose prognosis is completely different (Chapter 9). Molecular genetic techniques can be used for the separation.

early, and this may be a useful sign for the clinical diagnosis of the condition in young children with affected relatives or in parents of children with the disease (Garcia et al. 1998). Some affected patients do retain their tendon reflexes into adulthood.

Sensory abnormalities are mild and may be difficult to evidence when they are limited to subtle deficits of epicritic or deep sensation. Pain and touch sensation is not impaired until late, and dysaesthesiae or shooting pains are not a feature, although pain due to foot deformities or calluses may be severe in some patients. Muscle cramps are not uncommon.

Vasomotor disturbances are common, with frequent cyanosis and marbling of the skin. Palpable nerve enlargement is not rare in children but is difficult to assess objectively. Scoliosis, lordosis, hip dysplasia, metatarsal stress fractures and recurrent patellar dislocation may occur (Harding and Thomas 1980c, Thomas et al. 1997). The CSF protein level is elevated in over half the cases, but lumbar puncture is not indicated.

Progression of CMT I is slow, and arrests are common and often prolonged. Most patients remain active indefinitely but some severe cases exist. In an occasional patient, intercurrent infections or rapid growth may be associated with acceleration of the disease process. Pregnancy may cause significant deterioration (Gastaut et al. 2000), and exposure to vincristine can cause a severe regression (Igarashi et al. 1995). Rare cases of proven CMT 1 with rapid deterioration and response to steroid treatment are on record (Dyck et al. 1993). The interpretation of such cases of prednisone-responsive CMT 1 is difficult. They resemble chronic

AUTOSOMAL RECESSIVE DEMYELINATING TYPES OF CMT (CMT 4; AUTOSOMAL RECESSIVE HMSN TYPE I)

A few patients with a clinical picture similar to, but often more severe than, that of classical CMT 1 with an autosomal recessive transmission are on record (Harding and Thomas 1980a, Gabreëls-Festen et al. 1992, Gabreëls-Festen and Gabreëls 1993).

CMT 4 includes this group of autosomal recessive demyelinating neuropathies (Table 20.1). All are rather severe, early-onset disorders with moderately slow motor conduction velocities (usually around 20 m/s with a range 3–37 m/s). Affected children are likely to have similarly affected siblings with normal parents or to have consanguineous parents. Recent reports have shed light on clinical and molecular findings in a number of these conditions, and have provided some insight into their relative frequency. North African and Middle-Eastern populations appear to show a higher prevalence.

CMT 4A is caused by mutations in the ganglioside-induced differentiation-associated protein-1 (*GDAP1*) gene. Most patients show an early-onset severe phenotype with prominent foot deformities (Nelis et al. 2002). The clinical spectrum of this disorder has been expanded by the recognition that patients with *GDAP1* mutations may develop laryngeal and diaphragmatic paralysis in later life (Stojkovic et al. 2004). *GDAP1* mutations may cause demyelinating or axonal degenerative changes in nerve biopsies in different kindreds (Di Maria et al. 2004, Stojkovic et al. 2004).

CMT 4B1 and CMT 4B2 are characterized by the presence, on biopsy, of striking in- and outfoldings of myelin, although this finding is not invariable (Quattrone et al. 1996, Parman et al. 2004). Both disorders are associated with mutations of members of the myotubularin family. Cases of CMT 4B1 tend to have an early onset of mainly distal weakness followed by proximal weakness and wasting. Deep tendon reflexes are usually absent even in the early stages. Sensory changes are difficult to detect in infancy but are usually evident later in childhood. Most cases have pes cavus. Ptosis, and internal and external ophthalmoplegia are reported. Facial nerve weakness may give rise to pouting lips. Dysphagia, vocal cord paresis, dysarthria, ataxia and nocturnal hypoventilation may occur later. The clinical course is usually more severe than in CMT 1A. Scoliosis is frequent. Many adults are wheelchair-dependent and several have died in the fourth and fifth decades. CMT 4B1 is caused by mutations of the *MTMR2* (myotubularin) gene.

Apart from the myelin disturbance, CMT 4B2 is usually associated with congenital or juvenile glaucoma, although some kindreds with the causative *MTMR13* mutation lacked this feature (Hirano et al. 2004).

CMT 4C usually presents in the first decade and results in a high frequency of scoliosis. Some patients progress slowly, allowing ambulation up to the fifth decade, whereas others become wheelchair-dependent during their teenage years (Senderek et al. 2003). The disorder is due to mutations of the *KIAA1985* gene. Nerve conduction velocities range from 4 to 37 m/s. A remarkable difference in conduction slowing between nerves of the same limb may be seen (Gabreëls-Festen and Thomas 2005). Histopathologically, nerve biopsies characteristically reveal basal lamina onion bulbs and extended Schwann processes and occasional rings surrounding myelinated and unmyelinated fibres. Giant axons may also be seen (Vallat et al. 2005).

CMT 4D (HMSN-Lom) is the commonest of three recessively inherited polyneuropathies that are largely confined to inbred Gypsy populations. HMSN-Lom was originally identified in 'travellers' living in the city of Lom, Bulgaria. It is due to mutations of the *NDRG1* gene, which may code for a Schwann cell

signalling protein necessary for axonal survival. The clinical picture is similar to other autosomal recessive demyelinating neuropathies but deafness commonly supervenes after the first decade (Kalaydjieva et al. 2000). CMT 4E is a rare neuropathy attributed to homozygous mutations of the *EGR2* (early growth response) gene that can produce a Déjerine–Sottas or congenital hypomyelinating neuropathy phenotype (Warner et al. 1999). EGR2 regulates *periaxin* expression. Nerve conduction velocities are very low, often less than 5 m/s.

Patients with CMT 4F, which is caused by mutations of the *periaxin* gene, have usually had a severe CMT clinical phenotype (Boerkoel et al. 2001, Guilbot et al. 2001). Sensory involvement with dysaesthesiae and ataxia may be prominent. Nerve conduction velocities tend to be very slow (2–3 m/s). Nerve biopsies have shown a severe loss of myelinated fibres with many onion bulbs and some fibres with myelin outfoldings. Mice lacking periaxin show similar histopathological findings.

CMT 4G (HMSN-Russe) is another of the neuropathies seen in the European Gypsy population. It is similar to CMT 4D but without nerve deafness. It has been mapped to 10q22 but the gene has not yet been identified (Thomas et al. 2001). CMT 4H is very similar to CMT 4B1 but is due to a mutation of *FGD4*, which encodes the Rho GTPase guanine nucleotide exchange factor, frabin. Frabin may act on myotubularin (see CMT 4B1) (Stendel et al. 2007).

Other forms of CMT 4 are very rare or incompletely characterized at this time (Table 20.1).

It has been suggested that CMT 4A may constitute up to 25% of cases of autosomal recessive CMT, but only one GDAP1 mutation was detected in a recent study of 20 Turkish patients with probable autosomal recessive early-onset demyelinating neuropathy who were carefully studied with screening for nine possible causative genes. The other five proven mutations included two cases of *MTMR2*, and one each of *KIAA1985*, *NDRG1* and *PRX* mutations. Thus no mutation was detected in 14 of the 20 cases (Parman et al. 2004). In a similar study in Japan, 3 of 66 patients with CMT 4 were found to have *periaxin* mutations (Kijima et al. 2004).

CMT 2 / HMSN II

CMT 2 also produces a clinical picture consistent with the description of Charcot–Marie–Tooth disease. Its frequency in children is classically much lower than that of CMT 1 (Ouvrier 1992, Ouvrier et al. 1999, Ouvrier and Wilmhurst 2003). The high prevalence of the disease in Swedish children may be due to ethnic factors; however, the frequency of an asymptomatic or very mild form in young children makes the diagnosis difficult and may partly explain the discrepant figures.

PATHOLOGY

The pathology is characterized by the presence of signs of axonal degeneration with secondary involvement of the myelin sheath or Schwann cell. Myelinated fibres, especially those of large calibre, are reduced in number, and regenerative clusters may be seen. Onion bulbs are infrequent. The internodes are shortened and of irregular length on teasing. Acute axonal lesions are rare and the pathological abnormalities may be inconspicuous.

CLINICAL FEATURES

The clinical manifestations are similar to those of CMT 1 but often have a later onset, during the second or third decade, and a slower course. Atrophy of posterior tibial and calf muscles is commonly as marked as in the anterolateral compartment. Absent reflexes and foot deformity are less frequent than in type I, but foot ulcers may occur making certain subtypes, such as CMT 2B, difficult to distinguish from hereditary sensory and autonomic neuropathy (HSAN) type I (see below) (Elliott et al. 1997). Sensory manifestations are often difficult to demonstrate. There is no nerve hypertrophy and raised CSF protein is rare. Upper limb tremor is uncommon (Salisachs et al. 1979, Harding and Thomas 1980c, Westerberg et al. 1983).

Differentiation from type I is by electrophysiological investigation. Motor and sensory conduction velocities are normal or only mildly decreased to 60% or more of normal values (Berciano et al. 1986). In CMT patients over 2 years of age, a motor conduction velocity >38 m/s in the median nerve is compatible with the diagnosis of CMT 2, whereas values <38 m/s are more in favour of CMT 1 (Harding and Thomas 1980c).

HETEROGENEITY OF CMT 2

CMT 2 has been linked to at least 10 loci and 9 genes (Table 20.1). While CMT 2A was initially linked to a missense mutation in the kinesin family member *1B-ss* (*KIF1B*) gene in one pedigree, no such mutations have been identified in other affected kindreds. Mutations in the gene encoding a mitochondrial fusion protein, mitofusin 2 (*MFN2*), were recently detected in a number of such families (Kijima et al. 2004, Züchner et al. 2004).

CMT 2B is caused by missense mutations in the small GTP-ase late endosomal protein *RAB 7*, which may have a role in axonal transport (Houlden et al. 2004). It may be confused with HSAN type 1 because of the presence of moderate sensory loss with complicating ulcers in up to 50% of cases (Verhoeven et al. 2003).

The gene has not yet been found for CMT 2C, a condition clinically characterized by diaphragm, intercostal and vocal cord paralysis.

CMT 2D, which causes prominent weakness of the hands usually commencing in the teenage years, has been localized to chromosome 7p15 and is due to mutations of the GARS gene, which may also cause a syndrome of distal spinal muscular atrophy (SMA type 5)

CMT 2E is due to mutations of the neurofilament light protein (*NEFL*) gene. Nerve conduction velocities may span the demyelinating and axonal degenerative range. Cases with slow nerve conduction velocities have been classified as having CMT 1F, whereas those with velocities in the axonal range have been grouped as CMT 2E. Onset in those with slow nerve conduction is often before the age of 13 years and the nerve biopsy in one showed a mixed axonal/demyelinating picture (Jordanova et al. 2003).

Several genes usually associated with autosomal dominant demyelinating neuropathies may cause an axonal degenerative neuropathy. CMT 2I and 2J refer to axonal neuropathies caused by certain mutations of the *MPZ* gene, while CMT 2G and 2K are caused by dominant and recessive *GDAP1* alterations respectively.

Genes for two further forms of CMT 2 (L and F) have recently been identified. Both encode heat-shock proteins, which are stress proteins induced in response to a variety of physiological and environmental factors (Evgrafov et al. 2004; Tang et al. 2004, 2005).

The association of glomerular nephropathy with CMT 2 seems to be a nonfortuitous association with a dominant inheritance (Deniau et al. 1986). Accumulation of neurofilaments has been found in one typical case (Vogel et al. 1985).

AUTOSOMAL RECESSIVE FORMS OF CMT 2

Although autosomal recessive CMT of axonal degenerative types are known, few have been fully elucidated. *LMNA* mutations have been shown to cause CMT 2B1 as well as a variety of other disorders including autosomal dominant Emery–Dreifuss muscular dystrophy, limb–girdle muscular dystrophy type 1B and a dominant axonal neuropathy associated with muscular dystrophy, cardiac disease and leukonychia (Goizet et al. 2004). *LMNA* is the first gene found to cause both dominant and recessive CMT 2. Some mutations of the GDAP1 and *MPZ* genes occasionally cause an axonal degenerative picture.

The series of axonal neuropathies described by Ouvrier et al. (1981) and Gabreëls-Festen et al. (1991) included a number of autosomal recessive cases with a distinctive clinical phenotype at a time when recessive cases were not included in the Dyck classification of the hereditary neuropathies. The onset was in the first five years of life and there was rather rapid progression so that most patients were almost completely paralysed below the knees and elbows by their teens. Motor conduction velocities were unmeasurable in 5 patients because of absent motor responses, but were over 35 m/s in all other patients. Five of 10 patients tested from the Sydney series have now been shown to have mitofusin 2 (*MFN2*) gene mutations. Two were compound heterozygotes, i.e. recessively inherited; three had dominant (heterozygous) mutations. Another Sydney patient with a less severe phenotype was homozygous for a phe216ser mutation on exon 7 of the *MFN2* gene (personal observations, unpublished). Mitochondria undergo continued cycles of fission and fusion of their inner and outer membranes. *MFN2* is a large mitochondrial GTPase. It may function to tether mitochondria before fusion. The neuropathy may thus be due to a defect in mitochondrial fusion/fission that interferes with energy production and slows axonal transport. Many mutations are de novo. The clinical picture is probably not very different from that seen in some of the other recessive axonal neuropathies where the gene is actually known, but this is difficult to judge from the literature because, in many series, clinical and histopathological details have often been sketchy at best.

In addition to the axonal degenerative forms of CMT listed in Table 20.1, there are several other autosomal recessive axonal polyneuropathies that, for historical or other reasons, have not traditionally been included in CMT classifications. These include severe infantile axonal neuropathy with respiratory failure, giant axonal neuropathy (see below), and the Andermann syndrome, a neuropathy described in French Canadians that is associated with agenesis of the corpus callosum and which has recently been shown to be due to mutations of the gene *SLC12A6*, encoding the potassium-chloride co-transporter protein KCC3A (Casaubon et al. 1996, Howard et al. 2002).

SEVERE INFANTILE AXONAL NEUROPATHY WITH
RESPIRATORY FAILURE
Another recently characterized autosomal recessive axonal neuropathy that overlaps with spinal muscular atrophy has been labelled severe infantile axonal neuropathy with respiratory failure (SIANR) (Wilmshurst et al. 2000) or spinal muscular atrophy with respiratory disease (SMARD) (Grohmann et al. 2001) depending on the degree of abnormality in the peripheral nerves. This condition is described in Chapter 18.

CMT 3 / HMSN III
The terms CMT 3, HMSN type III and *Déjerine–Sottas disease* are applied to a heterogeneous group of inherited or sporadic neuropathies (Ouvrier et al. 1987, 1999) with various ages of onset and severity. The age of onset was widely different in the two patients originally reported by Déjerine and Sottas.

There is no universal agreement as to the limits or even the existence of this group especially with respect to the congenital types, but in our opinion it remains a useful clinical concept. Considerable genetic heterogeneity has been recognized. Mutations and deletions, often compound, of the *MPZ*, *PMP22*, *periaxin*, and *EGR2* genes, homozygosity for the CMT 1A genotype with or without duplication, and homozygosity for a CMT 2 syndrome caused by a myelin P₀ mutation have all been reported (Sghirlanzoni et al. 1992, Tyson et al. 1997).

Pathologically, nerve alterations are reminiscent of those in type I but they are more intense. There is a marked decrease of myelinated fibres, especially the larger ones. Onion bulbs are well formed but often consist of double basement membrane lamellae, and the ratio of the axon diameter to the total fibre diameter is higher than normal, indicating hypomyelination (Ouvrier et al. 1987). In some cases, there is massive interstitial collagen hypertrophy.

CLASSICAL PHENOTYPE
The most typical form (Ouvrier et al. 1987) has an early onset, with slow motor development and hypotonia commonly present during the first year of life. Ambulation is delayed in 30–50% of patients. Weakness is more profound and more diffuse than in type I cases and frequently involves the proximal muscles. Ataxia is consistently present and the weakness may be asymmetrical. Prominent eyes with thickening and eversion of the lips is a not uncommon feature, particularly with *PMP22* mutations (Ouvrier et al. 1987). Pupillary abnormalities and even an Argyll Robertson pupil are occasionally observed. In older patients, tendon

reflexes are abolished and nerve hypertrophy is frequent.

The course tends to be more severe than in CMT 1 and CMT 2, but not greatly so, although a few patients are incapable of independent walking by adolescence.

Nerve conduction velocities are severely diminished to below 10m/s or even cannot be measured as no evoked muscle response can be obtained. Parents have no clinical signs or slowing of NCVs, thus ruling out the possibility of a type I neuropathy, but EMG is said to reveal signs of mild neurogenic muscular involvement in some.

CONGENITAL HYPOMYELINATING NEUROPATHIES
The congenital hypomyelinating neuropathies are usually considered as a form of CMT 3, although an early onset may also be observed in some CMT 1 cases (Harati and Butler 1985). They are also a heterogeneous group and no agreement has been reached regarding their nosological situation. Guzzetta et al. (1982) distinguished two groups of congenital cases. A severe form may resemble acute Werdnig–Hoffmann disease with congenital hypotonia and paralysis, wasting and respiratory impairment that may be lethal in a few months or years (Goebel et al. 1976) and is aggravated by swallowing difficulties. A raised CSF protein level is constant, and nerve conduction velocities are unmeasurable or extremely low. Less severe cases exist that permit survival for many years but with severe motor impairment. Some sensory impairment may be observed in the course of such cases.

The pathological picture in most cases is that of complete absence of myelin (amyelinic form or amyelinating neuropathy) (Ouvrier et al. 1999) with formation of onion bulbs containing mainly layers of Schwann cells with little or no myelin. The molecular biological basis of the amyelinating cases is poorly defined. The pathological findings have been interpreted as indicating that the process is one of deficient myelin deposition rather than demyelination–remyelination. In some cases, there is proliferation of microfilaments in Schwann cells, along with demyelination (Ulrich et al. 1981). In others, unstable myelin with infolding of myelin lamellae has been described (Peudenier et al. 1993). Cases with congenital arthrogryposis have been reported (Balestrini et al. 1991, Boylan et al. 1992). Johnson et al. (1989) have described central hypomyelination in association with hypomyelination polyneuropathy. Similar cases have been caused by *SOX10* mutation in association with Hirschprung disease (Inoue et al. 2002) and by *GJA12* mutations responsible for the autosomal recessive form of Pelizaeus–Merzbacher-like disease (Uhlenberg et al. 2004).

Two remarkable cases of recovery from a congenital hypomyelinating neuropathy were reported by Ghamdi et al. (1997) and Levy et al. (1997).

UNCOMMON NEUROPATHIES WITH MOTOR AND SENSORY INVOLVEMENT
HEREDITARY NEUROPATHY WITH LIABILITY TO PRESSURE PALSIES (HNPP)
This is a rare, dominantly inherited disease, characterized by an

abnormal susceptibility to pressure palsies (Behse et al. 1972), usually with evidence of an underlying generalized neuropathy with moderate slowing of nerve conduction velocities and prolonged distal motor and sensory latencies. In most cases the disease is due to a deletion of the region of chromosome 17 that is duplicated in cases of CMT 1A, probably as a result of unequal crossing-over during meiosis (Mariman et al. 1994, Verhalle et al. 1994). Tyson et al. (1996) reported that the same DNA abnormalities may occasionally be found in cases of multifocal paralysis without pressure sensitivity, thus widening the spectrum of the disease. Affected subjects may develop symptoms during the first decade, although a later onset is more usual. The paralyses usually involve a single nerve trunk, especially the popliteal nerve, following prolonged maintenance of attitudes such as squatting or sitting cross-legged, or the cubital nerve following pressure on the elbow. Paralysis also occurs following a brief, unusual effort such as intense physical activity, especially sport. Many patients develop a carpal tunnel syndrome of early onset, which may be clinically manifested but is present on electrophysiological examination in most cases. A few cases have had evidence of CNS involvement with lesions resembling those of multiple sclerosis on MR images (Sanahuja et al. 2005). Recovery from palsies is usually complete over a period of days to weeks, but in some cases permanent generalized motor and sensory neuropathy eventually develops. Dunn et al. (1978) noted brachial plexus involvement in some patients. Although this suggested a relationship to hereditary brachial plexopathy, the two conditions are genetically distinct (Chance et al. 1994, Gouider et al. 1994).

The diagnosis is suggested by the disproportion between the minor degree of trauma and the occurrence of paralysis. The frequent presence of a similar history in relatives is virtually diagnostic. Electrophysiological examination confirms the suspicion of an underlying neuropathy by showing slowed conduction velocities outside the affected territory. Examination of family members may demonstrate a neuropathy even in the absence of attacks. Nerve biopsy, which is not necessary in most cases, can show segmental thickenings of myelin sheaths known as tomacula (Verhagen et al. 1993). Such findings have also been found in definite cases of familial brachial plexopathy (Martinelli et al. 1989) and in one patient with a clinical picture of recurrent polyneuropathy (Joy and Oh 1989). No treatment is known, but avoidance of repeated episodes that may leave sequelae may require changes in lifestyle.

HEREDITARY NEURALGIC AMYOTROPHY (BRACHIAL PLEXOPATHY)

This is also a dominantly transmitted condition, genetically distinct from hereditary neuropathy with liability to pressure palsies. The onset is usually in the second decade, but earlier onset can occur and brachial plexus paralyses at birth may be the first manifestation. Attacks closely resemble those observed in the non-hereditary type of plexopathy. Pain may be intense and precedes weakness usually by a few days. Weakness persists for variable periods. It is mainly proximal. Recovery takes place over a few weeks to months and is usually complete (van Alfen et al.

2000, van Alfen and van Engelen 2006). The frequency of recurrences is extremely variable (Airaksinen et al. 1985). Occasional patients may experience phrenic nerve involvement or episodes of lumbar plexopathy (Awerbuch et al. 1989, Thomson 1993). In several families a particular kind of mild dysmorphism with a long face and hypotelorism was present in affected members (Dunn et al. 1978). In some cases, involvement may be limited to a single branch of the brachial plexus, e.g. the long thoracic nerve with isolated palsy of the serratus anterior (Phillips 1986). The disease maps to chromosome 17q25 in most but not all affected kindreds (Pellegrino et al. 1996, Watts et al. 2002). Biopsies of involved nerves may show inflammatory infiltrates and/or acute axonal degeneration (Klein et al. 2002).

Diagnosis with a sporadic brachial plexopathy is not possible at the first episode unless affected relatives are known and/or dysmorphism is present.

Treatment is generally symptomatic but i.v. methylprednisolone may result in earlier improvement, especially in pain control (Klein and Windebank 2005).

MISCELLANEOUS TYPES OF HEREDITARY DEGENERATIVE MOTOR AND SENSORY NEUROPATHIES

Scapuloperoneal amyotrophy of neural origin (Dawidenkow syndrome)

This is a rare cause of the scapuloperoneal syndrome (Chapter 21). Evidence of neural involvement and nerve hypertrophy enable linkage of such cases to the hereditary motor and sensory neuropathies. Both axonal and demyelinating forms exist (Hyser et al. 1988). Such cases are to be distinguished from those of spinal cord origin (De Long and Siddique 1992).

HMSN type IV, better known as Refsum disease, and other metabolic neuropathies are described below. For a more complete description of the rare types of hereditary neuropathies, see Ouvrier et al. (1999).

THERMOSENSITIVE NEUROPATHY

Magy et al. (1997) reported on a remarkable family with intermittent episodes of extensive paralysis precipitated by body temperature elevations above 38.5°C with onset in childhood or adolescence and not allelic to CMT 1 or hereditary pressure-sensitive neuropathy.

Relapsing axonal neuropathy

The cases of relapsing axonal neuropathy reported in siblings by Quinlivan et al. (1994) are difficult to classify. Such cases may be difficult to distinguish from the rare infantile forms of Guillain–Barré syndrome. A similar family has been studied in Sydney (Wilmshurst et al. 2003).

HEREDITARY SENSORY AND AUTONOMIC NEUROPATHIES

Inherited peripheral sensory neuropathies are rare and their definitive diagnosis is difficult. Controversy over terminology confuses their classification (Axelrod and Pearson 1984), and some diagnostic tests may not be easily available outside specialized centres. The general management of sensory neuropathies is discussed by Klein and Dyck (2005a).

HSAN I (SENSORY RADICULAR NEUROPATHY, ACROPATHIE ULCEROMUTILANTE)

HSAN I differs from all other HSANs in that the symptoms appear late, usually after the first decade, rather than in infancy. The transmission is autosomal dominant. The gene for the classical form, the serine pamitoyltransferase longchain subunit 1 gene (*SPTLC1*) is involved in phospholipid biosynthesis and maps to 9q22.1–q22.3 (Dawkins et al. 2001). Pathological examination shows a marked reduction in the number of unmyelinated fibres. Small and large myelinated fibres are decreased to a smaller but quite significant extent. The dorsal root ganglia and the spinal dorsal roots supplying the lower limbs are degenerate. Symptoms appear in late childhood or adolescence with a progressive loss of sensation in the lower extremities, rapidly complicated by episodes of cellulitis and trophic ulcerations of the feet. Spontaneous stabbing pain may occur. There is loss of pain and temperature sensation with preservation of tactile sensation. Later, all sensation may disappear and the distal upper limbs may become involved. Neural deafness is frequently present. Peroneal weakness often eventually develops. Motor nerve conduction velocities are mildly slow, and sensory action potentials are absent. The course is slowly progressive. HSAN I is heterogeneous. *RAB7* mutations may cause a similar picture or a more typical CMT phenotype (CMT 2B). Another similar autosomal dominant entity with later onset and prominent symptoms of gastrooesophageal reflux and cough has been localized to 3p22–p24 (Kok et al. 2003). A form with early-onset dementia is on record (Wright and Dyck 1995).

HSAN II (CONGENITAL SENSORY NEUROPATHY)

This is an autosomal recessive condition with a congenital or early onset. Clinically, most patients have a universal absence of pain sensation resulting in burns and mutilations of the lips or fingertips and in painless fractures, especially of the metatarsals. Tactile sensation is also markedly impaired. Areas of normal sensation are preserved in some patients in whom the limbs and face are predominantly affected. Bladder sensation may be impaired with vesical distension (Verity et al. 1982). Deafness has been described in some patients (Verity et al. 1982). In most patients, the disease does not seem progressive or is only very slowly evolving (Ferrière et al. 1992). Some cases may run a faster course with clinical evidence of progression (Johnson and Spalding 1964) that is in agreement with nerve biopsy findings of fibre degeneration and regeneration. Motor conduction velocities are preserved or only slightly decreased, but sensory action potentials are unobtainable. Cortical evoked somatosensory potentials were lacking in the lower limbs in some patients. Nerve biopsy often shows grossly atrophic nerves. Myelinated axons are severely reduced in number, but unmyelinated fibres are usually normal or at least not greatly diminished. Linkage analysis of two large Canadian kindreds identified a novel gene, HSN2, which is located within

intron 8 of the *PRKWNK1* gene (Lafrenière et al. 2004). The function of HSN2 is unknown. A mutation in the same gene was subsequently identified in an affected Lebanese kindred.

HSAN III (FAMILIAL DYSAUTONOMIA, RILEY–DAY SYNDROME)

HSAN III is the most common of the sensory and autonomic neuropathies. The disorder is prevalent among Ashkenazi Jews, in whom the disease frequency is between 0.5 and 1 per 10,000 live births with an estimated carrier frequency of 1 in 50. Scattered case reports on non-Jewish patients can be found (e.g. Guzzetta et al. 1986). The disorder is transmitted as an autosomal recessive trait caused by mutations of the *IKBKAP* gene, which maps to chromosome 9q31 (Slaugenhaupt et al. 2005). Histopathological findings include loss of neurons in the posterior root, Lissauer tract and intermediolateral grey columns (Pearson and Pytel 1978) and loss of unmyelinated and myelinated fibres in peripheral nerves where catecholamine endings are lacking (Pearson et al. 1974). Substance P-immune reactivity in the substantia gelatinosa of the spinal cord and in the medulla is consistently depleted (Pearson et al. 1982). Sympathetic ganglia are hypoplastic.

Clinical manifestations are mainly referable to the autonomic nervous system. Onset is congenital, and hypotonia, sucking difficulties, a poor cry and vomiting are present from birth. Growth retardation becomes evident later in life. Patients do not have overflow tears. Skin blotching, motor incoordination, unstable temperature and blood pressure, cyclic vomiting and drooling are variably present. Relative indifference to pain is usual (Axelrod et al. 1981). Temperature perception, sweating and cutaneous innervation have been studied by Hilz et al. (2004). Bouts of apnoea and pneumonia are common and are a usual cause of death in infancy and childhood. Oesophageal dilatation and impaired gastric motility are frequent findings. Postural hypotension is almost always present. Scoliosis is a major problem. The gag reflex is often poor. Diagnostic criteria include the absence of fungiform papillae on the tongue, diminished or absent deep tendon reflexes, lack of overflow tears, miosis following instillation of 2.5% metacholine chloride in the eyes, and lack of an axon flare after intradermal histamine injection (Axelrod et al. 1974). None of these criteria is individually characteristic, and any of them can be found in other sensory neuropathies. Prenatal diagnosis is possible.

The course of familial dysautonomia is severe; in the early studies in the 1960s only 20% of patients survived to adulthood, although by the 1980s due to improvements in management this proportion had risen to 50% (Axelrod and Abularrage 1982). Digestive and respiratory complications are common and may be aggravated by the frequent occurrence of kyphoscoliosis. Emotional lability with repeated severe breath-holding spells is common. Intelligence remains normal.

Treatment is symptomatic. The risk of aspiration pneumonia should be minimized by attention to posture and by meticulous precautions during feeding that may necessitate gavage, gastrostomy or fundoplication. Diazepam is effective in association

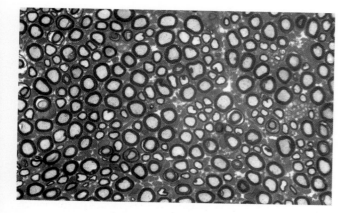

Fig. 20.4. Hereditary sensory neuropathy type IV. There is a patchy deficiency of small myelinated fibres. Unmyelinated fibres were very sparse on electron microscopic examination.

with chlorpromazine for the treatment of acute crises and of hypertension. The management of scoliosis is difficult and only partial surgical correction of the curve can be achieved in many patients (Kaplan et al. 1997). Families of affected children need considerable psychological support.

HSAN IV (CONGENITAL INSENSITIVITY TO PAIN WITH ANHIDROSIS)

In this rare disorder due to a mutation of the nerve growth factor receptor gene *TRK/NGF*, there is virtual absence of unmyelinated nerve fibres in peripheral nerves (Goebel et al. 1980) (Fig. 20.4). The Lissauer tract and dorsal spinal roots are also affected. The onset of the disease is congenital with episodes of unexplained fever often related to environmental temperature. Absence of sweating (anhidrosis) is usual. Insensitivity to pain is universal and leads to injuries, self-mutilation and osteomyelitis, especially of the lower extremities. Tongue-biting is frequent. Blotching of the skin and pupillary hypersensitivity to metacholine chloride occur (Axelrod and Pearson 1984). Mental retardation is the rule, measured IQ scores having varied from 41 to 78, the majority being in the sixties (Rosemberg et al. 1994). Motor and sensory nerve conduction velocities are normal or near-normal. A mild form without anhidrosis has been reported by Pavone et al. (1992).

HSAN V

HSAN type V presents as a congenital insensitivity to pain with decreased thermal sensitivity but with preservation of response to tactile and mechanical stimuli and retention of the deep tendon reflexes (Low et al. 1978). It is characterized pathologically by an almost complete disappearance of small myelinated fibres and a moderate decrease of unmyelinated fibres. Routine motor and sensory nerve conduction studies are normal. A possible locus for HSAN V on chromosome 1p11.2–p13.2 was identified in a large Swedish kindred with impaired sensation of deep pain and temperature but normal cognitive abilities. Analysis of functional candidate genes in the disease critical region revealed

a mutation in the coding region of the nerve growth-factor beta receptor (*NGFβ*) gene (Einarsdottir et al. 2004).

OTHER FORMS OF HSAN WITH INSENSITIVITY OR INDIFFERENCE TO PAIN

Several rare and/or controversial types of HSAN have been described. Additional types include HSAN with growth hormone deficiency (Liberfarb et al. 1993), progresssive panneuropathy with hypotension (Axelrod and Pearson 1984), HSAN type II without trophic changes (Bye et al. 1990), HSAN with neurotrophic keratitis (Donaghy et al. 1987), congenital sensory neuropathy with ichthyosis and anterior chamber syndrome (Quinlivan et al. 1993), deafness, sensory neuropathy and ovarian agenesis (Linssen et al. 1994), and HSAN with cataracts, mental retardation and skin lesions (Heckmann et al. 1995). HSAN associated with spastic paraplegia includes two distinct types, one affecting mainly the small sensory fibres (Cavanagh et al. 1979a), the other involving the large fibres with few neuropathic symptoms (Schady and Smith 1994). In addition, two different types of sensory neuropathy have been described in Navajo children (Appenzeller et al. 1976, Johnsen et al. 1993).

Some cases of sensory neuropathy can simulate child abuse (Makari et al. 1994).

The term *insensitivity to pain* in principle applies to patients in whom analgesia is the result of abnormalities of peripheral nerves, cutaneous nerve endings or central sensory pathways, whereas *indifference to pain* applies to those who have normal sensory pathways but fail to appreciate the painful nature of stimuli (Manfredi et al. 1981). Such a distinction may well be artificial, and Dyck et al. (1983) have emphasized the fact that precise analysis of cases of indifference to pain shows abnormalities of the peripheral sensory system when sophisticated methods are used. However, a case with a normal morphometric nerve study has been reported (Landrieu et al. 1990) and familial cases due to mutations in the gene of the Nav1.7 sodium channel have been recently described (Cox et al. 2006, Goldberg et al. 2007).

MISCELLANEOUS SENSORY AND AUTONOMIC NEUROPATHIES

Rare cases of involvement of the autonomic nervous system are marked by pain. A familial dominant syndrome of paroxysmal rectal pain of early onset, associated with unilateral or bilateral vasodilatation of the lower limbs and abdomen and often precipitated by defaecation has been described. Later, ocular and submaxillary pain may appear. Syncopes at the time of attacks often occur. This condition, now renamed *paroxysmal extreme pain* disorder, has been shown recently to result from mutations in the gene in the Nav1.7 receptor (Fertleman et al. 2007). The same gene is also mutated in *erythromelalgia*, characterized by attacks of distal pain and erythema precipitated by heat. Treatment with carbamazepine is often effective.

A polyneuropathy of variable severity with demyelination and interstitial fibrosis has been reported in association with chronic intestinal pseudo-obstruction and often ophthalmoplegia. The condition appears to be familial (Steiner et al. 1987). A leukoencephalopathy has been shown by MRI in similar cases for which the acronym 'POLIP' (*p*olyneuropathy, *o*phthalmoplegia, *l*eukoencephalopathy and *i*ntestinal *p*seudo-obstruction) has been proposed (Simon et al. 1990). Some such cases were shown to be associated with cytochrome *c* oxidase deficiency in muscle biopsy samples (Haftel et al. 2000).

The restless legs syndrome, which is a special type of sensory neuropathy frequent in adults, also exists in children (Kotagal and Silber 2004). The related syndrome of periodic limb movements in sleep has its onset before 10 years of age in 20% of cases.

COMPLEX NEUROPATHIES ASSOCIATED WITH CNS INVOLVEMENT AND METABOLIC NEUROPATHIES

Hereditary neuropathies may constitute a part of more complex neurological diseases involving the CNS (Table 20.2). Friedreich ataxia, a common cause of neuropathy with CNS involvement, is reviewed in Chapter 9.

HEREDITARY MOTOR AND SENSORY NEUROPATHIES WITH CNS INVOLVEMENT

Certain rare types of HMSN include affectation of the optic pathways and retina and, sometimes, more widespread disturbances. These are detailed by Klein and Dyck (2005b). HMSN type V features pyramidal tract signs associated with a motor and sensory neuropathy. There is variable clinical spasticity (Harding and Thomas 1984, Frith et al. 1994). Dyck (1984) recognized HMSN type VI associated with optic atrophy, and type VII with pigmentary retinopathy. The neuropathy in type VI is mainly sensory and the condition is heterogeneous (Ippel et al. 1995, Chalmers et al. 1996). Some cases of HMSN VI also feature mental retardation and pyramidal signs (McDermot and Walker 1987). The latter have also been reported by Pagès and Pagès (1983) in association with Leber optic atrophy. Sommer and Schröder (1989) indicate that in such cases the neuropathy is axonal in type and represents a distinct form. HMSN VII has been described in association with protanopia (defective red vision) (Khoubesserian et al. 1979). Polyneuropathy can also be associated with optico-acoustic degeneration (Rosenberg and Chutorian 1967) as well as with neural deafness in many different entities including CMT X, CMT 4D, and HSAN types I and II (Pinhas-Hamiel et al. 1993, Stojkovic et al. 1999, Kalaydjieva et al. 2000). Palmar–plantar keratodermia occurs in CMT in some cases (Tolmie et al. 1988), sometimes with cerebral dysgenesis (Sprecher et al. 2005). Wright and Dyck (1995) described early-onset dementia and deafness in association with HSAN I. Axonal neuropathy associated with juvenile parkinsonism and ophthalmoplegia is on record (van der Wiel and Staal 1981). A special form of congenital neuropathy, with associated osseous fragility, mental retardation and CNS involvement has been reported in one family by Neimann et al. (1973). A second family with two affected siblings has been observed in Paris (JA, unpublished). Agenesis of the corpus callosum was present together with severe degenerative CNS lesions and an apparently axonal neuropathy.

TABLE 20.2
Metabolic and degenerative CNS disorders in which a peripheral neuropathy may occur

Disease	References
Sulfatidosis (metachromatic leukodystrophy)	Bardosi et al. (1987)
Krabbe leukodystrophy	Tada et al. (1992)
Adrenomyeloneuropathy	Powers (1985)
Cockayne syndrome	Rapin et al. (2000)
Leigh disease	Jacobs et al. (1990), Chabrol et al. (1994)
Mitochondrial diseases, especially NARP	Rusanen et al. (1995)
Carbohydrate-deficient glycoprotein (CDG) syndrome	Jaeken and Carchon (1993)
Bassen–Kornzweig disease (abetalipoproteinaemia)	Wichman et al. (1985), Brin et al. (1986)
Hypobetalipoproteinaemia	Brown et al. (1974), Matsuo et al. (1994)
Tangier disease	Pollock et al. (1983)
Niemann–Pick A disease	Zafeiriou et al. (2003)
Cerebrotendinous xanthomatosis	Donaghy et al. (1990), Tokimura et al. (1992)
Refsum disease (adult and infantile forms)	Skjeldal et al. (1987), Dickson et al. (1989)
GM2 gangliosidosis	Specola et al. (1990)
Farber disease	Vital et al. (1976)
Chediak–Higashi disease	Lockman et al. (1967)
Peroxisomal diseases	MacCollin et al. (1990)
Adrenal insufficiency, achalasia and alachrymia	Tsao et al. (1994)
Ataxia–telangiectasia	Kwast and Ignatowicz (1990)
Xeroderma pigmentosum	Rapin et al. (2000), Tachi et al. (1988)
Lowe syndrome	Charnas et al. (1988)
Polyneuropathy, ophthalmoplegia, chronic intestinal pseudo-obstruction and leukoencephalopathy	Simon et al. (1990)
Trichothiodystrophy	Personal cases
Vitamin E deficiency or abnormal metabolism	Burck et al. (1981), Stumpf et al. (1987)
Vitamin B_1, B_6, B_{12} and folate deficiency	Chapter 22
Vitamin B_{12} deficiency or abnormal metabolism	Steiner et al. (1988)
Amyloidosis	Benson (2001)
Porphyria	This chapter

GIANT AXONAL NEUROPATHY

This condition is characterized pathologically by the presence of massive axonal enlargements filled with neurofilaments. Normal sized axons may be demyelinated and show 'onion bulb' structures. The disease probably represents a disorder of cytoplasmic intermediate filament formation affecting both the peripheral and central nervous system (Treiber-Held et al. 1994). It is transmitted as an autosomal recessive trait. The affected gene, *gigaxonin*, maps to chromosome 16q24.

The onset is in the first few years of life with motor deficit and areflexia. Progressive deterioration with ataxia, distal weakness and slow dementia ensue. Patients are usually wheelchair dependent by the late teens and many die in the third decade. Orthopaedic deformities include scoliosis and deformed feet.

Sensory abnormalities are usually present (Ouvrier 1989). Cranial nerves may be involved, and variable mental retardation is the rule. System degenerations may be associated (Ben Hamida et al. 1990), and diffuse involvement with endocrinological abnormalities has been reported (Takebe et al. 1981). Motor nerve conduction velocities are sometimes slowed, and sensory action potentials are often absent. The EEG is often disorganized with increased slow activity and/or spike discharges, and brainstem auditory evoked potentials are altered. On MRI, a high signal from white matter may be present on T_2 sequences. One remarkable feature is the presence of 'frizzy' or 'woolly' hair, although this is inconstant (Treiber-Held et al. 1994). The course is progressive with increasing disability, and no treatment is known. A recent review highlights the existence of milder variants, including the not-infrequent cases with absence of the characteristic 'woolly' hair (Bruno et al. 2004).

REFSUM DISEASE (HMSN IV, HEREDOPATHIA ATACTICA POLYNEURITIFORMIS)

Classical Refsum disease is rare in childhood, although some manifestations of the condition may appear early or even be congenital, e.g. bone deformities, especially short metatarsals (Skjeldal et al. 1987). Although Dyck classified Refsum disease as type IV of the hereditary motor and sensory neuropathies, the condition deserves a special place because of its well-established metabolic disturbance, its remarkable symptomatology and its partially treatable nature. The disease is caused by an abnormal accumulation of phytanic acid (a C16 branched-chain fatty acid) whose beta-oxidation is blocked due to phytanic oxidase deficiency. Most phytanic acid is of exogenous origin so that reduction of intake, sometimes in association with plasma exchanges (Gibberd et al. 1985, Dickson et al. 1989), results in lowering of abnormally high plasma levels when patients are placed on a phytol-free diet (Chapter 8). This treatment is accompanied by increased nerve conduction velocity, return of reflexes, and sensory and motor improvement.

The clinical manifestations of Refsum disease usually begin after 4–7 years of age but are often recognized much later as the progression of the disorder is slow. A few patients have presented in infancy with neurological features (Herbert and Clayton 1994). The picture is one of a chronic but sometimes fluctuating or remittent peripheral neuropathy in which the clinical expression is very variable (Skjeldal et al. 1987). A chronic relapsing picture and even an axonal neuropathy have been reported (Gelot et al. 1995). Ataxia is often marked. Atypical retinitis pigmentosa is present and hemeralopia (night blindness) may be the first symptom. Anosmia, deafness, ichthyosis and disorders of cardiac function are common. Nerve conduction velocities are usually markedly reduced, in keeping with the pathological findings of a hypertrophic demyelinating neuropathy with large onion bulb formation. The CSF protein level is >1 g/L but there is no excess of cells. The diagnosis can be confirmed by measurement of the plasma level of phytanic acid, which is considerably increased (300–1600 μmol/L instead of <10 μmol/L; 10–50 mg/dL vs <0.3 mg/dL). Mutations of the *PHYH* gene on chromosome 10p13 are responsible. This gene encodes for phytanoyl Co-A hydroxylase. Mutations of a second gene, *PEX7*, on chromosome 6q22–24 cause a mild form of the disorder (van den Brink et al. 2003).

OTHER NEUROPATHIES WITH KNOWN METABOLIC ABNORMALITY

A number of metabolic diseases feature a neuropathy that may be overshadowed by other neurological or systemic manifestations but may occasionally be the predominant or presenting feature. The main disorders in this group are shown in Table 20.2 and discussed in Chapter 8.

In some cases of metachromatic leukodystrophy, involvement of the peripheral nerves may be the only manifestation for periods of up to several months. Neuropathy with absence of deep tendon reflexes is common in Krabbe disease and has been reported in sialidosis type 1 (Steinman et al. 1980).

Neuropathy due to inherited *disorders of porphyrin metabolism* is very rare in childhood. It can be observed with four diseases: variegate porphyria due to deficiency of protoporphyrinogen oxidase, acute intermittent porphyria due to deficiency of porphobilinogen deaminase (mapping on chromosome 11q23–11qter), hereditary coproporphyrinuria due to deficient coproporphyrinogen oxidase, and delta-aminolaevulinic aciduria. These diseases are transmitted as autosomal dominant traits with variable penetrance. Prepubertal cases may occur. The symptoms and signs are similar to those in adult patients and are similar in the three types, except for the presence of photosensitivity in variegate porphyria and coproporphyria. The polyneuropathy can involve both the lower and the upper limbs (Windebank and Bonkovsky 2005). The weakness is both proximal and distal and may involve the respiratory muscles. Sensory involvement is minimal. Acute attacks of colicky abdominal pain, dysautonomic signs such as hypertension, and psychiatric disturbances may be observed. Most cases remain asymptomatic. Bouts of paralysis are often precipitated by administration of drugs, especially barbiturates but also several antibiotics, oral contraceptives, oestrogens, imipramine and methyldopa among others (Crimlisk 1997). Convulsions may be more frequent in children than in adults, and this is of considerable importance as antiepileptic drugs including phenytoin, carbamazepine, ethosuximide and sodium valproate, and also some anaesthetic agents can trigger attacks. Paraldehyde and chloral hydrate can be safely used, while gabapentin (Tatum and Zachariah 1995) and magnesium sulfate (Sadeh et al. 1991) have also been reported to be safe.

The diagnosis is confirmed by the finding of an increased urinary excretion of porphobilinogen and delta-aminolaevulinic acid. Between attacks, excretion of these compounds may be absent. Assay of erythrocyte porphobilinogen deaminase is the most accurate way of detecting acute intermittent porphyria, which is often signalled by a red discoloration of urine.

Treatment includes prevention of attacks by avoidance of precipitating drugs. During attacks, intravenous administration of glucose is indicated. If there is no improvement in 48 hours, intravenous haematin (2 mg/kg/day) should be given (Lamon et al. 1979). Side effects (thrombophlebitis, coagulopathy) are frequent. Haem arginate (Crimlisk 1997) seems both effective and well tolerated. Avoidance of skin trauma and light is important only in variegate porphyria, in which transient polyneuritis is accompanied by increased skin sensitivity.

Abetalipoproteinaemia (Bassen–Kornzweig disease) is an autosomal recessive disorder of the synthesis of the beta-lipoprotein due to a mutation of the microsomal triglyceride transfer protein (MTP) gene. As a consequence, fat absorption is deficient. Apparently, lipids are not transported from the intestinal mucosal cells into the lymphatic system, because beta-lipoproteins are necessary for the formation of chylomicrons. Fat-soluble vitamins are also poorly absorbed, and levels of vitamins A and E in the serum are quite low (Kane and Havel 1995). Neurological symptoms are the result of the deficit in vitamin E, resulting in peroxidation of the unsaturated myelin phospholipids. Pathologically, there is extensive demyelination of the posterior columns and spinocerebellar tracts, with severe depletion and segmental demyelination of large myelinated fibres in peripheral nerves and posterior roots. Involvement of the anterior horn cells and cerebellar cortex has been reported (Kane and Havel 1995).

The neurological picture is one of spinocerebellar degeneration with progressive ataxia, loss of tendon reflexes, disturbances of deep sensation and pes cavus in association with pigmentary retinal degeneration that gives rise to decreased visual acuity and night blindness. Paralysis of vertical gaze is a frequent feature. Muscle weakness and atrophy may supervene. Indeed, the picture is highly suggestive of a primary spinocerebellar degeneration and it is likely that many cases reported as Friedreich ataxia with retinitis pigmentosa were in fact cases of abetalipoproteinaemia. Neurological manifestations may appear as early as 2 years of age, and one third of patients are symptomatic by 10 years. About the same proportion of patients have mental retardation. A history of 'coeliac syndrome' during the first year of life with foul, bulky stools and abdominal distension is usually obtained, and most children exhibit growth retardation. The diagnosis rests on the presence of retinal lesions with an extinguished ERG, on the finding of low serum cholesterol and vitamin E levels, on the presence of acanthocytosis on blood smears, and ultimately on the absence of beta-lipoproteins. Electromyography may show evidence of denervation, while sensory nerve action potentials and conduction velocities are diminished. Abetalipoproteinaemia is a treatable condition, and supplementation of the diet with high-dose vitamin E (100 mg/kg/day orally) prevents the development or progression of eye and nervous disease (Kane and Havel 1995). Intramuscular vitamin E is not superior. Administration of vitamin A (200–400 IU/kg/day) and vitamin K_1 (5 mg every 2 weeks) is also advised.

Acanthocytosis is also observed in another dominantly inherited condition, known as amyotrophic choreoacanthocytosis, which includes symptoms of basal ganglia dysfunction, peripheral nerve involvement and other neurological features but is observed mostly in adults (Spencer et al. 1987), and in Hallervorden–Spatz disease (Chapter 9).

Hypobetalipoproteinaemia is a condition distinct from abetalipoproteinaemia (Mawatari et al. 1972), caused by *apo b* gene

mutations, which may produce acanthocytosis and neurological manifestations. These are usually limited to loss of deep tendon reflexes. Occasional cases may feature ataxia, hearing loss and retinitis pigmentosa (Matsuo et al. 1994).

Vitamin E deficiency may be due, in addition to absence of betalipoproteins, to biliary insufficiency that prevents normal emulsion of fat in the bowel lumen and results in poor absorption, in association with steatorrhoea (Guggenheim et al. 1982, Harding et al. 1982). A similar result has been observed in a case of intestinal lymphangiectasia (Gutmann et al. 1986). The clinical picture, indistinguishable from that observed with abetalipoproteinaemia, is observed in children with chronic liver disease, especially ductular hypoplasia (Sokol et al. 1985). The condition is amenable to the same therapy as abetalipoproteinaemia.

Rare cases of a similar syndrome *(ataxia with vitamin E deficiency; AVED; familial isolated vitamin E deficiency)* mimicking spinocerebellar degeneration have been described in children without liver disease or apparent fat malabsorption (Burck et al. 1981, Harding et al. 1985, Stumpf et al. 1987). For unknown reasons, these patients do not have retinopathy or ophthalmoplegia. This disorder is relatively frequent in Tunisia and results from mutations of the gene encoding the alpha-tocopherol transfer protein (Gotada et al. 1995, Hentati et al. 1996), which maps to chromosome 8 (Ben Hamida et al. 1993).

Tangier disease is a rare condition characterized by a decrease of high-density lipoproteins and a low cholesterol level. Accumulation of cholesterol esters in Schwann cells produces a sensorimotor neuropathy that may remain subclinical. Two main syndromes are seen: a pseudosyringomyelic syndrome and a multiple mononeuropathy.

Neuropathies are a major manifestation of the various types of amyloidosis but this condition is exceptional before adulthood (Benson 2001).

Several mitochondrial disorders can cause a neuropathy. These include the MELAS (mitochondrial encephalomyopathy, lactic acidosis and stroke-like episodes) and NARP (neuropathy, ataxia, retinitis pigmentosa) syndromes as well as cases of Leigh syndrome and other rare mitochondrial diseases (Goebel et al. 1986, Jacobs et al. 1990, Chabrol et al. 1994).

A neuropathy is also a frequent feature of the *carbohydrate-deficient glycoprotein syndrome* (Jaeken and Carchon 1993).

Vitamin deficiencies in association with other poorly defined nutritional factors are a major cause of endemic neuropathy in several developing countries (Chapter 22).

COMPLEX NEUROPATHIES OF OBSCURE ORIGIN
Large series of polyneuropathies in children include a variable proportion of unclassifiable cases that usually feature both peripheral and CNS involvement. This was the case in 16 of 61 patients of Evans (1979) who received a diagnosis of undefined 'degenerative disorder' or of 'spinocerebellar degeneration'.

ACQUIRED DIFFUSE NEUROPATHIES

Acquired neuropathies are most often inflammatory in origin

but various toxins and undetermined processes may also cause them.

Inflammatory disorders of the peripheral nervous system include two groups of diffuse diseases: the acute polyneuropathies, also termed polyradiculoneuritis, and the much less common chronic progressive polyneuropathies. Localized inflammatory neuropathies are relatively common, although their mechanisms are poorly known.

ACUTE INFLAMMATORY NEUROPATHY, ACUTE POLYRADICULONEURITIS, GUILLAIN–BARRÉ SYNDROME AND RELATED DISORDERS

The Guillain–Barré syndrome (GBS) is an acute inflammatory disease of peripheral nerves characterized clinically by progressive weakness that usually appears a few days after a viral illness or immunization. The nature of the relationship between nerve dysfunction and infection is not completely understood but an immunological mechanism plays an important role. The commonest form is characterized pathologically by acute demyelination, but acute motor axonal neuropathy (AMAN) and acute motor and sensory axonal neuropathy (AMSAN) due to an acute axonal degenerative process have been recognized increasingly frequently with a clear peak of incidence in summer, especially in China, Japan, Mexico, Korea and India but also in other countries (van der Meché et al. 1991, Thomas 1992, Feasby et al. 1993). The discovery of clinically similar cases of GBS, one with primary demyelinating lesions and the other with severe and probably primary axonal damage (Feasby et al. 1986, McKhann et al. 1993), supports the likelihood of two different mechanisms (Thomas 1992, Feasby et al. 1993).

PATHOLOGY

GBS is characterized by the presence of inflammatory lesions scattered throughout the peripheral nervous system from the anterior and posterior roots to distal twigs (Prineas 1981). In the demyelinating variety, the lesions consist of circumscribed areas of myelin loss associated with oedema and the presence of lymphocytes and macrophages. The initial site of lesions is predominantly at the Ranvier node. Myelin damage is produced mainly by macrophages that penetrate the basement membrane around nerve fibres and strip myelin away from the axon and the body of Schwann cells. Other cases develop vesicular myelin breakdown with the formation of a "soap-bubble appearance (Hafer-Macko et al. 1996). This appearance is associated with the presence of immunoglobulins and complement on the outside of the associated Schwann cell. In a minority of cases, macrophage-associated demyelination occurs despite a paucity of lymphocytes. These cases may be due to the action of an antibody rather than a T-cell autoimmune process (Honavar et al. 1991). Interruption of the axons with subsequent wallerian degeneration is present only in the most severe cases with intense inflammation. Proliferation of Schwann cells occurs later in the disease, probably as a first step in the remyelination process.

In the axonal forms, AMAN and AMSAN, wallerian-like degeneration predominates with little evidence of demyelination or lymphocyte infiltration. In AMAN, sensory axons are largely spared. Apart from the axonal degenerative changes, the motor neurons show chromatolysis (Griffin et al. 1995, Visser et al. 1995).

PATHOGENESIS

The pathological changes seen in the acute inflammatory demyelinating form of GBS (AIDP) resemble those of acute allergic neuritis produced in experimental animals by immunization with homogenates of peripheral nerves or heterologous myelin as well as by passive transfer of T cells activated to myelin proteins or peptides. In humans, the immunological mechanisms are still unclear and the respective roles of humoral and cellular factors are still in debate but humoral factors are probably important. Intraneural injection of sera from GBS patients produces demyelination in animals (Feasby et al. 1982). Antimyelin antibodies have been demonstrated in GBS patients by fixation of the C1 component of complement and are especially high at onset of the disease (Koski et al. 1986). Some antibodies have been found in myelin sheaths and on Schwann cells but no single antigen has been identified in AIDP cases. Activated complement components C3a and C5a have been found in CSF (Hartung et al. 1987). The most attractive hypothesis remains that a pathogenic agent may damage the Schwann cell with release of Schwann cell antigens triggering a cascade of events leading to segmental demyelination which, in turn, is responsible for multiple conduction blocks (Sumner 1981) that are the electrophysiological basis of the clinical manifestations of GBS.

Molecular mimicry involving antigens shared between cell wall/capsular lipopoly- or oligosaccharide of antecedent infective organisms and similar targets on the axons is a key element in the axonal forms of GBS. *Campylobacter jejuni* is the most frequently reported agent causing AMAN and AMSAN. Several *C. jejuni* serotypes are associated with GBS, particularly Penner type HS/O19. High titres of antibodies against gangliosides GM1 and GD1b are found in a large proportion of cases, especially those associated with *Campylobacter* infection (Gregson et al. 1993, Vriesendorp et al. 1993). More than 85% of Miller Fisher syndrome cases with ataxia, areflexia and ophthalmoplegia (see below) have anti-GQ1b antibodies (Yuki et al. 1993). The extraocular nerves, somatic nerve nodes of Ranvier and dorsal root ganglion cells bind anti-GQ1b antibodies, possibly explaining the specificity of the clinical manifestations. These antibodies are also found in AIDP with ophthalmoplegia. Antibodies to GQ1b and GM1 have been shown to block neuromuscular transmission in vitro. Anti-GM1 antibodies interfere with nodal ion-channel function (Takigawa et al. 1995). These findings may explain the rapid changes in strength sometimes seen early in the disorder and in response to immunoglobulin therapy.

EPIDEMIOLOGY

GBS occurs usually in children over 3–4 years of age but cases of early and even neonatal onset (Al-Qudah et al. 1988) are on record. The overall frequency of GBS is 1.9 cases per 100,000 population (Larsen et al. 1985). The incidence was approximately 0.8 per 100,000 per annum in Australian children aged less than 15 years (Morris et al. 2003). The disease usually follows infection or immunization by 2–4 weeks (Jones 1996). Among the identified viral agents, herpes viruses (cytomegalovirus, CMV; Epstein–Barr virus, EBV) have been frequently indicted (Dowling and Cook 1981), and immunization against rabies (Hemachudha et al. 1988) and against influenza (Poser and Behan 1982) have received considerable attention. Other viral agents such as that of non-A, non-B hepatitis (MacLeod 1987, De Klippel et al. 1993) and varicella-zoster virus (Sanders et al. 1987) are less frequently found, and a firm connection has been established only with CMV and EBV (Jones 1996). Poliovirus infection is not a cause (Rantala et al. 1994). *C. jejuni* infection, often with diarrhoea, is the most common infection preceding GBS and, even more so, the Miller Fisher variant (Vriesendorp et al. 1993, Jones 1996). In 100 patients studied by Winer et al. (1988), 38% had had respiratory symptoms and 17% gastrointestinal symptoms. Serological evidence of *C. jejuni* (14%) and CMV infection (11%) was significantly more frequent in patients than in controls.

CLINICAL FEATURES
The onset of GBS is usually fairly sudden with weakness generally affecting the lower limbs. The paralyses then follow an ascending course. Paralysis is generalized in half the cases, predominates in the distal parts of the limbs in 30%, and is symmetrical, although minor differences are not uncommon and gross asymmetry has been reported in rare patients (Jones 1996). Predominantly proximal involvement is present in 20% of cases. The facial nerve is involved in 50% of cases, often bilaterally (Hung et al. 1994). Ophthalmoplegia occurs in 3% of cases (Dehaene et al. 1986). Optic neuritis is uncommon (Behan et al. 1976). Papilloedema may also be associated with increased intracranial pressure (Morley and Reynolds 1966), but although altered consciousness is said to be not rare and CNS manifestations were found in 5 of 24 patients of Bradshaw and Jones (1992), objective evidence of CNS involvement is highly unusual (Willis and Van den Bergh 1988) and certainly uncommon in our experience. Sensory symptoms are present in about half the cases. Pain is often prominent at onset, while paraesthesiae and hypoaesthesiae are present only in a minority of older children. Deep tendon reflexes are abolished early in 83% of cases, even in nonparalytic territories (Winer et al. 1988). Loss of deep sensation is frequently found at examination later in the illness.

Paralysis of the respiratory muscles is a common complication of GBS and often requires respirator treatment (Ropper 1992). Mild respiratory impairment is even more frequent with resulting hypercarbia. In a Sydney study of 71 childhood cases from 1988 to 2004, 21 (30%) had evidence of respiratory involvement but only 5 required ventilation. Autonomic involvement is present in many patients and may be responsible for hypotension, hypertension, cardiac arrhythmia and even cardiac arrest (Winer et al. 1988). While often present in childhood cases, autonomic disturbances are rarely serious in our experience and few cases require treatment. Urinary retention or overflow incontinence may be present in up to 10% of cases. Ataxia of probable sensory origin is not uncommon and may dominate the clinical picture. Plantar responses are usually flexor but a Babinski response may be seen (Jones 1996).

The CSF is most often normal during the first days of the illness. Elevation of CSF protein appears between 2 and 15 days and reaches a peak by 4–5 weeks after clinical onset. The CSF total protein concentration and the IgG percentage seem to depend mainly on the degree of blood–brain barrier damage, which in turn correlates with the clinical course. Oligoclonal IgGs are frequently present in the CSF but come essentially from serum. Oligoclonal IgG banding in GBS is transitory and correlates with the development of blood–brain barrier damage, the presence of cranial nerve involvement and the severity of the disease (Segurado et al. 1986). In occasional cases, the CSF protein may remain normal (Sullivan and Reeves 1977). In contrast to protein, cell content of CSF usually remains normal in GBS, the classical albuminocytological dissociation, with fewer than 10 cells/mm^3. The presence of more than 50 mononuclear leukocytes/mm^3 should cast doubt on the diagnosis (Asbury and Cornblath 1990), but a lesser number of cells is acceptable and has no prognostic value.

ELECTROPHYSIOLOGY
Electrophysiological studies in AIDP (Cornblath et al. 1988, Ropper et al. 1990) show marked slowing of motor conduction velocities, along with prolonged distal latencies consistent with demyelination in about 50% of the patients. Some abnormalities of motor or sensory conduction velocities are present in 90% of patients but, because of the patchy distribution of lesions, the probability of finding abnormalities increases with the number of nerves studied, and the degree of involvement can vary with the nerve studied. In 20% of cases abnormalities are found in only one or two but not all nerves studied. The amplitude of the sensory action potentials and of the motor action potential is diminished. A conduction block could be demonstrated in at least one nerve in 74% of the cases of Bradshaw and Jones (1992). Measurement of F-wave latency may detect abnormalities of proximal nerves or roots that escape routine examination. In AMAN and AMSAN, motor conduction velocities are normal or near-normal but the amplitude of the compound muscle action potential is reduced or unmeasurable. In both forms of GBS, the amplitude of the mean compound muscle action potential bears a significant relationship to the prognosis (Cornblath et al. 1988). Signs of denervation and fibrillations indicate greater axonal involvement and may be of poor prognostic significance in adults but are less serious in children (Bradshaw and Jones 1992, Triggs et al. 1992).

Evoked potential studies have shown anomalies of both brainstem auditory evoked potentials and somatosensory evoked potentials (Ropper and Chiappa 1986).

COURSE
The initial phase of gradually increasing involvement lasts 10–30 days. Prolongation beyond 4 weeks excludes the diagnosis of

GBS and suggests a diagnosis of subacute GBS (Hughes et al. 1992, Rodriguez-Casero et al. 2005) or chronic inflammatory polyneuropathy. In some forms (Ropper 1986a) paralysis progresses very rapidly with complete quadriplegia in 2–5 days. Such patients often have severe respiratory involvement, and sequelae are more likely than in average cases.

A plateau phase then follows. A long plateau phase was found by some investigators (Billard et al. 1979) but not by others (Winer et al. 1988) to be associated with a relatively poor prognosis and the persistence of motor sequelae.

Death is said to occur in 2–3% of childhood cases, although in some adult series (Winer et al. 1988) mortality was as high as 15%, mostly in older adult patients. No deaths have occurred in the 71 patients seen by the present author (RO) since 1988.

Recovery is usually complete. Motor sequelae, often mild, occur in 5–25% of patients. Relapses and late recurrences occur in about 3% of patients (Wijdicks and Ropper 1990). Late recurrences that supervene several years after the first episode probably have a different mechanism from those seen after discontinuation of plasma exchange or corticosteroid therapy and are usually only partial (Ropper et al. 1988).

Factors giving an unfavourable prognosis include a rapid development of the paralysis, possibly a long duration of the plateau phase, a marked distal deficit, and the presence of fibrillation potentials and of a low amplitude of the mean compound motor unit potentials (Ropper 1986a). The prevalent impression that the disease has a better prognosis in children than in adults has been questioned by Kleyweg et al. (1989) and by Jansen et al. (1993) who found no difference in severity between 18 children and 50 adults and therefore recommended that the same treatments should be used in both groups. However, a large collaborative study (Korinthenberg and Mönting 1996) confirmed the lesser severity of the disease in children. Rantala et al. (1995) found three major risk factors for more severe cases: onset of symptoms within 8 days of the preceding infection, cranial nerve involvement, and a CSF protein level >800 mg/L during the first week of the disease.

TREATMENT

Symptomatic treatment is an essential part of the management of GBS. Careful monitoring of vital functions, avoidance of aspiration pneumonia, and tube feeding and respiratory assistance when needed have considerably lessened the mortality rate.

Corticosteroid treatment has been shown in controlled studies to have no beneficial effects and even to prolong hospitalization (Hughes 1991, Hughes et al. 2007). Plasmapheresis is clearly effective in adults (French Cooperative Group 1987, McKhann et al. 1988) when performed during the first week of the disease and repeated over a period of 7–14 days. This treatment has been shown to reduce the duration of hospitalization, to avoid respiratory insufficiency and to limit the extension of the paralyses. Such a treatment is probably indicated for severe cases when rapid extension is evident early. However, the exact indications are not yet firmly established. Plasmaphereses are difficult to use in children of less than 15 kg, although Khatri et al. (1990) and

Jansen et al. (1993) have reported favourable results with the use of a specially adapted technique. Epstein and Sladky (1990) found that plasmapheresis diminishes morbidity in childhood GBS by shortening the interval until recovery of independent walking. Results similar to those in adult patients have also been reported by Jansen et al. (1993). The demonstration that high-dose (2 g/kg) intravenous gammaglobulins (van der Meché and Schmitz 1992, Hartung et al. 1995) are also an effective therapy opened a new avenue for therapy. Doses of 0.4 g/kg/day for 5 days given during the first days of the disease give results similar to those of plasmapheresis (van der Meché and Schmitz 1992). Administration of the total dose in two days may be more effective than conventional fractionated therapy (Kanra et al. 1997) but has been shown to result in more treatment-related relapses (Korinthenberg et al. 2005). This technique has largely replaced plasmapheresis in children. Some reports have questioned the efficacy of immunoglobulin therapy. Castro and Ropper (1993) reported worsening in 7 of 15 adults, and relapses following initially good results have been reported (Irani et al. 1993). However, immunoglobulins appear to be an effective and safe treatment (van der Meché and Schmitz 1992, Jones 1996, Korinthenberg and Mönting 1996, Shahar et al. 1997). The exact indications are yet to be established; cases with rapid extension or impending respiratory insufficiency are obvious candidates but whether all incipient cases should be treated is not known. The present author (RO) would treat patients who are rapidly evolving or who are non-ambulant on presentation. Rantala et al. (1995) suggested early administration at the time of diagnosis when risk factors are present. A recent adult trial comparing i.v. immunoglobulin (IVIG) combined with i.v. methylprednisone (500 mg/day) to IVIG alone narrowly missed statistical significance for greater efficacy of the combination; the study group is now using the combination therapy routinely (Van Koningsveld et al. 2004).

DIAGNOSIS

GBS is a major cause of acute flaccid paralysis (Table 20.3). The diagnosis of GBS is easy in typical cases. Diagnostic criteria (Asbury and Cornblath 1990) include symmetrical weakness and areflexia, the presence of mild sensory symptoms and signs, progression of the symptoms lasting no more than four weeks after onset, absence of fever, sphincter dysfunction and evidence of CNS involvement. The last two criteria may not apply to all childhood cases (see above). Typical CSF and electrophysiological findings confirm the clinical diagnosis.

The conditions that may simulate GBS are common in children (Table 20.3) but only a few raise difficult problems. It is imperative to exclude conditions that require immediate specific treatment, especially spinal cord compression. Transverse myelitis can be distinguished by the finding of a sensory level and sphincter involvement. Rare cases of metabolic disease such as Leigh syndrome (Coker 1993) can closely simulate GBS. Poliomyelitis is now exceptional but some toxic neuropathies may be confused with acute polyneuritis. In adolescents the possibility of volatile solvent abuse neuropathy should be kept in mind.

TABLE 20.3
Causes of acute flaccid paralysis

Cause	References
Peripheral neuropathy	
Guillain–Barré syndrome (acute demyelinating neuropathy)	This chapter
Acute axonal neuropathy	This chapter
Neuropathies of infectious diseases (diphtheria, neuroborreliosis)	This chapter, Chapter 10
Acute toxic neuropathies	
Heavy metals	This chapter
Snake (elapid) toxins	This chapter
Wild berries, buckthorn	Villalobos and Santos (1996)
Arthropod bites	Créange et al. (1993)
Anterior horn cell disease	
Acute anterior poliomyelitis	Chapters 10, 19
Vaccinal poliomyelitis	Chapters 10, 19
Other neurotropic viruses (coxsackie, echoviruses, enteroviruses 70 and 71	Melnik (1984)
Acute myelopathy	
Cord compression (tumours, trauma, paraspinal abscess)	Chapter 13
Vascular malformation with thrombosis or bleeding	Chapter 14
Demyelinating diseases (multiple sclerosis, Devic syndrome, acute disseminated encephalomyelitis)	Chapters 10, 11
Systemic disease	
Acute porphyrias	This chapter
Critical illness neuropathy	This chapter
Acute myopathy in intensive care patients	Zochodne et al. (1993)
Disorders of neuromuscular transmission	
Myasthenia gravis	Chapter 21
Botulism	Chapters 1, 10
Insecticide (organophosphate) poisoning	Zwiener and Ginsberg (1988)
Tick paralysis	Smith (1992)
Snake bites	Saini et al. (1986)
Muscle disorders	
Polymyositis, dermatomyositis	Chapter 21
Trichinosis	Fourestié et al. (1993)
Periodic paralyses	Chapter 21
Corticosteroid and blocking agents	Hirano et al. (1992)
Mitochondrial diseases (infantile type)	Chapters 8, 21

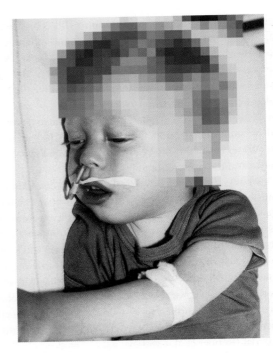

Fig. 20.5. Miller Fisher syndrome in a 20-month-old boy. Note ptosis of eyelids, unexpressive facies, open mouth and tube feeding (due to swallowing difficulties).

Diphtheritic neuropathy closely mimics GBS but is rare. Botulism and diphtheria can be excluded by the intrinsic eye involvement, which is never present in GBS. Tick paralysis can produce a very similar clinical picture but the finding of pupillary paralysis or of an engorged tick enables distinction. The clinical neurophysiological findings are also distinctive (Grattan-Smith et al. 1997).

CLINICAL VARIANTS OF THE GUILLAIN–BARRÉ SYNDROME AND RELATED DISORDERS

Miller Fisher syndrome is characterized by the triad of ophthalmoplegia, ataxia and areflexia (Fig. 20.5), which comes on rapidly and follows the same illnesses as classical GBS (Kohler et al. 1988). However, a history or serological evidence of *C. jejuni* infection is particularly common in this syndrome (Rees et al. 1995, Jones 1996), and antiganglioside GD1b antibodies are almost always present. CSF protein becomes elevated in most patients with few or no cells, and electrodiagnostic features indicate peripheral nerve involvement in some cases. Abnormalities of brainstem evoked potentials have been reported (Unishi et al. 1988), and some investigators have regarded the syndrome as a form of brainstem encephalitis (Al-Din et al. 1982, Petty et al. 1993) because of MRI anomalies. Similar anomalies of evoked potentials may occur in classical GBS and Miller Fisher syndrome (Ropper and Chiappa 1986), and the bulk of evidence indicates that Miller Fisher syndrome is a form of acute polyneuritis. The ataxia may be due to involvement of large sensory fibres (Weiss and White 1986). Transitional cases with variable peripheral motor weakness also link the Miller Fisher syndrome to GBS (Dehaene et al. 1986). The course is similar to that of GBS although recurrences are quite rare (Vincent and Vincent 1986).

Cases of sensory loss and areflexia without motor deficit probably represent GBS if the onset is rapid, the distribution widespread and symmetrical, and recovery complete with elevated CSF protein (Dawson et al. 1988). In rare instances, GBS may present mainly with painful manifestations (Mikati and DeLong 1985). Sensory neuropathy as described in adults is a different condition (Sterman et al. 1980).

The nosological situation of the case of childhood peripheral neuropathy with antibodies to P_0 myelin glycoprotein (Ben Jelloun-Dellagi et al. 1992) is unclear. Some cases of acute polyneuritis cranialis are probably variants of GBS provided that cranial nerves I and II are uninvolved and other features of GBS are present (Polo et al. 1992). They are very rare in childhood.

Rare instances of *acute pure pandysautonomia* (acute acquired dysautonomia) (Young et al. 1975, Pavesi et al. 1992) may be atypical aspects of acute polyneuritis. The clinical picture of such cases is highly polymorphic with various combinations of hypotension, disorders of sweating and lachrymation, diarrhoea or intestinal obstruction, pupillary abnormalities and vasomotor disturbances (McLeod and Tuck 1987, Takayama et al. 1987). Acute or subacute cholinergic dysautonomia is characterized by failure of postganglionic cholinergic fibres (including sympathetic efferents to sweat glands), sometimes preceded by a transient increase in function resulting in hypersalivation, increased sweating and more frequent bowel movements. Symptoms include blurred vision, absence of tears, dry mouth, dysphagia, abdominal distension, urinary retention and anhidrosis. Pupils are fixed and dilated, and heart rate is invariable. Paralytic ileus may occur. Pure pandysautonomia features in addition symptoms and signs of sympathetic failure with resulting postural hypotension, depressed pressor responses and a syncopal tendency. The course is variable, with substantial recovery in some cases. Treatment is symptomatic. Sensory dysfunction may be associated (Nass and Chutorian 1982, Kanda et al. 1990). In some cases, vasomotor dysfunction occurs in isolation, e.g. with unilateral flushing (Lance et al. 1988). Dopamine beta-hydroxylase deficiency is a rare cause of similar sympathetic failure (Mathias and Bannister 1992).

In some patients (mostly adults) the course of diffuse inflammatory polyneuropathy is longer than in classical GBS. In particular, the period of progression of the paralysis exceeds 4 weeks and may last up to 8 weeks (Hughes et al. 1992). These patients represent intermediate cases between GBS and the chronic inflammatory neuropathies and may warrant steroid therapy (Rodriguez-Casero et al. 2005).

CHRONIC INFLAMMATORY DEMYELINATING POLYNEUROPATHY (CIDP)

CIDPs are much rarer than GBS but cause up to 10% of cases of chronic childhood polyneuropathy (Ouvrier and Wilmshurst 2003). The diagnostic criteria for CIDP include: (1) a clinical course predominantly of weakness either monophasic, with an initial progressive phase lasting more than 8 weeks, or of a relapsing–remitting nature; (2) electrophysiological and pathological evidence of demyelination; and (3) the absence of systemic disease that may cause demyelinating neuropathy (Ouvrier 1992, Nevo and Topaloglu 2002). An immunological origin to the condition is likely. There is evidence for both cellular and humoral involvement but molecular mimicry is less clearly involved than in GBS (Hahn et al. 2005). Contrary to what is observed in GBS, it was thought that there is an increased frequency of certain HLA groups (A1, B8, DRW3) in patients with chronic inflammatory neuropathy (Stewart et al. 1978, Adams et al. 1979) but the results of later studies have not been consistent and a large Dutch study reported that the frequencies of certain HLA antigens implicated in CIDP were not significantly increased (van Doorn et

al. 1991). The disease has been seen in siblings (Gabreëls-Festen et al. 1986).

CLINICAL FEATURES

The disease occurs predominantly in children aged between 5 and 15 years, but cases with infantile or early childhood onset are on record (Sladky et al. 1986, Pearce et al. 2005). Typically, there is a slow subacute onset over several weeks of a sensory motor neuropathy involving the distal and proximal limbs but respecting the respiratory muscles and cranial nerves (Colan et al. 1980, Sladky et al. 1986). However, an acute onset as in GBS is possible. Cranial, especially facial, nerve involvement occurs in 10–40% of patients, and weakness of bulbar or respiratory muscles severe enough to necessitate assisted ventilation is present in about 10% of cases (Ouvrier 1992). Due to the usual predominance of weakness in the lower limbs, difficulties with ambulation are usually the first manifestation and in early cases may be responsible for delayed motor milestones. The weakness is not infrequently asymmetrical. It is associated with amyotrophy and sensory disturbances, although these are generally inconspicuous (McCombe et al. 1987b, Barohn et al. 1989). Action or postural tremor is present in some patients.

Two different courses are possible. In about one third of cases the disease is monophasic, although lasting several months. In the remaining cases there is a relapsing course with a variable number of exacerbations and remissions, often incomplete, which may extend over several years (Barohn et al. 1989).

The CSF shows a protein/cell dissociation as in GBS in 90% of patients. The presence of a monoclonal or of oligoclonal bands is frequent but the oligoclonal proteins seem to be plasma-derived (Segurado et al. 1986).

There is consistently electrophysiological evidence of demyelination with slowed motor and sensory conduction velocities, often varying in different segments of the same nerve, increased distal latencies and a neurogenic EMG. The precise parameters are a matter of ongoing debate. More recent requirements with emphasis on conduction block and temporal dispersion were found to have a sensitivity of 90% and a specificity of 97% for a cohort of adult CIDP patients (Nicholas et al. 2002). Paediatric criteria were proposed by Nevo and Topaloglu (2002).

Nerve biopsy (Fig. 20.6) shows endoneurial and subperineurial inflammatory oedema and mononuclear cell infiltration. In some cases, hypertrophic changes with marked enlargement of the roots may be present and can be demonstrated by MRI of the cauda equina (Crino et al. 1993). Segmental demyelination and remyelination with less prominent axonal degeneration and fibre loss are seen. Onion bulbs are present in about 50% of cases. The condition is aetiologically related to chronic dysimmune neuropathy (Maisonobe et al. 1996) but gammopathy-related cases are rarely, if ever, seen in childhood.

DIFFERENTIAL DIAGNOSIS

The main diagnostic difficulty is to distinguish CIDP from

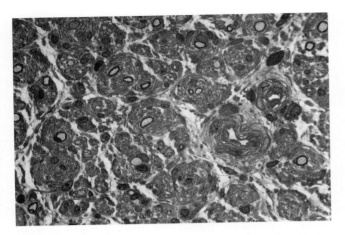

Fig. 20.6. Chronic inflammatory neuropathy. Note well-developed 'onion bulb' formation and paucity of myelinated fibres.

HMSN types I and III. It is indeed not clear whether steroid-responsive HMSN is actually a distinct condition (Baba et al. 1995), and so a course of steroids is worth trying in dubious cases (Gabreëls-Festen et al. 1986). Metabolic neuropathies, such as metachromatic leukodystrophy, may exhibit similar features with increased CSF protein.

CNS involvement in association with chronic demyelinating neuropathy has been described in some adult patients (Thomas et al. 1987, Ohtake et al. 1990) as well as in childhood (Rodriguez-Casero et al. 2003). Such cases raise the question of a relationship with multiple sclerosis. Systematic MRI in adult patients with chronic neuropathy has shown the occasional presence of areas of abnormal white matter signal (Feasby et al. 1990). The significance of this finding is unclear.

PROGNOSIS AND TREATMENT

The disorder does not usually threaten life, but its protracted course and the possible motor sequelae may make it a disabling condition. The prognosis in children is better than in adults and most achieve a full remission (Nevo et al. 1996, Simmons et al. 1997, Ryan et al. 2000, Connolly 2001). High-dose intravenous immunoglobulins (van Doorn et al. 1990, Hahn et al. 1996b) are effective therapy in adults and, in the opinion of the present author (RO) are the initial treatment of choice in children. The response is often rapid and remission may occur even with only one or two doses of IVIG (2 g/kg in total given over 2 or 5 days). Treatment with lower doses is maintained at 3–4 week intervals until a remission occurs or the patient is shown to be a non-responder. Plasma exchange is effective and has fewer side effects than protracted steroid therapy (Hahn et al. 1996a) but is difficult in young children. Otten et al. (1996) have reviewed immunoglobulin treatment in neurological disorders.

Therapy with corticosteroids is effective both in childen and in adults (Hahn et al. 2005) but the modalities of treatment are not fully codified. It is the author's practice to commence with 1 mg/kg/day of prednisone and to increase to 2 mg/kg/day if there is no response. Relapses following minimal decreases in

dosage may occur so that prolonged treatment with careful monitoring is sometimes necessary (Wertman et al. 1988). After remission occurs, the steroids are cautiously tapered to minimize side effects.

The development of steroid resistance is possible. In such cases, the use of a bolus of methylprednisolone and/or the addition of immunosuppressors should be tried. Azathioprine, methotrexate, cyclophosphamide, cyclosporine, mycophenylate and interferons have been utilized, but no systematic trials are available in children (Hahn et al. 2005). Treatment with corticosteroids has been suggested for the subacute form of inflammatory demyelinating polyneuropathy (Rodriguez-Casero et al. 2005).

LEPROSY

Leprosy is still a major health problem in several developing countries and together with vitamin deficiency is the main cause of neuropathy in many regions. The disease is due to infection with *Mycobacterium leprae* and is transmitted by intimate person-to-person contact with only a small proportion of any given population being susceptible. HLA-linked genes control the susceptibility to the organism and the course of the illness. Leprosy is a systemic disease with a marked predilection for superficial nerves, skin, the anterior third of the eye, the upper respiratory tract and the testes. Hosts with a low resistance to the organism develop lepromatous or nodular infection. Hosts with high resistance develop tuberculoid infection. In lepromatous leprosy, most infiltrates consist of macrophages heavily infected by *M. leprae*. In tuberculoid leprosy, the lesions contain only remnants of bacteria surrounded by well-organized granulomas with epithelioid and giant cells. Borderline cases intermediate between lepromatous and tuberculoid leprosy occur frequently, and unstable cases can oscillate between the two forms.

In lepromatous leprosy neural damage may produce a purely sensory polyneuritis with loss of touch, pain and temperature sensation in a characteristic distribution while deep sensitivity is preserved. Sensory loss first appears in cool areas of the body (ears, dorsal surface of the hands, forearms, feet and lateral aspect of the legs). Sensory motor neuropathy is less common (Sabin et al. 2005). Eventually, paralysis may develop in the territories of mixed limb and facial nerves. The ulnar nerve is most commonly affected, followed by the peroneal, median, radial, great auricular and other nerves. Claw hands and foot drop often develop. Pure mononeuritis is rare. In most patients the onset is insidious but an abrupt onset is possible. Shooting pains are uncommon. Enlargement of peripheral nerves may be present. The diagnosis may be difficult in non-endemic areas. Skin biopsies are helpful and a serological test is available (Young and Buchanan 1983). Nerve biopsy is useful both for diagnosis and for detection of persistent infection (Chimelli et al. 1997). Treatment uses sulfone derivatives, rifampicin and clofazimine (Sabin et al. 2005).

ENDOGENOUS AND EXOGENOUS TOXIC NEUROPATHIES

Toxic neuropathies of both endogenous and exogenous origin

are uncommon in childhood at least in symptomatic form (Gamstorp 1968, Evans 1979).

ENDOGENOUS TOXIC NEUROPATHIES

Subclinical neuropathy may not be rare in patients with *juvenile diabetes* as judged by electrophysiological findings. Ten per cent of children with chronic diabetes mellitus have symptoms and signs caused by peripheral neuropathy associated with diabetes (Gamstorp et al. 1966). Gallai et al. (1988) found decreased motor conduction velocity in the median nerve in 10%, in the posterior tibial nerve in 32%, and in the sural nerve in 44% of 50 juvenile diabetics with a mean age of 13 years. The neuropathy appeared to be more marked in poorly controlled diabetes. Compared with age-matched control subjects, impaired vibration perception was present in diabetic boys in the absence of clinical symptoms of peripheral or autonomic neuropathy (Olsen et al. 1994). Mildly impaired autonomic nervous system function was found in 30–50% of children with diabetes when measured soon after diagnosis (Verrotti et al. 1995, Donaghue et al. 1996). The percentage involved did not change over 3 years (Donaghue et al. 1996). In a large prospective study of nerve conduction and autonomic nervous system function in diabetic children, slowed sensory nerve conduction velocities and impaired autonomic function were present in 25% of children at the time of diagnosis (Solders et al. 1997). Clinically manifest diabetic neuropathy, however, is rare (Bastron and Thomas 1981, Fiçioglu et al. 1994), even though the study of spinal sensory evoked potentials also confirms that subclinical involvement of neural transmission in young diabetic patients is common (Cracco et al. 1984). Cranial nerve palsies are exceptional in juvenile diabetes. Autonomic involvement with gastrointestinal features is sometimes apparent. A neurogenic bladder may be relatively common but usually remains asymptomatic (Faerman et al. 1971). Further, asymptomatic diabetic children have diminished sensation of bladder filling (Barkai and Szabó 1993). Rare cases of mononeuritis multiplex have been recorded (Ouvrier et al. 1999). *Uraemic neuropathy* is also subclinical in a large majority of cases. Seventy-six per cent of uraemic children had a significant slowing of peroneal nerve conduction velocity without other evidence of neuropathy in the study by Mentser et al. (1978). Symptomatic patients may experience sensory abnormalities in the lower extremities that may evolve into a sensory motor polyneuropathy with flaccid paraplegia or quadriplegia. Any type of neuropathy (purely axonal, axonomyelinic or predominantly demyelinating) may be observed (Saïd et al. 1983). A purely motor type of uraemic neuropathy (McGonigle et al. 1985) may occur. The neuropathy of uraemia is usually reversed by successful renal transplant. A case of Miller Fisher syndrome with a relapsing course and fluctuations temporally related to uraemia and haemodialysis sessions has been observed (Galassi et al. 1990).

Polyneuropathy may also occur in hypothyroidism (Nemni et al. 1987).

EXOGENOUS TOXIC NEUROPATHIES

A vast number of chemicals can induce polyneuropathy (Table

TABLE 20.4
Some exogenous toxic causes of polyneuropathy

Agent	Reference
Drugs	
Isoniazid	Evans (1979)
Ethionamide	Argov and Mastaglia (1979)
Ethambutol	Idem
Nitrofurantoin	Toole and Parrish (1973)
Chlorambucil	Argov and Mastaglia (1979)
Vincristine	Casey et al. (1973)
Cisplatin	Gastaut and Pellissier (1985), Riggs et al. (1988)
Phenytoin	Lovelace and Horwitz (1968)
Lithium	Chang et al. (1988)
Thalidomide	Hess et al. (1986)
Metronidazole	Argov and Mastaglia (1979)
Amphotericin	Idem
Amitriptylin	Idem
Amiodarone	Bono et al. (1993)
Complication of bone marrow and solid transplants	Amato et al. (1993), Patchell (1994)
Heavy metals	
Mercury	Swaiman and Flager (1971)
Lead	Browder et al. (1973)
Arsenic	Evans (1979)
Thallium	Bank et al. (1972)
Organic chemicals	
N-hexane	Korobkin et al. (1975)
Triorthocresylphosphate	Evans (1979)
Carbon monoxide	Hopkins (1975)
Cyanate	Peterson et al. (1974)
Hydroxyquinolines	Baumgartner et al. (1970)
Pyridoxine abuse	Schaumburg et al. (1983)
Organophosphates	Zwiener and Ginsberg (1988)
Biological toxins	
Ciguatera toxin	Allsop et al. (1986)
Diphtheria	Solders et al. (1989)
Immunizations	Evans (1979)
Serum sickness	Chapter 11
Arthropod bites	Haller and Fabara (1972), Créange et al. (1993)
Tick paralysis	Grattan-Smith et al. (1997)

20.4). Only the most important ones, especially drugs, are discussed here. Isoniazid can cause a distal mixed sensory and motor neuropathy through interference with the metabolism of pyridoxine. Supplementation with pyridoxine is therefore indicated in patients treated for tuberculosis. Excessive doses of pyridoxine can cause a sensory neuropathy (Schaumburg et al. 1983). Vincristine is a relatively common cause of neuropathy in children with malignancies. The drug interferes with the formation of neurotubules. Abolition of reflexes starting with the ankle jerk is virtually constant following vincristine therapy. In more severe cases paraesthesiae develop, followed by sensory loss then by weakness that may be initially focal and may remain asymmetrical (Casey et al. 1973). Severe pain, in the parotid region, is frequent during vincristine treatment, and oculomotor palsies have been observed. An acute severe deterioration can occur in patients with Charcot–Marie–Tooth disease who are given vincristine (Igarashi et al. 1995).

Nitrofurantoin causes neuropathy mainly in children with renal insufficiency. Axonal involvement is the rule, and distal sensory symptoms are usually predominant. Differential diagnosis with uraemic neuropathy may be difficult. The resurgence of thalidomide has resulted in occasional cases of a toxic, mainly sensory, neuropathy in childhood (Fleming et al. 2005).

Most drug-induced neuropathies are reversible after discontinuation of treatment but recovery may be slow, especially when intoxication was prolonged. Phenytoin toxicity is almost always subclinical.

Accidental neuropathies due to heavy metals are rare. Insecticides should be suspected in rural communities along with arsenic. N-hexane neuropathy may result from solvent abuse ('glue-sniffing'), a practice that has become prevalent among adolescents and even children (Korobkin et al. 1975). A history of glue-sniffing should be routinely searched for in this age group. Nerve biopsy characteristically shows changes of demyelination with giant axons packed with neurofilaments.

Biological toxins are rarely a cause. Tick paralysis is seen in America and in Australia. It results in a flaccid, rapidly spreading paralysis involving the respiratory muscles, and may be lethal if the tick is not removed. Careful search is clearly imperative and removal leads to cure in a few hours to several days (Grattan-Smith et al. 1997). In Western Europe, paralysis following tick bite is due to Borrelia disease (Chapter 10).

NEUROPATHIES OF SYSTEMIC AND VASCULAR DISEASES

A neuropathy may be a manifestation of most vasculitides (Chapter 11) including lupus erythematosus (McCombe et al. 1987a), rheumatoid arthritis, polyarteritis nodosa, anaphylactoid purpura (Ritter et al. 1983) and other, less well-defined collagen disorders and vasculitides (Harati and Niakan 1986, Dyck et al. 1987). Such complications are rare in children. They may present as either mononeuritis multiplex or diffuse polyneuropathy (Parikh et al. 1995, Steinlin et al. 1995, Harel et al. 2002).

Neuropathy may occur in gravely ill patients with multiple visceral deficiency or following major surgery. The nature of these 'critical illness neuropathies' is obscure. They may entail compression, hypoxia (Pfeiffer et al. 1990) and other mechanisms. Similar cases have been observed in childhood (Heckmatt et al. 1993, Tsao et al. 1995, Williams et al. 2007). A neuropathy can occur in burn patients; it most frequently presents as mononeuritis multiplex, less often as a mononeuropathy (Marquez et al. 1993). A neuropathy with optic atrophy has been associated with malnutrition combined with tobacco toxicity in Cuba (Thomas et al. 1995).

LOCALIZED DISORDERS OF THE PERIPHERAL NERVES (EXCEPT CRANIAL NERVES)

INFLAMMATORY LOCALIZED NEUROPATHIES
These may involve a single nerve or branch or several nerves as in plexopathies. Transitional forms with the generalized neuropathies exist, e.g. neuropathy with liability to pressure palsies or cases of familial brachial plexopathy that may also affect the lumbar plexus and presumably are the result of a more or less diffuse process.

PAINFUL BRACHIAL NEUROPATHY OR PLEXOPATHY, PARSONAGE–TURNER SYNDROME, NEURALGIC AMYOTROPHY
Brachial plexopathy occurs from infancy, although paediatric cases are much rarer than in adults (Charles and Jayam-Trouth 1980). It may follow a nonspecific respiratory infection, a specific viral disease such as infectious mononucleosis (Watson and Ashby 1976, Dussaix et al. 1986) or parvovirus infection (Denning et al. 1987), or an immunization (Hamati-Haddad and Fenichel 1997).

The disorder usually begins with pain localized to the shoulder or involving the whole upper limb. Pain may last from hours to weeks and is often intense. It is followed by weakness that may be the first manifestation in 5% of cases. Paralysis affects the upper brachial roots in over half the patients and the whole plexus in one third, but may be limited to the hand and fingers in a small proportion. Amyotrophy sets in rapidly and objective sensory signs may be present (England and Sumner 1987).

Recovery is virtually constant but it may take months or years and some residua may rarely persist (Zeharia et al. 1990, van Alfen et al. 2006).

The diagnosis requires exclusion of spinal cord compression and transverse myelitis, which often demands an imaging study of the cervical cord. The CSF is usually normal although a mild inflammatory reaction may be present at onset. EMG and nerve conduction studies are useful for determining the extent of involvement of the ipsilateral and, occasionally, the contralateral plexus.

Treatment is based on analgesics and physiotherapy. Steroids do not modify the long-term outcome but may have a favourable effect in some cases. Rare cases in childhood may have a different phenotype with only mild or no pain but more extensive paralysis with less recovery than in adults (van Alfen et al. 2000, Kotsopoulos et al. 2007).

Involvement of only one nerve from the brachial plexus may be seen. The long thoracic nerve is commonly affected with consequent paralysis of the serratus anterior, producing a unilateral winged scapula.

OTHER LOCALIZED INFLAMMATORY NERVE DISORDERS
Lumbosacral plexopathy is the counterpart in the lower limb of neuralgic amyotrophy but is even rarer in children. Occasional cases are on record in adolescents (Evans et al. 1981) and even in 2- to 3-year-old children (Sander and Sharp 1981, Thomson 1993). Pain is located in a femoral or sciatic distribution and children will limp or refuse to walk. Weakness of the leg follows in about a week. Recovery is almost universal although mild residual weakness may persist. When the lower plexus is involved it may be confused with sciatica due to disc or vertebral disease. In

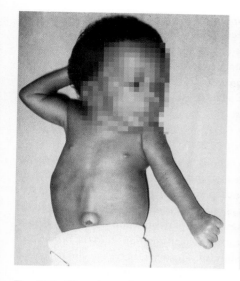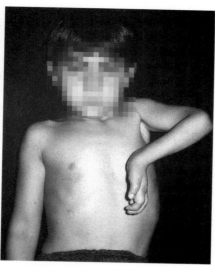

Fig. 20.7. Obstetric paralysis of the brachial plexus. *(Far left)* 1-month-old boy with proximal (Duchenne–Erb) palsy. The left arm is internally rotated, the forearm is extended and pronated. The intrinsic hand muscles are normal. *(Left)* 6-year-old boy with severe sequelae of total plexus involvement. Synkinetic contraction of proximal muscles is evident. The left hand is paralysed and atrophic. There is ipsilateral Horner syndrome. (Courtesy Dr J-P Padovani, Hôpital des Enfants Malades, Paris.)

some countries, schistosomiasis is an important cause (Marra 1983).

Sacral radiculomyelitis (Elsberg syndrome) is observed mainly in young adults and presents with a tetrad of acute urinary retention, sensory deficit in sacral dermatomes, paraesthesiae in the same territory and pleocytosis of the CSF (Herbaut et al. 1987). Most cases are due to genital herpes simplex virus but other viral agents, e.g. echovirus and cytomegalovirus, may be the cause (Vanneste et al. 1980, Michaelson et al. 1983). One case in a 6-year-old boy has been diagnosed at our institutions and a similar patient has been reported (Gerber and Cromie 1996).

TRAUMATIC NERVE INJURIES
BRACHIAL PLEXUS INJURY
The incidence of brachial plexus injury in neonates has decreased in recent years probably because of improved obstetric techniques. Since 1980, the incidence has varied from 0.37 to 0.87 per 1000 live births (Painter 1988, Evans-Jones et al. 2003). Women over 35 years of age, those with preeclampsia or diabetes mellitus, and those who had previously delivered children with brachial plexus injuries are more likely to have affected babies. In one series (Rossi et al. 1982), half of the affected children weighed more than 4000g at birth. Abnormal birth presentations are also a factor but the frequency of breech delivery varies with the series (Rossi et al. 1982, Painter 1988). Occasional cases of prenatal plexus injury due to deformation from uterine constraint, such as that of bicornuate uterus, are on record and are a possible cause of paralysis in siblings (Paradiso et al. 1997).

Pathology
Lesions affect the upper plexus (C5 and C6 roots) – the Duchenne–Erb type of plexus paralysis – in 55–72% of cases.

Lesions of the entire plexus occur on an average in 10% of patients; those of C5, C6 and C7 in 10–20%; and those of C8–T1 (Déjerine–Klumpke type) in less than 10%. Bilateral, but often asymmetrical, involvement is not rare. In most instances there is stretching of the upper cord of the plexus due to traction on the shoulder during delivery of the aftercoming head or to turning the head away from the shoulder in difficult cephalic presentations. Injury to the lower cord seems to result from traction on the abducted arm during vertex delivery or from traction on the trunk with breech presentation. The most common lesions are haemorrhages and oedema within the nerve sheath of primary plexus cords. Actual avulsion of the roots from the spinal cord with segmental damage of the grey matter or tearing of the nerves is uncommon but occurs when the degree of traction is severe enough.

Clinical manifestations
In the great majority of patients with upper plexus lesions, the paralysis is recognized from the first days of life. The affected arm hangs limply adducted and internally rotated, the elbow extended, the forearm pronated and the wrist variably flexed (Fig. 20.7). The grasp remains normal. The biceps and brachioradialis reflexes are absent. Weakness of the triceps and extensors of forearm and digits may complicate the picture when there is significant C7 involvement. In lower plexus lesions, intrinsic hand muscles are paralysed, the grasp is absent, and a Horner syndrome with ptosis and miosis is frequently present. If the Horner syndrome does not resolve, the iris fails to pigment and heterochromia iridis develops. Winging of the scapula and Horner syndrome generally herald a poor outcome. In some cases, there is significant sensory involvement with the possible appearance of whitlows on the fingers. Global palsy involving the upper and

lower roots of the plexus carries a very poor prognosis for recovery. Involvement of the diaphragm, due to a lesion of the fourth cervical root, is present in approximately 5% of cases and may produce symptoms of respiratory distress. This occurs most often in association with upper plexus palsy but may be present in isolation (Schifrin 1952).

Diagnosis
The diagnosis of plexus paralysis is readily apparent. Study of the somatosensory evoked potentials may help distinguish between an avulsed root and a more distal lesion of better prognosis (Jones 1979) in older patients. MRI of the spinal cord and roots may also be used for the same purpose. EMG may be helpful in determining the extent of paralysis but can be misleading (Yilmaz et al. 1999). Signs of denervation may occur earlier than happens in adults (Swoboda et al. 2003).

Prognosis and management
A majority of neonates with brachial plexus injury recover (DiTaranto et al. 2004, Strömbeck et al. 2007). This is partly due to the limited nature of the nerve damage but also to the plasticity of the newborn spinal cord (Korak et al. 2004). Gordon et al. (1973) studied 59 such infants: examination showed recovery in 46/52 at 4 months of age, in 48/52 at 12 months, and in 53/56 at 4 years, with only 3 patients lost to follow-up. Similarly, Greenwald et al. (1984) found that 23 of their 38 patients had recovered by 1 week, 35 by 3 months, and 36 at several years. Children with residual deficits may continue to improve even during preschool years. Sequelae may affect various muscles depending on the lesions but tend to predominate on the proximal limb (Rossi et al. 1982). Sequelae include weakness, amyotrophy and sensory deficits. Contractures are often more marked than weakness. They are due to faulty reinnervation and result in paradoxical synkinesias. In particular, attempts at any movement of the upper limb tend to provoke contraction of the deltoid and biceps with abduction of the flexed limb. In virtually all cases there is internal rotation of the arm and pronation of the forearm. Subluxation of the humeral head may contribute to the disability (Hernandez and Dias 1988).

The average case of plexus palsy in the newborn infant does not require more than range of motion exercises starting no sooner than 7–10 days after birth. Splinting is contraindicated as it may promote the development of contractures. For infants who have not significantly improved by age 6 months, the question of surgical therapy, including neural lysis, nerve anastomosis or grafting, arises (Gilbert and Tassin 1987, Gilbert et al. 1991). Laurent and Lee (1994) reported satisfactory results in 50 of 70 operated infants, but controversy persists in the absence of a prospective controlled study and no firm statement seems currently possible (Bodensteiner et al. 1994). Surgical intervention after 6–12 months of age is recommended by some groups but the precise indications are not agreed upon (Hunt 1988). Surgical procedures on joints and tendon transfers have variable results but may become indicated in older children to improve specific functions.

Postnatal injuries to the brachial plexus are mainly due to motor vehicle (especially motorcycle) and sports accidents and consequently affect principally adolescents. The prognosis of these injuries is often guarded. Traumatic lesions of the lumbosacral plexus are rare. Both neonatal (Hope et al. 1985) and childhood (Egel et al. 1995) cases have been reported with a favourable outcome.

SCIATIC NERVE INJURIES
Injury to the sciatic nerve is now less often the result of injections into the nerve or in its vicinity. Such accidents were particularly prone to occur in small preterm infants because of the small volume of the buttock allowing substances to diffuse right up to the nerve with resulting injury and dysfunction (Gilles and French 1961). Therefore, intramuscular injections into the buttocks of such infants are prohibited. The sciatic nerve can also be injured following injection of drugs into the umbilical artery. This is caused by thrombosis of the inferior gluteal artery and is accompanied by circulatory changes in the buttock (San Agustin et al. 1962, Wynne et al. 1978) or gangrenous skin areas in the leg. Similar changes may occur following injection of viscid substances into the buttocks.

Paralysis may affect the whole territory of the sciatic nerve or only one of its two main divisions, most commonly the peroneal nerve. Foot-drop, amyotrophy and growth disturbances of the leg are the most frequent manifestations. Surgical exploration of the nerve should be considered when no improvement occurs after a few weeks and/or when a granuloma is palpable at the site of injection. The prognosis is poor in severe cases especially as a result of trophic and growth disturbances.

Breech delivery is a rare cause of neonatal sciatic palsy (Jones et al. 1988).

Sciatic neuralgia due to disc herniation is rare in childhood, and pain in the territory of the lower lumbar and upper sciatic roots is more commonly due to tumours than to disc pathology.

In children above 10 years of age typical sciatica is occasionally observed. Spinal rigidity and scoliosis or kyphosis may be prominent manifestations (Kurihara and Kataoka 1980, Epstein et al. 1984).

Other causes of sciatic neuropathy in childhood include stretch injury after closed reduction of hip dislocation and due to braces, casts and prolonged abnormal lower extremity postures; compression by haematomas, tumours or lymphomas; and hypersensitivity vasculitis. In rare cases, a localized hypertrophy of the nerve, sometimes due to a perineuroma, or else no cause, is found (Jones et al. 1988, Ouvrier and Shield 1999).

CARPAL TUNNEL SYNDROME AND OTHER ENTRAPMENT SYNDROMES
Carpal tunnel syndrome is rare in childhood: Sainio et al. (1987) collected only 32 published cases and added 3 of their own. As in adults, the syndrome occurs most commonly in females. Motor symptoms tend to dominate the clinical picture in children with typical involvement of the thenar muscles but the latter can be congenitally hypoplastic (Cavanagh et al. 1979). Pain

and paraesthesiae are often less marked than in adults. Sensory and motor distal latencies are prolonged.

Mucopolysaccharidoses types IS, II and IV may cause the carpal tunnel syndrome through hypertrophy of the flexor retinaculum and related structures. Other rare causes include neuropathy with liability to pressure palsies (see pp. 766–7) and the Schwartz–Jampel syndrome (Cruz Martínez et al. 1984). Occasional familial idiopathic cases are on record (Danta 1975). An infant with suspected congenital insensitivity to pain associated with a family history of carpal tunnel syndrome was completely cured of self-mutilation of his hands by carpal tunnel release (Swoboda et al. 1998). Other rare entrapment neuropathies of the upper extremities have been reviewed by Dawson (1993) and by Ouvrier and Shield (1999).

Entrapment of the sciatic nerve due to a congenital iliac bony abnormality has been reported (Lester and McAlister 1970). Occasional childhood and adolescent cases of the thoracic outlet syndrome with cervical rib or fibrous band are known (Smith and Trojaborg 1987). Radial neuropathies in childhood have been reviewed by Escobar and Jones (1996).

MRI helps to diagnose the causes of such cases (Panegyres et al. 1993).

OTHER TRAUMATIC NERVE INJURIES

Neonatal injuries to the radial nerve as a result of subcutaneous fat necrosis of the upper arm (Eng et al. 1996) and of the median nerve as a result of attempts at catheterization of the radial or humeral artery have been reported (Chapter 1). Aicardi has seen two infants with transient paralysis of the femoral nerve after difficult puncture of the femoral vein and two similar cases following herniorrhaphy and appendectomy. In the latter procedure (for retrocaecal appendicitis), nerve injury was probably due to trauma of the nerve along the psoas muscle. Similar cases are reported in the literature (Stulz and Pfeiffer 1982).

Traumatic palsy of the peroneal nerve may be due to direct penetration or orthopaedic procedures in the region (Jones 1986) and has been reported following infiltration of intravenous fluid (Kreusser and Volpe 1984). Radial paralysis following constraint of the forearm for intravenous infusion is relatively common and always transient.

Lumbar plexus injuries are rare and occur only following major trauma to the pelvis, especially as a result of motor vehicle accidents. Rare cases have been seen following difficult breech delivery (Hope et al. 1985).

Glossopharyngeal neuralgia and hypoglossal nerve paralysis following tonsillectomy have been exceptionally recorded (Ekbom and Westerberg 1966, Sharp et al. 2002). Occipital neuralgia is not rare especially in adolescents (Dugan et al. 1962). The neck–tongue syndrome (Lance and Anthony 1980) consists of numbness of one side of the tongue with abnormal proprioception and sometimes twisting, on head turning. It may occur with degenerative or malformative abnormalities of the upper spine, although in many cases the cervical spine appears normal.

Nerve tumours are quite rare in children excepting the benign tumours of neurofibromatosis type I, which require no treatment. Detection of malignant nerve tumours is important, however, as effective treatment should not be delayed.

COMPLEX REGIONAL PAIN SYNDROME TYPE I (REFLEX SYMPATHETIC DYSTROPHY; REFLEX NEUROVASCULAR DYSTROPHY)

Reflex sympathetic dystrophy, now called complex regional pain syndrome type I, is a syndrome of unknown cause characterized by pain, tenderness, swelling, vasomotor disturbances and dystrophic skin changes typically affecting a single extremity (Schwartzman and McLellan 1987). Three diagnostic criteria have been suggested: (1) diffuse pain often not localized to anatomical nerve territories and out of proportion to the cause; (2) loss of function or impaired movements; (3) some objective evidence of autonomic dysfunction such as skin changes, oedema or osteoporosis. The disorder follows trauma, usually minor, in 40% of cases and typically occurs in young adolescent girls (Dietz et al. 1990, Gordon 1996). Pain may be so severe as to produce pseudoparalysis. In children, symptoms tend to be self-limited but a significant minority have protracted and disabling illness. Patients often appear to have a large psychological component to their condition that may also require attention (Bruehl and Carlson 1992). Affected children may have a special psychological profile (Sherry and Weisman 1988) but others have denied this (Lynch 1992). Bone scan may help in diagnosing the condition by usually showing localized decrease rather than the increased uptake seen in affected adults. Study by cutaneous thermography of local vasomotor reflex or by monitoring of near-surface blood flow may be of diagnostic value (Gordon 1996). Numerous forms of treatment have been used (Schwartzman and McLellan 1987, Kesler et al. 1988, Dietz et al. 1990) with variable results, including steroids, betablockers, calcitonin, vasodilators, transcutaneous nerve stimulation and physiotherapy (Gordon 1996). Infiltration of the regional sympathetic ganglia may be helpful, although involvement of the sympathetic system in the disorder has been contested. Sympathectomy may be used when infiltration proves helpful. Trophic changes may persist in long-standing cases.

Other rare autonomic disturbances of neural origin include Harlequin syndrome (Lance et al. 1988) and Ross syndrome (anhydrosis, Adie's pupil, syncope and other autonomic symptoms) (Drummond and Lance 1993), which have been occasionally reported in children.

LOCALIZED DISORDERS OF CRANIAL NERVES (EXCEPT OPTIC, OCULAR MOTOR AND AUDITORY NERVES)

The cranial nerves are affected together with the rest of the peripheral nerves in many diffuse nerve disorders. Certain conditions more specific to the cranial nerves, whether congenital or acquired, are described in this section.

Lesions of the optic, ocular motor and auditory nerves are described in Chapter 17.

TABLE 20.5
Facial nerve paralysis: features associated with weakness as a function of lesion location

Location	Taste	Hyperacousis	Lachrymation	Salivation
Motor nucleus	Normal	Present[1]	Normal	Normal
Facial nerve trunk between pons and internal auditory meatus	Normal	Present[1]	Impaired[2]	Impaired[3]
Geniculate ganglion	Impaired[3]	Present[1]	Impaired[2]	Impaired[2]
Facial nerve trunk between geniculate ganglion and emergence of stapedius nerve	Impaired[3]	Present[1]	Normal	Impaired[3]
Facial nerve trunk between stapedius nerve and chorda tympani	Impaired[3]	Absent	Normal	Impaired[3]
Lower facial nerve below chorda tympani	Normal	Absent	Normal	Normal

[1]Function subserved by the stapedius nerve.

[2]Function subserved by the greater superficial petrosal nerve (fibres originating from the solitary tract nucleus, coursing through the ganglion).

[3]Function subserved by the chorda tympani (fibres orginating from the solitary tract nucleus and joining the facial nerve through its anastomosis with the IXth cranial nerve).

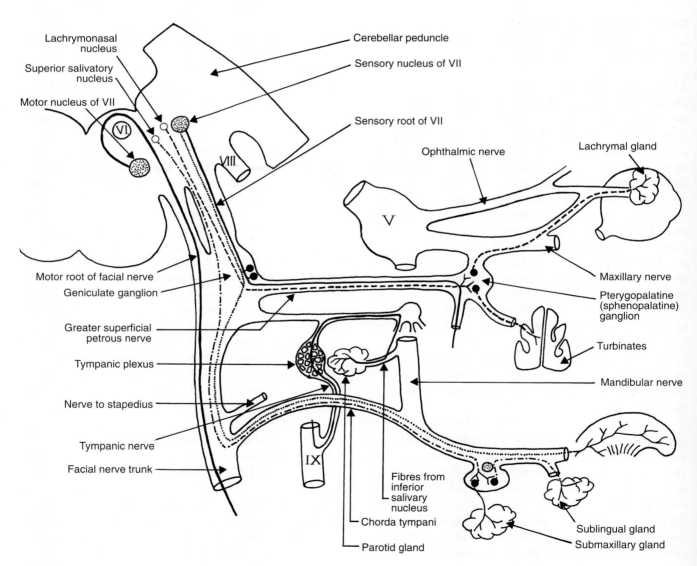

Fig. 20.8. Schematic representation of the facial nerve, indicating the distribution of sensory fibres and of autonomic fibres to lacrimal and salivary glands. (This schema helps explain the consequences to taste and hearing sensation, lacrimation and salivation of lesions at various levels—see also Table 20.5.)

ANOSMIA AND KALLMANN SYNDROME

Cranial trauma affecting the first cranial nerve may result in anosmia, which is often permanent. Anosmia may also occur in boys with cleft palate (Richman et al. 1988).

Congenital anosmia is a part of a usually but not exclusively X-linked syndrome of anosmia and eunuchoidism, sometimes associated with mild mental retardation, known as Kallmann syndrome, caused by mutations of the *Kal1* gene at Xp22.3 (Cadman et al. 2007) (Chapter 2). It results from an arrest of migration of axons from the olfactory placode that fail to reach the olfactory bulbs. Neurological defects are often present including mirror movements, cerebellar signs, hearing loss and abnormal eye movements (Schwankhaus et al. 1989). The syndrome is rarely associated with ichthyosis, short stature, chondrodystrophia punctata and ocular albinism, representing a contiguous gene syndrome associated with deletion of the entire short arm of the X chromosome (Gomez 1994). Multiple genes have been implicated in other forms of Kallmann syndrome (Cadman et al. 2007).

DISORDERS OF THE TRIGEMINAL NERVE

Except for traumatic and neoplastic lesions, disorders of the trigeminal nerve are uncommon in childhood. The most common disturbance, *jaw-winking* due to a congenital synkinesis (Marcus Gunn phenomenon), is described on page 702. Several types of congenital trigeminal anaesthesia occur, sometimes in association with the Goldenhaar or Moebius syndromes but also as an isolated defect (Rosenberg 1984). The presenting symptom is corneal inflammation and ulceration, which may require patching or tarsorrhaphy. Trigeminal neuralgia and neuropathy are very rare in childhood and are distinguished by the paroxysmal extreme pain in the former with less severe but chronic pain and altered sensation in the latter (Matoth et al. 2001). Underlying tumours must be excluded (Marshall and Rosman 1977). Surgery is effective if medical treatment fails (Resnick et al. 1998). The present author (RO) has observed several cases of tic in children, sometimes with Déjerine-Sottas disease or osteogenesis imperfecta (Hayes et al. 1999).

FACIAL NERVE PARALYSES

Facial paralysis of lower motor neuron type can be due to lesions located anywhere between the motor nucleus of the nerve and its terminal ramifications. Depending on the site of the lesion, variable symptoms and signs may accompany the facial weakness (Table 20.5, Fig. 20.8).

CONGENITAL FACIAL PARALYSES
Birth injury to the facial nerve
The facial nerve is the one most commonly involved in birth trauma or prenatal compression. Congenital unilateral facial nerve palsy is observed in approximately 0.3 per 1000 live births (McHugh et al. 1969) but is more common in large infants with an incidence of up to 6.5–7.5 per 1000 (Levine et al. 1984). In a majority of cases injury to the nerve is probably the result of pressure on the facial nerve distal to its emergence from the stylomastoid foramen against the sacral prominence of the

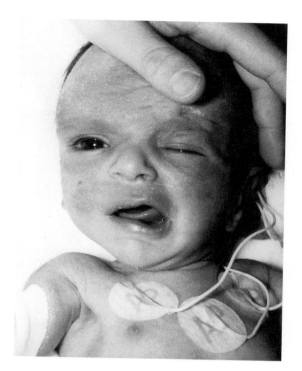

Fig. 20.9. Congenital facial palsy. 2-day-old infant born by forceps extraction. Note involvement of whole of right side of face, with failure of right eye to close.

maternal pelvis. This is suggested by the consistent relationship between fetal position and side of palsy, with left and right palsies observed subsequent to, respectively, left and right occipital positions. Paralysis resulting from application of forceps is comparatively rare.

The clinical expression of unilateral facial palsy even when it is complete is not always evident at birth, and partial involvement is not uncommon. In such cases, the orbicularis oculi is most often spared. This is because fibres that course upward just after leaving the foramen are not involved by compression over the parotid gland. The palpebral fissure is wider on the affected side and the eye fails to close completely (Fig. 20.9). Finding a periauricular ecchymosis or a haemotympanum helps diagnose traumatic palsy with a likely recovery (Shapiro et al. 1996).

In most cases, resolution of the paralysis is observed in a few weeks. Severe injuries with extensive disruption of the nerve seem to be rare. Surgical exploration of the nerve may be considered when no recovery is apparent after 3–6 months.

Congenital nontraumatic facial palsy
Congenital facial palsy can result from various anomalies of the nerve or its nucleus. Lesions of the inner ear may be associated with visible anomalies of the auricle and may be demonstrated by CT studies showing osseous abnormalities. More often, the nucleus or the nerve itself is abnormal or interrupted (Zucker 1990). Such patients present with unilateral complete paralysis and have no tendency to spontaneous recovery. Electrical stimulation at the stylomastoid foramen shows no muscle contraction,

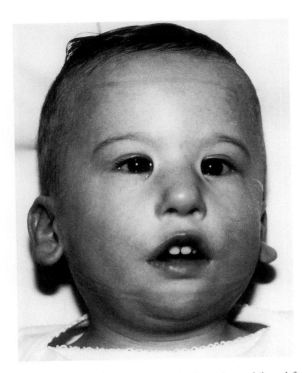

Fig. 20.10. Moebius syndrome. Mask-like facies due to bilateral facial paralysis. Note also bilateral internal strabismus due to involvement of both abducens nerves.

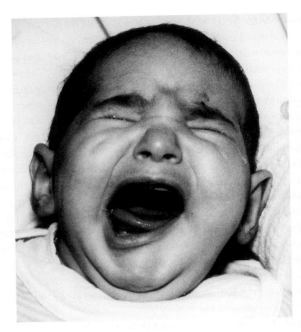

Fig. 20.11. Absence of depressor anguli muscle. Upper part of face is normal. Left corner of mouth fails to be lowered on crying.

in contrast to what obtains in traumatic palsy, and is of great value (Shapiro et al. 1996). Surgical exploration of the nerve may be indicated. Cleidocranial dysostosis and other bony dysplasias of the base of the skull are an unusual cause.

Moebius syndrome
Moebius syndrome is characterized by facial diplegia, typically associated with bilateral abducens palsy (Fig. 20.10) and, occasionally, with involvement of several cranial nerves, especially the lower cranial pairs, with frequent tongue involvement (Sudarshan and Goldie 1985). Affectation of the IIIrd nerves is uncommon. The syndrome often results in speech and sometimes feeding difficulties. Mental retardation is present in about 10–27% of affected children, although the immobile facies, drooling and speech difficulties often wrongly suggest subnormality. Unilateral Moebius syndrome has been reported (Towfighi et al. 1979). The mechanism of Moebius syndrome is probably multiple. A few cases may be of supranuclear origin; most are associated with abnormalities involving the rhombencephalon (Verzijl et al. 2005a) and may be due to absence of the brainstem nucleus (Towfighi et al. 1979). It seems more likely that many cases result from prenatal brainstem ischaemia with necrosis and sometimes calcification of the facial nuclei (Thakkar et al. 1977, Govaert et al. 1989, Fujita et al. 1991). Absence of the facial nerve has been shown pathologically and can be demonstrated by MRI studies (Verzijl et al. 2005b). Some cases may be due to congenital muscle aplasia or to other muscle disorders (Hanson and Rowland 1971). Some cases have been caused by the use of misoprostol

as an abortifacient (Marques-Dias et al. 2003). Bavinck and Weaver (1986) have speculated that Moebius syndrome and other regional malformations such as Klippel–Feil syndrome and the Poland anomaly might all be consequences of disrupted blood supply in the territory of the subclavian artery. Hamaguchi et al. (1993) separate three subgroups: children with only cranial nerve involvement, primarily of the VIth and VIIth pairs; patients with associated arthrogryposis; and those with absence or structural deformities of the extremities. The last type comprised 48% of 106 cases collected by Engler et al. (1979), who also encountered absence of the pectoralis major in 9% and micrognathia in 6% of their cases. Rare cases of familial Moebius syndrome are on record (Garcia-Erro et al. 1989). In some familial cases, other abnormalities such as Poland anomaly or arthrogryposis may be associated (Gadoth et al. 1979, Sudarshan and Goldie 1985).

Hypoplasia (or paralysis) of the depressor anguli oris muscle
This is a common minor anomaly (Nelson and Eng 1972). The corner of the mouth on the involved side fails to move downward on crying (Fig. 20.11). The lower lip may be slightly everted on the same side. This anomaly has been thought to be associated with other manifestations, especially congenital heart disease (Levin et al. 1982, Raymond and Holmes 1993), the so-called cardiofacial syndrome. Some are associated with the velo-cardiofacial syndrome of Shprintzen (Puñal et al. 2001). Nevertheless, the vast majority of children with this anomaly do not have other problems and a referral bias cannot be excluded. Beck et al. (1989) reported cases of isolated auriculotemporal syndrome in children, characterized by localized flushing of the face when eating.

Diagnosis of congenital facial palsies

The major causes of facial weakness are shown in Table 20.6. Congenital palsies represent about 8% of cases of childhood facial paralysis (Manning and Adour 1972), but it is not always easy to distinguish acquired from congenital cases or to separate nerve involvement from weakness due to muscle diseases.

For all cases with paralysis lasting more than a few weeks without improvement, imaging studies of the base of the brain are indicated. In cases of Moebius syndrome, brain CT or MRI should be performed.

ACQUIRED FACIAL PARALYSES

Paralysis of unknown cause – Bell palsy

Bell palsy is an acute idiopathic paralysis involving the territory of one facial nerve. The pathological changes include considerable oedema but there are few inflammatory signs. The pathogenesis is still uncertain but autoimmune demyelination probably plays a major role. The incidence of Bell palsy is 2.7 per 100,000 in the first decade of life and 10.1 per 100,000 in the second decade (Katusik et al. 1986). Both sides of the face are equally involved. Approximately 1–2% of patients have a family history of the disorder. A history of prior viral infection is frequently recorded but its significance is undecided. Multiple viral infections, especially herpes simplex, have been suspected. CSF studies in many cases have demonstrated pleocytosis, disordered blood–brain barrier and intrathecal immunoglobulin synthesis (Roberg et al. 1991). There is evidence that Bell palsy may be only the most striking manifestation of an autoimmune disorder affecting other cranial nerves, particularly the sensory trigeminal nerve, which may be involved in up to 50% of cases (Adour et al. 1978, Lapresle et al. 1980).

The first clinical manifestations may be pain or paraesthesiae in the ear or the face unilaterally but these are usually mild or absent. The paralysis reaches its maximum in a few hours and involves all muscles on one side of the face. The face is pulled to the side opposite the paralysis with efforts to use muscles of expression. The eye cannot be fully closed, and drinking may become difficult. Lachrymation is preserved in many cases but taste sensation is lost in about half the patients (see Table 20.5).

Weakness remains maximal for 2–4 weeks and then begins to lessen spontaneously (Adour 1982). Complete recovery is the rule in children especially when palsy is partial. Wong (1995) found complete recovery in 21 of 24 children. When denervation is complete, the onset of improvement may be delayed and recovery may not be total, reaching its maximum within 6 months (Adour 1982). Aberrant regeneration with 'crocodile tears' or auriculotemporal syndrome (Levin 1987) is exceptional in children. Recurrent paralysis is observed in around 6% of cases (Katusik et al. 1986). Electrical stimulation studies may be useful but are rarely necessary in childhood: incomplete denervation predicts complete recovery, whereas complete denervation may herald the persistence of some weakness. The CSF is abnormal in 10% (Weber et al. 1987) to 75% (Sandstedt et al. 1985) of patients, with increased protein and mononuclear cells, but lumbar puncture is rarely indicated. MR imaging is not usually

TABLE 20.6
Main causes of facial weakness in childhood*

Congenital
Congenital facial palsy due to birth injury
Congenital absence of depressor anguli oris muscle
Abnormalities of inner ear and/or facial nerve
Moebius syndrome of peripheral or central (nuclear) origin
Congenital or neonatal myasthenic syndromes
Congenital myotonic dystrophy
Other congenital myopathies or muscular dystrophies

Acquired
Diffuse neuromuscular diseases
    Muscular dystrophy (facioscapulohumeral type) and myopathies (*e.g.* nemaline myopathy)
    Acquired myasthenia and myasthenic syndromes
    Juvenile bulbar palsy (Fazio Londe and Van Laere types)
Involvement of facial nerve
    Inflammatory
        Bell palsy
        Idiopathic cranial neuropathy
        Miller Fisher syndrome and atypical forms of Guillain–Barré syndrome (Ropper 1986b)
        Herpes zoster (Ramsay Hunt syndrome)
        Lyme disease
        Otitis media and mastoiditis
        Infectious mononucleosis and other herpes viruses (Dowling and Cook 1981)
        Tuberculosis (tuberculoma or meningitis)
        Trichinosis (Lopez-Lozano *et al.* 1988)
        Sarcoidosis (Heerfordt syndrome)
        Multiple sclerosis
    Trauma and compression
        Fracture of petrous bone and other traumas
        Parotid gland tumours
        Osseous dysplasia of the base of the skull (*e.g.* cleidocranial dysostosis, osteopetrosis, hyperostosis cranialis interna) (Manni *et al.* 1990)
        Brainstem glioma and other intracranial tumours
        Langerhans histiocytosis (histiocytosis X)
        Intracranial hypertension
    Malformations
        Chiari malformation
        Syringobulbia
    Unknown mechanism
        Hyperparathyroidism
        Hypothyroidism
    Genetic
        Melkersson–Rosenthal syndrome
        Recurrent familial cranial neuropathy
    Vascular
        Arterial hypertension
        Vascular syndromes of the cranial nerve

*References given only for conditions not discussed in text.

indicated but, if performed, demonstrates contrast enhancement most commonly in the distal intracanalicular and labyrinthine segments of the facial nerve (Sartoretti-Scheffer et al. 1994).

The treatment of Bell palsy is purely symptomatic. Protection of an exposed cornea (by lubrication and patching) is essential. Corticosteroids are often advocated for adult patients but they are not indicated for children and there is indeed no proof of their efficacy (Burgess et al. 1984, Salinas et al. 2004, Chen and Wong

2005). It remains unclear whether antiviral agents are effective (Allen and Dunn 2004). It is important to exclude the possibility of otitis or mastoiditis and of any other lesional cause, and to rule out hypertension and Lyme disease (Clark et al. 1985), which may be the sole manifestation of the disease, although involvement of the chorda tympani is less frequent in Lyme disease.

Paralyses of known cause

Facial palsy is frequently the only manifestation of *Lyme disease*, especially in summer and autumn (Markby 1989, Grundfast et al. 1990). Christen et al. (1993) found that 32.9% of their cases were due to Lyme disease whereas viruses were apparently responsible for 18.4%. Facial palsy in neuroborreliosis may be unilateral; the occurrence of bilateral palsy a few days after involvement of one side is highly suggestive of borreliosis (Keane 1994, Kindstrand 1995). Stiff neck may be found in a quarter of cases. The CSF in such cases consistently shows pleocytosis and increased protein and may contain antibodies against *Borrelia burgdorferi* (Chapter 10).

Herpes zoster of the geniculate ganglion *(Ramsay Hunt syndrome)* is an uncommon cause of facial palsy in children. It may occur without any vesicular rash in the concha (Manning and Adour 1972). Other viruses may cause facial paralysis including Epstein–Barr, chicken pox and mumps viruses. A case due to Kawasaki disease has been described (Bushara et al. 1997).

Otitis media and mastoiditis, although now uncommon causes, should always be thought of, as antibiotic and/or surgical treatment may be required and as local signs may be extremely subtle. X-rays or CT of the temporal bone is indicated if there is any doubt about the possibility of a local otogenic process.

Tumours, especially rhabdomyosarcomas, may compress the nerve and should always be considered.

Hypertension is an infrequent cause of facial palsy (Lloyd et al. 1966) and should be systematically looked for (Chapter 14).

Traumatic paralysis is easy to suspect but demonstration may also require X-ray investigation (May et al. 1981). It may lead to aberrant regeneration and contractures.

Facial palsy is also the most common manifestation of neurosarcoidosis, a rare disorder in childen (Scott 1993).

Melkersson–Rosenthal syndrome is characterized by recurrent facial palsy, associated with swelling of the lips, face or eyelids and furrowing of the tongue (Wadlington et al. 1984, Ziem et al. 2000). Facial swelling and palsy may occur in isolation or simultaneously. Often swelling is the initial manifestation. Lingual involvement is inconstant. With repeated attacks, residual paralysis may appear and increase, leading to severe impairment.

Recurrent facial palsy may also be due to hypertension and to familial Bell palsy (Hageman et al. 1990).

Bilateral facial palsy is most commonly due to neuroborreliosis. Other causes in a mixed series of 43 children and adults (Keane 1994) included Guillain–Barré syndrome (6 cases), tumours of brainstem or meninges (9 cases), brainstem encephalitis and other miscellaneous causes. Ten cases were idiopathic (bilateral Bell palsy).

Hemifacial spasm has been reported in a few infants and children (Al Shahwan et al. 1994, Arzimanoglou 1996). The onset is usually in the first days of life with repeated attacks of unilateral tonic facial contracture lasting a minute or less and repeated many times daily. The syndrome is regularly associated with a small mass lesion in the cerebellum or in the region of the nucleus of the ipsilateral VIIth nerve that is hamartomatous or neoplastic in nature (Al Shahwan et al. 1994, Arzimanoglou 1996, Harvey et al. 1996). Harvey et al. (1996) have recorded mass paroxysmal discharges synchronous with the attack that may thus be regarded as a form of subcortical epilepsy. Their patient remained free of attacks following resection of a ganglioglioma. Such attacks differ from true peripheral hemifacial spasm, a rare condition in childhood, which is usually attributed to compression of the VIIth nerve trunk (Ronen et al. 1986). A case presenting in a newborn infant has been reported with a benign course (Zafeiriou et al. 1997).

LOWER CRANIAL NERVE PALSIES

Congenital lower cranial nerve palsies

Impairment of function of lower cranial nerves VII to XII may occur in cases of Chiari I and II malformation (Chapter 2). Involvement of the abductors of the vocal cords is particularly important as it often gives rise to severe respiratory insufficiency. Some cases are improved by treatment of the accompanying hydrocephalus.

Congenital traumatic laryngeal paralyses are probably related to intrauterine posture with rotation and lateral flexion of the head causing compression of the superior branch of the laryngeal nerve against the thyroid bone and that of the recurrent nerve against the cricoid cartilage. This produces a dual syndrome of the laryngeal nerve with both disturbances of swallowing due to sensory dysfunction of the superior laryngeal nerve and dysphonia due to involvement of the recurrent nerve (Chapple 1956). The prognosis of such cases is usually good (Narcy et al. 1978).

Hoarseness due to paralysis of the left recurrent nerve is in rare cases a presenting or accompanying symptom of congestive heart failure in infancy or a manifestation of a congenital anomaly of the great vessels of the base of the heart, the cardiovocal syndrome (Condon et al. 1985).

Congenital dysfunction of the vocal cords may occur in isolation and may be genetically transmitted. The posterior cricoarytenoid muscle, which is the sole abductor of the vocal cords and the only laryngeal muscle innervated solely by neurons of the ventral division of the ipsilateral nucleus ambiguus, is affected resulting in stridor and respiratory impairment. The condition may be familial (Cunningham et al. 1985). The course is towards spontaneous recovery in some cases, while other patients require a tracheostomy to maintain a free airway (Cohen et al. 1982).

Neurogenic stridor may also be of traumatic origin following forceps delivery or accidental trauma at birth (Maze and Bloch 1979). It may also be a feature of CNS involvement and occurs in association with nystagmus in connatal Pelizaeus–Merzbacher disease (Chapter 9).

Congenital dysphagia is rarely due to peripheral nerve involvement and is more often a part of pseudobulbar palsy that may be due to brain malformations or vascular and degenerative disorders. Severe dysarthria is often present in such cases (Van Dongen et al. 1987). Prolonged congenital dysphagia was reported by Mbonda et al. (1995). One of their four patients had associated paralysis of the adductors of the vocal cords. Cineradiographic study of swallowing showed major difficulties with the pharyngeal stage with only minimal involvement of the first oral stage. Two of the patients died; the others recovered in 20 and 40 months respectively. This syndrome is to be distinguished from benign transient pharyngeal dysfunction observed usually in preterm infants with recovery in a few weeks. EMG of the tongue and pharyngeal muscle confirms the peripheral involvement and helps predict the outcome.

Other lesions of the lower cranial nerves
Traumatic neonatal paralyses of the lower cranial nerves are uncommon. A few cases of glossopharyngeal paralysis variably associated with involvement of the IXth, Xth and XIth cranial nerves are on record (Greenberg et al. 1987), and hypoglossal palsy accompanied by brachial plexus injury has also been reported (Haenggeli and Lacourt 1989).

Intracranial disorders that produce raised intracranial pressure can be responsible for unilateral or, more commonly, bilateral vocal cord palsy often requiring tracheostomy. Spontaneous regression occurred in 4 of 7 cases reported by Chaten et al. (1991).

Isolated neuropathies probably related to viral or postviral diseases may raise serious diagnostic problems in children. Some may affect only one nerve, e.g. the hypoglossal nerve (Edin et al. 1976, Wright and Lee 1980), the recurrent nerve (Blau and Kapadia 1972) or the vagus nerve (Berry and Blair 1980). Others may involve both the IXth and Xth nerves, usually on one side, and produce an isolated temporary paralysis of the pharynx that may raise the suspicion of brainstem disease (Aubergé et al. 1979, Roberton and Mellor 1982, Suarez-Zeledon and Brian-Gago 1995). The onset is sudden, often following an upper respiratory infection, more rarely after a specific viral infection such as infectious mononucleosis (Wright and Lee 1980, Sugama et al. 1992, Connelly and De Witt 1994), with nasal reflux and/or dysphagia. Examination shows unilateral paresis of the soft palate and of the posterior pharyngeal wall. Spontaneous recovery occurs in a few days or weeks. Such cases are probably related to postinfectious abducens palsy (Chapter 17). XIIth nerve palsy is rare in children (Keane 1996).

Glossopharyngeal neuralgia is exceptional in children. Kandt and Daniel (1986) reported a case relieved by section of the glossopharyngeal nerve.

MULTIPLE CRANIAL NERVE PARALYSES
As indicated above, multiple involvement of cranial nerves may be more frequent than suspected, and Bell palsy is often the visible part of a subclinical multiple neuropathy. Such multiple nerve involvement in adults may be of vascular origin (Lapresle and Lasjaunias 1986). Affected nerves are few in such cases and belong to a localized arterial territory. In children, multiple cranial neuropathy is more often a manifestation of acute polyneuritis

akin to the Guillain–Barré syndrome (Ropper 1986a, Waddy et al. 1989). In occasional cases, a known virus is implicated, e.g. the varicella-zoster virus (Mayo and Booss 1989).

Idiopathic cranial polyneuropathy is observed mainly in adults (Hokkanen et al. 1978, Juncos and Beal 1987, Uldry and Régli 1988) but may also affect children. Various patterns of multiple cranial nerve involvement can obtain. The most commonly involved nerves are the facial nerves, the ocular motor nerves and the lower cranial nerves, but optic nerve involvement has been reported. The course of multiple cranial neuropathies is often recurrent, and such cases pose difficult diagnostic problems with myasthenia gravis, recurrent facial plasy, the syndrome of Tolosa–Hunt (Sorensen 1988), and some mitochondrial diseases. A migrating course is sometimes observed (Takahashi 1978). The condition may be familial (Sorensen 1988) but little is known about its mechanism.

A similar picture may be produced by tumours invading the base of the skull or basal meninges, hence the necessity of a careful radiological examination of such patients. Brainstem gliomas and encephalitis may also pose a diagnostic problem although they commonly produce signs of long tract involvement. Osseous diseases (hyperostosis cranialis interna) (Manni et al. 1990) may be a rare cause of multiple cranial nerve entrapment.

REFERENCES

Adams D, Festenstein H, Gibson JD, et al. (1979) HLA antigens in chronic relapsing idiopathic inflammatory polyneuropathy. *J Neurol Neurosurg Psychiatry* 42: 184–6.

Adour KK (1982) Diagnosis and management of facial paralysis. *N Engl J Med* 307: 348–51.

Adour KK, Byl FM, Hilsinger RL, et al. (1978) The true nature of Bell's palsy: analysis of 1000 consecutive patients. *Laryngoscope* 88: 787–801.

Airaksinen EM, Iivanainen M, Karli P, et al. (1985) Hereditary recurrent brachial plexus neuropathy with dysmorphic features. *Acta Neurol Scand* 71: 309–16.

Allen D, Dunn L (2004) Aciclovir or valaciclovir for Bell's palsy (idiopathic facial paralysis). *Cochrane Database Rev Syst* (3): CD001869.

Allsop JL. Martini L, Lebris H, et al. (1986) Neurologic manifestations of ciguatera. 3 cases with a neurophysiologic study and examination of one nerve biopsy. *Rev Neurol* 142: 590–7.

Al-Din AN, Anderson M, Bickestaff ER, Harvey I (1982) Brainstem encephalitis and the syndrome of Miller Fisher. *Brain* 105: 481–95.

Al-Qudah AA, Shahar E, Logan WJ, Murphy EG (1988) Neonatal Guillain–Barré syndrome. *Pediatr Neurol* 4: 255–6.

Al-Shahwan SA, Singh B, Riela AR, Roach ES (1994) Hemisomatic spasms in children. *Neurology* 44: 1332–3.

Amato AA, Barohn RJ, Sahenk Z, et al. (1993) Polyneuropathy complicating bone marrow and solid organ transplantation. *Neurology* 43: 1513–8.

Appenzeller O, Kornfeld M, Snyder R (1976) Acromutilating, paralyzing neuropathy with corneal ulceration in Navajo children. *Arch Neurol* 33: 733–8.

Argov Z, Mastaglia FL (1979) Drug-induced peripheral neuropathies. *BMJ* 1: 663–6.

Arzimanoglou A (1996) Hemifacial spasm or subcortical (infratentorial) epilepsy: a case report of a child with Goldenhar syndrome and a postmedullary junction lesion. In: Arzimanoglou A, Goutières F, eds. *Trends in Child Neurology.* Paris: John Libbey, pp. 43–51.

Asbury AK, Cornblath DR (1990) Assessment of current diagnostic criteria for Guillain–Barré syndrome. *Ann Neurol* 27 Suppl: S21–4.

Aubergé C, Ponsot G, Gayraud P, et al. (1979) [Acquired isolated velopalatine hemiparesis in children.] *Arch Fr Pediatr* 36: 283–6 (French).

Awerbuch GI, Nigro MA, Dabrowski E, Levin JR (1989) Childhood lumbosacral plexus neuropathy. *Pediatr Neurol* 5: 314–6.

Axelrod FB, Abularrage JJ (1982) Familial dysautonomia: a prospective study of survival. *J Pediatr* **101**: 234–6.

Axelrod FB, Pearson J (1984) Congenital sensory neuropathies: diagnostic distinction from familial dysautonomia. *Am J Dis Child* **138**: 947–54.

Axelrod FB, Nachtigall R, Dancis J (1974) Familial dysautonomia: diagnosis, pathogenesis and management. *Adv Pediatr* **21**: 75–96.

Axelrod FB, Iyer K, Fish I, et al. (1981) Progressive sensory loss in familial dysautonomia. *Pediatrics* **67**: 517–22.

Baba M, Takada H, Miura H, et al. (1995) "Pseudo" hypertrophic neuropathy of childhood. *J Neurol Neurosurg Psychiatry* **58**: 236–7.

Balestrini MR, Cavaletti G, D'Angelo A, Tredici G (1991) Infantile hereditary neuropathy with hypomyelination: report of two siblings with different expressivity. *Neuropediatrics* **22**: 65–70.

Bank WJ, Pleasure DE, Suzuki K, et al. (1972) Thallium poisoning. *Arch Neurol* **26**: 456–64.

Bardosi A, Creutzfeldt W, DiMauro S, et al. (1987) Myo-, neuro-, gastro-intestinal encephalopathy (MNGIE syndrome) due to partial deficiency of cytochrome-c-oxidase. A new mitochondrial multisystem disorder. *Acta Neuropathol* **74**: 248–58.

Barkai L, Szabó L (1993) Urinary bladder dysfunction in diabetic children with and without subclinical cardiovascular autonomic neuropathy. *Eur J Pediatr* **152**: 190–2.

Barohn RJ, Kissel JT, Warmolts JR, Mendell JR (1989) Chronic inflammatory demyelinating polyradiculoneuropathy: clinical characteristics, course and recommendation for diagnostic criteria. *Arch Neurol* **46**: 878–84.

Bastron JA, Thomas JE (1981) Diabetic polyneuropathy: clinical and electromyographic findings in 105 patients. *Mayo Clin Proc* **56**: 725–32.

Baumgartner G, Gawel MJ, Kaeser HE, et al. (1970) Neurotoxicity of halogenated hydroxyquinolines: clinical analysis of cases reported outside Japan. *J Neurol Neurosurg Psychiatry* **42**: 1073–83.

Bavinck JNB, Weaver DD (1986) Subclavian artery supply disruption sequence: hypothesis of a vascular etiology for Poland, Klippel–Feil and Möbius anomalies. *Am J Med Genet* **23**: 903–18.

Beck SA, Burks AW, Woody RC (1989) Auriculotemporal syndrome seen clinically as food allergy. *Pediatrics* **83**: 601–3.

Behan PO, Lessell S, Roche M (1976) Optic neuritis in the Landry–Guillain–Barré–Strohl syndrome. *Br J Ophthalmol* **60**: 58–9.

Behse F, Buchtal F, Carlsen F, Knappeis GG (1972) Hereditary neuropathy with liability to pressure palsies. *Brain* **95**: 777–94.

Ben Hamida M, Hentati F, Ben Hamida C (1990) Giant axonal neuropathy with inherited multisystem degeneration in a Tunisian kindred. *Neurology* **40**: 245–50.

Ben Hamida M, Belal S, Svingo G, et al. (1993) Friedreich's ataxia phenotype not linked to chromosome 9 and associated with selective autosomal recessive vitamin E deficiency in two inbred Tunisian families. *Neurology* **43**: 2179–83.

Ben Jelloun-Dellagi S, Dellagi K, Burger D, et al. (1992) Childhood peripheral neuropathy with antibodies to myelin glycoprotein P0. *Ann Neurol* **32**: 700–2.

Benson MD (2001) Amyloidosis. In: Scriver CR, Beaudet AL, Sly WS, Valle D, eds. *The Metabolic Basis of Inherited Disease, 8th edn.* New York: McGraw Hill, pp. 5345–78.

Berciano J, Combarros O, Figols J, et al. (1986) Hereditary motor and sensory neuropathy type II. Clinicopathological study of a family. *Brain* **109**: 897–914.

Berciano J, Combarros O, Calleja J, et al. (1989) The application of nerve conduction and clinical studies to genetic counselling in hereditary motor and sensory neuropathy type 1. *Muscle Nerve* **12**: 302–6.

Bergoffen J, Scherer SS, Wang S, et al. (1993) Connexin mutations in X-linked Charcot–Marie–Tooth disease. *Science* **262**: 2039–42.

Berry H, Blair RL (1980) Isolated vagus nerve palsy and vagal mononeuritis. *Arch Otolaryngol* **106**: 333–8.

Billard C, Ponsot G, Lyon G, Arthuis M (1979) [Acute polyradiculoneuritis in children. Clinical and genetic aspects. Pronostic factors apropos of 100 cases.] *Arch Fr Pediatr* **36**: 149–61 (French).

Blau JN, Kapadia R (1972) Idiopathic palsy of the recurrent laryngeal nerve: a transient cranial mononeuropathy. *BMJ* **4**: 259–61.

Bodensteiner JB, Rich KM, Landau WM (1994) Early infantile surgery for birth-related brachial plexus injuries: justification requires a prospective controlled study. *J Child Neurol* **9**: 109–10.

Boerkoel CF, Takashima H, Stankiewicz P, et al. (2001) Periaxin mutations cause recessive Déjerine–Sottas neuropathy. *Am J Hum Genet* **68**: 325–33.

Bono A, Beghi E, Bogliun G, et al. (1993) Antiepileptic drugs and peripheral nerve function: a multicenter screening investigation of 141 patients with chronic treatment. Collaborative Group for the Study of Epilepsy. *Epilepsia* **34**: 323–31.

Boylan KB, Ferriero DM, Greco CM, et al. (1992) Congenital hypomyelination neuropathy with arthrogryposis multiplex congenita. *Ann Neurol* **31**: 337–40.

Bradshaw DY, Jones HR (1992) Guillain–Barré syndrome in children: clinical course, electrodiagnosis, and prognosis. *Muscle Nerve* **15**: 500–6.

Brin MF, Pedley TA, Lovelace RE, et al. (1986) Electrophysiologic features of abetalipoproteinemia: functional consequences of vitamin E deficiency. *Neurology* **36**: 669–73.

Browder AA, Joselow MM, Louria DB (1973) The problem of lead poisoning. *Medicine* **52**: 121–39.

Brown BJ, Lewis LA, Mercer RD (1974) Familial hypobetalipoproteinemia: report of a case with psychomotor retardation. *Pediatrics* **54**: 111–3.

Bruehl S, Carlson C (1992) Predisposing psychological factors in the development of reflex sympathetic dystrophy. *Clin J Pain* **8**: 287–99.

Bruno C, Bertini E, Federico A, et al. (2004) Clinical and molecular findings in patients with giant axonal neuropathy. *Neurology* **62**: 13–6.

Burck U, Goebel HH, Kuhlendahl HD, et al. (1981) Neuromyopathy and vitamin E deficiency in man. *Neuropediatrics* **12**: 267–78.

Burgess LPA, Yim DWS, Lepore LM (1984) Bell's palsy: the steroid controversy revisited. *Laryngoscope* **94**: 1472–6.

Bushara K, Wilson A, Rust RS (1997) Facial palsy in Kawasaki syndrome. *Pediatr Neurol* **17**: 362–4.

Bye AM, Baker WdeC, Pollard J, Wise G (1990) Hereditary sensory neuropathy type II, without trophic changes. *Dev Med Child Neurol* **32**: 164–7.

Cadman SM, Kim SH, Hu Y, et al. (2007) Molecular pathogenesis of Kallmann's syndrome. *Horm Res* **67**: 231–42.

Casaubon LK, Melanson M, Lopes-Cendes I, et al. (1996) The gene responsible for a severe form of peripheral neuropathy and agenesis of the corpus callosum maps to chromosome 15q. *Am J Hum Genet* **58**: 28–34.

Casey EB, Jellife AM, Le Quesne PM, Millett Y (1973) Vincristine neuropathy. Clinical and electrophysiological observations. *Brain* **96**: 69–86.

Castro LHM, Ropper AH (1993) Human immunoglobulin infusion in Guillain–Barré syndrome: worsening during and after treatment. *Neurology* **43**: 1034–6.

Cavanagh NPC, Eames RA, Galvin RJ, et al. (1979a) Hereditary sensory neuropathy with spastic paraplegia. *Brain* **102**: 79–94.

Cavanagh NPC, Yates DAH, Sutcliffe J (1979b) Thenar hypoplasia with associated radiologic abnormalities. *Muscle Nerve* **2**: 431–6.

Chabrol B, Mancini J, Benelli C, et al. (1994) Leigh syndrome: pyruvate dehydrogenase defect. A case with peripheral neuropathy. *J Child Neurol* **9**: 52–5.

Chalmers RM, Bird AC, Harding AE (1996) Autosomal dominant optic atrophy with asymptomatic peripheral neuropathy. *J Neurol Neurosurg Psychiatry* **60**: 195–6.

Chance PF, Lensch MW, Lipe H, et al. (1994) Hereditary neurologic amyotrophy and hereditary neuropathy with liability to pressure palsies: two distinct genetic disorders. *Neurology* **44**: 2253–7.

Chang YC, Yip PK, Chiu YN, Lin HN (1988) Severe generalised polyneuropathy in lithium intoxication. *Eur Neurol* **28**: 39–41.

Chapple CC (1956) A duosyndrome of the laryngeal nerve. *Am J Dis Child* **91**: 14–8.

Charles LM, Jayam-Trouth A (1980) Brachial plexus neuropathy. Three cases in children. *Am J Dis Child* **134**: 299–300.

Charnas L, Bernar J, Pezeshkpour GH, et al. (1988) MRI findings and peripheral neuropathy in Lowe's syndrome. *Neuropediatrics* **19**: 7–9.

Chaten FC, Lucking SE, Young ES, Mickell JJ (1991) Stridor: intracranial pathology causing postextubation vocal cord paralysis. *Pediatrics* **87**: 39–43.

Chen WX, Wong V (2005) Prognosis of Bell's palsy in children—analysis of 29 cases. *Brain Dev* **27**: 504–8.

Chimelli L, Freitas M, Nascimento O (1997) Value of nerve biopsy in the diagnosis and follow-up of leprosy: the role of vascular lesions and usefulness of nerve studies in the detection of persistent bacilli. *J Neurol* **244**: 318–23.

Christen H-J, Hanefeld F, Eiffert H, Thomssen R (1993) Epidemiology and clinical manifestations of Lyme borreliosis in childhood. A prospective multicentre study with special regard to neuroborreliosis. *Acta Paediatr Suppl* **386**: 1–76.

Clark JR, Carlson RD, Sasaki CT, et al. (1985) Facial paralysis in Lyme disease. *Laryngoscope* **95**: 1341–5.

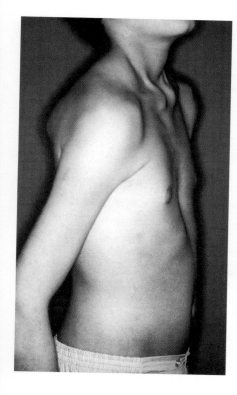
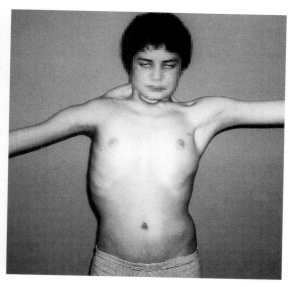

Fig. 21.3. Facioscapulohumeral dystrophy in a 13-year-old boy. *(Above)* Marked involvement of the scapular girdle, predominantly on right side. The eyes cannot be completely closed. *(Left)* Same patient, demonstrating atrophy of cervical muscles and amyotrophy of proximal arm with winged scapula. (Courtesy Dr F Renault, Hôpital Trousseau, Paris.)

peroneal syndromes. A range of myopathies and dystrophies can have skeletal muscle weakness and/or contractures and/or cardiac involvement, but there are usually additional clinical features. This group includes limb–girdle muscular dystrophies with cardiac involvement (e.g. LGMD 2A), the sarcoglycanopathies (LGMD2C–2F), LGMD 2I, Bethlem myopathy, myotonic dystrophy types 1 and 2, the dystrophinopathies, rigid spine syndrome and the myofibrillar myopathies. In scapulohumeral syndrome with dementia, also transmitted as an X-linked recessive disease, affected children, who are normal until age 5 years, develop first developmental delay, then mental retardation, weakness, contractures and cardiomyopathy (Bergia et al. 1986).

FACIOSCAPULOHUMERAL DYSTROPHY (FSHD)
FSHD is an autosomal dominant disorder characterized by a pattern of progressive muscle weakness involving the face, scapular stabilizers, upper arm, lower leg (peroneal muscles), and hip girdle (Tawil et al. 1998). Asymmetry of limb and/or shoulder weakness is common (Kilmer et al. 1995). Typically the initial symptoms are wasting of the shoulder girdle, winging of the scapulae, facial involvement with inability to purse the lips and to close the eyes tightly, and weakness of the zygomatic muscle with a transverse smile (Fig. 21.3). There may be more or less severe involvement of the biceps and triceps in the upper limbs, and the legs are variably involved, with peroneal muscle weakness with or without weakness of the hip girdle muscles. The deltoids are relatively spared until late in the disease. Respiratory function is usually normal (Tawil and Griggs 1997). Progression of the weakness is insidious and may be interrupted by periods of apparent arrest. Typically, individuals with FSHD become

symptomatic in their teens, but age of onset is variable. More than 90% of affected individuals demonstrate findings by age 20 years; some individuals remain asymptomatic throughout their lives. Onset may be early within some families (Bailey et al. 1986), and onset in infancy or early childhood with facial weakness has been observed. Additional manifestations include asymptomatic retinal vasculopathy (telangiectasia and microaneurysms) that can be demonstrated by fluorescein angiography in 40–60% of affected individuals and an abnormal audiogram with high-tone sensorineural hearing loss in around 60% of patients (Padberg et al. 1995). Serum CK is normal or only mildly elevated (3–5 times normal), and EMG is usually mildly myopathic. Muscle biopsy demonstrates chronic myopathic changes, although mononuclear inflammatory infiltrate may be present (Rothstein et al. 1971).

Over 95% of individuals with FSHD have a deletion within the D4Z4 repeat region of chromosome 4q35 (Wijmenga et al. 1992), which is detected by comparing the size of DNA fragments produced after digestion with the restriction enzyme EcoR1. Molecular testing is widely available in molecular diagnostic laboratories. Fragments of ≥42 kb are considered normal. About 95% of abnormal alleles are 34 kb or smaller (Upadhyaya et al. 1997). Fragments of 38–41 kb are borderline and need to be considered in association with the clinical findings. Individuals with smaller EcoR1 fragments (i.e. larger deletions) tend to be associated with earlier onset disease and more rapid progression (Zatz et al. 1995). About 10–30% of probands with FSHD have the disorder as the result of a de novo deletion; in the remainder of patients there is a family history consistent with autosomal dominant inheritance. A small group of affected

TABLE 21.1
Limb–girdle muscular dystrophies*

	Locus	Gene	Protein
X-linked recessive inheritance			
Duchenne/Becker muscular dystrophy (DMD/BMD)	Xp21.1	DMD	Dystrophin
Emery–Dreifuss muscular dystrophy (EDMD)	Xq28	EMD	Emerin
Autosomal dominant inheritance			
LGMD1A	5q31	TTID	Myotilin
LGMD1B (autosomal dominant EDMD)	1q11–q21	LMNA	Lamin A/C
LGMD1C (hyperCKaemia, rippling muscle disease)	3p25	CAV3	Caveolin-3
LGMD1D	6q23	?	?
LGMD1E (CMD1F)	7q	?	?
LGMD1F	7q32.1–32.2	?	?
LGMD1G	4p21	?	?
Autosomal recessive inheritance			
LGMD2A	15q15.1	CAPN3	Calpain 3
LGMD2B (Miyoshi myopathy)	2p13	DYSF	Dysferlin
LGMD2C	13q12	SGCG	γ-sarcoglycan
LGMD2D	17q12–q21.33	SGCA	α-sarcoglycan
LGMD2E	4q12	SGCB	β-sarcoglycan
LGMD2F	5q33	SGCD	δ-sarcoglycan
LGMD2G	17q12	TCAP	Telethonin
LGMD2H	9q31–q34	TRIM32	E3-ubiquitin ligase
LGMD2I	19q13.3	FKRP	Fukutin-related protein
LGMD2J	2q31	TTN	Titin
LGMD2K	9q34	POMT1	O-mannosyl transferase 1
LGMD2L	9q31-q33	FCMD	Fukutin
LGMD2M	11p13–p12	?	?
LGMD2N	14q24.3	POMT2	O-mannosyl transferase 2

*Adapted from: Gene table of monogenic neuromuscular disorders. *Neuromuscul Disord* 2008, **18**: 101–29.

families do not link to 4q35, indicating genetic heterogeneity (Gilbert et al. 1993).

A number of disorders may present with a pattern of weakness similar to that seen in FSHD. Myofibrillar myopathy, inclusion body myositis, mitochondrial myopathies and congenital myopathies are usually distinguishable on the basis of muscle histopathology. It may be more difficult to distinguish FSHD from some forms of limb–girdle muscular dystrophy (particularly LGMD 2A) and polymyositis. The myotonic dystrophies can present with an FSHD-like syndrome, but are usually distinguishable on EMG.

LIMB–GIRDLE MUSCULAR DYSTROPHIES (LGMDs)

The LGMDs are a heterogeneous group of disorders characterized by weakness and wasting of the pelvic and shoulder girdle muscles and a dystrophic muscle biopsy that shows ongoing degeneration of muscle fibres, fibre size variability and increased connective tissue. Even within a specific genetic subtype, the clinical course ranges from severe forms with rapid progression and onset in the first decade (similar to the clinical presentation of Duchenne muscular dystrophy), to milder forms with slower progression and later onset (similar to the range of severity seen in Becker muscular dystrophy) (for useful reviews see Gordon and Hoffman 2001, Zatz et al. 2003, Laval and Bushby 2004). Currently, 19 genetic loci for LGMD have been identified (Table

21.1). In addition, there are other forms of later-onset muscular dystrophy that are important to consider in the differential diagnosis in the clinical setting (Table 21.1).

CLINICAL CORRELATES AND APPROACH TO DIAGNOSIS

A detailed review of all of the different forms of LGMD is beyond the scope of this text. Nevertheless there are a few simple clinical clues that can aid the clinician in diagnosis (Table 21.2) and guide the approach to further diagnostic testing (Table 21.3). In general, inter- and intrafamilial variability is common. Calf hypertrophy can occur in all groups but is rare in LGMD 2B, where calf atrophy may occur. Cardiac involvement (cardiomyopathy) is common in DMD, EDMD, LGMD 1B, the sarcoglycanopathies and LGMD 2I, and is rare in LGMDs 2A and 2B. A severe (Duchenne-like) phenotype can be seen in the sarcoglycanopathies and in LGMDs 2A and 2I.

Often the different forms of LGMD cannot be distinguished on the basis of clinical presentation. The diagnosis often relies on protein studies on the patient muscle biopsy (immunohistochemistry and Western blot) to identify deficiency of the specific protein, followed by mutation analysis to confirm that the deficiency is due to a primary mutation in a specific gene (Table 21.3). It must be noted that protein analysis is not always specific – for example, dysferlin can be abnormally localized in up to 40% of LGMDs, although complete deficiency as demonstrated by immunohistochemistry (IHC) is usually due to a primary

TABLE 21.2
Clinical clues to the diagnosis of the limb–girdle muscular dystrophies

X-linked recessive inheritance	
Duchenne/Becker muscular dystrophy (DMD/BMD)	Hypertrophy of calves and other muscle groups. Static encephalopathy. Language delay
Emery–Dreifuss muscular dystrophy (EDMD)	Prominent contractures of the elbows, Achilles tendon and posterior cervical muscles. Initial scapulo-humero-peroneal weakness. Cardiac conduction defects. Dilated cardiomyopathy
Autosomal dominant inheritance	
LGMD1A	Late onset (>50 years). Peripheral neuropathy, cardiomyopathy, weakness may be distal>proximal. Nasal speech
LGMD1B (Autosomal dominant EDMD)	As for EDMD. Mutations in lamin A/C can also cause cardiomyopathy alone, partial lipodystrophy and peripheral neuropathy
LGMD1C	May present as asymptomatic hyperCKaemia, rippling muscle disease or myalgia
Autosomal recessive inheritance	
LGMD2A	Initially weakness may affect posterior compartment of lower limb. Scapular winging may occur. Variable onset (2–40 years)
LGMD2B (and Miyoshi myopathy)	Calf wasting often early feature. Lymphocytic infiltration on muscle biopsy. Proximal or distal (calf) onset
LGMD2C–F (sarcoglycanopathies)	Calf hypertrophy, DMD- or BMD-like
LGMD2G	Described to date only in Brazil
LGMD2H	Described to date only in Manitoba Hutterites
LGMD2I (MDC1C)	Calf and tongue hypertrophy prominent. Can be misdiagnosed as dystrophinopathy. Wide range of severity (congenital – late onset)
LGMD2J (TMD, CMD1G)	Described to date only in Finland. Tibialis anterior wasting
Common differential diagnoses: other forms of later-onset myopathy/muscular dystrophy	
Bethlem myopathy[1]	Distal contractures (e.g. finger flexors) and hyperlaxity
Facio-scapulo-humeral[1]	Distribution of weakness. Scapular winging. Facial weakness rare in other LGMDs
Myotonic dystrophy[1]	Paucity of facial expression. Cardiac conduction defects. Myotonia clinically and on EMG

[1]Autosomal dominant transmission.

TABLE 21.3
Limb–girdle muscular dystrophies: establishing protein/molecular diagnosis

X-linked recessive inheritance	
Duchenne/Becker muscular dystrophy (DMD/BMD)	IHC, WB, DNA diagnostic
Emery–Dreifuss muscular dystrophy (EDMD)	IHC, DNA research
Autosomal dominant inheritance	
LGMD1A	DNA research
LGMD1B (Autosomal dominant EDMD)	WB can show altered protein level. DNA research
LGMD1C	IHC and WB can show altered protein level. DNA research
Autosomal recessive inheritance	
LGMD2A	WB not specific, protein levels can be secondarily reduced. DNA research
LGMD2B (and Miyoshi myopathy)	IHC not specific, dysferlin levels often secondarily reduced. WB – dysferlin absent. DNA research
LGMD2C–F (sarcoglycanopathies)	IHC – often all members of the sarcoglycan complex reduced secondary to mutation in one gene. DNA research
LGMD2G	IHC, DNA research
LGMD2H	DNA research
LGMD2I (MDC1C)	IHC of α-dystroglycan. WB for laminin-α2 (secondarily reduced) and α-dystroglycan. DNA diagnostic (restriction enzyme study of *FKRP* for common mutation, C826A)
LGMD2J (TMD, CMD1G)	WB – secondary reduction in calpain. DNA research
Other forms of later onset myopathy/muscular dystrophy	
Bethlem myopathy[1]	May see reduction in collagen VI levels by IHC or WB – not sensitive. DNA research
Facio-scapulo-humeral[1]	DNA diagnostic
Myotonic dystrophy[1]	DNA diagnostic

Abbreviations: IHC = immunocytochemistry; WB = Western blotting.
DNA diagnostic: mutations analysis available as a diagnostic test from commercial labs.
DNA research: mutations analysis available currently mainly on a research basis.
[1]Autosomal dominant transmission.

dysferlin mutation (Bansal and Campbell 2004). Primary mutations in any one of the sarcoglycan complex can result in deficiency, evidenced by IHC, of all members of the sarcoglycan complex. Calpain deficiency demonstrated by Western blot is about 70% specific, but can occur in other dystrophies; conversely, patients with mutations in the calpain gene have been identified in whom Western blotting from calpain is normal. Laboratories willing to perform DNA diagnosis on a diagnostic (i.e. cost recovery) or research basis can be found at www.geneclinics.org.

PATHOGENESIS

As noted above, Duchenne muscular dystrophy is due to deficiency of the sarcolemmal membrane protein, dystrophin. Following the identification of dystrophin, researchers focused on the characterization of proteins related to, or that interact with, dystrophin, since there was a high probability that these proteins would also be involved in the pathogenesis of human neuromuscular diseases. This resulted in the cloning of genes for the dystrophin-associated proteins (DAPs), α, β-, δ- and γ-sarcoglycan, and the identification of mutations in each gene in different forms of AR-LGMD (LGMDs 2C–F). It is hypotheszed that deficiency of any one component of the DAP complex disrupts the binding of the extracellular matrix to the cytoskeleton, rendering the sarcolemmal membrane unstable and resulting in ongoing fibre necrosis (Zatz et al. 2003, Laval and Bushby 2004). LGMD 2I is associated with loss of α-dystroglycan at the cell

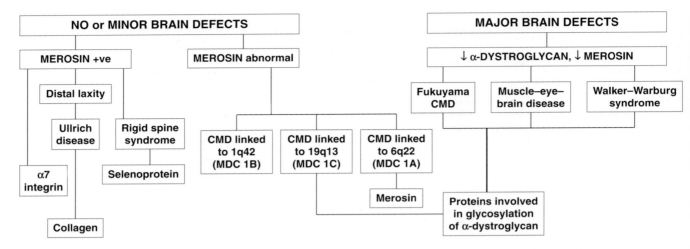

Fig. 21.4. Classification of congenital muscular dystrophies (courtesy of Dr Pascale Guicheney, INSERM Paris; adapted by permission).

TABLE 21.4
Working definition of congenital muscular dystrophy*

- Muscle weakness and hypotonia present from birth or first few months of life
- Congenital or early contractures, often involving the spine
- Histological changes compatible with a 'dystrophic' process combining active degeneration and regeneration, fibrosis, and lipomatosis
- Serum creatine kinase levels normal or elevated
- Intellect normal or impaired
- Brain on imaging/post-mortem normal or evidence of white matter changes, disorders of migration and cerebellar or brainstem abnormalities

*After Voit (2001).

membrane, again resulting in loss of the link between the extracellular matrix and the cytoskeleton. Glycosylation of α-dystroglycan by a variety of glycosyltransferases results in its normal localization to the muscle membrane (Muntoni et al. 2002). LGMD 2I is due to recessive mutations in the gene encoding the glycosyltransferase FKRP (fukutin-related protein). Aberrant *glycosylation of α-dystroglycan* also underlies a heterogeneous group of congenital muscular dystrophies with and without involvement of the central nervous system (e.g. Fukayama CMD, Walker–Warburg syndrome, muscle–eye–brain disease, CMD type 1C).

Mutations in the gene encoding the protein dysferlin result in LGMD 2B and Miyoshi myopathy (which initially predominantly involves the distal muscles). Dysferlin is localized to the sarcolemmal membrane but is not an integral component of the DAP complex. It is involved in vesicle fusion in skeletal muscle and has recently been implicated in muscle membrane repair (Bansal and Campbell 2004). This represents a different mechanism for muscle damage, i.e. inadequate repair rather than increased susceptibility to membrane damage (as is seen in dystrophies due to abnormalities of dystrophin and the DAP complex).

In addition, several muscular dystrophy genes have been identified that do not encode integral components of the DAP

complex, i.e.calpain, a calcium-sensitive intracellular protease; caveolin 3, a component of membrane lipid raft domains; lamin A/C and emerin, nuclear envelope proteins; the sarcomeric proteins telethonin and myotilin; and TRIM3, a putative ubiquitin ligase (Zatz et al. 2003). Abnormalities in these proteins may lead to disruption of cellular pathways, central to disease pathogenesis, rather than causing dystrophic changes in muscle by a direct effect on the structure and integrity of the sarcolemmal membrane.

CONGENITAL MUSCULAR DYSTROPHY

The term congenital muscular dystrophy (CMD) refers to a heterogeneous group of inherited disorders that are characterized by muscle weakness at birth or in the first few months of life, typically associated with a dystrophic pattern on muscle biopsy and an elevated creatine kinase level (although occasionally the biopsy can be myopathic rather than dystrophic and CK can be in the normal range). Infants are frequently hypotonic and may have joint contractures. The clinical course is usually static, although improvement or slow progression may be seen. There is variable involvement of the respiratory, cardiac and bulbar muscles (Dubowitz 1995, Jones and North 2003). The current working definition of CMD as described by Voit is shown in Table 21.4.

The genes currently known to cause CMD are shown in Table 21.5. Ten genes causing specific forms of CMD have now been identified. It is important to note that many individuals with CMD remain unclassified.

The original classification of CMD was based on clinical features. However, the classification is now based on a combination of clinical, biochemical and molecular genetic features as many types of CMD have overlapping phenotypes (Fig. 21.4). The congenital muscular dystrophies can be divided into two major groups: (1) those without brain defects (no CNS involvement); and (2) those with major brain defects. They are then subdivided based on the expression of the extracellular matrix protein, laminin-α2, commonly known as merosin, as well as additional clinical features such as distal laxity (common in colla-

TABLE 21.5
Genetics in the congenital muscular dystrophies (CMD)*

Disease	Mode of inheritance[1]	Gene location	Symbol (gene product)	Key reference
Laminin-α2 deficient CMD	AR	6q2	*LAMA2* (laminin-α2 chain of merosin)	Helbling-Leclerc et al. (1995)
Congenital muscular dystrophies associated with abnormal glycosylation of α-dystroglycan (includes Fukuyama CMD, muscle–eye–brain disease, Walker–Warburg syndrome[2])				
	AR	9q31–q33	*FCMD* (fukutin)	Kobayashi et al. (1998)
	AR	1p3	*POMGnT1* (O-mannose β-1, 2-N-acetylglucosaminyl transferase)	Yoshida et al. (2001)
	AR	9q34	*POMT1* (O-mannosyltransferase 1)	Beltran-Valero et al. (2002)
	AR	14q24.3	*POMT2* (O-mannosyltransferase 2)	
	AR	19q13	*FKRP* (fukutin-related protein)	Brockington et al. (2001a)
	AR	22q12	*LARGE* (like-glycosyl transferase)	
Rigid spine syndrome	AR	1p36	*SEPN1* (selenoprotein N1)	Moghadaszadeh et al. (2001)
Ullrich syndrome	AR	21q22.3	*COL6A1* (collagen type VI subunit α1)	Camacho et al. (2001)
		21q22.3	*COL6A2*	
		2q37	*COL6A3*	
Integrin α7 deficiency	AR	12q	*ITGA7* (integrin α7)	Hayashi et al. (1998)
CMD	AR	1q42	?	Brockington et al. (2000)

*Adapted from: Gene table of monogenic neuromuscular disorders. *Neuromuscul Disord* 2008, **18**: 101–29.

[1]AR = autosomal recessive.

[2]It is becoming increasingly evident that mutations in the genes encoding all the glycosyltransferases identified so far can result in a range of phenotypes including congenital muscular dystrophy with and without CNS involvement as well as limb–girdle muscular dystrophy (Godfrey et al. 2007).

gen VI disorders) and rigid spine (seen in disorders of selenoprotein N).

CONGENITAL MUSCULAR DYSTROPHIES WITHOUT MAJOR BRAIN DEFECTS: α-DEXTROGLYCANOPATHIES
Primary laminin-α2 (merosin) deficiency (MDC1A)
Children with primary laminin-α2 deficiency usually presents at birth or soon after with extreme general hypotonia, and feeding and respiratory difficulties. Severe muscle weakness affects the face, trunk and extremities, and approximately 50% of patients have contractures of single or multiple joints. The muscle weakness tends to be non-progressive or slowly progressive, however few patients achieve independent standing (Voit 2001, Jones and North 2003).

All patients with severe laminin-α2 abnormalities have cerebral white matter changes on cranial MRI reminiscent of a leukodystrophy, but intellect is usually normal or only mildly delayed (Fig. 21.5). The white matter changes become more marked during the first years of life, in parallel with increased brain myelination, but then persist over time. In some patients, additional structural abnormalities are present including occipital polymicrogyria/agyria and cerebellar or pontine hypoplasia. Epilepsy occurs in up to 30% of patients. Serum CK levels are often raised to between 1000 and 15000 IU/L. Patients with

later onset and milder weakness have been reported (Jones et al. 2001, Miyagoe-Suzuki et al. 2000). The muscle biopsy is usually severely dystrophic and immunohistochemistry typically shows laminin-α2 to be markedly reduced or absent. The disorder is autosomal recessive and due to mutations in the *LAMA2* gene on chromosome 6q (Helbling Leclerc et al. 1995). It is important to note that laminin-α2 immunohistochemistry and quantitation by Western blot can be abnormal secondary to disorders of glycosylation of α-dystroglycan (see below). In the latter disorders, laminin-α2 staining is usually patchy and reduced rather than completely deficient.

Rigid spine syndrome
This disorder is allelic to multiminicore disease (see below); the clinical picture is similar in patients with mutations in the gene encoding selenoprotein N (*SEPN1*) with predominantly axial weakness and the development of distinct rigidity of the spine. Such rigidity is not specific for this entity but is seen in other phenotypes such as Emery–Dreifuss muscular dystrophy. There is variability in the distribution of weakness, degree of scoliosis and limb contractures, and severity of functional disability. Respiratory failure requiring nocturnal ventilation is common and can occur in ambulant patients and hence monitoring for nocturnal hypercapnia is important. Intellect and cerebral imaging

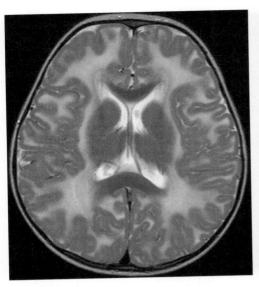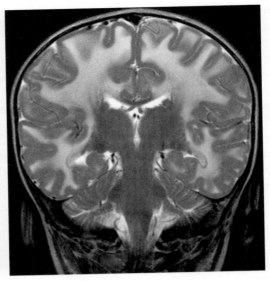

Fig. 21.5. Congenital muscular dystrophy with merosin deficiency. MRI showing diffuse high T$_2$ signal from white matter. *(Left)* Axial cut, *(right)* frontal cut.

are normal, and CK can be in the normal range (Voit 2001, Jones and North 2003).

Integrin α7 deficiency
This is a rare form of CMD and primary mutations in the integrin α7 gene (*ITGA7*) have been reported in only 3 patients to date (Hayashi et al. 1998).

Ullrich congenital muscular dystrophy (UCMD)
Ullrich first described this disorder as congenital hypotonic–sclerotic muscular dystrophy in 1930. Major clinical findings include generalized muscle weakness, wasting and hypotonia, striking contractures of the proximal joints with distal hyperextensibility from an early infantile stage, and a progressive course with slow progression of weakness and increase in the contractures (Higuchi et al. 2001). Other clinical features of the disease include dry skin and a 'sandpaper' rash, often mistaken for eczema (Bertini and Pepe 2002), high arched palate and prominence of the calcaneus. Intellectual development is normal. Bilateral congenital dislocation of the hips, torticollis and kyphoscoliosis can also occur (Camacho Vanegas et al. 2001, Higuchi et al. 2001, Bertini and Pepe 2002, Pepe et al. 2002). Often there is associated early rigidity of the spine and respiratory involvement. Some patients achieve independent ambulation, while others do not (Mercuri et al. 2002). UCMD is associated with mutations in any one of three genes that encode components of the collagen VI protein (*COL6A1*, *2* and *3*). Muscle biopsy displays the typical pathological changes of a muscular dystrophy (Higuchi et al. 2001) and collagen VI is variably reduced at the sarcolemmal membrane. Serum CK is either normal or slightly elevated.
   Bethlem myopathy (BM) (Higuchi et al. 2001) is a milder disorder of collagen VI associated with later onset and milder weakness in association with distal laxity and contractures. Originally

UCMD was considered to be an autosomal recessive disorder and Bethlem myopathy a milder autosomal dominant variant. However, recent genetic studies demonstrate that UCMD can be due to dominant mutations in up to 40% of cases, and that these mutations often occur de novo. In addition there appears to be a continuum in the clinical severity of collagen VI disorders so that it is not always possible to definitively classify patients as either UCMD or BM, and some cases with congenital-onset weakness can have a relatively mild clinical course (Baker et al. 2005, Lampe et al. 2005).

CONGENITAL MUSCULAR DYSTROPHIES WITH MAJOR BRAIN ANOMALIES: α-DYSTROGLYCANOPATHIES
A number of CMDs are caused by mutations in the genes encoding glycosyltransferases or putative glycosyltransferases (Table 21.5). Abnormal glycosylation of α-dystroglycan is a common feature, resulting in abnormal localization of α-dystroglycan to the muscle membrane. This results in reduced or absent staining of α-dystroglycan by immunohistochemistry. Laminin-α2 binds to α-dystroglycan at the membrane, and this causes a secondary reduction in laminin-·2; immunohistochemical staining can be normal or patchy, but on Western blotting the protein is often seen to be markedly reduced. CMDs due to abnormal glycosylation of α-dystroglycan are associated with variable involvement of the central nervous system (typically neuronal migration defects) and ocular manifestations, and include Fukuyama CMD, muscle–eye–brain disease, Walker–Warburg syndrome, MDC1C and MDC1D. There is considerable clinical overlap between the different conditions and there is genetic heterogeneity (Jones and North 2003, Godfrey et al. 2007).

Fukuyama congenital muscular dystrophy (FCMD)
FCMD occurs principally in Japan. The condition typically

manifests either prior to birth or in the neonatal period with reduced movement and severe dystrophic pathology. Few patients attain the ability to walk independently. Approximately half have evidence of ocular involvement. Common neuronal migration abnormalities include polymicrogyria, pachygyria and agyria of the cerebrum and cerebellum. Intellectual impairment and seizures are present in the majority. The majority of patients develop respiratory and cardiac involvement, and life expectancy is significantly reduced (Jones and North 2003, Muntoni and Voit 2004). FCMD is an autosomal recessively inherited condition caused by mutations in the gene, located on chromosome 9q31, encoding fukutin, a putative glycosyltransferase (Schachter et al. 2003, Muntoni et al. 2004).

Muscle–eye–brain disease (MEB)

MEB is similar in severity to FCMD. Clinical features include structural ocular involvement (microphthalmia, retinal defects and anterior chamber anomalies), type II lissencephaly (pachygyria, polymicrogyria, hypoplastic cerebellar vermis and cerebellar cysts) and CMD. Seizures are common and intellectual impairment is usually severe (Jones and North 2003, Barresi et al. 2004, Muntoni and Voit 2004). MEB is inherited in an autosomal recessive manner (Muntoni and Voit 2004). Disease-causing mutations were first identified in the gene encoding the glycosyltransferase protein O-mannose β-1, 2-N-acetylglucosaminyl-transferase (POMGnT1) gene on chromosome 1q33 (Kano et al. 2002). Recently, mutations in the POMGnT1 gene were reported in a patient with autistic features and stereotypic movements, further broadening the clinical spectrum (Haliloglu et al. 2004). MEB is genetically heterogeneous; mutations causing MEB have also been identified in the FKRP gene (see below), and it is likely that mutations in the genes encoding other glycosyltransferases will result in a similar phenotype (Beltran-Valero et al. 2004).

Walker–Warburg syndrome (WWS)

WWS is the most severe of the muscular dystrophies characterized by abnormal α-dystroglycan. Patients with WWS have CMD, severe ocular involvement (microphthalmia, optic nerve hypoplasia, retinal dysplasia and cataracts), type II lissencephaly with agyria, and cerebellar and brainstem hypoplasia, and usually die during infancy (Dubowitz 1995, Jones and North 2003, Currier et al. 2005). Other associated congenital malformations include hydrocephalus, Dandy–Walker malformation, cleft lip or palate and genital anomalies (Dubowitz 1995). WWS is inherited in an autosomal recessive manner and is genetically heterogeneous (Muntoni and Voit 2004, Beltran-Valero et al. 2004, Cohn 2005, van Reeuwijk et al. 2005, Godfrey et al. 2007) (Table 21.5).

MDC1D

There is one patient reported in the literature with CMD, severe mental retardation, abnormal glycosylation of α-dystroglycan and mutations in the LARGE gene, which encodes another glycosyltransferase. Serum CK was elevated. Brain MRI at 14 years of age showed extensive and symmetrical white matter changes in the periventricular region extending to the arcuate fibres.

There were also changes suggestive of an abnormal neuronal migration pattern (Longman et al. 2003).

MDC1C

MDC1C is associated with mutations in the FKRP gene (Brockington et al. 2001a). In the original description, patients had severe CMD and presented in the neonatal period with hypotonia, feeding difficulties and severe muscle weakness. Some developed muscle hypertrophy (calf and tongue), contractures and facial weakness. Several children had severe restrictive respiratory involvement and impaired cardiac function. Brain function and structure was normal. In most cases CK was elevated and the muscle dystrophic.

Subsequently children have been described with mutations in FKRP and abnormal brain structure and function (de Paula et al. 2003, Topaloglu et al. 2003, Beltran-Valero et al. 2004, Harel et al. 2004, Louhichi et al. 2004), and it appears that this phenotype is as frequent as the initial description of MDC1C. The patient can present with mental retardation and variable CNS abnormalities including cerebellar cysts or atrophy with or without white matter changes (Topaloglu et al. 2003, Louhichi et al. 2004). Mutations in FKRP have also been reported in one patient with MEB and one patient with WWS (Beltran-Valero et al. 2004). Mutations in FKRP also result in one of the most common forms of limb–girdle muscular dystrophy in Europe (LGMD 2I); patients with LGMD 2I can present with a Duchenne-like phenotype or can have a later onset and milder phenotype with a range of severity similar to that seen in Becker muscular dystrophy. Respiratory and cardiac involvement are common in LGMD 2I (Brockington et al. 2001b).

In combination, these data demonstrate the enormous variation in phenotype associated with FKRP mutations, ranging from those with normal intellect to those with severe CNS malformations and mental retardation, to those with severe CMD who never attain the ability to walk independently to those who remain asymptomatic and ambulatory in their 30s. It is speculated that this is due to the effects of the severity of the mutation on protein function (Beltran-Valero et al. 2004).

CONGENITAL MYOPATHIES

Congenital myopathies are characterized clinically by hypotonia and weakness, usually from birth, and by morphological changes on histological and/or electron microscopic examination. Histopathological signs of muscle dystrophy are not present, CK levels are normal or only mildly elevated, and the EMG is either normal or myopathic. There is wide variation in clinical severity within each form of myopathy, and marked clinical overlap with other neuromuscular disorders including the muscular dystrophies, metabolic myopathies and spinal muscular atrophies, as well as Prader–Willi syndrome, which can all present in the newborn period with marked hypotonia ('floppy infant').

Certain congenital myopathies are well defined clinically, morphologically and genetically (Table 21.6). Some are defined

TABLE 21.6
Congenital myopathies with identified gene loci

Disorder	Inheritance*	Protein and gene	Chromosome locus	References
Nemaline myopathy (NEM)	AD, AR	α-tropomyosin$_{slow}$ (TPM3)	1q22–q23	Laing et al. (1995), Tan et al. (1999)
	AD, AR, sporadic	Skeletal muscle α-actin (ACTA1)	1q42.1	Nowak et al. (1999)
	AD	β-tropomyosin (TPM2)	9p13.2	Donner et al. (2002)
	AD	?	15q	Gommans et al. (2003)
	AR	Nebulin (NE)	2q 21.2–2q22	Pelin et al. (1999)
	AR	Troponin T1 (TNNT1)	19q13.4	Johnston et al. (2000)
Central core disease	AD, AR, sporadic	Ryanodine receptor (RYR1)	19q13.1	Quane et al. (1993), Zhang et al. (1993), Ferreiro et al. (2002a)
Myotubular myopathy	X-linked	Myotubularin (MTM1)	Xq28	Laporte et al. (1996)
Centronuclear myopathy	AD	Dynamin 2 (DNM2)	19p13.2	Bitoun et al. (2005)
	AR	Ampiphysin (BIN1)	2q14	Nicot at al. (2007)
Congenital fibre-type disproportion	AD	Skeletal muscle α-actin (ACTA1)	1q42.1	Laing et al. (2004)
	AD	α-tropomyosin$_{slow}$ (TPM3)	1q22–q23	Clarke et al. (2008)
	AR	Selenoprotein N (SEPN1)	1p36	Clarke et al. (2006)
	X-linked	?	Xp22.13–11.4 Xq13.1–22.1	Clarke et al. (2005)
Multiminicore disease	AD, AR	Ryanodine receptor (RYR1)	19q13.1	Ferreiro et al. (2002), Pietrini et al. (2004)
	AR	Selenoprotein N (SEPN1)	1p36	Ferreiro et al. (2002b)
Hyaline body myopathy (myosin storage myopathy)	AD	Slow myosin heavy chain (MYH7)	14q12	Tajsharghi et al. (2003)
	AR	?	3p22.2–p21.32	Onengut et al. (2004)
Sarcotubular myopathy	AR	Tripartite motif-containing protein 32 (TRIM32)	9q31–33	Schoser et al. (2005)
Cap disease	AD	β-tropomyosin (TPM2)	9q13.2	Lehtokari et al. (2007), Tajsharghi et al. (2007)
Reducing body myopathy	X-linked	Four-and-a-half LIM domain (FHL1)		Schlessl et al. (2008)

*AD = autosomal dominant; AR = autosomal recessive.

TABLE 21.7
Putative congenital myopathies without defined genetic loci

Probable: some familial cases	Doubtful nosology or single cases
Cylindrical spirals myopathy	Lamellar body myopathy
Fingerprint body myopathy	Zebra body myopathy
Tubular aggregate myopathy	Broad A band myopathy

Adapted from: Goebel and Anderson (1999). See North (2004) for more detail regarding individual disorders.

by specific structural abnormalities but as yet have not been proven by genetic studies to represent distinct entities (Table 21.7).

Despite molecular genetic advances, muscle biopsy is usually required to establish a diagnosis, as unlike for the muscular dystrophies, the clinical features of individual disorders overlap considerably, and proceeding direct to DNA analysis is currently not practical.

There are currently no curative treatments for the congenital myopathies, but a multidisciplinary approach to the management of affected individuals can greatly improve both quality of life and longevity – in particular, physical and occupational therapy, orthopaedic intervention, respiratory care and management of feeding difficulties. Sometimes the course is relatively benign but many cases lead to severe disability and even death in childhood. Prenatal diagnosis is now available for several of these disorders. A useful website to check the availability of genetic testing is www.geneclinics.org.

NEMALINE MYOPATHY

The 'typical congenital' form of nemaline myopathy usually presents at birth or during the first year of life with hypotonia, weakness and feeding difficulties. Some children present later with delayed motor milestones, a waddling gait or speech abnormalities, while some cases do not manifest until adulthood. Facial weakness is common. There is often distal as well as proximal weakness. The respiratory muscles are always involved, and while hypoventilation may be subclinical, the need for active ventilatory support is not uncommon. Cardiac involvement is rare.

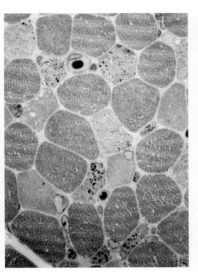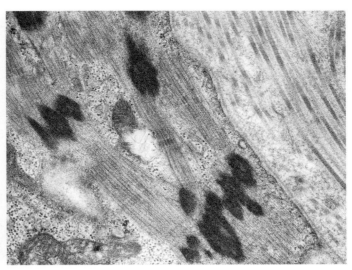

Fig. 21.6. Nemaline myopathy. *(Left)* Severe neonatal form. Semi-thin section stained with toluidine blue. Rod-like structures are visible in numerous, generally atrophic, angular fibres. *(Right)* Childhood form, electron microscopy (×47,000). Eosinophilic structures are made of Z-band protein irregularly organized. (Courtesy Dr M-C Routon, Hôpital Saint Vincent de Paul, Paris.)

The course of the disease is often static or only very slowly progressive, and most patients will be able to lead an active life (Ryan et al. 2001).

The severe congenital form of nemaline myopathy presents at birth with severe hypotonia and muscle weakness, little spontaneous movement, difficulties with sucking and swallowing, and respiratory insufficiency. Death due to respiratory insufficiency or recurrent pneumonia is common during the first weeks or months of life, although occasional patients survive and achieve the ability to walk (Ryan et al. 2001).

The diagnostic feature of nemaline myopathy is the presence of distinct rod-like inclusions, nemaline bodies, in the skeletal muscle fibres (Fig. 21.6). Rods are not visible on haematoxylin–eosin staining, but appear as red or purple structures against the blue-green myofibrillar background with the modified Gomori trichrome stain. Rods are considered to be derived from the lateral expansion of the Z-line. Additional pathological features include type I fibre predominance, fibre atrophy and/or fibre hypertrophy (Ryan et al. 2003).

Nemaline myopathy may be inherited in an autosomal dominant, autosomal recessive or sporadic fashion (including new dominant mutations). In the last nine years, mutations in five genes have been identified. These genes all encode protein components of the thin filament of muscle: α-tropomyosin$_{slow}$, nebulin, skeletal α-actin, β-tropomyosin, and troponin T (Table 21.6). Recessive mutations in nebulin probably account for up to 50% of cases. Sporadic or new dominant mutations in the skeletal α-actin gene (*ACTA1*) account for 20–25% of cases (and up to 50% of newborn lethal presentations).

CENTRAL CORE DISEASE (CCD)

CCD usually presents in infancy with weakness and hypotonia, primarily affecting the proximal musculature and lower extrem-

ities, and poor muscle bulk. Most patients achieve ambulation. The motor milestones are typically delayed, but muscle weakness is generally static or only slowly progressive. There may be mild facial and neck muscle weakness. The extraocular muscles are usually spared. Musculoskeletal deformities such as kyphoscoliosis, congenital hip dislocation, pes cavus, pes planus and thoracic deformities occur frequently. Significant respiratory insufficiency is unusual, cardiac abnormalities occur only rarely, and intellectual performance is not impaired (Shuaib et al. 1987). Although most patients display the 'typical' clinical phenotype, central cores may be found in individuals who are asymptomatic, in patients with mild weakness or skeletal deformity, and in patients with raised serum CK as their only manifestation of the disorder (Shuaib et al. 1987, Quinlivan et al. 2003). The clinical spectrum of CCD has recently been expanded with identification of children with dominant or recessive CCD presenting with arthrogryposis, severe weakness and respiratory failure in the neonatal period (Romero et al. 2003). Ophthalmoplegia and ptosis are also reported in a small number of severely affected children. Such patients may require ventilatory support from birth, but surviving children can demonstrate considerable improvement in respiratory and peripheral muscle strength with increasing age (Romero et al. 2003).

CCD has traditionally been regarded as an autosomal dominant disease with variable penetrance. De novo mutations are relatively common. Recessive inheritance is now also recognized, particularly in severe cases (Ferriero et al. 2002a, Romero et al. 2003). Most cases of central core disease are caused by mutations in the *RYR1* gene on chromosome 19q13.1 (Quane et al. 1993, Zhang et al. 1993, Ferriero et al. 2002a, Romero et al. 2003). The *RYR1* gene encodes the ryanodine receptor, which allows release of calcium from the sarcoplasmic reticulum into the sarcoplasm, triggering muscle contraction. CCD is allelic to malignant hyper-

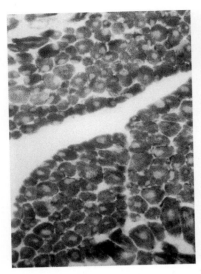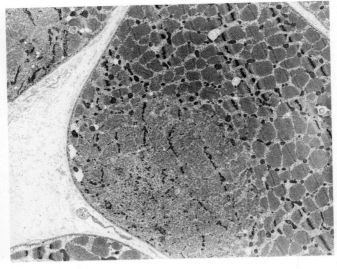

Fig. 21.7. Central core myopathy. *(Left)* Note uniformity of fibre type (type 1) and presence of clear central area devoid of enzymatic activity in virtually all fibres (NADH ×150). *(Right)* Electron microscopy shows that the 'core' region (which is lateral rather than central in this particular fibre) is devoid of normal muscle fibrils and of mitochondria and shows disorganization of myofilaments (×23,000). (Courtesy Drs M-C Routon and O Robain, Hôpital Saint Vincent de Paul, Paris.)

thermia, and thus anaesthetic precautions are essential in all patients and in anybody with undiagnosed muscle weakness with possible autosomal dominant inheritance. Some patients with malignant hyperthermia have cores on muscle biopsy, despite having normal muscle strength.

The characteristic abnormality of CCD is the presence of central cores: single, well-circumscribed circular regions in the centre of the majority of type 1 fibres (Fig. 21.7). Cores are zones of reduced oxidative enzyme activity staining negatively for phosphorylase and glycogen (Shy and Magee 1956, Quinlivan et al. 2003). Cores are devoid of mitochondria and sarcoplasmic reticulum (Quinlivan et al. 2003). In most cases there is type 1 fibre predominance.

MYOTUBULAR AND CENTRONUCLEAR MYOPATHIES

There are three groups of myotubular (centronuclear) myopathies based on clinical and genetic features. The X-linked recessive form is the best defined clinically and genetically. Onset is commonly in utero, and the pregnancy is complicated by polyhydramnios. There may be a history of miscarriages and neonatal deaths of male infants in the maternal line. Affected males present at birth with severe floppiness and weakness, facial diplegia, and difficulties with respiration and feeding. Additional features include thin ribs, contractures of the hips and knees, puffy eyelids, ophthalmoplegia and cryptorchidism. Many affected boys die in the neonatal period, but a minority survive long-term, often requiring permanent respiratory support (McEntagart et al. 2002). The gene for X-linked myotubular myopathy, *MTM1*, is located on Xq28 (Laporte et al. 1996) and is thought to be involved in a signal transduction pathway necessary for late myogenesis. The major differential diagnosis, congenital myotonic dystrophy, must be excluded by clinical or genetic testing.

The autosomal forms of myotubular myopathy are known as centronuclear myopathy and are extremely rare. The autosomal recessive form of centronuclear myopathy usually presents in infancy or early childhood with respiratory distress, hypotonia, a weak cry and difficulty sucking. Ophthalmoplegia, ptosis and facial diplegia are common. The clinical course is characterized by delayed motor milestones, slowly progressive weakness, and development of scoliosis. By adolescence many patients are confined to a wheelchair (Jeannet et al. 2004). The chromosomal locus for the recessive form of centronuclear myopathy is not known. The autosomal dominant and sporadic forms usually present in childhood, adolescence or adulthood, with a much milder phenotype and slowly progressive weakness and wasting; ptosis and limitation of eye movements occur frequently. Disease-causing mutations have recently been identified in the gene encoding dynamin 2 (Bitoun et al. 2005).

The characteristic histological feature is predominance of small type 1 fibres with centrally placed nuclei resembling fetal myotubes (North 2004). There is usually aggregation of mitochondria in the centre of the muscle fibre, associated with dense oxidative enzyme staining and a lack of staining with myosin adenosine triphosphatase (ATPase). A radial distribution of sarcoplasmic strands on the oxidative stains may be a characteristic finding in this condition (Jeannet et al. 2004). Obligate carriers of the X-linked form of myotubular myopathy are usually asymptomatic, but as many as 50% have typical changes on muscle biopsy.

MULTIMINICORE DISEASE

Multiminicore disease is a clinically heterogeneous disorder. Approximately 75% of patients have the 'classic' form of the disorder, which presents in the first year of life. Affected infants are hypotonic and weak, with joint hyperextensibility and delayed motor development. Weakness is predominantly axial; the neck flexors are usually the most affected muscles, resulting in poor or absent head control in infancy. Kyphoscoliosis and spinal rigidity are common and can progress rapidly during periods of rapid skeletal growth, particularly adolescence. This is frequently associated with progressive respiratory insufficiency, which may be rapid in onset (Ferreiro et al. 2000, Jungbluth et al. 2000). As many as two thirds of patients with the classic form of multiminicore disease develop respiratory insufficiency in late adolescence or early adulthood, although many remain ambulant (Ferreiro et al. 2000). Facial weakness is common, and the extraocular muscles are spared. Intelligence is normal. Multiminicore disease can also present with mild distal weakness of the upper limbs with hand amyotrophy and marked joint hyperlaxity. The lower extremities are mildly affected with proximal pelvic girdle weakness. Scoliosis and respiratory involvement are minimal or absent in this mild form (Ferreiro et al. 2000). Rarely, multiminicore disease can present with external ophthalmoplegia and proximal limb weakness (Jungbluth et al. 2000) or in the neonatal period with arthrogryposis multiplex congenita (Ferreiro et al. 2000).

Minicores are seen as multiple focal defects in oxidative enzyme activity in the majority of fibres on ATPase preparations; they occur in both type 1 and type 2 fibres (Ferreiro et al. 2000, Jungbluth et al. 2000). Associated features include increase in fibre size variability, central nuclei, hypotrophy of type I fibres and type I fibre predominance (Jungbluth et al. 2000). Dystrophic changes are occasionally seen in patients with multiminicore disease related to mutations in *SEPN1* (Ferreiro et al. 2002b).

Mutations in two genes have been found to be responsible for approximately 50% of cases of multiminicore disease. Recessive mutations in *SEPN1*, the gene for selenoprotein N, account for 30% of cases, particularly those with early, severe kyphoscoliosis and a significant risk of respiratory insufficiency (Ferreiro et al. 2004). Different mutations of the same gene cause rigid spine muscular dystrophy (Moghadaszadeh et al. 2001), desmin-related myopathy with Mallory body-like inclusions (Ferreiro et al. 2004), and congenital fibre-type disproportion (Clarke et al. 2006). The clinical picture in all these conditions is remarkably similar despite variations in muscle pathology. Recessive mutations in the muscle ryanodine (*RYR1*) gene are present in a minority of patients (Pietrini et al. 2004), and there is a single recent report of a dominant *RYR1* mutation causing adult-onset multiminicore disease (Ferreiro et al. 2002a). Patients with *RYR1*-related multiminicore disease are at increased risk of malignant hyperthermia (Guis et al. 2004).

CONGENITAL FIBRE-TYPE DISPROPORTION

The term congenital fibre-type disproportion (CFTD) was first coined by Brooke in 1973 in a report on a series of 12 children presenting with hypotonia, features of a congenital myopathy, and a distinct histological abnormality. The defining abnormality on light microscopy was a discrepancy in size between type 1 (slow twitch) and type 2 (fast twitch) muscle fibres, the former being

at least 12% smaller than the latter (Brooke and Engel 1969). This histological appearance has been termed *fibre-size disproportion (FSD)*. FSD can be associated with diverse clinical presentations and occurs as a secondary phenomenon in a wide range of skeletal and neuromuscular disorders, including CNS disorders, peripheral neuropathy, muscular dystrophy and other congenital myopathies such as nemaline myopathy, multiminicore disease and centronuclear myopathy. As a result, CFTD is a diagnosis of exclusion and is best reserved for patients who have clinical features of a congenital myopathy with reduction in type 1 fibre size relative to type 2 fibres as the only significant histological abnormality (Bodensteiner 1994, Clarke and North 2003).

The majority of patients with CFTD have congenital-onset hypotonia, weakness that improves with age, short stature, low body weight, multiple joint contractures (congenital hip dislocation and talipes equinovarus in particular), scoliosis, a long thin face, a high-arched palate and a tented upper lip (Brooke 1973, Iannaccone et al. 1987). Less commonly, patients with CFTD have slowly progressive weakness from childhood, ophthalmoplegia, pharyngeal or cardiac involvement, intellectual disability and severe progressive motor involvement with kyphoscoliosis and respiratory insufficiency (Iannaccone et al. 1987, Haltia et al. 1988, Torres and Moxley 1992, Akiyama and Nonaka 1996, Banwell et al. 1999).

CFTD is genetically heterogeneous, with families reported consistent with autosomal dominant and recessive inheritance. De novo dominant mutations have been identified in the gene encoding skeletal α-actin (*ACTA1*), also associated with nemaline myopathy, in patients with severe congenital-onset weakness and respiratory muscle involvement (Laing et al. 2004). Recessive mutations have been identified in the gene encoding selenoprotein N (*SEPN*), also associated with multiminicore disease (see above) (Clarke et al. 2006). In addition, a locus on the X chromosome has been identified in a family in whom the males have a severe lethal myopathy, and carrier females have facial weakness and ptosis (Clarke et al. 2005).

HYALINE BODY MYOPATHY (MYOSIN STORAGE MYOPATHY)

This rare congenital myopathy is characterized by proximal or generalized weakness with onset in infancy, childhood or rarely adulthood (Masuzugawa et al. 1997, Tajsharghi et al. 2003). Hyaline bodies are large areas devoid of sarcomeres, in the periphery of the muscle fibres, which contain a finely granular material, and show myofibrillar ATPase activity after acid preincubation. Associated pathological features include fibre-type disproportion and type 1 fibre predominance.

Autosomal dominant hyaline body (myosin storage) myopathy has recently been shown to be caused by mutations in the gene for slow myosin heavy chain MYH7 (Tajsharghi et al. 2003), mutations that also cause familial hypertrophic cardiomyopathy (Bonne et al. 1998) and Laing distal myopathy (Meredith et al. 2004). Recessive hyaline body myopathy has been linked to a locus on chromosome 3 (Onengüt et al. 2004).

SARCOTUBULAR MYOPATHY

This is a rare recessive disorder characterized by vacuolar changes in myofibres on light microscopy (Jerusalem et al. 1973). The vacuoles are membrane-bound and appear to arise from the sarcotubular system. Clinically the disorder presents as congenital-onset, non-progressive proximal weakness, with variable involvement of neck flexor, facial and respiratory muscles. Siblings have also been reported with exercise-induced myalgia and proximal weakness of markedly differing onset and severity (Muller-Felber et al. 1999). Disease-causing mutations been identified in the *TRIM32* gene, which is also associated with a form of limb girdle muscular dystrophy (LGMD 2H).

MARINESCO–SJÖGREN SYNDROME (MSS)

MSS (Chapter 9) is a long-recognized autosomal recessive multisystem disorder featuring ataxia due to cerebellar dysplasia, cataracts from infancy on, mild to moderate mental retardation, myopathy, muscle weakness and short stature. Additional reported features include skeletal abnormalities and hypergonadotropic hypogonadism. The disorder is usually marked in its later stages by muscle involvement characterized by generalized hypotonia and weakness and a myopathic EMG (Zimmer et al. 1992). Electron microscopy studies on muscle biopsies revealed a dense membranous structure surrounding myonuclei as being a characteristic ultrastructural feature in MSS (Sewry et al. 1988). Identification of disease-causing mutations in the *SIL1* gene, a key regulator of the major functions of the endoplasmic reticulum, implicates MSS as a disease of endoplasmic reticulum dysfunction and suggests a role for this organelle in multisystem disorders (Senderek et al. 2005).

MYOTONIC DISEASES AND RELATED CONDITIONS

Myotonia designates a disturbance in muscle relaxation following contraction of voluntary muscles and a slow, tonic response to mechanical and electrical stimulation. Myotonia is characterized electromyographically by repetitive response of motor units producing the classical 'dive bomber' aspect (crescendo–decrescendo). Myotonia is related to instability of the muscle cell membrane and is purely of muscular origin. It can occur in association with several genetic diseases and syndromes, including myotonic dystrophy, the most common myotonic disorder, as well as the 'channelopathies' or ion channel disorders.

MYOTONIC DYSTROPHY (DYSTROPHIA MYOTONICA, STEINERT DISEASE)

Myotonic dystrophy is a relatively common disease with an incidence of 13.5 per 100,000 live births. It is transmitted as an autosomal dominant trait and is characterized by the association of myotonia with a dystrophic process of muscles. Myotonic dystrophy is a multisystem disorder that affects skeletal and smooth muscle as well as the eye, heart, endocrine system and central nervous system. The clinical findings span a continuum from mild to severe and have been categorized into three somewhat overlapping phenotypes: mild, classical, and congenital.

CLINICAL FEATURES OF THE CLASSICAL FORM

The clinical presentation of myotonic dystrophy is variable. Individuals with mild myotonic dystrophy type 1 (DM1) may have only cataract, mild myotonia or diabetes mellitus. They may have fully active lives and a normal or minimally shortened life span. The age of onset for classical myotonic dystrophy is typically in the twenties or thirties, and less commonly after age 40 years. However, classical DM1 may be evident in childhood, when subtle signs such as myotonic facies and myotonia are observed. Myotonia is demonstrated by percussion of muscle, e.g. the thenar eminence or tongue, the thumb remaining opposed, the tongue being dimpled for several seconds after percussion of its side. Relaxation myotonia is demonstrated by shaking hands with the patient: release of grip is performed by the patient by forcing the flexors of the fingers open by flexion of the wrist.

The distribution of muscular atrophy and weakness is characteristic. Atrophy begins in the face – especially the masseters and temporal muscles, giving all the patients a similar appearance with a long, thin face and hollowed temporal fossae – and in the sternomastoid muscles. The shoulder girdle is then involved, and, characteristically, the brachioradialis and the muscles of the anterior compartment of the leg are also wasted. In some patients, there is only minimal weakness, even in the presence of visible atrophy, but when it is present before 20 years of age it is likely to be relentlessly progressive, severe distal weakness developing by middle adult life. Rarely, after several decades of disease, myotonic dystrophy progresses to the point of wheelchair confinement. Respiratory muscle compromise and increased aspiration may occur in individuals with advanced disease (Thornton 1999).

Smooth muscle involvement may be present with decreased gastrointestinal motility, and constipation is a well-recognized feature. In adults, baldness, testicular atrophy, hyperinsulinism and disturbances in growth hormone secretion may occur (Hudson et al. 1987). Cardiac conduction defects are the most important complication because of the risk of early mortality due to conduction block or cardiac arrhythmia. Reports vary of 50–90% of patients having abnormal ECG, arrhythmias or other cardiac disturbances (Hawley et al. 1991, Morgenlander et al. 1993). Posterior cataracts are not seen before 8–10 years of age, even by slit-lamp examination, but occur later and may be the first and occasionally the presenting feature of the disease. Intellectual impairment is rare in patients with the adult form of myotonic dystrophy; but personality may be affected with avoidant, obsessive–compulsive and passive–aggressive personality traits (Delaporte 1998). Hypersomnia and sleep apnoea are other well recognized, though later, manifestations of the disease (Rubinsztein et al. 1998). Lifespan may be reduced due to pneumonia and respiratory failure or cardiovascular complications such as arrhythmia (de Die-Smulders et al. 1998).

CLINICAL FEATURES OF THE CONGENITAL FORM

The congenital form of the disease has a completely different

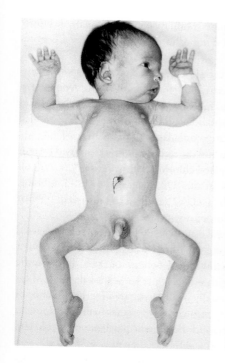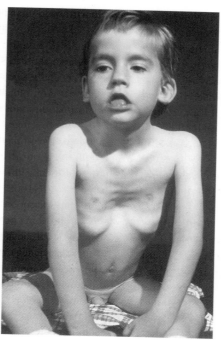

Fig. 21.8. Dystrophia myotonica (Steinert disease). *(Far left)* Neonatal form. Note equinovarus feet. *(Left)* Child with neonatal onset of mild form. Note tent-shaped upper lip, open mouth, mild ptosis and pectus excavatum. (Courtesy Dr F Renault, Hôpital Trousseau, Paris.)

presentation (Hageman AT et al. 1993). The onset is prenatal; hydramnios is present in about half the cases. Birth is often by breech delivery and the infant may be small for gestational age. Multiple congenital contractures are common. Hypotonia, weakness and facial diplegia with tented upper lip are the most striking features (Fig. 21.8). Respiratory insufficiency due to diaphragmatic and intercostal muscle involvement occurs in about half the patients and often leads to an early death. Surviving infants gradually improve and are usually able to walk, although they later develop a progressive myopathy, as in the classical form. Myotonia is never observed, even by EMG, before 3–4 years of age, often much later. In less severely affected patients who survive the neonatal period, mental impairment is present in the majority of cases and is often associated with ventricular dilatation and cerebral atrophy (Regev et al. 1987). Severe and relatively mild forms of congenital myotonic dystrophy may occur in the same sibship.

DIAGNOSIS AND TREATMENT
There are two main genetic variants of myotonic dystrophy – DM1 and DM2. DM1 is caused by expansion of a CTG trinucleotide repeat in the gene for myotonin protein kinase, *DMPK*. CTG repeat length exceeding 35 repeats is abnormal. Molecular genetic testing detects mutations in nearly 100% of affected individuals and is clinically available for diagnosis and prenatal diagnosis. As is usual with disorders associated with DNA expansion, anticipation and sex bias in genetic transmission are observed. The length of the repeat usually increases in successive generations, especially when maternally transmitted. There is a good correlation between the length of the expansion and the clinical severity and age of onset, the longer repeats being associated with congenital forms (Jaspert et al. 1995, Takahashi et al. 1996). Classical DM1 is associated with a repeat size of 100–1000, congenital

myotonic dystrophy is associated with repeat size >2000. Congenital DM1 is inherited from the mother in the vast majority of cases. The expanded CTG repeat leads to the abnormal processing of RNA transcripts that affect the alternative splicing and levels of expression of other genes, resulting in disease manifestations (e.g. chloride channel leading to myotonia, insulin receptor leading to diabetes) (Ranum and Day 2004).

Myotonic dystrophy type 2 (DM2, previously termed proximal myotonic myopathy) is much rarer and seen mostly in adults. It is also transmitted in an autosomal dominant fashion and is caused by a CCTG repeat expansion in intron 1 of the *ZNF9* gene encoding zinc finger protein 9 (Thornton et al. 1994, Udd et al. 1997, Liquori et al. 2001). DM2 is also characterized by clinical and electrophysiological evidence of myotonia, cataracts, frontal balding in males, cardiac conduction defects and endocrinopathies. Unlike with DM1, there is no severe congenital form of DM2.

Occasionally myotonic dystrophy needs to be differentiated from other forms of hereditary distal myopathy including inclusion body myositis, myofibrillar myopathy and Miyoshi myopathy. In infants the differential diagnosis is more difficult, although the overall appearance of the infant, especially the facial involvement, is suggestive. Patients with congenital myopathies and congenital muscular dystrophies may look very similar to those with myotonic dystrophy. Examination of the mothers, especially for myotonia, is the best diagnostic clue, although an occasional mother may have no myotonia, even by EMG, until months or years after the birth of an affected infant. If the DMPK CTG repeat length is in the normal range and if DM2 has been excluded by molecular genetic testing of *ZNF9*, further testing with EMG, serum CK and/or muscle biopsy is often warranted to evaluate for other causes of muscle disease.

Surveillance is important for patients with myotonic dystrophy, including ECG and/or Holter monitoring annually to detect cardiac conduction defects and measurement of fasting serum glucose and glycosylated haemoglobin levels to screen for diabetes. Myotonia is rarely severe enough to warrant treatment (Ricker et al. 1999). Agents used include procainamide, quinine and mexiletine.

ION CHANNEL DISORDERS

This section reviews the various ion channel disorders that affect skeletal muscle and variably produce myotonia, weakness or a mixture of both (Hudson et al. 1995). This group of disorders will be considered as follows:

1. Disorders of the chloride channel (*CLCN1*) – myotonia congenita, autosomal dominant and recessive forms
2. Disorders of the sodium channel (*SCN4A*) – paramyotonia congenita, hyperkalaemic periodic paralysis, other potassium-aggravated myotonias, a subset of patients with hypokalaemic periodic paralysis (~10%), normokalaemic periodic paralysis
3. Disorders of the calcium channel (*CACNA1S*) – a subset of patients with hypokalaemic periodic paralysis (~70%)
4. Malignant hyperthermia (*RYR1*).

CHLORIDE CHANNEL DISORDERS: MYOTONIA CONGENITA

Myotonia congenita is a genetic disorder, transmitted as either an autosomal dominant or autosomal recessive trait and also often occurring sporadically (Kuhn et al. 1979). It is characterized by myotonia and muscle hypertrophy. The clinical presentation varies from case to case from mild myotonia, which may not be known to the patient even in adulthood, to stiffness that severely interferes with everyday life. In general, the autosomal dominant form (Thomsen disease) is more benign than the recessive type. The disorder is often present from birth or infancy, although onset may not occur until adulthood. After rest, muscles are stiff and movement is difficult to initiate. The stiffness disappears with activity (known as the 'warm-up effect'), and movement may become normal. Many patients have generalized muscle hypertrophy as a consequence of continuous muscle contraction. Stiffness is painless and increased by exposure to cold. Myotonic contraction can be elicited by percussion of muscles. Serum CK may be normal or mildly elevated (3–4 times upper limit of normal).

The recessive form (Becker disease) (Sun and Streib 1983) begins slightly later than the dominant type – between 3 and 12 years of age. Muscle stiffness is prominent and always associated with weakness, and distal atrophy may coexist with hypertrophy. The disease is often progressive to age 30. Neither form of myotonia congenita is associated with the systemic features seen in myotonic dystrophy (e.g. cataracts, cardiac conduction defects or endocrine dysfunction).

The diagnosis is established clinically and confirmed by EMG, which records repetitive discharges when the needle is inserted in the muscle and on voluntary contraction. Muscle biopsy is rarely necessary and demonstrates absence of type 2B fibres (Heine 1986).

Malignant hyperthermia may occur in patients with myotonia congenita (Heiman-Patterson et al. 1988). Depolarizing muscle relaxants (including suxamethonium), adrenaline, beta-adrenergic agonists, propranolol and colchicine should be avoided as they may aggravate myotonia (Farbu et al. 2003).

Both the dominant and the recessive forms are caused by mutations in the voltage-gated chloride channel gene (*CLCN1*) on chromosome 7q (Koch et al. 1992; Ptácek et al. 1993, 1994b). Sequence analysis of the *CLCN1* gene detects more than 95% of mutations in both forms of myotonia congenita.

The main differential diagnoses are other disorders associated with myotonia. These include myotonic dystrophy and the other channelopathies, paramyotonia congenita, and the periodic paralyses associated with either hyper- or hypokalaemia. Myotonic dystrophy can usually be differentiated by the presence of muscle weakness and systemic/extramuscular manifestations. In paramyotonia congenita and the periodic paralyses, both cold and exercise can result in stiffness followed by muscle weakness, and muscle pain may accompany myotonia. In contrast, in myotonia congenita, pain is not usually a feature and muscle stiffness tends to improve with exercise (Shapiro and Ruff 2002).

Muscle stiffness in myotonia congenita may respond to a variety of agents including mexiletine (Kwiecinski et al. 1992), tocainide (may cause bone marrow suppression) (Rudel et al. 1980), procainamide, quinine or phenytoin (Gutmann and Phillips 1991). Beneficial effects have also been reported with carbamazepine, dantrolene and acetazolamide (Shapiro and Ruff 2002). Myotonia is alleviated temporarily by exercise.

SODIUM CHANNEL DISORDERS

Several types of myotonia and periodic paralyses are caused by point mutations in SCN4A gene encoding the voltage-gated skeletal muscle sodium channel and are inherited as autosomal dominant traits.

PARAMYOTONIA CONGENITA (EULENBERG DISEASE)

In this disease, myotonia is present from infancy and involves especially the eyelids, facial muscles and hand muscles, and sometimes the pharyngeal muscles. Characteristically, patients may be unable to reopen the eyes after several forceful closures in rapid succession. The myotonia may be augmented by exercise (i.e. paradoxical myotonia) and is very sensitive to cold (Johnsen and Friis 1980). Many patients also experience episodes of weakness and may develop muscular atrophy. Weakness is of two types: generalized attacks of weakness that can be brought on by cold; and localized weakness that is also precipitated by cold but may also occur in hot surroundings, provoked by exercise alone. This second type, when brought on by cold, may persist for hours after rewarming (Haas et al. 1981). The condition is also associated pathologically with absence of type 2B fibres (Heine 1986). It is caused mainly by mutations of codons 1313 and 1448 of *SCN4A* (Lerche et al. 1996).

HYPERKALAEMIC PERIODIC PARALYSIS (ADYNAMIA EPISODICA HEREDITARIA)

The diagnostic criteria for hyperkalaemic periodic paralysis (Jurkat-Rott and Lehmann-Horn 2005) include:

- A history of at least two attacks of flaccid limb weakness (may also include weakness of the muscles of the eyes, throat and trunk)
- Hyperkalaemia (serum potassium concentration >5 mmol/L) or an increase of serum potassium concentration of at least 1.5 mmol/L during an attack of weakness and/or onset/worsening of an attack as a result of oral potassium intake
- Normal serum potassium concentration and muscle strength between attacks
- Disease manifestations before the age of 20 years
- Absence of paramyotonia, i.e. muscle stiffness aggravated by cold and exercise
- Absence of cardiac arrhythmia between attacks
- Normal psychomotor development
- Typically, at least one affected first-degree relative
- Exclusion of other hereditary forms of hyperkalaemia and acquired forms of hyperkalaemia (drug abuse, renal and adrenal dysfunction).

The disorder may occur at an early age, even in infancy. Attacks of flaccid muscle weakness are often triggered by moderate exercise, are often brief and sometimes occur several times daily; occasionally attacks may last for several hours. Deep tendon reflexes are often diminished or absent during an attack. Some patients can delay the paralysis by sustained mild exercise. Attacks may be precipitated or worsened by potassium-rich food, rest after exercise, a cold environment, emotional stress, glucocorticoids and pregnancy (Lehmann-Horn et al. 2004). Myotonia of a mild degree is present between attacks in approximately 50% of individuals and is most readily observed in the eyelids, thenar and finger extensors; it is often associated with the weakness and is not aggravated by cold or exercise (distinguishing it from paramyotonia) (Subramony et al. 1986). The presence of myotonia suggests a diagnosis of hyperkalaemic periodic paralysis rather than other forms of familial periodic paralysis.

The diagnosis may be confirmed by demonstration of ECG changes such as peaked T waves, and also by the finding of elevated potassium concentration (by 1.5–3 mmol/L) during the attacks, although many patients have concentrations still within the normal range. The presence of myotonia on EMG supports the diagnosis, but is detectable in only around 50% of cases (Lehmann-Horn et al. 2004). Serum CK may be elevated to 5–10 times normal concentration between attacks. Oral administration of 2–5 g potassium chloride after exercise may provoke an attack. Mutations in SCN4A account for 60–70% of cases, suggesting genetic heterogeneity. DNA mutation analysis is available as a clinical diagnostic test.

The differential diagnosis includes other causes of hyperkalaemia, such as adrenal insufficiency, hypoaldosteronism, medications (e.g. spironolactone, ACE inhibitors) and rhabdomyolysis. It has been reported in an adolescent with Gordon syndrome (hypertension, tubular acidosis and hyperkalaemia possibly related to a lack of sensitivity to atrial natriuretic peptide) (Pasman et al. 1989). *Andersen–Tawil syndrome* is characterized by episodic flaccid muscle weakness, prolonged QT interval and ventricular arrhythmia and dysmorphic features (low-set ears, hypertelorism, micrognathia, clinodactyly, syndactyly, short stature and scoliosis). It is due to dominant mutations in the potassium channel gene, *KCNJ2* (Plaster et al. 2001).

Attacks can be prevented or aborted by ongoing mild exercise or carbohydrate loading at the onset of weakness (e.g. 2 g/kg glucose). Since attacks may be provoked by bed rest, patients should be advised to rise early and eat a full breakfast. Other preventative measures include frequent carbohydrate-rich meals and avoidance of foods rich in potassium, fasting and exposure to cold. If the attacks are frequent, the patient may benefit from regular thiazide diuretics or acetazolamide, aiming to keep the dose as low as possible (e.g. starting dose of 25 mg hydrochlorothiazide daily or second daily), and monitoring serum sodium and potassium levels (Jurkat-Rott and Lehmann-Horn 2005).

OTHER POTASSIUM-AGGRAVATED MYOTONIAS

These disorders are characterized by the development of stiffness following strenuous exercise or ingestion of potassium; all are associated with mutations in *SCN4A*. *Myotonia fluctuans* is the mildest form and resembles Thomsen disease with stiffness that is sometimes painful, precipitated by inactivity and resolving with continued exercise. Muscle weakness is not a significant feature (Heine et al. 1993, Ricker et al. 1994). In *acetazolamide-responsive myotonia* (atypical myotonia congenita) muscle pain may be induced by exercise (Ptácek et al. 1994b). *Myotonia permanens* is a severe disorder associated with continuous myotonic activity on EMG. This results in generalized muscle hypertrophy and may be confused with Schwartz–Jampel syndrome (Lehmann-Horn et al. 2004). *Normokalaemic periodic paralysis* resembles both hypo- and hyperkalaemic periodic paralysis; however, the serum potassium levels during attacks are normal. It has been reported in association with a specific mutation in the *SCN4A* gene (codon 675) (Vicart et al. 2004).

CALCIUM CHANNEL DISORDERS

HYPOKALAEMIC PERIODIC PARALYSIS (HYPOPP)

This autosomal dominant disorder is characterized by two different forms, the paralytic form and the myopathic form; these may occur separately or together (Greenberg 1997, Lehmann-Horn et al. 2004). The *pure paralytic form* is the most common and has its onset between 5 and 16 years of age in 60% of cases. Attacks of paralysis are at first infrequent and are often precipitated by meals rich in carbohydrate or by exercise following rest, and thus commonly occur in the early morning. Exposure to cold may also be a trigger. The intensity and extent of weakness are very variable. In some patients only the proximal limb muscles are affected, while others have diffuse paralysis; facial muscles are rarely affected, and extraocular and respiratory muscles are not involved. Some individuals have only one episode in a lifetime; more commonly, crises occur repeatedly on a daily, weekly, monthly or, less often, yearly basis. Most attacks last from 4 to 6 hours, and some for a whole day or more. In severe cases, tendon reflexes are absent and muscles can be swollen. The attacks tend initially to increase in frequency, then decrease after 25–30 years and may even disappear. The *myopathic form* of HypoPP develops in approximately 25% of affected individuals, and results in a progressive fixed muscle weakness that begins as exercise intolerance predominantly in the lower limbs at extremely variable ages. It occurs independent of the paralytic symptomatology and may be the sole manifestation of HypoPP, but is not usually observed in the paediatric age range. In such cases vacuolization of muscle fibres is present histologically, together with centralization of nuclei and unequal fibre diameter.

The diagnosis rests on the characteristics of paralysis and the family history. Potassium concentration during attacks may be as low as 1.5 mmol/L but is often only slightly lowered (<3.5 mmol/L). ECG changes are present, including bradycardia, prolonged P-R and Q-T intervals, and flattening of T waves. There is no evidence of myotonia clinically or on EMG. Attacks can be provoked by oral administration of 2 g/kg of glucose with 10–20 units of insulin subcutaneously. Hypokalaemia and weakness usually results within 2 or 3 hours. A negative test does not exclude the diagnosis. The adrenalin test (2 μg/min by intra-arterial route for 5 minutes) is positive if the action potential simultaneously recorded in a hand muscle is decreased by more than 30% 10 minutes after injection. Molecular genetic testing is available clinically and identifies mutations in the *CACNA1S* gene (the dihydropyridine receptor, a subunit of the DHP-sensitive calcium channel, whose gene maps to 1q31–32) in about 70% of cases (Ptácek et al. 1994a). About 12% of patients have mutations in the *SCN4A* gene (Jurkat-Rott et al. 2000). Mutations in these two genes are not found in around 20% of patients, raising the possibility of further genetic heterogeneity.

HypoPP is the most frequent cause of periodic paralysis, but needs to be differentiated from causes of secondary hypokalaemia. These are mainly caused by urinary or gastrointestinal losses of potassium, as occurs with primary hyperaldosteronism, renal tubular defects, thiazide treatment, amphotericin B therapy, gastrointestinal fluid loss due to vomiting, draining of intestinal fistulae, or liquorice intoxication and prolonged diarrhoea (Comi et al. 1985). In Oriental patients, hypokalaemic periodic paralysis is often associated with hyperthyroidism (Oh et al. 1990), which occurs only rarely in Western countries. Hypermagnesaemia due to disturbances in the renal tubular system may be a rare cause of periodic paralysis (Emser 1982). Periodic attacks of paralysis have been reported in one patient with multiple deletions of mitochondrial DNA (Prelle et al. 1993).

Treatment of acute attacks in patients with normal renal function is by oral potassium chloride administration, 5–10 g per dose, which may be repeated. Prevention of attacks may be achieved by a low sodium regimen and potassium supplementation. Acetazolamide is beneficial in many families (Links et al. 1988). HypoPP can rarely be associated with an increased risk of malignant hyperthermia (Lambert et al. 1994).

MALIGNANT HYPERTHERMIA
Malignant hyperthermia (MH) is an autosomal dominant pharmacogenetic disorder of skeletal muscle calcium regulation (Moroni et al. 1995). It is characterized by the occurrence of muscular rigidity and necrosis associated with a rapid rise in body temperature, triggered by the administration of anaesthetics (e.g. halothane, isoflurane, sevoflurane, desflurane, enflurane) either alone or in conjunction with depolarizing muscle relaxants (succinylcholine). The triggering agent increases sarcoplasmic calcium concentrations, resulting in uncontrolled muscle contraction and hyperthermia, which may be fatal if untreated. Malignant hyperthermia is still the most frequent cause of death during anaesthesia. During an attack individuals experience acidosis, hypercapnia, tachycardia, hypoxaemia, rhabdomyolysis (and increase in CK), hyperkalaemia with a risk of cardiac arrhythmia or even arrest, and myoglobinuria with a risk of renal failure. In nearly all cases, the first manifestations of MH, tachycardia and tachypnea occur in the operating room, but MH may also occur in the early postoperative period. Death results unless the individual is promptly treated. As the first exposure to these substances elicits an event in only 50% of MH-susceptible patients, a previous history of tolerance of halothane or succinylcholine does not ensure that these agents can be used safely in future anaesthesia.

The disorder is inherited as an autosomal dominant trait, so a family history of accidents during anaesthesia is of extreme diagnostic importance. The syndrome may occur in two different settings: in patients with a specific inherited predisposition, and in those with certain muscular diseases. Central core disease and multiminicore myopathy are associated with an increased risk of MH (McCarthy et al. 2000, Guis et al. 2004). Malignant hyperthermia has not been clearly associated with other congenital myopathies, although possible cases have been documented in nemaline myopathy (Asai et al. 1992), Schwartz–Jampel syndrome (Seay and Ziter 1978), Thomsen disease (Heiman-Patterson et al. 1988) and myoadenylate deaminase deficiency (Fishbein et al. 1985). Because the underlying diagnosis is unknown in many patients undergoing muscle biopsy, MH precautions should be taken in all patients prior to definitive diagnosis. Several cases of MH have occurred in patients with King–Denborough syndrome, characterized by multiple minor dysmorphisms such as pectus carinatum, kyphoscoliosis, cryptorchidism, small mandible and short size (King and Denborough 1973, Stewart et al. 1988). Such children often have mildly elevated CK levels, which may also be found in siblings without dysmorphism.

Siblings and relatives of patients with MH should be screened for high CK levels, and this should also be done in patients with suggestive dysmorphisms or recognized muscular disorders, and in patients who have experienced hyperthermia and/or tachycardia during anaesthesia. Contracture testing, the standard diagnostic test for MH since the mid-1970s, relies on the in vitro measurement of contracture response of biopsied muscle to graded concentrations of caffeine and the anaesthetic halothane. The sensitivity of the test approaches 100%, with specificity between 80% and 97% (Allen et al. 1998). The in vitro contracture test requires a fresh muscle biopsy and is not well standardized in children. To date, three MHS genes have been identified;

MHS1 is associated with mutations in the *RYR1* gene encoding ryanodine receptor type 1 and accounts for 50–70% of cases (McCarthy et al. 2000). In rare cases mutations have been identified in *CACNA2D1*, encoding dihydropyridine-sensitive L-type calcium channel alpha-2/delta subunits, and in *CACNA1S*, encoding skeletal muscle calcium channel (Monnier et al. 1997). Three additional loci have been mapped but the genes have not been identified. Molecular genetic testing for *RYR1* and *CACNA1S* is clinically available.

The differential diagnosis of MH includes sepsis, hyperthermia, phaeochromocytoma crisis, ischaemic encephalopathy following surgery and thyrotoxicosis. Rhabdomyolysis following anaesthesia can occur in patients with dystrophinopathy but is distinct from MH in terms of the pathophysiology. Patients with myotonic syndromes can also develop muscle rigidity following succinylcholine administration.

NEUROLEPTIC MALIGNANT SYNDROME

The neuroleptic malignant syndrome shares several features with MH induced by anaesthetics (Levenson 1985, Moore et al. 1986). The syndrome has occurred following the use of many antipsychotic agents including phenothiazines, butyrophenones, thioxanthenes, benzamides, sulpiride, clozapine and risperidone (Kashihara and Ishida 1988, Hasan and Buckley 1998, Adnet et al. 2000). Rigidity, high fever and raised CK level are major features. Sweating, tachpnoea, tachycardia, hypertension and altered consciousness develop over a few hours or days. Renal failure secondary to rhabdomyolysis is an ominous sign (Adnet et al. 2000). Early recognition, withdrawal of neuroleptic drugs and active supportive therapy especially for acute renal failure are vital to a good outcome. Bromocriptine offers the greatest benefit and should be given promptly. Dantrolene may also be useful, while levodopa and benzodiazepines are sometimes used (Ty and Rothner 2001). Mortality has been reduced to less than 20% in recent years (Adnet et al. 2000). A compilation of case reports in childhood and adolescents has been published by Ty and Rothner (2001). *Serotonin syndrome* (secondary to SSRIs) can display similar signs. Both syndromes occur in non-anaesthetized individuals.

The relationship between *exertional heat illness* and MH susceptibility in humans is based on anecdotal evidence; some individuals who have experienced exertional heat illness have been found to be MH-susceptible based on contracture testing; however, this test may have false positives and so the relationship has been questioned. Tobin et al. (2001) reported a 12-year-old boy who died following exercise; he had a previous clinical MH episode and had a classic *RYR1* mutation associated with MH. Wappler et al. (2001) found that 10 out of 12 young men with exercise-induced rhabdomyolysis were MH-susceptible on contracture testing, and 3 had *RYR1* mutations. Further molecular genetic testing may well clarify this possible association.

Treatment for episodes of MH includes termination of anaesthesia, body cooling, treatment of acidosis, and intravenous injection of dantrolene at a dose of 1–2 mg/kg, which may be repeated every 5–10 minutes up to a total dose of 10 mg/kg (Gronert 1980). Treatment with dantrolene significantly reduces morbidity and mortality. Preventive measures for individuals known to be MH susceptible include avoidance of potent volatile anaesthetic agents and succinylcholine. Individuals with any form of myotonia should not receive succinylcholine. Individuals with central core disease, dystrophinopathies, paramyotonia or myotonia fluctuans should not receive trigger anaesthetics. It is recommended that individuals with MH should carry proper identification as to their susceptibility (e.g. identification bracelets). They are generally advised to avoid extremes of heat but not to restrict athletic activity unless they have overt rhabdomyolysis.

CRAMPS AND ABNORMAL MUSCLE CONTRACTIONS

DEFINITIONS AND CLINICAL FEATURES

Cramps are involuntary painful contractions of a muscle or part of a muscle. When cramps occur in normal individuals they are usually confined to the distal lower extremities and are characterized on EMG by the repetitive firing of normal motor unit potentials. Such 'normal' cramps are not associated with other symptoms or signs or neurological disease, and are often precipitated by vigorous exercise or by excessive loss of fluids and electrolytes. Stretching the involved muscle usually relieves the cramp. Benign cramps often respond to simple interventions such as replacement of fluids and correction of metabolic disturbances, regular stretching exercises, avoidance of caffeine and other stimulants, and treatment with calcium, magnesium or quinine. Night cramps are also physiological events, although they occur much more frequently in partially denervated muscles. Cramps induced by exercise occur in patients with disorders of muscle energy metabolism. These cramps are electrically silent (Rowland 1985).

Muscle spasms are also involuntary and often painful muscle contractions that are more prolonged in duration and less explosive in onset than cramps and can result in the assumption of unusual postures.

Myokymias are rippling fascicular contractions that occur spontaneously in healthy children and adults, especially about the eyes but also in other muscles. They are a physiological phenomenon unless they are excessively diffuse and intense.

NONPHYSIOLOGICAL CRAMPS

Pathological cramps can occur in association with a variety of metabolic disorders and secondary to disorders of the anterior horn cell, peripheral motor axon or of the muscle itself (Table 21.8). Exercise-induced myalgia, with or without tenderness, exercise intolerance, weakness, cramps (contractures) and myoglobinuria can occur in metabolic myopathies and in association with congenital myopathies, muscular dystrophies, inflammatory myopathies, and toxic and endocrine myopathies (discussed separately in this chapter). Pathological cramps may be the first presenting feature, or can be associated with weakness, muscle atrophy, increased CK, erythrocyte sedimentation rate or lactate, and electrophysiological changes that suggest a site of primary pathology in the motor unit. A muscle biopsy is useful for the

TABLE 21.8
Causes of pathologic cramps and myalgia*

Metabolic and toxic disorders
Fluid and electrolyte imbalance
Uraemia and haemodialysis
Hepatic insufficiency
Hypothyroidism and hyperthyroidism
Cushing syndrome and adrenal insufficiency
Cholinesterase inhibitor intoxication
Other toxins, e.g. alcohol, lipid-lowering agents, vincristine,
  organophosphates

Primary disorders of muscle
Metabolic myopathies
    Disorders of glycogen metabolism
    Disorders of lipid metabolism/fatty acid oxidation
    Carnitine palmitoyltransferase deficiency
    Disorders of β-oxidation
    Mitochondrial cytopathies – all subtypes
Inherited myopathies
    Muscular dystrophies (dystrophinopathies; limb–girdle
      muscular dystrophies, e.g. caveolin 3)
    Congenital myopathies (central core and nemaline myopathy)
Muscle channelopathies
Myotonic dystrophy
Myotonia congenita and paramyotonia congenita
Periodic paralyses
Infective or inflammatory myopathies (including autoimmune)
Disorders of peripheral nerve/motor axon
Radioculopathy or plexopathy
Peripheral neuropathy
Peripheral nerve hyperexcitability syndromes (e.g. Isaacs syndrome)
Motor neuron disorders
Spinal muscular atrophy
Amyotrophic lateral sclerosis
Poliomyelitis

*Adapted from Harper (2004).

diagnosis of structural myopathies/dystrophies and in the diagnosis of metabolic myopathies.

Certain conditions are characterized exclusively or predominantly by an abnormal intensity or frequency of cramps and myalgia. Some patients develop excessive cramps in their second or third decade. The cramps may occur at rest or be induced by exercise, involve mainly the lower limbs and last up to 36 hours. Cramps are often made worse by cold, and myalgia is commonly present in addition. The muscle pain and stiffness may begin in childhood or adult life and can result in progressive and severe disability. Some patients may have brief episodes, reminiscent of myotonia, that affect the mouth and tongue and may interfere with speech. Symptoms are unrelated to fasting and there is no history of myoglobinuria. Neurological examination is normal and there is no weakness. This syndrome of myalgia and cramps is often associated with the presence in muscles of tubular aggregates that consist of densely packed, double-walled tubules originating from the sarcoplasmic reticulum (Rosenberg et al. 1985). Such aggregates are nonspecific and can be found in several muscle disorders, but their association with myalgia and cramps appears to be greater than expected (Niakan et al. 1985). The majority of reported patients are male, and the disorder is usually sporadic, although a few familial cases with autosomal

dominant (Martin et al. 1997) or possible recessive inheritance (Bendahan et al. 1996) have been described. One patient with adult-onset myalgia/cramps and tubular aggregate myopathy responded dramatically to steroids (Gilchrist et al. 1991). The patient was eventually tapered off steroids without symptoms and a repeat biopsy showed no tubular aggregates. There are no other reports of response to treatment in tubular-aggregate myopathy. Other genetic cramp disorders include hereditary persistent distal cramps (Jusic et al. 1972).

OTHER ABNORMAL MUSCLE CONTRACTIONS
RIPPLING MUSCLE DISEASE

Rippling muscle disease (RMD) (Ricker et al. 1989, Burns et al. 1994, Stephan et al. 1994) is characterized by 'mounding' produced by percussion of muscles and rolling movements that occur after contraction followed by stretching. The muscle contractions are electrically silent. Other clinical symptoms include muscle stiffness, cramps and pain, especially during or following exercise. Although calf hypertrophy has been reported in RMD, muscle weakness and wasting is usually absent. Linkage to chromosome 1q41 has been found in one family (Stephan et al. 1994), but the majority of cases are due to autosomal dominant mutations in the gene encoding caveolin-3, which is also associated with LGMD 1C (Betz et al. 2001). RMD associated with caveolin-3 mutation has been described with presentation in early childhood with toe walking (Madrid et al. 2005).

Sarcoplasmic Reticulum Adenosine Triphosphatase Deficiency (Brody Disease or Lambert–Brody Syndrome)

This is a rare genetic myopathy that usually begins in childhood with progressive exercise-induced stiffness and myalgia (Karpati et al. 1986, Danon et al. 1988). The main clinical manifestation is difficulty in muscle relaxation, which is different from myotonia in being electrically silent and increasing with continued exercise. Relaxation can take several minutes or more. The diagnosis can be confirmed only by demonstration of the biochemical defect, as conventional histological examination shows only atrophy of type 2 fibres. Autosomal recessive (Karpati et al. 1986) and autosomal dominant (Danon et al. 1988) kindreds have been described. The autosomal recessive form is now known to be due to mutations in the SERCA1 gene, which encodes the calcium-activated ATPase in sarcoplasmic reticulum of fast twitch muscles (Odermatt et al. 1996).

PERIPHERAL NERVE HYPEREXCITABILITY (PNH) SYNDROMES (CONTINUOUS MUSCLE FIBRE ACTIVITY, NEUROMYOTONIA, ISAACS SYNDROME, STIFF PERSON SYNDROME AND RELATED DISORDERS)

The terminology and nosology of this group of disorders are confusing, and there is particular difficulty in interpretation of older reports. These syndromes are rare in childhood and reports are limited mostly to single cases. Very few have been subjected to current genetic, biochemical or immunological investigations. Hart et al. (2002) point out that many terms are used to describe the clinical manifestations of PNH such as undulating myokymia, neuromyotonia, Isaacs syndrome and cramp–fasciculation syndrome. Their study of 60 patients with acquired PNH, including several children, selected by the presence or absence of doublet or multiplet myokymic motor unit discharges, showed that the EMG features reflect quantitative rather than qualitative differences between the diverse clinical syndromes. Furthermore, their study suggested that the EMG findings can change with time and that clinical or EMG evidence for PNH can be the end result of many different pathogenic processes. They suggest that classification be based on clinical associations and pathogenesis. Hence hereditary forms would be defined by the underlying genetic disorder and acquired forms as autoimmune, toxic or degenerative.

PNH (continuous muscle fibre activity, neuromyotonia) refers to a clinical phenomenon of abnormal, continuous muscle fibre activity that is of primary neural origin. Characteristic clinical accompaniments are muscle rippling or twitching, cramps, stiffness or delayed relaxation following voluntary muscle contraction (pseudomyotonia). One electrical accompaniment is the neuromyotonic discharge, which is a burst of rapidly firing (150–300 Hz) motor unit action potentials, often starting or stopping abruptly, with waning of the wave amplitude but not the waxing and waning pattern of myotonia. The discharges may occur spontaneously or be initiated by needle movement, voluntary effort or percussion of a nerve amongst other things (AAEM 2001a). PNH is a feature of several rare diseases and syndromes for which pathogenetic mechanisms are progressively being defined. Reference is made in the following discussion to some, but not all, childhood case reports predating modern methods of determining pathogenesis and nosology.

ISAACS SYNDROME

Isaacs syndrome is a rare disorder of continuous motor unit activity that in most cases is an acquired antibody-mediated channelopathy associated with antibodies against voltage-gated potassium channels (Hart 2000). There is an association with other autoimmune disorders and neoplasms, notably myasthenia gravis and thymoma. It usually presents in adolescence or adulthood but there are rare reports of onset even in infancy with stiffness and respiratory difficulty and with a fatal outcome (Thomas et al. 1994). A finding of diagnostic importance in one infant was that the EMG of the quadriceps muscle was silent at rest although other muscles showed continuous activity, indicating that several muscles may need to be examined. A few hereditary cases are on record including onset with stiffness and rigidity from early childhood (McGuire et al. 1984). These apparent early childhood onset case reports predated autoimmune and genetic studies to clarify nosology as noted above.

The main clinical features are muscle stiffness, cramps and sweating; myokymia may also be seen. The limbs and trunk are most affected. Deep tendon reflexes may be abolished, particularly if there is an associated neuropathy. Paraesthesiae may be reported even without associated neuropathy (Hart 2000). The EMG shows continuous fibre activity that appears to originate in the distal part of axons as it is not abolished by proximal nerve blocks. There is electrical evidence of a polyneuropathy in up to a third of patients (Hart 2000).

Treatment by carbamazepine or phenytoin suppresses the abnormal activity in some but not all cases. Gabapentin may also be useful (Dhand 2006). Immunotherapy may help in patients not benefiting from first-line drugs (Hart 2000).

STIFF PERSON SYNDROME (SPS)

SPS is ordinarily a sporadic disease of adults with rare case reports in adolescents (Daras and Spiro 1981, Udani et al. 1997, Garzo et al. 1998, Mikaeloff et al. 2001). Progressive rigidity develops primarily in trunk and proximal limb muscles with painful muscle spasms and this, along with rigidity of the hips and spine, results in a lumbar lordotic posture (Dalakas et al. 2000). There is excessive sensitivity to external stimuli. Rigidity is permanently present except in sleep. Variants are described including one with myoclonic jerks, one associated with breast cancer, another with a progressive encephalomyelitis and another involving predominately distal lower limb muscles with truncal sparing (Barker et al. 1998, Shaw 1999). EMG of affected muscles shows continuous muscle fibre activity.

There is an association with diabetes mellitus and other autoimmune disorders and up to 80% have autoantibodies to glutamic acid decarboxylase (GAD), which concentrates in GABA-ergic nerve terminals and in pancreatic cells (Shaw 1999, Rakocevic et al. 2004).

Benzodiazepines and baclofen are the most useful drugs, while intravenous immune globulin has been shown to be well tolerated and effective for those with anti-GAD65 antibodies (Shaw 1999, Dalakas 2005).

Reports of SPS in early childhood are rare, and according to Murinson (2004) there are no reported cases of GAD antibody positive SPS in infancy or pre-adolescence. The child described by Udani et al. (1997) had onset of episodic breath-holding and spasms of the trunk and limb muscles at 3 months of age, with clinical and EMG features suggestive of SPS with response to high-dose diazepam and baclofen. Another patient presenting at 4 years of age had some features consistent with SPS but later developed progressive dystonia (Wong et al. 2005). Autoantibodies to glutamic acid decarboxylase (anti-GAD) were not detected in him but they were in his neurologically asymptomatic sister with diabetes mellitus. The patient and his asymptomatic mother had a torsion dystonia gene (DYT1) mutation but his sister did not. Others (Greene and Dauer 2006) argued that this case represented severe torsion dystonia rather than an overlap syndrome. Onset at 6 years of age of a stiff limb variant of SPS was documented with continuous muscle fibre activity at rest, abolished by intravenous diazepam and clinically responding to oral diazepam (Markandeyulu et al. 2001).

HYPEREKPLEXIA

Hyperekplexia (see Chapter 16), sometimes referred to as the stiff baby syndrome [or previously as congenital stiff man (person) syndrome], has severe stiffness and excessive startle in response to external stimuli in common with SPS. The two disorders also share some brainstem physiological reflexes (Khasani et al. 2004). However, the common form of hyperekplexia is familial, has its onset in the newborn period with the stiffness at least improving after infancy, and is usually associated with mutations in the gene encoding the α1-subunit of the inhibitory glycine receptor (GLRA1) on chromosome 5q31.2, although genetic heterogeneity has been demonstrated (Rees et al. 2006). Onset in adolescence with a family history of a mild form, but without mutation analysis, is reported (Dooley and Andermann 1989). Less commonly hyperekplexia can occur as a sporadic disorder as in the 16-year-old GAD-negative patient studied by Khasani et al. (2004). In such cases the potential for overlapping features with SPS can be appreciated. The family with a recessively inherited syndrome of rapidly progressive rigidity of histologically abnormal skeletal muscles, early respiratory deficiency and death before 18 months of age reported by Lacson et al. (1994) has some features in common with hyperekplexia and SPS but is clearly different.

SCHWARTZ–JAMPEL SYNDROME (DYSTONIC CHONDRODYSTROPHY)

Schwartz–Jampel syndrome (SJS) is an hereditary (autosomal recessive) condition that features a neuromyotonic muscle abnormality, chondrodysplasia and short stature (Schwartz and Jampel 1962). The skeletal abnormalities are present in infancy and include coxa vara or valga, vertebral flattening, pectus carinatum and dwarfism, reminiscent of Morquio syndrome. Continuous activity is most prominent in the face and results in blepharophimosis, pursing of the mouth and puckering of the chin. The limbs are stiff, and contracture of the pharyngeal muscles can produce an abnormally high-pitched voice. Giedion et al. (1997) identified distinct subgroups by reviewing the clinical and radiological findings of 81 patients reported in the literature as well as 5 of their own. They found that a group of the patients had mild skeletal changes that may be secondary consequences of myotonia (SJS type 1A); the original descriptions of Schwartz and Jampel (1962) correspond to type 1A. Another group appeared to have primary bone dysplasia with myotonia. Within the latter group, there were differences in age of manifestation, clinical course and pattern of bone changes. SJS type 1B is similar to type 1A but recognizable at birth with more pronounced bone dysplasia resembling Kniest dysplasia (Spranger et al. 2000). SJS type 2 is manifest at birth with increased mortality and bone dysplasia. Thus SJS should be considered in the differential diagnosis of neonates with Kniest-like chondrodysplasia, congenital bowing of shortened femora and tibiae, and facial manifestations consisting of a small mouth, micrognathia, and possibly pursed lips.

Creatine kinase is normal or only mildly increased. EMG demonstrates the abnormal muscle fibre activity. Muscle histology is usually normal. Treatment of the myotonia with carbamazepine or mexiletine is rarely completely effective (Cao et al. 1978, Spaans 1991, Spranger et al. 2000).

Nicole et al. (1995) mapped the SJS1 locus to chromosome

1p36.1–p34 and subsequently identified disease-causing mutations in the gene encoding perlecan (*HSPG2*), a heparan sulphate proteoglycan highly expressed in basement membranes and cartilage; mice homozygous for a null mutation in the *HSPG2* gene developed severe chondrodysplasia and deterioration of basement membranes in regions of increased mechanical stress (Nicole et al. 2000). Giedion et al. (1997) reported that genetic analysis of the family with 2 siblings affected by SJS type 2 showed evidence against linkage to chromosome 1p36.1–p34, indicating genetic heterogeneity.

METABOLIC MYOPATHIES

Disorders of glycogen or lipid metabolism or mitochondrial functions may involve muscle, either as the sole or predominant participant, or as part of a multisystem syndrome. The myopathy may be permanent with usually progressive weakness, or it may be intermittent with episodes of myalgia, rhabdomyolysis and myoglobinuria often triggered by exercise or other factors. Although the clinical features may be easily identified, the underlying metabolic defect may be difficult to establish due to the complexity of the required laboratory analyses. Despite detailed knowledge of the biochemical and genetic basis of some of these disorders, effective treatments are frustratingly few and far between.

DISORDERS OF GLYCOGENOLYSIS AND GLYCOLYSIS – THE GLYCOGEN STORAGE DISORDERS (GSDS)

Disorders of glycogenolysis and glycolysis can present in two distinct ways. Some feature permanent and progressive weakness: these include glycogenoses types II, III and IV and occasional other rare types such as muscle phosphoglucomutase deficiency (DiMauro et al. 1982, Sugie et al. 1988) and muscle fructose diphosphatase deficiency (Kar et al. 1980). Others present with intermittent attacks of weakness, muscle pain and/or myoglobinuria including myophosphorylase deficiency (McArdle disease), deficits in phosphofructokinase, phosphoglycerate kinase (Aasly et al. 2000), phosphoglycerate mutase, lactate dehydrogenase and glucose-6-phosphate dehydrogenase (Bresolin et al. 1989), and abnormal hexosaminidase (Poulton and Nightingale 1988). Some cases are difficult to classify into either clinical presentation. These include the fatal infantile forms of phosphofructokinase deficiency (Danon et al. 1981, Servidei et al. 1986).

ACID MALTASE DEFICIENCY (GSD-II)

Acid maltase (acid ‑-glucosidase), a lysosomal enzyme present in all tissues, hydrolyses maltose to yield glucose. It has been traditional to divide acid maltase deficiency into three forms (infantile, childhood and adult) but to separate the childhood and adult forms may be an artificial construct (Winkel et al. 2005). All are transmitted as autosomal recessive disorders due to various mutations in the same gene, *GAA* (chromosome 17q25.2–q25.3). The *infantile form* of acid maltase deficiency, known as *Pompe disease* or type IIa glycogenosis, has symptom onset at a mean age of 1–2 months, with profound hypotonia, feeding problems, failure to thrive, severe delay in motor development, weakness, macroglossia, a progressive cardiomyopathy and cardiac failure. Occasionally cardiac problems are the presenting feature. Areflexia is present in one third of patients at presentation as a result of anterior horn cell involvement. Only rarely do type IIa patients achieve the ability to roll. The CK level may be normal but is usually elevated. Giant QRS complexes of left or biventricular hypertrophy and a very short P-R interval, inverted T waves and ST depression are a diagnostic clue. The mean age at death from cardiac failure is 6–7 months, with death before 1 year of age in 90% and only a few surviving beyond 18 months of age (van den Hout et al. 2003).

In the *childhood form*, usually only skeletal muscle is involved and patients present with slowly progressive proximal limb weakness. Mild hypertrophy of the calves may occur and may lead to confusion with one of the muscular dystrophies. Many deteriorate only slowly but there appears to be a subgroup with early onset (<2 years of age), who progress rapidly and become wheelchair dependent and require ventilator assistance before 15 years of age (Hagemans et al. 2005a).

The *adult form*, known as type IIb glycogenosis, has features similar to those of the juvenile form, with which it overlaps, with over 50% of patients reporting mild problems in childhood. A significant number require a wheelchair and assisted ventilation (Hagemans et al. 2005b).

In all types, the diagnosis depends on the demonstration of glycogen storage giving a vacuolar myopathy, and on demonstration of α-glucosidase deficiency (<10%) in muscle, leukocytes or fibroblasts. In the infantile form the deficiency is severe, less so in the later onset forms. A large number of mutations have been found in the α-glucosidase gene. Prenatal diagnosis is possible on trophoblasts or amniotic cells. Enzyme replacement therapy with recombinant human α-glucosidase is under investigation with early encouraging results (Van den Hout et al. 2004).

DEBRANCHER DEFICIENCY (GSD-III) AND BRANCHER DEFICIENCY (GSD-IV)

These forms are usually characterized by predominant hepatic involvement. Four clinical myopathy phenotypes of the autosomal recessive debrancher deficiency (GSD IIIa) (*AGL* gene, chromosome 1p21), including early childhood and juvenile onset generalized myopathy, have been described (Kiechl et al. 1999). While distal wasting and atrophy are often prominent, sometimes there is pseudohypertrophy (Marbini et al. 1989). Cardiomyopathy may be associated. High protein diet may be helpful (Kiechl et al. 1999).

Glycogen storage disease type IV (GSD-IV) is an autosomal recessive disorder due to mutations in the glycogen branching enzyme gene (*GBE1*, chromosome 3p12). An amylopectin-like polysaccharide is accumulated. Although most types present with hepatic disease, neuromuscular forms are recognized, with onset varying from perinatal to congenital, juvenile or adult (Bruno et al. 2004). The perinatal form presents as fetal akinesia deformation sequence (FADS) with multiple joint contractures, hydrops

fetalis, and perinatal death (Bruno et al. 2004). Cervical cystic hygroma seen by ultrasound may be a clue early in pregnancy (L'hermine-Coulomb et al. 2005). The congenital form includes hypotonia, hyporeflexia, cardiomyopathy, ventilator dependence and cardiorespiratory death in early infancy (Bruno et al. 2004, Giuffrè et al. 2004). The childhood form is dominated by myopathy or cardiomyopathy. The adult form can present as an isolated myopathy (Bruno et al. 2004).

McARDLE DISEASE (GSD-V)

McArdle disease (myophosphorylase deficiency) is the prototype of those glycogenoses that manifest with intermittent symptoms. Myophosphorylase deficiency leads to inability to mobilize muscle glycogen stores during exercise. It shows autosomal recessive inheritance, although a multigeneration family is reported (Chui and Munsat 1976). McArdle disease is caused by many different mutations of the *PYGM* gene (chromosome 11q13) without recognized genotype–phenotype correlation (Tsujino et al. 1993). The incidence of the disease is 1 per 50,000 births (DiMauro and Tsujino 1994).

The onset, frequently not recognized as such for many years, is usually in the first two decades. The cardinal clinical features are exercise intolerance with muscle pain and cramps soon after initiating exercise. Episodic weakness after exercise can be associated with rhabdomyolysis leading to myoglobinuria and, if severe, acute renal failure. In children, however, easy fatiguability can be the only symptom, and most children reduce their overall level of physical activity as a result of pain. Precipitants other than exercise, e.g. convulsions or fever (Ito et al. 2003), may trigger attacks. Permanent weakness may be observed after many years, particularly if there are repeated attacks of rhabdomyolysis. Some patients experience the so-called 'second wind phenomenon' (Braakhekke et al. 1986) whereby exercise may be pursued normally. This phenomenon largely results from a switch from glucose to free fatty acid as a substrate of muscle metabolism.

Rare patients have a different phenotype such as that of a congenital myopathy presenting with delayed milestones (Cornelio et al. 1983) or as slowly progressive proximal weakness with onset in childhood, without any cramp, myalgia or myoglobinuria (Abarbanel et al. 1987). A fatal infantile type has been described (Milstein et al. 1989). Occasionally, asymptomatic patients may be discovered fortuitously as a result of high CK levels (Gospe et al. 1998, Bruno et al. 2000).

The CK is moderately increased in most patients at rest but may rise dramatically after exercise, particularly in the context of myoglobinuria. Myopathic EMG abnormalities may be seen. The ischaemic forearm exercise test has been used as a screening test and may demonstrate failure of the lactate level to rise but an increase in ammonia. However, an abnormal result is not pathognomonic for myophosphorylase deficiency, and as the test may lead to pain and cramps and rarely focal rhabdomyolysis and a compartment syndrome, its use in children should be extremely limited and then only in the hands of those experienced in its use. While DNA mutation analysis of leukocytes may avoid the need for muscle biopsy (el-Schahawi et al. 1996), the variety of presentations and the relative nonspecificity or vagueness of symptoms in childhood means that muscle biopsy will usually, for the present at least, precede molecular genetic confirmation. Muscle biopsy shows a moderate increase in subsarcolemmal glycogen, and the absence of phosphorylase can be demonstrated histochemically. Muscle fibre degeneration may be seen following a recent episode. Definitive diagnosis requires the biochemical demonstration of decreased myophosphorylase activity (Servidei et al. 1988). Phosphorus magnetic resonance spectroscopy has been used to study muscle metabolism in McArdle disease and other metabolic disorders (Argov and Bank 1991) as well as in asymptomatic family members (Gruetter et al. 1990).

The rarity of the disorder has precluded large-scale controlled therapeutic trials to date. A systematic review of published controlled trials revealed that the only interventions for which there may be some modest benefit are low-dose creatine (60 mg/kg/day for adults) and oral sucrose taken 30 minutes before exercise (Quinlivan and Beynon 2004). Reports of benefit from other strategies including high protein diet remain anecdotal (Slonim and Goans 1985). Regular moderate exercise, preceded by 5 to 15 minutes of low-level 'warm up' exercise to promote the 'second wind' is recommended (Haller 2000, Ollivier et al. 2005).

PHOSPHOFRUCTOKINASE DEFICIENCY (GSD-VII OR TARUI DISEASE)
This disorder is due to mutations in the M subunit of phosphofructokinase (PFKM gene, chromosome 12q13.3). In muscle, only M subunits are present, while M and L subunits are found in erythrocytes, and hence in addition to muscle symptoms, deficit in M subunit may present with bouts of haemolysis. Impaired glycolysis leads to cramps on exercise and myoglobinuria (Di Mauro and Tsujino 1994) similar to McArdle disease. However, these patients are unable to achieve a spontaneous second wind under conditions that consistently produce one in patients with McArdle disease (Haller and Vissing 2004). A neonatal form is marked by hypotonia, weakness, respiratory insufficiency and joint deformities. Cerebral involvement is present and death supervenes during the first year (Servidei et al. 1986).

PHOSPHORYLASE B KINASE (PBK) DEFICIENCY (GSD-VIII)
Phosphorylase kinase deficient glycogen storage disorders are genetically and phenotypically heterogenous because mutations affect different subunits and isoforms of the enzyme. Muscle involvement is described with mutations of the beta subunit (PHKB gene, chromosome 16q12–q13). PBK deficiency is uncommon; onset of symptoms may be in infancy or early childhood with weakness and delayed motor milestones or later in childhood or adolescence with exercise intolerance, cramps and episodic myoglobinuria (Van den Berg and Berger 1990, DiMauro and Tsujino 1994). There may be liver involvement. Severe myopathy presenting in the neonatal period has been described (Sahin et al. 1998, Buhrer et al. 2000). CK levels and muscle histology are sometimes normal, which is likely to cause diagnostic difficulty (Wilkinson et al. 1994).

OTHER GLYCOGENOSES
Myopathy presenting with intolerance to exercise and associated myoglobinuria has been reported in phosphoglycerate mutase deficiency (GSD-X) (PGAM-M gene, chromosome 7p12–p13) (Vita et al. 1994, Hadjigeorgiou et al. 1999), lactate dehydrogenase deficiency (GSD-XI) (LDHA gene, chromosome 11p15.4) (DiMauro and Tsujino 1994) and phosphoglycerate kinase deficiency (GSD-IX) (PGK1 gene, chromosome Xq13) (Sugie et al. 1989, Aasly et al. 2000). In 28 families with phosphoglycerate kinase deficiency reviewed by Morimoto et al. (2003), 13 patients had muscle involvement and in 7 of them it was muscle alone, whereas usually there is also either haemolytic anaemia or developmental delay.

MYOADENYLATE DEAMINASE DEFICIENCY
Myoadenylate deaminase deficiency (MADA) (AMPD1 gene, chromosome 1p13–p21), an autosomal recessive familial trait, has been found in muscle samples of patients with infantile hypotonia, with progressive myopathies of childhood onset, and in a wide range of other neuromuscular disorders as well as in asymptomatic individuals. The significance of the deficit is still unclear (Mercelis et al. 1987, Walsh 2006). The diagnosis should be considered in patients with exertional myalgia and fatigue and muscle cramps with swelling or tenderness (Ashwal and Peckham 1985, Sabina 2000). The diagnosis is supported by ischaemic exercise test showing normal lactate production but failure of the blood ammonia level to rise, but this is not a test that should be routinely performed in children. Confirmation requires demonstration of the enzyme deficit in muscle biopsy. MADA has previously been divided into primary and secondary types but genetic studies have demonstrated the same underlying molecular defect in both forms (Verzijl et al. 1998).

DISORDERS OF LIPID UTILIZATION AND METABOLISM
(see also Chapter 8)

Fatty acids are very important fuels for striated muscle. They are especially important for sustained exercise and under fasting conditions. Carnitine is an essential cofactor in the transfer of long-chain fatty acids into the mitochondrion where fatty acids of long, medium and short chain are metabolized by beta-oxidation.

CARNITINE DEFICIENCY
Carnitine deficiency is often secondary to other metabolic disorders (Chapter 8) but can occur as a primary defect.

PRIMARY MUSCLE CARNITINE DEFICIENCY
Primary muscle carnitine deficiency is an autosomal recessive myopathy with progressive proximal limb weakness. A cardiomyopathy is often associated. Muscle biopsy shows lipid storage and reduced carnitine content. Dietary treatment with L-carnitine is effective in some cases. Corticosteroids may occasionally be helpful. Myopathy may also be part of primary systemic carnitine deficiency (Chapter 8).

DEFICITS IN CARNITINE–PALMITOYL TRANSFERASE (CPT)
This system consists of two enzymes (Meola et al. 1987, Zierz 1994) and entry of long-chain fatty acid into mitochondria is limited if there is a defect in the specific transfer system. *CPT I deficiency* is rare and has been identified in a few patients who presented with episodes of severe hypoglycaemia without ketonaemia that were triggered by fasting or intercurrent illnesses. *CPT II deficiency*, an autosomal recessive disorder, may present as a lethal neonatal form that may be limited to muscle (Land et al. 1995), in infancy with hepatic and cardiac involvement and nonketotic hypoglycaemia, or as a clinically quite different later onset form (Sigauke et al. 2003). The late-onset form is dominated by episodic weakness, myalgia and myoglobinuria and very high CK levels that usually, but not invariably, return to normal between attacks. There is no 'second wind' phenomenon. The onset is usually in late childhood or early adulthood, but onset as early as the first or second years of life has been described (Hurvitz et al. 2000, Gempel et al. 2001). Prolonged exercise, fasting, fever or infections are potential triggers. The severity of the disease is variable and partial deficiencies may be observed (Kieval et al. 1989). Respiratory muscles may be involved, and the other potentially serious metabolic consequences of myoglobinuria have to be taken care of during attacks. Death during an attack in childhood has been reported (Kelly et al. 1989). There is a marked reduction or complete absence of the CPT II enzyme in muscle and also in leukocytes, platelets and cultured fibroblasts.

Many mutations have been described in the *CPTII* gene on chromosome 1p32 (Sigauke et al. 2003). A similar clinical picture to that of CPT II deficiency may be seen with mitochondrial trifunctional protein (long-chain 3-hydroxyacyl-CoA dehydrogenase) deficiency (Schaefer et al. 1996, Miyajima et al. 1997).

Treatment consists mainly of avoidance of fasting or other triggering factors and a high-carbohydrate low-fat diet is said to reduce the frequency of attacks (Tein et al. 1990, Orngreen et al. 2003). Valproic acid has triggered acute rhabdomyolysis in CPT II deficiency and should be avoided (Kottlors et al. 2001).

OTHER DEFECTS OF LIPID METABOLISM
Defects of mitochondrial (beta) oxidation are clinically heterogeneous but myopathic presentations occur in older children and adults (Vockley et al. 2002). Recurrent myalgia, rhabdomyolysis and myoglobinuria precipitated by exercise and fasting may occur in very long chain acyl-coenzyme A dehydrogenase (VLCAD) deficiency, in which there appears to be some genotype–phenotype correlation (Andresen et al. 1999). Short chain acyl-coenzyme A dehydrogenase (SCAD), usually presents within the early months of life and may later show a myopathic picture with progressive external ophthalmoplegia clinically, and with multicores in muscle (Tein et al. 1999). Other disorders with reports of significant muscle involvement include, but are certainly not limited to, multiple acyl-CoA-dehydrogenase defect (electron transfer flavoprotein ubiquinone reductase: glutaric aciduria type II) (Jackson and Turnbull 1993, Olsen et al. 2004, Domizio et al. 2005), and long-chain 3-hydroxyacyl-CoA de-

hydrogenase (trifunctional protein) deficiency (Tein et al. 1995, Korenke et al. 2003).

Rare cases of multisystem, including muscle, triglyceride storage disease with ichthyosis, steatorrhoea and Jordan's anomaly of leukocytes are on record (Lefèvre et al. 2001, Nagai et al. 2003).

The management of patients with disorders of lipid metabolism is discussed in Chapter 8.

MITOCHONDRIAL MYOPATHIES
Mitochondrial cytopathies are relatively rare but within this group of disorders involvement of the CNS and neuromuscular systems is common. The distinction between purely myopathic and more complex forms is to some extent artificial because of the ubiquitous cellular presence of mitochondria. Skewed heteroplasmy, whereby skeletal muscle might have a predominance of pathogenic mitochondrial mutations compared to other tissues, may account for apparent preferential muscle tissue involvement and presentation as a myopathy, but there may be other explanations (DiMauro and Gurgel-Giannetti 2005). The protean clinical manifestations, along with the complexity of investigations required to establish a definitive aetiopathological diagnosis, have made these disorders difficult for clinicians to deal with. Nevertheless, there are a number of recognizable syndromes and their genetic, biochemical, pathological and clinical features are increasingly understood (Schapira and Cock 1999, DiMauro and Gurgel-Giannetti 2005, DiMauro and Hirano 2005).

Mitochondrial dysfunction may occur at various steps in the mitochondrial metabolism of lipids and other metabolites. These aspects have been reviewed in Chapter 8. This section deals only with myopathies due to mitochondrial diseases causing dysfunction of the electron transfer system (respiratory chain).

CLINICAL FEATURES
Mitochondrial myopathies may present from birth to adulthood and are extremely variable in their symptoms, severity and outcome (Harding et al. 1988, DiMauro 1993). Some are part of complex encephalomyopathies (Chapter 8), while others are purely or essentially limited to striated muscle. If the presentation is that of a clinically pure myopathic process with predominantly proximal muscle weakness, symptoms such as fatigue, myalgia, exercise intolerance (mild exercise giving disproportionate tachycardia and dyspnoea), and episodic exercise-related myoglobinuria, although not diagnostic, may give a clue. These symptoms may occur without fixed weakness. Ptosis and progressive external ophthalmoplegia are highly important clues (Moraes et al. 1989), as is the presence of cardiomyopathy. Other evidence of multisystem involvement as well as myopathy is common and facilitates recognition of syndromes such as Kearns–Sayre syndrome. A maternal pattern of inheritance, deafness and ophthalmoplegia were prominent clues to respiratory chain dysfunction in the study of Jackson et al. (1995). Failure to thrive, retinitis pigmentosa, diabetes, intellectual impairment, seizures and cerebellar ataxia also add valuable clues. Hypotonia may be prominent but less valuable in the differential diagnosis.

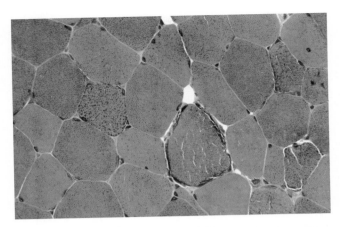

Fig. 21.9. Ragged red fibres in a case of Kearns–Sayre syndrome. Note subsarcolemmal deposits of red material representing mitochondria in most affected fibres, while similar but less marked changes are beginning to appear in other fibres. (Courtesy Prof. B Lake, Great Ormond Street Hospital, London.)

INVESTIGATION

If an obvious syndrome is not recognized clinically, early investigation clues to a respiratory chain defect come from an elevated blood or CSF lactate or imaging abnormalities in the basal ganglia (Jackson et al. 1995). For some of the recognizable syndromes, which are usually not predominantly myopathic (e.g. MELAS, MERRF, NARP), mutations may be found in circulating lymphocytes thereby avoiding the need for a biopsy.

Even in the absence of significant weakness, histological and histochemical assessment of muscle tissue often gives the initial or the confirmatory clue to a mitochondrial disorder. The characteristic morphological abnormality, seen best with Gomori trichrome staining, is the so-called ragged red fibre due to the accumulation of subsarcolemmal mitochondria. Electronmicroscopy may show abnormal mitochondrial structures that may contain paracrystalline inclusions (Fig. 21.9). However, ragged red fibres (Fig. 21.10) may be permanently or temporarily absent in proven mitochondrial diseases. Further assessment involves histochemical staining for the enzymes succinate dehydrogenase (SDH), which will demonstrate mitochondrial proliferation, and cytochrome *c* oxidase (COX). COX is encoded for by both nuclear and mitochondrial DNA (mtDNA), and a mosaic pattern of reactivity suggests a heteroplasmic mtDNA disorder while an overall decrease suggests a nuclear DNA mutation (Taylor et al. 2004). Ragged red fibres are usually COX-negative (Byrne et al. 1985) but they can also be COX-positive (Taylor et al. 2004, DiMauro and Hirano 2005). An excess of lipids or of glycogen is seen in some cases. Biochemical analysis of respiratory chain complex activity can point to defects in a single respiratory chain complex or multiple complexes, but can only be carried out in specialized centres. Further delineation is undertaken by molecular genetic studies of mt DNA and nuclear DNA locations relevant not only to the respiratory chain but also to mitochondrial abundance, structure and even movement (DiMauro and Hirano 2005).

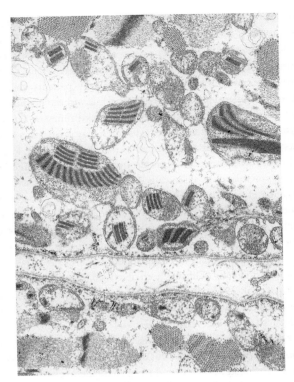

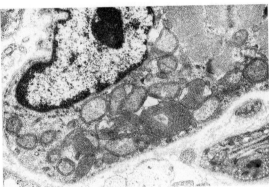

Fig. 21.10. Mitochondrial myopathy (electron microscopy, ×28,500). *(Top)* 13-year-old patient with typical history. Note classical 'parking lot' inclusions within mitochondria. *(Bottom)* 5-year-old patient. Note proliferation of the cristae within mitochondria. 'Parking lots' and paracrystalline arrays do not generally become apparent before 7–8 years of age. (Courtesy Prof. B Lake, Great Ormond Street Hospital, London.)

CLINICAL MYOPATHIC SYNDROMES

Marked clinical heterogeneity, lack of phenotype–genotype correlations and the multisystem nature of mitochondrial disorders have meant that while a number of encephalopathic syndromes that involve muscle have been defined (e.g. MERRF, MELAS), there are very few predominantly or entirely myopathic phenotypes. Some exceptions are discussed below.

Cytochrome c oxidase (COX)

One remarkable form of COX deficiency presents with severe congenital lactic acidosis, weakness and hypotonia that can be isolated or be associated with tubular and/or cardiac involvement.

Infants become symptomatic by a few weeks to 3 months of age and usually run a rapidly downward course with respiratory insufficiency (Zeviani et al. 1985, Darin et al. 2003). A reversible form of COX deficiency presenting in the newborn period with little spontaneous movement, ptosis, areflexia, increased CK and increased serum lactate but not CSF lactate is documented (Zeviani et al. 1987). Similar reversibility has been documented with childhood presentation of exercise intolerance, generalized muscle weakness with painful muscle cramps and fatigue (but without myoglobinuria), due to a mutation in the mtDNA *COXIII* gene leading to COX deficiency (Horváth et al. 2004). COX deficiency manifesting acutely at 7 years of age by ptosis, ophthalmoplegia and respiratory arrest with recovery following coenzyme Q10 administration has been reported (Nozaki et al. 1990).

Coenzyme Q10 (CoQ10) deficiency
Deficiency of CoQ10 (ubiquinone) in muscle is seen with an encephalopathic presentation with cerebellar ataxia dominating, but with some weakness (Musumeci et al. 2001). Conversely, some cases have a myopathic presentation with exercise intolerance, progressive proximal muscle weakness and exercise-related myoglobinuria. Ragged red fibres, lipid storage, reduced CoQ10 levels and reduced activity of respiratory chain complexes I + III and II + III are seen (Di Giovanni et al. 2001). The myopathy may be isolated (Lalani et al. 2005), but there may also be encephalopathic features such as seizures and ataxia. The importance of recognizing this disorder is that the response to oral CoQ10 therapy is often very good (Lalani et al. 2005), although this is not always the case (Aure et al. 2004).

Mitochondrial DNA depletion
The mitochondrial depletion syndrome (Elpeleg 2003), while often multisystemic, can be tissue specific, and a myopathic form presents in infancy or early childhood with progressive weakness, hypotonia, areflexia, early onset of respiratory failure and death in the first decade (Mancuso et al. 2002). Mutations in the thymidine kinase 2 (*TK2*) gene on chromosome 16 have been identified in some patients (Saada et al. 2001, Mancuso et al. 2002). Mutations in the *SUCLA2* gene are also reported to be associated with mitochondrial DNA depletion and progressive muscle weakness, but in these families the multisystem features are also quite prominent (Elpeleg et al. 2005).

Other mitochondrial myopathies
Development of sideroblastic anaemia during adolescence may give a clue to the syndrome entitled myopathy and sideroblastic anaemia (MLASA), which commences with exercise intolerance during childhood. Mutations have been found in the pseudo-uridine synthase 1 (*PUS1*) gene (Bykhovskaya et al. 2004). Childhood-onset exercise intolerance is also a prominent early feature resulting from mutations in the mt DNA cytochrome *b* gene (Andreu et al. 1999). Progressive external ophthalmoplegia (PEO) is seen in the Kearns–Sayre syndrome as part of a multisystem disorder and is associated with the mtDNA point mutation mt

3243 in 80% of cases (Hirano and Pavlakis 1994). Multiple mtDNA deletions due to mutations in the *ANT1*, *Twinkle* and *POLG1* genes are seen with inherited forms of PEO without other system involvement, although most of these cases present in adulthood (Agostino et al. 2003).

TREATMENT
The treatment of mitochondrial diseases is reviewed in Chapter 8.

MYOGLOBINURIA

Myoglobinuria secondary to rhabdomyolysis (Table 21.9) is a phenomenon with a wide range of aetiologies but with potentially fatal physiological consequences irrespective of the acquired or inherited cause (Warren et al. 2002). The development of pigmenturia, sometimes with muscle pain and swelling, in a child with or without a pre-existing neuromuscular disorder requires urgent medical attention. Life-threatening acute renal failure and cardiac arrhythmias mainly due to hyperkalaemia may occur. Bulbar muscle dysfunction, respiratory insufficiency and encephalopathic features including seizures can also eventuate. Apart from identifying myoglobin as the cause of the dark urine (positive urine dipstick tests for blood but no red blood cells), an extremely high CK level, often >100 times the upper limit of normal, is the cardinal clue to the nature of the problem. Although dipstick urine testing is sensitive, depending on timing, a negative test does not rule out myoglobinuria, and similarly, the CK may not be elevated early in an acute clinical setting (Coco and Klasner 2004).

Sporadic exogenous causes such as direct or indirect injury, animal toxins (e.g. snake bite) and drugs are usually but not always obvious. The long list of drugs includes those of abuse and those associated with the neuroleptic malignant syndrome (Coco and Klasner 2004). Even after extensive investigation no cause can be found in many cases, but children have been classified into two broad groups on the basis of precipitating factors (Tein et al. 1990): exertion triggered myoglobinuria, in which a metabolic cause is often found; and 'toxic' myoglobinuria, precipitated by fever and infection. The latter group is younger, have more severe homeostasis consequences in the acute episode, and often no metabolic defect can be recognized. However, in the paediatric series of Watemberg et al. (2000) it was the older children who were more likely to develop acute renal failure. The groups are not homogenous in that fasting and infection may precipitate an episode where there is a metabolic basis (e.g. CPT II deficiency), while infection can be a precipitant in cases otherwise triggered by exertion (Tein et al. 1990). Fasting is not usually a contributing factor in the glycogenoses. If there is no specific clinical clue to an aetiological diagnosis, muscle pathology may point in the direction of lipid, glycogen or mitochondrial pathways.

INFLAMMATORY MYOPATHIES

The inflammatory myopathies are a heterogeneous group of acquired muscle disorders. Some are due to known specific agents;

TABLE 21.9
Main causes of myoglobinuria*

Genetic – usually recurrent myoglobinuria

Disorders of glycogen metabolism
  Phosphorylase (PPL – McArdle syndrome)
  Phosphorylase b kinase (PBK)
  Phosphofructokinase (PFK)
  Phosphoglycerate kinase (PGK)
  Phosphoglycerate mutase (PGAM)
  Lactate dehydrogenase (LDH)
Disorders of fatty acid metabolism (list not definitive)
  Carnitine palmitoyltransferase II (CPT II)
  Mitochondrial trifunctional protein (Miyajima et al. 1997,
    Spiekerkoetter et al. 2004)
  Very long chain acyl-coenzyme A dehydrogenase (VLCAD) deficiency
    (Andresen et al. 1999)
Disorders of pentose phosphate pathway
  Glucose-6-phosphate dehydrogenase
Disorders of purine nucleotide cycle
  Myoadenylate deaminase (debated)
Disorders of respiratory chain and other disorders of mitochondria (list
  not exhaustive)
  CoQ10 (ubiquinone) deficiency
Multiple mitochondrial DNA (mtDNA) deletions (Ohno et al. 1991)
Mutation in the mtDNA cytochrome *b* gene (Andreu et al. 1999)
Mutation in the *COXI* gene (Karadimas et al. 2000 – complex 1V)
Cytochrome *c* oxidase deficiency (Keightley et al. 1996, McFarland et al.
  2004)

Nongenetic – usually nonrecurrent myoglobinuria

Mechanical trauma (Bayswater syndrome)
Toxins – including animal toxins, drugs (therapeutic and drugs of
  dependence), alcohol
Salt/water imbalance
Nonketotic hyperosmolar states (Watemberg et al. 2000)
Extreme hyperthermia
Hypothermia
Infections, especially viral
Exertion (Lin et al. 2005)

Other disorders with predisposition (Tein et al. 1990)

Dystrophinopathies (Figarella-Branger et al. 1997)
Myotonic dystrophy
Myotonia congenita
Schwartz–Jampel syndrome
Malignant hyperthermia including central core myopathy and
  King–Denborough syndrome
Neurolept malignant syndrome
Inflammatory myopathy
Dystonia

Others where biochemical abnormality unknown

* Modified from Tein et al. (1990). This list is not definitive.

---

some have autoimmune mechanisms. This latter group, the largest of the acquired, non-infective inflammatory myopathies, can be split into three major subgroups: dermatomyositis, polymyositis and sporadic inclusion-body myositis. They are clinically, pathologically and immunologically different, and they owe their importance to their treatment possibilities. In childhood, dermatomyositis has a distinctive clinical presentation, is relatively common and usually there are no major diagnostic difficulties. Polymyositis however is rare and prone to misdiagnosis as nonspecific secondary inflammation can be seen in dis-orders such as the dystrophies. Sporadic inclusion-body myositis is rare in childhood. Dalakas (2004) has reviewed advances in understanding of these complex disorders.

DERMATOMYOSITIS

Dermatomyositis (DM) is a systemic humorally mediated microangiopathy mainly affecting small vessels, capillaries, arterioles and venules (Dalakas 2006a). The microangiopathy accounts for all pathological changes in muscle, small nerves, gastrointestinal tract, connective tissue and skin. Although the trigger is not known, the immunopathogenesis hinges on activation of complement to deposit membranolytic attack complex on the endomysium of small blood vessels.

Unlike in adults, an association with malignancy in childhood DM is extremely rare (Martini et al. 2005). DM may occur in patients with X-linked agammaglobulinaemia, usually in association with involvement of the CNS (Chapter 11) and as a result of graft-versus-host reaction (Urbano-Márquez et al. 1986). A DM-like syndrome triggered by *Toxoplasma gondii* has been reported (Topi et al. 1979, Schroter et al. 1987, Harland et al. 1991).

CLINICAL FEATURES AND DIAGNOSIS

Onset is commonly between 5 and 15 years of age. Presentation is acute to subacute in one third of cases, with fever, muscle pain or arthralgia. In the remaining patients, the onset is insidious with weakness, fatigue, anorexia and sometimes mild fever. In one series the median interval between onset of symptoms and diagnosis was 3 months with a range of 0.5–20.0 months (Pachman et al. 1998). Long diagnostic delay may occur, particularly when presentation is with predominantly systemic or behavioural change and when cutaneous manifestations or weakness do not occur or are not recognized. The skin manifestations are variable. Reddish lavender (heliotrope or violaceous) discolouration involves the upper eyelids, and the periorbital and malar regions. Periorbital oedema may occur (Fig. 21.11). A similar rash, often scaly, may appear on the extensor surfaces of the knuckles, elbows, knees and malleoli of the ankles. Occasionally the skin lesions, which may be light sensitive, are more widespread involving the trunk as well. The rash may be evanescent and is easily missed if not looked for carefully. Small skin infarcts are sometimes seen. Symmetrical muscle weakness affects mainly the proximal muscles, and neck extension is accompanied in many cases by vague muscle pain and stiffness, and sometimes involves the bulbar muscles. Dysphagia and hoarseness occurred in over 40% of children at the time of diagnosis in one large series (Pachman et al. 1998). Joint contractures may develop early. Loss of ambulation occurs rapidly in some cases.

Gastrointestinal symptoms are present in about 20% of patients, and bowel ulcerations are potentially fatal (Bowyer et al. 1983). In a few children, retinal exudates are present. Asymptomatic abnormalities of lung function tests may occur (Trapani et al. 2001) but respiratory distress from parenchymal involvement is less common in children (Al-Mayouf et al. 2001) than in adults (Arakawa et al. 2003). ECG abnormalities are common

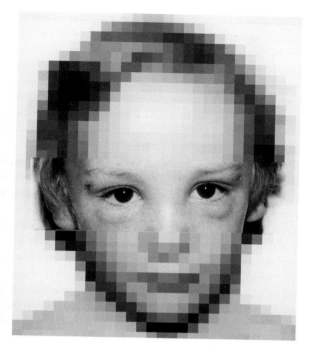

Fig. 21.11. Dermatomyositis in 11-year-old boy. Eyelid oedema is evident and was associated with heliotrope discoloration.

(Pachman 1990). Associated CNS vasculopathy or vasculitis has been reported in rare cases (Ramanan et al. 2001).

Chronicity manifests as generalized muscle wasting and severe contractures. The skin over the knuckles becomes thickened and discoloured. Generalized, partial or localized lipodystrophy may occur (Ramanan and Feldman 2002). Calcinosis of subcutaneous tissue occurs in 25–50% of cases but is usually not seen until late, and delay in diagnosis and treatment increases the likelihood of its development (Pachman et al. 1998). It may be located under the discoloured areas of skin or be more extensive along fascial planes (calcinosis universalis). Extrusion of calcium from indolent purulent ulcerative lesions ('milk of calcium') presents a difficult management problem. Often when the muscle inflammation burns out after many years it is the calcification and joint contractures that remain as the dominant long-term problem (Ramanan and Feldman 2002).

The early diagnosis of DM is sometimes difficult before a rash or definite weakness appears and it should always be suspected in a child with reduced motor activity and misery (Dubowitz 1995). However, the clinical diagnosis is often very clear because of a typical rash, proximal muscle weakness and an elevated CK level or positive inflammatory markers. Normal CK does not exclude DM. EMG, required only in difficult diagnostic cases, may show increased insertion activity with myopathic potentials, fibrillations and positive sharp waves at rest. Muscle ultrasound and MRI have been used in the diagnosis and further assessment (Collison et al. 1998, Maillard et al. 2004). Screening for a variety of autoantibodies, even those with fairly high specificity such as the anti-Jo-1 antibody, is usually undertaken but in paediatric practice this adds little to the diagnosis

or management of most cases. The complex topic has been reviewed by Garlepp and Mastaglia (2000).

Confirmation of the diagnosis should be by muscle biopsy even in clinically typical cases. Capillary loss leads to muscle fibre damage, ischaemic microinfarcts, inflammation and distinctive perifascicular atrophy (Dalakas 2004). Perivascular infiltrates are usually found but they may be missed in a small specimen. Further characterization of the disorder requires immunocytochemical study of muscle for detection of abnormalities such as deposition of membrane attack complex (Sakuta et al. 2005).

TREATMENT

A systematic review has highlighted the lack of high-quality randomized controlled trials to assess the efficacy and toxicity of immunotherapy in inflammatory myositis, even in adults (Choy et al. 2005), but corticosteroids are the accepted initial treatment. Without treatment mortality is about 30%, but treatment reduces this to less than 10% (Bowyer et al. 1983). Approaches to management differ but the principle is to give enough corticosteroid initially to significantly improve muscle strength, followed by progressive dosage reduction to minimize side effects while at the same time ensuring ongoing improvement. Traditionally, initial prednisolone doses of approximately 2 mg/kg/day have been used with tapering over periods up to 2 years, which corresponds to the average duration of the active phase of the disorder. Some have effectively used smaller doses of 1.0–1.5 mg/kg/day (Miller et al. 1983, Dubowitz 1995) with gradual tapering of the dose once response begins and with total duration of treatment as short as 3–6 months. Recognizable improvements in performance of the activities of daily living and in measured muscle strength typically occur by 2–4 weeks after commencement of therapy. The rate of tapering is determined by the requirement for continuing improvement with minimization of side effects. Some authors suggest reduction rates of 5–10 mg per month, but in the final analysis the rate should be determined by the benefit–side effect ratio judged on an ongoing basis. Relapses requiring increasing the dose temporarily are common (Spencer et al. 1984), and treatment should not be reduced too early or too rapidly. Occasional patients will return to normal with only pulses of intravenous high-dose methylprednisolone, greatly reducing the side-effect burden of long-term oral corticosteroid, but most will deteriorate with this approach alone (Lang and Dooley 1996). It is worth trying in resistant cases (Laxer et al. 1987).

Some 10–20% of affected children do not respond satisfactorily to corticosteroids and other immunosuppressive approaches are required. Intravenous immunoglobulin was effective in controlled studies in adults (Dalakas 1998) and is suggested by some as the second-line treatment (Dalakas 2006b). Methotrexate (Hanissian et al. 1982), cyclosporine (Heckmatt et al. 1989), azathioprine and cyclophosphamide (Riley et al. 2004) are used in steroid-resistant cases with variable success. There are no controlled studies of their relative merits in juvenile DM. Plasmapheresis used in steroid-resistant cases was not effective (Miller et al. 1992).

The treatment of calcinosis remains unsatisfactory and is often a major ongoing problem even after muscle weakness has improved or at least become stable. Alendronate has been reported to be effective in one child (Mukamel et al. 2001) but the value of this and other similar agents remains anecdotal.

Despite the beneficial effects of current treatments, good long-term outcome is not guaranteed. In a multicentre study of 65 patients with juvenile DM, at an average of about 7 years' follow-up, 47 (72%) had no or minimal disability (Huber et al. 2000). However the disease remains chronically active in a substantial number of patients and treatment side effects such as growth failure are commonly seen (Ramanan and Feldman 2002). A multidisciplinary approach by medical and allied health professionals experienced in treating this disorder is required. Physiotherapy, particularly aimed at the prevention of contractures, is an essential part of therapy as life-long disability is often related to contractures and calcinosis.

It remains to be seen if more specific targeted immunotherapies offer significant improvements in outcome (Dalakas 2004).

Clinical and some nonspecific pathological features of myositis are not the province of DM alone. Despite better understanding of the immunopathogenesis of inflammatory myopathies, *mixed connective tissue disorder* and other *overlap syndromes* continue to complicate separation of these disorders into clearly definable subsets. Criteria for the diagnosis of childhood scleromyositis with myalgia–myositis, arthralgia–arthritis, sclerotic fingers and Raynaud's phenomenon have been reported (Blaszczyk et al. 1991).

POLYMYOSITIS

Polymyositis (PM) as defined by recently elucidated immunopathological mechanisms is probably very rare in childhood, and even in adults is said to be overdiagnosed (van der Meulen et al. 2003). Presentation is similar to that of dermatomyositis (DM) but it is differentiated from DM not just by the absence of skin changes but also by histopathological and immunological characteristics. Muscle biopsy shows fibre necrosis and inflammatory infiltrates but not the perifascicular atrophy characteristic of DM. Even the histopathological inflammatory response is not enough for the diagnosis, as similar inflammation may be seen in a number of disorders, particularly the muscular dystrophies. Various childhood limb–girdle muscular dystrophies have been misdiagnosed as PM. One tenet of recently proposed new diagnostic criteria is that the diagnosis of PM should be reconsidered if the onset is below 18 years of age (Dalakas 2004).

In contrast to the humoral basis of DM, PM is a cell-mediated immune response directed against muscle fibres. In PM – and in sporadic inclusion body myositis (sIBM) – there are endomysial infiltrates composed of CD8+ T cells and macrophages invading muscle fibres that express major histocompatibility-I (MHC-I) antigen (Amato and Griggs 2003). This MHC-I/CD8 complex is considered to be a specific immune marker for PM (and sIBM). The T cells migrate through endothelial cell walls, recognize antigens on muscle cells and a necrotic process is triggered (Dalakos 2004).

The clinical picture and course of PM in children is reported to be similar to that in adults (Mastaglia and Ojeda 1985a,b). However, until there are large studies of suspected childhood-onset PM confirmed by strict clinical and immunohistopathological criteria, its true incidence, clinical features, response to therapy and outcome in childhood will remain unclear. Treatment strategies similar to those for DM are appropriate.

SPORADIC INCLUSION BODY MYOSITIS (sIBM)
This disorder is rare in childhood (Riggs et al. 1989, Griggs et al. 1995). It presents like a slow-onset myositis with early involvement of finger flexors or the quadriceps muscles (Dalakas 2004), and has been misdiagnosed as muscular dystrophy (Riggs et al. 1989) and polymyositis. Muscle biopsy shows both inflammatory and degenerative features with endomysial inflammation, sarcoplasmic rimmed vacuoles and intracellular accumulation of amyloid-related proteins (Dalakas 2006b). On electron microscopy, the vacuoles are shown to include membranous bodies and intranuclear and cytoplasmic filamentous inclusions. The vacuoles are not pathognomonic and can be seen in other disorders such as hereditary IBM and Emery–Dreifuss dystrophy (Fidzianska et al. 2004). The immunopathology is identical to that of PM but anti-inflammatory treatment is relatively ineffective (Dalakas 2004).

INFANTILE AND CONGENITAL MYOSITIS
Reports of inflammatory myopathy in infancy are rare (Shevell et al. 1990, Nagai et al. 1992). Some cases have responded to corticosteroid therapy at usual doses, but the existence of an infantile PM entity cannot be accepted until confirmed by recently accepted criteria, or until other unique characteristics are defined. Nonspecific inflammation is insufficient for a confirmed diagnosis.

TRANSIENT ACUTE MYOSITIS OF VIRAL, BACTERIAL, PARASITIC OR PROTOZOAN ORIGIN
Viral myositis
Epidemic pleurodynia (Bornholm disease) due to coxsackie virus B infection is a well-recognized disease involving the intercostal muscles. Myalgias are a regular feature of some other viral diseases, especially of influenza.

A picture of *acute diffuse polymyositis* is uncommon, and severe cases with myoglobinuria are rare (DiBona and Morens 1977, Gamboa et al. 1979). A possible role of viral infections as triggers of myositis has been suggested, as raised antibody titres to coxsackie virus B have been found in some patients (Dubowitz 1995). Other viruses (adenoviruses, parainfluenza viruses) rarely produce myositis. Association with rotavirus gastroenteritis has been reported (Hattori et al. 1992).

In some epidemics of influenza A or B, muscular involvement may be prominent, and in rare cases influenza virus has been isolated from muscle (Gamboa et al. 1979). *Benign acute childhood myositis* (Mackay et al. 1999) is an easily recognizable syndrome of mid-childhood affecting boys more than girls. Typically there is a concurrent or preceding (1–4 days) upper respiratory infec-

myotonic dystrophy (Shore 1975) and are one of the correlates of a poor outcome (Connolly et al. 1992). A case of arthrogryposis with ragged red muscle fibres and complex I deficiency (Laubscher et al. 1997) suggests that mitochondrial cytopathy should be looked for in some cases.

PERIPHERAL NERVE CAUSES

Peripheral nerve causes of multiple congenital contractures are rare (Yuill and Lynch 1974, Charnas et al. 1988, Boylan et al. 1992). In the transient neonatal form of myasthenia, FADS with congenital contractures can be seen particularly in those with maternal antibodies directed against fetal acetylcholine receptors. Although rare, this is an important cause to recognise not only because of the recurrence risk but also because it is potentially treatable (Polizzi et al. 2000). Mild congenital contractures can also be seen in the rapsyn early-onset congenital myasthenia syndrome (Burke et al. 2004) (see Table 21.10, p. 844) and in some acetylcholine receptor subunit mutations (Brownlow et al. 2001).

As multiple joint contractures are a sign rather than a disease, understanding the inheritance pattern depends on recognition of the specific syndrome (Hall 1997). All forms of inheritance are possible. These include dominantly inherited forms of distal arthrogryposis, autosomal recessive syndromes, and X-linked types including a rapidly lethal one mapping to Xp11.3–q11.2 (Hall et al. 1982b, Kobayashi et al. 1995).

OTHER MUSCLE ABNORMALITIES

CONGENITAL AGENESIS/HYPOPLASIA

Congenital agenesis or hypoplasia of muscle is common and may involve a whole muscle or parts of muscle, including, in decreasing order of frequency, the pectoralis, trapezius, sternocleidomastoid, serratus anterior and quadriceps femori. One common condition is the *Poland syndrome* in which absence of the sternal head of the pectoralis major is associated with ipsilateral brachysyndactyly of fingers and hypoplasia of the upper limb. Focal agenesis of muscles is usually asymptomatic. Vascular abnormalities may be a cause in some cases (Lee et al. 1995). The *prune belly syndrome* is characterized by absence or hypoplasia of abdominal wall muscles that may be primary or secondary (Moerman et al. 1984). *Thenar hypoplasia* (Cavanagh syndrome) may be either unilateral or bilateral (Sonel et al. 2002). Differentiation from carpal tunnel syndrome for which it is sometimes misdiagnosed, is important so as to prevent unnecessary intervention. Clinical clues are derived from the lack of sensory symptoms, the life-long duration of the problem and associated radiological abnormalities (Rhomberg et al. 2002). These include a slender first metacarpal and hypoplasia of carpal bones, especially the scaphoid. Familial cases have been reported (Selmar et al. 1986).

TRAUMA

Trauma to muscle may result from excessive strain (Cameron 1983) or overuse as in *compartmental syndromes*. The rectus abdominis syndrome (Rutgers 1986) and the anterior compartment syndrome of the leg (Sloane et al. 1994) are of clinical importance for diagnosis and treatment. Deltoid, gluteal or vastus lateralis fibrotic contracture results from repeated intramuscular injections usually in the neonatal period or in infancy (Chen et al. 1988). Fibrotic retractions produce, after a variable latent period, limitation of joint movements and abnormal gait or postures and may require surgical lengthening of affected muscle. The best treatment is preventive by avoidance of intramuscular injections in very young children.

CONGENITAL MUSCULAR TORTICOLLIS

Congenital muscular torticollis is due to shortening of sternomastoid muscle from fibrosis, sometimes with a palpable 'sternomastoid tumour' that is usually in the middle or lower two thirds of the muscle. The aetiology is unclear but trauma, vascular and intrauterine malposition theories have been proposed. Significant associations are breech presentation, difficult labour, plagiocephaly and other face or skull asymmetries and hip dysplasia (Cheng et al. 2002). It should be distinguished from neurological, vertebral or ocular causes of torticollis which include, inter alia, superior oblique palsy, posterior fossa tumours and osteoarticular lesions of the cervical column (Sarnat and Morrissy 1981, Morrison and MacEwen 1982). With early physiotherapy intervention including positioning and manual stretching a satisfactory outcome is usually achieved, and surgical intervention is required for only the very few who respond poorly to the physiotherapy (Cheng et al. 2002).

MUSCLE HYPERTROPHY

Muscle hypertrophy may be caused by many myopathic or neurogenic disorders. It may also be due to intensive exercise. Familial hypertrophy of masticatory muscles has been reported (Martinelli et al. 1987). While the dystrophinopathies and other muscular dystrophies are the commonest causes, muscle hypertrophy may also be seen in hypothyroidism (Kocher–Debré–Sémélaigne and Hoffmann syndromes), and myotonia congenita. Extraordinary hypertrophy has been described in a child with a mutation in the *myostatin* gene (Schuelke et al. 2004).

MYASTHENIA AND DISORDERS OF THE NEUROMUSCULAR JUNCTION

Diseases of the neuromuscular junction are characterized clinically by weakness and increased fatiguability on muscular exercise, particularly in cranial nerve innervated territory. The group includes two autoimmune diseases, juvenile myasthenia gravis and the Lambert–Eaton syndrome, congenital myasthenic syndromes, and various types of neuromuscular blockade due to drugs, toxins or other exogenous factors. Infant botulism is discussed in Chapters 10 and 12.

JUVENILE (AUTOIMMUNE) MYASTHENIA GRAVIS

Juvenile myasthenia gravis (JMG) is the commonest cause of neuromuscular block in children and adolescents. Approximately 10% of all cases of myasthenia gravis occur in this age range.

MECHANISMS, PATHOLOGY, PATHOGENESIS

Typical JMG is due to binding of autoantibodies to acetylcholine receptors (AChR-MG) on striated muscle postsynaptic membrane. Available receptors are considerably reduced in number due to the action of these autoantibodies, whose presence has been demonstrated in serum and at the neuromuscular junction of human patients (Andrews et al. 1993, Drachman 1994). Some cases of autoimmune MG do not have detectable AChR antibodies and these have been referred to as seronegative myasthenia gravis (SN-MG). The term 'seronegative' is misleading in that some of these patients, including children, have IgG antibodies against the muscle-specific receptor tyrosine kinase (MuSK) (Evoli et al. 2003, Sanders et al. 2003). This has been termed MuSK-MG. Although there is good evidence for the pathogenicity of AChR antibodies, the pathogenetic role of MuSK antibodies remains unclear (Selcen et al. 2004, Vincent et al. 2005). Other antibodies of uncertain significance may be present, including those directed against titin, the ryanodine receptor and the intracellular AChR-associated protein, rapsyn (Richman and Agius 2003).

The mechanism responsible for the production of autoantibodies is unknown. A role of the thymus is suggested by the association of AChR-MG with thymus lymphoid hyperplasia and thymus tumours and by the effects of thymectomy. Thymus histology, if abnormal, is only minimally so in MuSK-MG (Lauriola et al. 2005, Vincent and Leite 2005). A genetic susceptibility is suggested by the relative frequency of clinical or EMG manifestations in relatives of myasthenic patients and by increased frequency of some HLA groups (Kerzin-Storrar et al. 1988).

Other autoimmune disorders cosegregate, particularly thyroid disease (hyper- or hypothyroidism), rheumatoid arthritis, lupus erythematosus and diabetes (Ichiki et al. 1992, Robertson et al. 1998). Malignant disease was present in 5% of children in one series (Rodriguez et al. 1983).

CLINICAL FFEATURES

Symptoms may occur any time after 1 year of age but the disease is most prevalent in adolescent girls (Andrews et al. 1994). Variability in muscle function with good strength after rest and deterioration after exercise or towards the end of the day, i.e. fatiguability, is the hallmark of myasthenic weakness. Occasionally this history of fatigue is either not present or difficult to obtain. The onset may be insidious or sudden, usually with involvement of the extraocular muscles with diplopia, ophthalmoplegia and ptosis. These signs can be symmetrical, asymmetrical or unilateral (Afifi and Bell 1993). Usually there is weakness of facial muscles, particularly the orbicularis oculi. Proximal limb muscle weakness may be present at the outset or develop later. The time frame for involvement for different muscle groups varies considerably but early severe involvement of respiratory and oropharyngeal muscles is not uncommon and requires urgent attention. There may be diagnostic difficulties in rare cases in which involvement of the lower limbs is the first manifestation (Drachman 1994). Deep tendon reflexes are retained. JMG should be considered in a child presenting with respiratory failure without an adequate pulmonary explanation, even if there are no other signs of JMG.

A history suggestive of JMG can usually, but not invariably, be confirmed by demonstration of muscle fatigue on examination. Initial muscle strength may be normal or near normal, and strength should be tested before and after exercise.

The natural course of JMG is variable. It tends to be slowly progressive but with fluctuation on a baseline of reduced function. With chronicity the symptoms and weakness may fluctuate less. *Myasthenic crises* with increased weakness and especially with involvement of respiratory muscles may occur spontaneously or following febrile illnesses and may require assisted ventilation. Death, usually from medical co-morbidity, may occur (Thomas et al. 1997).

The proportion of cases in which involvement remains limited to the extraocular muscles (*ocular myasthenia*) varies considerably from one report to another but is likely to be between 20% and 50% (Afifi and Bell 1993, Sommer et al. 1997, Anlar et al. 2005) and up to 80% in young Chinese children (Wong et al. 1992). In adults at least, the risk of generalization is less if disease is mild, the repetitive nerve stimulation test is normal, and AChR antibodies are low or absent at the time of diagnosis (Sommer et al. 1997).

Rodriguez et al. (1983) observed spontaneous remissions in 30% of patients after a 15-year follow-up, but in patients with extremity weakness the remission rate was significantly lower. Patients with prepubertal onset are much more likely than older patients to have spontaneous remission (Andrews et al. 1994).

For MuSK-MG in adults there is a female predominance and the clinical picture is dominated by cranial and bulbar muscle weakness and frequent episodes of respiratory crises (Evoli et al. 2003). Any differences between MuSK-MG and AChR-MG in childhood are yet to be clarified.

DIAGNOSIS

The diagnosis of the JMG is primarily a clinical one supported by three main types of investigation:

(1) *Anticholinesterase administration.* The effect of injection of one of these drugs is observed on one or more weak muscles. Edrophonium chloride (Tensilon) given intravenously has a rapid onset effect (30 seconds) but with short duration (5 minutes). While this may be appropriate for cooperative children and adults, some children become upset and it is difficult to satisfactorily observe the response. For this reason, intramuscular neostigmine with its effect starting after 10–15 minutes and reaching a maximum at 30 minutes is often preferred. Some authors indicate that neostigmine should not be given intravenously because of possible induction of fatal cardiac arrhythmia (Sarnat and Menkes 2006). Parenteral administration of atropine is usually undertaken before the anticholinesterase to neutralize the muscarinic effects of the drug. Assessing the response, particularly in young children, can be aided by taking photographs (Fig. 21.13) or preferably by videotaping the procedure. The maximum dose of Tensilon varies with age from 1 mg in infants to up to 10 mg in an adolescent. A test dose (e.g. 1 or 2 mg for an older child)

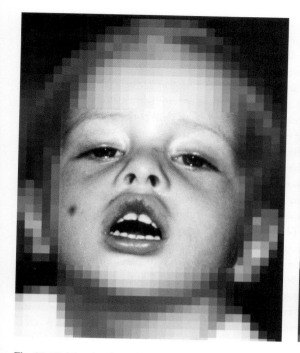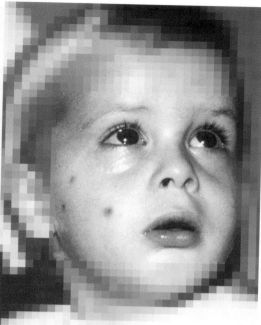

Fig. 21.13. Myasthenia gravis in 3-year-old boy. *(Left)* Note asymmetrical ptosis, open mouth and lack of expression. *(Right)* Three minutes after i.v. administration of 8 mg of edrophonium chloride (Tensilon): complete disappearance of all previous abnormalities.

is given first, the rest being injected after 30–60 seconds if there is no response. The dose of neostigmine is usually 0.04 mg/kg up to 1.5 mg total in an older child. In definite JMG a response is usually seen with doses at the lower end of the range. In rare cases serious side effects may occur with either drug so the test should always be performed with resuscitation equipment available. A negative anticholinesterase test does not exclude JMG, and a positive result is sometimes only obtained on repeat testing. Conversely, a positive test is not pathognomonic, and should not be the only basis for diagnosis (Drachman 1994).

(2) *Repetitive nerve stimulation (RNS)* provides electrical evidence of neuromuscular block (Oh et al. 1992). Compound muscle action potentials are recorded from surface electrodes placed preferably over a weak muscle, with the nerve stimulated at rates of 3 Hz and 5 Hz. A decrement in amplitude of more than 10% from the third to the fifth response is considered positive. This test is distressing for young children especially and should be used sparingly. Technical difficulties are also an issue in young children and it is important to be sure that the pattern of the decrement is of a myasthenic type before calling the test positive. In one childhood series (Afifi and Bell 1993) RNS was positive in 33% of cases when distal nerves were stimulated and in 66% when proximal and distal nerves were stimulated. The abnormality is corrected after injection of anticholinesterase. Single-fibre EMG to demonstrate increased 'jitter' in contraction of pairs of fibres is more sensitive than classical RNS but difficult to perform in children. A normal RNS does not exclude JMG.

(3) *Antibody testing.* AChR antibodies can be found in about 80% of adults with MG (Vincent and Leite 2005) but positivity is in the 60–80% range in childhood (Afifi and Bell 1993, Andrews et al. 1993). In prepubertal children the positivity figure drops to around 50% (Andrews et al. 1993). The antibody titre declines in successfully treated patients. Of those seronegative for AChR antibodies about 40–50% are seropositive for MuSK antibodies (MuSK-MG) (Evoli et al. 2003, Sanders et al. 2003, McConville et al. 2004). The prevalence of these antibodies in children is not clear but they can be present in early childhood-onset disease (Evoli et al. 2003, Vincent and Leite 2005).

The choice of a diagnostic test largely depends on the clinical presentation and experience of each institution with positivity rates for each test varying from one series to another. The anticholinesterase and RNS tests are the least sensitive and specific, while the presence of AChR antibodies is specific for myasthenia gravis (Drachman 1994).

Hyperthyroidism occurs in 3–8% of patients with JMG, and either hyperthyroidism or hypothyroidism may aggravate myasthenic weakness. Tests of thyroid function should be performed routinely (Drachman 1994). Evidence for other coexisting autoimmune disorders should be sought by careful history, clinical examination and laboratory tests where indicated. Imaging of the thymus looking for thymoma is routine in adults. There is one report of JMG developing following removal of a thymoma in a child presenting with a mediastinal mass at just under 5 years of age (Furman et al. 1985), but nevertheless thymoma is very rare in childhood. The cost–benefit ratio of routine screening in the pre-adolescent age group is not favourable.

Differential diagnosis includes other neuromuscular disorders in which fatiguability can sometimes be marked, and rare cases of myasthenic syndromes, especially resulting from the use of agents such as penicillamine, carnitine and aminoglycosides. Structural lesions of the midbrain such as tumours may be responsible for fatiguable ptosis, ophthalmoplegia and oropharyngeal weakness and thus mimic myasthenia. Imaging studies should be performed if the diagnosis of MG is not definitive and particularly if signs are confined to cranial nerve territory.

TREATMENT

The main therapeutic options for JMG are enhancement of neuromuscular transmission with anticholinesterase agents, short-term immunotherapies, including plasma exchange and intravenous immune globulin, and drug-induced immunosuppression on a long-term basis as well as surgical thymectomy (Drachman 1994). Better understanding in the future of the aetiopathogenetic role of the various antibodies is likely to inform a more tailored approach to therapy than exists currently. Already there is evidence, for instance, that adults with MuSK-MG may respond less well to immunosuppression and thymectomy than patients with AChR-MG (Evoli et al. 2003, Sanders et al. 2003).

Anticholinesterase agents

Anticholinesterase agents are usually the first line of treatment but they are symptomatic rather than curative. These drugs increase the half-life of acetylcholine released into the synaptic cleft by inhibiting its hydrolysis by acetylcholinesterase, thus increasing the probability of acetylcholine molecules reaching the reduced number of receptors (Drachman 1994). While an initial good response is usually seen, effectiveness may wane over time. Pyridostigmine is the most commonly used oral agent, while neostigmine may be useful parenterally during crises or when oral intake is otherwise not possible. Ambenomium is used in some countries. The clinical effect of pyridostigmine commences after about 30 minutes and peaks at about 2 hours post-dose.

Pyridostigmine up to 7 mg/kg/day is given in 3–5 doses. The initial dosage of neostigmine is 0.2–0.5 mg/kg every 4 hours in children younger than 5 years and 0.25 mg/kg in older children, not to exceed 15 mg per dose. The dosage should be slowly increased, and timing should be tailored to the child's individual needs. The family can be given latitude to alter the dose accordingly, but within set limits. For adolescents, doses of pyridostigmine beyond 120 mg given five times per day rarely give extra benefit, and the risk of increased muscle weakness (cholinergic crises) increases. Cramping abdominal pain or diarrhoea is often the first symptom of excessive dose, but diaphoresis, nausea, vomiting, bradycardia and miosis may supervene. Theoretically, administration of edrophonium can separate cholinergic crisis (over-treatment) from myasthenic crises (under-treatment) but the differentiation may be impossible, and in severe cases assisted ventilation and weaning from drugs may be necessary. The sustained-release preparation of pyridostigmine should be used only for troublesome symptoms overnight or on awakening as there is evidence from animal studies that sustained exposure to anticholinesterase agents may damage the endplate region of the neuromuscular junction (Hudson et al. 1978).

Pre-adolescent children in whom the remission rate is high and some older children with purely ocular myasthenia can often, but not always, be successfully managed with anticholinesterase agents alone.

Most older children and adolescents will also require therapy directed against the immune system abnormality. The timing and agents used are tailored for individual patients, based upon institutional experience and with the long-term cost–benefit ratio in mind (Richman and Agius, 2003), rather than on any current evidence-based approach for children. Even for adults many questions about the optimum approach to immunotherapy remain. The aim is to induce then maintain immunological remission. Corticosteroids, sometimes also with intravenous immunoglobulin or plasmapheresis, are effective for induction. Maintenance of the remission with slow reduction of the corticosteroids may be accomplished with other drugs such as azathioprine or with thymectomy (Richman and Agius 2003). Early thymectomy is often used without corticosteroids, particularly in adolescents, if urgent control is not required for life-threatening or severe weakness.

Corticosteroids

Corticosteroids induce remission in most children with JMG, but long-term use particularly in adolescents should be based only on a considered decision that benefit outweighs potential side effects. Initiating high-dose corticosteroid therapy can be associated with deterioration in subsequent weeks and gradually increasing the dose over several weeks lessens the risk. A prednisolone dose of 1–2 mg/kg/day is usually given until a good response is sustained, followed by progressive, but only slow, tapering. Switching to an alternate-day schedule may be successful in maintaining remission while minimizing side effects. If high dosage is required initially for severe disease, intravenous immunoglobulin or plasmaphoresis may be used to manage any acute deterioration (Richman and Agius 2003).

Other long-term immunotherapy

Other long-term immunotherapy may be required as an alternative for cases that do not respond to steroids or as a steroid-sparing strategy. Azathioprine may be used in conjunction with steroids or in isolation. A randomized, double-blinded trial in adults has demonstrated that azathioprine as an adjunct to alternate-day prednisolone in antibody-positive generalized MG reduces the maintenance dose of prednisolone and is associated with fewer treatment failures, longer remissions and fewer side effects (Palace et al. 1998). Cyclosporine can be considered if azathioprine is not tolerated while cyclophosphamide has been used for very severe disease (Richman and Agius 2003). The role in children of promising newer agents such as mycophenolate mofetil (Chaudhry et al. 2001) and tacrolimus (Sanders et al. 2006) is not known. High-dose pulse methylprednisolone has been used successfully in children with refractory disease (Sakano et al. 1989).

Plasma exchange

Plasma exchange can produce rapid but short-lived improvement and has been used for the treatment of myasthenic crises, and for pre- and postoperative support. *Intravenous immunoglobulin (IVIG)* is superior to plasma exchange in terms of ease of use and side-effect profile in children. Benefit may be seen in 3 or 4 days but lasts less than 3 months. Although some suggest that the benefits of plasma exchange in adults are slightly better (Qureshi et al. 1999), for others IVIG has been equally effective (Gajdos et al. 1997). Reports of IVIG use specifically in children are few (Sakano et al. 1989). A dose of 2 g/kg (given over two successive days) showed no significant superiority over 1 g/kg as a single infusion for MG exacerbation in an adult randomized dose comparison trial (Gajdos et al. 2005). A consensus panel suggested that IVIG appears to have a role for acute intervention or as a chronic maintenance therapy when all other treatment modalities have failed (Howard 1998).

Thymectomy

Thymectomy is used as the main long-term strategy, particularly in children where potential adverse effects of long-term treatment with anticholinesterases, corticosteroids or other immunotherapies are pertinent. It frequently results in significant and lasting improvement, although other long-term therapy remains necessary for some time as the benefit from thymectomy may not be evident for up to a year, and the full effect for even longer after the procedure. It is usually indicated for moderate or severe disease, particularly if there are oropharyngeal or respiratory symptoms at presentation or soon after. Intervention with short-term agents such as IVIG, plasma exchange or corticosteroids may be required for stabilization before or after surgery.

For children, thymectomy significantly increases the remission rate up to 67% (Adams et al. 1990). Of 79 patients with juvenile-onset myasthenia (onset 12–18 years), 65 received thymectomy, usually in association with immunosuppressive treatment. Thirty-nine (60%) of these went into remission, as against only 4 of 14 non-operated patients (Lindner et al. 1997). Patients are more likely to be improved or in remission if thymectomy is performed early, particularly within the first year following the onset of symptoms (Andrews et al. 1994, DeFilippi et al. 1994, Richman and Agius 2003). There is some evidence in adults that long-term immunosuppressive treatment and thymectomy may prevent generalization of ocular myasthenia (Sommer et al. 1997), but because of the possibility of spontaneous remission in younger children, such therapy should be considered only in severe cases. Adults with MuSK-MG, in which there is little or no thymus abnormality, have not responded to thymectomy (Evoli et al. 2003).

The results from the trans-cervical approach for thymectomy appear to be as good as those for the traditional trans-sternal approach, with the added benefits of less discomfort and shorter hospital stay (Calhoun et al. 1999). Even less invasive video-assisted techniques are being assessed.

Wittbrodt (1997) reviewed drugs prescribed for coexisting conditions that may impair neuromuscular transmission. Those commonly prescribed agents listed that have a probable association with exacerbation of MG were aminoglycoside antibiotics, ciprofloxacin, lithium, phenytoin, trimethadione, procainamide,

quinidine sulphate and beta-adrenergic receptor-blocking drugs (including eye drops). Commonly prescribed agents listed with a possible association with exacerbation of MG were ampicillin, anticholinergic drugs, erythromycin, radiocontrast agents and verapamil. Most of these possible associations are based only on case reports. Penicillamine may induce a variant of MG (Wittbrodt 1997); D,L-carnitine has been reported to induce a myasthenia-like syndrome (Bazzato et al. 1981). In a patient deteriorating while on high-dose corticosteroids, the possibility of steroid-induced myopathy needs consideration.

TRANSIENT NEONATAL MYASTHENIA (NMG)
Approximately 5–10% of infants born to myasthenic mothers are affected by transient NMG (Hoff et al. 2003). Antibodies directed against acetylcholine receptors are transferred from the maternal to the fetal circulation. In one study, 13 of 30 newborn infants of myasthenic mothers were AChR antibody positive. All 5 newborns who were clinically affected were in the AChR antibody-positive group, and no AChR antibody-negative mothers had an affected baby (Batocchi et al. 1999), although some cases have been noted (Riemersma et al. 1996). Importantly, many patients with MG have antibodies directed not only against the main adult immunogenic region of the AChR but also against the fetal isoform (Polizzi et al. 2000). The adult to fetal antibody ratio has been found to predict, either before or during pregnancy, the occurrence of NMG for the first child at least (Gardnerova et al. 1997). There is no relation between the severity of maternal disease and involvement of the infant.

The clinical features of transient myasthenia are usually distinctive (Papazian 1992). The onset is delayed to a few hours after birth, sometimes as long as 3 days, and is marked by hypotonia, feeding difficulties due to poor sucking and/or swallowing, poor crying and facial diplegia. Ptosis is present in only a minority of cases. Respiratory distress requiring mechanical ventilation may occur. These features permit an easy diagnosis when myasthenia is known in the mother, but the mother may be undiagnosed or asymptomatic. The diagnosis can be confirmed by intramuscular or subcutaneous injection of neostigmine, and RNS can also be used to assist diagnosis but is technically difficult at this age and is also painful. Diagnostic, followed by therapeutic, use of neostigmine particularly prior to feeding time, is often preferable because of the longer time available for assessment (e.g. 0.1 mg per dose prior to feeding but with adjustment of dose depending on need).

In severe forms with respiratory distress and/or profound hypotonia, exchange transfusion has been used (Pasternak et al. 1981, Bassan et al. 1998). The role of IVIG is not clear (Bassan and Spirer 1999, Tagher et al. 1999). Symptoms usually resolve by 4–6 weeks but occasionally can take up to several months (Morel et al. 1988).

For a small number of infants of mothers with autoimmune MG (some of whom are asymptomatic), multiple congenital contractures and hypotonia dominate, although in some less severe cases there is a mixture of contractures and NMG features (Barnes et al. 1995). There is a high incidence of polyhydramnios, fetal or neonatal death and other, including CNS, abnor-

TABLE 21.10
Congenital myasthenia syndromes

Disorder	Neurophysiology	Clinical	Genetics	References
Presynaptic				
Congenital myasthenic syndrome with episodic apnoea (CMS-EA)	Decremental response	Episodic apnoea or respiratory failure anytime after birth, often triggered by infection. Ophthalmoplegia unusual. Responds well to anticholinesterase and tends to improve with age	Mutations in the gene encoding for choline acetyltransferase (*CHAT*)	Engel et al. (2003)
Other syndromes with decreased acetylcholine quantal release		One resembles the Lambert–Eaton myasthenic syndrome. Another may show mild ataxia or cerebellar nystagmus		Bady et al. (1987), Milone et al. (2006)
Synaptic				
Endplate acetylcholinesterase deficiency (EP AChE deficiency)	Repetitive and decrementing CMAP with single nerve stimulus	Often severe with ophthalmoplegia and weakness, particularly of axial muscles. Slow pupillary light response. Deterioration or no response to anticholinesterases	Mutations in the gene *COLQ* encoding for the collagenic tail of acetylcholinesterase	Engel et al. (2003)
Postsynaptic	Receptor deficiency, kinetic abnormality or disordered clustering of receptors			
AChR deficiency	Single response	Mild to severe cases. Early onset. Ptosis, ophthalmoplegia, oropharyngeal symptoms, limb weakness. May improve with antiAChE and 3,4-DAP. Moderately disabled	Mutations in AChR subunit genes, especially ε subunit	Burke et al. (2004)
AChR kinetic abnormalities				
Slow-channel syndrome (SCCMS)	Repetitive CMAP from single nerve stimulus	Variable age of onset and severity. Selective weakness of cervical, scapular and finger extensor muscles. Mild ophthalmoplegia. May deteriorate with anti-AChE drugs. Quinidine and fluoxetine have been used but potential serious side effects	Usually autosomal dominant. Autosomal recessive inheritance reported	Croxen et al. (2002), Engel et al. (2003), Harper et al. (2003)
Fast-channel syndrome (FCCMS)		Variable phenotype mild to severe. Responds well to anti-AChE alone or with 3,4-DAP but report of death in 2 children started on 3,4-DAP. Relation to 3,4-DAP not proven	Various mutations in AChR subunit genes	Engel et al. (2003), Beeson et al. (2005)
AChR aggregation abnormalities: endplate rapsyn deficiency				
Rapsyn-EO (early onset)	Often normal RNS	Mild arthrogryposis, hypotonia, oropharyngeal dysfunction, episodic apnoea or respiratory failure from birth, facial dysmorphism in some, ophthalmoplegia rare. Response to anti-AChE alone or with 3,4-DAP		Burke et al. (2004)
Rapsyn-LO (late onset)		Onset in adolescence or adulthood. Misdiagnosed as seronegative MG. Responds to anti-AChE		Burke et al. (2004)
Others				
Muscle-specific receptor tyrosine kinase (MuSK)	Decremental response	Neonatal onset. Ptosis and respiratory distress	Mutation in the gene encoding for muscle-specific receptor tyrosine kinase (*MuSK*)	Chevessier et al. (2004)
SCN4A (Nav1.4) sodium channel	Decremental response	Ptosis, weakness, recurrent respiratory and bulbar paralysis	Mutation in the gene encoding the voltage-gated sodium channel SCN4A (*Nav1.4*)	Engel et al. (2003)

AChR = acetylcholine receptor; anti-AChE = anti-acetylcholinesterase; CMAP = compound muscle action potential; 3,4-DAP = 3,4-diaminopyridine; RNS = repetitive nerve stimulation; MG = myasthenia gravis.

malities (Polizzi et al. 2000). The recurrence rate is extremely high but the outcome may be improved by maternal treatment (Vincent et al. 1995, Polizzi et al. 2000). There is a high association with the presence of fetal isoform AChR antibodies, although this is not invariable, and it is likely that antibodies to other proteins may also be involved (Polizzi et al. 2000). Mild joint contractures may also be seen in some of the congenital myasthenic syndromes (see below).

CONGENITAL MYASTHENIA SYNDROMES (Table 21.10)

The congenital myasthenia syndromes (CMS) are not antibody-mediated but are genetically determined disorders compromising neuromuscular transmission and usually presenting in the newborn period or the first year or two of life. Anatomically, CMS may arise from molecular defects of proteins at presynaptic, synaptic or postsynaptic levels, and many of the responsible gene mutations are known (Engel et al. 2003). Occasionally presentation can be in later childhood or even adult life, when misdiagnosis as seronegative autoimmune MG becomes a major issue (Burke et al. 2004). Autosomal recessive inheritance is usual but most patients with the slow channel syndrome show autosomal dominant inheritance.

The clinical picture is heterogeneous. Reduced fetal movements and arthrogryposis may be the first problem. Feeding difficulties with poor suck and cry, ptosis and ophthalmoplegia, and facial and generalized weakness often dominate the neonatal period. Mild facial dysmorphism and high-arched palate is reported (Goldhammer et al. 1990, Burke et al. 2004). Later, delay in motor milestones, fluctuaing ptosis and ophthalmoplegia (Mullaney et al. 2000), oropharyngeal dysfunction requiring artificial tube feeding and with the risk of aspiration, weakness and fatiguability may occur. Scoliosis may also be seen. Life-threatening episodes of respiratory insufficiency with sudden apnoea and cyanosis can be a major issue from birth or later in infancy. Often these episodes are precipitated by minor infections or other intercurrent illnesses and they are the hallmark of what is now called CMS with episodic apnoea (CMSEA), previously known as familial infantile myasthenia (Engel et al. 2003). Response to treatment with anticholinesterase and 3-4 diaminopyridine (which increases acetylcholine quantal release) depends on the defect. Ephedrine is reported to help some patients (Beeson et al. 2005).

While understanding of these syndromes is still incomplete, recent advances are allowing better classification and genotype–phenotype correlations (Beeson et al. 2005).

LAMBERT–EATON SYNDROME AND OTHER DEFECTS IN NEUROMUSCULAR TRANSMISSION

LAMBERT–EATON MYASTHENIA SYNDROME (LEMS)

Lambert–Eaton myasthenia syndrome (LEMS) consists of fatiguable muscle weakness, hyporeflexia, autonomic disturbance and a characteristic response to repetitive nerve stimulation due to autoimmune presynaptic impairment of neuromuscular transmission. About half of adults affected have small-cell lung cancer (Wirtz et al. 2004), with the syndrome mediated by P/Q-type voltage-gated calcium-channel antibodies to calcium channels in the tumour. The trigger for those without this tumour is unknown. Electrophysiological characterization with RNS depends on demonstration of initially low compound muscle action potentials, an initial decrement at low rates of stimulation (e.g. 2–5 Hz) and with post-exercise (maximum voluntary contraction) or post-tetanic potentiation of at least 25% but preferably 100% for greater accuracy (AAEM 2001b). Others suggest that a 60% increment is appropriate for diagnosis (Oh et al. 2005).

LEMS is extremely rare in children. Patients with an age at onset as young as 8 (Tim et al. 2000) and 11 years (Maddison et al. 2001, Wirtz et al. 2004) are reported in large studies, but details are not included. A case reported as a congenital form (Bady et al. 1987) is a type of presynaptic congenital myasthenia resembling LEMS (Milone et al. 2006). Two children with P/Q-type calcium channel antibodies but without tumour responded to cyclosporine (Tsao et al. 2002). Another child developed an AChR-negative LEMS-like syndrome at 9½ years with electrophysiological characteristics of a presynaptic defect, autoantibodies in the context of multiple other autoimmune disorders, and a family history of autoimmune disorders (Hoffman et al. 2003).

IVIG and 3-4 diaminopyridine are useful for symptomatic treatment of LEMS (Tim et al. 2000, Maddison and Newsom-Davis 2005). Immunosuppressive therapy requirements depend on the underlying disorder.

Some sporadic and familial (probably autosomal recessive) cases of *juvenile limb–girdle myasthenia* have been described. There is proximal weakness fluctuating over time and with some response to anticholinesterases, but little if any ocular involvement. The CK level is often increased, and electrophysiological studies are consistent with a postsynaptic defect. Muscle biopsy often shows tubular aggregates. Known CMS gene defects have been eliminated and further studies are underway (Husain et al. 1989, Beeson et al. 2005).

OTHER NEUROMUSCULAR BLOCKS

Drugs potentially interfering with neuromuscular transmission are discussed earlier in the section on JMG and the topic has been reviewed by Wittbrodt (1997). Toxins of several venomous animals have been instrumental in understanding the structure and function of the neuromuscular junction (Vincent et al. 2000). Agents that impair neuromuscular transmission at a presynaptic level include arthropod venoms and some insect bites, while at the postsynaptic level several snake venoms are active. Magnesium intoxication acts antagonistically to calcium at the neuromuscular junction. A prolonged myasthenic syndrome has been reported in patients treated with muscle relaxants (Benzing et al. 1990). Electrophysiological abnormalities are an indication of the acetylcholinesterase inhibition secondary to organophosphate poisoning (Besser et al. 1989).

REFERENCES

AAEM (2001a) American Association of Electrodiagnostic Medicine glossary of terms in electrodiagnostic medicine. *Muscle Nerve* 24 Suppl 10: S1–50.

AAEM Quality Assurance Committee. American Association of Electrodiagnostic Medicine (2001b) Literature review of the usefulness of repetitive nerve stimulation and single fiber EMG in the electrodiagnostic evaluation of patients with suspected myasthenia gravis or Lambert–Eaton myasthenic syndrome. *Muscle Nerve* 24: 1239–47.

Aasly J, van Diggelen OP, Boer AM, Bronstad G (2000) Phosphoglycerate kinase deficiency in two brothers with McArdle-like clinical symptoms. *Eur J Neurol* 7: 111–3.

Abarbanel JM, Potashnik R, Frisher S, et al. (1987) Myophosphorylase deficiency: the course of an unusual congenital myopathy. *Neurology* 37: 316–8.

Adams C, Theodorescu D, Murphy G, Shandling B (1990) Thymectomy in juvenile myasthenia gravis. *J Child Neurol* 5: 216–8.

Adnet P, Lestavel P, Krivosic-Horber R (2000) Neuroleptic malignant syndrome. *Br J Anaesth* 85: 129–35.

Afifi AK, Bell WE (1993) Tests for juvenile myasthenia gravis: comparative diagnostic yield and prediction of outcome. *J Child Neurol* 8: 404–11.

Agostino A, Valletta L, Chinnery PF, Ferrari G, et al. (2003) Mutations of ANT1, Twinkle, and POLG1 in sporadic progressive external ophthalmoplegia (PEO). *Neurology* 60: 1354–6.

Akiyama C, Nonaka I (1996) A follow-up study of congenital non-progressive myopathies. *Brain Dev* 18: 404–8.

Allen GC, Larach MG, Kunselman AR (1998) The sensitivity and specificity of the caffeine–halothane contracture test: a report from the North American Malignant Hyperthermia Registry. The North American Malignant Hyperthermia Registry of MHAUS. *Anesthesiology* 88: 579–88.

Alman BA, Raza SN, Biggar WD (2004) Steroid treatment and the development of scoliosis in males with Duchenne muscular dystrophy. *J Bone Joint Surg Am* 86-A: 519–24.

Al-Mayouf SM, Al-Eid W, Bahabri S, Al-Mofada S (2001) Interstitial pneumonitis and air leakage in juvenile dermatomyositis. *Rheumatology* 40: 588–90.

Alyaarubi S, Rodd C (2005) Treatment of malabsorption vitamin D deficiency myopathy with intramuscular vitamin D. *J Pediatr Endocrinol Metab* 18: 719–22.

Amato AA, Griggs RC (2003) Unicorns, dragons, polymyositis, and other mythological beasts. *Neurology* 61: 288–90.

Anderson JL, Head SI, Rae C, Morley JW (2002) Brain function in Duchenne muscular dystrophy. *Brain* 125: 4–13.

Andresen BS, Olpin S, Poorthuis BJ, et al. (1999) Clear correlation of genotype with disease phenotype in very-long-chain acyl-CoA dehydrogenase deficiency. *Am J Hum Genet* 64: 479–94.

Andreu AL, Hanna MG, Reichmann H, et al. (1999) Exercise intolerance due to mutations in the cytochrome b gene of mitochondrial DNA. *N Engl J Med* 341: 1037–44.

Andrews PI, Massey JM, Sanders DB (1993) Acetylcholine receptor antibodies in juvenile myasthenia gravis. *Neurology* 43: 977–82.

Andrews PI, Massey JM, Howard JF, Sanders DB (1994) Race, sex, and puberty influence onset, severity, and outcome in juvenile myasthenia gravis. *Neurology* 44: 1208–14.

Anlar B, Senbil N, Köse G, Degerliyurt A (2005) Serological follow-up in juvenile myasthenia: clinical and acetylcholine receptor antibody status of patients followed for at least 2 years. *Neuromuscul Disord* 15: 355–7.

Arakawa H, Yamada H, Kurihara Y, et al. (2003) Nonspecific interstitial pneumonia associated with polymyositis and dermatomyositis: serial high-resolution CT findings and functional correlation. *Chest* 123: 1096–103.

Argov Z, Bank WJ (1991) Phosphorus magnetic resonance spectroscopy (31P MRS) in neuromuscular disorders. *Ann Neurol* 30: 90–7.

Asai T, Fujise K, Uchida M (1992) Anaesthesia for cardiac surgery in children with nemaline myopathy. *Anaesthesia* 47: 405–8.

Ashwal S, Peckham N (1985) Myoadenylate deaminase deficiency in children. *Pediatr Neurol* 1: 185–8.

Aure K, Benoist JF, Ogier de Baulny H, et al. (2004) Progression despite replacement of a myopathic form of coenzyme Q10 defect. *Neurology* 63: 727–9.

Bach JR, O'Brien J, Krotenberg R, Alba AS (1987) Management of end stage respiratory failure in Duchenne muscular dystrophy. *Muscle Nerve* 10: 177–82.

Bady B, Chauplannaz G, Carrier H (1987) Congenital Lambert–Eaton myasthenic syndrome. *J Neurol Neurosurg Psychiatry* 50: 476–8.

Bailey RO, Marzulo DC, Harris MB (1986) Infantile facioscapulohumeral muscular dystrophy: new observations. *Acta Neurol Scand* 74: 51–8.

Baker EM, Khorasgani G, Gardner-Medwin D, et al. (1996) Arthrogryposis multiplex congenita and bilateral parietal polymicrogyria in association with intrauterine death of a twin. *Neuropediatrics* 27: 54–6.

Baker NL, Mörgelin M, Peat R, et al. (2005) Dominant collagen VI mutations are a common cause of Ullrich congenital muscular dystrophy. *Hum Mol Genet* 14: 279–93.

Banker BQ (1994) Congenital deformities. In: Engel AG, Franzini-Armstrong C, eds. *Myology, Basic and Clinical. 2nd edn.* New York: McGraw-Hill, pp. 1905–37.

Bansal D, Campbell KP (2004) Dysferlin and the plasma membrane repair in muscular dystrophy. *Trends Cell Biol* 14: 206–13.

Banwell BL, Becker LE, Jay V, et al. (1999) Cardiac manifestations of congenital fibre-type disproportion myopathy. *J Child Neurol* 14: 83–7.

Banwell BL, Mildner RJ, Hassall AC, et al. (2003) Muscle weakness in critically ill children. *Neurology* 61: 1779–82.

Barker RA, Revesz T, Thom M, et al. (1998) Review of 23 patients affected by the stiff man syndrome: clinical subdivision into stiff trunk (man) syndrome, stiff limb syndrome, and progressive encephalomyelitis with rigidity. *J Neurol Neurosurg Psychiatry* 65: 633–40.

Barnes PR, Kanabar DJ, Brueton L, et al. (1995) Recurrent congenital arthrogryposis leading to a diagnosis of myasthenia gravis in an initially asymptomatic mother. *Neuromuscul Disord* 5: 59–65.

Barohn RJ, Levine EJ, Olson JO, Mendell JR (1988) Gastric hypomotility in Duchenne's muscular dystrophy. *N Engl J Med* 319: 15–8.

Barresi R, Michele DE, Kanagawa M, et al. (2004) LARGE can functionally bypass alpha-dystroglycan glycosylation defects in distinct congenital muscular dystrophies. *Nat Med* 10: 696–703.

Bassan H, Spirer Z (1999) Intravenous immunoglobulin in neonatal myasthenia gravis. *J Pediatr* 135: 790.

Bassan H, Muhlbaur B, Tomer A, Spirer Z (1998) High-dose intravenous immunoglobulin in transient neonatal myasthenia gravis. *Pediatr Neurol* 18: 181–3.

Batocchi AP, Majolini L, Evoli A, et al. (1999) Course and treatment of myasthenia gravis during pregnancy. *Neurology* 52: 447–52.

Bazzato C, Coli U, Landini S, et al. (1981) Myasthenia-like syndrome after D,L-but not L-carnitine. *Lancet* 1: 1209 (letter).

Beals RK (2005) The distal arthrogryposes: a new classification of peripheral contractures. *Clin Orthop Relat Res* 435: 203–10.

Beeson D, Hantai D, Lochmuller H, Engel AG (2005) 126th International Workshop: congenital myasthenic syndromes, 24–26 September 2004, Naarden, the Netherlands. *Neuromuscul Disord* 15: 498–512.

Beltran-Valero DB, Currier S, Steinbrecher A, et al. (2002) Mutations in the O-mannosyltransferase gene POMT1 give rise to the severe neuronal migration disorder Walker–Warburg syndrome. *Am J Hum Genet* 71: 1033–43.

Beltran-Valero DB, Voit T, Longman C, et al. (2004) Mutations in the FKRP gene can cause muscle–eye–brain disease and Walker–Warburg syndrome. *J Med Genet* 41: e61.

Bendahan D, Pouget J, Pellissier JF, et al. (1996) Magnetic resonance spectroscopy and histological study of tubular aggregates in a familial myopathy. *J Neurol Sci* 139: 149–55.

Benzing G, Iannacone ST, Bove KE, et al. (1990) Prolonged myasthenic syndrome after one week of muscle relaxants. *Pediatr Neurol* 6: 190–6.

Bergia B, Sybers HD, Butler IJ (1986) Familial lethal cardiomyopathy with mental retardation and scapuloperoneal muscular atrophy. *J Neurol Neurosurg Psychiatry* 49: 1423–6.

Berkelhammer C, Bear RA (1985) A clinical approach to common electrolyte problems: 4. Hypomagnesemia. *Can Med Assoc J* 132: 360–8.

Bertini E, Pepe G (2002) Collagen type VI and related disorders: Bethlem myopathy and Ullrich scleroatonic muscular dystrophy. *Eur J Paediatr Neurol* 6: 193–8.

Besser R, Gutmann L, Dillmann U, et al. (1989) End-plate dysfunction in acute organophosphate intoxication. *Neurology* 39: 561–7.

Betz RC, Schoser BG, Kasper D, et al. (2001) Mutations in CAV3 cause mechanical hyperirritability of skeletal muscle in rippling muscle disease. *Nat Genet* 28: 218–219.

Biggar WD, Harris VA, Eliasoph L, Alman B (2006) Long-term benefits of deflazacort treatment for boys with Duchenne muscular dystrophy in their second decade. *Neuromuscul Disord* 16: 249–55.

Bitoun M, Maugenre S, Jeannet P-Y, et al. (2005) Mutations in dynamin 2 cause dominant centronuclear myopathy. *Nat Genet* 37: 1207–9.

Blaszczyk M, Jablonska S, Szymanska-Jagiello W, et al. (1991) Childhood scleromyositis: an overlap syndrome associated with PM-Scl antibody. *Pediatr Dermatol* 8: 1–8.

Bodensteiner JB (1994) Congenital myopathies. *Muscle Nerve* 17: 131–44.

Bolton CF (2005) Neuromuscular manifestations of critical illness. *Muscle Nerve* 32: 140–63.

Bonne G, Carrier L, Richard P, et al. (1998) Familial hypertrophic cardiomyopathy: from mutations to functional defects. *Circ Res* 83: 580–93.

Bonne G, Yaou RB, Béroud C, et al. (2003) 108th ENMC International Workshop, 3rd Workshop of the MYO-CLUSTER project: EUROMEN, 7th International Emery–Dreifuss Muscular Dystrophy (EDMD) Workshop, 13–15 September 2002, Naarden, The Netherlands. *Neuromuscul Disord* 13: 508–15.

Bönnemann CG, Wong J, Jones KJ, et al. (2002) Primary γ-sarcoglycanopathy (LGMD 2C): broadening of the mutational spectrum guided by the immunohistochemical profile. *Neuromuscul Disord* 12: 273–80.

Bowyer SL, Blane, C.E., Sullivan, D.B., Cassidy, J.T. (1983) Childhood dermatomyositis: factors predicting functional outcome and development of dystrophic calcification. *J Pediatr* 103: 882–8.

Boylan KB, Ferriero DM, Greco CM, et al. (1992) Congenital hypomyelination neuropathy with arthrogryposis multiplex congenita. *Ann Neurol* 31: 337–40.

Braakhekke JP, De Bruin MI, Stegeman DF, et al. (1986) The second wind phenomenon in McArdle's disease. *Brain* 109: 1087–101.

Breningstall GN, Grover WD, Barbera S, Marks HG (1988) Neonatal rhabdomyolysis as a presentation of muscular dystrophy. *Neurology* 38: 1271–2.

Bresolin N, Bet L, Moggio M, et al. (1989) Muscle glucose-6-phosphate dehydrogenase deficiency. *J Neurol* 236: 193–8.

Brockington M, Sewry CA, Herrmann R, et al. (2000) Assignment of a form of congenital muscular dystrophy with secondary merosin deficiency to chromosome 1q42. *Am J Hum Genet* 66: 428–35.

Brockington M, Blake DJ, Prandini P, et al. (2001a) Mutations in the fukutin-related protein gene (FKRP) cause a form of congenital muscular dystrophy with secondary laminin alpha2 deficiency and abnormal glycosylation of alpha-dystroglycan. *Am J Hum Genet* 69: 1198–209.

Brockington M, Yuva Y, Prandini P, et al. (2001b) Mutations in the fukutin-related protein gene (FKRP) identify limb girdle muscular dystrophy 2I as a milder allelic variant of congenital muscular dystrophy MDC1C. *Hum Mol Genet* 10: 2851–9.

Brooke MH (1973) Congenital fibre type disproportion. In: Kakulas BA, ed. *Clinical Studies in Myology. Proceedings of the 2nd International Congress on Muscle Diseases, Perth, Australia, Nov. 22–29, 1971.* Amsterdam: Excerpta Medica ICS, pp. 147–59.

Brooke MH, Engel WK (1969) The histographic analysis of human muscle biopsies with regard to fibre types: IV. Children's biopsies. *Neurology* 19: 591–605.

Brooke MH, Fenichel GM, Griggs RC, et al. (1989) Duchenne muscular dystrophy: patterns of clinical progression and effects of supportive therapy. *Neurology* 39: 475–81.

Brownlow S, Webster R, Croxen R, et al. (2001) Acetylcholine receptor delta subunit mutations underlie a fast-channel myasthenic syndrome and arthrogryposis multiplex congenita. *J Clin Invest* 108: 125–30.

Bruno C, Bertini E, Santorelli FM, DiMauro S (2000) HyperCKemia as the only sign of McArdle's disease in a child. *J Child Neurol* 15: 137–8.

Bruno C, van Diggelen OP, Cassandrini D, et al. (2004) Clinical and genetic heterogeneity of branching enzyme deficiency (glycogenosis type IV). *Neurology* 63: 1053–8.

Buckley AE, Dean J, Mahy IR (1999) Cardiac involvement in Emery Dreifuss muscular dystrophy: a case series. *Heart* 82: 105–8.

Buhrer C, van Landeghem F, Bruck W, et al. (2000) Fetal-onset severe skeletal muscle glycogenosis associated with phosphorylase-b kinase deficiency. *Neuropediatrics* 31: 104–6.

Burglen L, Amiel J, Viollet L, et al. (1996) Survival motor neuron gene deletion in the arthrogryposis multiplex congenita–spinal muscular atrophy association. *J Clin Invest* 98: 1130–2.

Burke G, Cossins J, Maxwell S, et al. (2004) Distinct phenotypes of congenital acetylcholine receptor deficiency. *Neuromuscul Disord* 14: 356–64.

Burns RJ, Bretag AH, Blumbergs PC, Harbord MG (1994) Benign familial disease with muscle mounding and rippling. *J Neurol Neurosurg Psychiatry* 57: 344–7.

Bushby KMD, Gardner-Medwin D (1993) The clinical, genetic and dystrophin characteristics of Becker muscular dystrophy. I. Natural history. *J Neurol* 240: 98–104.

Bushby KMD, Gardner-Medwin D, Nicholson LVB, et al. (1993) The clinical, genetic and dystrophin characteristics of Becker muscular dystrophy. II.

Correlation of phenotype with genetic and protein abnormalities. *J Neurol* 240: 105–12.

Bushby KMD, Hill A, Steele JG (1999) Failure of early diagnosis in symptomatic Duchenne muscular dystrophy. *Lancet* 353: 557–8.

Bykhovskaya Y, Casas K, Mengesha E, et al. (2004) Missense mutation in pseudouridine synthase 1 (PUS1) causes mitochondrial myopathy and sideroblastic anemia (MLASA). *Am J Hum Genet* 74: 1303–8.

Byrne E, Dennett X, Trounce I, Henderson R (1985) Partial cytochrome oxidase (aa3) deficiency in chronic progressive external ophthalmoplegia. Histochemical and biochemical studies. *J Neurol Sci* 71: 257–71.

Caldwell CJ, Swash M, Van der Walt JD, Geddes JF (1995) Focal myositis: a clinicopathological study. *Neuromuscul Disord* 5: 317–21.

Calhoun RF, Ritter JH, Guthrie TJ, et al. (1999) Results of transcervical thymectomy for myasthenia gravis in 100 consecutive patients. *Ann Surg* 230: 555–9.

Camacho Vanegas O, Bertini E, Zhang RZ, et al. (2001) Ullrich scleroatonic muscular dystrophy is caused by recessive mutations in collagen type VI. *Proc Natl Acad Sci USA* 98: 7516–21.

Cameron PF (1983) Strained abdominal muscles as a cause of acute abdominal pain in children and young adults and its treatment with Paramax. *Br J Clin Pract* 37: 178–80.

Cao A, Cainchetti C, Calisti L et al. (1978) Schwartz–Jampel syndrome: clinical electrophysiological and histopathological study of a severe variant. *J Neurol Sci* 35: 175–87.

Chan W, Wong GWK, Fan DSP, et al. (2002) Ophthalmopathy in childhood Grave's disease. *Br J Ophthalmol* 86: 740–2.

Charnas L, Trapp B, Griffin J (1988) Congenital absence of peripheral myelin: abnormal Schwann cell development causes lethal arthrogryposis multiplex congenita. *Neurology* 38: 966–74.

Chaudhry V, Cornblath DR, Griffin JW, et al. (2001) Mycophenolate mofetil: a safe and promising immunosuppressant in neuromuscular diseases. *Neurology* 56: 94–6.

Chen SS, Chien CH, Yu HS (1988) Syndrome of deltoid and/or gluteal fibrotic contracture: an injection myopathy. *Acta Neurol Scand* 78: 167–76.

Cheng JCY, Tang SP, Chen TMK, et al. (2002) The clinical presentation and outcome of treatment of congenital muscular torticollis in infants—a study of 1,086 cases. *J Pediatr Surg* 35: 1091–6.

Chevessier F, Faraut B, Ravel-Chapuis A, et al. (2004) MUSK, a new target for mutations causing congenital myasthenic syndrome. *Hum Mol Genet* 13: 3229–40.

Chiba S, Hatanaka Y, Ohkubo Y, et al. (1999) Focal myositis: magnetic resonance imaging findings and peripheral arterial administration of prednisolone. *Clin Rheumatol* 18: 495–8.

Choy EHS, Hoogendijk JE, Lecky B, Winer JB (2005) Immunosuppressant and immunomodulatory treatment for dermatomyositis and polymyositis. *Cochrane Database Syst Rev* (3): CD003643.

Chui LA, Munsat TL (1976) Dominant inheritance of McArdle syndrome. *Arch Neurol* 33: 636–41.

Clarke N, North KN (2003) Congenital fiber type disproportion – pathology in search of a disease. *J Neuropathol Exp Neurol* 62: 977–89.

Clarke NF, Smith R, Bahlo M, North KN (2005) A novel X-linked form of congenital fibre type disproportion. *Ann Neurol* 58: 767–72.

Clarke NF, Kidson W, Quijano-Roy S, et al. (2006) SEPN1: Associated with congenital fibre type disproportion and insulin resistance. *Ann Neurol* 59: 546–52.

Clarke NF, Kolski H, Dye DE, et al. (2008) Mutations in TPM3 are a common cause of congenital fiber type disproportion. *Ann Neurol* 63: 329–37.

Coco TJ, Klasner AE (2004) Drug-induced rhabdomyolysis. *Curr Opin Pediatr* 16: 206–10.

Cohn RD (2005) Dystroglycan: important player in skeletal muscle and beyond. *Neuromuscul Disord* 15: 207–17.

Collison CH, Sinal SH, Jorizzo JL, et al. (1998) Juvenile dermatomyositis and polymyositis: a follow-up study of long-term sequelae. *South Med J* 91: 17–22.

Comi G, Testa D, Cornelio F, et al. (1985) Potassium depletion myopathy: a clinical and morphological study of 6 cases. *Muscle Nerve* 8: 17–21.

Comi G, Prelle A, Bresolin N, et al. (1994) Clinical variability in Becker muscular dystrophy. Genetic, biochemical and immunohistochemical correlates. *Brain* 117: 1–14.

Connolly MB, Roland EH, Hill A (1992) Clinical features for prediction of survival in neonatal muscle disease. *Pediatr Neurol* 8: 285–8.

Cooper ST, North KN (2006) Methodological approach to protein diagnosis of dystrophinopathies. In: Chamberlain JS, Rando TA, eds. *Duchenne Muscular Dystrophy. Advances in Therapeutics*. New York: Taylor & Francis, pp. 112–7.

Cornelio F, Bresolin N, DiMauro S, et al. (1983) Congenital myopathy due to phosphorylase deficiency. *Neurology* 33: 1383–5.

Cotton S, Voudouris NJ, Greenwood KM (2001) Intelligence and Duchenne muscular dystrophy: full-scale, verbal, and performance intelligence quotients. *Dev Med Child Neurol* 43: 497–501.

Cotton SM, Voudouris NJ, Greenwood KM (2005) Association between intellectual functioning and age in children and young adults with Duchenne muscular dystrophy: further results from a meta-analysis. *Dev Med Child Neurol* 47: 257–65.

Croxen R, Hatton C, Shelley C, et al. (2002) Recessive inheritance and variable penetrance of slow-channel congenital myasthenic syndromes. *Neurology* 59: 162–8.

Currier SC, Lee CK, Chang BS, et al. (2005) Mutations in POMT1 are found in a minority of patients with Walker–Warburg syndrome. *Am J Med Genet A* 133: 53–7.

Dalakas MC (1998) Controlled studies with high-dose intravenous immunoglobulin in the treatment of dermatomyositis, inclusion body myositis, and polymyositis. *Neurology* 51 Suppl 5: 37–45.

Dalakas MC (2004) Inflammatory disorders of muscle: progress in polymyositis, dermatomyositis and inclusion body myositis. *Curr Opin Neurol* 17: 561–7.

Dalakas MC (2005) The role of IVIg in the treatment of patients with stiff person syndrome and other neurological diseases associated with anti-GAD antibodies. *J Neurol* 252 Suppl 1: I19–25.

Dalakas MC (2006a) Therapeutic targets in patients with inflammatory myopathies: present approaches and a look to the future. *Neuromuscul Disord* 16: 223–36.

Dalakas MC (2006b) The role of high-dose immune globulin intravenous in the treatment of dermatomyositis. *Int Immunopharmacol* 6: 550–6.

Dalakas MC, Fujii M, Li M, McElroy B (2000) The clinical spectrum of anti-GAD antibody-positive patients with stiff-person syndrome. *Neurology* 55: 1531–5.

Danon MJ, Oh SJ, DiMauro S (1981) Lysosomal glycogen storage disease with normal acid maltase. *Neurology* 31: 51–7.

Danon MJ, Karpati G, Charuk J, Holland P (1988) Sarcoplasmic reticulum adenosine triphosphatase deficiency with probable autosomal dominant inheritance. *Neurology* 38: 812–5.

Daras M, Spiro AJ (1981) 'Stiff-man syndrome' in an adolescent. *Pediatrics* 67: 725–6.

Darin N, Moslemi A-R, Lebon S, et al. (2003) Genotypes and clinical phenotypes in children with cytochrome-c oxidase deficiency. *Neuropediatrics* 34: 311–7.

Darwish H, Sarnat H, Archer C, et al. (1981) Congenital cervical spinal atrophy. *Muscle Nerve* 4: 106–10.

Deconinck N, Van Parijs V, Beckers-Bleukx G, Van den Bergh P (1998) Critical illness myopathy unrelated to corticosteroids or neuromuscular blocking agents. *Neuromuscul Disord* 8: 186–92.

de Die-Smulders CE, Howeler CJ, Thijs C (1998) Age and causes of death in adult-onset myotonic dystrophy. *Brain* 121: 1557–63.

DeFilippi VJ, Richman DP, Ferguson MK (1994) Transcervical thymectomy for myasthenia gravis. *Ann Thorac Surg* 57: 194–7.

de la Peña LS, Billings PC, Fiori JL et al. (2005) Fibrodysplasia ossificans progressiva (FOP), a disorder of ectopic osteogenesis, misregulates cell surface expression and trafficking of BMPRIA. *J Bone Miner Res* 20: 1168–76.

Delaporte C (1998) Personality patterns in patients with myotonic dystrophy. *Arch Neurol* 55: 635–40.

Delatycki M, Rogers JG (1998) The genetics of fibrodysplasia ossificans progressiva. *Clin Orthopaed Relat Res* 346: 15–8.

de Paula F, Vieira N, Starling A, et al. (2003) Asymptomatic carriers for homozygous novel mutations in the FKRP gene: the other end of the spectrum. *Eur J Hum Genet* 11: 923–30.

de Visser M, de Voogt WG, la Rivière GV (1992) The heart in Becker muscular dystrophy, facioscapulohumeral dystrophy, and Bethlem myopathy. *Muscle Nerve* 15: 591–6.

Dhand UK (2006) Isaacs' syndrome: clinical and electrophysiological response to gabapentin. *Muscle Nerve* 34: 646–50.

DiBona FJ, Morens DM (1977) Rhabdomyolysis associated with influenza A. Report of a case with unusual fluid and electrolyte abnormalities. *J Pediatr* 91: 943–5.

Di Giovanni S, Mirabella M, Spinazzola A, et al. (2001) Coenzyme Q10 re-

verses pathological phenotype and reduces apoptosis in familial CoQ10 deficiency. *Neurology* 57: 515–8.

DiMauro S (1993) Mitochondrial encephalomyopathies. In: Rosenberg RN, Prusiner SB, DiMauro S, eds. *The Molecular and Genetic Basis of Neurological Disease*. Boston: Butterworth-Heinemann, pp. 665–94.

DiMauro S, Gurgel-Giannetti J (2005) The expanding phenotype of mitochondrial myopathy. *Curr Opin Neurol* 18: 538–42.

DiMauro S, Hirano M (2005) Mitochondrial encephalomyopathies: an update. *Neuromuscul Disord* 15: 276–86.

DiMauro S, Tsujino S (1994) Phosphorylase deficiency. In: Engel AG, Franzini-Armstrong C, eds. *Myology, Basic and Clinical. 2nd edn*. New York: McGraw-Hill, pp. 1557–61.

DiMauro S, Miranda AF, Olarte M, et al. (1982) Muscle phosphoglycerate mutase deficiency. *Neurology* 32: 584–91.

Di Muzio A, Capasso M, Verrotti A, et al. (2004) Macrophagic myofasciitis: an infantile Italian case. *Neuromuscul Disord* 14: 175–7.

Di Rocco M, Callea F, Pollice B, et al. (1995) Arthrogryposis, renal dysfunction and cholestasis syndrome: report of five patients from three Italian families. *Eur J Pediatr* 154: 835–9.

Domizio S, Romanelli A, Brindisino P, et al. (2005) Glutaric aciduria type II: a case report. *Int J Immunopathol Pharmacol* 18: 805–8.

Donley DK, Evans BK (1989) Reversible neuromuscular syndrome in malnourished children. *Dev Med Child Neurol* 31: 797–803.

Donner K, Ollikainen M, Ridanpaa M, et al. (2002) Mutations in the β-tropomyosin (TPM2) gene – a rare cause of nemaline myopathy. *Neuromuscul Disord* 12: 151–8.

Dooley JM, Andermann F (1989) Startle disease or hyperekplexia: adolescent onset and response to valproate. *Pediatr Neurol* 5: 126–7.

Doriguzzi C, Palmucci L, Mongini T, et al. (1993) Exercise intolerance and recurrent myoglobinuria as the only expression of Xp21 Becker type muscular dystrophy. *J Neurol* 240: 269–71.

Drachman DB (1994) Myasthenia gravis. *N Engl J Med* 330: 1797–810.

Dubowitz V (1995) *Muscle Disorders in Childhood, 2nd edn*. London: WB Saunders.

Dubowitz V (2002) Therapeutic possibilities in muscular dystrophy: the hope versus the hype. *Neuromuscul Disord* 12: 113–6.

Dubowitz V, Crome L (1969) The central nervous system in Duchenne muscular dystrophy. *Brain* 92: 505–8.

Duyff RF, Van den Bosch J, Laman DM, et al. (2000) Neuromuscular findings in thyroid dysfunction: a prospective clinical and electrodiagnostic study. *J Neurol Neurosurg Psychiatry* 68: 750–5.

Eagle M, Baudouin SV, Chandler C, et al. (2002) Survival in Duchenne muscular dystrophy: improvements in life expectancy since 1967 and the impact of home nocturnal ventilation. *Neuromuscul Disord* 12: 926–9.

Elpeleg O (2003) Inherited mitochondrial DNA depletion. *Pediatr Res* 54: 153–9.

Elpeleg O, Miller C, Hershkovitz E, et al. (2005) Deficiency of the ADP-forming succinyl-CoA synthase activity is associated with encephalomyopathy and mitochondrial DNA depletion. *Am J Hum Genet* 76: 1081–6.

el-Schahawi M, Tsujino S, Shanske S, DiMauro S (1996) Diagnosis of McArdle's disease by molecular genetic analysis of blood. *Neurology* 47: 579–80.

Emanuel BS, Zackai EH, Tucker SH (1983) Further evidence for Xp21 location of Duchenne muscular dystrophy (DMD) locus: X;9 translocation in a female with DMD. *J Med Genet* 20: 461–3.

Emser W (1982) Hypermagnesemic periodic paralysis: treatment with digitalis and lithium carbonate. *Arch Neurol* 39: 727–30.

Engel AG, Ohno K, Sine SM (2003) Congenital myasthenic syndromes: a diverse array of molecular targets. *J Neurocytol* 32: 1017–37.

Evoli A, Tonali PA, Padua L, et al. (2003) Clinical correlates with anti-MuSK antibodies in generalized seronegative myasthenia gravis. *Brain* 126: 2304–11.

Farbu E, Softeland E, Bindoff LA (2003) Anaesthetic complications associated with myotonia congenita: case study and comparison with other myotonic disorders. *Acta Anaesthesiol Scand* 47: 630–4.

Fedrizzi E, Botteon G, Inverno M, et al. (1993) Neurogenic arthrogryposis multiplex congenita: clinical and MRI findings. *Pediatr Neurol* 9: 343–8.

Ferreiro A, Estournet B, Château D, et al. (2000) Multi-minicore disease. Searching for boundaries: phenotype analysis of 38 cases. *Ann Neurol* 48: 745–57.

Ferreiro A, Monnier N, Romero NB, et al. (2002a) A recessive form of central core disease, transiently presenting as multi-minicore disease, is associated with a homozygous mutation in the ryanodine receptor type 1 gene. *Ann Neurol* 51: 750–9.

Ferreiro A, Quijano-Roy S, Pichereau C, et al. (2002b) Mutations in the selenoprotein N gene, which is implicated in rigid spine muscular dystrophy, cause the classical phenotype of multiminicore disease: reassessing the nosology of early-onset myopathies. *Am J Hum Genet* 71: 739–49.

Ferreiro A, Ceuterick-de Groote C, Marks JJ, et al. (2004) Desmin-related myopathy with Mallory body-like inclusions is caused by mutations of the selenoprotein N gene. *Ann Neurol* 55: 676–86.

Fidzianska A, Rowinska-Marcinska K, Hausmanowa-Petrusewicz I (2004) Coexistence of X-linked recessive Emery–Dreifuss muscular dystrophy with inclusion body myositis-like morphology. *Acta Neuropathol* 104: 197–203.

Figarella-Branger D, Baeta Machado AM, Putzu GA, et al. (1997) Exertional rhabdomyolysis and exercise intolerance revealing dystrophinopathies. *Acta Neuropathol* 94: 48–53.

Finder JD, Birnkrant D, Carl J, et al. (2004) Respiratory care of the patient with Duchenne muscular dystrophy: ATS consensus statement. *Am J Respir Crit Care Med* 170: 456–65.

Fischer AQ, Carpenter DW, Hartlage PL, et al. (1988) Muscle imaging in neuromuscular disease using computerized real-time sonography. *Muscle Nerve* 11: 270–5.

Fishbein WN, Muldoon SM, Deuster PA, Armbrustmacher VW (1985) Myoadenylate deaminase deficiency and malignant hyperthermia susceptibility: is there a relationship? *Biochem Med* 34: 344–54.

Furman WL, Buckley PJ, Green AA, et al. (1985) Thymoma and myasthenia gravis in a 4-year-old child. Case report and review of the literature. *Cancer* 56: 2703–6.

Gajdos P, Chevret S, Clair B, et al. (1997) Clinical trial of plasma exchange and high-dose intravenous immunoglobulin in myasthenia gravis. *Ann Neurol* 41: 789–96.

Gajdos P, Tranchant C, Clair B, et al. (2005) Myasthenia Gravis Clinical Study Group: Treatment of myasthenia gravis exacerbation with intravenous immunoglobulin: a randomized double-blind clinical trial. *Arch Neurol* 62: 1689–93.

Galloway HR, Dahlstrom JE, Bennett GM (2001) Focal myositis. *Australas Radiol* 45: 347–9.

Gamboa ET, Eastwood AB, Hays AP, et al. (1979) Isolation of influenza virus from muscle in myoglobinuric polymyositis. *Neurology* 29: 1323–35.

García-Cabezas MA, García-Alix A, Martín Y, et al. (2004) Neonatal spinal muscular atrophy with multiple contractures, bone fractures, respiratory insufficiency and 5q13 deletion. *Acta Neuropathol* 107: 475–8.

Gardner-Medwin D, Sharples P (1989) Some studies of the Duchenne and autosomal recessive types of muscular dystrophy. *Brain Dev* 11: 91–7.

Gardnerova M, Eymard B, Morel E, et al. (1997) The fetal/adult acetylcholine receptor antibody ratio in mothers with myasthenia gravis as a marker for transfer of the disease to the newborn. *Neurology* 48: 50–4.

Garlepp MJ, Mastaglia FL (2000) Autoantibodies in inflammatory myopathies. *Am J Med Sci* 319: 227–33.

Garzo C, Perez-Sotelo M, Traba A, et al. (1998) Stiff-man syndrome in a child. *Mov Disord* 13: 365–8.

Gempel K, von Praun C, Baumkötter J, et al. (2001) "Adult" form of muscular carnitine palmitoyltransferase II deficiency: manifestation in a 2-year-old child. *Eur J Pediatr* 160: 548–51.

Giedion A, Boltshauser E, Briner J, et al. (1997) Heterogeneity in Schwartz–Jampel chondrodystrophic myotonia. *Eur J Pediatr* 156: 214–23.

Gilbert JR, Stajich JM, Wall S, et al. (1993) Evidence for heterogeneity in facioscapulohumeral muscular dystrophy (FSHD). *Am J Hum Genet* 53: 401–8.

Gilchrist JM, Ambler M, Agatiello P (1991) Steroid-responsive tubular aggregate myopathy. *Muscle Nerve* 14: 233–6.

Giuffrè B, Parinii R, Rizzuti T, et al. (2004) Severe neonatal onset of glycogenosis type IV: clinical and laboratory findings leading to diagnosis in two siblings. *J Inherit Metab Dis* 27: 609–19.

Godfrey C, Clement E, Mein R, et al. (2007) Refining genotype phenotype correlations in muscular dystrophies with defective glycosylation of dystroglycan. *Brain* 130: 2725–35.

Goebel HH, Anderson JR (1999) Structural congenital myopathies (excluding nemaline myopathy, myotubular myopathy and desminopathies): 56th European Neuromuscular Centre (ENMC) sponsored International Workshop. December 12–14, 1997, Naarden, The Netherlands. *Neuromuscul Disord* 9: 50–7.

Goldhammer Y, Blatt I, Sadeh M, Goodman RM (1990) Congenital myasthenia associated with facial malformations in Iraqi and Iranian Jews. A new genetic syndrome. *Brain* 113: 1291–306.

Gommans IM, Davis M, Saar K, et al. (2003) A locus on chromosome 15q for a dominantly inherited nemaline myopathy with core-like lesions. *Brain* 126: 1545–51.

Goodman M, Solomons CL, Miller PD (1978) Distinction between the common symptoms of the phosphate-depletion syndrome and glucocorticoid-induced disease. *Am J Med* 65: 868–72.

Gordon ES, Hoffman EP (2001) The ABC's of limb–girdle muscular dystrophy: alpha-sarcoglycanopathy, Bethlem myopathy, calpainopathy and more. *Curr Opin Neurol* 14: 567–73.

Gospe S, Lazaro RP, Lava NS, et al. (1989) Familial X-linked myalgia and cramps: a nonprogressive myopathy associated with a deletion in the dystrophin gene. *Neurology* 39: 1277–80.

Gospe SM, El-Schahawi M, Shanske S, et al. (1998) Asymptomatic McArdle's disease associated with hyper-creatinekinase-emia and absence of myophosphorylase. *Neurology* 51: 1228–9.

Grain L, Cortina-Borja M, Forfar C, et al. (2001) Cardiac abnormalities and skeletal muscle weakness in carriers of Duchenne and Becker muscular dystrophies and controls. *Neuromuscul Disord* 11: 186–91.

Greenberg DA (1997) Calcium channels and neurological disease. *Ann Neurol* 42: 275–82.

Greene PE, Dauer W (2006) Stiff child syndrome with mutation of DYT1 gene. *Neurology* 66: 1456.

Griggs RC, Bushby K (2005) Continued need for caution in the diagnosis of Duchenne muscular dystrophy. *Neurology* 64: 1498–9.

Griggs RC, Moxley RT, Mendell JR, et al. (1993) Duchenne dystrophy: randomized, controlled trial of prednisone (18 months) and azathioprine (12 months). *Neurology* 43: 520–7.

Griggs RC, Askanas V, DiMauro S, et al. (1995) Inclusion body myositis and myopathies. *Ann Neurol* 38: 705–13.

Gronert GA (1980) Malignant hyperthermia. *Anesthesiology* 53: 395–423.

Gruetter R, Kaelin P, Boesch C, et al. (1990) Non-invasive 31P magnetic resonance spectroscopy revealed McArdle disease in an asymptomatic child. *Eur J Pediatr* 149: 483–6.

Gubbay AJ, Isaacs D (2000) Pyomyositis in children. *Pediatr Infect Dis J* 19: 1009–12.

Guis S, Figarella-Branger D, Monnier N, et al. (2004) Multiminicore disease in a family susceptible to malignant hyperthermia: histology, in vitro contracture tests, and genetic characterization. *Arch Neurol* 61: 106–13.

Gutmann L, Phillips LH (1991) Myotonia congenita. *Semin Neurol* 11: 244–8.

Haas A, Ricker K, Rüdel R, et al. (1981) Clinical study of paramyotonia congenita with and without myotonia in a warm environment. *Muscle Nerve* 4: 388–95.

Hadjigeorgiou GM, Kawashima N, Bruno C, et al. (1999) Manifesting heterozygotes in a Japanese family with a novel mutation in the muscle-specific phosphoglycerate mutase (PGAM-M) gene. *Neuromuscul Disord* 9: 399–402.

Hageman AT, Gabreëls FJ, Liem KD (1993) Congenital myotonic dystrophy; a report on thirteen cases and a review of the literature. *J Neurol Sci* 115: 95–101.

Hageman G, Gooskens RHMJ, Willemse J (1985) A cerebral cause of arthrogryposis: unilateral cerebral hypoplasia. *Clin Neurol Neurosurg* 87: 119–22.

Hageman G, Willemse J, van Ketel BA, et al. (1987a) The heterogeneity of the Pena–Shokeir syndrome. *Neuropediatrics* 18: 45–50.

Hageman G, Willemse J, van Ketel BA, Verdonck AFMM (1987b) The pathogenesis of fetal hypokinesia. A neurological study of 75 cases of congenital contractures with emphasis on fetal lesions. *Neuropediatrics* 18: 22–33.

Hageman G, Ippel EPF, Beemer FA, et al. (1988a) The diagnostic management of newborns with congenital contractures: a nosologic study of 75 cases. *Am J Med Genet* 30: 883–904.

Hageman G, Jennekens FGI, Vete UK, Willemse J (1988b) The heterogeneity of distal arthrogryposis. *Brain Dev* 6: 273–83.

Hageman G, Ramaekers VT, Hilhorst BGJ, Rozeboom AR (1993) Congenital cervical spinal muscular atrophy: a non-familial, non-progressive condition of the upper limbs. *J Neurol Neurosurg Psychiatry* 56: 365–8.

Hagemans MLC, Winkel LPF, Hop WCJ, et al. (2005a) Disease severity in children and adults with Pompe disease related to age and disease duration. *Neurology* 64: 2139–41.

Hagemans MLC, Winkel LPF, Van Doorn PA, et al. (2005b) Clinical manifestation and natural course of late-onset Pompe's disease in 54 Dutch patients. *Brain* 128: 671–7.

Haliloglu G, Gross C, Senbil N, et al. (2004) Clinical spectrum of muscle–eye–

brain disease: from the typical presentation to severe autistic features. *Acta Myol* 23: 137–9.

Hall JG (1997) Arthrogryposis multiplex congenita: etiology, genetics, classification, diagnostic approach, and general aspects. *J Pediatr Orthopaed B* 6: 159–66.

Hall JG, Reed SD, Greene G (1982a) The distal arthrogryposes: delineation of new entities—review and nosologic discussion. *Am J Med Genet* 11: 185–239.

Hall JG, Reed SD, Scott CI, et al. (1982b) Three distinct types of X-linked arthrogryposis seen in 6 families. *Clin Genet* 21: 81–97.

Hall JG, Reed SD, Driscoll EP (1983) The syndromes of arthrogryposis congenita. Part I. Amyoplasia: a common, sporadic condition with congenital contractures. *Am J Med Genet* 15: 571–90.

Haller RG (2000) Treatment of McArdle disease. *Arch Neurol* 57: 923–4.

Haller RG, Vissing J (2004) No spontaneous second wind in muscle phosphofructokinase deficiency. *Neurology* 62: 82–6.

Haltia M, Somer H, Rehunen S (1988) Congenital fibre type disproportion in an adult: a morphometric and microchemical study. *Acta Neurol Scand* 78: 65–71.

Hanissian AS, Masi AT, Pitner G, et al. (1982) Polymyositis and dermatomyositis in children: an epidemiologic and clinical comparative analysis. *J Rheumatol* 9: 390–4.

Harding AE, Petty RKH, Morgan-Hughes JA (1988) Mitochondrial myopathy: a genetic study of 71 cases. *J Med Genet* 25: 528–35.

Harel T, Goldberg Y, Shalev SA, et al. (2004) Limb–girdle muscular dystrophy 2I: phenotypic variability within a large consanguineous Bedouin family associated with a novel FKRP mutation. *Eur J Hum Genet* 12: 38–43.

Harland CC, Marsden JR, Vernon SA, Allen BR (1991) Dermatomyositis responding to treatment of associated toxoplasmosis. *Br J Dermatol* 125: 76–8.

Harper CM (2004) Muscle pain, cramps and fatigue. In: Engel A, Franzini-Armstrong C, eds. *Myology, 3rd edn.* New York: McGraw-Hill, pp. 1473–534.

Harper CM, Fukodome T, Engel AG (2003) Treatment of slow-channel congenital myasthenic syndrome with fluoxetine. *Neurology* 60: 1710–3.

Hart IK (2000) Acquired neuromyotonia: a new autoantibody-mediated neuronal potassium channelopathy. *Am J Med Sci* 319: 209–16.

Hart IK, Maddison P, Newsom-Davis J, et al. (2002) Phenotypic variants of autoimmune peripheral nerve hyperexcitability. *Brain* 125: 1887–95.

Hasan S, Buckley P (1998) Novel antipsychotics and the neuroleptic malignant syndrome: a review and critique. *Am J Psychiatry* 155: 1113–6.

Hattori H, Torii S, Nagafuji H, et al. (1992) Benign acute myositis associated with rotavirus gastroenteritis. *J Pediatr* 121: 748–9.

Hawley RJ, Milner MR, Gottdiener JS, Cohen A (1991) Myotonic heart disease: a clinical follow-up. *Neurology* 41: 259–62.

Hayashi YK, Chou FL, Engvall E, et al. (1998) Mutations in the integrin alpha7 gene cause congenital myopathy. *Nat Genet* 19: 94–7.

Heckmatt JZ, Pier N, Dubowitz V (1988) Real-time ultrasound imaging of muscles. *Muscle Nerve* 11: 56–65.

Heckmatt JZ, Hasson N, Saunders C, et al. (1989) Cyclosporin in juvenile dermatomyositis. *Lancet* 1: 1063–6.

Heiman-Patterson T, Martino C, Rosenberg H, et al. (1988) Malignant hyperthermia in myotonia congenita. *Neurology* 38: 810–2.

Heine R (1986) Evidence of myotonic origin of type 2B muscle fibre deficiency in myotonia and paramyotonia congenita. *J Neurol Sci* 76: 357–9.

Heine R, Pika U, Lehmann-Horn F (1993) A novel SCN4A mutation causing myotonia aggravated by cold and potassium. *Hum Mol Genet* 2: 1349–53.

Helbling-Leclerc A, Zhang X, Topaloglu H, et al. (1995) Mutations in the laminin alpha 2-chain gene (LAMA2) cause merosin-deficient congenital muscular dystrophy. *Nat Genet* 11: 216–8.

Hendriksen JGM, Vles JSH (2006) Are males with Duchenne muscular dystrophy at risk for reading disabilities? *Pediatr Neurol* 34: 296–300.

Hernandez RJ, Strouse PJ, Craig CL, Farley FA (2002) Focal pyomyositis of the perisciatic muscles in children. *Am J Roentgenol* 118: 1267–71.

Higuchi I, Shiraishi T, Hashiguchi T, et al. (2001) Frameshift mutation in the collagen VI gene causes Ullrich's disease. *Ann Neurol* 50: 261–5.

Hirano M, Pavlakis SG (1994) Mitochondrial myopathy, encephalopathy, lactic acidosis, and stroke-like episodes (MELAS): current concepts. *J Child Neurol* 9: 4–13.

Hoff JM, Daltveit AK, Gilhus NE (2003) Myasthenia gravis: consequences for pregnancy, delivery, and the newborn. *Neurology* 25: 1362–6.

Hoffman EP, Fischbeck KH, Brown RH, et al. (1988) Characterization of dystrophin in muscle-biopsy specimens from patients with Duchenne's or Becker's muscular dystrophy. *N Engl J Med* 318: 1363–8.

Hoffman EP, Kunkel LM, Angelini C, et al. (1989) Improved diagnosis of Becker muscular dystrophy by dystrophin testing. *Neurology* 39: 1011–7.

Hoffman WH, Helman SW, Sekul E, et al. (2003) Lambert–Eaton myasthenic syndrome in a child with an autoimmune phenotype. *Am J Med Genet A* 119: 77–80.

Horváth R, Lochmuller H, Hoeltzenbein M, et al. (2004) Spontaneous recovery of a childhood onset mitochondrial myopathy caused by a stop mutation in the mitochondrial cytochrome c oxidase III gene. *J Med Genet* 41: e75.

Howard JF (1998) Intravenous immunoglobulin for the treatment of acquired myasthenia gravis. *Neurology* 51 Suppl 5: S30–6.

Huber AM, Lang B, LeBlanc CM, et al. (2000) Medium- and long-term functional outcomes in a multicenter cohort of children with juvenile dermatomyositis. *Arthritis Rheumatol* 43: 541–9.

Hudson AJ, Huff MW, Wright CG, et al. (1987) The role of insulin resistance in the pathogenesis of myotonic muscular dystrophy. *Brain* 110: 469–88.

Hudson AJ, Ebers GC, Bulman DE (1995) The skeletal muscle sodium and chloride channel diseases. *Brain* 118: 547–63.

Hudson CS, Rash JE, Tiedt TN, Albuquerque EX (1978) Neostigmine-induced alterations at the mammalian neuromuscular junction. II. Ultrastructure. *J Pharmacol Exp Ther* 205: 340–55.

Hurvitz H, Klar A, Korn-Lubetzki I, et al. (2000) Muscular carnitine palmitoyltransferase II deficiency in infancy. *Pediatr Neurol* 22: 148–50.

Husain F, Ryan NJ, Hogan GR (1989) Concurrence of limb–girdle muscular dystrophy and myasthenia gravis. *Arch Neurol* 46: 101–2.

Hyser CL, Griggs RC, Mendell JR, et al. (1987) Use of serum creatine kinase, pyruvate kinase and genetic linkage for carrier detection in Duchenne and Becker dystrophy. *Neurology* 37: 4–10.

Iannaccone ST, Bove KE, Vogler CA, et al. (1987) Type 1 fibre size disproportion: morphometric data from 37 children with myopathic, neuropathic, or idiopathic hypotonia. *Pediatr Pathol* 7: 395–419.

Ichiki S, Komatsu C, Ogata H, Mitsudome A (1992) A case of myasthenia gravis complicated with hyperthyroidism and thymic hyperplasia in childhood. *Brain Dev* 14: 164–6.

Illum N, Reske-Nielsen E, Skovby F, et al. (1988) Lethal autosomal recessive arthrogryposis multiplex congenita with whistling face and calcifications of the nervous system. *Neuropediatrics* 19: 186–92.

Isaacson G, Chan KH, Heffner RR (1991) Focal myositis. A new cause for the pediatric neck mass. *Arch Otolaryngol Head Neck Surg* 117: 103–5.

Ito Y, Saito K, Shishikura K, et al. (2003) A 1-year-old infant with McArdle disease associated with hyper-creatine kinase-emia during febrile episodes. *Brain Dev* 25: 438–41.

Jackson MJ, Schaefer JA, Johnson MA, et al. (1995) Presentation and clinical investigation of mitochondrial respiratory chain disease. A study of 51 patients. *Brain* 118: 339–57.

Jackson S, Turnbull DM (1993) Lipid disorders of muscle. In: Rosenberg RN, Prusiner SB, DiMauro S, eds. *The Molecular and Genetic Basis of Neurological Disease.* Boston: Butterworth-Heinemann, pp. 651–61.

Jagadha V, Becker LE (1988) Brain morphology in Duchenne muscular dystrophy: a Golgi study. *Pediatr Neurol* 4: 87–92.

Jaspert A, Fahsold R, Grehl H, Claus D (1995) Myotonic dystrophy: correlation of clinical symptoms with the size of the CTG trinucleotide repeat. *J Neurol* 242: 99–104.

Jeannet PY, Bassez G, Eymard B, et al. (2004) Clinical and histologic findings in autosomal centronuclear myopathy. *Neurology* 62: 1484–90.

Jeppesen J, Green A, Steffensen BF, Rahbek J (2003) The Duchenne muscular dystrophy population in Denmark, 1977–2001: prevalence, incidence and survival in relation to the introduction of ventilator use. *Neuromuscul Disord* 13: 804–12.

Jerusalem F, Engel AG, Gomez MR (1973) Sarcotubular myopathy. A newly recognized, benign, congenital, familial muscle disease. *Neurology* 23: 897–906.

Johnsen T, Friis ML (1980) Paramyotonia congenita (von Eulenburg) in Denmark. *Acta Neurol Scand* 62: 78–87.

Johnston JJ, Kelley RI, Crawford TO, et al. (2000) A novel nemaline myopathy in the Amish caused by a mutation in troponin TI. *Am J Hum Genet* 67: 814–21.

Jones KJ, North K (2003) Congenital muscular dystrophies. In: Royden Jones H, De Vivo DC, Darras BT, eds. *Neuromuscular Disorders of Infancy, Childhood, and Adolescence. A Clinician's Approach.* Philadelphia: Butterworth Heinemann, pp. 633–47.

Jones KJ, Morgan G, Johnston H, et al. (2001) The expanding phenotype of laminin alpha2 chain (merosin) abnormalities: case series and review. *J Med Genet* **38**: 649–57.

Jungbluth H, Sewry C, Brown SC, et al. (2000) Minicore myopathy in children: a clinical and histopathological study of 19 cases. *Neuromuscul Disord* **10**: 264–73.

Jurkat-Rott K, Lehmann-Horn F (2005) Hyperkalemic periodic paralysis type 1. Online at: http://www.geneclinics.org/servlet/access?db=geneclinics&site=gt&id=8888891&key=OkH4IV0Ch5nuY&gry=&fcn=y&fw=IdAS&filename=/profiles/hyper-pp/index.html.

Jurkat-Rott K, Mitrovic N, Hang C, et al. (2000) Voltage-sensor sodium channel mutations cause hypokalemic periodic paralysis type 2 by enhanced inactivation and reduced current. *Proc Natl Acad Sci USA* **97**: 9549–54.

Jusic A, Dogan S, Stojanovic V (1972) Hereditary persistent distal cramps. *J Neurol Neurosurg Psychiatry* **35**: 379–84.

Kaminsky HJ, Ruff RL (1994) Endocrine myopathies (hyper- and hypofunction of adrenal, thyroid, pituitary, and parathyroid glands and iatrogenic corticosteroid myopathy. In: Engels AG, Franzini-Armstrong C, eds. *Myology, Basic and Clinical. 2nd edn*. New York: McGraw-Hill, pp. 1726–52.

Kano H, Kobayashi K, Herrmann R, et al. (2002) Deficiency of alpha-dystroglycan in muscle–eye–brain disease. *Biochem Biophys Res Commun* **291**: 1283–6.

Kar NC, Pearson CM, Verity MA (1980) Muscle fructose 1,6-diphosphatase deficiency associated with an atypical central core disease. *J Neurol Sci* **48**: 243–56.

Karadimas CL, Greenstein P, Sue CM, et al. (2000) Recurrent myoglobinuria due to a nonsense mutation in the COX I gene of mitochondrial DNA. *Neurology* **55**: 644–9.

Karasawa T, Takizawa I, Morita K, et al. (1981) Polymyositis and toxoplasmosis. *Acta Pathol Jpn* **31**: 675–80.

Karpati G, Charuk J, Carpenter S, et al. (1986) Myopathy caused by a deficiency of Ca(2+)-adenosine triphosphatase in sarcoplasmic reticulum (Brody's disease). *Ann Neurol* **20**: 38–49.

Kashihara K, Ishida K (1988) Neuroleptic malignant syndrome due to sulpiride. *J Neurol Neurosurg Psychiatry* **51**: 1109–11.

Kasturi L, Sawant SP (2005) Sodium valproate-induced skeletal myopathy. *Indian J Pediatr* **72**: 243–4.

Keightley JA, Hoffbuhr KC, Burton MD, et al. (1996) A microdeletion in cytochrome c oxidase (COX) subunit III associated with COX deficiency and recurrent myoglobinuria. *Nat Genet* **12**: 410–6.

Kelly KJ, Garland JS, Tang TT, et al. (1989) Fatal rhabdomyolysis following influenza infection in a girl with familial carnitine palmityl transferase deficiency. *Pediatrics* **84**: 312–6.

Kerzin-Storrar L, Metcalfe RA, Dyer PA, et al. (1988) Genetic factors in myasthenia gravis: a family study. *Neurology* **38**: 38–42.

Khasani S, Becker K, Meinck H-M (2004) Hyperekplexia and stiff-man syndrome: abnormal brainstem reflexes suggest a physiological relationship. *J Neurol Neurosurg Psychiatry* **75**: 1265–9.

Kho N, Czarnecki L, Kerrigan JF, Coons S (2002) Pena–Shokier [sic] phenotype: case presentation and review. *J Child Neurol* **17**: 397–9.

Kiechl S, Kohlendorfer U, Thaler C, et al. (1999) Different clinical aspects of debrancher deficiency myopathy. *J Neurol Neurosurg Psychiatry* **67**: 364–8.

Kieval RI, Sotrel A, Weinblatt ME (1989) Chronic myopathy with a partial deficiency of the carnitine palmityltransferase enzyme. *Arch Neurol* **46**: 575–6.

Kilmer DD, Abresch RT, McCrory MA, et al. (1995) Profiles of neuromuscular diseases. Facioscapulohumeral muscular dystrophy. *Am J Phys Med Rehabil* **74** (5 Suppl): S131–9.

Kinali M, Mercuri E, Main M, et al. (2002) An effective, low-dosage, intermittent schedule of prednisolone in the long-term treatment of early cases of Duchenne dystrophy. *Neuromuscul Disord* **12** Suppl 1: S169–74.

Kinali M, Messina S, Mercuri E, et al. (2006) Management of scoliosis in Duchenne muscular dystrophy: a large 10-year retrospective study. *Dev Med Child Neurol* **48**: 513–8.

King JO, Denborough M (1973) Anesthetic-induced malignant hyperpyrexia in children. J Pediatr **83**: 37–40.

Kluger G, Kochs A, Holthausen H (2000) Heterotopic ossification in childhood and adolescence. *J Child Neurol* **15**: 406–14.

Kobayashi H, Baumbach L, Matise TC, et al. (1995) A gene for a severe lethal form of X-linked arthrogryposis (X-linked infantile spinal muscular atrophy) maps to human chromosome Xp11.3–q11.2. *Hum Mol Genet* **4**: 1213–6.

Kobayashi K, Nakahori Y, Miyake M, et al. (1998) An ancient retrotransposal insertion causes Fukuyama-type congenital muscular dystrophy. *Nature* **394**: 388–92.

Koch MC, Steinmeyer K, Lorenz C, et al. (1992) The skeletal muscle chloride channel in dominant and recessive human myotonia. *Science* **257**: 797–800.

Koenig M, Hoffman EP, Bertelson CJ, et al. (1987) Complete cloning of the Duchenne muscular dystrophy (DMD) cDNA and preliminary genomic organization of the DMD gene in normal and affected individuals. *Cell* **50**: 509–17.

Korenke GC, Wanders RJ, Hanefeld F (2003) Striking improvement of muscle strength under creatine therapy in a patient with long-chain 3-hydroxyacyl-CoA dehydrogenase deficiency. *J Inherit Metab Dis* **26**: 67–8.

Kottlors M, Jaksch M, Ketelsen UP, Weiner S (2001) Valproic acid triggers acute rhabdomyolysis in a patient with carnitine palmitoyltransferase type II deficiency. *Neuromuscul Disord* **11**: 757–9.

Krahn M, de Munain L, Streichenberger N, et al. (2006) CAPN3 mutations in patients with idiopathic eosinophilic myositis. *Ann Neurol* **59**: 905–11.

Krassas GE, Segni M, Wiersinga WM (2005) Childhood Graves' ophthalmopathy: results of a European questionnaire study. *Eur J Endocrinol* **153**: 515–21.

Kuhn E, Fiehn W, Seiler D, Schröder JM (1979) The autosomal recessive (Becker) form of myotonia congenita. *Muscle Nerve* **2**: 109–17.

Kwiecinski H, Ryniewicz B, Ostrzycki A (1992) Treatment of myotonia with antiarrhythmic drugs. *Acta Neurol Scand* **86**: 371–5.

Lacomis D, Giuliani MJ, van Cort A, Kramer DJ (1996) Acute myopathy of intensive care: clinical, electromyographic, and pathological aspects. *Ann Neurol* **40**: 645–50.

Lacson AG, Seshia SS, Sarnat HB, et al. (1994) Autosomal recessive, fatal infantile hypertonic muscular dystrophy among Canadian natives. *Can J Neurol Sci* **21**: 203–12.

Laing NG, Wilton SD, Akkari PA, et al. (1995) A mutation in the alpha tropomyosin gene TPM3 associated with autosomal dominant nemaline myopathy NEM1. *Nat Genet* **10**: 249.

Laing NG, Clarke NF, Dye D, et al. (2004) Actin mutations are one cause of congenital fibre type disproportion. *Ann Neurol* **56**: 689–94.

Lalani S, Vladutiu G, Plunkett K, et al. (2005) Isolated mitochondrial myopathy associated with muscle coenzyme Q10 deficiency. *Arch Neurol* **62**: 317–20.

Lambert C, Blanloeil Y, Horber RK, et al. (1994) Malignant hyperthermia in a patient with hypokalemic periodic paralysis. *Anesth Analg* **79**: 1012–4.

Lampe AK, Dunn DM, von Niederhausern AC, et al. (2005) Automated genomic sequence analysis of the three collagen VI genes: applications to Ullrich congenital muscular dystrophy and Bethlem myopathy. *J Med Genet* **42**: 108–20.

Land JM, Mistry S, Squier M, Hope P, et al. (1995) Neonatal carnitine palmitoyltransferase-2 deficiency: a case presenting with myopathy. *Neuromuscul Disord* **5**: 129–37.

Lang B, Dooley J (1996) Failure of pulse intravenous methylprednisolone treatment in juvenile dermatomyositis. *J Pediatr* **128**: 429–32.

Laporte J, Hu L-J, Kretz C, et al. (1996) A gene mutated in X-linked myotubular myopathy defines a new putative tyrosine phosphatase family conserved in yeast. *Nat Genet* **13**: 175–82.

Laubscher B, Janzer RC, Krühenbühl S, Deonna T (1997) Ragged-red fibers and complex I deficiency in a neonate with arthrogryposis congenita. *Pediatr Neurol* **17**: 249–51.

Lauriola L, Ranelletti F, Maggiano N, et al. (2005) Thymus changes in anti-MuSK-positive and -negative myasthenia gravis. *Neurology* **64**: 536–8.

Laval SH, Bushby KM (2004) Limb–girdle muscular dystrophies – from genetics to molecular pathology. *Neuropathol Appl Neurobiol* **30**: 91–105.

Laxer RM, Stein LD, Petty RE (1987) Intravenous pulse methyl-prednisolone treatment of juvenile dermatomyositis. *Arthritis Rheum* **30**: 328–34.

Lee WT, Wang PJ, Young C, et al. (1995) Thenar hypoplasia in Klippel–Feil syndrome due to aberrant radial artery. *Pediatr Neurol* **13**: 343–5.

Lefèvre C, Jobard F, Caux F, et al. (2001) Mutations in CGI-58, the gene encoding a new protein of the esterase/lipase/thioesterase subfamily, in Chanarin–Dorfman syndrome. *Am J Hum Genet* **69**: 1002–12.

Lehmann-Horn F, Rudel R, Jurkat-Rott K (2004) Non-dystrophic myotonias and periodic paralyses. In: Engel AG, Franzini-Armstrong C, eds. *Myology: Basic and Clinical, 3rd edn*. New York: McGraw-Hill, pp. 1257–300.

Lehtokari VL, Ceuterick-de Groote C, de Jonghe P, et al. (2007) Cap disease caused by heterozygous deletion of the beta-tropomyosin gene TPM2. *Neuromuscul Disord* **17**: 433–42.

Lerche H, Mitrovic N, Dubowitz V, Lehmann-Horn F (1996) Paramyotonia congenita: the R1448P Na+ channel mutation in adult human skeletal muscle. *Ann Neurol* **39**: 599–608.

Levenson JL (1985) Neuroleptic malignant syndrome. *Am J Psychiatry* **142**: 1137–45.

Levy CE, Lash AT, Janoff HB, Kaplan FS (1999) Conductive hearing loss in individuals with fibrodysplasia ossificans progressiva. *Am J Audiol* **8**: 29–33.

Lewis CA, Boheimer N, Rose P, Jackson G (1985) Myopathy after short term administration of procainamide. *BMJ (Clin Res Ed)* **292**: 593–4.

L'hermine-Coulomb A, Beuzen F, Bouvier R, et al. (2005) Fetal type IV glycogen storage disease: clinical, enzymatic, and genetic data of a pure muscular form with variable and early antenatal manifestations in the same family. *Am J Med Genet* **139**: 118–22.

Lin AC, Lin CM, Wang TL, Leu JG (2005) Rhabdomyolysis in 119 students after repetitive exercise. *Br J Sports Med* **39**: e3.

Lindner A, Schalke B, Toyka KV (1997) Outcome in juvenile-onset myasthenia gravis: a retrospective study with long-term follow-up of 79 patients. *J Neurol* **244**: 515–20.

Links TR, Zwarts MJ, Oosterhuis HJGH (1988) Improvement of muscle strength in familial hypokalaemic periodic paralysis with azetazolamide. *J Neurol Neurosurg Psychiatry* **51**: 1142–5.

Liquori CL, Ricker K, Moseley ML, et al. (2001) Myotonic dystrophy type 2 caused by a CCTG expansion in intron 1 of ZNF9. *Science* **293**: 864–7.

Liu GT, Heher KL, Katowitz JA, et al. (1996) Prominent proptosis in childhood thyroid eye disease. *Ophthalmology* **103**: 779–84.

Longman C, Brockington M, Torelli S, et al. (2003) Mutations in the human LARGE gene cause MDC1D, a novel form of congenital muscular dystrophy with severe mental retardation and abnormal glycosylation of alpha-dystroglycan. *Hum Mol Genet* **12**: 2853–61.

Louhichi N, Triki C, Quijano-Roy S, et al. (2004) New FKRP mutations causing congenital muscular dystrophy associated with mental retardation and central nervous system abnormalities. Identification of a founder mutation in Tunisian families. *Neurogenetics* **5**: 27–34.

Mackay MT, Kornberg AJ, Shield LK, Dennett X (1999) Benign acute childhood myositis: laboratory and clinical features. *Neurology* **53**: 2127–31.

Maddison P, Newsom-Davis J (2005) Treatment for Lambert–Eaton myasthenic syndrome. *Cochrane Database Syst Rev* (2): CD003279.

Maddison P, Lang B, Mills K, et al. (2001) Long term outcome in Lambert–Eaton myasthenic syndrome without lung cancer. *J Neurol Neurosurg Psychiatry* **70**: 212–7.

Madrid RE, Kubisch C, Hays AP (2005) Early-onset toe walking in rippling muscle disease. *Neurology* **65**: 1301–3.

Maillard SM, Jones R, Owens C, et al. (2004) Quantitative assessment of MRI T2 relaxation time of thigh muscles in juvenile dermatomyositis. *Rheumatology* **43**: 603–8.

Makela-Bengs P, Jarvinen N, Vuopala K, et al. (1998) Assignment of the disease locus for lethal congenital contracture syndrome to a restricted region of chromosome 9q34, by genome scan using five affected individuals. *Am J Hum Genet* **63**: 506–16.

Mancuso M, Salviati L, Sacconi S, et al. (2002) Mitochondrial DNA depletion: mutations in thymidine kinase gene with myopathy and SMA. *Neurology* **59**: 1197–202.

Marbini A, Gemignani F, Saccardi F, Rimoldi M (1989) Debrancher deficiency neuromuscular disorder with pseudohypertrophy in two brothers. *J Neurology* **236**: 418–20.

Markandeyulu V, Joseph TP, Solomon T, et al. (2001) Stiff-man syndrome in childhood. *J R Soc Med* **94**: 296–7.

Martin JJ, Ceuterick C, Van Goethem G (1997) On a dominantly inherited myopathy with tubular aggregates. *Neuromuscul Disord* **7**: 512–20.

Martinelli P, Fabbri R, Gabellini AS, et al. (1987) Familial hypertrophy of masticatory muscles. *J Neurol* **234**: 251–3.

Martini G, Calabrese F, Biscaro F, Zulian F (2005) A child with dermatomyositis and a suspicious lymphadenopathy. *J Rheumatol* **32**: 744–6.

Massa G, Casaer P, Ceulemans B, Van Eldere S (1988) Arthrogryposis multiplex congenita associated with lissencephaly: a case report. *Neuropediatrics* **19**: 24–6.

Massey GV, Kuhn JG, Nogi J, et al. (2004) The spectrum of myositis ossificans in haemophilia. *Haemophilia* **10**: 189–93.

Mastaglia FL, Laing NG (1996) Investigation of muscle disease. *J Neurol Neurosurg Psychiatry* **60**: 256–74.

Mastaglia FL, Ojeda VJ (1985a) Inflammatory myopathies. Part 1. *Ann Neurol* **17**: 215–27.

Mastaglia FL, Ojeda VJ (1985b) Inflammatory myopathies. Part 2. *Ann Neurol* **17**: 317–23.

Mastaglia FL, Ojeda VJ, Sarnat HB, Kakulas BA (1988) Myopathies associated with hypothyroidism: a review based upon 13 cases. *Aust N Z J Med* **18**: 799–806.

Masuzugawa S, Kuzuhara S, Narita Y, et al. (1997) Autosomal dominant hyaline body myopathy presenting as scapuloperoneal syndrome: clinical features and muscle pathology. *Neurology* **48**: 253–7.

McCarthy TV, Quane KA, Lynch PJ (2000) Ryanodine receptor mutations in malignant hyperthermia and central core disease. *Hum Mutat* **15**: 410–7.

McConville J, Farrugia ME, Beeson D, et al. (2004) Detection and characterization of MuSK antibodies in seronegative myasthenia gravis. *Ann Neurol* **55**: 580–4.

McEntagart M, Parsons G, Buj-Bello A, et al. (2002) Genotype–phenotype correlations in X-linked myotubular myopathy. *Neuromuscul Disord* **12**: 939–46.

McFarland R, Taylor RW, Chinnery PF, et al. (2004) A novel sporadic mutation in cytochrome c oxidase subunit II as a cause of rhabdomyolysis. *Neuromuscul Disord* **14**: 162–6.

McGuire SA, Tomosovic JJ, Ackerman N (1984) Hereditary continuous muscle fiber activity. *Arch Neurol* **41**: 395–6.

Medori R, Brooke MH, Waterston RH (1989) Genetic abnormalities in Duchenne and Becker dystrophies: clinical correlations. *Neurology* **39**: 461–5.

Medsger TA (1990) Tryptophan-induced eosinophilia–myalgia syndrome. *N Engl J Med* **322**: 926–8.

Melacini P, Fanin M, Danieli GA, et al. (1996) Myocardial involvement is very frequent among patients affected with subclinical Becker's muscular dystrophy. *Circulation* **94**: 3168–75.

Mennen U, van Heest A, Ezaki MB, et al. (2005) Arthrogryposis multiplex congenita. *J Hand Surg (Br)* **30**: 468–74.

Meola G, Scarpini E, Velicogna M, et al. (1986) Cytogenetic analysis and muscle differentiation in a girl with severe muscular dystrophy. *J Neurol* **233**: 168–70.

Meola G, Bresolin N, Rimoldi M, et al. (1987) Recessive carnitine palmityl transferase deficiency: biochemical studies in tissue cultures and platelets. *J Neurol* **235**: 74–9.

Mercelis R, Martin JJ, De Barsy T, et al. (1987) Myoadenylate deaminase deficiency: absence of correlation with exercise intolerance in 452 muscle biopsies. *J Neurol* **234**: 385–9.

Mercuri E, Yuva Y, Brow SC, et al. (2002) Collagen VI involvement in Ullrich syndrome: a clinical, genetic, and immunohistochemical study. *Neurology* **58**: 1354–9.

Meredith C, Herrmann R, Parry C, et al. (2004) Mutations in the slow skeletal muscle fibre myosin heavy chain gene (MYH7) cause Laing early-onset distal myopathy (MPD1). *Am J Hum Genet* **75**: 703–8.

Merlini L, Granata C, Dominici P, Bonfiglioni S (1986) Emery–Dreifuss muscular dystrophy: report of five cases in a family and review of the literature. *Muscle Nerve* **9**: 481–5.

Mikaeloff Y, Jambaque I, Mayer M, et al. (2001) Benefit of intravenous immunoglobulin in autoimmune stiff-person syndrome in a child. *J Pediatr* **139**: 340.

Miller FW, Leitman SF, Cronin ME, et al. (1992) Controlled trial of plasma exchange and leukapheresis in polymyositis and dermatomyositis. *N Engl J Med* **326**: 1380–4.

Miller G, Heckmatt JZ, Dubowitz V (1983) Drug treatment of juvenile dermatomyositis. *Arch Dis Child* **58**: 445–50.

Milone M, Fukuda T, Shen XM, et al. (2006) Novel congenital myasthenic syndromes associated with defects in quantal release. *Neurology* **66**: 1223–9.

Milstein JM, Herron TM, Haas JE (1989) Fatal infantile muscle phosphorylase deficiency. *J Child Neurol* **4**: 186–8.

Miyagoe-Suzuki Y, Nakagawa M, Takeda S (2000) Merosin and congenital muscular dystrophy. *Microsc Res Tech* **48**: 181–91.

Miyajima H, Orii KE, Shindo Y, et al. (1997) Mitochondrial trifunctional protein deficiency associated with recurrent myoglobinuria in adolescence. *Neurology* **49**: 833–7.

Moerman P, Fryns J-P, Goddeeris P, Lauweryns JM (1984) Pathogenesis of the prune-belly syndrome: a functional urethral obstruction caused by prostatic hypoplasia. *Pediatrics* **73**: 470–5.

Moghadaszadeh B, Petit N, Jaillard C, et al. (2001) Mutations in SEPN1 cause congenital muscular dystrophy with spinal rigidity and restrictive respiratory syndrome. *Nat Genet* **29**: 17–8.

Mohammadianpanah M, Omidvari S, Mosalaei A, Ahmadloo N (2004) Cisplatin-induced hypokalemic paralysis. *Clin Ther* 26: 1320–3.

Monnier N, Procaccio V, Stieglitz P, Lunardi J (1997) Malignant-hyperthermia susceptibility is associated with a mutation of the alpha 1-subunit of the human dihydropyridine-sensitive L-type voltage-dependent calcium-channel receptor in skeletal muscle. *Am J Hum Genet* 60: 1316–25.

Moore A, O'Donohoe NV, Monaghan H (1986) Neuroleptic malignant syndrome. *Arch Dis Child* 61: 793–5.

Mora M, Cartegni L, Di Blasi C, et al. (1997) X-linked Emery–Dreifuss muscular dystrophy can be diagnosed from skin biopsy or blood sample. *Ann Neurol* 42: 249–53.

Moraes CT, DiMauro S, Zeviani M, et al. (1989) Mitochondrial DNA deletions in progressive external ophthalmoplegia and Kearns–Sayre syndrome. *N Engl J Med* 320: 1293–9.

Morel E, Eymard B, Vernet-der Garabedian B, et al. (1988) Neonatal myasthenia gravis: a new clinical and immunologic appraisal on 30 cases. *Neurology* 38: 138–42.

Morgenlander JC, Nohria V, Saba Z (1993) EKG abnormalities in pediatric patients with myotonic dystrophy. *Pediatr Neurol* 9: 124–6.

Morimoto A, Ueda I, Hirashima Y, et al. (2003) A novel missense mutation (1060G→C) in the phosphoglycerate kinase gene in a Japanese boy with chronic haemolytic anaemia, developmental delay and rhabdomyolysis. *Br J Haematol* 122: 1009–13.

Moroni I, Gonano EF, Comi GP, et al. (1995) Ryanodine receptor gene point mutation and malignant hyperthermia susceptibility. *J Neurol* 242: 127–33.

Morrison DL, MacEwen GD (1982) Congenital muscular torticollis: observations regarding clinical findings, associated conditions, and results of treatment. *J Pediatr Orthop* 2: 500–5.

Moser H (1984) Duchenne muscular dystrophy: pathogenetic aspects and genetic prevention. *Hum Genet* 66: 17–40.

Moskovic E, Fisher C, Westbury G, Parsons C (1991) Focal myositis, a benign inflammatory pseudotumour: CT appearances. *Br J Radiol* 64: 489–93.

Mukamel M, Horev G, Mimouni M (2001) New insight into calcinosis of juvenile dermatomyositis: a study of composition and treatment. *J Pediatr* 138: 763–6.

Mullaney P, Vajsar J, Smith R, Buncic JR (2000) The natural history and ophthalmic involvement in childhood myasthenia gravis at the hospital for sick children. *Ophthalmology* 107: 504–10.

Muller-Felber W, Schlotter B, Topfer M, et al. (1999) Phenotypic variability in two brothers with sarcotubular myopathy. *J Neurol* 246: 408–11.

Muntoni F, Voit T (2004) The congenital muscular dystrophies in 2004: a century of exciting progress. *Neuromuscul Disord* 14: 635–49.

Muntoni F, Brockington M, Blake DJ, et al. (2002) Defective glycosylation in muscular dystrophy. *Lancet* 360: 1419–21.

Muntoni F, Brockington M, Torelli S, Brown SC (2004) Defective glycosylation in congenital muscular dystrophies. *Curr Opin Neurol* 17: 205–9.

Murinson BB (2004) Stiff-person syndrome. *Neurologist* 10: 131–7.

Musumeci O, Naini A, Slonim AE, et al. (2001) Familial cerebellar ataxia with muscle coenzyme Q10 deficiency. *Neurology* 56: 849–55.

Nagai K, Oshima Y, Hirota H, et al. (2003) Specific cardiomyopathy caused by multisystemic lipid storage in Jordans' anomaly. *Intern Med* 42: 587–90.

Nagai T, Hasegawa T, Saito M, et al. (1992) Infantile polymyositis: a case report. *Brain Dev* 14: 167–9.

Narkis G, Landau D, Manor E, et al. (2004) Homozygosity mapping of lethal congenital contractural syndrome type 2 (LCCS2) to a 6 cM interval on chromosome 12q13. *Am J Med Genet A* 130: 272–6.

Naschitz JE, Misselevich I, Rosner I, et al. (1999) Lymph-node-based malignant lymphoma and reactive lymphadenopathy in eosinophilic fasciitis. *Am J Med Sci* 318: 343–9.

Nevo Y, Kutai M, Jossiphov J, et al. (2004) Childhood macrophagic myofasciitis—consanguinity and clinicopathological features. *Neuromuscul Disord* 14: 246–52.

Niakan E, Harati Y, Danon MJ (1985) Tubular aggregates: their association with myalgia. *J Neurol Neurosurg Psychiatry* 48: 882–6.

Nicole S, Ben Hamida C, Beighton P, et al. (1995) Localization of the Schwartz–Jampel syndrome (SJS) locus to chromosome 1p34–p36.1 by homozygosity mapping. *Hum Molec Genet* 4: 1633–6.

Nicole S, Davoine C-S, Topaloglu H, et al. (2000) Perlecan, the major proteoglycan of basement membranes, is altered in patients with Schwartz–Jampel syndrome (chondrodystrophic myotonia). *Nat Genet* 26: 480–3.

Nicot AS, Toussaint A, Tosch V, et al. (2007) Mutations in amphiphysin 2 (BIN1) disrupt interaction with dynamin 2 and cause autosomal recessive centronuclear myopathy. *Nat Genet* 39: 1134–9.

Nolan MA, Jones OD, Pedersen RL, Johnston HM (2003) Cardiac assessment in childhood carriers of Duchenne and Becker muscular dystrophies. *Neuromuscul Disord* 13: 129–32.

Nonaka D, Birbe R, Rosai J (2005) So-called inflammatory myofibroblastic tumour: a proliferative lesion of fibroblastic reticulum cells? *Histopathology* 46: 604–13.

North KN (2004) Congenital myopathies. In: Engel AG, Franzini-Armstrong C, eds. *Myology. 3nd edn.* New York: McGraw-Hill, pp. 1473–535.

North KN, Miller G, Ianaccone S, et al. (1996) Cognitive dysfunction as the major presenting feature of Becker muscular dystrophy. *Neurology* 46: 461–5.

Nowak KJ, Wattanasirichaigoon D, Goebel HH, et al. (1999) Mutations in the skeletal muscle ··actin gene in patients with actin myopathy and nemaline myopathy. *Nat Genet* 23: 208–12.

Nozaki H, Hamano SI, Jeoka Y, et al. (1990) Cytochrome c oxidase deficiency with acute onset and rapid recovery. *Pediatr Neurol* 6: 330–2.

Odermatt A, Taschner PEM, Khanna VK, et al. (1996) Mutations in the gene-encoding SERCA1, the fast-twitch skeletal muscle sarcoplasmic reticulum Ca(2+) ATPase, are associated with Brody disease. *Nat Genet* 14: 191–4.

Oh SJ, Kim DE, Kuruoglu R, et al. (1992) Diagnostic sensitivity of the laboratory tests in myasthenia gravis. *Muscle Nerve* 15: 720–4.

Oh SJ, Kurokawa K, Claussen GC, Ryan HF (2005) Electrophysiological diagnostic criteria of Lambert–Eaton myasthenic syndrome. *Muscle Nerve* 32: 515–20.

Oh VMS, Taylor EA, Yeo SH, Lee KD (1990) Cation transport across lymphocyte plasma membranes in euthyroid and thyrotoxic men with and without hypokalaemic periodic paralysis. *Clin Sci* 78: 199–206.

Ohno K, Tanaka M, Sahashi K, et al. (1991) Mitochondrial DNA deletions in inherited recurrent myoglobinuria. *Ann Neurol* 29: 364–9.

Ollivier K, Hogrel J-Y, Gomez-Merino D, et al. (2005) Exercise tolerance and daily life in McArdle's disease. *Muscle Nerve* 31: 637–41.

Olsen RK, Pourfarzam M, Morris AA, et al. (2004) Lipid-storage myopathy and respiratory insufficiency due to ETFQO mutations in a patient with late-onset multiple acyl-CoA dehydrogenase deficiency. *J Inherit Metab Dis* 27: 671–8.

Onengüt S, Ugur SA, Karasoy H, et al. (2004) Identification of a locus for an autosomal recessive hyaline body myopathy at chromosome 3p22.2–p21.32. *Neuromuscul Dis* 14: 4–9.

Ono S, Inouye K, Mannen T (1987) Myopathology of hypothyroid myopathy. Some new observations. *J Neurol Sci* 77: 237–48.

Orngreen MC, Ejstrup R, Vissing J (2003) Effect of diet on exercise tolerance in carnitine palmitoyltransferase II deficiency. *Neurology* 61: 559–61.

Pachman LM (1990) Juvenile dermatomyositis: a clinical overview. *Pediatr Rev* 12: 117–25.

Pachman LM, Hayford JR, Chung A, et al. (1998) Juvenile dermatomyositis at diagnosis: clinical characteristics of 79 children. *J Rheumatol* 25: 1198–204.

Padberg GW, Brouwer OF, de Keizer RJW (1995) On the significance of retinal vascular disease and hearing loss in facioscapulohumeral muscular dystrophy. *Muscle Nerve* 2: S73–80.

Palace J, Newsom-Davis J, Lecky B (1998) A randomized double-blind trial of prednisolone alone or with azathioprine in myasthenia gravis. Myasthenia Gravis Study Group. *Neurology* 50: 1778–83.

Papazian O (1992) Transient neonatal myasthenia gravis. *J Child Neurol* 7: 135–41.

Pasman JW, Gabreëls FJ, Semmekrot B, et al. (1989) Hyperkalemic periodic paralysis in Gordon's syndrome: a possible defect in atrial natriuretic peptide function. *Ann Neurol* 26: 392–5.

Pasternak JF, Gageman J, Adams MA, et al. (1981) Exchange transfusion in neonatal myasthenia. *J Pediatr* 99: 644–6.

Pelin K, Hilpela P, Donner K, et al. (1999) Mutations in the nebulin gene associated with autosomal recessive nemaline myopathy. *Proc Natl Acad Sci USA* 96: 2305–10.

Pena SDJ, Shokeir MHK (1974) Syndrome of camptodactyly, multiple ankyloses, facial anomalies and pulmonary hypoplasia: a lethal condition. *J Pediatr* 85: 373–5.

Pepe G, Bertini E, Bonaldo P, et al. (2002) Bethlem myopathy (BETHLEM) and Ullrich scleroatonic muscular dystrophy: 100th ENMC International Workshop, 23–24 November 2001, Naarden, The Netherlands. *Neuromuscul Disord* 12: 984–93.

Perlman JM, Burns DK, Twickler DM, Weinberg AG (1995) Fetal hypokinesia syndrome in the monochorionic pair of a triplet pregnancy secondary to severe disruptive cerebral injury. *Pediatrics* **96**: 521–3.

Pietrini V, Marbini A, Galli L, Sorrentino V (2004) Adult onset multi/minicore myopathy associated with a mutation in the RYR1 gene. *J Neurol* **251**: 102–4.

Pillen S, van Engelen B, van den Hoogen F, et al. (2006) Eosinophilic fasciitis in a child mimicking a myopathy. *Neuromuscul Disord* **16**: 144–8.

Plaster NM, Tawil R, Tristani-Firouzi M, et al. (2001) Mutations in Kir2.1 cause the developmental and episodic electrical phenotypes of Andersen's syndrome. *Cell* **105**: 511–9.

Polizzi A, Huson SM, Vincent A (2000) Teratogen update: maternal myasthenia gravis as a cause of congenital arthrogryposis. *Teratology* **62**: 332–41.

Poulton KR, Nightingale S (1988) A new metabolic muscle disease due to abnormal hexokinase activity. *J Neurol Neurosurg Psychiatry* **51**: 250–5.

Prelle A, Moggio M, Checcarelli N, et al. (1993) Multiple deletions of mitochondrial DNA in a patient with periodic attacks of paralysis. *J Neurol Sci* **117**: 24–7.

Ptáček LJ, Johnson KJ, Griggs RC (1993) Genetics and physiology of the myotonic muscle disorders. *N Engl J Med* **328**: 482–9.

Ptáček LJ, Tawil R, Griggs RC, et al. (1994a) Dihydropyridine receptor mutations cause hypokalemic periodic paralysis. *Cell* 77: 863–8.

Ptáček LJ, Tawil R, Griggs RC, et al. (1994b) Sodium channel mutations in acetazolamide-responsive myotonia congenita, paramyotonia congenita, and hyperkalemic periodic paralysis. *Neurology* **44**: 1500–3.

Quane KA, Healy JMS, Keating KE, et al. (1993) Mutations in the ryanodine receptor gene in central core disease and malignant hyperthermia. *Nat Genet* **5**: 51–5.

Quinlivan R, Beynon RJ (2004) Pharmacological and nutritional treatment for McArdle's disease (glycogen storage disease type V). *Cochrane Database Syst Rev* (3): CD003458.

Quinlivan RM, Muller CR, Davis M, et al. (2003) Central core disease: clinical, pathological, and genetic features. *Arch Dis Child* **88**: 1051–5.

Quinlivan R, Roper H, Davie M, et al. (2005) Osteoporosis in Duchenne muscular dystrophy; its prevalence, treatment and prevention. *Neuromuscul Disord* **15**: 72–9.

Qureshi AI, Choudhry MA, Akbar MS, et al. (1999) Plasma exchange versus intravenous immunoglobulin treatment in myasthenic crisis. *Neurology* **52**: 629–32.

Rakocevic G, Raju R, Dalakas MC (2004) Anti-glutamic acid decarboxylase antibodies in the serum and cerebrospinal fluid of patients with stiff-person syndrome: correlation with clinical severity. *Arch Neurol* **61**: 902–4.

Ramanan AV, Feldman BM (2002) Clinical outcomes in juvenile dermatomyositis. *Curr Opin Rheumatol* **14**: 658–62.

Ramanan AV, Sawhney S, Murray KJ (2001) Central nervous system complications in two cases of juvenile onset dermatomyositis. *Rheumatology* **40**: 1293–8.

Rando TA, Disatnik MH, Yu Y, Franco A (1998) Muscle cells from mdx mice have an increased susceptibility to oxidative stress. *Neuromuscul Disord* **8**: 14–21.

Ranum LP, Day JW (2004) Myotonic dystrophy: RNA pathogenesis comes into focus. *Am J Hum Genet* **74**: 793–804.

Rees MI, Harvey K, Pearce BR, Chung SK (2006) Mutations in the gene encoding GlyT2 (SLC6A5) define a presynaptic component of human startle disease. *Nat Genet* **38**: 801–6.

Regev R, De Vries LS, Heckmatt JZ, Dubowitz V (1987) Cerebral ventricular dilatation in congenital myotonic dystrophy. *J Pediatr* **111**: 372–6.

Reimers CD, de Koning J, Neubert U, et al. (1993) Borrelia burgdorferi myositis: report of eight patients. *J Neurol* **240**: 278–83.

Renault F, Quesada R (1993) Muscle complications of malnutrition in children: a clinical and electromyographic study. *Neurophysiol Clin* **23**: 371–80.

Rhomberg M, Herczeg E, Piza-Katzer H (2002) Pitfalls in diagnosing carpal tunnel syndrome. *Eur J Pediatr Surg* **12**: 67–70.

Rich MM, Teener JW, Raps EC, et al. (1996) Muscle is electrically inexcitable in acute quadriplegic myopathy. *Neurology* **46**: 731–6.

Richman DP, Agius MA (2003) Treatment of autoimmune myasthenia gravis. *Neurology* **61**: 1652–61.

Ricker K, Moxley RT, Rohkamm R (1989) Rippling muscle disease. *Arch Neurol* **46**: 405–8.

Ricker K, Moxley RT, Heine R, Lehmann-Horn F (1994) Myotonia fluctuans: a third type of muscle sodium channel disease. *Arch Neurol* **51**: 1095–102.

Ricker K, Grimm T, Koch MC, et al. (1999) Linkage of proximal myotonic myopathy to chromosome 3q. *Neurology* **52**: 170–1.

Riemersma S, Vincent A, Beeson D, et al. (1996) Association of arthrogryposis multiplex congenita with maternal antibodies inhibiting fetal acetylcholine receptor function. *J Clin Invest* **98**: 2358–63.

Riggs JE, Schochet SS, Gutmann L, Lerfald SC (1989) Childhood onset inclusion body myositis mimicking limb–girdle muscular dystrophy. *J Child Neurol* **4**: 283–5.

Riley P, Maillard SM, Wedderburn LR, et al. (2004) Intravenous cyclophosphamide pulse therapy in juvenile dermatomyositis. A review of efficacy and safety. *Rheumatology* **43**: 491–6.

Robertson NP, Deans J, Compston DAS (1998) Myasthenia gravis: a population based epidemiological study in Cambridgeshire, England. *J Neurol Neurosurg Psychiatry* **65**: 492–6.

Robinson RO (1990) Arthrogryposis multiplex congenita: feeding, language and other health problems. *Neuropediatrics* **21**: 177–88.

Rodolico C, Pastura C, Sinicropi S, et al (2005) Juvenile limb–girdle myasthenia gravis. *Neuropediatrics* **36**: 353–6.

Rodriguez M, Gomez MR, Howard FM, Taylor WF (1983) Myasthenia gravis in children: long-term follow-up. *Ann Neurol* **13**: 504–10.

Romero NB, Monnier N, Viollet L, et al. (2003) Dominant and recessive central core disease associated with RYR1 mutations and foetal akinesia. *Brain* **126**: 2341–9.

Rosenberg NL, Neville HE, Ringel SP (1985) Tubular aggregates: their association with neuromuscular diseases including the syndrome of myalgias/cramps. *Arch Neurol* **42**: 973–6.

Rothstein TL, Carlson CB, Sumi SM (1971) Polymyositis with facioscapulohumeral distribution. *Arch Neurol* **25**: 313–9.

Rowland LP (1985) Cramps, spasms and muscle stiffness. *Rev Neurol* **141**: 261–73.

Rubinsztein JS, Rubinsztein DC, Goodburn S, Holland AJ (1998) Apathy and hypersomnia are common features of myotonic dystrophy. *J Neurol Neurosurg Psychiatry* **64**: 510–5.

Rudel R, Dengler R, Ricker K, et al. (1980) Improved therapy of myotonia with the lidocaine derivative tocainide. *J Neurol* **222**: 275–8.

Rutgers MJ (1986) The rectus abdominis syndrome: a case report. *J Neurol* **233**: 180–1.

Ryan MM, Schnell C, Strickland CD, et al. (2001) Nemaline myopathy: a clinical study of 143 cases. *Ann Neurol* **50**: 312–20.

Ryan MM, Ilkovski B, Strickland CD, et al. (2003) Clinical course correlates poorly with muscle pathology in nemaline myopathy. *Neurology* **60**: 665–73.

Saada A, Shaag A, Mandel H, et al. (2001) Mutant mitochondrial thymidine kinase in mitochondrial DNA depletion myopathy. *Nat Genet* **29**: 342–4.

Sabina R (2000) Myoadenylate deaminase deficiency. A common inherited defect with heterogeneous clinical presentation. *Neurol Clin* **18**: 185–94.

Sahin G, Gungor T, Rettwitz-Volk W, et al. (1998) Infantile muscle phosphorylase-b-kinase deficiency. A case report. *Neuropediatrics* **2**: 48–50.

Sakano T, Hamasaki T, Kinoshita Y, et al. (1989) Treatment for refractory myasthenia gravis. *Arch Dis Child* **64**: 1191–3.

Sakuta R, Murakami N, Jin Y, et al. (2005) Diagnostic significance of membrane attack complex and vitronectin in childhood dermatomyositis. *J Child Neurol* **20**: 597–602.

Samaha FJ, Quinlan JG (1996) Myalgia and cramps: dystrophinopathy with wide-ranging laboratory findings. *J Child Neurol* **11**: 21–4.

Sanchez-Arjona MB, Rodriguez-Uranga JJ, Giles-Lima M, et al. (2006) Spanish family with myalgia and cramps syndrome. *J Neurol Neurosurg Psychiatry* **76**: 286–9.

Sanders DB, El-Salem K, Massey JM, et al. (2003) Clinical aspects of MuSK antibody positive seronegative MG. *Neurology* **60**: 1978–80.

Sanders DB, Aarli JA, Cutter GR (2006) Long-term results of tacrolimus in cyclosporine- and prednisone-dependent myasthenia gravis. *Neurology* **66**: 954–5.

Sarnat HB, Menkes JH (2006) Diseases of the motor unit. In: Menkes JH, Sarnat HB, Maria BL, eds. *Child Neurology. 7th edn.* Philadelphia: Lippincott, Williams & Wilkins, pp. 969–1024.

Sarnat HB, Morrissy RT (1981) Idiopathic torticollis: sternocleidomastoid myopathy and accessory neuropathy. *Muscle Nerve* **4**: 374–80.

Scarlett RF, Rocke DM, Kantanie S, et al. (2004) Influenza-like viral illnesses and flare-ups of fibrodysplasia ossificans progressiva. *Clin Orthopaed Relat Res* **423**: 275–9.

Schachter H, Vajsar J, Zhang W (2003) The role of defective glycosylation in congenital muscular dystrophy. *Glycoconj J* **20**: 291–300.

Schaefer J, Jackson S, Dick DJ, Turnbull DM (1996) Trifunctional enzyme deficiency: adult presentation of a usually fatal beta-oxidation defect. *Ann Neurol* 40: 597–602.

Schapira AH, Cock HR (1999) Mitochondrial myopathies and encephalomyopathies. *Eur J Clin Invest* 29: 886–98.

Schessl J, Zou Y, McGrath MJ, et al. (2008) Proteomic identification of FHL1 as the protein mutated in human reducing body myopathy. *J Clin Invest* 118: 904–12.

Scheuerbrandt G, Lundin A, Lövgren T, Mortier W (1986) Screening for Duchenne muscular dystrophy: an improved screening test for creatine kinase and its application in an infant screening program. *Muscle Nerve* 9: 11–23.

Schoser BGH, Frosk P, Engel AG, et al. (2005) Commonality of TRIM32 mutations causing sarcotubular myopathy and LGMD2H. *Ann Neurol* 57: 591–5.

Schroter HM, Sarnat HB, Matheson DS, Seland TP (1987) Juvenile dermatomyositis induced by toxoplasmosis. *J Child Neurol* 2: 101–4.

Schuelke M, Wagner KR, Stolz LE, et al. (2004) Myostatin mutation associated with gross muscle hypertrophy in a child. *N Engl J Med* 350: 2682–8.

Schwartz O, Jampel RS (1962) Congenital blepharophimosis associated with a unique generalized myopathy. *Arch Ophthalmol* 68: 52–7.

Seay AR, Ziter FA (1978) Malignant hyperpyrexia in a patient with Schwartz–Jampel syndrome. *J Pediatr* 93: 83–4.

Selcen D, Fukuda T, Shen X, Engel AG (2004) Are MuSK antibodies the primary cause of myasthenic symptoms? *Neurology* 62: 1945–50.

Sells JM, Jaffe KM, Hall JG (1996) Amyoplasia, the most common type of arthrogryposis: the potential for good outcome. *Pediatrics* 97: 225–31.

Selmar P, Skov T, Skov BG (1986) Familial hypoplasia of the thenar eminence: a report of three cases. *J Neurol Neurosurg Psychiatry* 49: 105–6.

Senderek J, Krieger M, Stendel C, et al. (2005) Mutations in SIL1 cause Marinesco–Sjögren syndrome, a cerebellar ataxia with cataract and myopathy. *Nat Genet* 37: 1312–4.

Serratrice G, Pellissier JF, Roux H, Quilichini P (1990) Fasciitis, perimyositis, myositis, polymyositis, and eosinophilia. *Muscle Nerve* 13: 385–95.

Servidei S, Bonilla E, Diedrich RG, et al. (1986) Fatal infantile form of muscle phosphofructokinase deficiency. *Neurology* 36: 1465–70.

Servidei S, Shanske S, Zeviani M, et al. (1988) McArdle's disease: biochemical and molecular genetic studies. *Ann Neurol* 24: 774–81.

Sethna NF, Rockoff MA, Worthen HM, Rosnow JM (1988) Anesthesia-related complications in children with Duchenne muscular dystrophy. *Anesthesiology* 68: 462–5.

Sewry CA, Voit T, Dubovitz V (1988) Myopathy with unique ultrastructural feature in Marinsco–Sjögren syndrome. *Ann Neurol* 24: 576–80.

Shapiro B, Ruff R (2002) Disorders of skeletal muscle membrane excitability: myotonia congenita, paramyotonia congenita, periodic paralysis, and related disorders. In: Katirji B, Kaminski H, Preston D, et al., eds. *Neuromuscular Disorders in Clinical Practice*. Boston: Butterworth-Heinemann, pp. 987–1020.

Sharma KR, Mynhier MA, Miller RG (1993) Cyclosporine increases muscular force generation in Duchenne muscular dystrophy. *Neurology* 43: 527–32.

Shaw P (1999) Stiff-man syndrome and its variants. *Lancet* 353: 86–7.

Shevell M, Rosenblatt B, Silver K, et al. (1990) Congenital inflammatory myopathy. *Neurology* 40: 1111–4.

Shore EM, Xa M, Feldman GJ, et al (2006) A recurrent mutation in the BMP type 1 receptor ACVR1 causes inherited and sporadic fibrodysplasia ossificans progressiva. *Nat Genet* 38: 525–27.

Shore RN (1975) Myotonic dystrophy: hazards of pregnancy and infancy. *Dev Med Child Neurol* 17: 356–61.

Shuaib A, Paasuke RT, Brownell AKW (1987) Central core disease. Clinical features in 13 patients. *Medicine* 66: 389–96.

Shy GM, Magee KR (1956) A new congenital non-progressive myopathy. *Brain* 79: 610–21.

Sigauke E, Rakheja D, Kitson K, Bennett MJ (2003) Carnitine palmitoyltransferase II deficiency: a clinical, biochemical, and molecular review. *Lab Invest* 83: 1543–54.

Sills E (1982) Diffuse fasciitis with eosinophilia in childhood. *Johns Hopkins Med J* 151: 203–7.

Simon DB, Ringel SP, Sufit RL (1982) Clinical spectrum of fascial inflammation. *Muscle Nerve* 5: 525–37.

Sloane AE, Vajsar J, Laxer RM, et al. (1994) Spontaneous non-traumatic anterior compartment syndrome with peroneal neuropathy and favorable outcome. *Neuropediatrics* 25: 268–70.

Slonim AE, Goans PJ (1985) Myopathy in McArdle's syndrome. Improvement

with a high-protein diet. *N Engl J Med* 312: 355–9.

Smith AG, Urbanits S, Blaivas M, et al. (2000) Clinical and pathologic features of focal myositis. *Muscle Nerve* 23: 1569–75.

Smith R (1998) Fibrodysplasia (myositis) ossificans progressiva: clinical lessons from a rare disease. *Clin Orthop Relat Res* 346: 7–14.

Smith R, Athanasou NA, Vipond SE (1996) Fibrodysplasia (myositis) ossificans progressiva: clinicopathological features and natural history. *Q J Med* 89: 445–56.

Sommer N, Sigg B, Melms A, et al. (1997) Ocular myasthenia gravis: response to long term immunosuppressive treatment. *J Neurol Neurosurg Psychiatry* 62: 156–62.

Sonel B, Senbil N, Yavus Gurer YK, Evcik D (2002) Cavanagh's syndrome (congenital thenar hypoplasia). *J Child Neurol* 17: 51–4.

Spaans F (1991) Schwartz–Jampel syndrome with dominant inheritance. *Muscle Nerve* 14: 1142–4 (letter).

Spencer CH, Hanson V, Singsen BH, et al. (1984) Course of treated juvenile dermatomyositis. *J Pediatr* 105: 399–408.

Spiegel DA, Meyer JS, Dormans JP, et al. (1999) Pyomyositis in children and adolescents: report of 12 cases and review of the literature. *J Pediatr Orthop* 19: 143–50.

Spiekerkoetter U, Bennett MJ, Ben-Zeev B, et al. (2004) Peripheral neuropathy, episodic myoglobinuria, and respiratory failure in deficiency of the mitochondrial trifunctional protein. *Muscle Nerve* 29: 66–72.

Spranger J, Hall BD, Hane B, et al. (2000) Spectrum of Schwartz–Jampel syndrome includes micromelic chondrodysplasia, kyphomelic dysplasia, and Burton disease. *Am J Med Genet* 94: 287–95.

Stephan DA, Buist NRM, Chittenden AB, et al. (1994) A rippling muscle disease gene is localized to 1q41: evidence for multiple genes. *Neurology* 44: 1915–20.

Stewart CR, Kahler SO, Gilchrist JM (1988) Congenital myopathy with cleft palate and increased susceptibility to malignant hyperthermia: King syndrome? *Pediatr Neurol* 4: 371–4.

Subramony SH, Wee AS, Mishra SK (1986) Lack of cold sensitivity in hyperkalemic periodic paralysis. *Muscle Nerve* 9: 700–3.

Sugie H, Kobayashi J, Sugie Y, et al. (1988) Infantile muscle glycogen storage disease: phosphoglucomutase deficiency with decreased muscle and serum carnitine levels. *Neurology* 38: 602–5.

Sugie H, Sugie Y, Nishida M, et al. (1989) Recurrent myoglobinuria in a child with mental retardation: phosphoglycerate kinase deficiency. *J Child Neurol* 4: 95–9.

Sullivan EA, Kamb ML, Jones JL, et al. (1996) The natural history of eosinophilia–myalgia syndrome in a tryptophan-exposed cohort in South Carolina. *Arch Intern Med* 156: 973–5.

Sun SF, Streib EW (1983) Autosomal recessive generalized myotonia. *Muscle Nerve* 6: 143–8.

Sunohara N, Arahata K, Hoffman EP, et al. (1990) Quadriceps myopathy: forme fruste of Becker muscular dystrophy. *Ann Neurol* 28: 634–9.

Swoboda KJ Specht L, Jones RH, et al. (1997) Infantile phosphofructokinase deficiency with arthrogryposis: clinical benefit of a ketogenic diet. *J Pediatr* 131: 932–4.

Tabarki B, Coffinieres A, Van Den Bergh P, et al. (2002) Critical illness neuromuscular disease: clinical, electrophysiological, and prognostic aspects. *Arch Dis Child* 86: 103–7.

Tagher RJ, Baumann R, Desai N (1999) Failure of intravenously administered immunoglobulin in the treatment of neonatal myasthenia gravis. *J Pediatr* 134: 233–5.

Tajsharghi H, Thornell LE, Lindberg C, et al. (2003) Myosin storage myopathy associated with a heterozygous missense mutation in MYH7. *Ann Neurol* 54: 494–500.

Tajsharghi H, Ohlsson M, Lindberg C, Oldfors A (2007) Congenital myopathy with nemaline rods and cap structures caused by a mutation in the beta-tropomyosin gene (TPM2). *Arch Neurol* 64: 1334–8.

Takahashi S, Miyamoto A, Oki J, Okuno A (1996) CTG trinucleotide repeat length and clinical expression in a family with myotonic dystrophy. *Brain Dev* 18: 127–30.

Tan P, Briner J, Boltshauser E, et al. (1999) Homozygosity for a nonsense mutation in the alpha-tropomyosin gene TPM3 in a patient with severe congenital nemaline myopathy. *Neuromuscul Disord* 9: 573–9.

Tanamy MG, Magal N, Halpern GJ, et al. (2001) Fine mapping places the gene for arthrogryposis multiplex congenita neuropathic type between D5S394 and D5S2069 on chromosome 5qter. *Am J Med Genet* 104: 152–6.

Tarnopolsky MA, Mahoney DJ, Vajsar J, et al. (2004) Creatine monohydrate enhances strength and body composition in Duchenne muscular dystrophy. *Neurology* 62: 1771–7.

Tawil R, Griggs RC (1997) Facioscapulohumeral muscular dystrophy. In: Rosenberg RN, Pruisner SB, DiMaurio S, et al., eds. *The Molecular and Genetic Basis of Neurological Disease. 2nd edn.* Boston: Butterworth-Heinemann, pp. 931–8.

Tawil R, Figlewicz DA, Griggs RC, Weiffenbach B (1998) Facioscapulohumeral dystrophy: a distinct regional myopathy with a novel molecular pathogenesis. FSH Consortium. *Ann Neurol* 43: 279–82.

Taylor RW, Schaefer AM, Barron MJ, et al. (2004) The diagnosis of mitochondrial muscle disease. *Neuromuscul Disord* 14: 237–45.

Tein I, DiMauro S, DeVivo DC (1990) Recurrent childhood myoglobinuria. *Adv Pediatr* 37: 77–117.

Tein I, Donner EJ, Hale DE, et al. (1995) Clinical and neurophysiologic response of myopathy and neuropathy in long-chain L-3-hydroxyacyl-CoA dehydrogenase deficiency to oral prednisone. *Pediatr Neurol* 12: 68–76.

Tein I, Haslam RHA, Rhead WJ, et al. (1999) Short-chain acyl-CoA dehydrogenase deficiency: a cause of ophthalmoplegia and multicore myopathy. *Neurology* 52: 366–72.

Thomas CE, Mayer SA, Gungor Y, et al. (1997) Myasthenic crisis: clinical features, mortality, complications, and risk factors for prolonged intubation. *Neurology* 48: 1253–60.

Thomas NH, Heckmatt JZ, Rodillo E, et al. (1994) Continuous muscle fibre activity (Isaacs' syndrome) in infancy: a report of two cases. *Neuromuscul Disord* 4: 147–51.

Thornton C (1999) The myotonic dystrophies. *Semin Neurol* 19: 25–33.

Thornton CA, Griggs RC, Moxley RT (1994) Myotonic dystrophy with no trinucleotide repeat expansion. *Ann Neurol* 35: 269–72.

Tim RW, Massey JM, Sanders DB (2000) Lambert–Eaton myasthenic syndrome: electrodiagnostic findings and response to treatment. *Neurology* 54: 2176–8.

Tobin JR, Jason DR, Challa VR, et al. (2001) Malignant hyperthermia and apparent heat stroke. *JAMA* 286: 168–9.

Topaloglu H, Brockington M, Yuva Y, et al. (2003) FKRP gene mutations cause congenital muscular dystrophy, mental retardation, and cerebellar cysts. *Neurology* 60: 988–92.

Topi GC, D'Alessandro L, Catricala C, Zardi O (1979) Dermatomyositis-like syndrome due to Toxoplasma. *Br J Dermatol* 101: 589–91.

Torres CF, Moxley RT (1992) Early predictors of poor outcome in congenital fibre-type disproportion myopathy. *Arch Neurol* 49: 855–6.

Torres CF, Forbes GB, Decancq GH (1986) Muscle weakness in infants with rickets: distribution, course and recovery. *Pediatr Neurol* 2: 95–8.

Towbin JA (2003) A noninvasive means of detecting preclinical cardiomyopathy in Duchenne muscular dystrophy? *J Am Coll Cardiol* 42: 317–8.

Trapani S, Camiciottoli G, Vierucci A, et al. (2001) Pulmonary involvement in juvenile dermatomyositis: a two-year longitudinal study. *Rheumatology* 40: 216–20.

Tsao CY, Mendell JR, Friemer ML, Kissel JT (2002) Lambert–Eaton myasthenic syndrome in children. *J Child Neurol* 17: 74–6.

Tsujino S, Shanske S, DiMauro S (1993) Molecular genetic heterogeneity of myophosphorylase deficiency (McArdle's disease). *N Engl J Med* 329: 241–5.

Ty EB, Rothner AD (2001) Neuroleptic malignant syndrome in children and adolescents. *J Child Neurol* 16: 157–63.

Udani VP, Dharnidharka VR, Gajendragadkar AR, Udani SV (1997) Sporadic stiffman syndrome in a young girl. *Pediatr Neurol* 17: 58–60.

Udd B, Krahe R, Wallgren-Pettersson C, et al. (1997) Proximal myotonic dystrophy—a family with autosomal dominant muscular dystrophy, cataracts, hearing loss and hypogonadism: heterogeneity of proximal myotonic syndromes? *Neuromuscul Disord* 7: 217–28.

Upadhyaya M, Maynard J, Rogers MT, et al. (1997) Improved molecular diagnosis of facioscapulohumeral muscular dystrophy (FSHD): validation of the differential double digestion for FSHD. *J Med Genet* 34: 476–9.

Urbano-Márquez A, Estruch R, Grau JM, et al. (1986) Inflammatory myopathy associated with chronic graft-versus-host disease. *Neurology* 36: 1091–3.

Van den Berg IET, Berger R (1990) Phosphorylase b kinase deficiency in man: a review. *J Inherit Metab Dis* 13: 442–51.

van den Hout HMP, Hop W, van Diggelen OP, et al. (2003) The natural course of infantile Pompe's disease: 20 original cases compared with 133 cases from the literature. *Pediatrics* 112: 332–40.

Van den Hout JM, Kamphoven JH, Winkel LP, et al. (2004) Long-term intravenous treatment of Pompe disease with recombinant human alpha-glucosidase from milk. *Pediatrics* 113: 448–57.

van der Heyden JJ, Verrips A, ter Laak HJ, et al. (2004) Hypovitaminosis D-related myopathy in immigrant teenagers. *Neuropediatrics* 35: 290–2.

van der Meulen MFG, Bronner IM, Hoogendijk JE, et al. (2003) Polymyositis: an overdiagnosed entity. *Neurology* 61: 316–21.

van Ommen GJB, Scheuerbrandt G (1993) Neonatal screening for muscular dystrophy. Consensus recommendation of the 14th workshop sponsored by the European Neuromuscular Center (ENMC). *Neuromuscul Disord* 3: 231–9.

van Reeuwijk J, Janssen M, van den Elzen C, et al. (2005) POMT2 mutations cause alpha-dystroglycan hypoglycosylation and Walker–Warburg syndrome. *J Med Genet* 42: 907–12.

Verzijl HT, van Engelen BG, Luyten JA, et al. (1998) Genetic characteristics of myoadenylate deaminase deficiency. *Ann Neurol* 44: 140–3.

Vicart S, Sternberg D, Fournier E, et al. (2004) New mutations of SCN4A cause a potassium-sensitive normokalemic periodic paralysis. *Neurology* 63: 2120–7.

Vincent A, Leite M (2005) Neuromuscular junction autoimmune disease: muscle specific kinase antibodies and treatments for myasthenia gravis. *Curr Opin Neurol* 18: 519–25.

Vincent A, Newland C, Brueton L, et al. (1995) Arthrogryposis multiplex congenita with maternal autoantibodies specific for a fetal antigen. *Lancet* 346: 24–5.

Vincent A, Beeson D, Lang B, et al. (2000) Molecular targets for autoimmune and genetic disorders of neuromuscular transmission. *Eur J Biochem* 267: 6717–28.

Vincent AC, McConville J, Newsom-Davis J (2005) Is "seronegative" MG explained by autoantibodies to MuSK? *Neurology* 64: 399. (Comment on *Neurology* 2004, 62: 1920–1.)

Vita G, Toscano A, Bresolin N, et al. (1994) Muscle phosphoglycerate mutase (PGAM) deficiency in the first caucasian patient: biochemistry, muscle culture and 31P-MR spectroscopy. *J Neurol* 241: 289–94.

Vockley J, Singh RH, Whiteman DAH (2002) Diagnosis and management of defects of mitochondrial beta-oxidation. *Curr Opin Clin Nutr Metab Care* 5: 601–9.

Voit T (2001) Congenital muscular dystrophy. In: Karpati G, Hilton-Jones D, Griggs RC, eds. *Disorders of Voluntary Muscle, 7th edn.* Cambridge: Cambridge University Press, pp. 525–40.

Voit T, Krogmann O, Lenard HG, et al. (1988) Emery–Dreifuss muscular dystrophy: disease spectrum and differential diagnosis. *Neuropediatrics* 19: 62–71.

Vuopala K, Leisti J, Herva R (1994) Lethal arthrogryposis in Finland—a clinico-pathological study of 83 cases during thirteen years. *Neuropediatrics* 25: 308–15.

Wagner KR, Hamed S, Hadley DW, et al. (2001) Gentamicin treatment of Duchenne and Becker muscular dystrophy due to nonsense mutations. *Ann Neurol* 49: 706–11.

Walsh RJ (2006) Metabolic myopathies. *Continuum* 12: 76–120.

Walton JN, Gardner-Medwin D (1981) Progressive muscular dystrophy and the myotonic disorders. In: Walton JN, ed. *Disorders of Voluntary Muscle, 4th edn.* Edinburgh: Churchill Livingstone, pp. 481–524.

Wappler F, Fiege M, Steinfath M, et al. (2001) Evidence for susceptibility to malignant hyperthermia in patients with exercise-induced rhabdomyolysis. *Anesthesiology* 94: 95–100.

Warren JD, Blumbergs PC, Thompson PD (2002) Rhabdomyolysis: a review. *Muscle Nerve* 25: 332–47.

Watemberg N, Leshner RL, Armstrong BA, Lerman-Sagie T (2000) Acute pediatric rhabdomyolysis. *J Child Neurol* 15: 222–7.

Wedel DJ (1992) Malignant hyperthermia and neuromuscular disease. *Neuromuscul Disord* 2: 157–64.

Wessel HB (1990) Dystrophin: a clinical perspective. *Pediatr Neurol* 6: 3–12.

Wijmenga C, Hewitt JE, Sandkuijl LA, et al. (1992) Chromosome 4q DNA rearrangements associated with facioscapulohumeral muscular dystrophy. *Nat Genet* 2: 26–30.

Wilkinson DA, Tonin P, Shanske S, et al. (1994) Clinical and biochemical features of 10 adult patients with muscle phosphorylase kinase deficiency. *Neurology* 44: 461–6.

Wingard DW, Gatz EE (1978) Some observations in stress susceptible patients. In: Aldrete JA, Britt BA, eds. *Second International Symposium on Malignant Hyperthermia.* New York: Grune & Stratton, pp. 363–72.

Winkel LPF, Hagemans MLC, van Doorn PA, et al. (2005) The natural course of non-classic Pompe's disease; a review of 225 published cases. *J Neurol* **252**: 875–84.

Wirtz PW, van Dijk JG, van Doorn PA, et al. (2004) The epidemiology of the Lambert–Eaton myasthenic syndrome in the Netherlands. *Neurology* **63**: 397–8.

Witkowski JA (1989) Dystrophin-related muscular dystrophies. *J Child Neurol* **4**: 251–71.

Wittbrodt ET (1997) Drugs and myasthenia gravis. An update. *Arch Intern Med* **157**: 399–408.

Witters I, Moerman P, Fryns JP (2002) Fetal akinesia deformation sequence: a study of 30 consecutive in utero diagnoses. *Am J Med Genet* **113**: 23–8.

Wong V, Hawkins BR, Yu YL (1992) Myasthenia gravis in Hong Kong Chinese. 2. Paediatric disease. *Acta Neurol Scand* **86**: 68–72.

Wong VC, Lam CW, Fung CW (2005) Stiff child syndrome with mutation of DYT1 gene. *Neurology* **65**: 1465–6.

Yazawa M, Ikeda SI, Owa M, et al. (1987) A family of Becker's progressive muscular dystrophy with severe cardiomyopathy. *Eur Neurol* **27**: 13–9.

Yoshida A, Kobayashi K, Manya H, et al. (2001) Muscular dystrophy and neuronal migration disorder caused by mutations in a glycosyltransferase, POMGnT1. *Dev Cell* **1**: 717–24.

Yuill GM, Lynch PG (1974) Congenital non-progressive peripheral neuropathy with arthrogryposis multiplex. *J Neurol Neurosurg Psychiatry* **37**: 316–23.

Zatz M, Marie SK, Passos-Bueno MR, et al. (1995) High proportion of new mutations and possible anticipation in Brazilian facioscapulohumeral muscular dystrophy families. *Am J Hum Genet* **56**: 99–105.

Zatz M, de Paula F, Starling A, Vainzof M (2003) The 10 autosomal recessive limb–girdle muscular dystrophies. *Neuromuscul Disord* **13**: 532–44.

Zeviani M, Nonaka I, Bonilla E, et al. (1985) Fatal infantile myopathy and renal dysfunction caused by cytochrome c oxidase deficiency: immunological studies in a new patient. *Ann Neurol* **17**: 414–7.

Zeviani M, Peterson P, Servidei S, et al. (1987) Benign reversible muscle cytochrome c oxidase deficiency: a second case. *Neurology* **37**: 64–7.

Zhang Y, Chen HS, Khanna VK, et al. (1993) A mutation in the human ryanodine receptor gene associated with central core disease. *Nat Genet* **5**: 46–50.

Zierz S (1994) Carnitine palmitoyl transferase deficiency. In: Engel AG, Franzini-Armstrong C, eds. *Myology, Basic and Clinical. 2nd edn.* New York: McGraw-Hill, pp. 1577–85.

Zimmer C, Gosztonyi G, Cervos-Navarro J, et al. (1992) Neuropathy with lysosomal changes in Marinesco–Sjögren syndrome: fine structural findings in skeletal muscle and conjunctiva. *Neuropediatrics* **23**: 329–35.

PART X

NEUROLOGICAL MANIFESTATIONS
OF SYSTEMIC DISEASES

A degree of neurological involvement is common in many systemic diseases, some of which have already been discussed or alluded to elsewhere in this book. Such involvement represents a significant part of the work of neurologists and serves to remind us that the nervous system is critically dependent on the rest of the organism. A complete coverage of this vast field is not the aim of this part, which is limited to the most important disorders that can produce major neurological disturbances and have not been previously dealt with. These include neurological syndromes due to disturbances of the electrolyte and acid-base metabolism to which the nervous system is extremely sensitive, nutritional diseases involving the CNS, which represent a major cause of neurological disease in developing countries, and CNS involvement in endocrine and visceral diseases. Both the peripheral and the central nervous system can be affected in several of these conditions.

22
ELECTROLYTE AND ACID-BASE METABOLISM DISTURBANCES, NUTRITIONAL DISORDERS AND OTHER SYSTEMIC DISEASES

DISORDERS OF WATER AND ELECTROLYTE METABOLISM

COMPLICATIONS OF ACUTE DEHYDRATION
Acute dehydration can be seen at all ages but is more common in infancy because of the frequency of gastroenteritis. Although its frequency has considerably decreased in industrialized countries because of better control of diarrhoeal diseases, it remains a major cause of disease and death in developing countries. Other causes of dehydration include renal and adrenal disease, central nervous system disease, heat exhaustion, limited intake often due to dependence on a third party for access to water, and diabetes insipidus. Acute dehydration can act on the CNS by at least two different mechanisms, which are not mutually exclusive. One is volume loss that may lead to circulatory insufficiency and vascular collapse with resulting hypoxic brain damage, and the second is electrolyte imbalance with hyper- or hyponatraemia.

HYPOVOLAEMIA AND VASCULAR COLLAPSE AS A CAUSE OF NEUROLOGICAL COMPLICATIONS OF DEHYDRATION
There is evidence that in many cases of diarrhoeal disorders of infants, hypovolaemia and resulting circulatory insufficiency play a major role in the genesis of neurological complications. Such disturbances can result in vascular collapse that is observed in infants with either hyper- or hyponatraemic dehydration. The resulting acute hypoxic–ischaemic encephalopathy involves diffuse areas of the brain, predominantly the territory fed by the carotid arteries and relatively sparing that fed by the posterior circulation (Fig. 22.1). The occurrence of convulsive seizures is better correlated to indices of volume loss such as a high urea level (Andrew 1991) than to sodium level or to the more or less rapid fall of natraemia. The neurological features include coma and convulsive seizures that occur on or a few hours after starting treatment. Sequelae of acute hypoxic encephalopathy include diplegia, microcephaly, mental retardation and seizures. Cortical blindness is not uncommon following the acute phase but useful recovery is usually observed.

Hypovolaemia with slowed venous circulation is one of the major causal factors of the venous and sinus thromboses that often occur with acute dehydration. They are probably responsible for the subarachnoid haemorrhage not uncommonly present in such cases (Sébire et al. 2005) and can also produce focal neurological symptoms and signs (Barron et al. 1992).

HYPERNATRAEMIA
Hypernatraemia is usually present in cases of severe dehydration and can be responsible for the neurological complications observed in such cases.

An increased concentration of sodium in body fluids results in shrinkage of the brain as fluid is drawn from the cells into the hyperosmolar vascular compartment, which becomes engorged and overdistended. Subdural haemorrhage has been experimentally produced in this way (Luttrell and Finberg 1959) but the clinical relevance in children remains uncertain (Andrew 1991). Small haemorrhages in the choroid plexus have been found by imaging (Mocharla et al. 1997), and haemorrhage (of whatever source) is probably the cause of elevated CSF protein in dehydration.

Other consequences of hypernatraemia may occur in the absence of structural alteration of the CNS. Clinical manifestations include varying degrees of impaired consciousness, fever and spasticity. About one third of infants experience convulsions, which usually do not start until 24–48 hours following onset of rehydration. These have been attributed to oedema resulting from rapid return of fluid into the brain on lowering plasma osmolality. Fluid is attracted into the cells because of increased intracellular chloride level and the release by the brain tissue of intracellular osmotically active particles, both Cl^- and K^+ ions and nonionic compounds such as polyalcohols and methylamines during the hypertonic phase of dehydration, which produces intracellular osmolality and consequently limits the degree of cellular dehydration (Lee et al. 1994, Pasantes-Morales et al. 2002). Seizures may well be due also to the return to basal value, during rehydration, of the convulsive threshold that had been

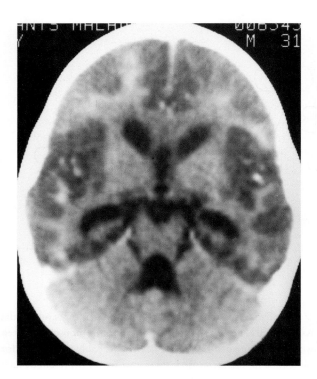

Fig. 22.1. Extensive ischaemic cortical necrosis in 18-month-old boy who suffered acute dehydration with vascular collapse and cardiac arrest at age 13 months.

TABLE 22.1
Main causes of hyper- and hyponatraemia

Hypernatraemia

Limited water intake (often due to inability to access fluid in neurological disorders)

Dehydration due to loss of water through diarrhoea, renal disease or other excessive losses of water with relative electrolyte conservation through hyperpnoea, fever or high ambient temperature

Salt intoxication

Endocrinological diseases

Neurological diseases with dysregulation of osmotic set point

Hyponatraemia

Water intoxication through excess administration of solute-free fluids

Water retention due to congestive heart failure or hepatic disease

Inappropriate secretion of antidiuretic hormone due to neurological (hypothalamic) disease

Postoperative hyponatraemia

Several neurological diseases (e.g. trauma, tumours, infections, haemorrhage) and non-neurological diseases (e.g. pneumonia)

Excessive salt losses: renal (diabetes insipidus, diuretics), or through evaporation/transpiration (cystic fibrosis, heat exhaustion)

maintained during the initial phase at a supranormal level as a result of the hypertonicity of body fluids. This may result in 'unmasking' the convulsive effects of vascular or hypoxic brain damage.

Hypernatraemia may be due to excessive evaporative losses of pure water or excess of salt caused by heat or hyperpnoea, salt poisoning or sodium retention as observed in hyperaldosteronism or Cushing disease (Table 22.1). Hypernatraemia is virtually always associated with dehydration, and it is difficult to determine which neurological features are due to the various factors. Rare cases of hypernatraemia are attributed to 'central' neurological causes (a disordered function of the hypothalamus). Hypernatraemia may be part of the syndrome of idiopathic hypothalamic dysfunction, in association with obesity, poor thermoregulation and disturbances of pituitary functions (North et al. 1994). A similar syndrome is more often caused by hypothalamic lesions including neoplasms. True central hypernatraemia without chronic dehydration is rare, and most such cases are due to abnormal thirst resulting in adipsic hypernatraemia (Radetti et al. 1991), or to hyperosmolar alimentation in patients on tube feeding receiving concentrated formulas, or occur in unconscious patients unable to have proper access to water. In all three cases there is associated latent dehydration. The condition of central diabetes insipidus is a primary failure of antidiuretic hormone secretion that may lead to hypernatraemia. It is most often due to brain tumours, especially craniopharyngioma, to malformations of the midline of the brain such as septo-optic dysplasia, and to CNS infections; no cause was found in 5 of the 35 cases studied

by Wang et al. (1994). The persistently increased diuresis in the face of marked hyperosmolality distinguishes diabetes insipidus from primary 'central' hypernatraemia.

HYPONATRAEMIA

Hyponataemia is uncommon in acute dehydration, but can occur in children hospitalized for dehydration who are given excessive diluted water load (*Lancet* 1992, Hoorn et al. 2004) or when intense vomiting was the cause. Severe alkalosis is usually associated in the latter cases. Vascular collapse and hypoxic encephalopathy may supervene if dehydration is severe enough, and death or severe neurological complications can ensue, so this is an emergency situation (Moritz and Ayus 2005).

Hyponatraemia may result from primay sodium deficiency, dilution secondary to oedema with hypervolaemia, or from excess secretion or release of antidiuretic hormone (Diederich et al. 2003, Bhardwaj 2006). It is most commonly due to mismanagement of fluid therapy. It is apt to occur in patients with inappropriate secretion of antidiuretic hormone, due to CNS disorders such as meningitis head trauma, brain tumours or encephalitis, as a side effect of some drugs such as vincristine or carbamazepine, or as a consequence of postoperative release of antidiuretic hormone (Table 22.1). Neurological disorders can also be responsible for another syndrome, the *cerebral salt wasting syndrome*, which, in contrast to excess arginin–vasopressin secretion, is associated with volume depletion. This syndrome should be distinguished from the preceding conditions because treatment requires fluid replacement and not fluid restriction, which should be avoided. Hyponatraemia is also observed in children with water retention due to heart or liver failure, in patients who receive excessive amounts of solute-poor fluids in the face of impaired renal function, and in cases of excess salt depletion as occurs with adrenal insufficiency, malnutrition or the use of diuretics. Oral water intoxication as a result of compulsive water drinking may occur in psychotic patients. Ingestion of 3-4 methylene dioxymeth-amphetamine (MDMA, 'ecstasy') may be associated with severe hyponatraemia (Parr et al. 1997) and should be thought of in cases of unexplained coma or abnormal behaviour, especially in adolescents.

The *hyponatraemia hypertensive syndrome* is characterized by arterial hypertension associated with low sodium plasma levels. It is observed mainly in adults with severe renal disease and is uncommon in chidren, although cases are on record in infants (Dahlem et al. 2000) and even in neonates (Daftary et al. 1999). Neurological manifestations are headache, nausea and vomiting incoordination, disturbances of consciousness and, especially, convulsive seizures. These are usually brief and are often associated with low body temperature, apnoea, and an opisthotonic posture (Finberg 1991). Any neurological symptom in patients who are dependent on a third party for their fluid requirements should lead to the suspicion of abnormal electrolyte concentrations.

Treatment by fluid restriction may be sufficient for most asymptomatic cases and in some symptomatic patients. In many symptomatic patients, hypertonic sodium solution should be immediately administered. Active correction of hyponatraemia with sodium-rich solutions is advised, but correction should be slow and cautious to avoid rapid shifts in osmolality. Prevention of hyponatraemia requires strict limitation of hypotonic solutions and the use of 0.9% sodium (Moritz and Ayus 2005) to limit the risk of central myelinolysis.

CENTRAL MYELINOLYSIS AND RELATED CONDITIONS

Central pontine myelinolysis, the most common location of central myelinolysis, is characterized pathologically by symmetrical demyelination of the central basis pontis. The clinical picture is marked by confusion and quadriplegia, sometimes with cranial nerve dysfunction. The disease was reported in chronically ill children with debilitating conditions (Kotagal et al. 1984), with kernicterus or following liver transplantation, or with viral gastroenteritis (Gregorio et al. 1997) and used to be considered fatal in most cases. More recently, neuroimaging techniques have enabled in vivo diagnosis in patients who went on to recover, and cases with milder expression or paucisymptomatic cases are not rare (Menger and Jörg 1999, Stanescu et al. 2002). The extent of apparent demyelination does not correlate with the clinical features and course. Although the mechanisms of the condition are not precisely known, it seems to be usually associated with rapid correction of hyponatraemia or with rapid shifts in osmolarity (Aylin et al. 2003, Martin 2004), so the condition is often referred to as *osmotic demyelination syndrome* and is a major reason for using slow correction of hyponatraemia. However, the safe rates for correction of hyponatraemia are still debated. Other uncommon causes have been indicted such as hypoglycaemia (Rajbhandari et al. 1998) and acute folate depletion (Ramaekers et al. 1997), and idiopathic cases have been reported (Menakaya et al. 2001).

Extrapontine structures such as the basal nuclei and/or central white matter can also be involved (Haspolat et al. 2004).

TABLE 22.2
Main causes of hypocalcaemia

Cause	References
Hypoparathyroidism	Winer et al. (2003), Armelisasso et al. (2004)
Pseudohypoparathyroidism	Chapter 9
Vitamin D deficiency	Pettifor (2005)
DiGeorge syndrome	Garcia-Garcia et al. (2000)
Renal disease	Locatelli et al. (2002), Morii et al. (2004)
Transient neonatal hypoparthyroidism	Bainbridge et al. (1987), Ip (2003)
Maternal hyperparathyroidism	Thomas et al. (1999)
Hypomagnesaemic tetany of infancy	Yamamoto et al. (1985)
Preterm birth	Hsu and Levine (2004)
Post-term birth and critically ill newborn infants	Cardenas-Rivero et al. (1989)

OTHER ELECTROLYTE DISTURBANCES

Chloride deficiency obtains with profuse vomiting such as occurs in infants with pyloric stenosis and results in metabolic alkalosis. The latter decreases ionization of calcium and can result in normocalcaemic tetany.

Chloride deficiency rarely results from intestinal losses in children with chloride diarrhoea and in children who have ingested a chloride-deficient formula for periods of one month or more. Clinical features include lethargy, failure to thrive, weakness and delayed milestones, reversible on chloride administration. Head growth is slowed or arrested. Although chloride supplementation rapidly reverses the symptoms, cognitive sequelae may persist (Willoughby et al. 1987). In rare cases chloride deprivation may occur as a result of a maternal chloride deficiency in breast-fed infants.

Calcium and phosphorus disturbances occur preferentially in the neonatal period (Chapter 1) or as a complication of parathyroid disease. They may also be associated with endocrinological conditions such as pituitary and adrenal insufficiency, and often with severe hyponatraemia and hyperkalaemia that can necessitate emergency treatment.

Hypercalcaemia may occur with hyperparathyroidism, either acquired or congenital. Neonatal severe hyperparathyroidism features marked muscular hypotonia in association with failure to thrive and vomiting. The condition is observed in children with chronic renal failure (Sanchez 2003). It has been recorded in association with maternal hypoparathyroidism (Daoud et al. 2000). Conversely, *hypocalcaemia* with neonatal seizures may occur in infants born to mothers with hyperparathyroidism (Jaafar et al. 2004). Other causes of hypocalcaemia are listed in Table 22.2.

Primary *hypomagnesaemia* with secondary hypocalcaemia has been considered in Chapter 1. This condition occurs mainly in males, but study of large pedigrees does not support an X-linked disease but rather sex-limitation of an autosomal recessive disorder. It can produce focal neurological deficits (Leicher et al. 1991). Chronic magnesium deficiency was described in a child with nephropathy in association with carpopedal spasm, convulsions and mitochondrial myopathy (Riggs et al. 1992).

NUTRITIONAL DISORDERS OF THE NERVOUS SYSTEM

The nervous system may be affected by nutritional deficiencies whether they involve globally deficient nutrition as a result of grossly inadequate quantities of food, poor protein intake, dietary imbalances, or lack of specific necessary nutriments. In many cases, intercurrent parasitic or bacterial infections, poor hygiene, and educational and emotional deprivation combine to produce a complex clinical picture. The growing nervous system is particularly at risk under such circumstances.

The total complement of neurons in the cerebrum is virtually complete at birth, but the growth of dendritic and axonal trees and of glial cells and the process of myelination are all very active during the first two years of life. In fact, the weight of the infant brain almost trebles during the first year of life. In the cerebellum, proliferation of the granule cells continues postnatally for at least the first year. The cerebellum may thus be especially vulnerable and this might be a factor in the origin of the clumsiness frequently observed in individuals submitted to early malnutrition. The first two or three years of life thus constitute, together with the prenatal period, a 'critical period' as the brain growth spurt begins about mid-gestation and ends between the second and third year of life (Dobbing 1981, Ballabriga 1989). Dendritic development has been shown to be abnormal in malnourished infants (Benítez-Bribiesca et al. 1999). During this period, both brain insults and neglect are especially apt to result in brain growth disturbances and dysfunction. The effects of prenatal deprivation are reviewed by Volpe (2005). This section is devoted to the neurological consequences of postnatal nutritional deficiencies.

PROTEIN–ENERGY MALNUTRITION, PROTEIN–CALORIE MALNUTRITION (PCM)

Winick (1969) estimated that 300 million children in the world suffer varying degrees of malnutrition, and the figure may well have increased since (Muller and Krawinkel 2005). The sequelae of this problem may represent a large proportion of cases of mental retardation, learning difficulties and abnormal behaviour in many parts of the world.

CLINICAL FEATURES

PCM may present as one of two main syndromes. Deficiency of micronutrients, especially iron, iodine, vitamin A, phosphorus and zinc, are very often associated and represent another major nutritional problem. *Marasmus* is primarily due to caloric insufficiency and is observed in infants weaned before 1 year of age or when the amount of breast milk becomes markedly reduced. The major clinical manifestations are emaciation, loss of muscle mass and growth failure. *Kwashiorkor* results from a diet containing sufficient calories but deficient in proteins. Other factors such as infections, specific vitamin deficiencies and lack of

appropriate stimulation also play a role (Jelliffe and Jelliffe 1992). Kwashiorkor is most common in children weaned between 2 and 3 years of age. The clinical features include oedema, growth failure, muscle wasting and behavioural disturbances. Abnormal pigmentation of the hair and skin, anaemia and hepatomegaly may be associated. The clinical picture is quite variable. Recently, diagnostic difficulties have resulted from the diffusion of HIV infection, as wasting and lipodystrophies observed in this condition may prevent recognition of underlying PCM (Kotler 2004, Wanke 2004).

The neurological features of marasmus and kwashiorkor are similar. Indeed, the two conditions are often associated, as symptoms of kwashiorkor may develop in children already suffering from PCM. They include apathy which may be of such degree that children may manifest little interest in food despite severe wasting. Muscle wasting and hypotonia are common, and tendon reflexes may be decreased. This reflects involvement of peripheral nerves with reduction of nerve conduction velocities and segmental demyelination (Chopra et al. 1986, Chopra and Sharma 1992). Soft neurological signs are significantly more frequent in malnourished than in well-fed children (Agarwal et al. 1989). CT may show brain atrophy, and confirms the possibility of reversible atrophy, but shows appropriate-for-age myelination (Gunston et al. 1992). MRI has confirmed the frequent occurrence of global atrophy and showed ventricular dilatation in severe cases (Odabas et al. 2005b). Nonspecific EEG abnormalities have been reported (Agarwal et al. 1989), and increased latencies of auditory potential were found to be commonly present (Odabas et al. 2005a).

NEUROLOGICAL COMPLICATIONS OF THE TREATMENT OF PCM

Up to 20% of children with PCM experience neurological problems within 3–7 days after being started on a normal diet. In most cases this is limited to drowsiness, but rare cases of coma and even of fatality are on record. This syndrome may result from hepatic failure when a large protein load is presented to an atrophic liver.

In some patients with PCM, coarse tremor ('kwashi shakes'), myoclonus, bradykinesia and rigidity are observed one to several weeks after protein refeeding (Thame et al. 1999). Tan and Önbas (2004) reported massive myoclonus that might have been due to refeeding associated with central pontine myelinolysis in a child with kwashiorkor. The syndrome usually resolves in a few days or weeks. The tremor is usually generalized but localized jerking is occasionally seen and may be difficult to distinguish from epileptic jerking, especially from partial continuous epilepsy, as in two of my patients. The mechanism of this syndrome is unknown. A role of magnesium deficiency has been proposed, and magnesium therapy was said to accelerate recovery. The syndrome may also be observed in cases of renutrition following protracted diarrhoea (personal cases). Megaloblastic anaemia may be associated. A relationship between this syndrome and *infantile tremor syndrome* as observed in India (Garewal et al. 1988) remains to be explored; the latter is associated with vitamin B_{12} deficiency in 87% of cases and occurs in malnourished children in 82%. It usually leaves behind a significant degree of mental retardation despite control with vitamin B_{12} therapy.

Other complications of treatment include thrombosis of the superior vena cava following prolonged catheterization responsible for increased intracranial pressure (Chapter 13). In some cases, increased T_1 signal from the basal ganglia has been found on MRI in patients receiving total parenteral nutrition (Mirowitz et al. 1991). This may be related to manganese toxicity (Barron et al. 1994).

LONG-TERM NEURODEVELOPMENTAL EFFECTS OF PCM

Extreme PCM has been shown to result in reduced brain growth and behavioural abnormalities, both in experimental animals and in man (Winick 1969). In human beings, however, the role of malnutrition is more difficult to assess because malnourished infants also suffer several other adverse conditions such as crowding, poor hygiene, infections, deficient education and care, and such factors have a cumulative effect. However, there is little doubt that head growth, which reflects brain growth in humans (Bartholomeusz et al. 2002), is slowed in severely malnourished infants (Stoch et al. 1982), and that the younger the infant at the time of deprivation the greater the effect on head circumference. 'Catch-up' growth of the brain can occur if renutrition is provided during the first one or two years of life but not later, even though catch-up of size and weight occurs (Stoch et al. 1982). CT and MRI have confirmed the presence of atrophy in the temporoparietal region bilaterally in patients with kwashiorkor followed up to early adulthood. However, this is largely reversible (Gunston et al. 1992). Regrowth may be so rapid that splaying of the skull sutures occurs. Even though a small head does not necessarily mean a reduction in neuronal number, as neurons represent only a small fraction of human brain (Dobbing 1981), experience has shown that microcephaly is correlated with low IQ and learning difficulties (Gillberg and Rasmussen 1982) and that brain growth in low-birthweight infants is an excellent predictor of later IQ (Hack and Breslau 1986). There is also evidence that intellectual attainments in patients with PCM are inferior to those of normally fed children (Galler et al. 1987, Agarwal et al. 1995), even though other factors such as gender, education and home environment may play a role as great or greater than nutrition in this regard. Fine motor skills are also disturbed (Colombo et al. 1992). It is of note that malnutrition occurring in children older than 1–2 years of age has much less effect on the eventual IQ than earlier PCM. Disentangling the multiple factors responsible for developmental delay in malnourished children is difficult as lack of stimulation has been shown to be a possible cause. A study comparing four groups (supplemented, stimulated, supplemented and stimulated, and controls) showed a significantly greater benefit when both supplementation and stimulation were offered than when each was offered alone (Grantham-McGregor et al. 1991), and Colombo et al. (1992) found that neurodevelopment of adopted children who had had PCM reverted to normal levels, thus indicating both the reversibility of the condition and the value of environmental stimulation.

More subtle malnutrition can occur and remain undetected

in infants, especially preterm infants, following acute neonatal illnesses (Embleton et al. 2001, Hulst et al. 2006). Recent studies have shown that such infants have accumulated a deficit of energy during their acute disease and that a greater energy intake than currently advised results in better general and head growth (Brandt et al. 2003, Dabydeen et al. 2008) and may improve ultimate brain function and IQ in children with neonatal brain injury (Lucas et al. 1998, Brandt et al. 2003). These findings emphasize the need for systematic monitoring of calorie intake in such infants as an adequate energy intake could prevent some of the consequences of neonatal problems.

NONORGANIC FAILURE TO THRIVE

The complexity of the relationships between malnutrition and somatic and mental development is illustrated by the common problem of 'nonorganic failure to thrive' (Casey et al. 1984). The syndrome mainly manifests in infancy. Growth retardation is commonly found in children from underprivileged homes even in industrialized countries (King and Taitz 1985). Their failure to thrive is poorly understood and is probably not simply the result of food deprivation, as shown by the rapid growth gain on changing the environment. The parents of children with 'deprivation dwarfism' are found to differ in several respects from control parents. They have less emotional responsivity, the level of maternal acceptance of the child is lower, and they are less able to organize the physical home environment (Casey et al. 1984). Such parents fail to 'read' the child's needs and respond to them. Poor feeding skills can be an important cause of nonorganic growth failure, particularly in infants with early feeding difficulties (Ramsay et al. 1993), and children with neurological problems often have feeding difficulties that may be responsible for poor nutrition and growth (Morton et al. 1993).

The syndrome of psychosocial or psychosomatic dwarfism appears to be associated with reversible inhibition of somatotropin secretion (Green et al. 1984). Affected children may have behaviour problems, bizarre eating habits, self-mutilation and poor response to pain (Mouridsen and Nielson 1990). All symptoms are reversible when the child's domicile is changed to a more benign environment. However, persistent growth retardation continues into late childhood (Drewett et al. 1999, Boddy et al. 2000) and behavioural disturbances (Boddy et al. 2000, Dykman et al. 2001, Steward 2001) have been reported several years after recovery. Some investigators found a lower IQ in former patients than in controls (Dykman et al. 2001) but this was not the experience of others who found no difference in IQ and educational attainments from normal children (Drewett et al. 1999). This syndrome should be considered in the differential diagnosis of every child with short stature, low IQ, learning disabilities or bizarre behaviour in various combinations.

VITAMIN DEFICIENCIES

In addition to dietary deficiency, the action of vitamins in intermediary metabolism can be disturbed by abnormally high requirements – which may be of dietary origin, e.g. an excess of carbohydrates increases the need for B group vitamins – or by the action of inhibitory substances, or by an alteration of configuration of apoenzyme proteins that also results in a considerable increase in vitamin requirements. Some inborn errors of metabolism can be corrected by large doses of certain vitamins (Chapter 8).

THIAMINE (VITAMIN B₁) DEFICIENCY
Thiamine plays an important role in the decarboxylation of pyruvate and alpha-ketoglutarate, two steps of the Krebs cycle, and the conversion of 5-carbon to 6-carbon sugars by means of the enzyme transketolase. Therefore, thiamine deficiency decreases energy available to the brain and increases the concentration of the two keto acids.

The clinical features of thiamine deficiency are variable. Classical *beriberi*, as seen in Asia and Africa, is marked by the sudden onset of weakness due to acute peripheral neuropathy, neck stiffness, aphonia and cardiac failure. In industralized countries, cases of Wernicke encephalopathy are sometimes seen in patients receiving parenteral nutrition (Barrett et al. 1993), in those on dialysis (Jagadha et al. 1987), in children with malignant or debilitating diseases, especially when they are taking a high-carbohydrate diet (Pihko et al. 1989) and in children receiving antineoplasic chemotherapy (Vanhulle et al. 1997). The clinical picture is highly variable from sudden collapse and death to chronic cognitive impairment, through the classic picture of acute ataxia (Ogunlesi 2004), global confusion and ocular abnormalities. The diagnosis is often missed and it should be thought of in all appropriate settings as Wernicke encephalopathy is a preventable cause of death (Pihko et al. 1989, Barrett et al. 1993). Imaging may be of considerable help if it shows hypodense areas with contrast enhancement in the paraventricular region of both thalami and along the cerebral aqueduct. MRI better shows a low-intensity signal from these regions (Weidauer et al. 2003). Diffusion-weighted MRI can be useful in cases with negative MRI findings by showing increased diffusion in the same areas (Halavaara et al. 2003). In patients on parenteral nutrition, unusual location of haemorrhagic lesions in the superior vermis and lower brainstem without involvement of the mamillary bodies has been observed (Vortmeyer et al. 1992). The condition may occur even in children receiving conventional doses of vitamin B₁ if the requirements are increased by the carbohydrate intake. Treatment is with large amounts of intravenous thiamine. The condition should be differentiated from Leigh disease (Chapter 8), which does not affect the mamillary bodies in most cases, contrary to their almost constant involvement in thiamine deficiency. Thiamine deficiency may favour the occurrence of epileptic seizures in patients with a latent predisposition (Keyser and DeBruijn 1991).

PYRIDOXINE (VITAMIN B₆) DEFICIENCY AND PYRIDOXINE DEPENDENCY
Vitamin B₆ in the form of its aldehyde derivative pyridoxal-5-phosphate is essential for correct functioning of the CNS. It is, in particular, necessary for the decarboxylation of glutamic acid to GABA, an essential inhibitory neurotransmitter in cerebral cortex. *Pyridoxine deficiency* is responsible for heightened brain excitability and seizures. It has been observed during the first year of life in infants on a diet providing less than 0.1 mg/day such as powdered goat's milk (Johnson 1982). Less rarely, pyridoxine deficiency may occur in patients who have a jejunal bypass or in those who receive treatment with hydrazide drugs such as isoniazid or penicillamine. In such cases, however, peripheral neuropathy (Chapter 20) is more common than convulsions.

Pyridoxine dependency (Chapter 8) is a rare familial disease transmitted as an autosomal recessive trait, characterized by seizures, usually severe and repeated, which occurs soon after birth and frequently in utero (Haenggeli et al. 1991, Gospe and Hecht 1998). Neurological and general manifestations such as abdominal distension, vomiting and encephalopathic manifestations are frequent, so the term pyridoxine-dependent encephalopathy is appropriate, and raise a diagnostic problem with hypoxic–ischaemic encephalopathy (Baxter et al. 1996). Imaging may show progressive ventricular dilatation or abnormalities of the white matter (Gospe and Hecht 1998, Baxter 2001). The diagnosis formerly rested on administration of pyridoxine, which must be systematically given to all neonates and infants under 2 years of age with unexplained seizures. Recently, elevation of pipecolic acid in blood and urine was shown to allow a probable biochemical diagnosis (Gospe 2006). The diagnosis can now be confirmed by demonstration of mutations in the *antiquitin* gene (Mills et al. 2006, Plecko et al. 2007; see also Chapter 8), thus avoiding the need to wait for recurrence of seizures after discontinuation of pyridoxine treatment. Pyridoxine, when given early, may prevent deterioration and sequelae such as microcephly (Tan et al. 2004) and mental retardation.

In a rarer, late-onset form (Baxter et al. 1996, Baxter 2001), seizures manifesting pyridoxine dependency occur relatively late, up to 18–24 months. Such seizures are apt to occur repeatedly in bouts of status epilepticus but may also present as infantile spasms or myoclonic attacks (Goutières and Aicardi 1985). In some cases, the seizures may respond to anticonvulsants and remain controlled for periods of several weeks or even months, or may remain controlled for similar periods after receiving vitamin B₆ therapy.

Treatment of pyridoxine dependency requires doses of vitamin B₆ widely varying from 0.2 to 30 mg/kg/day. In cases with status epilepticus, intravenous administration of 50–100 mg should stop the seizures in less than 10 minutes. In the case of brief seizures, oral administration of 50 mg/day as a single dose produces rapid discontinuation of attacks. Intravenous doses of more than 200 mg may produce hypotonia and apnoea (Kroll 1985). However, coma and respiratory disturbances have been observed even after gastric tube administration of the drug in a patient who responded to very small doses (Grillo et al. 2001).

Cases of neonatal epileptic encephalopathy refractory to pyridoxine but responding dramatically to pyridoxal phophate have been reported (Kuo and Wang 2002, Clayton et al. 2003, Hoffmann et al. 2007). So, pyridoxal phosphate, when available, is the best therapeutic choice in cases of pyridoxine dependency, and has been shown to be life-saving and to be able to prevent brain damage (Hoffmann et al. 2007). Such cases have been

URAEMIC ENCEPHALOPATHY

The main neurological complication of renal insufficiency is uraemic encephalopathy marked by alteration in cognitive status, hypotonia, seizures, athetoid movements, nystagmus, asterixis and ataxia (Brouns and De Deyn 2004). Myoclonus is a suggestive symptom, as are peripheral cramps. Transient focal cerebral symptoms, including hemiparesis and cortical blindness, may be more closely related to hypertensive encephalopathy. Encephalopthy can also result from toxicity of some drugs used.

In children with moderate to severe chronic renal failure, a small head and developmental delay are commonly encountered (McGraw and Haka-Ikse 1985). Bock et al. (1989) found that children with the most severe renal insufficiency had a small head circumference early in life, motor developmental delay and progressive decrease in IQ in the absence of neurological signs.

Uraemic encephalopathy is reversible upon correction of renal insufficiency by haemodialysis or kidney transplantation. The latter is highly efficacious for uraemic polyneuropathy, whereas haemodialysis does not correct sensory deficits. Treatment of seizures is with standard anticonvulsant therapy, taking into account the changes in metabolism and excretion of drugs used to prevent rejection brought about by inducing anticonvulsive agents (Chapter 15). Benzodiazepines are effective against the myoclonus.

In a number of patients with renal failure, a syndrome of *reversible posterior leukoencephalopathy* has been repeatedly observed. It is marked clinically by headache, obtundation, often convulsions and sometimes visual failure and focal deficits. Imaging shows areas of increased T_2 and FLAIR signal predominating in the parieto-occipital areas but wnich may extend anteriorly and even involve the brainstem (Lamy et al. 2004). The syndrome is most often reversible but occasional sequelae may persist (Prasad et al. 2003). Hypertension appears to be the major cause of the syndrome, but it may also be associated with some chemotherapy agents (Tam et al. 2004) such as tacrolimus and cyclosporine.

Cognitive deficits, cortical atrophy and disseminated brain calcification are often associated with *nephropathic cystinosis* (Broyer et al. 1996) Social difficulties are prominent, whereas cognition and language remain relatively normal (Delgado et al. 2005). The effect of kidney transplantation in such cases is not yet known. Other neurological manifestations may be present with certain causes of renal failure such as haemolytic–uraemic syndrome (Chapter 10). The frequency and mechanism of sensorineural hearing loss in children with long-standing renal failure are disputed. Ototoxic drugs such as furosemide and aminoglycosides are likely to be an important factor (Mancini et al. 1996).

COMPLICATIONS OF THE TREATMENT OF CHRONIC RENAL FAILURE

Dialysis may be associated with aggravation of neurological manifestations as a result of the *dialysis dysequilibrium syndrome*. This syndrome is due to failure of the urea to equilibrate rapidly between brain and blood, thus resulting in a shift of extracellular water into the brain but the mechanisms appear to be complex (Trinh-Trang-Tan et al. 2005). It manifests with headache, nausea, vomiting, progressive obtundation and occasional convulsions. This complication can be avoided by gradual changes in blood electrolytes and earlier dialysis.

Repeated dialysis may be associated with a variety of symptoms probably related to deficiency of vitamins, other nutritional factors or electrolyte dysequilibrium. These include central pontine myelinolysis, Wernicke encephalopathy and the 'burning feet syndrome', a form of sensorimotor neuropathy that may respond to supplementation with group B vitamins.

Dialysis encephalopathy is characterized by personality changes, dysarthria, apraxia of speech, myoclonus and seizures. The EEG shows slowing of background tracings and multiple paroxysms (Hughes and Schreeder 1980). The disorder is fatal in a few years. However, the realization that aluminium toxicity was the cause, as a result of a high content of this metal in the dialysis bath, led to the almost complete disappearance of the syndrome with the use of aluminum-free water. Cases identical to dialysis encephalopathy have been seen in patients not on dialysis receiving large quantities of aluminium salts, who had levels of serum and bone aluminium considerably in excess of the average figures (Griswold et al. 1983). In such cases, reversal of symptoms was achieved by discontinuation of the use of gels and by aluminium chelation (Ackrill et al. 1980).

Acute hypercalcaemia in haemodialysis patients may mimic dialysis dementia (Rivera-Vásquez et al. 1980) and has an excellent prognosis on correction of serum calcium.

Symptomatic hypoglycaemia has been observed months to years following renal transplantation (Wells et al. 1988). It occurred in children receiving propranolol and responded to discontinuation of the drug.

Patients with renal transplants run the risks attendant on organ transplantation. These are mostly the result of immunosuppression and are dealt with below.

REJECTION ENCEPHALOPATHY

An acute neurological syndrome occurs in some renal transplant recipients (Brouns and De Deyn 2004). It is important to recognize that this syndrome is not due to disturbances in electrolytes, hypertension, fever or steroids, so steroid treatment may be continued.

It is also important to keep in mind that drugs such as most anticonvulsants accelerate the catabolism of steroids resulting in possible reduction of allograft survival. Treatment of seizures should be with non-enzyme-inducing drugs such as valproate or benzodiazepines.

HEPATIC DISEASE

HEPATIC ENCEPHALOPATHY

Hepatic encephalopathy constitutes the end stage of acute or chronic liver disease and culminates in hepatic coma. Liver failure may be due to acute hepatitis, drug toxicity, Wilson disease or metabolic diseases, or less commonly to chronic hepatitis or various terminal liver illnesses, including cystic fibrosis of the pancreas and deficiency in alpha 1 antitrypsin (Lee et al. 2005). Hyperammonaemia is an important factor of hepatic encephalopathy (Katayama 2004). However, the mechanism of ammonia toxicity is obscure and occasional patients with hepatic encephalopathy have normal or mildly elevated levels of ammonia in the blood and CSF. The toxicity of ammonia is well shown by the possible occurrence of encephalopathy in patients receiving essential amino acid hyperalimentation (Grazer et al. 1984) but does not account for all features of the encephalopathy of liver failure. Its role as a cause of the stuporous episodes sometimes observed during valproate therapy (Marescaux et al. 1982) remains unclear. It appears that increased ammonia levels induce and/or alter the expression of several genes that code for neurotransmitter-associated proteins, including those of monoamine oxidase (A isoform), nitric oxide synthase, and peripheral GABA receptors. Glutamine synthesis is increased in astrocytes with resulting swelling as a result of increased activation of glutamate receptors. Overall, increased inhibition results (Jones 2002, Butterworth 2003).

Neuropathological changes are limited. Gross examination of the brain shows no abnormalities. Microscopically, the main alteration is enlargement and increase in the number of protoplasmic astrocytes, the so-called Alzheimer type II astrocytes. These are seen throughout the cerebral cortex, basal ganglia and brainstem nuclei. Astrocyte swelling is thought to play a mjor role in the neurological manifestations possibly by interference with glial neuronal communication.

The onset of hepatic encephalopathy is sometimes fulminating but it is often heralded by malaise, anorexia and vomiting. Disorders of consciousness are the principal symptoms. Disorientation, anxiety, depression and slurred speech appear first. They are rapidly followed by drowsiness, lethargy, disorientation and inappropriate behaviour. Asterixis or 'flapping tremor' may be an early feature. Extrapyramidal rigidity and choreic movements are frequent in children. Ataxia, seizures, myoclonus and hyperventilation with resulting alkalosis frequently develop in advanced stages. Decerebrate posturing may occur in the terminal phase. Cerebral oedema is a major cause of death (Lidofsky et al. 1992). The EEG often shows diffuse bursts of high-voltage, slow-wave activity and sometimes triphasic spikes (Tasker et al. 1988). The course may be rapidly lethal or fluctuate considerably, and symptoms may be rapidly reversible if the course of the liver disease is favourable.

In cases of chronic liver failure, hyperintensity of the globus pallidus, the hypothalamus and the hypophysis is frequently found on T_1-weighted MRI. It is due to deposition of manganese, which is correlated to the severity of liver failure (Pujol et al. 1993, Genovese et al. 2000). Manganese toxicity, which is reversible by discontinuation of parenteral manganese in parenteral nutrition (Barron et al. 1994), may be an important factor in such cases.

The treatment of hepatic encephalopathy is beyond the scope of this book (see Devictor et al. 1993, Riordan and Williams 1997). Treatment of cerebral oedema is essential. Nonabsorbable antibiotics have an important role in the treatment and prevention of hepatic encephalopathy (Maddrey 2005) by limiting ammonia synthesis by intestinal flora. It is customary to stop protein intake and to sterilize the intestinal tract with antibiotics, although the relationship between diet and hepatic encephalopathy is complex. Hepatic transplantation is often necessary.

FULMINANT HEPATIC FAILURE
Fulminant hepatic failure has been observed repeatedly in epileptic patients receiving valproic acid or sodium valproate (Scheffner et al. 1988). This rare complication occurs mainly in infants and young children, who most commonly are mentally retarded and receiving valproic acid as part of a multidrug treatment (Dreifuss et al. 1989). In the USA the incidence has been estimated to be as high as 1 in 500 treated infants under 2 years, which seems vastly in excess of what is observed in western Europe. However, a dramatic decrease in fatal hepatotoxicity has been recently reported from the USA (Dreifuss et al. 1989). It is doubtful in this writer's opinion that this decrease is due to preventive measures. It is more likely that the recognition of metabolic disorders as a cause and the stricter criteria now required for attributing hepatic failure to valproate have restricted the apparent frequency. Valproate toxicity closely resembles Reye syndrome (Chapter 10) or cases of impaired fatty acid beta-oxidation (Chapter 8). It is likely that metabolites of the drug interfere with fatty acid or other metabolisms in patients with some latent enzyme defect. This has been observed in patients with deficiencies of enzymes of the urea cycle (Christmann et al. 1990) and of the respiratory chain, especially cytochrome c oxidase (Chabrol et al. 1994; and personal case) and medium-chain acyl-CoA dehydrogenase (Njølstad et al. 1997). A proportion of the cases may in fact be due to liver failure, which accompanies naturally some cases of poliodystrophy (Alpers disease, Chapter 9) due to mitochondrial mutations, especially of the *POLG1* gene (Horvath et al. 2006), or of other mitochondrial abnormalities, and may be precipitated by administration of the drug (Bicknese et al. 1992). Cases of liver failure induced by valproate cannot be prevented by determination of the blood levels of transaminases, which remain normal up to the onset of failure in many cases but may be moderately increased in patients on uncomplicated valproate therapy (Dreifuss et al. 1989). The preventive value of carnitine is not demonstrated. Parents should be warned that they should report any vomiting, lethargy or increase in seizure frequency. Other drugs, notably anticonvulsants such as phenytoin and carbamazepine, may occasionally produce fatal hepatitis (Pellock 1987).

OTHER COMPLICATIONS OF HEPATIC FAILURE AND ITS TREATMENT
Cognitive development and somatic growth in children with chronic liver disease are frequently impaired (Stewart et al. 1988), especially in liver disease of early onset. Part of the impairment

is perhaps due to vitamin E deficiency, which is frequent in disorders of biliary secretion.

ENDOCRINE DISEASE

THYROID DISEASES

Thyroid hormones are crucial to normal neural maturation and function. In the human fetus, thyroxine (T4) is synthesized from 10 to 14 weeks gestation. Therefore, early in gestation, neurological maturation, dependent on thyroid hormone, relies on T4 from the mother. The view that the placenta is impermeable to thyroid hormones, even in late gestation, is now being revised. Work with animals has shown that substantial amounts of T4 and T3 are present in all fetal tissues and that iodothyronines are transferred in significant quantity from mother to fetus early in gestation (Pharoah and Connolly 1995). In humans, T4 levels of 35–70 nmol/L have been found in cord blood of infants with complete failure of T4 synthesis (Vulsma et al. 1989). T4 but not T3 has been shown to be associated with measures of fetal neurological development, and the availability of circulating T4 is crucial to the normal maturation of neuronal cells (Pharoah and Connolly 1995). In this view, the timing of any T4 deficiency will determine the clinical picture. Early deficiency of exclusively maternal origin will be responsible for endemic cretinism. Later deficiency due to more or less severe failure of fetal thyroid hormone synthesis, with only partial maternal compensation, will result in congenital hypothyroidism of variable severity.

Absent or insufficient thyroxine results in impaired RNA and protein synthesis, reduced size and number of cortical neurons, hypoplasia of dendrites and axons, and retarded myelination (Smith 1981).

CONGENITAL HYPOTHYROIDISM

The diagnosis of congenital hypothyroidism, at least in many industrialized countries, is now usually made by screening in the neonatal period. Various screening techniques are utilized using TSH, thyroxine, or thyroxine/TSH ratio. There is still debate over the best method but there is consensus regarding the interest of an early diagnosis.

Transient hypothyroidism poses a special problem as the final diagnosis of hypothyroidism can be made only by repetition of the tests. This situation obtains mostly in preterm infants (Williams et al. 2005), especially those whose mothers had received an overload of iodine during pregnancy. Although most clinicians treat such infants with thyroxine until persistent thyroid deficiency is demonstrated or excluded, thyroxine therapy may not be necessary in all mild or borderline cases (Williams et al. 2005).

Most cases of *persistent hypothyroidism* detected by screening are sporadic. Only 2% are familial, and these are mostly due to disturbances in hormonosynthesis (Park and Chatterjee 2005). Most cases are associated with absence or defects of development of the gland, which, when present, is usually in ectopic position. The proportion of cases due to ectopic or absent gland varies with the populations studied (Schoen et al. 2004) but cases in which

a thyroid gland is found in normal position are more frequent than previously thought (Weber et al. 2005). Among cases with a gland of normal position and shape, only a minority are associated with a specific disorder of hormonosynthesis. Permanent deficiency was associated with goitre in 27 of 49 infants with an in situ thyroid gland studied by Gaudino et al. (2005), while 14 had a normal-sized and -shaped gland, and 8 had a hypoplastic thyroid. Deficits in thyroglobulin synthesis and other defects of iodine organification were present in 10 infants with goitre. One infant had Pendred syndrome, and 1 had a defect of sodium-iodide symporter, while in 7 no precise diagnosis could be made. Two infants with a hypoplastic gland had a mutation of the TSH receptor gene.

Hypothyroidism is thus a heterogeneous condition whose diagnosis requires both clinical skills and laboratory facilities.

In *neonatal nongoitrous hypothyroidism* the thyroid gland is absent, ectopic or too small to produce adequate amounts of hormones. However, cases with in situ thyroid are recognized. The diagnosis is difficult at birth, the reason why many countries have introduced systematic screening of TSH level in the neonatal period. Clinical diagnosis becomes more obvious over the following months. Untreated infants are placid or hypotonic with a grunting cry. They have a protuberant abdomen, often with umbilical hernia, and may have prolonged jaundice. They are pale and have coarse, lustreless hair and widely open fontanelles and sutures. One third of affected infants have neurological abnormalities including spasticity, incoordination and cerebellar ataxia (Smith et al. 1975). Sensorineural hearing loss is present in 10% of infants (Vanderschueren-Lodeweyckx et al. 1983) as a result of developmental cochlear abnormalities. Less severe forms with milder symptoms are even more difficult to diagnose yet may generate neurodevelopmental retardation.

Neonatal goitrous hypothyroidism is usually due to defects in the synthesis of thyroid hormones (Gaudino et al. 2005). Impairment of intelligence varies with the responsible defect. Pendred syndrome (Chapter 18), transmitted as an autosomal recessive anomaly, includes goitre, deafness and hypothyroidism (Sugiura et al. 2005).

EARLY TREATMENT OF NEONATAL HYPOTHYROIDISM

Administration of synthetic laevothyroxine is essential to avoid developmental retardation. The outcome depends on the date of onset, the cause and the dose used. Infants with prenatal onset of thyroid insufficiency as shown by low T4 levels and retarded bone age at birth tend to have lower than normal scores on visuospatial, perceptual, motor and language subtests despite a normal global IQ (Rovet and Ehrlich 1995). Most children treated within the first four weeks of life do well, although subtle developmental difficulties may be present in later life (Gottschalk et al. 1994) even in infants detected by neonatal screening and immediately treated, although there are divergent opinions in this regard (Iliki and Larsson 1988, Kooistra et al. 1994, Simons et al. 1994). Rovet (2005) found the IQ of these children to be globally mildly decreased (by 6–9 points) as compared with their siblings. A recent report of very long term follow-up in adults screened as neonates between 1979 and 1985 found no difference in rates of employment and school difficulties from those in the rest of the population (Toublanc et al. 2005). An increased incidence of cerebral palsy in preterm infants with transient hypothyroxinaemia has been reported by Reuss et al. (1996).

In infants treated after 3 months of age, developmental delay and a cerebellar ataxic syndrome (Wiebel 1976) are common.

CHILDHOOD-ONSET HYPOTHYROIDISM
The prognosis for hypothyroidism that develops during childhood is clearly better. In such patients, in addition to cognitive deterioration and slow movements, there is sometimes muscle hypertrophy that is often associated with a degree of myotonia or, at least, of reduced speed of contraction and relaxation, constituting the Kocher–Debré–Sémelaigne syndrome (Tullu et al. 2003).

ENDEMIC CRETINISM
Endemic cretinism is a major worldwide problem of public health with an estimated 800 million people at risk in many countries (Hetzel 1994). Although the condition is still mostly encountered in developing countries, cases continue to be seen in Europe (Delange 2002). There are two forms of the condition, myxoedematous and nervous cretinism, but neurological signs are common to both types (Halpern et al. 1991) and include mental retardation and a nonprogressive neurological syndrome of bilateral spasticity, extrapyramidal features, notably dystonia, and parkinsonian gait. Goiter can be present (Dunn 2001). Deafness is usually associated. Calcification of the basal ganglia is present in 30% of patients (Ma et al. 1993).

Endemic cretinism is a consequence of iodine deficiency in the mothers of affected children (Cao et al. 1994, Hetzel 1994, Pharoah and Connolly 1995), with consequent deficit of maternal T4 during pregnancy. The exact timing of deficiency, however, is still unclear. Pharoah and Connolly (1995) considered that the first trimester is critical. Cao et al. (1994) believe that iodine supplementation begun before the end of the second trimester prevents neurological consequences. It is likely that there is a wide spectrum of manifestations from fetal wastage to mild cognitive or neurological deficits and/or deafness, depending on the degree of maternal iodine deficiency, so preventive administration of iodine could significantly improve the health of at-risk populations (Pharoah and Connolly 1995). This is best achieved by iodization of salt, which should be better implemented in many places (Delange 2001).

HASHIMOTO THYROIDITIS
Hashimoto thyroiditis is an immunological disorder usually associated with hypothyroidism. It may be associated with an acute encephalopathy featuring confusion, ataxia, quadriparesis and seizures followed by progressive brain atrophy (Vasconcellos et al. 1999, Duffey et al. 2003) which may be related to immunological abnormalities. Status epilepticus has been reported and the disorder can occur in children (Sybesma et al. 1999, von Maydell et al. 2002). The diagnosis depends on the demonstration of elevated levels of antithyroid autoantibodies. Treatment with corticosteroids is efficacious (Takahashi et al. 1994).

HYPERTHYROIDISM
Hyperthyroidism is much less common than hypothyroidism. CNS involvement may be marked by irritability and nervousness; by abnormal movements, especially chorea in the adult patient, that may be permanent or paroxysmal (Pozzon et al. 1992); and rarely by seizures as a manifestation of thyrotoxic crisis (Li Voon Chong et al. 2000). Exophthalmos may be accompanied by ocular motor nerve palsies. Several reports of papilloedema, sometimes associated with other neurological symptoms and signs, are on record. Myasthenia gravis may be more common in patients with thyrotoxicosis, and one type of periodic paralysis is associated with thyrotoxicosis in Oriental populations (Chapter 21).

OTHER ENDOCRINE DISORDERS
The neurological symptoms of *parathyroid disease* are directly related to calcium and phosphorus metabolism, as has been described elsewhere (Chapters 1, 9). They include CNS manifestations and may present as neuromuscular syndromes (Tonner and Schelte 1993), psychiatric disease in adults, and compression of neural structures by bone abnormalities.

Pituitary diseases have been considered in Chapter 13.

Neonatal hypopituitarism is often missed, with the risk of death or cerebral damage because of growth hormone deficiency and hypoglycaemia. Costello and Gluckman (1988) studied 12 patients. Six had *septo-optic dysplasia* (Chapter 2), 1 agenesis of the corpus callosum, 1 an empty fossa visualized by CT, and 1 pituitary hypoplasia. Two had idiopathic hypopituitarism, and 1 a dominant growth hormone deficiency. These infants were not small at birth and most had early seizures. Hyperbilirubinaemia was common and hypoglycaemia was documented in 11 patients. A microphallus was noted in 7 males. Bell et al. (2004) reviewed 169 cases drawn from a neonatal growth hormone registry; hypoglycaemia was the most common feature and was the only anomaly in 9 infants. In over one third of patients, stuctural brain abnormalities or midfacial defects and other hormonal deficits were present, but body length was usually normal. Midline brain and/or facial defects and micropenis in males are clues to the diagnosis, allowing early treatment. Scott et al. (2004) stressed the importance of thinking of hypopituitarism in prolonged unconjugated hyperbilirubinaemia. Immediate treatment with growth hormone is imperative to prevent neurodevelopmental sequelae (Scommegna et al. 2004).

Isolated hypogonadotrophic hypogonadism is found in older patients but is associated with developmental abnormalities that permit an early diagnosis. These include anosmia, hyposmia, mirror movements, ocular motor abnormalities, cerebellar dysfunction and pes cavus deformity. Delayed sexual maturation becomes apparent in adolescence. The mechanism of associated abnormalities is poorly known.

ADRENAL INSUFFICIENCY
This can produce neurological disturbances by disrupting water

and electrolyte metabolism or by inducing hypoglycaemia. Papilloedema and pseudotumour cerebri may occur, and this may be likened to pseudotumour following withdrawal of corticosteroids (Chapter 13).

HAEMATOLOGICAL DISORDERS

HEREDITARY HAEMOGLOBINOPATHIES
SICKLE CELL DISEASE (DREPANOCYTOSIS)
Sickle cell disease is a genetic disorder affecting predominantly Black African populations but also observed in other ethnic groups including Greeks, Orientals and Latin Americans. It is transmitted as an autosomal recessive trait that may manifest mildly in heterozygotes. Neurological complications occur in up to one third of cases and constitute a major cause of disability in this disorder. Neurological complications usually appear before 5 years of age. They are, at least in part, the consequence of vascular disease.

The mechanism of neurological accidents is probably twofold (Huttenlocher et al. 1984). Occlusive disease of large vessels at the base of the brain is common (13–17%) and may be one cause of increased collateral circulation or moyamoya syndrome. The second mechanism involves reduction in capillary flow, which may be a direct consequence of the sickling phenomenon and produces diffuse signs such as stupor or coma.

From a pathological viewpoint, there is intimal proliferation and sometimes thrombosis of vessels. Microinfarcts are frequently present and are usually disseminated. Large vessels are more involved than small ones.

Neurological symptoms may be isolated or appear at the time of sickle cell crises, which may be precipitated by dehydration, hypoxia or intercurrent disease including operations. Their description, diagnosis and therapy are discussed in Chapter 14. Hyperventilation should be avoided in patients with sickle cell disease as it may result in neurological impairment precipitated by the reduction of blood flow that occurs during the test (Allen et al. 1976). This may also be the cause of severe headache observed in up to 28% of patients (Pavlakis et al. 1989). Other neurological complications of sickle-cell disease include spinal infarction and mononeuropathies. Neurological manifestations associated with or following the severe acute chest syndrome are probably due, at least in part, to fat embolism and community acquired pneumonia (Vichinsky et al. 2000). Reversible posterior leukoencephalopathy has been reported (Henderson et al. 2003). An unusual necrotizing encephalitis has been observed in the same set of circumstances (Lee et al. 2002). Children with sickle cell disease are at an increased risk of *pneumococcal meningitis* that may be due to decreased phagocytic potential of the reticuloendothelial system. Salmonella infection with meningitis or osteomyelitis is facilitated in patients with sickle cell disease (Martino and Winfield 1990–1991). Intracerebral haemorrhage is much less common than infarction but does occur in some chidren (Van Hoff et al. 1985).

Academic difficulties, cognitive deficits and behavioural problems are common in children with sickle cell disease. These are due in part to abnormal brain circulation with patent or latent infarcts. However, it is difficult to disentangle the roles of biological and environmental risk factors present in most affected children (Schatz et al. 2004).

Children with sickle cell trait (heterozygotes) have a low incidence of neurological accidents, of the order of 6%.

THALASSAEMIA
Thalassaemia rarely gives rise to overt neurological disorder. About 20% of patients have myalgia, proximal weakness and a myopathic EEG pattern (Logothetis et al. 1972). *Spinal compression* due to bone marrow hyperplasia as a result of extramedullary haematopoiesis has been occasionally observed (Issaragrisil et al. 1981). Two *syndromes of mental retardation associated with alpha-thalassaemia* have been reported in children (Gibbons and Higgs 1996). One (also termed ATR-16) is due to various telomeric mutations (deletions, truncations or translocations) in the tip of chromosome 16p13.3 involving the genes *HBA-1* and *HBA-2*. This abnormality cannot be detected by routine cytogenetic analysis (Wilkie et al. 1990). Another alpha-thalassaemia mental retardation syndrome (ATR-X) featuring specific dysmorphic features has been recognized (Wilkie et al. 1991). It is not associated with a chromosomal deletion but rather is due to mutations in the gene *XH2* coding for helicase-2, a protein that regulates the expression of several proteins, and is transmitted as an X-linked character (Gibbons and Higgs 1996, Cardoso et al. 2000, Wada et al. 2000).

Neurological symptoms are uncommon in other haemoglobinopathies. They have been observed, however, in *haemoglobin SC disease* (Fabian and Peters 1984).

HAEMOLYTIC ANAEMIAS DUE TO DEFICIENCY OF GLYCOLYTIC ENZYMES
Pyruvate kinase deficiency can produce neurological complications only as a result of kernicterus.

Erythrocyte phosphoglycerate kinase deficiency is a sex-linked recessive disorder that may give rise to a slowly progressive extrapyramidal disorder that features dystonia, hyperlordosis, resting tremor and other extrapyramidal signs. It has been recognized that neuromuscular manifestations associated with glycerol kinase deficiency are not directly due to the enzymatic deficit but rather are the consequence of a contiguous gene syndrome due to a microdeletion affecting the glycerol kinase locus as well as neighbouring loci, so the clinical picture may include sex-linked muscular dystrophy and/or congenital adrenogenital hypoplasia (Darras and Francke 1988).

Triose phosphate isomerase deficiency is regularly associated with a progressive neurological disease that features extrapyramidal manifestations of a dystonic type, tremor, cerebellar symptoms, pyramidal tract signs and involvement of the anterior horn cell (Poll-Thé et al. 1985, Valentin et al. 2000). Isolated axonal neuropathy has been recorded (Wilmhurst et al. 2004). Cortical function is preserved. Spinal cord disease has also been reported in hereditary spherocytosis (McCann and Jacob 1976), which is a disorder related to erythrocyte membrane abnormality rather than to glycolysis.

OTHER ANAEMIAS

All anaemias may be accompanied by minor neurological symptoms such as irritability, listlessness and fatigue. A bruit can be heard over the head in some patients. Headache, and papilloedema due to increased intracranial pressure may be encountered in severe cases (Yager and Hartfield 2002). *Iron deficiency* is the most common cause of anaemia worlwide. In addition to anaemia, multiple neurological manifestations have been described in children with iron deficiency including develomental delay, breath-holding spells, pseudotumour cerebri and cranial nerves palsies. Although a role of iron deficiency is possible, a co-incidence cannot be excluded as these conditions are common and nonspecific. Strokes were reported in 6 children with iron deficiency (Hartfield et al. 1999). A role of iron deficiency was also suspected as a causal factor for arterial and venous thrombosis in children with cyanotic cardiac diseases. Again, it is difficult to rule out a multifactorial origin. Superior sagittal sinus thrombosis has been reported in patients receiving androgen therapy for the treatment of aplastic anaemia (Shiozawa et al. 1982). Symptoms subsided slowly upon withdrawal of treatment. Subacute combined degeneration of the posterior and lateral columns of the spinal cord is a classical complication of *pernicious anaemia*. In children, the most likely cause is a congenital defect of vitamin B_{12} absorption, which is also associated with mental retardation and abnormalities of brain myelination (Salameh et al. 1991). Atypical presentation such as ataxia is possible (Facchini et al. 2001). Congenital deficiency of intrinsic factor is rare. Deficiency of B_{12} due to an unbalanced vegetarian diet has been described above. Iron-deficiency anaemia may have a bearing on the neurological development of affected infants and children (Lozoff et al. 1991). A severe encephalopathy with seizures has been observed in an infant born to a mother with pernicious anaemia; it responded well to vitamin B_{12}, underlying the need to take into account maternal health status (Korenke et al. 2004).

POLYCYTHAEMIA

Polycythaemia, whether primary or secondary, can be associated with neurological symptoms (Newton 1990). The latter type is much more common in infants and especially in neonates (Chapter 1). Vertigo, headaches, tinnitus and seizures may be encountered in older patients. Cerebrovascular accidents as a result of increased viscosity due to high haematocrit are possible and may not always be transient, especially in newborn infants. Neurological sequelae were present in 38% of newborn infants with polycythaemia in one series (Black et al. 1982), but the genesis of neurological involvement is probably multifactorial as infants with polycythaemia are often born post-term and also suffer from hypoglycaemia and hypoxia. Seizures, visual disturbances and, rarely, intracranial haemorrhage have been reported (Wiswell et al. 1986, Nelson 2006). Exchange transfusion does not improve the outcome and may increase the incidence of necrotic enteritis (Dempsey and Barrington 2006). Peripheral neuropathy has been reported in adults with polycythaemia vera. It has not been recognized in children.

DISORDERS OF COAGULATION AND PLATELETS

Haemophilia is a major cause of intracranial haemorrhage that may occur at any age. Bleeding may be extradural, subdural or intraparenchymal. CT indicates the extent and origin of the haemorrhage, which is best treated by medical means (coagulation factors) whenever possible. Surgery, when indicated, should be deferred until factor VIII replacement therapy has been completed.

Other causes of bleeding include factor IX deficiency and Von Willebrand disease.

In infants, factor XIII deficiency is an important cause of idiopathic intracranial bleeding (Larsen et al. 1990).

Thrombocytopenic purpura, whether acute or chronic, is a relatively uncommon cause of intracranial haemorrhage. Intracranial bleeding can occur, however, and is one of the indications for splenectomy in this disease.

Alloimmunization against platelet antigens (usually PA1 antigen) produces prenatal or neonatal thrombocytopenia that may be responsible for intracranial haemorrhage (Matsui et al. 1995). Treatment with maternal platelets and immunoglobulins (Massey et al. 1987) is indicated. Effective prevention by immunoglobulin administration during pregnancy (1 g/kg/week) and delivery by caesarian section is possible (Menell and Bussel 1994).

NEUROLOGICAL COMPLICATIONS OF BONE MARROW AND ORGAN TRANSPLANTATION

Transplantation is extensively used in the treatment of haematological malignancies such as leukaemia and other haematological conditions. It is increasingly being employed as a replacement therapy of chronically impaired essential organs such as the kidneys, liver and intestine, and for several immunological deficiency diseases. Bone marrow and stem cell transplants are now commonly used to temporarily compensate for deficiencies resulting from aggressive therapies necessary following intensive chemotherapy or total body irradiation especially as rescue for pancytopenia. Some of the complications of transplantation occur in all types; others depend on the organ transplanted. Complications of transplantations raise highly complex issues that are beyond the scope of this book and will therefore be only briefly discussed. These are becoming increasingly common as the indications for the procedure are widening (Bashir 2001, Krouwer and Wijdicks 2003). The frequency of neurological and other complications tends to decrease with technical improvements even though new complications are being described.

Complications result from various mechanisms. One is rejection of the graft by the host (Gilman and Serendy 2006), also termed *rejection syndrome* or *host-versus-graft disease*, or the inverse phenomenon of graft-versus-host syndrome. As a consequence of these problems, another mechanism of complication arises from the necessity of using immunosuppression to avoid rejection. Immunosuppression, in turn, may require the use of neurotoxic drugs and may facilitate infections, resulting in increased sensitivity to bacteria or viruses. Both mechanisms may be responsible for neurological complications.

Toxicity of antimitotic as well as of immunosuppressive drugs is a common problem. Their effect can be direct or through interference with concomitant treatments received by patients. Direct toxicity of drugs is a frequent problem, and the central and/or peripheral nervous system can be involved with most antimitotic agents including methotrexate and platinum salts, which can generate encephalopathy or peripheral neuropathies as well as psychiatric syndromes. The toxic effects of drugs can be indirect; for instance, cyclosporine is often associated with arterial hypertension and may be responsible for the syndrome of transient posterior leukoencephalopathy (Chapter 14), and it has been implicated in a recently described irreversible leukoencephalopathy (Minn et al. 2007). The role of hypertension in this complication is compounded by the association of direct toxicity of other agents such as the immunomodifying drug tacrolimus or other agents used with organ transplantation such as FK506 (Wijdicks et al. 1994). Indirect neurological effects may also result from the involvement of other systems, especially haematological disturbances with haemorrhages, thrombocytopenia or leukopenia. Interference of certain drugs with other therapeutic agents, for example enzyme-inducing antiepileptic drugs, can cause ineffectiveness of corticosteroids by increasing their catabolism.

Increased sensitivity to infections results in increased frequency and/or severity of viral or bacterial diseases. Opportunistic infections in the CNS are due to organisms different from those causing infections in immunocompetent patients. They include bacterial diseases due to organisms of low pathogenicity for individuals with normal immunity such as *Listeria monocytogenes*, *Aspergillus* and *Nocardia*; viral diseases especially with herpes viruses, including cytomegalovirus, and JC virus which is responsible for progressive leukoencephalopathy; and fungal or parasitic diseases such as those caused by *Cryptococcus* and *Toxoplasma gondii* that also have a predilection for the CNS. Another problem resulting from immunosuppression is the develoment of malignancies attributed to induced impairment of immunosurveillance, especially CNS lymphomas (Walker and Brochstein 1988).

BONE MARROW TRANSPLANTATION
This technique is increasingly used primarily for the treatment of malignant disorders and other disorders such as severe immunodeficiencies, some metabolic and some immunological and/or haematological disorders. Early complications of the procedure include mucositis and the often fatal hepatic veno-occlusive disease, in addition to infections and acute graft-versus-host syndrome (Copeland 2006). CNS complications were observed in 46% of patients in one early childhood series (Wiznitzer et al. 1984). Infection, cerebrovascular accidents and metabolic encephalopathy were the main causes (Graus et al. 1996). Peripheral nervous system involvement was present in 24% of children treated by Amato et al. (1993). Metabolic encephalopathy was the most frequent complication in a large series including adults and children (Patchell 1994). Myasthenia gravis has been reported in isolation and in association with myositis and peripheral neuropathy (Adams et al. 1995). A syndrome of acute parkinsonism with white matter demyelination has been observed, es-

pecially in patients receiving amphotericin for the treatment of aspergillosis (Mott et al. 1995). Polymyositis in association with other features of graft-versus-host syndrome is on record (Klein et al. 2007). An encephalopathy was observed in 6% of 405 paediatric patients following allogenic *transplantation of bone marrow stem cells*. In 2 of 6 children it manifested with symptoms of thrombocytopenic purpura and had a poor prognosis (Woodard et al. 2004).

LIVER TRANSPLANTATION
Liver transplantation is a powerful treatment for acute and chronic hepatic failure and has achieved considerable success. It should be performed before there is evidence of cerebral oedema as the results are poor in its presence. However, transplantation and the immunological abnormalities that its treatment implies may give rise to neurological complications. Some can result directly from drug toxicity; others are complications related to immunological problems (Walker and Brochstein 1988, Ghaus et al. 2001). An acute encephalopathy with cortical blindness, seizures and coma has been reported (Stein et al. 1992). Cerebral oedema is the most common pathological basis for these complications.

The presence of infection, haemorrhage or noncholestatic liver disease is a predictive factor for CNS complications following transplantation (Pujol et al. 1994).

KIDNEY TRANSPLANTATION
The complications of renal transplantation are mainly the result of immunodeficiency. The high incidence of minor neurological and cognitive deficits reported eatly in the experience of renal transplants seems likely to have been due to the fact that many children had other associated anomalies.

GASTROINTESTINAL DISORDERS

GLUTEN ENTEROPATHY
Gluten enteropathy is a disorder of intestinal malabsorption characterized by villous atrophy, absence of surface mucosa and crypt hyperplasia. Neurological complications reported in adults include cerebellar dysfunction, myelopathy, disordered mentation, and a syndrome of ataxia and myoclonus similar to the Ramsay Hunt syndrome (Bhatia et al. 1995). Peripheral neuropathy has sometimes been attributed to coeliac disease but the evidence seems unconvincing (Rosenberg and Vermeulen 2005). The picture of Ramsay Hunt syndrome has not been reported in children, but cerebellar ataxia, although uncommon, is known to supervene (Gordon 2000). The possibility of neurological complications should be kept in mind, however, as it may represent a disorder treatable with gluten restriction (Kaplan et al. 1988). The role played by vitamins B_6, B_{12} and E in this disorder is not determined.

GLUTEN ENTEROPATHY ASSOCIATED WITH EPILEPSY AND CEREBRAL CALCIFICATION (see also Chapter 15)
Multiple cases of this association have been reported (Tortorella

et al. 1993, Gobbi 2005). The enteropathy may be overt with typical features of the coeliac syndrome or revealed only by villous atrophy on intestinal biopsy. In some cases, coeliac disease can be latent and even intestinal biopsy may be normal but the presence of antibodies to gliadin and of endomysial antibodies can suggest the condition (Gobbi 2005, Ranua et al. 2005). However, antibodies can be present in normal individuals so their presence does not prove their causal role. Usually, folate levels in plasma are low. Brain calcification is often bilateral, located in the parieto-occiptal regions and reminiscent of that seen in Sturge–Weber syndrome. In a few cases there may be frontal calcified areas or unilateral occipital calcification. Contrary to what obtains in Sturge–Weber cases, hypodensities may underlie the calcified areas (Toti et al. 1996). The epilepsy was initially reported as severe (Gobbi et al. 1988) but cases with a favourable course are not rare; however, secondary refractoriness may develop. Exclusion of gluten when started early may result in control or reduction of seizures. Lat-onset treatment is not effective (Gobbi 2005). Whether gluten-free diet can prevent the development of epilepsy and calcification is not known. The histopathological basis of the syndrome is imperfectly known (Gobbi 2005). Biopsy in a few cases showed angiomatous areas similar to those in Sturge–Weber syndrome, separated by fibrous tissue. The relationship between the components of the syndrome is not understood. Epilepsy seems to be more common in patients with coeliac disease than in the general population.

OTHER CAUSES OF MALABSORPTION

Other causes of malabsorption can produce neurological disease, in particular optic neuropathy associated with peripheral neuropathy, sometimes observed in patients with resection or exclusion of significant lengths of intestine (Pallis and Lewis 1980).

WHIPPLE DISEASE

Whipple disease is uncommon in childhood (Tan et al. 1995). The disease is primarily intestinal. Neurological complications occur in some cases. In older patients, neurological involvement most commonly consists of myoclonus, cerebellar ataxia, ataxia and ophthalmoplegia (Louis et al. 1996). Oculomasticatory and oculofacioskeletal myorhythmias are pathognomonic; dementia may develop. In a childhood case (Duprez et al. 1996), MRI revealed disseminated multiple white matter lesions. Diagnosis can be made by the discovery of bacilli-like structures in biopsy samples of the jejunal mucosa. The condition is due to infection of the gut by the bacillus *Tropheryma whipplei*, as shown by microscopic examination of jejunal biopsy. However, this may be absent in some instances and the best diagnostic method is by polymerase chain reaction on intestinal biopsy specimen (Sloan et al. 2005). Long-term treatment with antibiotics (cotrimoxazole) is effective against the gastrointestinal disease. When neurological signs are present, streptomycin and penicillin are recommended for at least two weeks (Muir-Padilla and Myers 2005).

INTUSSUSCEPTION

Intussusception in some infants may present initially with disturbances of consciousness (obtundation or even coma) that may suggest a primary neurological disease. This may be due to electrolytic disturbances, shock, or release of enterotoxins, gut hormones or peptides. In such unexplained cases of 'intussusception encephalopathy', one should enquire for abdominal symptoms and vomiting, and abdominal film or ultrasound should be obtained (Goetting et al. 1990).

BONE DISORDERS

Several bone disorders may be associated with neurological symptoms and signs, through various mechanisms that include compression of nerves at the skull base, venous compression with resulting hydrocephalus, narrowing of the foramen magnum or of the vertebral canal with resulting compression of the medulla, spinal cord or nerve roots, and craniosynostosis (Saland 2004). Several of these disorders are mentioned elsewhere in this book.

Fibrous dysplasia of bone is characterized by proliferation of fibrous tissue in osseous tissue. Onset is in childhood or adolescence in over half the cases. Up to 34% of cases may exhibit the association of skin pigmentation (Wilson and Hall 2002).

Osteopetrosis, especially in its severe infantile form, is often associated with neurological problems (Lehman et al. 1977, Abinun et al. 1999). Compression of the optic nerves in their bony canal is most common and frequently leads to visual impairment and blindness. Nystagmus and strabismus may occur. Compression of the facial nerve with facial paralysis is not uncommon, and anosmia and trigeminal nerve involvement have been reported. Not uncommonly, patients with infantile osteopetrosis exhibit mental retardation, and brain atrophy is apparent on CT. The reasons for cognitive involvement, sometimes associated with signs of upper neuron affectation, are not understood, but neurological assessment is essential before considering medullary transplant. Ceroid–lipofuscin storage was found in several cases (Chapter 9) but the mechanism remains unclear.

REFERENCES

Abinun M, Newson T, Rowe PW, et al. (1999) Importance of neorological assessment before bone marrow transplantation for osteopetrosis. *Arch Dis Child* 80: 273–4.
Ackrill P, Ralston AJ, Day JP, Hodge KC (1980) Successful removal of aluminium from a patient with dialysis encephalopathy. *Lancet* 2: 692–3.
Adair JC, Call GK, O'Connell JB, Baringer JR (1992) Cerebrovascular syndromes following cardiac transplantation. *Neurology* 42: 819–23.
Adams C, August CS, Maguire H, Sladky JT (1995) Neuromuscular complications of bone marrow transplantation. *Pediatr Neurol* 12: 58–61.
Agarwal KN, Das D, Agarwal DK, et al. (1989) Soft neurological signs and EEG pattern in rural malnourished children. *Acta Paediatr Scand* 78: 873–8.
Agarwal KN, Agarwal DK, Upadhyay SK (1995) Impact of chronic undernutrition on higher mental functions in Indian boys 10–12 years. *Acta Paediatr* 84: 1357–61.
Al Essa M, Sakati NA, Dabbagh O, et al. (1998) Inborn error of vitamin B12 metabolism: a treatable cause of of chilhood dementia/paralysis. *J Child Neurol* 13: 239–43.
Allen JP, Imbus CE, Powars DR, Harwood LJ (1976) Neurologic impairment induced by hyperventilation in children with sickle cell anemia. *Pediatrics* 58: 124–6.
Altman DI, Perlman JM, Volpe JJ, Powers NJ (1993) Cerebral oxygen metabolism in newborns. *Pediatrics* 92: 99–104.

mato AA, Barohn RJ, Sahenk Z, et al. (1993) Polyneuropathy complicating bone marrow and solid organ transplantation. *Neurology* 43: 1513–8.

ndrew RD (1991) Seizure and acute osmotic change: clinical and neurophysiological aspects. *J Neurol Sci* 101: 7–18.

rmelisasso C, Vaccario ML, Pontecorvi A, Mazza S (2004) Tonic–clonic seizures in a patient with primary hypoparathyroidism: a case report. *Clin EEG Neurosci* 35: 97–9.

cluru VL (1986) Spontaneous intracerebral hematomas in juvenile diabetic ketoacidosis. *Pediatr Neurol* 2: 167–9.

ylin OF, Uner C, Senhil N, et al. (2003) Central pontine and extrapontine myelinolysis owing to dysequilibrium syndrome. *J Child Neurol* 18: 292–6.

inbridge R, Mughal Z, Mimoun F, Tsang RL (1987) Transient congenital hypoparathyroidism: how transient is it? *J Pediatr* 111: 866–8.

allabriga A (1989) Some aspects of clinical and biochemical changes related to nutrition during brain development in humans. In: Evrard P, Minkowski A, eds. *Developmental Neurobiology. Nestlé Nutrition Workshop Series no. 12.* New York: Raven Press, pp. 271–86.

rrett TG, Forsyth JM, Nathavitharana KA, Booth IW (1993) Potentially lethal thiamine deficiency complicating parenteral nutrition in children. *Lancet* 341: 901.

rrett TG, Bundey SE, McLeod AF (1995) Neurodegeneration and diabetes: UK nationwide study of Wolfram (DIDMOAD) syndrome. *Lancet* 316: 1458–63.

rron TF, Gusnard DA, Zimmerman RA, Clancy RR (1992) Cerebral venous thrombosis in neonates and children. *Pediatr Neurol* 8: 112–6.

rron TF, Devenyi AG, Mamourian AC (1994) Symptomatic manganese neurotoxicity in a patient with chronic liver disease: correlation of clinical symptoms with MRI findings. *Pediatr Neurol* 10: 145–8.

rtholomeusz H, Courchesne E, Karns C (2002) Relationship between head circumference and brain volume in healthy normal toddlers, children and adults. *Neuropediatrics* 33: 239–41.

shir RM (2001) Neurologic complications of organ transplant. *Curr Therap Options Neurol* 3: 543–54.

axter P (2001) Pyridoxine dependent and pyridoxine responsive seizures. In: Baxter P, ed. *Vitamin Responsive Conditions in Child Neurology. International Review of Child Neurology Series.* London: Mac Keith Press for the International Child Neurology Association, pp. 109–65.

axter P, Griffiths P, Kelly T, Gardner-Medwin D (1996) Pyridoxine-dependent seizures: demographic, clinical, MRI and psychometric features, and effect of dose on intelligence quotient. *Dev Med Child Neurol* 38: 998–1006.

ell JJ, August GP, Blethen SL, Baptista J (2004) Neonatal hypoglycemia in a growth hormone registry: incidence and pathogenesis. *J Pediatr Endocrinol Metab* 17: 629–35.

enítez-Bribiesca I, De la Rosa-Alvarez I, Mansilla-Olivares A (1999) Dendritic spine pathology in infants with severe protein–calorie malnutrition. *Pediatrics* 104: e21.

rretta JS, Holbrook CT, Haller JS (1986) Chronic renal failure presenting as proximal muscle weakness in a child. *J Child Neurol* 1: 50–2.

hardwaj A (2006) Neurological impact of vasopressin dysregulation and hyponatremia. *Ann Neurol* 59: 229–36.

hatia KP, Brown P, Gregory R, et al. (1995) Progressive myoclonic ataxia associated with coeliac disease. The myoclonus is of cortical origin but the pathology is in the cerebellum. *Brain* 118: 1087–93.

cknese AR, May W, Hickey WF, Dodson WE (1992) Early childhood hepatocerebral degeneration misdiagnosed as valproate hepatotoxicity. *Ann Neurol* 32: 767–75.

ack VD, Lubchenco LO, Luckey DW, et al. (1982) Developmental and neurologic sequelae of neonatal hyperviscosity syndrome. *Pediatrics* 69: 426–31.

ock GH, Conners CK, Ruley J, et al. (1989) Disturbances of brain maturation and neurodevelopment during chronic renal failure. *J Pediatr* 114: 231–8.

oddy J, Skuse D, Andrews B (2000) The developmental sequelae of non-organic failure to thrive. *J Child Psychol Psychiatry* 41: 1013–4.

andt I, Sticker EJ, Lentze MJ (2003) Catch-up growth of head circumference of very low birth weight, small for gestational age preterm infants and mental development to adulthood. *J Pediatr* 142: 463–8.

in MF, Pedley TA, Lovelace RE, et al. (1986) Electrophysiologic features of abetalipoproteinemia: functional consequences of vitamin E deficiency. *Neurology* 36: 669–73.

ouns R, De Deyn PP (2004) Neurological complications in renal failure: a review. *Clin Neurol Neurosurg* 107: 1–16.

Brown AF (2004) Aetiology of cerebral oedema in diabetic ketoacidosis. *Emerg Med* 21: 754–5.

Broyer M, Tete MJ, Guest G, et al. (1996) Clinical polymorphism of cystinosis encephalopathy. Results of treatment with cysteinamine. *J Inher Metab Dis* 19: 65–75.

Butterworth RF (2003) Pathogenesis of hepatic encephalopathy: update on molecular mechanisms. *Int J Gastroenterol* 22 Suppl 2: S11–6.

Cao XY, Jiang XM, Dou ZH, et al. (1994) Timing of vulnerability of the brain to iodine deficiency in endemic cretinism. *N Engl J Med* 331: 1739–44.

Caraballo RH, Sakar D, Mozzi M, et al. (2004) Symptomatic occipital lobe epilepsy following neonatal hypoglycemia. *Pediatr Neurol* 31: 24–9.

Cardenas-Rivero N, Chemow B, Stoiko MA, et al. (1989) Hypocalcemia in critically ill children. *J Pediatr* 114: 946–51.

Cardoso C, Mignon C, Lutz Y, et al. (2000) ATR-X mutation cause impaired nuclear location and altered DNA binding properties of the XNP/ATR-X protein. *J Med Genet* 37: 46–51.

Carton H, Kayembe K, Kabeya M, et al. (1986) Epidemic of spastic paraparesis in Bandudu (Zaïre). *J Neurol Neurosurg Psychiatry* 49: 620–7.

Casey PH, Bradley R, Wortham B (1984) Social and nonsocial home environments of infants with nonorganic failure-to-thrive. *Pediatrics* 73: 348–53.

Chabrol B, Mancini J, Chretien D, et al. (1994) Valproate-induced hepatic failure in a case of cytochrome c oxidase deficiency. *Eur J Pediatr* 153: 133–5.

Chen CH, Lo MC, Hwang KL, et al. (2001) Infective endocarditis with neurologic complications: 10-year experience. *J Microbiol Immunol Infect* 34: 118–24.

Chopra JS, Sharma A (1992) Protein energy malnutrition and the nervous system. *J Neurol Sci* 110: 8–20.

Chopra JS, Dhand UK, Mehta S, et al. (1986) Effect of protein calorie malnutrition on peripheral nerves. A clinical, electrophysiological and histopathological study. *Brain* 109: 307–23.

Christaens FJ, Mowasingh LD, Christophe C, et al. (2003) Unilateral cortical necrosis following status epilepticus wth hypoglycemia. *Brain Dev* 25: 107–12.

Christmann D, Hirsch E, Mutschler V, et al. (1990) [Late diagnosis of congenital argininemia during administration of sodium valproate.] *Rev Neurol* 146: 764–6 (French).

Clayton PT, Surtees RA, DeVile C, et al. (2003) Neonatal epileptic encephalopathy. *Lancet* 361: 1614.

Clayton PT (2006) B6-responsive disorders: a model of vitamin dependency. *J Inherit Metab Dis* 29: 317–26.

Colombo M, de la Perra A, López I (1992) Intellectual and physical outcome of children undernourished in early life is influenced by later environmental conditions. *Dev Med Child Neurol* 36: 611–22.

Copeland EA (2006) Hematopoietic stem-cell transplantation. *N Engl J Med* 354: 1813–26.

Cornblath M, Schwartz R (1991) *Disorders of Carbohydrate Metabolism in Infancy, 3rd edn.* Oxford: Blackwell.

Costello JM, Gluckman PD (1988) Neonatal hypopituitarism: a neurological perspective. *Dev Med Child Neurol* 30: 190–9.

Curless RG, Katz DA, Perryman RA, et al. (1994) Choreoathetosis after surgery for congenital heart disease. *J Pediatr* 124: 737–9.

Dabydeen L, Thomas JE, Aston TJ, et al. (2008) High-energy and -protein diet increases brain and corticospinal tract growth in term and preterm infants after perinatal brain injury. *Pediatrics* 121: 148–56.

Daftary AS, Patole SK, Whitehall J (1999) Hypertension–hyponatremia syndrome in neonates: case report and review of literature. *Am J Perinatol* 16: 385–9.

Dahlem P, Groothoff JW, Aronson DC (2000) The hyponatraemic hypertensive syndrome in a 2-year-old child with behavioural symptoms. *Eur J Pediatr* 159: 500–2.

Daniels SR, Bates SR, Kaplan S (1987) EEG monitoring during paroxysmal hyperpnea of tetralogy of Fallot: an epileptic or hypoxic phenomenon? *J Child Neurol* 2: 98–100.

Daoud P, Mirc M, Tarazourte MF, et al. (2000) [Neonatal hyperparathyroidism secondary to unknown maternal hypoparathyroidism.] *Arch Pediatr* 7: 45–8 (French).

Darras BT, Francke U (1988) Myopathy in complex glycerol kinase deficiency patients is due to 3′ deletions of the dystrophin gene. *Am J Hum Genet* 43: 126–30.

Delange F (2001) Iodine deficiency as a cause of brain damage. *Postgrad Med* 77: 217–20.

Delange F (2002) Iodine deficiency in Europe; an update. *Eur J Nuclear Med Imaging* **29** Suppl 2: S414–6.

Delgado G, Schatz A, Nichols S, Applebaum M (2005) Behavioural profiles of children with infantile nephropathic cystinosis. *Dev Med Child Neurol* **47**: 403–7.

Dempsey EM, Barrington K (2006) Short and long term outcomes following partial exchange transfusion in the polycythaemic newborn: a systematic study. *Arch Dis Child Fetal Neonatal Ed* **91**: F2–6.

Devictor D, Tahiri C, Rousset A, et al. (1993) Management of fulminant hepatic failure in children—analysis of 56 cases. *Crit Care Med* **21** Suppl: S348–9.

Diederich S, Franzen NF, Bohr V, Oelkers W (2003) Severe hyponatremia due to hypopituitarism with adrenal insufficiency: report of 28 cases. *Eur J Endocrinol* **149**: 177–8.

Dobbing J (1981) *Scientific Foundation of Pediatrics, 2nd edn.* London: Heinemann.

Dreifuss FE, Langer DH, Moline KA, Maxwell JE (1989) Valproic acid hepatic fatalities. II. US experience since 1984. *Neurology* **39**: 201–7.

Drewett RF, Corbbett SS, Wright CM (1999) Cognitive and educational attainments at school age of children who failed to thrive in infancy: a population-based study. *J Child Psychol Psychiatry* **40**: 551–61.

Duffey P, Yee S, Reed IN (2003) Hashimoto's encephalopathy: postmortem findings. *Neurology* **61**: 1124–6.

Dunn JT (2001) Endemic goiter and cretinism: an update on iodine status. *J Pediatr Endocrinol Metab* **14** Suppl 6: 1469–73.

Du Plessis AJ (1997) Neurologic complications of cardiac disease in the newborn. *Clin Perinatol* **24**: 807–28.

Du Plessis AJ, Chang AC, Wessell DL, et al. (1995) Cerebrovascular accidents following the Fontan operation. *Pediatr Neurol* **12**: 230–6.

Du Plessis AJ, Bellinger DC, Gauvreau K, et al. (2002) Neurologic outcome of choreoathtoid encephalopathy after cardiac surgery. *Pediatr Neurol* **27**: 9–17.

Duprez TP, Grandin CB, Bonnier C, et al. (1996) Whipple disease confined to the central nervous system in childhood. *AJNR* **17**: 589–91.

Dusser A, Goutières F, Aicardi J (1986) Ischemic strokes in children. *J Child Neurol* **1**: 131–6.

Dykman RA, Casey PH, Ackerman PT, Melkerson WB (2001) Behavioral and cognititve status in school-aged children with a history of failure to thrive during infancy. *Clin Pediatr* **40**: 69–70.

Ehyai A, Fenichel GM, Bender HW (1984) Incidence and prognosis of seizures in infants following cardiac surgery with profound hypothermia and circulatory arrest. *JAMA* **252**: 3165–7.

el Bahri-Ben Mrad F, Gouider M, Fredj M, et al. (2000) Childhood diabetic neuropathy: a clinical and electrophysiological study. *Funct Neurol* **15**: 35–40.

Ellison PH, Farina MA (1980) Progressive central nervous system deterioration: a complication of advanced chronic lung disease of prematurity. *Ann Neurol* **8**: 43–6.

Embleton NE, Pang N, Cooke RJ (2001) Postnatal manutrition and growth retardation: an inevitable consequence of current recommendations in preterm infants? *Pediatrics* **107**: 270–3.

Emery ES, Homans AC, Colletti R (1987) Vitamin B12 deficiency: a cause of abnormal movements in infants. *Pediatrics* **99**: 255–6.

Fabian RH, Peters BH (1984) Neurological complications of hemoglobin SC disease. *Arch Neurol* **41**: 289–92.

Facchini SA, Jami MM, Neuberg RW, Sorrel AD (2001) A treatable cuase of ataxia in children. *Pediatr Neurol* **24**: 135–8.

Ferguson SC, Blane A, Wardlaw J, et al. (2005) Influence of an early-onset age of type I diabetes on cerebral structure and cognitive function. *Diabetes Care* **28**: 1431–7.

Fernández-Mayoralas DM, Muñoz-Jareño N, Manzana-Palomo A, Campos-Castelló J (2004) Acute hemiparesis in a boy with type 1 diabetes. *Eur J Paediatr Neurol* **8**: 161–4.

Ferrieri P, Gewitz MH, Gerber MA, et al. (2002) Unique features of infective endocarditis in childhood. *Pediatrics* **109**: 931–43.

Finberg L (1991) Water intoxication. A prevalent problem in the inner city. *Am J Dis Child* **145**: 981–2.

Freed DH, Robertson CM, Sauve RS, et al. (2006) Intermediate-term outcomes of the arterial switch operation for transposition of great arteries in neonates: alive but well? *J Thorac Cardiovasc Surg* **132**: 845–52.

Freedom RM (1989) Cerebral vascular disorders of cardiovascular origin in infants and children. In: Edwards BS, Hoffman HJ, eds. *Cerebral Vascular Disease in Children and Adolescents.* Baltimore: Williams & Wilkins, pp. 423–8.

Frye RE, Donner C, Golja A, Rooney CM (2003) Folinic acid-responsive seizures presenting as breakthrough seizures in a 3-month-old baby. *J Child Neurol* **18**: 562–9.

Galler JR, Ramsay FC, Salt P, Archer E (1987) Long-term effects of early kwashiorkor compared with marasmus. III: Motor skills. *J Pediatr Gastroenterol Nutr* **6**: 844–59.

Garcia-Garcia E, Camacho-Alonso J, Gomez-Rodriguez MJ, et al. (2000) Transient congenital hypoparathyroidism and 22q11 deletion. *J Pediatr Endocrinol Metab* **13**: 659–61.

Garewal G, Narang A, Das KC (1988) Infantile tremor syndrome: a vitamin B12 deficiency syndrome in infants. *J Trop Med* **34**: 174–8.

Gaudino R, Garel C, Czernichow P, Leger J (2005) Proportion of various types of thyroid disorders among newborns with congenital hypothyroidism and normally located gland: a regional cohort study. *Clin Endocrinol* **62**: 644–8.

Genovese E, Maghaic C, Maggiori G (2000) MR imaging of CNS involvement in children affected by chronic liver disease. *AJNR* **21**: 845–51.

Gessain A (1996) Virological aspects of tropical spastic paresis/HTLV-I-associated cord myelopathy and HTLV-I infection. *J Neurovirol* **2**: 299–306.

Ghaus N, Bohlega S, Rezeig M (2001) Neurological complications in liver transplantation. *J Neurol* **248**: 1042–8.

Gibbons RJ, Higgs DR (1996) The alpha-thalassemia/mental retardation syndromes. *Medicine* **75**: 45–52.

Gillberg C, Rasmussen P (1982) Abnormal head circumference and learning disability. *Dev Med Child Neurol* **24**: 198–9 (letter).

Gilman AL, Serendy J (2006) Diagnosis and treatment of chronic graft-versus-host disease. *Semin Hematol* **43**: 70–80.

Giuliano F, Bannwarth S, Monnot S, et al. (2005) Wolfram syndrome in French population: characterization of novel mutations and polymorphisms in the WFS1 gene. *Hum Mutat* **25**: 99–100.

Glass P, Wagner AE, Papero PH, et al. (1995) Neurodevelopmental status at age five years of neonates treated with extracorporal membrane oxygenation. *J Pediatr* **127**: 447–57.

Glauser TA, Rorke LB, Weinberg PM, Clancy RR (1990) Congenital brain anomalies associated with the hypoplastic left heart syndrome. *Pediatrics* **85**: 984–90.

Gobbi G (2005) Coeliac disease, epilepsy and cerebral calcification. *Brain Dev* **27**: 189–200.

Gobbi G, Bouquet F, Greco L, et al. (1988) Coeliac disease, epilepsy, and cerebral calcifications. *Lancet* **340**: 439–43.

Goetting MG, Tiznado-Garcia E, Bakdash TF (1990) Intussusception encephalopathy: an underrecognized cause of coma in children. *Pediatr Neurol* **6**: 419–21.

Goldberg CS, Schwarrtz EM, Brumberg JA, et al. (2000) Neurodevelopmental outcome of patients after the Fontan operation: a comparison of children with hypoplastic left heart syndrome and other functional single ventricle lesions. *J Pediatr* **137**: 546–52.

Gordon N (2000) Cerebellar ataxia and gluten sensitivity: a rare but possible cause of ataxia even in childhood. *Dev Med Child Neurol* **42**: 283–6.

Gospe SM (2006) Pyridoxine-dependent seizures: new genetic and biochemical clues to help with diagnosis and treatment. *Curr Opin Neurol* **19**: 148–53.

Gospe SM, Hecht ST (1998) Longitudinal MRI findings in pyridoxine dependent seizures. *Neurology* **51**: 74–8.

Gottschalk B, Richman R, Lewandowski L (1994) Subtle speech and motor deficits of children with congenital hypothyroid treated early. *Dev Med Child Neurol* **36**: 216–20.

Goutières F, Aicardi J (1985) Atypical presentations of pyridoxine-dependent seizures: a treatable cause of intractable epilepsy in infants. *Ann Neurol* **17**: 117–24.

Grantham-McGregor SM, Powell CA, Walker SP, Himes JH (1991) Nutritional supplementation, psychosocial stimulation, and mental development of stunted children: the Jamaican Study. *Lancet* **338**: 1–5.

Grattan-Smith PJ, Wilcken B, Procopis PG, Wise GA (1997) The neurological syndrome of infantile cobalamin deficiency: developmental regression and involuntary movements. *Mov Disord* **12**: 39–46.

Graus F, Saiz A, Sierra J, et al. (1996) Neurologic complications of autologous and allogeneic bone marrow transplantation in patients with leukaemia: a comparative study. *Neurology* **46**: 1004–9.

Grazer RE, Sutton JM, Friedstrom S, McBarron FD (1984) Hyperammonemic encephalopathy due to essential amino acid hyperalimentation. *Arch Intern Med* 144: 2278–9.

Graziani LJ, Gringlas M, Baumgart S (1997) Cerebrovascular complications and neurodevelopmental sequelae of neonatal ECMO. *Clin Perinatol* 24: 655–75.

Green WH, Campbell M, David R (1984) Psychosocial dwarfism: a critical review of the evidence. *J Am Acad Child Psychiatry* 23: 39–48.

Greenblatt JM, Hoffman LC, Reiss A (1994) Folic acid in neurodevelopment and child psychiatry. *Prog Neuropsychopharmacol Biol Psychiatry* 18: 647–60.

Gregorio L, Sutton CL, Lee DA (1997) Central pontine myelinolysis in a previously healthy 4-year-old child with acute rotavirus gastroenteritis. *Pediatrics* 99: 738–43.

Grillo F, Da Silva RJ, Barbento JH (2001) Pyridoxine-dependant seizures responding to extremely low dose pyridoxine. *Dev Med Child Neurol* 43: 413–5.

Griswold WR, Reznik V, Mendoza SA, et al. (1983) Accumulation of aluminum in a nondialyzed uremic child receiving aluminum hydroxide. *Pediatrics* 71: 56–8.

Grosse Aldenhövel HB, Gallenkamp U, Sulemana CA (1991) Juvenile onset diabetes mellitus, central diabetes insipidus and optic atrophy (Wolfram syndrome)—neurological findings and prognostic implications. *Neuropediatrics* 22: 103–6.

Gunston GD, Burkimsher D, Malan H, Sive AA (1992) Reversible cerebral shrinkage in kwashiorkor: an MRI study. *Arch Dis Child* 67: 1030–2.

Hack M, Breslau N (1986) Very low birth weight infants: effects of brain growth during infancy on intelligence quotient at 3 years of age. *Pediatrics* 77: 196–202.

Hadders-Algra M, Bos AF, Martijn A, Prechtl HFR (1994) Infantile chorea in an infant with severe bronchopulmonary dysplasia: an EMG study. *Dev Med Child Neurol* 36: 177–82.

Haenggeli CA, Girardin E, Paunier L (1991) Pyridoxine-dependent seizures, clinical and therapeutic aspects. *Eur J Pediatr* 150: 452–5.

Hahn JS, Vaucher Y, Bejar R, Coen RW (1993) Electroencephalographic and neuroimaging findings in neonates undergoing extracorporeal membrane oxygenation. *Neuropediatrics* 24: 19–24.

Halavaara J, Brander A, Lyytinen J, et al. (2003) Wernicke's encephalopathy: is diffusion-weighted MRI useful? *Neuroradiology* 45: 519–23.

Halpern JP, Boyages SC, Maberly GF, et al. (1991) The neurology of endemic cretinism. A study of two endemias. *Brain* 114: 825–41.

Hamrick SE, Gremmels DB, Keet CA, et al. (2003) Neurodevelopmental outcome of infants supported by extracorporeal membrane oxygenation after cardiac surgery. *Pediatrics* 111: 671–5.

Hartfield DS, Lowry NJ, Keene DL, Yager JY (1999) Iron deficiency as a cause of stroke in infants and children. *Pediatr Neurol* 16: 50–3.

Haspolat S, Duman O, Senol U, Yegin O (2004) Extrapontine myelinolysis in infancy: report of a case. *J Child Neurol* 19: 913–5.

Henderson JN, Noetzel MJ, McKinstry RC et al. (2003) Reversible posterior leukoencephalopathy syndrome and silent cerebral infarction are associated with severe acute chest syndrome in children with sickle cell disease. *Blood* 101: 415–9.

Hetzel BS (1994) Iodine deficiency and fetal brain damage. *N Engl J Med* 331: 1770–1.

Hoffmann GF, Schmitt B, Windfuhr M, et al. (2007) Pyridoxal 5'-phosphate may be curative in early-onset epileptic encephalopathy. *J Inherit Metab Dis* 30: 96–9.

Hoorn EJ, Geary D, Robb M et al. (2004) Acute hyponatremia related to intravenous fluid administration in hospitalized children: an observational study. *Pediatrics* 113: 1279–84.

Horvath R, Hudson G, Ferrari G, et al. (2006) Phenotypic spectrum associated with mutations of the mitochondrial polymerase gamma gene. *Brain* 129: 1674–84.

Hövels-Gürich HH, Konrad K, Wiesner M, et al. (2002a) Long term behavioural outcome after neonatal arterial switch operation for transposition of the great arteries. *Arch Dis Child* 87: 506–10.

Hövels-Gürich HH, Seghaye MC, Schnitker R, et al. (2002b) Long-term neurodevelopmental outcomes in school-aged children after neonatal arterial switch operation. *J Thorac Cardiovasc Surg* 124: 448–58.

Howlett WP, Brubaker GR, Mlingi N, Rosling H (1990) Konzo, an epidemic upper motor neuron disease studied in Tanzania. *Brain* 113: 223–35.

Hsu SC, Levine MA (2004) Perinatal calcium metabolism: physiology and pathophysiology. *Semin Neonatol* 9: 23–36.

Hughes JR, Schreeder MT (1980) EEG in dialysis encephalopathy. *Neurology* 30: 1148–54.

Hulst JM, Joosten KF, Tibboel D, van Goudoever JB (2006) Causes and consequences of inadequate substrate supply to pediatric ICU patients. *Curr Opin Clin Nutr Metab Care* 9: 297–303.

Huttenlocher PR, Moohr JW, Johns L, Brown FD (1984) Cerebral blood flow in sickle cell cerebrovascular disease. *Pediatrics* 73: 615–21.

Hyland K, Arnold LA (2002) Value of lumbar puncture in the diagnosis of infantile epilepsy and folinic acid-responsive seizures. *J Child Neurol* 17 Suppl 3: S48–53.

Iliki A, Larsson A (1988) Psychomotor development of children with congenital hypothyroidism diagnosed by neonatal screening. *Acta Paediatr Scand* 77: 142–7.

Ip P (2003) Neonatal convulsions revealing maternal hyperparathyroidism: an unusual case of late neonatal hypoparathyroidism. *Arch Gynecol Obstet* 268: 227–9.

Issaragrisil S, Piankigagum A, Wasi P (1981) Spinal cord compression in thalassemia: report of 12 cases and recommendations for treatment. *Arch Intern Med* 141: 1033–6.

Jaafar R, Yun Boo N, Rasat R, Latiff HA (2004) Neonatal seizures due to maternal primary hyperparathyroidism. *J Pediatr Child Health* 40: 329.

Jackson CE, Amato AA, Barohn RJ (1996) Isolated vitamin E deficiency. *Muscle Nerve* 19: 1161–5.

Jagadha V, Deck JHN, Halliday WC, Smyth HS (1987) Wernicke's encephalopathy in patients on peritoneal dialysis or hemodialysis. *Ann Neurol* 21: 78–84.

Jarayam S, Soman A, Tarvade S, Londhe V (2005) Cerebellar ataxia due to isolated vitamin E deficiency. *Indian J Med Sci* 59: 20–3.

Jarjour IT, Ahdab-Barmada M (1994) Cerebrovascular lesions in infants and children dying after extracorporeal membrane oxygenation. *Pediatr Neurol* 10: 13–9.

Jelliffe DB, Jelliffe EFP (1992) Causation of kwashiorkor: toward a multifactorial consensus. *Pediatrics* 90: 110–3.

Johnson GM (1982) Powdered goat's milk: pyridoxine deficiency and status epilepticus. *Clin Pediatr* 21: 494–5.

Jones EA (2002) Ammonia, the GABA neurotransmitter system, and hepatic encephalopathy. *Metab Brain Dis* 17: 279–81.

Kaplan JG, Pack D, Horoupian D, et al. (1988) Distal axonopathy associated with chronic gluten enteropathy: a treatable disorder. *Neurology* 38: 642–5.

Karavanaki K, Baum JD (2003) Coexistence of impaired indices of autonomic neuropathy and diabetic neuropathy in a cohort of children with type 1A diabetic mellitus. *J Pediatr Endocrinol Metab* 16: 79–90.

Katayama K (2004) Ammonia metabolism and hepatic encephalopathy. *Hepatol Res* 305: 73–80.

Keating JP, Schears GJ, Dodge PR (1991) Oral water intoxication in infants. An American epidemic. *Am J Dis Child* 145: 985–90.

Kello AB, Gilbert C (2003) Causes of severe visual impairment and blindness in children in schools for the blind in Ethiopia. *Br J Ophthalmol* 87: 526–30; comment 1432.

Kershaw MJ, Newton T, Barrett TG, et al. (2005) Childhood diabetes presenting with hyperosmolar dehydration but without ketoacidosis: a report of three cases. *Diabet Med* 22: 625–7.

Keyser A, De Bruijn SFTM (1991) Epileptic manifestations and vitamin B1 deficiency. *Eur Neurol* 31: 121–5.

King JM, Taitz LS (1985) Catch up growth following abuse. *Arch Dis Child* 60: 1152–4.

Klein R, Franck P, Ehl S, et al. (2007) Polymyositis—an unusual presentation of cGvHD in children. *Pediatr Transplant* 11: 225–7.

Koh THHG, Aynsley-Green A, Tarbit M, Eyre JA (1988) Neural dysfunction during hypoglycaemia. *Arch Dis Child* 63: 1353–8.

Kohlschütter A (1993) Vitamin E and neurological problems in childhood: a curable neurodegenerative process. *Dev Med Child Neurol* 35: 642–6.

Kohrman MH, Carney PR (2000) Sleep-related disorders in neurologic disease during childhood. *Pediatr Neurol* 23: 107–13.

Kooistra L, Laane C, Vulsma T, et al. (1994) Motor and cognitive development in children with congenital hypothyroidism: a long-term evaluation of the effects of neonatal treatment. *J Pediatr* 124: 903–9.

Korenke GC, Hunneman DH, Eber S, Hanefeld F (2004) Severe encephalopathy with epilepsy in an infant caused by subclinical maternal pernicious anaemia: case report and review of the literature. *Eur J Pediatr* 163: 196–201.

Korinthenberg R, Kachel W, Koelfen W, et al. (1993) Neurological findings in newborn infants after extracorporeal membrane oxygenation, with special reference to the EEG. *Dev Med Child Neurol* 35: 249–57.

Kotagal S, Rolfe U, Schwarz KB, Escober W (1984) "Locked-in" state following Reye's syndrome. *Ann Neurol* 15: 599–601.

Kotler D (2004) Challenges to diagnosis of HIV-associated wasting. *J Acquir Immune Syndr* 37 Suppl 5: S280–3.

Krane EJ, Rockoff MA, Wallman JK, Wolfsdorf JI (1985) Subclinical brain swelling in children during treatment of diabetic ketoacidosis. *N Engl J Med* 312: 1147–51.

Kroll JS (1985) Pyridoxine for neonatal seizures: an unexpected danger. *Dev Med Child Neurol* 27: 377–9.

Krouwer HG, Wijdicks EF (2003) Neurologic complications of bone marrow transplantation. *Neurol Clin* 21: 319–52.

Kumar S (2004) Vitamin B12 deficiency presenting with an acute reversible extrapyramidal syndrome. *Neurology India* 52: 507–9.

Kuo MF, Wang HS (2002) Pyridoxal-phosphate-responsive epilepsy with resistance to pyridoxine. *Pediatr Neurol* 26: 146–7.

Kurlan R, Krall RL, Deweese JA (1984) Vertebrobasilar ischemia after total repair of tetralogy of Fallot. Significance of subclavian steal created by Blalock–Taussig anastomosis. *Stroke* 15: 359–62.

Lamy C, Oppenheim C, Méder JF, Mas JL (2004) Neuroimaging in posterior reversible encephalopathy syndrome. *J Neuroimaging* 14: 89–96.

Lancet (1992) Excess water administration and hyponatraemic convulsions in infancy. *Lancet* 339: 153–5 (editorial).

Larsen PD, Wallace JW, Frankel LS, Crisp B (1990) Factor XIII deficiency and intracranial hemorrhages in infancy. *Pediatr Neurol* 6: 277–8.

Lee, J.H., Arcinue, E., Ross, B.D. (1994) Brief report: organic osmolytes in the brain of an infant with hypernatremia. *N Engl J Med* 331: 439–42.

Lee KH, McKie VC, Sekul EA, et al. (2002) Unusual encephalopathy after acute chest syndrome in sickle cell disease: acute necrotizing encephalitis. *J Pediatr Hematol Oncol* 24: 585–8.

Lee WS, McKiernan P, Kelly DA (2005) Etiology, outcome, and prognostic indicators of childhood fulminant hepatic failure. *J Pediatr Gastroenterol Nutr* 40: 375–81.

Lehman RAW, Reeves JD, Wilson WB, Wesenberg RI (1977) Neurological complications of infantile osteopetrosis. *Ann Neurol* 2: 378–84.

Leicher CR, Mezoff AG, Hyams JS (1991) Focal cerebral deficits in severe hypomagnesemia. *Pediatr Neurol* 7: 380–1.

Lidofsky SD, Bass NM, Prager MC, et al. (1992) Intracranial pressure monitoring and liver transplantation for fulminant hepatic failure. *Hepatology* 16: 1–7.

Li Voon Chong JS, Lecky BA, MacFarlane IA (2000) Recurrent encephalopathy and generalized seizures associated with relapses of tyrotoxicosis. *Int J Clin Pract* 54: 621–2.

Limperopoulos C, Majnemer A, Shevell MI, et al. (2002) Predictors of developmental disabilities after open heart surgery in young children with congenital heart defects. *J Pediatr* 141: 51–8.

Lindenbaum J, Healton EB, Savage DG, et al. (1988) Neuropsychiatric disorders caused by cobalamin deficiency in the absence of anemia or macrocytosis. *N Engl J Med* 318: 1720–8.

Locatelli F, Cannata-Andía JB, Drüeke TB, et al. (2002) Management of disturbances of calcium and phosphate metabolism in chronic renal insufficiency, with emphasis on the control of hyperphosphataemia. *Nephrol Dial Transplant* 17: 723–31.

Logothetis J, Constantoulakis M, Economidou J, et al. (1972) Thalassemia major (homozygous beta thalassemia): a survey of 138 cases with emphasis on neurologic and muscular aspects. *Neurology* 22: 294–304.

Louis ED, Lynch T, Kaufmann P, et al. (1996) Diagnostic guidelines in central nervous system Whipple's disease. *Ann Neurol* 40: 561–8.

Lozoff B, Jimenez E, Wolf AW (1991) Long-term developmental outcome of infants with iron deficiency. *N Engl J Med* 325: 687–94.

Lucas A, Morley R, Cole T (1998) Randomized trial of early diet in preterm babies and later intelligence quotients. *BMJ* 317: 1481–7.

Ludolph AC, Hugon J, Dwivedi MP, et al. (1987) Studies on the aetiology and pathogenesis of motor neuron diseases. 1. Lathyrism: clinical findings in established cases. *Brain* 110: 149–65.

Luttrell CN, Finberg L (1959) Hemorrhagic encephalopathy induced by hypernatremia. I: Clinical, laboratory and pathological observations. *Arch Neurol Psychiatry* 81: 424–32.

Ma T, Lian ZC, Qi SP, et al. (1993) Magnetic resonance imaging of brain and the neuromotor disorder in endemic cretinism. *Ann Neurol* 34: 91–4.

Maddrey WC (2005) Role of antibiotics in the management of hepatic encephalopathy. *Rev Gastroenterol Disord* 5 Suppl 1: S3–9.

Mahle WT, Wernovsky G (2004) Neurodevelopmental outcomes in hypoplasic

left heart syndrome. *Semin Thorac Cardiovasc Surg Pediatr Card Surg Annu* 7: 39–47.

Manni R, Tartara A, Marchioni E, et al. (1987) A clinical, EEG and CT study in 21 cases of chronic respiratory failure. *J Neurol* 234: 83–5.

Mancini ML, Dello Strologo L, Bianchi PM, et al. (1996) Sensorineural hearing loss in patients reaching chronic renal faillure in childhood. *Pediatr Nephrol* 10: 38–40.

Marescaux C, Warter JM, Micheletti G, et al. (1982) Stuporous episodes during treatment with sodium valproate: report of seven cases. *Epilepsia* 23: 297–305.

Mariotti C, Gellera C, Rimoldi M, et al. (2004) Ataxia with isolated vitamin E deficiency: neurological phenotype, clinical follow-up and novel mutations in TTPA gene in Italian families. *Neurol Sci* 25: 130–7.

Martin RJ (2004) Central pontine and extrapontine myelinolysis: the osmotic demyelination syndromes. *J Neurol Neurosurg Psychiatry* 75 Suppl 3: iii22–8.

Martino AM, Winfield JA (1990–1991) Salmonella osteomyelitis with epidural abscess. A case report with review of osteomyelitis in children with sickle cell anemia. *Pediatr Neurosurg* 16: 321–5.

Massey GV, McWilliams NB, Mueller DG, et al. (1987) Intravenous immunoglobulin in treatment of neonatal isoimmune thrombocytopenia. *J Pediatr* 111: 133–5.

Matsui K, Ohsaki E, Koresawa M, et al. (1995) Perinatal intracranial hemorrhage due to severe neonatal alloimmune thrombocytopenic purpura (NAITP) associated with anti-Yukb (HPA-4a) antibodies. *Brain Dev* 17: 352–5.

McCann SR, Jacob HS (1976) Spinal cord disease in hereditary spherocytosis: report of two cases with a hypothesized common mechanism for neurologic and red cell abnormalities. *Blood* 48: 259–63.

McConnell JR, Fleming WH, Chu WK, et al. (1990) Magnetic resonance imaging of the brain in infants and children before and after cardiac surgery. A prospective study. *Am J Dis Child* 144: 374–8.

McGraw ME, Haka-Ikse K (1985) Neurologic–developmental sequelae of chronic renal insufficiency. *J Pediatr* 106: 579–83.

Medlock MD, Cruse RS, Winek SJ, et al. (1993) A 10-year experience with postpump chorea. *Ann Neurol* 34: 820–6.

Menakaya JO, Wassmer E, Bradshaw K, et al. (2001) Idiopathic central pontine myelinolysis in childhood. *Dev Med Child Neurol* 43: 697–700.

Menell JS, Bussel JB (1994) Antenatal management of the thrombocytopenias. *Clin Perinatol* 21: 591–614.

Menger H, Jörg EJ (1999) Outcome of central pontine and extrapontine myelinolysis (n = 44). *J Neurol* 246: 700–5.

Menni F, de Lonlay P, Sevin C, et al. (2001) Neurologic outcome of 90 neonates and infants with persistent hyperinsulinemic hypoglycemia. *Pediatrics* 107: 476–9.

Miller G, Mamourian AC, Tesman JR, et al. (1994) Long-term MRI changes in brain after pediatric open heart surgery. *J Child Neurol* 9: 390–7.

Mills PB, Surtees RA, Champion MP, et al. (2005) Neonatal epileptic encephalopathy caused by mutations in the PNPO gene encoding pyridox(am)ine-5′-phosphate oxidase. *Hum Molec Genet* 14: 1077–86.

Mills PB, Struys E, Jakobs C, et al. (2006) Mutations in antiquitin in individuals with pyridoxine-dependent seizures. *Nat Med* 12: 307–9.

Minn AY, Fisher PG, Barnes PD, Dahl GV (2007) A syndrome of irreversible leukoencephalopathy following pediatric allogeneic bone marrow transplantation. *Pediatr Blood Cancer* 48: 213–7; erratum 372.

Mirowitz SA, Westrich TJ, Hirsch JD (1991) Hyperintense basal ganglia on T1-weighted MR images in patients receiving parenteral nutrition. *Radiology* 181: 117–20.

Mocharla R, Schernayder SM, Glasiez CM (1997) Fatal cerebral edema and intracranial hemorrhage associated with hypernatremic dehydration. *Pediatr Radiol* 27: 785–7.

Morii H, Inoue T, Nishijima T, et al. (2004) Management of calcium and bone abnormalities in hemodialysis patients. *Semin Nephrol* 24: 444–8.

Moritz ML, Ayus JC (2005) Preventing neurological complications from dysnatremias in children. *Pediatr Nephrol* 20: 1687–700.

Morton RE, Bonas R, Fourie B, Minford J (1993) Videofluoroscopy in the assessment of feeding disorders of children with neurological problems. *Dev Med Child Neurol* 35: 388–95.

Mott SH, Packer RJ, Vezina LG, et al. (1995) Encephalopathy with parkinsonian features in children following bone marrow transplantations and high-dose amphotericin B. *Ann Neurol* 37: 810–4.

Mouridsen SE, Nielsen S (1990) Reversible somatotropin deficiency (psychosocial dwarfism) presenting as conduct disorder and growth hormone deficiency. *Dev Med Child Neurol* 32: 1093–8.

Muir AB, Quisling RG, Yang MC, Rosenbloom AM (2004) Cerebral edema in childhood diabetic ketoacidosis: natural history, radiographic findings, and early identification. *Diabetes Care* **27**: 1541–6.

Muir-Padilla J, Myers JB (2005) Whipple disease: a case report and review of the literature. *Arch Pathol Lab Med* **129**: 933–6.

Muller O, Krawinkel M (2005) Malnutrition and health in developing countries. *CMAJ* **173**: 279–86.

Nelson KB (2006) Thrombophilias, perinatal stroke, and cerebral palsy. *Clin Obstet Gynecol* **49**: 875–84.

Newburger JW, Silbert AR, Buckley LP, Fyler DC (1984) Cognitive functions and age at repair of transposition of the great arteries in children. *N Engl J Med* **310**: 1495–9.

Newton IK (1990) Neurologic complications of polycythemia and their impact on therapy. *Oncology* **4**: 59–64.

Nicolai J, van Kraven-Mastenbroek VH, Wevers RA, et al. (2006) Folinic acid-responsive seizures initially responsive to pyridoxine. *Pediatr Neurol* **34**: 164–7.

Nield TA, Langenbacher D, Poulsen MK, Platzker AC (2000) Neurodevelopmental outcome of infants supported by extracorporeal life support: relationship to primary diagnosis. *J Pediatr* **136**: 338–44.

Nijst TQ, Wevers RA, Schoonder-Waldt HC, et al. (1990) Vitamin B12 and folate concentrations in serum and cerebrospinal fluid of neurological patients with special reference to multiple sclerosis and dementia. *J Neurol Neurosurg Psychiatry* **53**: 951–4.

Njølstad PR, Skjeldal OH, Agsterribe E, et al. (1997) Medium-chain acyl-CoA dehydrogenase deficiency and fatal valproate toxicity. *Pediatr Neurol* **16**: 160–2.

North KN, Ouvrier RA, McLean CA, Hopkins IJ (1994) Idiopathic hypothalamic dysfunction with dilated unresponsive pupils: report of two cases. *J Child Neurol* **9**: 320–5.

Odabas D, Caksen H, Sar S, et al. (2005a) Auditory brainstem potentials in children with protein–energy malnutrition. *Int J Pediatr Otorhinolaryngol* **69**: 923–8.

Odabas D, Caksen H, Sar S, et al. (2005b) Cranial MRI findings in children with protein–energy malnutrition. *Int J Neurosci* **115**: 829–37.

Ogunlesi TA (2004) Thiamine deficiency: a cause of childhood ataxia not to be ignored. *Ann Trop Med* **24**: 257–60.

Olson DM, Shewmon DA (1989) Electroencephalographic abnormalities in infants with hypoplastic left heart syndrome. *Pediatr Neurol* **5**: 93–8.

Orchard TJ, Lloyd CE, Maser RE, Kuller LH (1996) Why does diabetic autonomic neuropathy predict IDDM mortality? An analysis from the Pittsburgh Epidemiology of Diabetes Complications Study. *Diabetes Res Clin Pract* **34** Suppl: S167–71.

Ozer EA, Turker M, Bakiler AR, et al. (2001) Involuntary movements in infantile cobalamin deficiency appearing after treatment. *Pediatr Neurol* **25**: 81–3.

Palacio S, Hart RG (2002) Neurologic manifestations of cardiogenic emboli: an update. *Neurol Clin* **20**: 179–93.

Pallis CA, Lewis PD (1980) Neurology of gastrointestinal disease. In: Vinken PJ, Bruyn GW, eds. *Handbook of Clinical Neurology, vol. 39. Neurological Manifestations of Systemic Disorders, Part II.* Amsterdam: North Holland, pp. 449–68.

Palmer CA (2002) Neurologic manifestations of renal disease. *Neurol Clin* **20**: 23–34.

Park SM, Chatterjee VK (2005) Genetics of congenital hypthyroidism. *J Med Genet* **42**: 379–89.

Parr MJ, Low HM, Botterill P (1997) Hyponatraemia and death after "ecstasy" ingestion. *Med J Aust* **166**: 136–7.

Pasantes-Morales H, Franco R, Ordaz B, Ochoa LD (2002) Mechanisms counteracting swelling in brain cells during hyponatremia. *Arch Med Res* **33**: 237–44.

Patchell RA (1994) Neurological consequences of organ transplantation. *Ann Neurol* **36**: 688–703.

Pavlakis SG, Prohovnik K, Pianelli S, De Vivo DC (1989) Neurologic complications of sickle cell disease. *Adv Pediatr* **36**: 247–76.

Pellock JM (1987) Carbamazepine side-effects in children and adults. *Epilepsia* **28** Suppl 3: S64–70.

Perlman JM, Volpe JJ (1989) Movement disorder of premature infants with severe bronchopulmonary dysplasia: a new syndrome. *Pediatrics* **84**: 215–8.

Pettifor JM (2005) Rickets and vitamin D deficiency in children and adolescents. *Endocrinol Metab Clin North Am* **34**: 537–553.

Pharoah POD, Connolly KJ (1995) Iodine and brain development. *Dev Med Child Neurol* **37**: 744–8.

Phornphutkul C, Rosenthal R, Nadas AS, Berenberg W (1973) Cerebrovascular accidents in infants and children with cyanotic congenital heart disease. *Am J Cardiol* **32**: 329–34.

Pihko H, Saarinen U, Paetau A (1989) Wernicke encephalopathy. A preventable cause of death. Report of 2 children with malignant disease. *Pediatr Neurol* **5**: 237–42.

Pirzada NA, Morgenlander JC (1997) Peripheral neuropathy in patients with chronic renal failure. A treatable source of discomfort and disability. *Postgrad Med* **102**: 249–50, 255–7, 261.

Pitsavas S, Andreou C, Bascialla F, et al. (2004) Pellagra encephalopathy following B-complex vitamin treatment without niacin. *Int J Psychiatry Med* **34**: 91–5.

Plecko B, Paul K, Paschke E, et al. (2007) Biochemical and molecular characterization of 18 patients with pyridoxine dependent epilepsy and muations of the antiquitin (ALDH7A1) gene. *Hum Mutat* **28**: 19–26.

Pocecco M, Ronfani L (1998) Transient focal neurologic deficits associated with hypoglycaemia in children with insulin-dependent diabetes mellitus. Italian Collaborative Paediatric Diabetologic Group. *Acta Paediatr* **87**: 542–4.

Poll-Thé BT, Aicardi J, Girot R, Rosa R (1985) Neurological findings in triose phosphate isomerase deficiency. *Ann Neurol* **17**: 439–43.

Pozzon GB, Battistella PA, Rigon F, et al. (1992) Hyperthyroid-induced chorea in an adolescent girl. *Brain Dev* **14**: 126–7.

Prasad N, Gujati S, Gupta RK, et al. (2003) Is reversible posterior leukoencepahalopathy with severe hypertension completely reversible in all patients? *Pediatr Nephrol* **18**: 1161–6.

Pujol A, Pujol J, Graus F, et al. (1993) Hyperintense globus pallidus on T1-weighted MRI in cirrhotic patients is associated with severity of liver failure. *Neurology* **43**: 65–9.

Pujol A, Graus F, Rimola A, et al. (1994) Predictive factors of in-hospital CNS complications following liver transplantation. *Neurology* **44**: 1226–30.

Puntis JW, Green SH (1985) Ischaemic spinal cord injury after cardiac surgery. *Arch Dis Child* **60**: 517–20.

Radetti G, Rizza F, Mengarda G, Pittschieler K (1991) Adipsic hypernatremia in two sisters. *Am J Dis Child* **145**: 321–5.

Raja R, Johnston JK, Fitts JA, et al. (2003) Post-transplant seizures in infants with hypoplastic left heart syndrome. *Pediatr Neurol* **28**: 370–8.

Rajbhandari SM, Powell T, Davies-Jones GAB, Ward JD (1998) Central pontine myelinolysis and ataxia: an unusual manifestation of hypoglycaemia. *Diabet Med* **15**: 259–61.

Ramaekers VT, Blau N (2004) Cerebral folate deficiency. *Dev Med Child Neurol* **46**: 843–51.

Ramaekers VT, Calomme M, Vanden Berghe D, Makropoulos W (1994) Selenium deficiency triggering intractable seizures. *Neuropediatrics* **25**: 217–23.

Ramaekers VT, Reul J, Kusenbach G, et al. (1997) Central pontine myelinolysis associated with acquired folate depletion. *Neuropediatrics* **28**: 125–30.

Ramsay M, Gisel EG, Boutary M (1993) Non-organic failure to thrive: growth failure secondary to feeding-skills disorders. *Dev Med Child Neurol* **35**: 285–97.

Rando TA, Horton JC, Layzer RB (1992) Wolfram syndrome: evidence of a diffuse neurodegenerative disease by magnetic resonance imaging. *Neurology* **42**: 1220–4.

Ranua J, Luoma K, Auvinen A, et al. (2005) Celiac disease-related antibodies in an epilepsy cohort and matched reference population. *Epilepsy Behav* **6**: 388–92.

Reuss ML, Paneth N, Pinto-Martin JA, et al. (1996) The relation of transient hypothyroxinemia in preterm infants to neurologic development at two years of age. *N Engl J Med* **334**: 821–27.

Riggs JE, Klingberg WG, Flink EB, et al. (1992) Cardioskeletal mitochondrial myopathy associated with chronic magnesium deficiency. *Neurology* **42**: 128–30.

Riordan SM, Williams R (1997) Treatment of hepatic encephalopathy. *N Engl J Med* **337**: 473–9.

Rivera-Vásquez AB, Noriega-Sánchez A, Ramírez-González R, Martinez-Maldonado M (1980) Acute hypercalcemia in hemodialysis patients: distinction from 'dialysis dementia'. *Nephron* **25**: 243–6.

Robinson RO, Samuels M, Pohl KRE (1988) Choreic syndrome after cardiac surgery. *Arch Dis Child* **63**: 1466–9.

Rogers BT, Msall ME, Buck GM, et al. (1995) Neurodevelopmental outcome of infants with hypoplastic left heart syndrome. *J Pediatr* **126**: 496–8.

Román G (1998) Tropical myeloneuropathy revisited. *Curr Opin Neurol* **11**: 539–44.

Román GC, Spencer PS, Schoenberg BS (1985) Tropical myeloneuropathies. The hidden endemias. *Neurology* 35: 1158–70.

Rosenberg NR, Vermeulen M (2005) Should coeliac diseases be considered in the work up of patients with chronic peripheral neuropathy? *J Neurol Neurosurg Psychiatry* 76: 1415–9.

Rovet JF (2005) Children with congenital hypothyroidism and their siblings: do they really differ? *Pediatrics* 115: e52–7.

Rovet JF, Ehrlich RM (1995) Long-term effects of L-thyroxine therapy for congenital hypothyroidism. *J Pediatr* 126: 380–6.

Salameh MM, Banda RW, Mohdi AA (1991) Reversal of severe neurological abnormalities after vitamin B12 replacement in the Imerslund–Grasbeck syndrome. *J Neurol* 238: 349–50.

Saland JM (2004) Osseous complications of pediatric transplantation. *Pediatr Transplant* 8: 400–15.

Salhab WA, Wyckoff MH, Laptook AR, Perlman JR (2004) Initial hypoglycemia and neonatal brain injury in term infants with severe fetal acidemia. *Pediatrics* 114: 361–6.

Sanchez CP (2003) Secondary hyperparathyroidism in children with chronic renal failure: pathogenesis and treatment. *Pediatr Drugs* 5: 763–76.

Schatz J, Finke R, Roberts CW (2004) Interactions of biomedical and environmental risk factors for cognitive development: a preliminary study of sickle cell disease. *J Dev Behav Pediatr* 25: 304–10.

Schaumburg H, Kaplan J, Windebank A, et al. (1983) Sensory neuropathy from pyridoxine abuse: a new megavitamin syndrome. *N Engl J Med* 309: 445–8.

Scheffner D, König S, Rauterberg-Ruland I, et al. (1988) Fatal liver failure in 16 children with valproate therapy. *Epilepsia* 29: 530–42.

Schillingford AJ, Wernowsky G (2004) Academic performance and behavioral difficulties after neonatal and infantile heart surgery. *Pediatr Clin North Am* 51: 1625–39.

Schoen EJ, Clapp W, To TT, Fireman BH (2004) The key role of newborn thyroid scintigraphy with isotope iodide (123I) in defining and managing congenital hypothyroidism. *Pediatrics* 114: e683–8.

Scolding NJ, Kellar-Wood HF, Shaw C, et al. (1996) Wolfram syndrome: hereditary diabetes mellitus with brainstem and optic atrophy. *Ann Neurol* 39: 352–60.

Scommegna S, Galeazzi D, Picone S, et al. (2004) Neonatal identification of pituitary aplasia: a life-saving diagnosis. Review of five cases. *Horm Res* 62: 10–6.

Scott R, Aladangady N, Maalouf E (2004) Neonatal hypopituitarism presenting with poor feeding, hypoglycemia and prolonged unconjugated hyperbilirubinemia. *J Matern Fetal Neonatal Med* 16: 131–3.

Sébire G, Tabarki B, Saunders DE, et al. (2005) Cerebral venous sinus thrombosis in children: risk factors, presentation, diagnosis and outcome. *Brain* 128: 477–89.

Shintani S, Tsuruoka S, Shiigai T (1993) Hypoglycaemic hemiplegia: a repeat SPECT study. *J Neurol Neurosurg Psychiatry* 56: 700–1.

Shiozawa Z, Yamada H, Mabuchi C, et al. (1982) Superior sagittal sinus thrombosis associated with androgen therapy for hypoplastic anemia. *Ann Neurol* 12: 578–80.

Simons WF, Fuggle PW, Grant DB, Smith I (1994) Intellectual development at 10 years in early treated congenital hypothyroidism. *Arch Dis Child* 71: 232–4.

Sloan LM, Rosenblatt JE, Cockerill FR (2005) Detection of Tropheryma whipplei DNA in clinical specimens by LightCycler real-time PCR. *J Clin Micobiol* 43: 3516–8.

Smadja D, Bellance R, Cabre P, et al. (1995) [Involvements of the peripheral nervous system and skeletal muscles in HTLV1-related paraplegia. Study of 70 cases seen in Martinique.] *Rev Neurol* 151: 190–5 (French).

Smith CJ, Crock PA, King BR, et al. (2004) Phenotype–genotype correlations in a series of Wolfram syndrome families. *Diabetes Care* 27: 2003–9.

Smith DW, Klein AM, Henderson JR, Myrianthopoulos NC (1975) Congenital hypothyroidism—signs and symptoms in the newborn period. *J Pediatr* 87: 958–62.

Smith R (1981) Thyroid hormones and brain development in children. In: Hetzel BS, Smith RM, eds. *Fetal Brain Disorders—Recent Approaches to the Problem of Mental Deficiency.* Amsterdam: Elsevier, pp. 149–85.

Spallino L, Stirling HF, O'Reagan M, et al. (1998) Transient hypoglycemic hemiparesis in children with insulin dependent diabetes mellitus. *Diabetes Care* 21: 1576–8.

Stanescu I, Zahar JR, Brugières P, et al. (2002) [Paucisymptomatic and reversible myelinolysis after an anaphylactic shock.] *Rev Neurol* 158: 1118–20 (French).

Stein DP, Lederman RJ, Vogt DP, et al. (1992) Neurological complications following liver transplantation. *Ann Neurol* 31 : 644–9.

Steinschneider M, Sherbany A, Pavlakis S, et al. (1990) Congenital folate malabsorption: reversible clinical and neurophysiologic abnormalities. *Neurology* 40: 1315.

Steward DK (2001) Behavioral characteristics of infants with nonorganic failure to thrive during a play interaction. *MCN Am J Matern Child Nurs* 26: 79–85.

Stewart SM, Uauy R, Kennard BD, et al. (1988) Mental development and growth in children with chronic liver disease of early and late onset. *Pediatrics* 82: 167–72.

Stieh J, Kramer HH, Harding P, Fischer G (1999) Gross and fine motor development is impaired in children with cyanotic congenital heart disease. *Neuropediatrics* 30: 77–82.

Stoch MB, Smythe PM, Moodie AD, Bradshaw D (1982) Psychosocial outcome and CT findings after gross undernourishment during infancy: a 20-year developmental study. *Dev Med Child Neurol* 24: 419–36.

Stollhoff K, Schulte FJ (1987) Vitamin B12 and brain development. *Eur J Pediatr* 146: 201–5.

Streletz LJ, Bej MD, Graziani LJ, et al. (1992) Utility of serial EEGs in neonates during extracorporeal membrane oxygenation. *Pediatr Neurol* 8: 190–6.

Sugiura M, Sato E, Nakashima T, et al. (2005) Long-term follow-up in patients with Pendred syndrome: vestibular, auditory and other phenotypes. *Eur Arch Otorhinolaryngol* 262: 737–43.

Sybesma CA, v Pinxteren-Nagler E, Sinnige LG, et al. (1999) Hashimoto encephalopathy in a 12-year-old girl. *Eur J Paediatr* 158: 867–8.

Takahashi S, Mitamura R, Itoh Y, et al. (1994) Hashimoto encephalopathy: etiologic considerations. *Pediatr Neurol* 11: 328–31.

Tam CS, Galanos J, Seymour JF, et al. (2004) Reversible posterior leukoencephalopathy syndrome complicating cytotoxic therapy for hematologic malignancies. *Am J Hematol* 77: 72–6¬.

Tan H, Önbas O (2004) Central pontine myelinolysis manifesting with massive myoclonus. *Pediatr Neurol* 31: 64–6.

Tan H, Kardas F, Buynkavei M, Karakelloglu C (2004) Pyridoxine-dependent seizures and microcephaly. *Pediar Neurol* 31: 211–3.

Tan TQ, Vogel H, Tharp BR, et al. (1995) Presumed central nervous system Whipple's disease in a child: a case report. *Clin Infect Dis* 20: 883–9.

Tasker RC, Boyd S, Harden A, Matthew DJ (1988) Monitoring in non-traumatic coma. Part II: Electroencephalography. *Arch Dis Child* 63: 895–9.

Thame M, Gray R, Forrester T (1999) Parkinsonian-like tremors in the recovery phase of kwashiorkor. *West Indian Med J* 43: 102–3.

Thomas AF, McVie R, Levine SN (1999) Disorders of maternal calcium metabolism implicated by abnormal calcium metabolism in the neonate. *Am J Perinatol* 16: 515–20.

Thomas PK (1997) Tropical neuropathies. *J Neurol* 244: 475–82.

Tonner DR, Schelte JA (1993) Neurological complications of thyroid and parathyroid disease. *Med Clin North Am* 77: 251–63.

Torres OA, Miller VS, Buist NM, Hyland K (1999) Folinic acid-responsive neonatal seizures. *J Child Neurol* 14: 529–32.

Tortorella G, Magaudda A, Mercuri E, et al. (1993) Familial unilateral and bilateral occipital calcifications and epilepsy. *Neuropediatrics* 24: 341–2.

Tory K, Sallay P, Tóth-Heyn P, et al. (2001) Signs of autonomic neuropathy in childhood uremia. *Pediatr Nephrol* 16: 25–8.

Toti P, Balestri P, Cano M, et al. (1996) Celiac disease with cerebral calcium and silica deposits: X-ray spectroscopic findings, an autopsy study. *Neurology* 46: 1088–92.

Toublanc JE, Rives S, Boileau P (2005) [Scholarly and occupational outcomes of the first patients screened in France for congenital hypothyroidism.] *Bull Acad Natl Med* 189: 87–95; discussion 95–8 (French).

Trinh-Trang-Tan MM, Cartron JP, Bankir L (2005) Molecular basis for the dialysis disequilibrium syndrome: altered aquaporin and urea transporter expression in the brain. *Nephrol Dial Transplant* 20: 1984–8.

Tullu MS, Udgirkar VS, Muronjan MN, et al. (2003) Kocher–Debré–Sémelaigne syndrome: hypothyroidism with muscle pseudohypertrophy. *Indian J Pediatr* 70: 671–3.

Tyler HR, Clark DB (1957) Cerebrovascular accidents in patients with congenital heart disease. *Arch Neurol Psychiatry* 77: 483–97.

Valentin C, Pissard S, Martin J, et al. (2000) Triose phosphate isomerase deficiency in 3 French families: two novel null alleles, a frameshift mutation (TPI Alfortville) and an alteration in the initiation codon (TPI Paris). *Blood* 96: 1130–5.

Vanderschueren-Lodeweyckx, M., Debruyne F, Dooms L, et al. (1983) Sensorineural hearing loss in sporadic congenital hypothyroidism. *Arch Dis Child* **58**: 419–22.

Van Hoff J, Ritchley AK, Shaywitz BA (1985) Intracranial hemorrhage in children with sickle cell disease. *Am J Dis Child* **139**: 1229–32.

Vanhulle C, Dacher JN, Delangre T, et al. (1997) [Antineoplastic chemotherapy and Wernicke's encephalopathy.] *Arch Pediatr* **9**: 243–6 (French).

Vannucci RC, Vannucci SJ (2001) Hypoglycemic brain injury. *Semin Neonatol* **6**: 147–155.

Vasconcellos E, Piña-Garza JE, Fakhouri T, Fenichel G (1999) Pediatric manifestations of Hashimoyo's encephalopathy. *Pediatr Neurol* **20**: 394–8.

Vichinsky EP, Neumayr LD, Earles AN, et al. (2000) Causes and outcome of the acute chest syndrome in sickle cell disease. *N Engl J Med* **342**: 1855–65.

Volpe J (2005) *Neurology of the Newborn, 4th edn.* London: Saunders.

von Maydell B, Kopp M, von Komarowski G, et al. (2002) Hashimoto encephalopathy – is it underdiagnosed in pediatric patients? *Neuropediatrics* **33**: 86–9.

Vortmeyer AO, Hagel C, Laas R (1992) Haemorrhagic thiamine deficient encephalopathy following prolonged parenteral nutrition. *J Neurol Neurosurg Psychiatry* **55**: 826–9.

Vulsma T, Gons MH, De Vijlder JJM (1989) Maternal–fetal transfer of thyronine in congenital hypothyroidism due to a total organification defect or thyroid agenesis. *N Engl J Med* **321**: 13–6.

Wada T, Kubota T, Fukushima Y, Saitoh S (2000) Molecular genetic study of Japanese patients with X-linked alpha-thalassemia syndrome *Am J Med Genet* **18**: 242–8.

Walker RW, Brochstein JA (1988) Neurologic complications of immunosuppressive agents. *Neurol Clin* **6**: 261–78.

Wang LC, Cohen ME, Duffner PK (1994) Etiologies of central diabetes insipidus in children. *Pediatr Neurol* **11**: 273–7.

Wanke C (2004) Pathogenesis and consequences of HIV-associated wasting. *J Acquir Immune Defic Syndr* **37** Suppl 5: S277–9.

Wayne EA, Dean HJ, Booth F, Tenenbein M (1990) Focal neurologic deficits associated with hypoglycemia in children with diabetes. *J Pediatr* **117**: 575–7.

Weber G, Vigone MC, Passoni A, et al. (2005) Congenital hypothyroidism with gland in situ: diagnostic re-evaluation. *J Endocrinol Invest* **28**: 516–22.

Weidauer S, Nichtweiss M, Lanfermann H, Zanella FE (2003) Wernicke encephalopathy: MR findings and clinical presentation. *Eur Radiol* **13**: 1001–9.

Wells TG, Ulstrom RA, Nevins TE (1988) Hypoglycemia in pediatric renal allograft recipients. *J Pediatr* **113**: 1002–7.

Wevers RA, Hansen SI, Van Hellenberg Hubar JL, et al. (1994) Folate deficiency in cerebrospinal fluid associated with a defect in folate binding protein in the central nervous system. *J Neurol Neurosurg Psychiatry* **57**: 223–6.

Wiebel J (1976) Cerebellar–ataxic syndrome in children and adolescents with hypothyroidism under treatment. *Acta Paediatr Scand* **65**: 201–5.

Wijdicks EF, Wiesner RH, Dahlke LJ, Krom RA (1994) FK506-induced neurotoxicity in liver transplantation. *Ann Neurol* **35**: 498–501.

Wilkie AOM, Zeitlin HC, Lindenbaum RH, et al. (1990) Clinical features and molecular analysis of the alpha thalassemia mental retardation syndromes. II. Cases without detectable abnormality of the alpha globulin complex. *Am J Hum Genet* **46**: 1127–40.

Wilkie AOM, Gibbons RJ, Higgs DR, Pembrey ME (1991) X linked alpha thalassemia/mental retardation: spectrum of clinical features in three related males. *J Med Genet* **28**: 738–41.

Williams FL, Mires GJ, Barnett HC, et al. (2005) Transient hypothyroxinemia in preterm infants: the role of cord sera thyroid hormone levels adjusted for prenatal and intrapartum factors. *J Clin Endocrinol Metab* **90**: 4599–606.

Willison HJ, Muller DPR, Matthews S, et al. (1985) A study of the relationship between neurological function and serum vitamin E concentrations in patients with cystic fibrosis. *J Neurol Neurosurg Psychiatry* **48**: 1097–102.

Willoughby A, Moss HA, Hubbard VS, et al. (1987) Developmental outcome in children exposed to chloride-deficient formula. *Pediatrics* **79**: 851–7.

Wilmhurst JM, Wise GA, Pollard JD, Ouvrier RA (2004) Chronic axonal neuropathy with triose phosphate isomerase deficiency. *Pediatr Neurol* **30**: 146–8.

Wilson LC, Hall CR (2002) Albright hereditary osteodystrophy and hypoparathyroidism. *Semin Musculoskelet Radiol* **6**: 273–83.

Winer KK, Ko CW, Reynolds JC, et al. (2003) Long-term treatment of hypoparathyroidism: a randomized controlled study comparing parathyroid hormone-(1-34) versus calcitriol and calcium. *J Clin Endocrinol Metab* **88**: 4214–20.

Winick M (1969) Malnutrition and brain development. *J Pediatr* **74**: 667–79.

Wiswell TE, Cornish JD, Northam RS (1986) Neonatal polycythemia: frequency of clinical manifestations and other associated findings. *Pediatrics* **78**: 26–30.

Wiznitzer M, Packer RJ, August CS, Burkey E (1984) Neurological complications of bone marrow transplantation in childhood. *Ann Neurol* **16**: 569–76.

Woodard P, Helton K, McDaniel H, et al. (2004) Encephalopathy in pediatric patients after allogeneic hematopoieetic stem cell transplantation is associated with a poor prognosis. *Bone Marrow Transplant* **33**: 1151–7.

Wright M, Nolan T (1994) Impact of cyanotic heart disease on school performance. *Arch Dis Child* **71**: 64–70.

Yager JY, Hartfield DS (2002) Neurologic manifestations of iron deficiency in childhood. *Pediatr Neurol* **27**: 85–92.

Yamamoto T, Kobata H, Yagi R, et al. (1985) Primary hypomagnesemia with secondary hypocalcemia. Report of a case and review of the world literature. *Magnesium* **5**: 153–64.

PART XI

DEVELOPMENTAL AND NEUROPSYCHIATRIC DISORDERS OF CHILDHOOD

Christopher Gillberg

Neuropsychiatric disorders of childhood include those conditions presenting mainly with emotional and/or behavioural symptoms, but for which an exclusive or partial biological basis has been documented or presumed to exist. As a result of this emphasis on biological factors, they are described in different chapters of the book.

Many of the mental retardation syndromes present initially only with psychiatric or developmental problems, or with a combination of both. Among these are the so-called 'behavioural phenotype syndromes' (i.e. syndromes with a known or presumed genetic cause – such as Prader–Willi syndrome and Williams syndrome – in which behaviour in some key respects is similar from one case to another). The major behavioural syndromes are studied in Chapter 4, which also includes Rett syndrome (in the previous edition dealt with in the chapter on heredodegenerative disorders as it was considered at the time as a neurodegenerative condition). In mental retardation of unknown origin, it is perhaps even more common to encounter developmental, emotional and behavioural presenting problems rather than major neurological or other physical deficits.

Autism and the different autistic-like conditions (including Asperger syndrome) have gradually come to be accepted as mainly biologically determined syndromes. Unfortunately, the term 'pervasive developmental disorders' has come into use in some quarters to cover autism and autistic-like conditions. Autism, however, need not be pervasive (and Asperger syndrome usually is not). It is conceptually confusing to use such a term but not to include severe or profound mental retardation under this label.

Tourette syndrome and other severe tic disorders are now conceptualized more and more as a biologically determined spectrum of problems that includes a prominent movement disorder and major psychiatric manifestations, the most striking being obsessive–compulsive disorder (OCD). Tourette syndrome is described in Chapter 9 because the movement disorder is often the first obvious manifestation. However, these psychiatric disturbances are not specific for Tourette syndrome and can be associated with other conditions or exist in isolation. Obsessions and compulsions are phenomena that are now believed to be biological in nature. They are part and parcel of Tourette syndrome and OCD, and are also common in several of the neuropsychiatric disorders referred to in these chapters.

Most of the various symptom constellations comprising attentional, motor control and perceptual deficits (e.g. attention deficit hyperactivity disorder and specific developmental disorders, including dyslexia) have a clear or surmised biological basis (and a very strong correlation with emotional and behavioural disorders). They are therefore an important part of child neuropsychiatry. These are common problems, affecting 5–10% of the general population of school-age children.

A number of 'minor' developmental problems presenting as sleep disorders, speech disorders and disorders of bladder and bowel control also often cause or are in other ways associated with psychiatric problems.

Finally, child neuropsychiatry encompasses a number of 'borderline' problems, such as behavioural and emotional problems associated with known neurological disorders (epilepsy, hydrocephalus, cerebral palsy, etc.) and a number of psychiatric disorders not yet documented to have a biological basis but in which biological factors play an essential role (anorexia nervosa, schizophrenia, etc.).

In the following chapters, all of the above-mentioned problems and syndromes will be briefly surveyed or at least referred to in more general terms. Before that, however, some comments on normal mental and behavioural development will be made.

PART XI

DEVELOPMENTAL AND NEUROPSYCHIATRIC DISORDERS OF CHILDHOOD

23

DEVELOPMENT: NORMAL/DELAYED/DISORDERED

Martin Bax and Christopher Gillberg

CLINICAL PRESENTATION OF DEVELOPMENTAL DELAY

Many children who present to child neurologists, child psychiatrists or community paediatricians superficially have no physical or neurological signs but have delay in one or other aspect of development. The largest group of these children is those with 'intellectual' disability. The term intellectual or (general) learning disability is used in many English-speaking countries now in preference to 'mental retardation', although this is not the case in America at the time of writing. Similar complications pertain in the nomenclature of *specific* learning disorders. These include dyslexia, dysgraphia and dyscalculia, and some would also include developmental coordination disorder (DCD), some of the language disorders and attention deficit hyperactivity disorder (ADHD) under this umbrella term. A full discussion of this issue is given by Whitmore et al. (1999). These classifications of children are not diagnostic in the real sense (at least initially), but rather *syndromic* descriptions where there is a lack of clear clues to pathogenesis and aetiology.

Developmental delay may persist, in which case the child has permanent developmental dysfunction, or the child may 'recover'. A good example of this 'recovery' situation is in the development of walking. Ninety-eight per cent of children walk by the age of 18 months; for those who do not, this may be due to a variety of causes such as a motor disorder, e.g. cerebral palsy, or it may represent an extreme of normal variation in the development of upright gait. The genetically inherited trait of bottom shuffling whereby a child moves by sitting and 'punting' on their bottom may result in them not walking until as late as 30 months and yet subsequently walking may be normal. At around 18 months a child may show a number of other features that deviate from typical development. For example they may not have downward parachute reactions, the feet may be poorly developed and the lower limbs may show a relative hypotonia compared to other children so that the examiner may think that there is some significant pathology; in such a case distinguishing the child from one who has diplegia may present problems (Robson and Mac Keith 1971). It is hard too to make a judgement as to whether the absence of walking at the age of 2 years may pose any social disadvantage for the child. If these phenomena are observed with the relatively simple function of walking, one can predict similar difficulties with other functions such as vision.

DEVELOPMENTAL ASSESSMENT

Normal development of the infant was very extensively studied during the 20th century and the pioneering work of, inter alia, Arnold Gesell, Myrtle McGraw and Albrecht Peiper was followed by many people who made clinical applications of their work allowing distinctions to be made by examining the child for differences between normal and abnormal behaviour (Egan 1971, Sheridan 1973, Illingworth 1988). A developmental schema with some examination data at seven stages from birth to 4.5 years is presented overleaf. These stages have been described as benchmarks but it is important to be aware that development is a gradual process and not steplike. The programme is derived from Bax et al. (1980), where further data are given.

Vision and hearing are discussed in Chapters 17 and 18 respectively. Speech and language represent the most complex area of development and are closely linked to intelligence. Language is often described as the inner symbolization of thought. Thought usually takes place in some semantic form, although it may take other forms such as graphic or mathematical. Language may be expressed through speech or sign language, or via digital methods ranging from the classic Morse code to computer-based programmes. In the young child, intelligibility of speech, vocabulary, length of utterance and grammar of expressed language, and understanding of language (receptive language) are assessed in the context of the child's age. Obviously the assessment of language in the young child (15 months to 3 years) is the most difficult area, particularly for the busy neurologist assessing what may be a complex and multifaceted disorder. In the study reported by Bax et al. (1980) comparing clinical assessment with the results of standard language testing (using the Reynell scales), it was found that an experienced clinician using simple pictures and objects could reliably identify children whose speech and language were more than 1.5 SD below the mean and in whom a further speech and language evaluation was necessary. It should be stressed that all children whose language development is causing concern should have also have a full audiometric assessment (see Chapter 18). Environmental/social deprivation should also be considered

SUMMARY OF DEVELOPMENT FROM BIRTH TO 4.5 YEARS

A. the first 6 months

GROSS MOTOR FUNCTION AND POSTURE

Newborn
Prone: arms and legs flexed, pelvis high, knees under abdomen
Ventral suspension: head held just below body
Supine: arms and legs semiflexed, head to one side
Pull-to-sit: complete head lag
Held upright: legs extended, stepping and placing reflex

4 weeks
Prone: pelvis lower, lifts head off couch
Ventral suspension: lifts head momentarily
Supine: arms and legs semiflexed
Pull-to-sit: lifts head momentarily
Held sitting: rounded back, lifts head momentarily
Held upright: stepping and placing reflex, legs extended

6 weeks
Prone and ventral suspension: holds head in line with body for a few
  seconds
Supine and pull-to-sit: holds head up for a few seconds, intermittent
  asymmetric tonic neck reflex

12 weeks
Prone: lifts head and upper chest off couch, pelvis flat, legs extended
Ventral suspension: maintains head 45–90° to body
Pull-to-sit: little or no head lag
Held sitting: lumbar curve still present, some head wobble
Held upright: sags at knees, stepping and placing reflexes hard to elicit

FINE MOTOR

4 weeks
Grasp reflex
Drops objects immediately
Hands mainly fisted
Sweeping movements towards objects

12 weeks
Little or no grasp reflex
Opens and closes hands
Watches objects for a few seconds
Holds bottle for a few moments, but seldom capable of regarding it at
  same time
Hand regard begins – watches movement of own hands

20 weeks
Accurate reaching
Palmar grasp on ulnar side of hand
Hand regard less common

LANGUAGE

4–6 weeks
Coos, gurgles
Phonemes – oo, ugh

LANGUAGE (cont'd)

12 weeks
Long streams of babble
'Babble conversations' with mother

16–24 weeks
Babbling – ebe, ele, da, ba, ka, mum

SOCIAL BEHAVIOUR AND UNDERSTANDING

4 weeks
Can imitate tongue protrusion
Gazes at bright lights, faces, coloured objects
Recognizes mother

12 weeks
Laughs at playful activities
Recognizes familiar situation – bathing, feeding
Dislikes being left

20 weeks
Looks for dropped toy
Holds bottle
Smiles at mirror image

VISION

4 weeks
Pupils react to light
Focuses at 23 cm away
Looks at faces, bright light, coloured objects
Prefers mother's face to stranger's
Appreciates depth
Follows moving objects and faces up to 45° from midline

12 weeks
Visually very alert
Looks at small objects
Smooth convergence and binocular vision developed
Discriminates between colours
Follows moving objects through 180° vertically and horizontally

HEARING

4 weeks
Turns eyes and head to sound
Prefers voice sounds to pure tones
Startles, blinks, cries to loud sounds
Quietens to mother's voice or rattle
Recognizes mother's voice

12 weeks
Eyes and head move together to sound

5–6 months
Downward localization of sound

B. 6 months to 4.5 years

6 MONTHS

Gross motor
Supine – raises head in anticipation of being picked up
Prone – lifts head, chest and upper abdomen off couch with extended arms
Held standing bears weight on legs and bounces up and down
Sits with minimal support, head firmly erect
Rolls front to back
Hand regard less common

Fine manipulation and vision
Picks up cube with palmar grasp, often places in mouth
Transfers objects from one hand to the other
Looks at pellet – attempts to scoop up with palmar grasp

6 MONTHS (cont'd)

Fine manipulation and vision (cont'd)
Holds bottle
Visually very alert
Follows dropped toy to the ground
Follows object at 1m through 180° arc
Looks at 6mm mounted ball at 3m

Vocalization and hearing
Vocalizes tunefully using consonants, e.g. da, mum, nan
Localizes sound to left and right
In response to sounds at 45° turns head, horizontally and then towards
  sound

6 MONTHS (cont'd)

Social behaviour and play
Friendly towards strangers
Excited by approach of familiar people
Laughs at peep-bo game
Smiles at mirror image

12 MONTHS

Gross motor
Rises from lying to sitting
Crawls on hands and knees
Pulls to standing
Walks with one hand held

Fine manipulation and vision
Points at objects with index finger
Picks up 3 mm pellet with pincer grasp between thumb and tip of index
    finger
Compares (matches) two objects
Releases toy on request
Watches and follows mounted 3 mm ball at 3 m

Language and hearing
Long tuneful babble in sentence-like pattern
Imitates sound
First naming words
Understands several words, e.g. dog, dad, teddy
Understands simple commands if accompanied by gesture, e.g. waves
    bye-bye
Localizes sound above and below ear level

Social behaviour and play
Imitates sounds and actions, e.g. claps hands
Drinks from cup
Eats food with fingers
Looks for hidden toy
Wary of strangers, closely attached to familiar adults
Joint attention
Protoimperative pointing to objects wanted

18 MONTHS

Gross motor
Walks (from 13 months) with feet slightly apart
Holds arms nearly to sides (low guard)
Runs

Fine manipulation and vision
Picks up 3 mm pellet with neat pincer grip
Casting (throwing objects down, hoping they will be picked up and given
    back) and mouthing ceased
Builds tower of three or four cubes
Feeds self with spoon
Drinks from cup unaided
Identifies small detail in pictures

Language and hearing
Identifies familiar objects by use, e.g. toothbrush, comb
Identifies familiar objects when named
Obeys simple instructions
Points to parts of the body
Uses 6–20 recognizable words
Names familiar animals

Social understanding and play
'Domestic mimicry' – copies mother's actions
Meaningful play with toys
Plays with toys alone but near familiar people
Emotionally dependent on familiar adult
Likes sitting on knee and looking at books for a few minutes
Protodeclarative pointing to show interest

2 YEARS

Gross motor
Runs
Kicks ball
Goes up and down stairs (on standard 15–20 cm treads) holding rail or
    hand (two feet per step)

2 YEARS (cont'd)

Fine manipulation and vision
Builds tower of 6 or 7 cubes
Holds pencil in fist and draws circular scribble
Handedness developing
May recognize and name familiar in pictures at 3 m

Language and hearing
Obeys simple commands
Identifies common objects and parts of body
Uses 50 or more words
Starting to use 2- or 3-word phrases
Identifies named toys or pictures in hearing test

Social behaviour and play
Plays make-believe games with toys, etc., makes cup of tea
Plays near other children but not with them
Constantly demands parents' attention
Tantrums when unable to make him/herself understood and when
    demands are refused
Puts on and takes off shoes and socks
Clean and dry by day

3 YEARS

Gross motor
Goes upstairs one foot per step, downstairs two feet per step
Stands on one foot momentarily
Rides tricycle

Fine manipulation and vision
Builds tower of nine cubes
Copies train made of cubes
Imitates bridge
Holds pencil in preferred hand with tripod grip
Copies circle and imitates cross
Threads large beads on shoe lace
Cuts with scissors

Language and hearing
Large vocabulary
Holds conversation
Uses sentences with most prepositions and personal pronouns
Uses why, where, who
Knows names and sex
Still has some consonantal omissions and substitutions
Performs speech discrimination test

Social behaviour and play
Eats with fork and spoon
Dresses him/herself, except buttons
Plays imaginative games with other children
Dry at night
Able to be left in familiar surroundings – understands mother's temporary
    absence

4.5 YEARS

Gross motor
Goes downstairs one foot per step
Walks along narrow line
Hops on each foot (may need hand held)

Fine manipulation and vision
Copies steps made of 3 cubes
Mature tripod grip of pencil
Copies cross and square
Draws a recognizable man with six parts

Language and hearing
Long sentences grammatically correct
Phonetically correct except s, f, th, r (English)
Repeats a short story
Cooperates with audiogram

Social behaviour and play
Complicated make-believe play alone and with other children
Dresses him/herself fully
Appreciates meaning of time of day

when looking for an underlying cause for a child's immature speech. Some children with delay in speech and language development may 'catch up' by school age, but about 7% of 5-year-olds (Tomblin et al. 1997) will have specific language impairment (SLI) and some will have global intellectual disability and autism spectrum disorders. Speech disorders can occur in the absence of any language delay in certain neurological conditions. Classically the child with athetoid cerebral palsy may have dysarthric speech that is unintelligible and may make the language component very difficult to assess. Dysarthric speech may also be a feature of genetic disorders such as the childhood ataxias and congenital suprabulbar palsy and of acquired conditions such as post-encephalitis, post-traumatic brain injury and posterior fossa tumours.

Specific language disorder is diagnosed when a child's language development is substantially below his/her age level but the child is developing normally in other respects. The ICD-10 Research Diagnostic Criteria for Specific Developmental Language Disorders (WHO 1993) specify scores below the 2 SD limit on standardized language testing together with language skills at least 1 SD below nonverbal IQ. However, some researchers regard the discrepancy criterion as over-restrictive as there are some children who have all the linguistic characteristics of SLI but do not have a large mismatch between verbal and nonverbal ability (Stark and Tallal 1981). From a clinical viewpoint there is an argument that the diagnosis of SLI should not be restricted to children with normal nonverbal IQ. Bishop (1997) asserts that "we should expect to see this kind of developmental problem in children of all IQ levels. Furthermore, language-impaired children of low IQ benefit just as much from speech–language therapy as those of average IQ." A comprehensive account of specific language impairment can be found in Bishop (1997) and Bishop and Leonard (2000).

Children with speech and language problems often have impaired phonological awareness and are more likely to have literacy difficulties in school than those without language problems (Catts et al. 2002). They are also more likely to demonstrate neurodevelopmental/neuropsychiatric disorders, as recently reported by Gillberg's group (Miniscalco et al. 2006, 2007). They found that 'language delay' (including late onset of speech, poverty of speech and comprehension problems) observed by the health visitor/child health nurse in children aged 30 months predicted a very high rate (70%) of neurodevelopmental/neuropsychiatric disorder (including autism spectrum disorders and ADHD) at age 7–8 years. Interestingly, all the children with remaining problems at school age had major difficulties regarding narrative skills. This underlines the crucial importance of observation and interview regarding children's language development at age 2–3 years so that early-onset neurodevelopmental/neuropsychiatric disorders can be diagnosed and remedied at a very young age.

THE INTERNATIONAL CLASSIFICATION OF FUNCTIONING, DISABILITY AND HEALTH (ICF – WHO 2001)

When the child's developmental delay or failure to develop 'normally' is perceived as being permanent, the child is recognized

TABLE 23.1
Conceptual framework of the International Classification of Impairments, Disabilities and Handicaps (ICIDH, WHO 1980)

Impairment: In the context of health experience an impairment is any loss or abnormality of psychological, physiological or anatomical structure or function

Disability: In the context of health experience a disability is any restriction or lack (resulting from an impairment) of ability to perform an activity in the manner or within the range considered normal for a human being

Handicap: In the context of health experience a handicap is a disadvantage for a given individual, resulting from an impairment or disability, that limits or prevents the fulfilment of a role that is normal (depending on age, sex, and social and cultural factors) for that individual

TABLE 23.2
Conceptual framework of the International Classification of Functioning, Disability and Health (ICF, WHO 2001)

In the context of health:

Body functions are the physiological functions of body systems (including psychological functions)

Body structures are anatomical parts of the body such as organs, limbs and their components

Impairments are problems in body function or structure such as significant deviation or loss

Activity is the execution of a task or action by an individual

Participation is involvement in a life situation

Activity limitations are difficulties an individual may have in executing activities

Participation restrictions are problems an individual may experience in involvement in life situations

Environmental factors make up the physical, social and attitudinal environment in which people live and conduct their lives

as requiring not only health services but also special education and social services. An attempt to define and categorize disability was first made by the World Health Organization (WHO) in 1980 (Table 23.1); this has been refined and developed into the more complex definition used currently (WHO 2001) (Table 23.2, Fig. 23.1). Rightfully this same disability definition extends across all ages but the circumstances for children are somewhat different to those for adults. The disabled adult demands full participation in the development of services for disabled people but may be limited by the profound degree of disabilities originating from childhood. The nature of the participation that the severely physically and intellectually disabled person is capable of may be limited but the paediatrician is left with the task of trying to assess the functional consequences of the biological phenomenon they study and the consequences of pathological states they are able to describe. The clinician is anxious to see that the child participates as much as possible. Nevertheless, the consequences of the child's clinical assessment and diagnosis may be such that in many countries a diagnosis of one sort may lead to quite different services from a diagnosis of another sort even when the underlying disorder is the same. For example, individuals with cerebral palsy and severe learning disability (mental retardation) may have

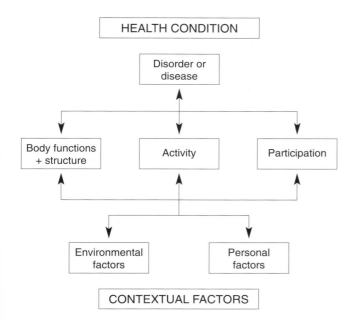

Fig. 23.1. Interactions between the components of the ICF (WHO 2001).

very different services provided by education and social services, and this can have profound consequences for the children and their families.

CLASSIFICATION OF THE NEURODEVELOPMENTAL DISORDERS

For those who started to study child development in the 1930s and 1940s it was obvious to divide development into various functions. Classically these included motor (gross and fine), hearing, speech and language and to this might be added intellectual (perceptual) development and behaviour. As a result of findings of delayed development under these categories we see 'syndromic' diagnoses emerge such as 'cerebral palsy'. The clumsy child may be diagnosed as having 'minimal cerebral dysfunction', but may have additional problems such as hearing difficulties, visual disorder that may or may not be correctable by glasses, speech problems that can be divided into categories such as stuttering and dysarthria, language problems, behavioural problems in which there are huge sets and subsets of behaviour that might develop such as sleep disorders, abnormal activity levels, temper tantrums, antisocial behaviours, enuresis and so on. There are psychological tests, for example the Griffiths, subdivided into various functions (such as gross motor, hearing and speech, and practical reasoning). There are also specific tests for all sorts of diagnoses, e.g. the Diagnostic Interview for Social and Communication Disorders (DISCO) in autism (Leekam et al. 2002, Wing et al. 2002).

Early efforts to use functional methods to classify disorders include those of Denhoff and Robinault (1960) who defined neuromotor, intellectual, consciousness, neurosensory, behavioural and perceptual dysfunction. To some extent the categories could be linked with neuropathological findings, although these were few and many conditions were not diagnosable. However,

because of the great difficulties of either aetiological or neuropathological diagnosis, in fact syndromic classifications have been and still are used extensively in this group of disorders.

CHALLENGES IN DEVELOPMENTAL DIAGNOSIS

Recent developments both in genetic research and in brain imaging have led to the possibility of more precise aetiological diagnoses for children with delay in one or more areas of development. In the last two decades enormous numbers of genetic disorders have been identified that account for the 'mental retardation' or 'learning disability' in some of these conditions (such as phenylketonuria and Angelman syndrome). Identification of the cause has led to the possibility of prevention. This is an aim in all genetic disease but not likely to be possible within the next decade in most instances.

Cerebral palsy (CP) provides an illustrative example of the problems currently encountered in the field of neurodevelopmental diagnoses. In a population identified as having CP the commonest finding on MRI is periventricular leukomalacia (PVL) (Bax et al. 2006). However, in reviewing PVL it has been found that CP is not the most common diagnosis following this white matter damage. The most common diagnosis in children with PVL is visual disorder. One of the difficulties of assessing visual function in a child with previously diagnosed CP such as spastic diplegia is that it is hard to tell whether the motor problem which is easy to identify, or the visual problems that the child may or may not have, is the important issue and this throws into question the basis for classifying a group of children under the diagnostic heading of 'cerebral palsy'.

Autism is another example of conceptually difficult issues in neurodevelopmental diagnosis. As originally described, autism was perceived as a syndromic condition with social, language and behavioural features. It is now known that these diagnostic features may arise in a great number of genetic conditions, for example tuberous sclerosis, Moebius syndrome and fragile X syndrome. In many genetic disorders autistic features may be seen but equally other behaviours relating to a specific phenotype may be noted. In Rett syndrome, the majority of affected individuals have marked autistic features, but the development over time of these is not typical of 'classic' autism. So should autism be diagnosed in Rett syndrome when criteria for autism are met? Or should autistic features be seen as part and parcel of Rett syndrome in the early years of development? Is it, as indeed has been proposed by the developers of the current diagnostic manuals (DSM-IV-TR and ICD-10), a separate subgroup of autism?

BEHAVIOURAL PHENOTYPES
Identification by genetic studies of many causes of mental retardation has made it possible to recognize specific behavioural features of individual conditions that had previously been grouped together. A classic example is the Prader–Willi syndrome where the child initially presents with failure to thrive and slow development of suck and swallow and consequently delayed

feeding. Paradoxically, the situation alters at around the age of 2 years so that subsequently, by about age 5, they present with gross overeating and obesity. Overactive behaviour is seen in a number of genetic syndromes, as are unusual social behaviours. Laughter, normal in the young child, can be abnormal in Angelman syndrome and also occurs in Rett syndrome where affected adults frequently laugh at night. Nyhan (1968) coined the phrase 'behavioural phenotype' and he recognized what is now known as Lesch–Nyhan syndrome, a striking and disturbing disorder characterized by self-mutilation. More recently the definition has been proposed that a behavioural phenotype is a characteristic pattern of motor, cognitive, linguistic and social observations that are consistently associated with a biological disorder. In some cases the behavioural phenotype may constitute a psychiatric disorder, while in others behaviours that are not usually regarded as symptoms of psychiatric diagnosis may occur. A characteristic pattern refers to a grouping or an occurrence of behaviours that have a typical distinctive nature. This may to some extent inform the appropriate interventions. There is rarely, if ever, a single pathognomonic behaviour. There are many syndromes with more prominent or significant behaviours. Once the behavioural phenotype is recognized as consistently associated with a biological disorder it is reasonable to anticipate that certain behaviours may ensue that have been described as common or typical of the disorder. For example, in Prader–Willi syndrome at around the age of 7 or 8 in some 60–70% of the children face picking will occur; this is a distressing and disturbing behaviour (although milder forms of face picking can be seen in typically developing young children). Sleep disorder is usually regarded as a psychiatric condition and occurs in many behavioural phenotypes but commonly forms only part of the behavioural picture.

INTELLECTUAL DISABILITY/MENTAL RETARDATION

One of the most common forms of developmental delay is mental retardation/learning disability, i.e. functional adaptation impairment stemming from a consistent level of tested IQ <70. (Other common forms are speech and language delay and developmental coordination disorder, both types affecting about 5% of the general population of children.)

Intellectual development and the development of intelligence are often considered synonymous. Intelligence is "the broadest and most pervasive cognitive trait, and is conceived of as being involved in virtually every kind of cognitive skill" and "it is a quintessentially high-level skill at the summit of a hierarchy of intellectual skills" (Butcher 1970). Intelligence is also "what intelligence tests measure – a sample of current intellectual performance" (Madge and Tizard 1980). Tested IQ is a *relatively* stable variable: more than 90% of all children show less than 30 points IQ variation from age 2 to 18 years if several tests are performed during this period (Honzik et al. 1948), and more than 80% show less than 15 points variation if only one retest is undertaken (Vernon 1976). Stability over time is further increased if the first IQ test is undertaken after age 6 years. Before age 2 years,

developmental tests have strong predictive validity only in the case of severely and profoundly mentally retarded children.

The remarkable stability of IQ over time was demonstrated in the long-term follow-up study from Dunedin (Moffitt et al. 1993). Almost 800 children were followed with IQ tests at ages 7, 9, 11 and 13 years. Only 13% showed IQ changes that exceeded what was expected from sources of measurement errors. However, even in this rather small subgroup, IQ changes tended not to be major and to return to previous levels at continued follow-up.

Cognitive development is rapid during the first few years of life and continues at a fast rate throughout childhood to adolescence. Thereafter the rate is much slower, and most people reach a point (perhaps in early adult life) beyond which they do not increase their intelligence capacity. In adults, IQ is defined by tests that yield normally distributed results in the general population and have a mean of 100. In children IQ can be conceptualized in similar terms, but can also be expressed as a developmental quotient (DQ) in which mental age is divided by chronological age and multiplied by 100. When used in this way a child with an IQ of 50 around age 8 years can be seen as having roughly 50% of normal development for chronological age, and therefore as performing similarly to a normal 4-year-old.

Spearman (1927) found that people who did well on one cognitive task usually also did well on most of the other cognitive tasks. He hypothesized that a 'general' (g) factor, or 'mental energy' was in operation. Children with emotional and behavioural problems, as we shall see, very often have cognitive profiles that are extremely uneven and cannot be predicted by a specific g-factor level.

Both genetic and environmental factors play a part in determining individual differences in IQ, but their relative contribution is not clearly established. That there are strong genetic determinants for IQ is now widely accepted. The overall effects of environment on the development of intelligence in individuals falling within the normal range of intelligence are probably less significant except in grossly abnormal situations such as extreme psychosocial deprivation and long-term near starvation (Madge and Tizard 1980).

Previous discussion emphasizes that mental retardation is not a disease, disorder or specific disability nor even a syndrome. It is a blanket description for a wide variation of genetic, social and specific medical conditions sharing the one common feature that affected individuals score consistently below an IQ of 80.

CLASSIFICATION

Mental retardation is sub-grouped according to the level of measured IQ, and two levels are now usually recognized: severe mental retardation with IQ <50, and mild mental retardation with IQ in the 50–70 range. 'Borderline intellectual functioning' is where the IQ is in the 71–84 range and many children in this category can be perceived as 'normal'. In recent years there has been great emphasis on the social model as opposed to the medical model. Some writers have even implied that all disability relates to society's response to an individual rather than any biological component. Nevertheless, in many situations in which a child experiences difficulties a full assessment will show that there are in fact biological components for these difficulties, although their impact will be very much affected by the tolerance and understanding given to the child by the community in which s/he is brought up. Deciding therefore to what extent a biological component is affecting the child requires a consideration of his/her environmental situation. A good example of this is the overactive child, where there is now known to be a strong genetic component (Taylor 2007). The cut-off point for this effect will very much depend on the educational environment to which the child is exposed. In population studies from several European countries reported by Whitmore et al. (1999), children perceived as having minor neurodevelopmental problems such as clumsiness, overactivity or a mild degree of developmental delay were found to be more likely to have difficulties in school such as reading and behavioural problems. These associations occur in 5–10% of the normal population but again it should be emphasized that children with similar assessments may or may not experience problems. Children often fall into the mild to borderline retardation group and the notion of vulnerability is an important one in terms of the prevention of potential problems – both educational and behavioural – developing for the child in school.

PREVALENCE

The prevalence rates reported in this section refer to IQ studies only and not the full range of neurodevelopmental difficulties.

Mild mental retardation is more common than severe mental retardation, but claims that it is as much as six times more common – such as in the DSM-IV (American Psychiatric Association 1994) – seem to have relatively weak support in the modern literature.

Swedish studies have suggested that clear mental retardation occurs in less than 1% of school-age children. Hagberg et al. (1981) found that 0.7% of 10- to 13-year-olds in one Swedish urban area had IQ scores <70 and were in need of extra educational support. Slightly less than half of these children had severe mental retaration (IQ <50) and the rest had mild mental retardation (IQ 50–70). Hagberg's group acknowledged that a number of borderline cases might have been missed and that tested IQ in the Swedish population of children tended towards a higher mean than 100. On follow-up during the teenage period, almost 1% of the population were classified as mentally retarded. Mild mental retardation was about twice as common as severe mental retardation. Gillberg et al. (1983) found that 1% of the whole 7- to 8-year-old population had tested IQ <73 and needed special education. They also found that a further 1% of children in this age-group had tested IQs close to 73 without clearly and constantly falling below this level and also required special education.

These prevalence figures are considerably lower than reported in earlier studies from Sweden and from other Western countries. One possible explanation is that the IQ tests used were standardized long ago and that for some reason they now yield a 'falsely high' IQ score. Another contributory factor could be the early stimulation in nurseries, day-care centres and similar

settings, which could lead to a 'transiently higher' IQ score in early childhood. This is supported by the finding of Hagberg et al. (1981) that 'new' mental retardation cases continue to be diagnosed even in adolescence after the impact of early stimulation has to some extent subsided.

Interestingly, a study from a rural Swedish county (Landgren et al. 1996) suggested that mild mental retardation may occur in as many as 1.5% of all 7-year-old children, a finding that is in fair accord both with the older studies and with the results of a Swedish urban study by Fernell (1996), who found a prevalence of 12.8/1000. The findings from these newer studies can probably be explained by lower socioeconomic status in the communities studied and by the fact that testing is now more acceptable. Nearly 90% of the children with mild mental retardation in Fernell's study had symptoms in their preschool years, mainly motor problems, speech/language disorders and a relative inability to perform certain tasks. These symptoms also occur in children with ADHD, autism spectrum disorders, and deficits in attention, motor control and perception, which should be taken into consideration when selecting screening tests for developmental delay.

The rate of diagnosed severe mental retardation is already 0.3–0.4% at age 3 years, because it is usually recognized in the first few years of life. The rate is then relatively stable for a number of years, and eventually begins to drop a little because of the increased mortality rate. Diagnosed mild mental retardation is at a very low rate during the first years of life, because milder degrees of retardation become progressively more difficult to recognize. Most cases of mild mental retardation are diagnosed from age 3 to 7 years, but the prevalence will continue to increase throughout the school years, at least if screening tests are not performed at a young age.

The rate of mental retardation will also depend upon cultural factors, such as early stimulation, social deprivation, tolerance (in both the positive and negative senses of the word) and access to and provision of special education services.

Boys are affected by mental retardation more often than girls. The boy/girl ratio is in the range of 1.3:1 to 1.9:1. Some mental retardation conditions are much more common in boys than in girls (e.g. the fragile X syndrome and autism) but in a few instances (e.g. Rett syndrome) the reverse is true.

BACKGROUND FACTORS IN SEVERE MENTAL RETARDATION

In a study of the aetiology of severe mental retardation in Sweden, Hagberg and Kyllerman (1983) found a definite or highly probable cause in just over 80% of cases (Fig. 23.2). (This percentage will undoubtedly have risen in recent years as more and more genetic causes of mental retardation are identified. This increase in diagnostic possibility occurs also in mild mental retardation). Two thirds of these were of prenatal origin and about one sixth each were of peri- and postnatal origin. The *prenatal factors* were chromosomal in more than half the cases (trisomy 21 being much the most common type). In a further 20%, multiple anomalies were present in the absence of chromosomal abnormalities. Prenatal

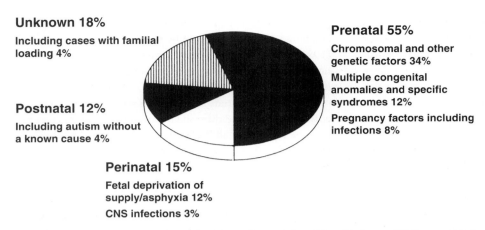

Unknown 18%
Including cases with familial
loading 4%

Prenatal 55%
Chromosomal and other
genetic factors 34%
Multiple congenital
anomalies and specific
syndromes 12%
Pregnancy factors including
infections 8%

Postnatal 12%
Including autism without
a known cause 4%

Perinatal 15%
Fetal deprivation of
supply/asphyxia 12%
CNS infections 3%

Fig. 23.2. Aetiological panorama of severe mental retardation. (Adapted from Hagberg and Kyllerman 1983.)

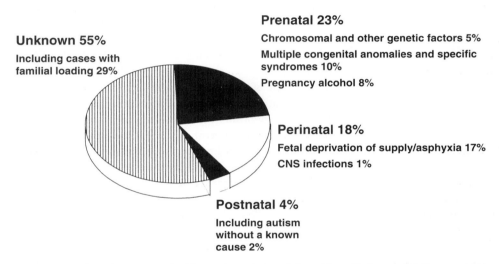

Prenatal 23%
Chromosomal and other genetic factors 5%
Multiple congenital anomalies and specific
syndromes 10%
Pregnancy alcohol 8%

Unknown 55%
Including cases with
familial loading 29%

Perinatal 18%
Fetal deprivation of supply/asphyxia 17%
CNS infections 1%

Postnatal 4%
Including autism
without a known
cause 2%

Fig. 23.3. Aetiological panorama of mild mental retardation. (Adapted from Hagberg and Kyllerman 1983.)

infections accounted for 13% of cases, while clear genetic disorders without demonstrable chromosomal abnormality constituted less than 10%. The *perinatal factors* were fetal deprivation and asphyxia in most cases, and perinatal CNS infections in a minority. The *postnatal factors* were very variable and could not be easily grouped. Of the 18% of severe mental retardation cases of unknown aetiology, slightly less than one in four had a familial clustering.

The prevalence and background factors in severe mental retardation were studied in a suburban municipality of Stockholm (Fernell 1998). The study area had a high proportion of non-European nationals. The total prevalence of severe mental retardation was 4.5 per 1000, being 3.7 per 1000 and 5.9 per 1000 in the European and in the non-European populations, respectively. The majority of cases (66%) had a definite prenatal origin. Down syndrome was the cause in 20%. In 10% of affected families there were at least two affected siblings with severe mental retardation. The reported prevalence was higher than in previous Swedish studies. Many cases were attributed to genetic factors.

Consanguineous marriages were assumed to be a factor of importance in the distribution of aetiologies.

BACKGROUND FACTORS IN MILD MENTAL RETARDATION

In mild mental retardation it is more difficult to arrive at a correct aetiological diagnosis. In the study by Hagberg and Kyllerman (1983) a definite or highly probable cause was found in just under 45% of cases (Fig. 23.3).

More than half of the known or probable causes were of *prenatal* origin. However, the pattern was very different from that seen in severe mental retardation. Fetal alcohol exposure was the single most common factor, accounting for one third of the prenatal cases. Identifiable chromosomal abnormalities were much less common than in the severely retarded group, but syndromes with multiple congenital anomalies were relatively common. *Perinatal factors* were relatively common, and almost all of these were associated with fetal deprivation and asphyxia. Only 1 out of 91 cases of mild mental retardation appeared to have been caused by perinatal CNS infection. *Postnatal factors* were a rare cause for mild mental retardation. Of the 55% of mild mental retardation cases without a known or probable cause, more than half showed familial clustering.

EXECUTIVE FUNCTION DISORDERS

Executive function refers to the ability to sequentially arrange events in an orderly way and to postpone to a later time the need for gratification. Executive functions and dysfunctions are seen not only very specifically in certain genetic conditions but also in the normal child. Believed to be a function of the frontal cortex or lobes, activities may be quite simple such as turning on the spinal reflex system to initiate walking in an appropriate and timed sequence. Behavioural functions can be controlled, but in circumstances associated with brain or neurological damage these functions may be lost. It is unclear what the early markers of executive function might be in the infant and young child but school-age children usually have remarkable skills in this area. It is well known that executive functions are deficient in many of the syndromes on the autistic spectrum (Happé 1994). They are also usually dysfunctional in syndromes comprising attention deficits (such as ADHD) and motor control problems (including DCD).

DEVELOPMENT OF SOCIAL COMPETENCE

The normal infant is already socially responsive and ready to interact immediately after birth. Newborn infants have been demonstrated to fixate, give gaze contact and even to imitate slightly after intensive coaxing. This should not be taken to mean that the newborn baby has good social interaction skills, typical of older children. It does imply that the old notion of a 'normal autistic phase' in early development was mistaken.

The necessary basic skills for developing a superficially acceptable 'social competence' are, in a sense, there from the beginning. Gaze contact, imitation, detection of eye direction and turn-taking are all necessary if the kinds of behaviours associated with gossiping, interaction at cocktail parties or small talk at the bus station – best termed 'superficial social competence skills' – are ever to develop. It is likely that such skills can be strengthened through training and practice. This is evidenced by the observation that girls tend to be better at such things than boys (girls often get more training in these areas than boys when they are young). On the other hand, there could already be qualitative biological differences between boys and girls in this respect from infancy.

Around the age of 8–14 months, most girls and boys begin to show clear signs that they want to share other people's attention, indicating joint points of reference (such as the lamp above the table). Not only do they indicate the objects as such; in doing so they also look at people as if to check whether they too are interested and perhaps looking at the same thing. It is possible that this drive for shared attention (Mundy and Sigman 1989) is present in even younger infants. It is also possible that

precursors of mentalizing ability (see below) might be necessary for the appearance of signs of shared attention, and that shared attention may be the first outward reflection of the presence of mentalizing skills.

Parallel to the emergence of shared attention behaviours, there is usually also the typical interest in 'peep-bo' games and objects that appear out of sight. This is not necessarily connected with shared attention, and the child may participate in these types of games in an imitative fashion without really sharing a joint external reference point with the other person.

Similar to the notion of shared attention is the concept of social referencing (Walden and Ogan 1988). A four-level sequence of development leading to the ability to participate in social referencing has been proposed by Plutschik and Kellerman (1983). First emerges the ability to discriminate among emotional expressions, for instance on the mother's or father's face. Then follows the gradual recognition of the meaning of these various expressions. After that comes emotional responsiveness. Finally, the ability to refer to another person and interactive regulation of behaviour appear. It is this final stage that is usually referred to as social referencing. The first links in this chain of development are already observable at or before age 6 months.

Possibly separate from superficial social competence skills, there appear towards the end of the child's first year obvious signs that s/he is developing mentalizing skills (or a *'theory of mind'*), that is, an ability to impute mental states such as knowing and believing to other people and to oneself. For instance, if a 12-month-old baby turning the pages of a picture book is stopped in this activity by another person firmly putting his/her hand over the child's, the child will often look the other person in the eye rather than just try to get rid of the hand. It seems reasonable to assume that underlying this kind of gaze contact would be the presumption on the part of the child that the other person has an intention in doing what s/he is doing. In other words, the child has a mentalizing ability, or a theory of mind. As s/he grows older s/he will become aware that there are a variety of mental states in other people and that there is not necessarily a correspondence between superficial social competence skills and these states of mind. The child even begins to be able to think: "He thinks she thinks". S/he will then also be able gradually to develop a more sophisticated understanding of complex social cues and interactions and of other people's many-faceted feelings. A theory of mind would also be necessary for the development of a good 'human' intelligence. Without theory of mind the child will not be able to ask meaningful questions of other people (either verbally or non-verbally) and his/her use of language and 'communication' will not be appropriate for acquiring new skills. Rote memory skills need not be affected at all, however, and some children who appear to lack a theory of mind may be thought of as *'idiots savants'* (see Frith 1989) and show remarkable skill in one or a few areas.

Mentalizing ability is a prerequisite for developing empathy (the ability to reflect intuitively and correctly about other people's thoughts and feelings). Empathy, in turn, is necessary for the development of sympathy and compassion (terms often semantically confused with empathy). However, empathy is not all that is necessary to develop these 'talents'. For instance, sociopaths/psychopaths may basically have good empathic skills (necessary when deliberately trying to deceive people), yet generally show little compassion or sympathy with anybody but themselves.

Many children show signs of compassion and sympathy before age 2 years, for instance in approaching and wanting to hug, kiss and comfort someone who has been hurt or is crying.

Executive functions and the drive for central coherence probably need to be relatively well developed in order for empathy skills to emerge in a smooth and harmonious fashion. When deficient, even with a relatively well-developed theory of mind, empathy would tend to be 'unfocused', 'piecemeal', flimsy and shallow.

It is common knowledge that we are all different in our superficial social competence skills and in respect of empathy skills and compassion. Perhaps all these three variables are to a considerable extent biologically determined, discrete or only partly overlapping functions that are all distributed in much the same way as IQ along a spectrum from superior skills to severe dysfunction. Maybe, in the lowermost portion of each spectrum there exists a small group affected by environmentally caused dysfunction (such as in the case of brain damage in individuals with very low IQ). If this were the case, there would be similar types of social dysfunction caused either by brain damage/dysfunction or by simply being at the lowermost end of the normal distribution.

DISORDERS OF SOCIAL COMPETENCE

Social dysfunctions of various kinds are the hallmarks of many of the neuropsychiatric disorders of childhood. Autism and Asperger syndrome are now the best known of such conditions. Both seem to share severe problems of empathy. People with autism are generally deficient in superficial social competence skills, empathy, and to some extent compassion. IQ is often low as well. People with Asperger syndrome are invariably deficient in empathy and, to some extent, compassion. IQ is often normal or high. Such people are likely to be diagnosed with Asperger syndrome if superficial social competence skills are also impaired. However, there could be Asperger cases with relatively well developed superficial skills of this kind who would then be accepted as belonging in a normal group in spite of severe empathy deficits. Girls in particular might have relatively good social competence skills and yet be severely deficient in the development of empathy skills. A diagnosis of Asperger syndrome in such girls will probably not be thought of, much less made. Children with deficits in attention, motor control and perception often have slight dysfunction in all three areas (and sometimes in overall intelligence as well). Psychopaths need only be deficient in compassion and must – almost by definition – have some, or even good, empathy skills. It appears that an analysis in terms of superficial social competence skills, empathy, compassion and IQ in patients showing social dysfunction might be useful and have far-reaching practical implications. So far, most psychiatric/neuropsychiatric evaluations

do not make use of this model for analysis. In Chapter 24 the presentation of neuropsychiatric problems in childhood also relies on a more conservative phenotypical structure, and various syndromes are described mainly as they show in outward symptoms and signs. Nevertheless, an awareness of the briefly surveyed expansion of our knowledge as regards children's social and cognitive development is likely to be helpful when trying to understand children affected with neuropsychiatric problems in more depth.

CENTRAL COHERENCE DISORDERS

Central coherence refers to the drive for seeing the bigger picture on the basis of an environment of details, and to be able to change perspective from whole to detail and vice versa. It appears that most young children are hard wired for this drive for central coherence, i.e. they are 'driven' to seek out meaning, pattern and coherence from details presented to them (Frith 1989, Happé 1994). However, some children appear to have an inborn drive for detail instead. This can be seen as the basis for various kinds of adaptation disorders, but can also be construed as a difference in cognitive style that may have some advantages.

Children with autism and children with nonverbal learning disability often have a very pronounced drive for detail rather than drive for central coherence. Individuals with autism spectrum disorders often have normal or superior fact learning and seriation skills compared to peers matched for developmental/mental age (e.g. Yirmiya and Shulman 1996, O'Shea et al. 2005), but have difficulty with procedural learning and with making sense of the facts that they know. This could be seen as one example of how the drive or lack of drive for central coherence can lead to both advantages and deficits depending on what type of function is being studied.

Clinically, it is not only children in the autism spectrum who have a decreased drive for central coherence. Many children with attention disorders, including the large subgroup with deficits in attention, motor control and perception, have a similar cognitive style.

In the future, it would probably be more reasonable to diagnose 'overarching' disorder (such as social communication disorder or 'autism', attention disorder or 'ADHD') and then to provide a neurocognitive profile (such as 2nd centile theory of mind, 5th centile executive function, 7th centile central coherence, 50th centile full-scale IQ) than just stating that a person suffers from 'autism' or 'ADHD' without further qualification.

REFERENCES

American Psychiatric Association (1994) *Diagnostic and Statistical Manual of Mental Disorders, 4th edn: DSM-IV.* Washington DC: American Psychiatric Association.

Bax M, Hart H, Jenkins S (1980) Assessment of speech and language development in the young child. *Pediatrics* 29: 40–5.

Bax M, Tydeman C, Flodmark O (2006) Clinical and MRI correlates of cerebral palsy. The European Cerebral Palsy Study. *JAMA* 296: 1650–2.

Bishop DVM (1997) *Uncommon Understanding. Development and Disorders of Language Comprehension in Children.* Hove, East Sussex: Psychology Press.

Bishop DVM, Leonard LB, eds. (2000) *Speech and Language Impairments in*

Children. Causes, Characteristics, Intervention and Outcome. Hove, East Sussex: Psychology Press.

Butcher HJ (1970) *Human Intelligence: Its Nature and Assessment.* London: Methuen.

Catts HW, Fey ME, Tomblin JB, Zhang X (2002) A longitudinal investigation of reading outcomes in children with language impairments. *J Speech Lang Hear Res* 45: 1142–57.

Denhoff E, Robinault I (1960) *Cerebral Palsy and Related Disorders: a Developmental Approach to Dysfunction.* London and New York: McGraw-Hill.

Egan D (1971) *Developmental Examination of Infants and Pre-school Children. Clinics in Developmental Medicine No. 112.* London: Spastics International Medical Publications.

Fernell E (1996) Mild mental retardation in schoolchildren in a Swedish suburban municipality: prevalence and diagnostic aspects. *Acta Paediatr* 85: 584–8.

Fernell E (1998) Aetiological factors and prevalence of severe mental retardation in children in a Swedish municipality: the possible role of consanguinity. *Dev Med Child Neurol* 40: 608–11.

Frith U (1989) *Autism: Explaining the Enigma.* Oxford: Basil Blackwell.

Gillberg C, Svenson B, Carlström G, et al. (1983) Mental retardation in Swedish urban children: some epidemiological considerations. *App Res Ment Retard* 4: 207–18.

Hagberg B, Hagberg G, Lewerth A, Lindberg U (1981) Mild mental retardation in Swedish school children. I. Prevalence. *Acta Paediatr Scand* 70: 441–4.

Hagberg B, Kyllerman M (1983) Epidemiology of mental retardation – a Swedish survey. *Brain Dev* 5: 441–9.

Happé FG (1994) Current psychological theories of autism: the "theory of mind" account and rival theories. *J Child Psychol Psychiatry* 35: 215–29.

Honzik MP, MacFarlane JW, Allen L (1948) The stability of mental test performance between two and eighteen years. *J Exp Educ* 17: 309–24.

Illingworth RS (1988) *Basic Developmental Screening 0–4 years.* Oxford: Blackwell Scientific.

Landgren M, Pettersson R, Kjellman B, Gillberg C (1996) ADHD, DAMP and other neurodevelopmental/psychiatric disorders in 6-year-old children: epidemiology and co-morbidity. *Dev Med Child Neurol* 38: 891–906.

Leekam SR, Libby SJ, Wing L, et al. (2002) The Diagnostic Interview for Social and Communication Disorders: algorithms for IC-10 childhood autism and Wing and Gould autistic spectrum disorder. *J Child Psychol Psychiatry* 43: 327–42.

Madge N, Tizard J (1980) Intelligence. In: Rutter M, ed. *Developmental Psychiatry.* London: Heinemann Medical, pp. 245–65.

Miniscalco C, Nygren G, Hagberg B, et al. (2006) Neuropsychiatric and neurodevelopmental outcome of children at age 6 and 7 years who screened positive for language problems at 30 months. *Dev Med Child Neurol* 48: 361–6.

Miniscalco C, Hagberg B, Kadesjö B, et al. (2007) Narrative skills, cognitive profiles and neuropsychiatric disorders in 7–8-year-old children with late developing language. *Int J Lang Commun Disord* 42: 665–81.

Moffitt TE, Caspi A, Harkness AR, Silva PA (1993) The natural history of change in intellectual performance: Who changes? How much? Is it meaningful? *J Child Psychol Psychiatry* 34: 455–506.

Mundy P, Sigman M (1989) Specifying the nature of the social impairment in autism. In: Dawson G, ed. *Autism: New Perspectives on Nature, Diagnosis and Treatment.* New York: Guilford, pp. 3–31.

Nyhan WL (1968) Clinical features of the Lesch–Nyhan syndrome. Introduction—clinical and genetic features. *Fedn Proc* 27: 1027–33.

O'Brien G, Yule W, eds. (1995) *Behavioural Phenotypes. Clinics in Developmental Medicine No. 138.* London: Mac Keith Press.

O'Shea AB, Fein DA, Cillessen AH, et al. (2005) Source memory in children with autism spectrum disorders. *Dev Neuropsychol* 27: 337–60.

Plutschik R, Kellerman H, eds. (1983) *Emotion: Theory, Research and Experience. Vol 2. Emotions in Early Development.* Orlando, FL: Academic Press.

Robson P, Mac Keith RC (1971) Shufflers with spastic diplegic cerebral palsy: a confusing clinical picture. *Dev Med Child Neurol* 13: 651–9.

Sheridan M (1973) *From Birth to Five Years: Children's Developmental Progress.* Windsor: NFER.

Spearman C (1927) The doctrine of two factors. Reprinted in: Wiseman S, ed. (1967) *Intelligence and Ability: Selected Readings.* Harmondsworth: Penguin, pp. 58–68.

Stark RE, Tallal P (1981) Selection of children with specific language deficits. *J Speech Hear Disord* 46: 114–22.

Taylor E (2007) *People with Hyperactivity: Understanding and Managing their Problems. Clinics in Developmental Medicine No. 171.* London: Mac Keith Press.

Tomblin JB, Records NL, Buckwalter P, et al. (1997) Prevalence of specific language impairment in kindergarten children. *J Speech Lang Hear Res* 40: 1245–60.

Vernon PE (1976) Development of intelligence. In: Hamilton V, Vernon MD, eds. *The Development of Cognitive Processes.* London and New York: Academic Press, pp. 507–47.

Walden TA, Ogan TA (1988) The development of social referencing. *Child Dev* 59: 1230–40.

Whitmore K, Hart H, Willems G (1999) *A Neurodevelopmental Approach to Specific Learning Disorders. Clinics in Developmental Medicine No. 145.* London: Mac Keith Press.

WHO (1980) *International Classification of Impairments, Disabilities, and Handicaps (ICIDH).* Geneva: World Health Organization.

WHO (1993) *The ICD-10 Classification of Mental and Behavioural Disorders. Diagnostic Criteria for Research.* Geneva: World Health Organization.

WHO (2001) *International Classification of Functioning, Disability and Health (ICF).* Geneva: World Health Organization.

Wing L, Leekam SR, Libby SJ, et al. (2002) The Diagnostic Interview for Social and Communication Disorders: background, inter-rater reliability and clinical use. *J Child Psychol Psychiatry* 43: 307–25.

Yirmiya N, Shulman C (1996) Seriation, conservation, and theory of mind abilities in individuals with autism, individuals with mental retardation, and normally developing children. *Child Dev* 67: 2045–59.

24
AUTISM AND AUTISTIC-LIKE CONDITIONS

Christopher Gillberg

There are descriptions in the literature (e.g. Haslam 1809, Malson 1964, Frith 1989, Fitzgerald 2005) of people living several hundred years ago, who, according to our present-day terminology, would have fulfilled criteria for infantile autism (Rutter 1978a,b; APA 1980), childhood autism (WHO 1993), autistic disorder or Asperger's disorder (APA 1994). Obviously autistic syndromes are not 'new' conditions typical of contemporary Western societies (as has been proposed by Tinbergen and Tinbergen 1983), even though current concepts and definitions are less than 30 years old.

AUTISM DEFINITIONS AND DIAGNOSTIC CRITERIA

PREVIOUS DEFINITIONS AND CONCEPTS
The US child psychiatrist Leo Kanner (1943) and the Austrian paediatrician Hans Asperger (1944) were among the first to describe the type of empathy disorders encompassed in the 'autistic continuum' (Wing 1989), highlighting the specificity of the social interaction deficit, which has, ever since, been regarded as the core symptom of autism. Before them, however, Ssucharewa (1926), a Russian clinical assistant working in a 'psychoneurological clinic', described 'schizoid personality disorder' in children in a way that makes it clear that she was referring to the disorder now known as Asperger syndrome. Before her, Jean Itard and John Haslam described young people with severely debilitating conditions that would nowadays be diagnosed as autistic disorder or childhood autism.

Whether to regard Kanner's 'early infantile autism' and Asperger's 'autistic psychopathy' as synonymous, as different sections on an autism spectrum, as partly biologically and psychologically overlapping disabilities or as clearly different conditions has been the subject of considerable debate. Here they will be described separately, even though they can probably – at least regarding some key features – be conceptualized as existing on a continuum or a spectrum, or as belonging in the same general class of 'autistic syndromes' or 'disorders of empathy'.

A number of labelled conditions and syndromes, some of which can be regarded as synonymous and others that can be seen as partly overlapping entities, are shown in Table 24.1.

The word autism not only refers to the syndrome of autism but is also used in its original Bleulerian sense to describe the particular quality of thought encountered as a first-rank symptom in schizophrenia (Bleuler 1911). In the following, unless otherwise specified, 'autism' will be used throughout when referring to the syndrome of autism (outlined below).

CURRENT DEFINITIONS OF AUTISM
All currently accepted definitions of autism include the three main criteria (suggested by Wing and Gould 1979) that have to be met for a diagnosis to be made. These are: (1) severe restriction in the ability to reciprocate socially; (2) severe restriction in the ability to communicate reciprocally (including language comprehension and spoken language problems as well as communication problems affecting body language, facial expressions, mime and gesture); (3) severe restriction in the ability to vary behaviour and to engage in imaginative activities, leading to extreme restriction in the behavioural repertoire. The various specific symptoms associated with each criterion tend to be slightly differently emphasized by different diagnostic manuals, but the basic symptom categories are the same throughout. Some authors also require an onset before age 30–36 months to make the diagnosis of autism. It is often difficult to separate (1) from (2), social and communication problems often being felt to represent/reflect the same type of underlying social–cognitive dysfunction. The need for the overlap of (3) with (1) and (2) for a diagnosis of an autism spectrum disorder is sometimes felt to be artificial, and community-based studies suggest that the 'triad' of social impairment may not be as cohesive as originally suggested.

The criteria currently most used in the field are those of the DSM-IV-TR (APA 2000). This set of criteria is outlined in Table 24.2. The ICD-10 criteria for childhood autism (WHO 1993) are also in use. They are almost identical to those of the DSM-IV-TR.

Wing (1989) has argued that the specificity of infantile autism or 'Kanner autism' is in doubt. She has demonstrated that a number of mental retardation and brain damage syndromes show the same triad of social, communicative and behavioural impairments, and that a case for separating out a diagnosis of 'pure' Kanner autism sometimes cannot be made. Even when the phenomenology is concordant with Kanner's description, background factors and outcome tend to vary considerably (Wing and Gould 1979, Gillberg and Steffenburg 1987, Gillberg et al.

TABLE 24.1
Synonyms and partly overlapping labels in the spectrum of autism disorders

Label	References
Infantile autism	Rutter (1978a,b), American Psychiatric Association (1980)
Autistic disorder	American Psychiatric Association (1987, 1994)
Early infantile autism	Kanner (1943)
Childhood autism	Wing (1981b)
Autistic syndrome	Gillberg and Coleman (2000)
Triad of social impairments	Wing and Gould (1979)
Pervasive developmental disorder	American Psychiatric Association (1987)
Childhood schizophrenia	Bender (1947)
Autistic psychopathy	Asperger (1944)
Asperger syndrome	Wing (1981b)
Atypical child syndrome	Rank (1949)
Symbiotic psychosis	Mahler (1952)

1987, Billstedt et al. 2005, Gillberg and Cederlund 2005). Wing has also shown that, in cognitively impaired individuals, the presence of one of the problems included in the triad dramatically increases the risk that one or both of the other two types of problems will be present as well.

However, more recent research has demonstrated that the triad is not as cohesive as previously believed, and there are many cases in which the social–communication problems typical of autism do not coincide with the obsessive–compulsive and ritualistic phenomena believed to be necessary for the diagnosis of autistic disorder to be made. Conversely, there are individuals who have the typical ritualistic phenomena encountered in autism, who do not show the typical social–communication problems (Posserud et al. 2006). This research calls into question the uniqueness of the autistic syndrome and suggests that we might be dealing with a dyad – or even monad – of social–communication impairment on the one hand, and obsessive-compulsive and ritualistic phenomena on the other.

Gillberg and Coleman (2000) have advocated a similar line of reasoning when referring to the 'autistic syndromes'. It has gradually become accepted that autism is a behavioural symptom constellation signalling underlying nervous system dysfunction. The evidence for a specific 'nuclear autism' disease entity is lacking. Also, recent community-based studies (e.g. Posserud et al. 2006) have shown that autistic features are common in the general population of children, and that the triad is in doubt, insofar as it is unclear whether the social and communicative problems can be validly separated, there are many children who show social–communication deficits who do not have the ritualistic behaviours expected in autism, and there are many others who have the ritualistic behaviours without the social–communication problems.

PERVASIVE DEVELOPMENTAL DISORDERS
The term 'pervasive developmental disorders' (PDD) was introduced in the 1980s to cover the whole range of conditions variously labelled as 'autism', 'infantile autism', 'childhood autism', 'atypical autism', 'autistic disorder', etc. The terminology represented a positive move away from the old categories under which autism was seen to represent a form of early-onset psychosis. PDD is still used as the umbrella concept in the DSM-IV-TR, and is particularly often applied to cases that are 'atypical' in one way or another ('pervasive developmental disorder not otherwise specified – PDDNOS'). However, it is a very misleading term, and one that will not be used further in this context. First, most people with autism spectrum problems (particularly those classified as having Asperger syndrome) do not have pervasive problems. There are specific developmental problems within the autism spectrum (see below), but they are usually not pervasive. Further, it is illogical to use the term pervasive for this group of conditions, and not include the most pervasive of all conditions (severe and profound mental retardation/learning disability) under this heading. Finally, the addition of the term 'NOS' in cases considered 'atypical' is not helpful to individuals with autistic problems or their carers. It only helps making autism a more diffuse condition in the minds of lay people and doctors not specializing in the field.

AUTISM SPECTRUM
There is now growing acceptance of the concept of an autism spectrum. Some authors prefer to use the term autism spectrum disorder when referring to conditions that have the symptom triad described in the previous section, and subgroup according to IQ, language skills, etc., rather than making the type of – implicitly more fine-grained – diagnoses of autistic disorder, Asperger syndrome or atypical autism/PDDNOS.

PREVALENCE OF AUTISTIC DISORDER AND OTHER AUTISM SPECTRUM DISORDERS

Recent studies suggest that in industrialized countries the prevalence of *autistic disorder* – defined according to DSM-III, DSM-III-R or DSM-IV – is at least in the range of 1–2 per 1000, not including Asperger syndrome cases (for overviews, see Gillberg and Wing 1999, Wing and Potter 2002, Fombonne 2003, Gillberg et al. 2006). Older reports suggested a lower prevalence rate (around 0.2–0.5 per 1000).

Several studies have now shown that *autism spectrum disorders* – including autistic disorder, Asperger syndrome and atypical autism/PDDNOS – exist at rates very much higher than previously believed. The total prevalence for autism spectrum disorders in the general population of school-age children is usually reported to be in the range of 0.5–1.2% (e.g. Kadesjö et al. 1999, Yeargin-Allsopp et al. 2003, Gillberg et al. 2006), Asperger syndrome often accounting for more cases than 'classic' autistic disorder.

Hertzig et al. (1990) proposed that the increased prevalence could be accounted for by the use of more inclusive criteria in later diagnostic manuals such as the DSM-III-R. However, there is no good evidence from population studies to support this

TABLE 24.2
Diagnostic criteria for autism

Label	Diagnostic criteria
Infantile autism (DSM-III: American Psychiatric Association 1980)	Onset before age 30 months Pervasive lack of responsiveness to other people Gross deficits in language development and, if speech is present, peculiar patterns such as echolalia, metaphorical language and pronominal reversals Bizarre responses to environment, e.g. resistance to change, peculiar interests (+ Absence of clear signs suggestive of schizophrenia)
Autistic disorder (DSM-III-R: American Psychiatric Association 1987)	Onset during infancy or childhood Qualitative impairment in reciprocal social interaction as manifested by at least two of the following: • marked lack of awareness of the existence of feelings of others • no or abnormal seeking of comfort at times of distress • no or impaired imitation • no or abnormal social play • gross impairment in ability to make peer friendships Qualitative impairment in verbal and nonverbal communication, and in imaginative activity, as manifested by at least one of the following: • no mode of communication, such as communicative babbling, facial expression, gesture, mime or spoken language • markedly abnormal nonverbal communication, as in the use of eye-to-eye gaze, facial expression, body posture or gestures to initiate or modulate social interaction • absence of imaginative activity, e.g. play-acting of adult roles, fantasy characters or animals; lack of interest in stories about imaginary events • marked abnormalities in speech production, including volume, pitch, stress, rate, rhythm and intonation • marked abnormalities in the use of speech, including stereotyped and repetitive speech • marked impairment in the ability to initiate or sustain a conversation with others, despite adequate speech Markedly restricted repertoire of activities and interests, as manifested by at least one of the following: • stereotyped body movements, e.g. hand flicking, twisting, spinning, head banging or complex whole-body movements • persistent preoccupation with parts of objects • marked distress over changes in trivial aspects of environment, e.g. when a vase is moved from its usual position • unreasonable insistence on following routines in precise detail, e.g. insisting that exactly the same route always be followed when shopping • markedly restricted range of interest and a preoccupation with one narrow interest, e.g. lining up objects, amassing facts about meteorology, or pretending to be a fantasy character At least 8 of the 16 specified items above must be fulfilled

Autistic disorder DSM-IV: (American Psychiatric Association 1994)	A. A total of six (or more) items from (1), (2), and (3) with at least two from (1), and one each from (2) and (3):
	(1) qualitative impairment in social interaction, as manifested by at least two of the following:
	  (a) marked impairment in the use of multiple nonverbal behaviours such as eye-to-eye gaze, facial expression, body postures and gestures to regulate social interaction
	  (b) failure to develop peer relationships appropriate to developmental level
	  (c) a lack of spontaneous seeking to share enjoyment, interests or achievements with other people (e.g. by a lack of showing, bringing or pointing out objects of interest)
	  (d) lack of social or emotional reciprocity
	(2) qualitative impairments in communication as manifested by at least one of the following:
	  (a) delay in, or total lack of, the development of spoken language (not accompanied by an attempt to compensate through alternative modes of communication such as gesture or mime)
	  (b) in individuals with adequate speech, marked impairment in the ability to initiate or sustain a conversation with others
	  (c) stereotyped and repetitive use of language or idiosyncratic language
	  (d) lack of varied, spontaneous make-believe play or social imitative play appropriate to developmental level
	(3) restricted repetitive and stereotyped patterns of behaviour, interests and activities, as manifested by at least it one of the following:
	  (a) encompassing preoccupation with one or more stereotyped and restricted patterns of interest that is abnormal either in intensity or focus
	  (b) apparently inflexible adherence to specific, nonfunctional routines or rituals
	  (c) stereotyped and repetitive motor mannerisms (e.g. hand or finger flapping or twisting, or complex whole-body movements)
	  (d) persistent preoccupation with parts of objects
	B. Delays or abnormal functioning in at least one of the following areas, with onset prior to age 3 years:
	  (1) social interaction,
	  (2) language as used in social communication,
	  (3) symbolic or imaginative play
	C. The disturbance is not better accounted for by Rett syndrome or Childhood Disintegrative Disorder

Childhood autism (WHO 1993)	Qualitative impairments in reciprocal social interaction Qualitative impairments in communication Restricted, repetitive and stereotyped patterns of behaviour, interests and activities Developmental abnormalities must have been present in the first 3 years for the diagnosis to be made
Autism (Denckla 1986)	Social impairment Delayed and deviant language Repetitive, stereotypic or ritualistic behaviour

notion. To the contrary, there is limited evidence that the reasons for the relatively high recent figures are an increasing awareness of the existence of autism generally and particularly in severely and profoundly mentally retarded people, and the fact that a higher incidence of autism has been observed in recent years among children of immigrants from remote countries (Akinsola and Fryers 1986, Gillberg et al. 1987).

GENDER RATIOS IN AUTISTIC DISORDER

In the older literature on classic autism cases, boys tend to outnumber girls by at least 3:1 (Wing 1981b). Among cases with severe and profound mental retardation/learning disability, the ratio is lower, and in those with higher IQ it tends to be considerably higher. However, it is possible that (a) the old studies may have inflated the boy:girl ratio, (b) girls with autism may often be misdiagnosed as having mental retardation/learning disability or a less specific variant of a psychiatric/behavioural disorder, and (c) many girls may have been missed altogether by the screening procedure.

ASSOCIATED DISABILITIES IN AUTISTIC DISORDER

Mental retardation/learning disability is present in 65–88% of autistic disorder cases, but in only about 1% or so of cases diagnosed as suffering from Asperger syndrome. This is probably an artificial effect of current diagnostic boundaries, which favour a diagnosis of autistic disorder/childhood autism in individuals with social–communication problems who have an IQ <70 and support a diagnosis of Asperger syndrome in individuals with IQs in the normal range. Overall, across the full range of autism spectrum disorders, the rate of associated mental retardation is probably in the order of 15%.

Epilepsy occurs in 30–40% of autistic disorder cases before 30 years of age (Gillberg 1991c, Danielsson et al. 2005). Slightly less than half this proportion comprises various epilepsy types (including infantile spasms) with onset in early childhood. The other half is mostly adolescent-onset epilepsy. However, new cases of epilepsy may occur even after the age of 20 years in individuals who were diagnosed as suffering from autism in early childhood. Partial complex seizures and generalized tonic–clonic seizures are the most common types of epilepsy encountered, but there is often a mixture of seizure types, and any type of seizure disorder can occur in association with autism. Landau–Kleffner syndrome, a rare disorder comprising verbal auditory agnosia and epileptic EEG activity, sometimes presents with overwhelming autistic symptomatology. The seizures that occur in autism at or after adolescence are often relatively benign, whereas those with onset in the first 5 years often run a more malign course and sometimes signal a relatively poor outcome.

Visual problems are common in autism (but may be difficult to diagnose). On the basis of results from one Swedish study (Steffenburg 1991), about half of those children with autism who function at a level sufficient to permit a comprehensive ophthal-

mological assessment have refraction errors or squints or both. Some studies (Hobson 1993, Ek et al. 1998) suggest that children who are blind may have a high rate of autistic disorder, particularly if the blindness is associated with so-called retinopathy of prematurity.

Hearing deficits and deafness are clearly more common in autism than in the general population (Rosenhall et al. 2003). A hearing deficit of 25 dB or more is present in about 20% of children with typical autism (Steffenburg 1991). It is clinically important to recognize this association so that appropriate hearing aids may be provided rather than 'auditory problems' being attributed to the autism spectrum disorder per se and not being considered as a 'real' hearing deficit.

Dysphasia and related disorders are probably overrepresented in autism spectrum disorders. A considerable proportion of people with autism have expressive dysphasia 'superimposed' on their autistic-type speech and language abnormalities. When dysphasia is associated with autism, the types of alternative communication modes that are used for other children with dysphasia may be used, but in those who do not have dysphasia, such interventions are generally much less helpful.

Motor control abnormalities of a severe degree are uncommon in classical autism in childhood. However, follow-up into adulthood (von Knorring 1991, Billstedt et al. 2005) reveals that many patients develop disturbances of gait, ataxic movements and overall motor clumsiness with increasing age. Hypotonia and mild ataxia sometimes occur in early childhood autism cases (Gillberg and Coleman 2000). Also, children with spastic tetraplegia exhibit social interaction and communication deficits in a relatively large proportion of cases, even when the effects of concomitant severe mental retardation are taken into account. Catatonic features are fairly common in young adults with autism spectrum disorders, and may occasionally be so severe – particularly in relatively high-functioning individuals – that a separate diagnosis of catatonia should be considered.

In children with Asperger syndrome, motor clumsiness is often seen, and is part of the diagnostic criteria under certain manuals. The clumsiness may not actually be more pronounced than in autistic disorder, but the higher functioning of individuals with Asperger syndrome contributes to the impression of poor motor skills, because of the much higher expectations of normal motor skills in this group.

Some studies suggest that infant motor control problems (including poor facial movements) may be the first obvious sign of abnormal/unusual development in autism (Teitelbaum et al. 1998).

ASSOCIATED SPECIFIC MEDICAL CONDITIONS IN AUTISTIC DISORDER

A large number of specific medical conditions have been found to be associated with autism or autistic symptoms at a rate higher than that found in the general population. Conversely, in autism there is a high rate of associated medical conditions such as fragile X syndrome, other chromosomal abnormalities, tuberous

TABLE 24.3
Associated medical conditions in autism documented in at least two studies

Medical condition	Important reference
Fragile X syndrome	Hagerman (1989)
Other sex chromosome anomalies	Hagerman (1989)
Marker chromosome syndrome	Gillberg et al. (1991b)
Down syndrome	Lowenthal et al. (2007)
22q11 deletion syndrome	Niklasson et al. (2001)
22q13.3 syndrome	Phelan (2008)
Other chromosome anomalies	Hagerman (1989)
Tuberous sclerosis	Hunt and Dennis (1987)
Neurofibromatosis	Gillberg and Forsell (1984)
Hypomelanosis of Ito	Åkefeldt and Gillberg (1991)
Rett syndrome	Gillberg and Coleman (1992)
Angelman syndrome	Steffenburg et al. (1996)
Moebius syndrome	Ornitz et al. (1977)
Phenylketonuria	Friedman (1969)
Lactic acidosis	Coleman and Blass (1985)
Rubella embryopathy	Chess et al. (1971)
Herpes encephalitis	Gillberg (1986)
Cytomegalovirus infection	Stubbs (1978)
Williams syndrome	Reiss et al. (1985)
Duchenne muscular dystrophy	Komoto et al. (1984)
Retinopathy of prematurity	Jacobsson et al. (1998)
Smith–Lemli–Opitz syndrome	Sikora et al. (2006)
Thalidomide embryopathy	Strömland et al. (1994)

sclerosis, neurofibromatosis, Moebius syndrome and Rett syndrome. Table 24.3 shows some of the correlations between autism and specific medical conditions that have been reported in the literature to date.

SOCIAL COGNITION AND LEARNING SKILLS IN AUTISTIC DISORDER

Several sets of psychological functions are often impaired in autism. These include (1) mentalizing (also referred to as 'theory of mind' and 'empathy'); (2) executive functions; and (3) drive for central coherence (Happé 1994). Of these, (1) and (3) appear to be, perhaps, more 'autism-specific', and (2) less so.

Several recent studies suggest a specific drive for lower face processing (with the resulting impression of 'gaze avoidance'), abnormal facial emotional recognition, and unusual brain activation in connection with face processing in autism. Procedural learning skills appear to be much reduced, whereas fact and rote memory learning may actually exceed the level encountered in individuals who are not in the autism spectrum (Baron-Cohen and Belmonte 2005). Neuropsychological, physiological and autopsy studies support the notion of 'decreased neural connectivity' in autism spectrum disorders (Frith 2004). These characteristics may or may not be linked to the other mentioned neuropsychological peculiarities associated with autism spectrum disorders.

Attachment behaviours, originally believed to be severely abnormal in autism, are usually not primarily affected (Sigman and Mundy 1989, Dissanayake and Crossley 1996). However, the capacity for social referencing/shared attention – superficially seemingly linked, but theoretically separate from attachment – is usually reduced in autism.

Mentalizing (which requires a 'theory of mind') is the ability to attribute mental states (such as knowing, believing, etc.) to other people. It has been clearly demonstrated that young children with autism have severe problems in this domain as compared to typically developing children and children with mental retardation who do not have autistic features. Mentalizing is needed for the capacity to develop empathy skills, and may indeed be thought of as, in many respects, synonymous with empathy. Empathy is crucially reduced in autism.

Gillberg (1992) has proposed that autism and autistic-like conditions could be seen as 'disorders of empathy' and that 'empathy quotients' (EQs) (conceptually similar to IQs, but referring to theory of mind skills rather than overall cognitive skills) are specifically low in such disorders.

Executive functions comprise initiation of responses to the environment, maintaining the response, maintaining a strategy for the achievement of a future goal, and shifting to a new set of responses. Attentional ability, planning, sequencing, impulse control and time conceptualization are all examples of such executive functions, which are usually impaired in autism. However, they are also commonly impaired in other disorders, such as attention deficit hyperactivity disorder (ADHD).

Drive for central coherence – i.e. seeking to find a coherent theme or 'picture' behind a set of details – is usually weak in autism. Individuals with autism spectrum disorders are often obsessed with detail, and may be better than other people at registering detail and learning concrete facts.

Decreased connectivity across brain areas and brain functions is likely to play an important part in the pathogenesis of autism (Minshew and Williams 2007). Many 'functions' appear to be at 'normal levels' in autism, but they do not appear to communicate with each other in the way that they do in people who do not have autism.

It is not clear 'where in the brain' these cognitive psychological abilities are located. However, it is generally assumed that executive functions involve the frontal lobes (Harris 1995a,b). One PET (positron emission tomography) study of mentalizing abilities in males with and without Asperger syndrome suggested that such functions may be located in the medial portion of the left frontal lobe (Happé et al. 1996).

GENETIC FACTORS IN AUTISTIC DISORDER

There is overwhelming evidence that, in a majority of cases, genetic factors are in operation in autism. Several well-designed twin studies have all shown a very strong concordance for autism in monozygotic twins and a low rate of concordance in dizygotic twins – similar to that found in non-twin siblings (Bolton and Rutter 1990). Family studies of population-based series of autism cases have demonstrated a 50- to 100-fold autism risk increase for siblings of children with autism as compared with children in the general population. Family studies (e.g. Bowman 1988,

Bolton et al. 1994, Cederlund and Gillberg 2004) show that, in certain families, Asperger syndrome, autistic-like conditions (including one that is sometimes referred to as a 'lesser variant of autism') and autism 'proper' cluster in such a way as to suggest the presence of a strong heritability for some kind of autism-associated traits. Folstein and Rutter (1977) have suggested that it is not autism as such that is inherited, rather that some kind of cognitive disorder is transmitted that in certain cases will turn into autism if environmental insults are added. Other authors (e.g. Gillberg et al. 1992) have argued that a genetically transmitted social or 'social cognitive' deficit factor might be present in some families of children with autism. The family studies favour the notion of an 'Asperger trait' running in some kinships. If combined with brain damage, such as in the case of intrauterine rubella infection, this trait might produce autism (Gillberg 1991a). Most family studies show support for the notion of a language-associated cognitive deficit running in certain families, but a few have not found any evidence for this (e.g. Steffenburg 1990). Several different hereditary factors, interacting with other factors, could produce the same end result. Thus, there might be Asperger-associated heredity in some families and dyslexia-associated heredity in others.

In many families of children with autism, there are high rates of affective disorders, social phobia, obsessive–compulsive behaviours and 'broader autism phenotype symptoms' (Murphy et al. 2000, Wassink and Piven 2000).

It is now generally believed that in a majority of cases of autism there are susceptibility genes – one, two, or several, in each individual case – that predispose to the development of the behavioural phenotype, and that may, or may not, be sufficient to account for the full syndrome of autism, or may combine with (biological) environmental risk factors to push a susceptible individual 'over the border'. Some of the responsible genes are in the process of being identified (Philippe et al. 1999, Delorme et al. 2005). Specific mutated genes (e.g. *neuroligin 4*) have been identified as being crucial in certain families, but by and large, the bulk of the genetic variance has yet to be accounted for (Jamain et al. 2003).

THE PATHOGENETIC CHAIN OF EVENTS IN AUTISM

Reduced optimality in the pre-, peri- and neonatal periods has been found to be considerably more 'pathological' in autism than in a number of other developmental disorders such as mental retardation without autistic traits, syndromes associated with deficits in attention, motor control and perception and teenage psychosis (Gillberg and Gillberg 1991). These disorders are in turn associated with reductions of optimality greater than those that are to be expected in normal children. Bleeding in pregnancy, high maternal age, pre- and post-term birth, clinical dysmaturity and hyperbilirubinaemia are among the factors that contribute to a high prevalence of reduced optimality scores in autism (Gillberg and Gillberg 1983, Bryson et al. 1988, Coleman 2005). The added negative effects of several factors that deviate

from the optimal state in pregnancy and the newborn period could lead to a suboptimal environment for the developing nervous system that could cause brain dysfunction showing later as autistic symptomatology. However, the interpretation of reduced optimality is not straightforward.

Clear brain-damage risks (such as haemolytic anaemia caused by blood-group incompatibility, severe and protracted asphyxia, thalidomide embryopathy, herpes encephalitis, alcohol in utero, etc.) are also associated with some cases of autism (e.g. Folstein and Rutter 1977, Gillberg and Coleman 2000, Coleman 2005). Such findings imply that typical autism can arise on the basis of (nonspecific?) brain damage.

In an overview of all studies providing detailed information about associated medical disorders (Gillberg and Coleman 1996), the rate of such conditions in typical autism cases was estimated at about one in four individuals. In a study by Steffenburg (1991) of a total population cohort of children with severe autism, about one third had a clear associated medical condition, less than 10% had a 'pure' hereditary form, and the majority of the remainder had major signs of brain dysfunction revealed by comprehensive neurobiological work-up. The aetiology of the disorder was unknown in more than half of all affected individuals. Genetic factors alone or interacting with pre-, peri- or postnatal brain damaging factors may account for much or all of the variance in this 'idiopathic' group. In a study of a clinical cohort of cases with Asperger syndrome, Gillberg and Cederlund (2005) found that 70% of those affected had a close relative with either the same diagnosis or a milder variant of a 'broader autism phenotype'.

Several theories regarding the aetiology of autism have been proposed over the last 20 years. It is clear that autism can be the end result of a number of different conditions, ranging from tuberous sclerosis and the fragile X chromosome abnormality to metabolic disorders. Do these aetiologies share a common feature, namely that they impinge on the same brain structures or functional systems? In recent years, the brainstem, the temporal lobes and the prefrontal areas of the frontal lobes of the brain have been most often implicated in studies of neurophysiology/neuroradiology in autism (Coleman 2005). A few studies have drawn attention to the possible role of the cerebellum and the basal ganglia. The target areas for the brain's dopaminergic nerve fibres arising in the brainstem are the mesolimbic structures in the temporal lobes and prefrontal areas and in the basal ganglia. The dopamine system has been reported to be abnormal in autism (Gillberg and Svennerholm 1987, Barthélémy et al. 1988, Nordin et al. 1998). One theory proposes that the diverse aetiologies all affect this functional dopamine system in the brain and that when dopamine systems become dysfunctional, many of the typical autism symptoms ensue (Gillberg and Coleman 2000). Support for this theory is also provided by recent observations that babies born to mothers addicted to the cocaine derivative 'crack' show many of the characteristic features of autism from the first few months of life (Gillberg and Coleman 2000). Crack affects the brain's dopamine systems. However, alternative theories, such as hyperserotoninaemia problems, locus ceruleus dysfunction and endorphin imbalance, have been advanced

TABLE 24.4
Neuropsychiatric assessment in autism

(1) History

Detailed, structured assessment in relation to autism using standard questionnaire (including handedness)

Review of optimality in pre-, peri- and neonatal periods (medical records required)

Review of postnatal, potentially brain-damaging events (medical records usually needed)

Review of previous medical illness, growth patterns, etc.

Detailed psychiatric history:
- family factors and psychosocial milieu
- temperament and attention span of child
- heredity (especially autism, Asperger syndrome, 'autistic-like conditions' (including so-called 'lesser variants of autism'), learning disorders, mental retardation, 'childhood psychosis', childhood schizophrenia, affective disorders, obsessive–compulsive disorders, psychiatric disorders generally including anorexia nervosa and elective mutism, tuberous sclerosis, neurofibromatosis, geniuses, kinship)

(2) General physical examination

Measurement of cranial circumference, height, weight, auricle length and interpupillary distance

Assessment with respect to minor physical anomalies: meticulous physical examination (often needs repeating), including search for diagnostic skin changes (tuberous sclerosis, neurofibromatosis, hypomelanosis of Ito)

Assessment of heartbeat variation

In boys, inspection of external genitalia (prepuce, penile and testicular size and volume)

(3) Age-appropriate neurodevelopmental neurological examination

(4) Psychological evaluation

Has to be performed by an experienced clinical psychologist who knows how to do cognitive testing in children with autism and knows which test is appropriate according to child's age, developmental level, language and degree of cooperation

(5) Laboratory examinations (see Table 24.5)

(Cook 1990). The various theories need not be exclusive. It does not seem likely that one pathogenetic chain of events will ever be discovered to account for all autism cases.

In summary, autism is best conceptualized as a behavioural disorder – not so specific as previously believed – with multiple aetiologies. Autism is a sign that there is something wrong in the nervous system. It is best regarded as belonging with the other major neurodisabling conditions such as mental retardation, cerebral palsy and epilepsy. It often occurs in conjunction with other disorders and there should no longer be a need to discuss whether a child has, for example, 'autism or a hearing deficit', in a case where it is clear that both diagnoses apply.

MEDICAL WORK-UP IN AUTISTIC DISORDER

Studies by Steffenburg (1991) and others have demonstrated that a comprehensive medical work-up should be performed in all cases of autism. Steffenburg found a clear aetiology in about one third of cases (and signs of major nonspecific brain dysfunction in another 50%). More than half of the clear aetiologies would not have been disclosed without a detailed medical work-up of the kind suggested in Tables 24.4 and 24.5. These tables

list the essentials in the work-up of a child under 10 years of age who receives a diagnosis of autistic disorder (usually with mild, moderate or severe associated learning disability) for the first time. In older children, and in children for whom a clear aetiology is suspected, the work-up may be differently tailored.

If there is a nearby laboratory testing CSF amino acids (phenylalanine in particular), CSF monoamines and CSF endorphins, these tests should be considered if the child has a lumbar puncture anyway (to exclude progressive encephalitis/encephalopathy).

Even in those many cases for which a clear aetiology cannot be established, the medical work-up may be important for psychological reasons. The parents need to know that their doctor has done what is currently the best possible work-up in the field of autism. The fact that so many cases turn out to have demonstrable signs of brain dysfunction – even when no exact cause can be established – is often helpful rather than, as some seem to fear, contributing to pessimistic attitudes in parents and others working to help the affected child. The disorder becomes less mysterious, and some of the child's problems take on a less baffling, less threatening character.

NEUROPSYCHOLOGICAL WORK-UP IN AUTISTIC DISORDER

All children with autism also need a neuropsychological work-up. This must include some kind of cognitive/intellectual testing or evaluation. No single measure in childhood will be able to predict outcome in autism better than an IQ test: IQ <50 around age 5–8 years almost invariably means a relatively poor outcome, whereas IQ >70 at this age predicts that outcome may be relatively good (see below). The test used will vary from one culture to another. It should be performed by a psychologist both clinically and theoretically experienced with testing and evaluating children with autism.

At least four different cognitive/developmental scales seem to be useful in autism: the WISC-IV (Wechsler 2003), the Leiter International Scale (Leiter 1980), the Vineland Adaptive Behaviour Scales (Sparrow and Cicchetti 1985) and the Griffiths Developmental Scale II (Griffiths 1970). For language evaluation, the Reynell Developmental Language Scales (Reynell 1969) and the Peabody Picture Vocabulary Test (Dunn 1970) can be useful. A more recently developed neuropsychological test battery, the NEPSY (Korkman et al. 1997), may prove worthwhile in the evaluation of childhood autism, but so far no systematic studies exist.

The *WISC-IV* can be used only for children aged 6 years or over but is particularly useful in relatively high-functioning individuals with autism (those with IQ levels >50). The 'typical' profile is one in which Verbal scores are lower than Performance scores. However, in Asperger syndrome, the pattern is reversed in half or more of cases (Gillberg and Cederlund 2005). Also, scores tend to be exceptionally low (relative to the child's other scores) for Picture Arrangement (even though this tended to be more true of previous versions of the WISC) and Comprehension (tests that, to a considerable degree, require 'common sense'

TABLE 24.5
TABLE 24.5
Relevant laboratory analyses in all medium- and low-functioning, and certain high-functioning cases with autism and autistic-like conditions

Analysis	Finding	Reference
Chromosomal and DNA (e.g. *FMR1*, 22q11, 22q13, 15q, *neuroligin*)	Fragile Xq27.3	Hagerman (1989)
	XYY	Gillberg et al. (1984)
	Deletions, e.g. 15q12, 22q11	Kerbeshian et al. (1990), Phelan (2008)
	Marker chromosome (15q)	Gillberg et al. (1991b)
	Other	Hagerman (1989), Jamain et al. (2003)
CT/MRI	Tuberous sclerosis	Gillberg et al. (1987)
	Intrauterine infections	Chess et al. (1971)
	Neurofibromatosis	Gillberg and Forsell (1984)
	Hypomelanosis of Ito	Åkefeldt and Gillberg (1991)
	Other	Tsai (1989)
CSF protein[1]	Progressive encephalopathy	Wing and Gould (1979)
EEG	Tuberous sclerosis	Steffenburg (1990)
	Subclinical epilepsy	Gillberg and Schaumann (1983)
	Epileptic discharges	Gillberg and Schaumann (1983)
	Landau–Kleffner syndrome	Rapin (1995), Neville (1997), Gillberg and Coleman (2000), Rosenhall et al. (2003)
Auditory brainstem response	Brainstem dysfunction	Gillberg and Coleman (2000)
Ophthalmology	Poor vision, fundus signs	Steffenburg (1990)
Otolaryngology (including hearing test)	Poor hearing, anatomical defects	Smith et al. (1988)
Blood:		
Phenylalanine	High	Friedman (1969)
Uric acid	High	Gillberg and Coleman (2000)
Lactic acid	High	Coleman and Blass (1985)
Pyruvic acid	High	Gillberg and Coleman (2000)
Herpes titre	Seroconversion	Gillberg (1986)
24-hour urine:		
Metabolic screening including mucopolysaccharidosis	Abnormal	Gillberg and Coleman (2000)
Uric acid	High	Gillberg and Coleman (2000)
Calcium	Low	Gillberg and Coleman (2000)

[1]If there is a nearby laboratory testing CSF amino acids (phenylalanine in particular), CSF monoamines and CSF endorphins, these tests should be considered since the child has to have a lumbar puncture anyway (to exclude progressive encephalitis/encephalopathy).

and the ability to reflect on other people's inner thoughts and to take account of context, and on which results can be improved by early training, as indexed by poor results in young children with Asperger syndrome but much better results in adolescents and young adults in this group), and exceptionally high for Block Design, at least in 'classic' autistic disorder (Block Design is a WISC subtest that does not require the child to take account of context other than that provided by the visible patterns on the cubes, but that does make some demands on visuomotor skills, which are sometimes impaired in Asperger syndrome). Object Assembly results are often poor in Asperger syndrome. In high-functioning individuals with this diagnosis, test results are often similar to those seen in ADHD (poor results on one or more of Arithmetic, Digit Symbol and Digit Span).

The *Leiter* is a nonverbal test that is easy to administer (for a skilled psychologist), even to non-speaking children with autism. Many of the subtests of the Leiter reflect underlying abilities akin to those tested in the Block Design test of the WISC. Therefore, some children with autism will receive a high Leiter IQ even when overall IQ (verbal and nonverbal) is below normal. Nevertheless, the Leiter has been shown to have relatively good correlation with other IQ tests in many cases of autism and is widely used in the field.

The *Vineland Adaptive Behaviour Scales* are not ordinary tests but rather a structured interview with the closest carer. The examiner comes up with a social quotient, which, in autism, fairly well indicates the intelligence level also. The Vineland is therefore especially useful in patients considered 'untestable'.

The *Griffiths* scale seems to be relatively useful in young children with autism (aged 2–7 years) for discriminating between those with IQ <50 and those >50 (Dahlgren Sandberg et al. 1993). For a more detailed evaluation, the Griffiths scale appears inadequate and usually has to be followed up with a WISC-IV test during the early school years.

QUESTIONNAIRES, OBSERVATION SCHEDULES, AND DIAGNOSTIC INTERVIEWS

In making the diagnosis of autism spectrum disorders, various questionnaires and other evaluation tools are available. Currently the two most used instruments are the CARS (Childhood Autism Rating Scale—Schopler et al. 1980, 1988) and the ABC (Autism Behavior Checklist – Krug et al. 1980). The ASSQ (Autism Spectrum Screening Questionnaire – Ehlers and Gillberg 1993) is a screening instrument for high-functioning individuals that has come to be used extensively in recent years. The ADOS (Autism Diagnostic Observation Schedule – Lord et al. 1994) is in widespread clinical use, but requires training and certification. In addition, many clinics now use the DISCO (Diagnosis of Social and Communication Disorders – Leekam et al. 2002) or the ADI-R (Autism Diagnostic Interview, Revised – Lord et al. 1994), both of which require diploma training and were originally developed for (clinical) research purposes. For preliminary clinical diagnosis of higher-functioning individuals, the ASDI (Asperger Syndrome/Autism Spectrum Diagnostic Interview – Gillberg et al. 2001) is used in many centres.

The *CARS* has good reliability and validity, at least in cases with clear-cut and severe autism. It is a mixed interview observation schedule that is best completed after interview with a carer and observation of the individual with autism. Scores range from 15 to 60 with 'autism cut-off' at 30 and severe cases being identified by levels of 36 and above. In high-functioning individuals it works less well, and a considerable proportion would be missed if the recommended cut-off of 30 is used. The CARS is less useful for work-up of individuals with Asperger syndrome.

The *ABC* comprises an interview containing 57 statements that can be used to elicit information about the child in about 30 minutes; it should not be used as the sole instrument for making a diagnosis of autism. The suggested cut-off point (above 67 for autism) leads to many false-negative cases (Nordin et al. 1998). The ABC should be used rather as a screen for amount of autistic symptomatology than for the diagnosis of autism per se. Again, it is not generally useful for individuals with Asperger syndrome.

The *ADOS* (and its prelinguistic version, the PL-ADOS) is an observation schedule that is very good for systematic observation in a research setting and may be helpful in difficult differential diagnostic decisions but which, by and large, does not lend itself to use in general diagnostic practice, particularly given the special training required for using it.

The *DISCO* is an investigator-based interview with good validity and reliability. It is very useful across the range of diagnostic categories in the autism spectrum, but suffers from being very time-consuming and the need for highly specialized training.

The *ADI-R* is another investigator-based interview, similar in style to the DISCO, but more specifically focused on core autistic disorder symptomatology. It too requires expensive training before use.

EDUCATIONAL EVALUATION

For the educational evaluation, which is an important part of the

TABLE 24.6
Important components of management/treatment regimes in autism and autistic-like conditions

Early diagnosis
Specific treatments such as diets
Rehabilitation team well acquainted with basic problems of autism
Home-based treatment programme
Structured environment, including 'ritualizing' of everyday routines
Continuity as regards people, place and approach
Graded change
Physical exercise
Education focusing on activities of daily life and interest patterns which can form the basis for future work
Pharmacotherapy for a minority (not specifically for autism)
Applied behaviour analysis
Long-term (lifetime) perspective

neuropsychological work-up, the PEP-R (Psycho-Educational Profile—Revised – Mesibov et al. 1989) is useful. It provides a concise picture of the child's current educational status in a number of areas and forms the basis for goal-directed educational interventions in the individual case. The PEP is intended to be used at regular intervals in an educational treatment programme in order to promote and evaluate intervention effects.

INTERVENTIONS: TREATMENTS, MANAGEMENT AND EDUCATION

There can be no clear dividing line between various kinds of intervention, i.e. education, management and treatment, in autism. A few cases can be rationally treated (e.g. by diet in phenylketonuric autism, and, perhaps, by neurosurgery in tuberous sclerosis with autism and epilepsy), others may be helped by way of classic interventions, such as pharmacotherapy or psychotherapy or both. However, in the majority of cases, such measures do not produce significant change. On the other hand, education and 'management', in a broad sense of that word, can lead to worthwhile improvements. The crucial elements in any management/treatment programme for autism (or autistic-like conditions) are outlined in Table 24.6.

PSYCHOEDUCATION

Perhaps the most important part of intervention in the whole field of autism is that of psychoeducation. 'Educating' the family (those affected, siblings, mother and father, grandparents) about what autism is and what it is not is essential for improvement of quality of life. Making those affected and their near and dear truly knowledgeable about the condition should be a primary goal of all 'autism programmes'. When the family has sufficient knowledge, they themselves can access new knowledge as it unfolds, through booklets, books, DVDs, videos and the internet. Changing the attitudes of people in society generally can go a long way in furnishing an 'autism-friendly' environment, where carers and teachers know as much as possible about the underlying neuropsychology and communication styles and needs of people affected by autism.

SPECIFIC TREATMENTS (INCLUDING PREVENTION)

DIET-BASED TREATMENTS

Phenylketonuria, if untreated, can cause autism. If it is appropriately treated with a diet from the first few days of life, autistic symptoms never develop. In fact, one is here dealing with prevention rather than cure, since the autistic symptoms are never allowed to appear before treatment is started.

Other diet-based treatments are possible for autism. Coleman and Blass (1985) described lactic acidosis associated with autism and showed that in such cases dietary treatment could lead to disappearance of autistic symptoms. Gluten- and casein-free diets have not been shown to have generally positive effects in autism (Millward et al. 2008).

PHARMACOTHERAPY

Pharmacotherapy plays a minor, but important, role in the treatment of autism. No medication is available for which benefits outweigh side effects in a majority of cases of autism. Nevertheless, some drugs, adequately tested in controlled studies, have positive effects in a sufficient number of cases to warrant recommendation for treatment trials if there is a clinically felt need for pharmacological intervention. This is sometimes the case when thorough educational measures have not led to expected gains; when overactivity, destructiveness and/or self-injurious behaviour cause such turmoil that other interventions cannot be used at all; or when adolescent aggravation of symptoms (see below) prevents developmental progress. Drugs should never be used as the sole kind of intervention but should always be accompanied by educational and psychosocial approaches. Antiepileptic pharmacotherapy is quite often indicated in autism with epilepsy.

In the treatment of epilepsy in autism, *lamotrigine, carbamazepine* and *valproic acid* are drugs of first choice in many cases. These substances may also sometimes be tried when there are severe mood swings in autism.

Neuroleptics (particularly haloperidol and risperidone) have been examined in a number of double-blind placebo-controlled studies (Campbell 1989, McCracken et al. 2002, Troost et al. 2005). They seem to exert some positive effects on the basic problems associated with autism (social withdrawal, communication, learning and rigid behaviour patterns). However, it is difficult to recommend their use in the long term because of the high incidence of severe or moderate extrapyramidal side effects (25–30% in most series) in the case of haloperidol, and severe weight gain in risperidone. Neuroleptics can be of some value in breaking up 'vicious circles', particularly in adolescent symptom aggravation, self-injury, violent behaviours, hyperactivity and sleep problems. Risperidone has shown some beneficial effects for these types of problems over periods of more than 6 months, and can sometimes be helpful if there is no indication of weight gain during the early phases of treatment.

Sedative drugs are not indicated for more than short-term use (days/weeks). They are most often considered in the treatment of sleep problems. They often have paradoxical effects, the child reacting with even more hyperactivity and difficulty settling down in the evening. Benzodiazepines usually have extremely negative effects on behaviour and cognition in autism (Gillberg 1991c) and should, if possible, be avoided.

In the treatment of epilepsy in autism, many drugs have detrimental side effects on behaviour and learning (Gillberg 1991c). There are no well-controlled double-blind studies in the field, but a systematic survey of the literature and clinical experience suggest that valproic acid and carbamazepine may be less negative than other drugs with respect to behavioural side effects. The side effects of phenobarbitone (irritability, hyperactivity, aggressive outbursts and decreased learning) are well known, but the benzodiazepines (clonazepam in particular) are often even worse. It is not uncommon for a child with complex partial seizures to appear autistic while on clonazepam but nonautistic as soon as s/he is taken off the drug.

Stimulant medication (methylphenidate and amphetamine in particular) has, by and large, been avoided in the treatment of autism. However, recently a new trend has emerged in this field, so that some children with mild mental retardation and autism who also have severe attention deficits are indeed treated with central stimulants, usually with few side effects (Di Martino et al. 2004). Some studies suggest that stimulants may, indeed, be very helpful in the treatment of attention deficits and hyperactivity/impulsivity associated with Asperger syndrome (Gillberg et al. 1997).

The *serotonin reuptake inhibitors* (such as fluvoxamine, fluoxetine and sertraline) are currently being evaluated, and although some promising results have been reported, it is as yet too early to determine their possible role in the treatment of autism. The same holds for the *noradrenalin reuptake inhibitor*, atomoxetine.

Lithium may be an adjunct in controlling mood swings (and perhaps violent behaviours) occurring particularly during the adolescent period. Serum concentration should be kept at the lowest possible level (0.4–0.7 mmol/L).

Naltrexone and other opiate blockers have been tried in autism after the report of associated endogenous opioid dysfunction (Gillberg 1995). Naltrexone seems to be a relatively safe drug, perhaps particularly if there is concomitant hyperactivity, but it is not widely used. Self-injurious behaviours in autism have been reported to be associated with particularly high levels of CSF endorphins (Gillberg et al. 1985), but evidence that naltrexone reduces self-injury is lacking.

Fenfluramine, an anorexogenic drug with serotonin-lowering properties, despite early enthusiastic reports, has little place in the treatment of most cases of autism (Gualtieri 1987).

Vitamin B_6 has been shown to have at least some positive effects in relatively well-designed studies (e.g. Lelord et al. 1981). It is given in doses of 300–900 mg/day, supplemented with magnesium in cases with severe nonspecific behaviour problems (including restlessness, aggressiveness, sleep problems and self-injurious behaviour).

Fish oils – usually omega-3 fatty acids – have become popular in the treatment of all sorts of neuropsychiatric disorders including autism. The scientific rationale for this is so far meagre or lacking altogether, but several studies are currently underway.

For a good overview of drug treatment in autism, the reader is referred to Campbell (1989), Buitelaar and Willemsen-Swinkels (2000) and Malone et al. (2005).

NON-DRUG MEDICAL/BIOLOGICAL TREATMENTS
Physical exercise
Physical exercise is effective in reducing major behaviour problems (self-injury, aggressiveness, hyperactivity and sleep problems) in autism (McGimsey and Favell 1988, Haracopos 1989) and should be used much more than is currently the case. Jogging programmes (two half-hour sessions a day for instance) can be very helpful (Celiberti et al. 1997).

Psychotherapy
In a wide sense of the word, there can be no treatment for autism without psychotherapeutic elements. However, classical analytically oriented psychotherapy for children with autism has never been shown to have lasting positive effects and should not be used, unless as part of a systematic research trial, since there have been reports of negative effects both on the child and on the family (Gillberg 1989).

From around the time of puberty, some high-functioning people with autism who have good verbal ability appear to benefit from *individual talks* with somebody well acquainted with the various aspects of autism, when many of them begin to realize the extent to which they differ from other people.

Family therapy usually has no place in autism. However, regular contact with the family and teaching the family to become the child's best advocate (see below) should be essential parts of any good treatment/management programme.

Interventions using *Applied Behaviour Analysis (ABA)* seem to have positive effects in some cases of autism, but large-scale studies of long-term effects are lacking. Several small-scale studies do indicate positive gains for young children with autism, particularly when there is some expressive spoken language development before age 3 years. However, it should be noted that children with autism and some spoken language development by age 3 years have a relatively better outcome in themselves, and it is unclear what the specific effects have been of the intervention used.

Early diagnosis
To give autism a name as soon as possible can have far-reaching positive consequences. An early diagnosis can mean (1) the discovery of treatable underlying conditions, (2) the identification of genetic disorders requiring genetic counselling, (3) getting the family out of a vicious circle including elements of self-blame, practical problems, loss of sleep and inappropriate behaviour management techniques, and (4) appropriate interventions and education for the child (Howlin 2005). Also, siblings can be better informed so that they may better understand the atypical child's strange behaviour (Bågenholm and Gillberg 1992).

Home-based approaches
Howlin and Rutter (1987) and Schopler (1989) have shown that home-based approaches to autism can have beneficial effects for both child and family. Parents should be regarded as co-therapists. All parents need to receive as much education as possible about autism, including symptoms, aetiology and available treatments. Seminars for groups of parents are often useful. The family should be informed about the existence of available autism support groups. An integrated education/behaviour modification programme for the child, including elements of 'graded change' (Howlin and Yates 1989), should be planned in collaboration with the parents. Activities of daily life (such as feeding, hygiene and sleeping) should be the focus of home-based interventions. 'Institutional handling' of problems in this field usually does not generalize to the home situation without proper training at home.

EDUCATION
For at least 200 years it has been recognized that education has particular merit in relation to autism. Education in autism is a vast and growing area (Schopler 1989), beyond the scope of this volume. However, some brief comments are warranted.

Children with autism need a structured environment with as much predictability as possible. Their own need to insist on routine and 'sameness' should be met by adults introducing useful routines that can be accepted by child and adult alike. Once routines have been established by adults, the child with autism is more likely to stop introducing new, bizarre routines, and even to abandon some of the old ones. Whereas typical children – and indeed most mentally retarded children without autism – learn 'automatically' as they seek new experiences and interact with other people, children with autism do not get anything for free and need to learn through training. Training needs to be planned, and this requires an evaluation tool. The PEP (see above) is a useful instrument for pinpointing individual skills and deficits in autism. The PEP can then also be used in the follow-up of management to document that the child has actually developed 'according to plan'.

Some principles of education in autism are essential. First, there is a need to individualize: in spite of similarities, people with autism are, first and foremost, individuals with different personalities, different IQs and different social backgrounds.

Second, there is a need for structure and continuity in relation to time, place and teacher. In other words, the same thing should be taught at the same time in the same room by the same person. This style of structure might have to be applied with some rigour in the early stages of education, whereas the long-term goal is, wherever possible, to be able gradually to introduce a little more flexibility.

Third, children with autism can usually harbour only one thought at a time, which means that instruction about several things cannot be given at once.

Fourth, and interconnected with the third point, is their deficient sense of time in most cases. This should be met, for instance, by ensuring that one task is finished before the next task is introduced.

Last, but not least, education has to take account of the fact that children with autism – even those labelled as high-functioning – usually have extremely deficient comprehension of spoken language and poor understanding of abstract symbols, but often relatively good visual or visuospatial skills. Spoken language has to be reduced to a minimum in interactions with people with autism, and one must find ways of ensuring that they actually understand any communication used. Long sentences must be avoided in most cases, as must use of metaphorical language. Token and sign language can often be as difficult to cope with as spoken language. Instead, pictures containing photos of concrete situations that the child knows well are often very helpful. Picture Exchange Communication Systems (PECS) have been used successfully with many low- and middle-functioning individuals with autistic disorder and similar conditions.

Some of the higher-functioning individuals with autism may need specific help in training mentalizing abilities (Ozonoff and Miller 1995, Howlin 1997, Wellman et al. 2002).

Special education and intervention facilities for people with autistic disorder

There is a need for special preschools, special classrooms, special job facilities and services planning work, and special group homes for people with autism and autistic-like conditions. Such facilities are also needed for people with other kinds of social and communication disorders, most of whom are likely to have some kind of minor or major intellectual impairment. For some children with autism the best option would be placement in a class specifically for children with autism, for others it would be better to attend a class for the communication-impaired with or without autism, while for some a class for the mentally retarded would be more suitable. Many children with autism do not need any special services, but they and their families might need the help of an expert autism team to guide them through childhood, adolescence and adult life.

The most important thing is that real options should exist for the child and family and that no extreme philosophy of segregation or integration should govern the kind of help and service that can be provided.

OUTCOME IN AUTISTIC DISORDER AND OTHER AUTISM SPECTRUM DISORDERS

Most follow-up studies of autism agree that psychosocial outcome is variable but often quite poor.

LIFE EXPECTANCY

The mortality rate in autism seems to be slightly increased (Gillberg 1991b, Billstedt et al. 2005). Almost 8% of people with autism surviving the first 2 years of life die before age 40 years. Of those who survive much longer, a small number can hold half-sheltered jobs. Another 25% show considerable progress, but still remain dependent on other people for many things. About 10% (recruited almost exclusively from the group with tested IQ >60 in childhood) function independently and hold ordinary jobs, but may still be perceived as somewhat odd in their style of social

interaction. At most, about 5% in different follow-up studies have been considered 'cured', or rather as having grown out of symptoms associated with autism.

However, as regards individuals with Asperger syndrome (see also below), the evidence is still wanting, and much of what has been published to date suggests that outcome may be very good in some cases. One study of 100 individuals with the disorder, diagnosed in childhood and followed through adolescence and into early adult life, showed more than half had acceptable or very good outcomes. Nevertheless, slightly under 50% showed a restricted or in some cases poor outcome with considerable psychosocial adjustment problems in early adult life (Gillberg and Cederlund 2005).

DETERIORATION

About 10–20% of all children with classic autism deteriorate in adolescence, and about 60% become totally dependent on other people for their everyday lives. Some of these, it appears, never return to their preadolescent level of functioning. Another 30% show symptom aggravation in adolescence. This aggravation may run a periodic course, but will usually become less of a problem by 25–30 years of age. The symptoms encountered in these pubertal change cases are often similar to those seen in the same child in the preschool period, i.e. overactivity, violent behaviours, self-injurious behaviour, sleep problems, incoherent language, and bladder and bowel incontinence. A trial of risperidone – or lithium in cases of severe mood swings – can be indicated in some such cases, and may occasionally be helpful. Epilepsy is sometimes the first sign that deterioration may follow, although some cases with the combination of epilepsy and symptom aggravation do not later develop deterioration. The reason for deterioration is not known (even though in some instances progressive neurological/neurometabolic disorders are suspected), and usually there is no treatment available. Neuroleptics are often tried but sometimes with little effect. Physical exercise frequently yields positive results.

REGRESSIVE AUTISM

There is also a subgroup of children with autism who deteriorate during the first few years of life (Rapin 1996). Although previously a matter of considerable debate, it is now clear that a relatively small group of children (perhaps around 10–20%) with classic autism symptoms have a period of deterioration around 16–24 months of age. Some of these are normal before deterioration, others show mild autism symptoms before the onset of regression. It is possible that this type – sometimes referred to as 'regressive autism' – constitutes a separate clinical entity or one that is more closely linked to childhood disintegrative disorder (see below) than to Kanner's variant of autism. Deterioration may be temporally linked with the appearance of seizure activity on EEG (or clinical seizures), but in many cases no such association is found.

SOCIAL STYLE SUBTYPES OF AUTISM

In adulthood, three broad groups of people with autism can be discerned (Wing 1989): those who remain autistic in many respects; those who are passive and friendly; and those who appear active and odd. The second (passive) group quite often is not recognized as having autism unless a clear diagnosis of autism had been made in early childhood. The third group too is often not recognized as having autism, but, because of the conspicuous problems they show (e.g. undressing or masturbating in public, touching other people in unexpected ways), they more often are brought to a psychiatrist who might be able to discern the original nature of the disorder. These three styles of social interaction can often be recognized already in early childhood. A fourth group – formal, rigid and stilted – can often be recognized in later childhood, and may usually be diagnosed with Asperger syndrome. It is possible that this subgrouping occurs not just in autism but that people in general may also fall into these four categories, but only in the presence of autism will they appear more 'clear-cut'.

OUTCOME IN AUTISM: CONCLUDING REMARKS
The natural history in the individual case will also depend on the natural history of the particular associated medical condition (e.g. tuberous sclerosis, fragile X syndrome). Finally, symptomatology in autism changes over the years, even in the subgroup that remains 'autistic'. Many clinicians are surprised when faced with a 10-year-old child given a diagnosis of autism at age 4 years. The child may no longer be gaze-avoidant (in fact s/he might never have been clearly gaze-avoidant, but perhaps only 'gaze-odd'), and may accept the company of other people and even try to interact with them in a number of different ways. In these circumstances it is common for clinicians to confront the parents with the self-assured remark, "This child does not have autism," sometimes followed by, "and I do not think s/he ever had autism!" Autism symptomatology is not a 'once and for all' thing.

ATYPICAL AUTISM/AUTISTIC-LIKE CONDITIONS

In clinical practice cases with most but not all of the symptoms typical of autism are not unusual. Also, some people with profound mental retardation show all three elements of the triad of symptoms considered necessary and sufficient to diagnose autism (see above), but are difficult to classify as autism cases because it is difficult to decide whether the social, language and behavioural 'symptoms' are out of keeping with the degree of overall mental development. Finally, there is a group of children with deficits in attention, motor control and perception (DAMP, see Chapter 25) who show varying degrees of social, communication and behavioural problems, but who do not fit the full clinical picture of autism or Asperger syndrome.

At present no adequate diagnostic category is available for all these cases. 'Pervasive developmental disorder not otherwise specified' is used for some of these cases by the DSM-IV (roughly corresponding to 'atypical autism' in the ICD-10). This term is often seriously misleading, particularly when one is dealing with children of normal intelligence. 'Autistic-like conditions' (Nordin and Gillberg 1996) has been proposed by others to cover the

group of 'autism-like' problems that do not fit readily into the classification systems. Some clinicians use the term 'autistic traits'.

Many children with so-called autistic traits fulfil currently accepted criteria for the full syndrome of autism (or for Asperger syndrome, see below) but for some reason do not receive the correct diagnosis of autism (or Asperger syndrome). This appears to be particularly common in cases where obvious brain dysfunction has been diagnosed at an early stage in the development of the child's problems, for instance when there is hydrocephalus, infantile spasms, tuberous sclerosis or some other well-known neurological disorder.

The prevalence of autistic traits is possibly much higher than that of autism proper. Wing's studies of mentally retarded individuals under 15 years of age in London and my own studies in the general 7-year-old population in Göteborg suggest that at least 2–6 per 1000 children exhibit severe autistic traits. A more recent study from Bergen, Norway (Posserud et al. 2006) found that more than 3% of all 7- to 9-year-olds had several autistic features.

Some children do not show overt evidence of autism until after age 3 years. These cases can be classified as 'autistic disorder' according to the DSM-III-R, but doubt remains whether they represent the same type of condition as autism with early onset. In some, a case can be made for diagnosing childhood disintegrative disorder (Heller dementia).

CHILDHOOD DISINTEGRATIVE DISORDER – HELLER DEMENTIA INFANTILIS
Heller (1930) described children who appeared to develop normally up until about the age of 2–4 years but who then dramatically regressed, became confused and hyperactive, and were left, months later, in a more or less aloof and demented state (Burd et al. 1989, Volkmar and Rutter 1995). Many of these children are clinically indistinguishable from those with autism once the regression period is over after 2–20 months. Others follow a gradually more downhill course. Some have neurodegenerative conditions, but less is known about the aetiology of childhood disintegrative disorder than about that of autism. Long-term outcome appears to be even worse than in autism.

ASPERGER SYNDROME
In 1944, the Austrian paediatrician Hans Asperger described what he considered to be an unusual personality variant in young children, most of whom were boys. He alluded to 'autistic psychopathy' but, after an influential paper by Wing (1981a), the particular combination of problems that Asperger described is now generally referred to as Asperger syndrome. Asperger syndrome is believed by many to be on a continuum with autism and autistic-like conditions, but it is not yet clear whether it represents autism in people of generally good intelligence or a specific cognitive profile involving at least some areas of superior functioning.

DIAGNOSIS
Diagnostic criteria have been proposed (Table 24.7) but have not yet been validated. These should not be taken to imply that Asperger syndrome is clearly distinct from autism (the criteria for

Asperger syndrome obviously overlap with those for autism). The symptom criteria of the ICD-10 (WHO 1993) and DSM-IV (APA 1994) are virtually identical. These diagnostic manuals regard normal early language development and intellectual functioning and normal curiosity about the environment in the first 3 years of life as prerequisites for a diagnosis of Asperger's disorder/Asperger syndrome. However, Asperger himself included cases with abnormal language development and mild mental retardation in his series of cases. The DSM-IV and ICD-10 further draw a distinct line between autistic disorder and Asperger's, and this is out of keeping with clinical experience suggesting that some individuals meet criteria for autistic disorder early on and later fit the clinical picture of Asperger syndrome much better (and vice versa). Several studies have shown that the ICD-10 and DSM-IV criteria for Asperger syndrome do not apply to other than an extremely tiny fraction of all individuals with autism spectrum disorders, and that Asperger's own cases do not meet these criteria (Miller and Ozonoff 1997, Leekam et al. 2002). In clinical practice, these criteria are of little use. Instead, the criteria by Gillberg and Gillberg (1989) are often used.

The most distinctive feature of Asperger syndrome in very young children may be a decreased ability of subjects to conceptualize the mental states of other people, similar to that seen in autism. This inability is nowhere near as pronounced as in autism, and some reflection on other people's 'inner' needs can usually be prompted by reminding the subject of their existence, but the degree of empathy to be expected is generally low. A partial lack of a 'theory of mind' in Asperger syndrome has been supported by studies in experimental psychology (for a review, see Frith 1991). However, in later childhood most individuals with the syndrome pass simple theory of mind tests, but show clear deficits in executive functions.

Asperger syndrome is sometimes evident in the first year of life as a restricted interest in social interaction, but usually it is not until the second to fourth year that parents become concerned. Often there is worry about the apparent lack of need for playmates and the relatively late language development, often superseded by the development of formally impeccable, pedantic and prematurely adult-type language. Some cases do not attract attention until well into school age and then only because of extremely limited interests, motor clumsiness and lack of empathy. There is usually an odd prosody with a flat or staccato intonation or a shrill, monotonous quality. In certain cases there is an exceptional tendency to cluttering. Speech therapists often refer to the speech and language problems as 'semantic–pragmatic disorder' (Bishop 1989).

Because of their socially abnormal behaviour, peculiar, restricted interest patterns and unusual language characteristics, children with Asperger syndrome are variously described as odd, original, eccentric, 'the little professor', hilarious, cold, naive, lacking in common sense or immature. Some become the subject of teasing or bullying at school, but most manage fairly well in this respect, possibly as a result of their 'untouchability'.

Asperger syndrome is usually associated with normal or above-normal intelligence, but occasional typical cases in children with subnormal intelligence have been described. Associated impairments/medical conditions are much less common than in autism, but the available evidence suggests that the rate of epilepsy may be slightly higher than in the general population, and associated chromosomal abnormalities (e.g. fragile X, XYY) may not be altogether uncommon. Cases of Asperger syndrome in children with mild cerebral palsy have also been described (Gillberg 1989).

EPIDEMIOLOGY
Asperger syndrome is about 10 times more frequent in boys than in girls. It is possible that a similar core condition might be present in girls but with a slightly different phenotype. The overall prevalence has been estimated to be at least 3 per 1000 children born (Ehlers and Gillberg 1993), but could be higher.

Most cases are thought to be caused by genetic factors. In many instances there is a close relative with similar problems or sometimes clear-cut autism. Brain damage without a genetic predisposition can probably also cause Asperger syndrome (Wing 1981a, Cederlund and Gillberg 2004). Perinatal brain insults, postnatal brain infections and congenital hypothyroidism have been reported as causing brain damage in children who later received a diagnosis of Asperger syndrome.

In a study by Happé et al. (1996) it appeared that portions of the left medial frontal lobe may be specifically dysfunctional in Asperger syndrome and that this impairment might underlie the difficulties individuals with the syndrome have when solving mentalizing tasks. People with Asperger syndrome and other high-functioning individuals with autism spectrum disorders may have a fairly specific dysfunction of the gyrus fusiformis resulting in difficulties processing other people's facial expressions. It also seems likely that such people have a particular way of 'processing faces', and that they are driven to look at the lower rather than the upper portion of the face (Ashwin et al. 2005).

DIFFERENTIAL DIAGNOSIS
The distinction of Asperger syndrome from sociopathy, severe antisocial behaviour ('psychopathy'), borderline conditions and various types of manipulating personality disorders is based on the fact that because of their limitations in conceiving of other people's minds, Asperger subjects do not have a well-developed capacity for lying, luring or manipulating other people. 'Borderline conditions' (a dubious notion anyway) are supposed to be characterized by intense swings in relationships with other people (love–hate: "cannot live with you, cannot live without you"). This is the opposite of Asperger syndrome, in which stability of relationship and behaviour over time is usually highly characteristic.

MEDICAL AND PSYCHOLOGICAL WORK-UP
The work-up in a child or adolescent suspected of having Asperger syndrome is similar to that in high-functioning autism (see above). A screen for visual and hearing problems should be made in all cases. If there is academic failure, the WISC-R (with typically relatively lower results on Comprehension and Picture Arrangement) and a more exhaustive neuropsychological work-up might be appropriate.

TABLE 24.7
TABLE 24.7
Diagnostic criteria for Asperger syndrome/disorder

Asperger syndrome (Gillberg and Gillberg 1989)
1. Severe impairment in reciprocal social interaction (at least two of the following):
   - inability to interact with peers
   - lack of desire to interact with peers
   - lack of appreciation of social cues
   - socially and emotionally inappropriate
2. All-absorbing narrow interests (at least one of the following):
   - exclusion of other activities
   - repetitive adherence
   - more rote than meaning
3. Imposition of routines and interests (at least one of the following):
   - on self, in aspects of life
   - on others
4. Speech and language problems (at least three of the following):
   - delayed development
   - superficially perfect expressive language
   - formal, pedantic language
   - odd prosody, peculiar voice characteristics
   - impairment of comprehension including misinterpretations of literal/implied meanings
5. Nonverbal communication problems (at least one of the following):
   - limited use of gestures
   - clumsy/gauche body language
   - limited facial expression
   - inappropriate expression
   - peculiar, stiff gaze
6. Motor clumsiness, poor performance on neurodevelopmental examination

Asperger's disorder (ICD-10: WHO 1993)
A. There is no clinically significant general delay in spoken or receptive language or cognitive development. Diagnosis requires that single words should have developed by 2 years of age or earlier and that communicative phrases be used by 3 years of age or earlier. Self-help skills, adaptive behaviour, and curiosity about the environment during the first 3 years should be at a level consistent with normal intellectual development. However, motor milestones may be somewhat delayed and motor clumsiness is usual (although not a necessary diagnostic feature). Isolated special skills, often related to abnormal preoccupations, are common, but are not required for diagnosis
B. There are qualitative abnormalities in reciprocal social interaction (criteria as for autism)
C. The individual exhibits an unusually intense, circumscribed interest or restricted, repetitive, and stereotyped patterns of behaviour, interests, and activities (criteria as for autism; however, it would be less usual for these to include either motor mannerisms or preoccupations with part-objects or nonfunctional elements of play materials)
D. The disorder is not attributable to the other varieties of pervasive developmental disorder: simple schizophrenia; schizotypal disorder; obsessive–compulsive disorder; anancastic personality disorder; reactive and disinhibited attachment disorders of childhood

Asperger syndrome (DSM-IV: American Psychiatric Association 1994)
A. Qualitative impairment in social interaction, as manifested by at least two of the following:
   (1) marked impairment in the use of multiple nonverbal behaviours such as eye-to-eye gaze, facial expression, body postures, and gestures to regulate social interaction
   (2) failure to develop peer relationships appropriate to developmental level
   (3) a lack of spontaneous seeking to share enjoyment, interests, or achievements with other people (e.g. by lack of showing, bringing, or pointing out objects of interest to other people)
   (4) lack of social or emotional reciprocity
B. Restricted repetitive and stereotyped patterns of behaviour, interests, and activities, as manifested by at least one of the following:
   (1) encompassing preoccupation with one or more stereotyped and restricted patterns of interest that is abnormal either in intensity or focus
   (2) apparently inflexible adherence to specific, nonfunctional routines or rituals
   (3) stereotyped and repetitive motor mannerisms (e.g. hand or finger flapping or twisting, or complex whole-body movements)
   (4) persistent preoccupation with parts of objects
C. The disturbance causes clinically significant impairments in social, occupational or other important areas of functioning
D. There is no clinically significant general delay in language (e.g. single words used by age 2 years, communicative phrases used by age 3 years)
E. There is no clinically significant delay in cognitive development or in the development of age-appropriate self-help skills, adaptive behaviour (other than in social interaction), and curiosity about the environment in childhood
F. Criteria are not met for another specific pervasive developmental disorder or for schizophrenia

INTERVENTIONS

Specific treatment for Asperger syndrome is not available. The best approach is to make a proper diagnosis, to give oral and written information to those concerned, to offer educational and other measures intended to improve school adjustment, and to follow up (yearly if appropriate, more often if necessary). Attempts should be made to find areas of interest that might eventually provide a basis for a good education and adult hobbies, and to actively avoid areas that may hold potential danger (e.g. 'violent' sports). Medication makes little difference in most cases and may have harmful side effects. The new serotonin reuptake inhibitors (e.g. sertraline and fluoxetine) may be effective in reducing ritualistic behaviours and may improve mood. Psychotherapy is usually not indicated, but supportive talks on a regular basis with somebody knowledgeable in the field can be helpful, particularly in the teenage period when some insight into the situation is often gained and the experience of being different from one's peers can become overwhelming. For younger children with Asperger syndrome, group sessions can also be of value (Mesibov and Stephens 1990).

Parents often ask about the genetic risk for themselves, for the affected child and for his/her siblings. There is a risk that more cases of Asperger syndrome will occur in the family (Bowman 1988). At least half of all children with Asperger syndrome have a parent with the same (or very similar) condition (Gillberg et al. 2005). This should be acknowledged truthfully, while at the same time emphasizing the relatively benign character of the problems. However, the possibility that Asperger syndrome might be genetically linked to classic autism makes counselling in this respect somewhat difficult. Recent estimates for siblings are not available. In a study of 23 children with Asperger syndrome (Gillberg 1989), one boy had a brother with autism (and another brother with mild Asperger syndrome) and one girl had a sister with selective mutism (and Asperger traits). In another, more recent study, 70 of 100 males with Asperger syndrome had a first-degree relative with autistic features, a small proportion of whom had classic autistic disorder.

Adult psychiatrists need to be aware of the existence of Asperger syndrome. In stressful situations, young adults with the syndrome are often referred to psychiatrists because of obsessiveness, feelings of helplessness and chaotic reactions. Because of limited facial expression, mimicry and gestures they may be diagnosed as depressed or paranoid and accordingly treated with antidepressants or neuroleptic drugs, which usually do little to alter the course of the disorder. Quite often, stress relief combined with the appreciation that this is only part of a life-long condition will go a long way in reducing acute symptoms.

OUTCOME

Only a fraction of all children with Asperger syndrome apply for paediatric or psychiatric help specifically as a consequence of their 'Asperger problems'. Therefore, follow-up of cases seen in clinics will not necessarily yield a true picture of outcome. So far, the only studies of outcome available refer either to such populations or to groups assessed in adult psychiatric clinics and diagnosed retrospectively as possibly having had symptoms and signs of Asperger syndrome from early childhood (Tantam 1988). The overall impression is that many children with Asperger syndrome diagnosed in childhood, although not outgrowing the basic problems, manage fairly well in adult life, at least with respect to education, employment and marriage (Gillberg et al. 2005). Equally obvious, however, is the tendency for some to have severe psychiatric problems (often diagnosed as depression, paranoia, non-regressive schizophrenia, or 'borderline' psychosis or personality disorder), to attempt suicide or develop alcoholism (Wing 1981a), or to commit criminal offences (usually directly associated with one or other extreme interest, e.g. gunpowder, poisonous chemicals, fire) (Baron-Cohen 1988, Everall and Le Couteur 1990, Scragg and Shah 1994).

SELECTIVE MUTISM

Some children do not speak to more than a very limited number of people from early childhood, throughout the early school years and often into adolescence and adult life. It is not that they cannot speak, indeed some of them can be verbally demanding and talkative when in their home environment. They do, however, refuse to say a word to most people outside of the immediate family (perhaps excluding even one or more members of the family). A few have one or two friends with whom they will communicate verbally. Some are mute most of the time but will occasionally give up their complete silence to whisper a few words. This group of children who can speak but who do so with only a very limited number of people are referred to as having '(s)elective mutism' (Kolvin and Fundudis 1981). Many 'shy' children are temporarily silent on entering preschool or school. If their silence is of a transient nature, they should not be considered for a diagnosis of selective mutism.

The child with selective mutism probably can have normal language development but often shows delay and deviance; there are frequently minor associated developmental disorders such as enuresis and slight motor delay; it appears that there may be a markedly increased rate of epilepsy; IQ tends to be lower than in the general population of children; typical symptoms usually appear before the child's fourth birthday; there is often a family history of psychiatric disorder, 'shyness' and selective mutism; and the outcome is variable but probably restricted, although it may be excellent in individual cases. Many features of selective mutism are similar to those encountered in relatively high-functioning autistic-like conditions.

Children with selective mutism are usually shy, avoidant and sometimes clearly withdrawn. Also, many are described as being strong-willed and have outbursts of rage if demands or changes of routine are made. Gillberg (1989) noted the association of selective mutism and Asperger traits (see above).

Selective mutism is rare, occurring in severe forms (with a duration of more than 1 year) in 0.6–2 per 1000 children (Kolvin and Fundudis 1981, Kopp and Gillberg 1997, Kristensen 2002). The boy/girl ratio appears to be equal, or with a slight preponderance in females.

The psychological and medical work-up should include a cognitive test and a thorough clinical examination aimed at detecting hearing deficits and symptoms and signs suggestive of autistic disorder. The possibility of associated medical conditions should be entertained. I know of two cases with the combination of elective mutism and neurofibromatosis.

Treatment in elective mutism has to focus on training of basic social skills and activities of daily life, to enable the child/adolescent to accept the company of others and to express – at least in writing – his/her academic skills. Psychotherapeutic or psychopharmacological approaches have not been successful according to clinical experience.

CHILDHOOD SCHIZOPHRENIA

Autism and autistic-like conditions were long considered synonymous with childhood schizophrenia. Since about 1970, however, childhood schizophrenia has been regarded as a clearly separate condition, implying a severe disorder of affect and thought, showing before 10 years of age with typical schizophrenic thought disorder, hallucinations and emotional bluntness. It appears to be very rare, maybe occurring in no more than 2–3 per 100,000 children. Some authors have even questioned the existence of typical schizophrenia in early childhood. In recent years, however, US authors have reintroduced the term when referring to early-onset conditions on the autism spectrum (e.g. Asarnow et al. 1988). Others regard it as a more distinct syndrome with symptom onset at any age between 5 and 12 years (Caplan et al. 1989, Werry et al. 1991, Murray 1994, Remschmidt et al. 1994). The male:female ratio in this very early onset variant of schizophrenia is reported to be in the range of 2:1–3:1. From the age of 13 years and up, authors in the USA and elsewhere agree that schizophrenia is more common and that the male:female ratio is closer to equality, as seen in adulthood (Harris 1995a,b). Stayer et al. (2004) have drawn attention to the risk of overdiagnosing schizophrenia in young children who behave in disruptive and confused ways.

Neuroleptics are likely to be more effective than in autism, and outcome is supposedly better. However, no good population-based follow-up studies exist, and the matter cannot be regarded as settled.

REFERENCES

Åkefeldt A, Gillberg C (1991) Hypomelanosis of Ito in three cases with autism and autistic-like conditions. *Dev Med Child Neurol* 33: 737–43.

Akinsola HA, Fryers T (1986) A comparison of patterns of disability in severely mentally handicapped children of different ethnic origins. *Psychol Med* 16: 127–33.

APA (1980) *Diagnostic and Statistical Manual of Mental Disorders, 3rd edn (DSM-III).* Washington, DC: American Psychiatric Association.

APA (1987) *Diagnostic and Statistical Manual of Mental Disorders, 3rd edn— Revised (DSM-III-R).* Washington, DC: American Psychiatric Association.

APA (1994) *Diagnostic and Statistical Manual of Mental Disorders, 4th edn (DSM-IV).* Washington, DC: American Psychiatric Association.

APA (2000) *Diagnostic and Statistical Manual of Mental Disorders, 4th edn, Text Revision (DSM-IV-TR).* Washington, DC: American Psychiatric Association.

Asarnow JW, Goldstein MJ, Ben-Meir S (1988) Parental communication deviance in childhood onset schizophrenia spectrum and depressive disorders. *J Child Psychol Psychiatry* 29: 825–38.

Ashwin C, Wheelwright S, Baron-Cohen S (2005) Laterality biases to chimeric faces in Asperger syndrome: what is 'right' about face-processing? *J Autism Dev Disord* 35: 183–96.

Asperger H (1944) Die autistischen Psychopathen im Kindesalter. *Archiv Psychiatrie Nervenkrankh* 117: 76–136.

Bågenholm A, Gillberg C (1992) [Autism and mental retardation. More attention should be paid to sibling relations when helping families with severely handicapped children in the future.] *Läkartidningen* 89: 555–60 (Swedish).

Baron-Cohen S (1988) An assessment of violence in a young man with Asperger's syndrome. *J Child Psychol Psychiatry* 29: 351–60.

Baron-Cohen S, Belmonte MK (2005) Autism: a window onto the development of the social and the analytic brain. *Annu Rev Neurosci* 28: 109–26.

Barthélémy C, Bruneau N, Cottet-Eymard JM, et al. (1988) Urinary free and conjugated catecholamines and metabolites in autistic children. *J Autism Dev Disord* 18: 583–91.

Bender L (1947) Childhood schizophrenia. Clinical study of one hundred schizophrenic children. *Am J Orthopsychiatry* 17: 40–56.

Billstedt E, Gillberg IC, Gillberg C (2005) Autism after adolescence: population-based 13- to 22-year follow-up study of 120 individuals with autism diagnosed in childhood. *J Autism Dev Disord* 35: 351–60; erratum in: *J Autism Dev Disord* 2007 37: 1822.

Bishop DVM (1989) Autism, Asperger's syndrome and semantic–pragmatic disorders. Where are the boundaries? *Br J Disord Commun* 24: 107–21.

Bleuler E (1911) *Dementia Praecox or the Group of Schizophrenias.* Vienna: F Deuticke. (Translated by J Zinkin, 1950. New York: International Universities Press.)

Bolton P, Rutter M (1990) Genetic influences in autism. *Int Rev Psychiatry* 2: 67–80.

Bolton P, Macdonald H, Pickles A, et al. (1994) A case–control family history study of autism. *J Child Psychol Psychiatry* 35: 877–900.

Bowman EP (1988) Asperger's syndrome and autism: the case for a connection. *Br J Psychiatry* 152: 377–82.

Bryson SE, Clark BS, Smith IM (1988) First report of a Canadian epidemiological study of autistic syndromes. *J Child Psychol Psychiatry* 29: 433–45.

Buitelaar JK, Willemsen-Swinkels SH (2000) Medication treatment in subjects with autistic spectrum disorders. *Eur Child Adolesc Psychiatry* 9 Suppl 1: I85–97.

Burd L, Fisher W, Kerbeshian J (1989) Pervasive disintegrative disorder: are Rett syndrome and Heller dementia infantilis subtypes? *Dev Med Child Neurol* 31: 609–16.

Campbell M (1989) Pharmacotherapy in autism: an overview. In: Gillberg C, ed. *Diagnosis and Treatment of Autism.* New York: Plenum, pp. 203–18.

Caplan R, Guthrie D, Fish B, et al. (1989) The Kiddie Formal Thought Disorder Rating Scale: clinical assessment, reliability, and validity. *J Am Acad Child Adolesc Psychiatry* 28: 408–16.

Cederlund M, Gillberg C (2004) One hundred males with Asperger syndrome: a clinical study of background and associated factors. *Dev Med Child Neurol* 46: 652–60.

Celiberti DA, Bobo HE, Kelly KS, et al. (1997) The differential and temporal effects of antecedent exercise on the self-stimulatory behavior of a child with autism. *Res Dev Disabil* 18: 139–50.

Chess S, Korn SJ, Fernandez PB (1971) *Psychiatric Disorders of Children with Congenital Rubella.* New York: Brunner/Mazel.

Coleman M (2005) Advances in autism research. *Dev Med Child Neurol* 47: 148.

Coleman M, Blass JP (1985) Autism and lactic acidosis. *J Autism Dev Disord* 15: 1–8.

Cook EH (1990) Autism: review of neurochemical investigation. *Synapse* 6: 292–308.

Dahlgren Sandberg A, Nydén A, Gillberg C, Hjelmquist E (1993) The cognitive profile in infantile autism—a study of 70 children and adolescents using the Griffiths Mental Development Scale. *Br J Psychol* 84: 365–73.

Danielsson S, Gillberg IC, Billstedt E, et al. (2005) Epilepsy in young adults with autism: a prospective population-based follow-up study of 120 individuals diagnosed in childhood. *Epilepsia* 46: 918–23.

Delorme R, Betancur C, Wagner M, et al. (2005) Support for the association between the rare functional variant I425V of the serotonin transporter gene and susceptibility to obsessive compulsive disorder. *Mol Psychiatry* 10: 1059–61.

Di Martino A, Melis G, Cianchetti C, Zuddas A (2004) Methylphenidate for pervasive developmental disorders: safety and efficacy of acute single dose test and ongoing therapy: an open-pilot study. *J Child Adolesc Psychopharmacol* 14: 207–18.

Dissanayake C, Crossley SA (1996) Proximity and sociable behaviours in autism: evidence for attachment. *J Child Psychol Psychiatry* 37: 149–56.

Doll EA (1965) *Vineland Social Maturity Scale.* Circle Pines, MN: American Guidance Service.

Dunn LM (1970) *Peabody Picture Vocabulary Test.* Circle Pines, MN: American Guidance Service.

Ehlers S, Gillberg C (1993) The epidemiology of Asperger syndrome. A total population study. *J Child Psychol Psychiatry* 34: 1327–50.

Ek U, Fernell E, Jacobson L, Gillberg C (1998) Relation between blindness due to retinopathy of prematurity and autistic spectrum disorders: a population-based study. *Dev Med Child Neurol* 40: 297–301.

Everall IP, LeCouteur A (1990) Firesetting in an adolescent boy with Asperger's syndrome. *Br J Psychiatry* 157: 284–7.

Fitzgerald M (2005) Borderline personality disorder and Asperger syndrome. *Autism* 9: 452.

Folstein S, Rutter M (1977) Infantile autism: a genetic study of 21 twin pairs. *J Child Psychol Psychiatry* 18: 297–321.

Fombonne E (2003) The prevalence of autism. *JAMA* 289: 87–9.

Friedman E (1969) The autistic syndrome and phenylketonuria. *Schizophrenia* 1: 249–61.

Frith U (1989) *Autism: Explaining the Enigma.* Oxford: Basil Blackwell.

Frith U, ed. (1991) *Autism and Asperger Syndrome.* Cambridge: Cambridge University Press.

Frith U (2004) Is autism a disconnection disorder? *Lancet Neurol* 3: 577.

Gillberg C (1986) Onset at age 14 of a typical autistic syndrome. A case report of a girl with herpes simplex encephalitis. *J Autism Dev Disord* 16: 369–75.

Gillberg C (1989) Asperger syndrome in 23 Swedish children. *Dev Med Child Neurol* 31: 520–31.

Gillberg C (1991a) Clinical and neurobiological aspects of Asperger syndrome in six family studies. In: Frith U, ed. *Autism and Asperger Syndrome.* Cambridge: Cambridge University Press, pp. 122–46.

Gillberg C (1991b) Outcome in autism and autistic-like conditions. *J Am Acad Child Adolesc Psychiatry* 30: 375–82.

Gillberg C (1991c) The treatment of epilepsy in autism. *J Autism Dev Disord* 21: 61–77.

Gillberg C (1992) The Emanuel Miller Memorial Lecture 1991. Autism and autistic-like conditions: subclasses among disorders of empathy. *J Child Psychol Psychiatry* 33: 813–42.

Gillberg C (1995) Endogenous opioids and opiate antagonists in autism: brief review of empirical findings and implications for clinicians. *Dev Med Child Neurol* 37: 239–45.

Gillberg C, Cederlund M (2005) Asperger syndrome: familial and pre- and perinatal factors. *J Autism Dev Disord* 35: 159–66.

Gillberg C, Coleman M (1996) Autism and medical disorders: a review of the literature. *Dev Med Child Neurol* 38: 191–202.

Gillberg C, Coleman M (2000) *The Biology of the Autistic Syndromes, 3rd edn. Clinics in Developmental Medicine No. 153.* London: Mac Keith Press.

Gillberg C, Forsell C (1984) Childhood psychosis and neurofibromatosis—more than a coincidence? *J Autism Dev Disord* 14: 1–8.

Gillberg C, Gillberg IC (1983) Infantile autism: a total population study of reduced optimality in the pre-, peri-, and neonatal period. *J Autism Dev Disord* 13: 153–66.

Gillberg C, Gillberg IC (1991) Note on the relationship between population-based and clinical studies: the question of reduced optimality in autism. *J Autism Dev Disord* 21: 251–4 (letter).

Gillberg C, Schaumann H (1983) Epilepsy presenting as infantile autism? Two case studies. *Neuropediatrics* 14: 206–12.

Gillberg C, Steffenburg S (1987) Outcome and prognostic factors in infantile autism and similar conditions: a population-based study of 46 cases followed through puberty. *J Autism Dev Disord* 17: 273–87.

Gillberg C, Svennerholm L (1987) CSF-monoamines in autistic syndromes and other pervasive developmental disorders of early childhood. *Br J Psychiatry* 151: 89–94.

Gillberg C, Wing L (1999) Autism: not an extremely rare disorder. *Acta Psychiatr Scand* 99: 399–406.

Gillberg C, Winnergård I, Wahlström J (1984) The sex chromosomes—one key to autism? An XYY case of infantile autism. *Appl Res Ment Retard* 5: 353–60.

Gillberg C, Terenius L, Lönnerholm G (1985) Endorphin activity in childhood psychosis. Spinal fluid levels in 24 cases. *Arc Gen Psychiatry* 42: 780–3.

Gillberg C, Steffenburg S, Jakobsson G (1987) Neurobiological findings in 20 relatively gifted children with Kanner-type autism or Asperger syndrome.

Dev Med Child Neurol 29: 641–9.

Gillberg C, Steffenburg S, Wahlström J, et al. (1991) Autism associated with marker chromosome. *J Am Acad Child Adolesc Psychiatry* 30: 489–94.

Gillberg C, Gillberg IC, Steffenburg S (1992) Siblings and parents of children with autism: a controlled population-based study. *Dev Med Child Neurol* 34: 389–98.

Gillberg C, Melander H, von Knorring AL, et al. (1997) Long-term stimulant treatment of children with attention-deficit hyperactivity disorder symptoms. A randomized, double-blind, placebo-controlled trial. *Arch Gen Psychiatry* 54: 857–64.

Gillberg C, Gillberg C, Råstam M, Wentz E (2001) The Asperger Syndrome (and high-functioning autism) Diagnostic Interview (ASDI): a preliminary study of a new structured clinical interview. *Autism* 5: 57–66.

Gillberg C, Cederlund M, Lamberg K, Zeijlon L (2006) Brief report: "The autism epidemic". The registered prevalence of autism in a Swedish urban area. *J Autism Dev Disord* 36: 429–35.

Gillberg IC, Gillberg C (1989) Asperger syndrome—some epidemiological considerations: a research note. *J Child Psychol Psychiatry* 30: 631–8.

Griffiths RG (1970) *The Abilities of Young Children. A Comprehensive System of Mental Measurement for the First Eight Years of Life.* High Wycombe, Bucks: The Test Agency.

Gualtieri CT (1987) Reappraisal of "Fenfluramine and autism: careful reappraisal is in order." Reply. *J Pediatr* 110: 159–60 (letter).

Hagerman RJ (1989) Chromosomes, genes and autism. In: Gillberg C, ed. *Diagnosis and Treatment of Autism.* New York: Plenum Press, pp. 105–32.

Happé FGE (1994) Current psychological theories of autism: the "theory of mind" account and rival theories. *J Child Psychol Psychiatry* 35: 215–29.

Happé F, Ehlers S, Fletcher P, et al. (1996) 'Theory of mind' in the brain. Evidence from a PET scan study of Asperger syndrome. *Neuroreport* 8: 197–201.

Haracopos D (1989) Comprehensive treatment program for autistic children and adults in Denmark. In: Gillberg C, ed. *Diagnosis and Treatment of Autism.* New York: Plenum Press, pp. 251–61.

Harris JC (1995a) *Developmental Neuropsychiatry. I. The Fundamentals.* Oxford: Oxford University Press.

Harris JC (1995b) *Developmental Neuropsychiatry. II. Assessment, Diagnosis and Treatment of Developmental Disorders.* Oxford: Oxford University Press.

Haslam J (1809) *Observations on Madness and Melancholy.* London: Hayden.

Heller T (1930) Über Dementia infantilis. *Zeitschr Kinderforschung* 37: 661–7.

Hertzig ME, Snow ME, New E, Shapiro T (1990) DSM-III and DSM-III-R diagnosis of autism and pervasive developmental disorder in nursery school children. *J Am Aca Child Adolesc Psychiatry* 29: 123–6.

Hobson RP (1993) *Autism and the Development of Mind.* London: Lawrence Erlbaum.

Howlin P (1997) Prognosis in autism: do specialist treatments affect long-term outcome? *Eur Child Adolesc Psychiatry* 6: 55–72.

Howlin P (2005) The effectiveness of interventions for children with autism. *J Neural Transm Suppl* (69): 101–19.

Howlin P, Rutter M (1987) *Treatment of Autistic Children. Wiley Series on Studies in Child Psychiatry.* London: John Wiley.

Howlin P, Yates P (1989) Treating autistic children at home. A London based programme. In: Gillberg C, ed. *Diagnosis and Treatment of Autism.* New York: Plenum, pp. 307–22.

Hunt A, Dennis J (1987) Psychiatric disorder among children with tuberous sclerosis. *Dev Med Child Neurol* 29: 190–8.

Jacobsson L, Broberger U, Fernell E, et al. (1998) Children with blindness due to retinopathy of prematurity: a population-based study. Perinatal data, neurological and ophthalmological outcome. *Dev Med Child Neurol* 40: 155–9.

Jamain S, Quach H, Betancur C, et al. (2003) Mutations of the X-linked genes encoding neuroligins NLGN3 and NLGN4 are associated with autism. *Nat Genet* 34: 27–9.

Kadesjö B, Gillberg C, Hagberg B (1999) Brief report: autism and Asperger syndrome in seven-year-old children: a total population study. *J Autism Dev Disord* 29: 327–31.

Kanner L (1943) Autistic disturbances of affective contact. *Nerv Child* 2: 217–50.

Kerbeshian J, Burd L, Randall T, et al. (1990) Autism, profound mental retardation and atypical bipolar disorder in a 33-year-old female with a deletion of 15q12. *J Ment Defic Res* 34: 205–10.

Kolvin I, Fundudis T (1981) Elective mute children: psychological development and background factors. *J Child Psychol Psychiatry* 22: 219–32.

Komoto J, Udsui S, Otsuki S, Terao A (1984) Infantile autism and Duchenne muscular dystrophy. *J Autism Dev Disord* **14**: 191–5.

Kopp S, Gillberg C (1997) Selective mutism: a population-based study: a research note. *J Child Psychol Psychiatry* **38**: 257–62.

Korkman M, Kirk V, Kemp SL (1997) *A Developmental Neuropsychological Assessment.* San Antonio, TX: Psychological Corporation.

Kristensen H (2002) Non-specific markers of neurodevelopmental disorder/delay in selective mutism—a case–control study. *Eur Child Adolesc Psychiatry* **11**: 71–8.

Krug DA, Arick J, Almond P (1980) Behavior checklist for identifying severely handicapped individuals with high levels of autistic behavior. *J Child Psychol Psychiatry* **21**: 221–9.

Leekam SR, Libby SJ, Wing L, et al. (2002) The Diagnostic Interview for Social and Communication Disorders: algorithms for IC-10 childhood autism and Wing and Gould autistic spectrum disorder. *J Child Psychol Psychiatry* **43**: 327–42.

Leiter RG (1980) *Leiter International Performance Scale: Instruction Manual.* Chicago: Stoelting.

Lelord G, Muh JP, Barthélémy C, et al. (1981) Effects of pyridoxine and magnesium on autistic symptoms—initial observations. *J Autism Dev Disord* **11**: 219–30.

Lord C, Rutter M, Le Couteur A (1994) Autism Diagnostic Interview—Revised: a revised version of a diagnostic interview for caregivers of individuals with possible pervasive developmental disorders. *J Autism Dev Disord* **24**: 659–85.

Lowenthal R, Paula CS, Schwartzman JS, et al. (2007) Prevalence of pervasive developmental disorder in Down's syndrome. *J Autism Dev Disord* **37**: 1394–5.

Mahler MS (1952) On child psychoses and schizophrenia: autistic and symbiotic infantile psychoses. *Psychoanal Study Child* **7**: 286–305.

Malone RP, Gratz SS, Delaney MA, Hyman SB (2005) Advances in drug treatments for children and adolescents with autism and other pervasive developmental disorders. *CNS Drugs* **19**: 923–34.

Malson L, ed. (1964) *Les Enfants Sauvages—Mythe et Realité.* Paris: Union Generale d'Editions.

McCracken JT, McGough J, Shah B, et al. (2002) Risperidone in children with autism and serious behavioral problems. *N Engl J Med* **347**: 314-21.

McGimsey JF, Favell JE (1988) The effects of increased physical exercise on disruptive behavior in retarded persons. *J Autism Dev Disord* **18**: 167–9.

Mesibov GB, Stephens J (1990) Perception of popularity among a group of high-functioning adults with autism. *J Autism Dev Disord* **20**: 33–43.

Mesibov GB, Schopler E, Caison W (1989) The Adolescent and Adult Psychoeducational Profile: assessment of adolescents and adults with severe developmental handicaps. *J Autism Dev Disord* **19**: 33–40.

Miller JN, Ozonoff S (1997) Did Asperger's cases have Asperger disorder? A research note. *J Child Psychol Psychiatry* **38**: 247–51.

Millward C, Ferriter M, Calver S, Connell-Jones G (2008) Gluten- and casein-free diets for autistic spectrum disorder. *Cochrane Database Syst Rev* (2): CD003498.

Minshew NJ, Williams DL (2007) The new neurobiology of autism: cortex, connectivity, and neuronal organization. *Arch Neurol* **64**: 945–50; erratum 1464.

Murphy M, Bolton PF, Pickles A, et al. (2000) Personality traits of the relatives of autistic probands. *Psychol Med* **30**: 1411–24.

Murray RM (1994) Neurodevelopmental schizophrenia: the rediscovery of dementia praecox. *Br J Psychiatry* **25** (Suppl): 6–12.

Niklasson L, Rasmussen P, Oskarsdóttir S, Gillberg C (2001) Neuropsychiatric disorders in the 22q11 deletion syndrome. *Genet Med* **3**: 79–84.

Nordin V, Gillberg C (1996) Autism spectrum disorders in children with physical or mental disability or both. Part I: Clinical and epidemiological aspects. *Dev Med Child Neurol* **38**: 297–313.

Nordin V, Lekman A, Johansson M, et al. (1998) Gangliosides in cerebrospinal fluid in children with autism spectrum disorders. *Dev Med Child Neurol* **40**: 587–94.

Ornitz EM, Guthrie D, Farley AH (1977) The early development of autistic children. *J Autism Child Schizophr* **7**: 207–29.

Ozonoff S, Miller JN (1995) Teaching theory of mind. A new approach to social skills training for individuals with autism. *J Autism Dev Disord* **25**: 415–33.

Phelan MC (2008) Deletion 22q13.3 syndrome. *Orphanet J Rare Dis* **3**: 14.

Philippe A, Martinez M, Guilloud-Bataille M, et al. (1999) Genome-wide scan for autism susceptibility genes. Paris Autism Research International Sibpair Study. *Hum Mol Genet* **8**: 805–12; erratum 1353.

Posserud MB, Lundervold AJ, Gillberg C (2006) Autistic features in a total

population of 7–9-year-old children assessed by the ASSQ (Autism Spectrum Screening Questionnaire). *J Child Psychol Psychiatry* **47**: 167–75.

Rank B (1949) Adaptation of the psycho-analytic technique for the treatment of young children with atypical development. *Am J Orthopsychiatry* **19**: 130–9.

Rapin I, ed. (1996) *Preschool Children with Inadequate Communication. Developmental Language Disorder, Autism, Low IQ. Clinics in Developmental Medicine No. 139.* London: Mac Keith Press.

Reiss AL, Feinstein C, Rosenbaum KN, et al. (1985) Autism associated with Williams syndrome. *J Pediatr* **106**: 247–9.

Remschmidt HE, Schulz E, Martin M, et al. (1994) Childhood-onset schizophrenia: history of the concept and recent studies. *Schizophr Bull* **20**: 727–45.

Reynell J (1969) *Reynell Developmental Language Scales.* Windsor, Berks: NFER.

Rosenhall U, Nordin V, Brantberg K, Gillberg C (2003) Autism and auditory brain stem responses. *Ear Hear* **24**: 206–14.

Rutter M (1978a) Diagnosis and definition. In: Rutter M, Schopler E, eds. *Autism. A Reappraisal of Concepts and Treatment.* New York: Plenum Press, pp. 1–25.

Rutter M (1978b) Diagnosis and definition of childhood autism. *J Autism Child Schizophr* **8**: 139–61.

Schopler E (1989) Principles for directing both educational treatment and research. In: Gillberg C, ed. *Diagnosis and Treatment of Autism.* New York: Plenum Press, pp. 167–83.

Schopler E, Reichler RJ, DeVellis RF, Daly K (1980) Towards objective classification of childhood autism: Childhood Autism Rating Scale (CARS). *J Autism Dev Disord* **10**: 91–103.

Schopler E, Reichler RJ, Renner BR (1988) *The Childhood Autism Rating Scale (CARS). Revised.* Los Angeles: Western Psychological Services.

Scragg P, Shah A (1994) Prevalence of Asperger's syndrome in a secure hospital. *Br J Psychiatry* **165**: 679–82.

Sigman M, Mundy P (1989) Social attachments in autistic children. *J Am Acad Child Adolesc Psychiatry* **28**: 74–81.

Sikora DM, Pettit-Kekel K, Penfield J, et al. (2006) The near universal presence of autism spectrum disorders in children with Smith–Lemli–Opitz syndrome. *Am J Med Genet A* **140**: 1511–8.

Smith DE, Miller SD, Stewart M, et al. (1988) Conductive hearing loss in autistic, learning-disabled, and normal children. *J Autism Dev Disord* **18**: 53–65.

Sparrow SS, Cicchetti DV (1985) Diagnostic uses of the Vineland Adaptive Behavior Scales. *J Pediatr Psychol* **10**: 215–25.

Ssucharewa GE (1926) Die schizoiden Psychopathien im Kindesalter. *Monatsschr Psychiatrie Neurol* **60**: 235–61.

Stayer C, Sporn A, Gogtay N, et al. (2004) Looking for childhood schizophrenia: case series of false positives. *J Am Acad Child Adolesc Psychiatry* **43**: 1026–9.

Steffenburg S (1990) Neurobiological correlates of autism. MD thesis, University of Göteborg.

Steffenburg S (1991) Neuropsychiatric assessment of children with autism: a population-based study. *Dev Med Child Neurol* **33**: 495–511.

Steffenburg S, Gillberg C, Steffenburg U, Kyllerman M (1996) Autism in Angelman syndrome. A population-based study. *Pediatr Neurol* **14**: 131–6.

Strömland K, Nordin V, Miller M, et al. (1994) Autism in thalidomide embryopathy: a population study. *Dev Med Child Neurol* **36**: 351–6.

Stubbs EG (1978) Autistic symptoms in a child with congenital cytomegalovirus infection. *J Autism Child Schizophr* **8**: 37–43.

Tantam D (1988) Asperger's syndrome. *J Child Psychol Psychiatry* **29**: 245–55.

Teitelbaum P, Teitelbaum O, Nye J, et al. (1998) Movement analysis in infancy may be useful for early diagnosis of autism. *Proc Natl Acad Sci USA* **95**: 13982–7.

Tinbergen N, Tinbergen EA (1983) *Autistic Children. New Hope for a Cure.* London: Allen & Unwin.

Troost PW, Lahuis BE, Steenhuis MP, et al. (2005) Long-term effects of risperidone in children with autism spectrum disorders: a placebo discontinuation study. *J Am Acad Child Adolesc Psychiatry* **44**: 1137–44.

Tsai LY (1989) Recent neurobiological findings in autism. In: Gillberg C, ed. *Diagnosis and Treatment of Autism.* New York: Plenum Press, pp. 83–104.

Volkmar FR, Rutter M (1995) Childhood disintegrative disorder: results of the DSM-IV autism field trial. *J Am Acad Child Adolesc Psychiatry* **34**: 1092–5.

von Knorring A-L (1991) Outcome in autism. *Svensk Med* **23**: 34–6.

Wassink TH, Piven J (2000) The molecular genetics of autism. *Curr Psychiatry Rep* **2**: 170–5.

Wechsler D (2003) *WISC-IV Technical and Interpretive Manual.* London:

Harcourt Assessment.

Wellman HM, Baron-Cohen S, Caswell R, et al. (2002) Thought-bubbles help children with autism acquire an alternative to a theory of mind. *Autism* **6**: 343–63.

Werry JS, McClellan JM, Chard L (1991) Childhood and adolescent schizophrenic, bipolar, and schizoaffective disorders: a clinical and outcome study. *J Am Acad Child Adolesce Psychiatry* **30**: 457–65.

WHO (1993) *The ICD-10 Classification of Mental and Behavioural Disorders. Clinical Descriptions and Guidelines.* Geneva: World Health Organization.

Wing L (1981a) Asperger's syndrome: a clinical account. *Psychol Med* **11**: 115–29.

Wing L (1981b) Sex ratios in early childhood autism and related conditions. *Psychiatry Res* **5**: 129–37.

Wing L (1989) Autistic adults. In: Gillberg C, ed. *Diagnosis and Treatment of Autism.* New York: Plenum Press, pp. 419–32.

Wing L, Gould J (1979) Severe impairments of social interaction and associated abnormalities in children: epidemiology and classification. *J Autism Dev Disord* **9**: 11–29.

Wing L, Potter D (2002) The epidemiology of autistic disorders: is the prevalence rising? *Ment Retard Dev Disabil Res Rev* **8**: 151–61.

Yeargin-Allsopp M, Rice C, Karapurkar T, et al. (2003) Prevalence of autism in a US metropolitan area. *JAMA* **289**: 49–55.

25

ATTENTION DEFICIT HYPERACTIVITY DISORDER AND COEXISTING IMPAIRMENTS

Christopher Gillberg

The symptoms of attention deficit hyperactivity disorder (ADHD) have been with us as long as history has been recorded. The first description by a physician of ADHD probably dates back to an 1844 poem, 'The Story of Fidgety Phil' by German psychiatrist Heinrich Hoffmann. In 1902 the British paediatrician George Still described overactive children with discipline problems who seemed to have a syndrome of "moral dyscontrol". Still described 20 children (15 boys and 5 girls) who were oppositional–defiant, overly emotional, passionate, lawless and spiteful, had little inhibitory volition, and whose problems had started at or under the age of 7 years. The children had been raised in benign environments, with "good-enough" parenting. Still speculated that there might be a biological, possibly genetic, basis to the children's behaviour. He also discovered that some members of these children's families had psychiatric difficulties such as depression, alcoholism and conduct problems.

In 1937, Dr Charles Bradley reported remarkable improvement in the types of behaviour problems that Still had described in the school performance of children who were given the stimulant benzedrine. His work set the standard for treating ADHD with stimulants.

Over the past 70 years, a number of behavioural and learning disorders have been lumped together under the uninformative label of 'minimal brain dysfunction' (MBD). The roots of this unfortunate diagnostic etiquette are to be found about 1920, when, on the basis of studies of children with encephalitis, it was surmised that a characteristic syndrome of overactivity often developed as a consequence of brain damage sustained in utero or in early childhood. Reciprocally, the notion gradually emerged that overactivity was in itself a sign that the child was brain damaged. Subsequent empirical study has shown that (a) overactivity is not usually a sign of brain damage, and (b) brain damage does not usually lead to overactivity (Rutter 1982).

SYNONYMS

A comprehensive survey of all the many synonyms and partly overlapping concepts used in this field is beyond the scope of this book. However, a list of some of the most common diagnostic labels (Table 25.1) is appropriate, as an introduction to a description of the symptom profiles encountered in children who have been given the (often inappropriate) label of MBD over the past 50 years.

The array of labels testifies to the confusion in this field. However, in recent years, emerging consensus supports the use of the term ADHD, even though this diagnostic concept (from the Diagnostic and Statistical Manual of Mental Disorders, DSM-IV) clearly encompasses subtypes that are not necessarily as closely linked as would be suggested by a common denominator diagnostic label. There have been more than ten thousand empirical studies of ADHD. In contrast, studies of children and adults with deficits in attention, motor control and perception (DAMP), a subgroup of those with ADHD who also have developmental coordination disorder (DCD), are much fewer in number. An even smaller number of studies have been published on another subgroup within the 'ADHD spectrum', namely hyperkinetic disorder (HKD), which is still the term referred to in the International Classification of Diseases (ICD-10).

Further complication stems from the fact that many other neuropsychiatric syndromes (e.g. autism spectrum conditions, many of the behavioural phenotype syndromes and Tourette syndrome) often comprise elements of ADHD. At present, the most common practice seems to be to diagnose only one syndrome. For instance, if a boy of 10 years suffers from the combination of multiple motor and vocal tics, pervasive attention deficit problems and dyslexia, it is quite common to diagnose only Tourette syndrome, although a case could be made for diagnosing ADHD and dyslexia as well. This should become less of a problem once it becomes generally accepted that 'comorbidity' (i.e. the simultaneous coexistence in one individual of several different types of 'named' problems) is common in child neuropsychiatry.

DEFINITION OF ADHD

Some children show a persistent pattern of inattention, often associated with hyperactivity and impulsivity, from the first years

TABLE 27.1
Syndromes attributed to so-called 'minimal brain dysfunction' (MBD): synonyms and partly overlapping concepts

Diagnostic label	Comments
MBD (minimal brain dysfunction)	Once referred to as minimal brain *damage* (before c. 1960). Almost universally used until c. 1980. Still in *clinical* use in many countries. Usually refers to various combinations of attention and motor/learning problems. Inappropriate in that it infers brain dysfunction on phenotypical grounds and in its use of the word 'minimal'
ADD (attention deficit disorder)	DSM-III label (American Psychiatric Association 1980). Widespread use in USA. Semantically confusing (should be either 'deficit' or 'disorder'). Diagnostic criteria very loose and subjective. Pervasiveness not required. With or without motor/learning problems
ADHD (attention deficit–hyperactivity disorder)	DSM-III-R label (American Psychiatric Association 1987). Does not account for cases without clear hyperactivity. If categorized as 'severe', then pervasiveness required. With or without motor/learning problems
DAMP (deficits in attention, motor control and perception)	Accepted term in Nordic countries. Umbrella term to cover the various combinations of motor control, perceptual and attentional problems encountered in children without mental retardation or cerebral palsy
Hyperkinetic syndrome/disorder	Mostly used in the UK. Usually refers to a syndrome of pervasive hyperactivity. In the past, this diagnosis was often made only if there were no major associated conduct problems. The syndrome was then regarded as exceedingly rare. As used in the late 1980s, it has become obvious that it is not quite so rare, that conduct disorders often coincide, and that motor/speech/learning problems are the rule
MND (minor neurological dysfunction)	Sometimes used to describe summary score for minimal motor/neurological problems or 'soft neurological signs'
MCD (minimal cerebral dysfunction)	Rarely used. Refers mostly to overriding concept of cerebral dysfunction rather than to any specific clinical syndrome
Clumsy child syndrome	UK concept. Highlights only one aspect of what is usually a multifaceted syndrome
Motor/perceptual impairment	Common Scandinavian concept. Attention problems are common in this group
Organic brain syndrome	Central European concept. Highlights certain behavioural features, but essentially similar to MBD
OBD (organic brain dysfunction)	Used particularly by groups who stress the importance of neonatal reflexes in the genesis of learning and attention problems

of life. The terms attention deficit disorder (ADD – APA 1980) and ADHD (APA 1994) to cover this group of problems have been widely accepted in North America, and more recently in the rest of the world, and criteria for diagnosis have become increasingly operationalized. In the latest version of the DSM (the DSM-IV-TR, APA 2000), three subtypes of ADHD are recognized: (1) *mainly inattentive*, (2) *mainly hyperactive–impulsive*, and (3) *combined*, plus a residual category of ADHD not otherwise specified (Table 25.2). In clinical practice and research, doctors are now increasingly making multiple diagnoses in children who are reported to have ADHD. Even in general population (non-clinic) samples of ADHD, the rate of 'comorbidity' (i.e. meeting criteria for at least one further impairing condition) is more than 80% (Kadesjö and Gillberg 2001).

EPIDEMIOLOGY
ADHD occurs at a rate of 3–9% of all school-age children (Faraone et al. 2003). It is several times more common in boys than in girls. IQ tends to be skewed downwards, even though the majority of children receiving this diagnosis are of normal intelligence. About one in six to one in seven of all those with ADHD

have some degree of learning disability; this proportion is probably higher in those with the most severe forms of hyperactivity.

ADHD is valid from the behavioural point of view, although there is considerable symptom overlap with 'conduct disorder' and 'oppositional–defiant disorder' (ODD) (Gillberg 1995, Kadesjö et al. 2001). ADHD tends to signal a poor psychosocial outcome (Weiss et al. 2006), but it is possible that prognosis is better predicted by some of the often associated problems (such as specific learning disorders and conduct problems) rather than by the attention deficit symptoms per se (Hellgren et al. 1994).

The concept of attention deficit has become linked with that of hyperactivity. It is not clear, however, whether attention deficit underlies hyperactivity in the majority of cases: some findings suggest that it may not (Taylor et al. 1991). Attention deficits are quite often associated with normoactive behaviour, hypoactivity and fluctuating degrees of activity.

DEFINITION OF HYPERKINETIC DISORDER

The term hyperkinetic disorder has gradually come to refer to a

TABLE 25.2
DSM-IV-TR diagnostic criteria for ADHD*

A. Either (1) or (2):

(1) Six (or more) of the following symptoms of **inattention** have persisted for at least 6 months to a degree that is maladaptive and inconsistent with developmental level:

Inattention

(a) Often fails to give close attention to details or makes careless mistakes in schoolwork, work or other activities

(b) Often has difficulty sustaining attention in tasks or play activities

(c) Often does not seem to listen when spoken to directly

(d) Often does not follow through on instructions and fails to finish schoolwork, chores, or duties in the workplace (not due to oppositional behaviour or failure to understand instructions)

(e) Often has difficulty organizing tasks and activities

(f) Often avoids, dislikes or is reluctant to engage in tasks that require sustained mental effort (such as schoolwork or homework)

(g) Often loses things necessary for tasks or activities (e.g. toys, school assignments, pencils, books or tools)

(h) Is often easily distracted by extraneous stimuli

(i) Is often forgetful in daily activities

(2) Six (or more) of the following symptoms of **hyperactivity–impulsivity** have persisted for at least 6 months to a degree that is maladaptive and inconsistent with developmental level:

Hyperactivity

(a) Often fidgets with hands or feet or squirms in seat

(b) Often leaves seat in classroom or in other situations in which remaining seated is expected

(c) Often runs about or climbs excessively in situations in which it is inappropriate (in adolescents or adults, may be limited to subjective feelings of restlessness)

(d) Often has difficulty playing or engaging in leisure activities quietly

(e) Is often "on the go" or often acts as if "driven by a motor"

(f) Often talks excessively

Impulsivity

(g) Often blurts out answers before questions have been completed

(h) Often has difficulty awaiting turn

(i) Often interrupts or intrudes on others (e.g. butts into conversations or games)

B. Some hyperactive–impulsive or inattentive symptoms that caused impairment were present before age 7 years

C. Some impairment from the symptoms is present in two or more settings (e.g. at school or work and at home)

D. There must be clear evidence of clinically significant impairment in social, academic or occupational functioning

E. The symptoms do not occur exclusively during the course of a Pervasive Developmental Disorder, Schizophrenia or other Psychotic Disorder and are not better accounted for by another mental disorder (e.g. Mood Disorder, Anxiety Disorder, Disassociative Disorder or a Personality Disorder)

Code based on type:

314.01[1] **Attention Deficit Hyperactivity Disorder, Combined Type:**
if both Criteria A1 and A2 are met for the past 6 months

314.00 Attention Deficit Hyperactivity Disorder, Predominantly Inattentive Type:
if Criterion A1 is met but Criterion A2 is not met for the past 6 months

314.01[1] **Attention Deficit Hyperactivity Disorder, Predominantly Hyperactive–Impulsive Type:**
if Criterion A2 is met but Criterion A1 is not met for the past 6 months

Coding note: For individuals (especially adolescents and adults) who currently have symptoms that no longer meet full criteria, "In Partial Remission" should be specified

314.9 Attention Deficit Hyperactivity Disorder Not Otherwise Specified
This category is for disorders with prominent symptoms of inattention or hyperactivity–impulsivity that do not meet criteria for Attention Deficit Hyperactivity Disorder. Examples include:

1. Individuals whose symptoms and impairment meet the criteria for Attention Deficit Hyperactivity Disorder, Predominantly Inattentive Type but whose age at onset is 7 years or after

2. Individuals with clinically significant impairment who present with inattention and whose symptom pattern does not meet the full criteria for the disorder but have a behavioural pattern marked by sluggishness, daydreaming and hypoactivity

---

*Adapted from APA (2000).
[1]Some DSM-IV-TR diagnoses share the same code numbers in order to maintain compatibility with the ICD-9-CM classification system.

constellation of childhood symptoms that closely resemble those described under the ADHD label. However, only 30 years ago it was usually thought of as a rare 'disorder' characterized by extremes of hyperactivity. In respect of symptoms, hyperkinetic disorder in the ICD-10 (WHO 1993) is very similar to that of ADHD in the DSM-IV. However, the ICD-10 algorithm is such (requiring symptoms from all three subdomains of hyperactivity, impulsivity and inattention) that the actual number of children diagnosable under this label is much smaller.

EPIDEMIOLOGY

In the Isle of Wight population study in the 1960s, the 'pure' hyperkinetic syndrome was encountered in fewer than 1 in 2000 10- to 11-year-olds without 'neuroepileptic' disorders who attended normal schools (Rutter et al. 1970). In marked contrast, 7% of all children with neuroepileptic disorders and children excluded from school because of severe mental retardation were considered to suffer from a hyperkinetic syndrome. It was not until the early 1980s, when a reanalysis of the Isle of Wight material (Schachar et al. 1981) revealed that about 2% of the population showed hyperactive behaviour both at home and at school, that it became accepted that hyperactivity – even pervasive forms – is a common problem in school-age children.

DEFINITION OF DAMP

Surveying the literature on MBD in the 1970s it became apparent that the problems inferred were perceptual, motor and attention deficits in various combinations in children without mental retardation or cerebral palsy. The concept of DAMP with operationalization of criteria and an algorithm for diagnosis was therefore launched – before the advent of DSM ADHD or ICD-10 hyperkinetic disorder – to cover most of the syndromes previously referred to as 'MBD' but without any implicit aetiological meaning (Gillberg et al. 1989).

EPIDEMIOLOGY

The concept of DAMP as currently used refers to a condition meeting criteria for the combination of ADHD and DCD. About half of all children with ADHD have DCD, and about half of all children with DCD have ADHD. ADHD and DCD have been shown to have an interactive effect leading to a very high risk of language, academic and social interaction problems (Kadesjö and Gillberg 1999), and to share additive genes (Visscher et al. 2006). DAMP can be subdivided into severe cases, showing all five of (1) ADHD, (2) gross motor, (3) fine motor, (4) perceptual and (5) speech/language dysfunction, and mild–moderate cases showing ADHD plus one to three, but not all, of these other dysfunctions.

DIAGNOSIS

An adequate working diagnosis (i.e. a formulation in diagnostic terms that can serve as a basis for intervention suggestions) in the field of severe ADHD (with 'comorbidities' that are almost always present if criteria for ADHD with substantial degree of clinical impairment are met) requires the collaboration of the paediatrician (or a child psychiatrist) and a clinical psychologist, who should make independent evaluations and then combine their data. In mild-moderate cases, the paediatrician (or school doctor) will have to do most of the diagnostic work alone, considering the high prevalence of the disorder and the lack of diagnostic resources.

PAEDIATRIC/PSYCHIATRIC ASSESSMENT

The paediatric/psychiatric assessment needs to include a detailed developmental history and a behavioural and physical/motor evaluation of the child (e.g. the brief motor examination suggested by Gillberg et al. 1983). Questionnaires (including the Conners rating scales and scales for coexisting problems, such as the Five To Fifteen by Kadesjö et al. 2004) completed by both parents and teachers are usually very helpful but can never provide the sole basis for making a diagnosis of ADHD. Checklists covering the symptom criteria for ADHD, ODD, depression and anxiety should be included in the diagnostic process, but, again, they can never provide the only basis for making a diagnosis. Children who present with the combination of ADHD and DCD need to be assessed for the presence of autism spectrum disorder (Kadesjö and Gillberg 1999), by the use of either checklists such as the Autism Spectrum Screening Questionnaire (ASSQ – Ehlers and Gillberg 1993) or interviews such as the Asperger Syndrome Diagnostic Interview (ASDI – Gillberg et al. 2001). For a definitive diagnosis of ADHD to be made there is a need to demonstrate (a) considerable clinical impairment, (b) cross-situational symptomatology, (c) full symptom criteria for ADHD according to DSM-IV, (d) onset of symptoms in early childhood, and (e) the clinical 'gestalt' of ADHD. 'Comorbidity' (DCD, ODD, affective/anxiety disorders) is to be expected, and a dianosis of ADHD should be seen as a prompt to be looking for further neurodevelopmental or psychiatric problems.

NEUROPSYCHOLOGICAL ASSESSMENT

The neuropsychological assessment should include – at the very least – testing using an appropriate measure of cognitive function, such as one of the Wechsler scales. Attentional problems are often reflected in poor results on the Coding and Digit Span subtests of the Wechsler scales. As the child grows older the Information and Arithmetic subtests may yield gradually poorer results. In some cases this can be seen as a reflection of the gradually more important associated problem of dyslexia, which leads to a relative decline in skills for which good reading is essential. In other cases there is a tendency to depressed results on the majority of the subscales. Children with slightly lower than average IQ very often have the same 'ACID' (troughs on Arithmetic, Coding, Information and Digit Span) profile that is considered typical of ADHD (Ek et al. 2007). Clinical experience suggests that low IQ (with inappropriate environmental expectations of good attention and processing skills) can be 'misdiagnosed' as ADHD. In either case, it is important that children with the type of neuropsychological deficits considered typical of ADHD, regardless of whether or not criteria for ADHD are met, have their problems recognized and attended to.

FURTHER EXAMINATIONS

Hearing and vision should be properly assessed in all cases. There is a need for the assessment team to consider possible aetiology in each individual case. Behavioural phenotype syndromes, thyroid dysfunction and other physical disorders should be reviewed and ruled out or in. There needs to be a low threshold for referral for EEG examination (including in sleep), given the not uncommon occurrence of difficult-to-diagnose seizure disorders with attention/absence symptomatology. Karyotyping and specific genetic testing should be performed in cases with multiple physical anomalies or otherwise raising suspicion of specific genetic disorders.

BACKGROUND AND ASSOCIATED 'RISK' OR PATHOGENETIC FACTORS

The heritability of ADHD is about 80% (Spencer et al. 2007). There is an approximately five-fold elevated risk for ADHD in first-degree relatives. Several genome scans have led to the identification of chromosomal regions potentially relevant in ADHD; especially the evidence for linkage to chromosome 5p13 is convincing. Meta-analyses of a large number of candidate gene studies suggest association with gene variants of the dopaminergic receptors DRD4 and DRD5, the serotonergic receptor HTR1B, and the synaptosomal receptor protein SNAP-25 (Schimmelmann et al. 2006). It appears that the DRD4-associated variant of ADHD might have a better outcome, as suggested by studies in adults with persisting ADHD supporting the association with DRD5 in 'chronic' ADHD but not in milder or transient forms (Johansson et al. 2007). The established associations with dopamine genes account for only a small portion of all 'ADHD heritability', and it is likely that a whole host of other genes are involved in the pathogenesis of the disorder.

It is clear that not only genes but pre-, peri- and neonatal risk factors increase the likelihood that an individual will develop ADHD, whether in the context of a family history of ADHD or not. For instance there is good evidence of a higher than expected rate of ADHD following extremely preterm birth (Cooke and Foulder-Hughes 2003), fetal alcohol exposure (Aronson et al. 1997), smoking in pregnancy (Biederman 2005) and heavy metal exposure (Braun et al. 2006), and in various behavioural phenotype syndromes such as 22q11 deletion syndrome, fragile X syndrome and tuberous sclerosis (personal observations, unpublished).

The brain is slightly smaller in ADHD than in children and adolescents who do not have ADHD (Rapoport et al. 2001). Structural and functional imaging studies suggest that dysfunction in the fronto-subcortical pathways (and possibly cerebellar–brainstem, callosal and hippocampal pathways), and imbalances in the dopaminergic, noradrenergic and glutamatergic systems contribute to the pathophysiology of ADHD (Biederman and Faraone 2005, Plessen et al. 2006, Carrey et al. 2007).

According to Swedish studies, DAMP (i.e. ADHD with DCD) is 'idiopathic' in about 10% of cases, hereditary/familial in slightly more than half of cases (sometimes associated with pre- or perinatal risk), and mainly associated with pre-, peri- or postnatal risk factors in about one third (Gillberg and Rasmussen 1982). Some of the variance attributed to perinatal risk factor could actually be due to hereditary factors (Chapter 23).

CLINICAL PICTURE AND COURSE

As already outlined, the diagnosis of ADHD should always prompt the assessment of motor/perception dysfunction and 'non-ADHD' behavioural/emotional problems. According to three sets of Swedish studies (Gillberg et al. 1989, Landgren et al. 1996, Kadesjö and Gillberg 1998) there are about as many children with ADHD only as there are children with ADHD plus DCD. Follow-up studies suggest that children with the combination of problems have a different trajectory of development than those with ADHD without motor/perception dysfunction. Academic, speech–language, dyslexic, autistic-type and other learning problems are common in the former group, but not much overrepresented in the latter, in which ODD and conduct problems (and to some extent later antisocial and substance misuse problems) are instead the major threats to a good quality of life in adulthood. The identification of 'pervasively hyperkinetic' (as opposed to 'situationally hyperkinetic') children (Sandberg et al. 1978) has revealed that motor/perception and speech/language problems are almost universal in this group. This argues for the clinical separation of a diagnostic category with the combination of attention and motor/perception dysfunctions from groups with only one of the two types of dysfunction.

Situational attention deficit or hyperactivity can be a sign of psychological problems specific to a particular situation. Follow-up at age 13 years of children who had situational as compared to pervasive hyperkinesis at age 6–7 years (Gillberg and Gillberg 1988) has shown that outcome is much better in the former group and not very different to that of children without attention deficits of any kind. 'Isolated' motor/perception difficulties (often equivalent to DCD) sometimes cause considerable academic problems, particularly during the early school years. Nevertheless, limited systematic follow-up and clinical experience suggest that, in this group also, outcome can sometimes be considerably better than for those with the combination of attention problems and motor/perception difficulties (Hellgren et al. 1994). Longer term studies (e.g. Rasmussen and Gillberg 2000) point to the very poor outcome of ADHD in about 50% of those individuals who continue to meet criteria not only for ADHD but also for a variety of other psychiatric and personality disorders. The vast majority of individuals meeting full criteria for ADHD in childhood will have some problems in the domains of inattention (almost all) and hyperactivity/impulsivity (possibly under 50%) in adult life.

ADHD: THE INFANTILE PERIOD

Retrospective analysis of case histories of children suffering from

TABLE 25.3
Children with DAMP: outcome from age 7 to 16 years*

Area of dysfunction	% of children with dysfunction			
	7 yrs	10 yrs	13 yrs	16 yrs
Attention	100	55	49	40
Motor control	100	55	30	25
Perception/reading–writing	69	76	67	55
Psychiatric/behavioural	69	81	64	55
DAMP problem requiring specialist treatment	40	50	52	70
Accidents requiring hospital treatment	12	—	24	—

*Gillberg (1987) and unpublished results.

DAMP at age 4–6 years provides important clues to the clinical picture of DAMP in infancy. It seems that there may be at least two clinically distinct subgroups with respect to infant development: (1) the hyperactive group; and (2) the hypo- or normo-active group.

Infants in the hyperactive group usually show sleep problems, feeding difficulties, 'colicky' stomach pains and a generally high level of motor activity even from the first months of life. They often start walking before 10 months of age. From that time on (and sometimes even before), parents often have to change their domestic habits dramatically: anything moveable will have to be removed, not only from the level of the child's reach, but completely out of sight. This group needs to be evaluated at an early age. It is not uncommon for children with extremes of early-onset hyperactivity to have low IQ (including learning disability). Some of them have autism. In certain cases, extreme early hyperactivity can be the first indicator of Tourette syndrome or bipolar disorder, diagnostic signs of which may not appear until many years later.

Children in the hypoactive/normoactive group have often been thought to have low IQ. These infants are regarded by parents as 'good' (i.e. well-behaved), sometimes even 'exceptionally good'. Some of them show repetitive behaviours from a very early age (head rolling, even head banging, and repetitive sounds).

ADHD: THE PRESCHOOL YEARS

From about the age of starting to walk, the two subgroups, for a number of years, often appear to be indistinguishable from each other. Children of both groups appear hyperactive, or at least inattentive. Parents may worry because their child does not seem to listen, shouting being the only way of attracting their attention. Oppositional–defiant behaviours (and ODD) are often (about 50-60% of all cases with ADHD) at the forefront from about 3 years of age. Some of the symptoms currently under the diagnostic umbrella of ODD (such as 'loses temper') appear to be almost universal in ADHD. Motor coordination problems may surface already around age 2–4 years, but are often obscured by the high activity level and lack of appropriate fear, which is also very common. Speech is delayed in about half of cases, but only in about half of these is the delay severe enough to warrant consultation. (Conversely, children with early speech delay, say at about the age of 30 months, should always be considered for a diagnosis of ADHD or autism.) Toward the end of the preschool years the child's 'unwillingness' to draw and paint, and the constant clashes in games with age-peers, may become a major source of concern and of increasing scolding.

ADHD: THE EARLY SCHOOL YEARS

Some children with ADHD can manage fairly well through infancy and the preschool years but their behavioural and academic performance almost invariably deteriorates during the first few years at school. They have difficulties in concentrating, sitting still and listening, problems with impulse control, and major difficulties interacting in an age-appropriate fashion with peers. They may find it very problematic to participate in physical education and games, and sometimes they have almost insurmountable difficulties acquiring basic automatic reading and writing skills. All of these problems peak at around age 7–10 years in the vast majority of ADHD cases and cause emotional upset in the child, parents and teachers. Problems will be especially difficult to cope with if the diagnosis and its implications are not explained to those involved with the child (see below).

At age 6 years, those children with ADHD who also meet criteria for DAMP (i.e. who have DCD as well as ADHD), by definition, will have motor control problems and pervasive attention deficits. Pooled data presented in Table 25.3 show that at around age 10 years only about half of these children will have persistent obvious motor difficulties, and attentional problems will also have subsided to a similar degree. Unfortunately, these data also indicated increases in the prevalence of psychiatric/behavioural problems (from 69% to 81%) and of dyslexia/dysgraphia (from 69% to 76%) at this age. In age-peers without DAMP, such problems will be found at a very much lower level.

ADHD: PREADOLESCENCE AND ADOLESCENCE

Many preadolescent and adolescent children with ADHD experience persistent difficulties in concentrating. Some are described by their teachers or parents as daydreaming. Dyslexia is a very common complaint. The motor clumsiness is often less conspicuous than it used to be. There is a considerable risk for various types of psychiatric problems (such as depression, anxiety disorder or 'borderline personality disorder' and substance use disorder). If a child with ADHD (with or without DCD) attends a clinic for the first time in the teenage years, the psychiatric disorder is often seen as primary and a 'new' problem, not specifically associated with ADHD/DAMP. The child's problems then run the risk of not being put into perspective, and suggestions for intervention might be inappropriate.

COMORBID PROBLEMS IN ADHD

There are five main groups of 'comorbid' problems in ADHD: (1) DCD and other learning disorders; (2) anxiety/depression/bipolar disorders; (3) conduct and oppositional–defiant disorders; (4) tics and Tourette syndrome; and (5) autism spectrum conditions.

LEARNING DISORDERS INCLUDING DCD AND DYSLEXIA, DYSGRAPHIA AND DYSCALCULIA

A wide variety of academic problems are much overrepresented in ADHD. Some of these are probably a direct consequence of the attention deficits per se, whereas others are indistinguishable from conditions that can be diagnosed even in the absence of ADHD.

DEVELOPMENTAL COORDINATION DISORDER

The motor coordination problems are usually best described as immature performance on various neurological/motor tests such as diadochokinesis, finger tapping, alternating movements, standing and skipping on one leg, walking on the lateral sides of the feet, and various fine motor performance tests such as tracing in a maze, cutting out paper, etc. These problems are evident in everyday settings as overall clumsiness, poor table manners, difficulties in dressing and tying shoe-laces, and difficulties learning to draw, write, ride a bicycle, swim, ski and skate. Many such children are poor at games, particularly ball games, and especially if such games involve small balls. The Touwen manual for examination of the child with minor neurological dysfunction (Touwen 1979) is helpful to the clinician wanting to acquire the skills necessary to perform an age-appropriate neuromotor evaluation in this field. A number of other such manuals are available (Denckla 1985, Whitmore and Bax 1986, Gillberg 1987, Michelsson and Ylinen 1989). The perceptual problems appear on formal tests – such as the Performance part of the WISC-III (Block Design, Picture Completion and Object Assembly are often problematic) and the Southern California Sensory Integration Tests (Ayres 1974) – and on specific tests of perception that may vary from one country to another. There are often perceptual problems in several domains (visual, auditory, tactile, etc.), but most tests focus on visual–perceptual tasks and it is sometimes difficult to determine whether one is dealing with a pure visual–perceptual problem, a fine motor problem, a dysfunction of eye–hand coordination, or a combination of these. Perceptual problems often show in impaired perception of form, space and shape, in drawing and writing immaturities, and in severe problems in acquiring automatic reading skills. Disturbance of body image is also a common consequence of various perceptual difficulties.

SPEECH AND LANGUAGE DISORDERS

Children with ADHD often show various types of speech and language difficulties, some of which may be a consequence of the motor problems or reflect auditory perceptual problems, while others are related to some basic and specific language deficit. Those who have clear speech–language difficulties from a young age (documented before 4 years of age) have an extremely high rate of later dyslexia.

DYSLEXIA, DYSGRAPHIA, DYSCALCULIA

Dyslexia constitutes one of the most challenging problems in child neuropsychiatry in that it is an invisible disabling condition with possible consequences for the emotional well-being of the individual affected. Dyslexia is often referred to as 'reading disorder' (the DSM-IV terminology).

At least 5–10% of a school-age population of children are affected by dyslexia/dysgraphia. The figures are likely to be somewhat (though not much) lower in the adult population. The male:female ratio is similar to that in most neuropsychiatric disorders of childhood, at around 2:1 to 4:1 in different studies. However, there is a clear possibility that the male:female ratio in dyslexia may not be as high as suggested by clinical studies. In studies of children with 'pure' dyslexia, i.e. reading disorder without comorbidity, girls have been reported to have problems at least as often as boys. Boys tend to have much more associated disruptive behaviour problems, and it may be these, not the reading disorder, that get them referred to clinical specialists (Sanson et al. 1996).

Dyslexia and dysgraphia are often collectively referred to as dyslexia, which is quite inadequate, considering that spelling and other writing problems do not necessarily overlap with reading problems and vice versa. The twin study of Stevenson et al. (1987) suggests that spelling problems may have a considerably stronger genetic load than reading disorder, which would support the separation of these two problems. Nevertheless, the two are usually treated as one, and it is indeed very common for the two to occur together. Dyscalculia is less frequently associated with dyslexia. Dyscalculia and dyslexia often seem to reflect separate conditions. One study demonstrated the strong correlation of DAMP problems with dyscalculia but not with dyslexia (Rosenberg 1989).

Dyslexia (and dysgraphia) often develop during the school years in children with DAMP. Extrapolating the results of the Göteborg studies (Gillberg 1987), it would appear that almost half of all children with severe dyslexia have an ADHD/DAMP background. The majority of children still showing severe dyslexic/dysgraphic problems in the early teenage years had been diagnosed in the preschool period to have ADHD/DAMP. Clinical experience indicates that the true number of children with dyslexia/dysgraphia/dyscalculia who also have attention/motor/perception problems may be even greater, and that it is uncommon for a child to have isolated dyslexia/dysgraphia/dyscalculia without associated attention/motor or major behaviour problems (Sanson et al. 1996).

Dyslexia is often defined as a reading level 2 years below grade (or below the level expected on the basis of IQ results). It is extraordinary that this illogical definition has managed to survive almost uncriticized. It goes without saying that being 2 years behind at age 7 (minus 29%) is very different from being 2 years behind at age 13 (minus 15%). The only sound way of defining dyslexia would be on the basis of some sort of quotient conceptually similar to that used in defining overall intelligence. Another important diagnostic issue is whether to relate the reading problems to full scale IQ or to performance IQ only. It is self-evident that if verbal IQ measures are included, the determining overall IQ level for a child with dyslexia is likely to be lower than if only nonverbal subtests are included.

Dyslexia has a tendency to become chronic. Even though with appropriate remediation there is usually a gradual amelioration of some of the most severe reading and writing problems, many dyslexic children become slow readers and poor spellers in adult life. In a review of the best follow-up studies in the field, Schonaut and Satz (1983) concluded that outcome in dyslexia is variable but poor with respect to reading skills and psychosocial adjustment. However, it is still open to debate whether it is the dyslexia, the often associated behaviour problems or both that tend to predict poor psychosocial adjustment. There is some evidence that reading disorder without behaviour problems or ADHD has a relatively good outcome (Sanson et al. 1996), at least as regards psychosocial adjustment.

AFFECTIVE DISORDERS (INCLUDING BIPOLAR) AND ANXIETY

Depression and feelings of low self-esteem are already common during the early school years but appear to peak around age 10 years, when they frequently coincide with various kinds of behaviour problems. The child with ADHD often becomes increasingly aware of his/her 'otherness' during the school years. Feeling that 'there is nobody to help', the child often becomes depressed and even contemplates suicide (which is uncommon in groups without ADHD/DAMP). Many become very anxious and actually withdraw. Bullying is common, but the child with ADHD may also, him/herself, be the bully rather than the victim. In either case, depressive feelings are common. In the midst of depression there is also often much anger and resentment that may show outwardly as some kind of behaviour disorder/ODD or conduct disorder. The child's predicament may be mistaken for 'antisocial problems with an outlook to psychopathy'. Personal interview with the child will soon reveal, however, that this is (usually) not a hardened criminal-to-be, but rather an immature and sad child who needs to have certain basic attentional and learning problems recognized.

OPPOSITIONAL–DEFIANT AND CONDUCT PROBLEMS

The behaviour problems encountered in ADHD can be of any kind: a general oppositional–defiant attitude to adults, stealing, firesetting, lying, bullying, running away from home, or drug/alcohol abuse. In the preschool years there is often aggression towards other children in connection with inadvertent disruption of play and games. About 10% of children with ADHD/DAMP already show severe conduct problems on school entry. This figure increases to about 50% around age 10 years, but seems to decline to around 30% during the teenage years. Unfortunately, about the same proportion of young adults with a childhood presentation of typical ADHD still have severe conduct/antisocial problems.

TIC DISORDERS

Children with ADHD/DAMP often have tics, and some meet full criteria for Tourette syndrome. The association of ADHD and Tourette syndrome appears to be stronger if looked at from the perspective of the tic disorder: about half of all children with Tourette syndrome have major attention problems, and many of these meet criteria for ADHD. It is not uncommon for children and adolescents with Tourette syndrome to have an early childhood history compatible with a diagnosis of ADHD, including, as already mentioned, extremes of early onset hyperactivity/impulsivity.

AUTISM SPECTRUM CONDITIONS

At least half of all children with severe variants of ADHD with DCD (i.e. DAMP) show autistic traits. These comprise motor stereotypies, preoccupations with certain topics, objects or parts of objects, ritualistic phenomena, peculiarities of language (pronoun reversal, repetitive questioning and immaturities of grammar), and similar, but usually milder, reciprocal social interaction problems as in autism. Occasionally, the differentiation of severe DAMP from Asperger syndrome may be very difficult. Children with ADHD without DCD usually do not exhibit autistic-type features.

INTERVENTIONS

OVERALL PSYCHOEDUCATION

No single intervention or treatment is applicable for a group of disorders as heterogeneous as ADHD. Some Swedish studies of representative groups of children with ADHD receiving various kinds of intervention at age 6–7 years (Gillberg et al. 1993; Nydén et al. 2000, 2008) have suggested a positive effect of making the diagnosis and informing child, parents and teachers. Outcome in the 3-year perspective for school adjustment and achievement and for behaviour both at school and at home was better than for children who had not received information about the diagnosis. Psychological well-being was better in teenagers 9 years after diagnosis was significantly better in those who had been given a psychoeduactional programme (including much information about the meaning of the diagnosis) than in those who had not received this type of intervention.

The most important part of any intervention plan for a child with ADHD is the physical, behavioural and neuromotor/

neuropsychological examination, followed by oral and written information to parents, child, siblings and teachers, about the type of problems the child exhibits and their possible aetiology. This usually takes away much of the feeling of self-blame that has been strongly felt by both parents and children. Secondary behavioural/emotional problems tend to be minimized if information is given in this way.

SPECIAL EDUCATION

Many children with ADHD need special educational measures. Many will need individualized (i.e. one-on-one) education for some hours every day in order to be able to acquire new academic skills. A considerable minority need special physical education or the help of a physiotherapist. Most importantly, the physical education teacher has to be informed about the child's disability, so that s/he will not treat the child as one who is simply badly behaved.

Various approaches to the remediation of dyslexia and dysgraphia, and to a lesser extent dyscalculia (with or without ADHD), have been suggested. An almost unbelievable array of claims regarding the efficacy of various programmes has been made, but the fact remains that in order to achieve better reading and writing skills, reading and writing have to be trained. Several studies have demonstrated that if parents of preschool children can be encouraged to listen to their children reading on a regular basis, this has some preventive effect on the development of reading problems.

Increasing the speed of reading nonsense phonemes also appears to increase reading skills. Computer-based reading and spelling programmes are valuable aids for some children with dyslexia/dysgraphia. Computers have the added advantage of allowing the dysgraphic child to have as 'beautiful' a written output (on the screen or on the print-out) as the child without dysgraphia. Also, computers do not take offence (as teachers and parents can) when the child makes mistakes, which makes 'interactions' less emotionally stressful.

MEDICATION

A limited number of children with ADHD should be tried on medication treatment, usually with one of the stimulants. Both d-amphetamine (10–40 mg/day given in 2–5 doses with 3-hour intervals in order to last through the school day) and methylphenidate (20–80 mg/day given in the same fashion) have been shown to be effective in the amelioration of hyperactivity, concentration difficulties, some learning problems, feelings of low self-esteem and family interaction problems. Both drugs have also been shown to be relatively free of major side effects. 'Long-acting', 'slow-release' or 'differentially released' preparations of methylphenidate have also been shown to have good effects, and they can sometimes be dosed (18–54 mg/day or 10–60 mg/day depending on preparation) only once daily (or 'topped up' with one dose of short-acting methylphenidate). Relatively common side effects are loss of appetite, a tendency to increase the likelihood of tics (questioned by many and seen by some authorities to be the 'unmasking' of Tourette syndrome rather than a side

effect provoked in a child not genetically liable to tics) and stereotypies, reduced mimicry (sometimes mistaken for depression) and hallucinations – all of which cease promptly upon drug discontinuation. A recent placebo-controlled long-term study (over a period of 15 months) demonstrated remaining beneficial effects of amphetamine throughout the study period (Gillberg et al. 1997). The large-scale US MTA (Multimodal Treatment of ADHD) study of more than 500 children with ADHD has shown long-term methylphenidate treatment to be as effective as the combination of methylphenidate and cognitive behaviour therapy (CBT) and considerably more effective than CBT alone or 'treatment as usual' for 'core' ADHD symptoms (Arnold et al. 1997). However, the combination of methylphenidate and CBT was superior in the longer run in terms of ameliorating other problems such as depression and anxiety (Jensen et al. 2001, Hinshaw 2007).

Ultimate height may be decreased by 1–2 cm if the treatment is continued throughout puberty. The risk for increasing doses and developing drug dependence and abuse appears to be non-existent. Side effects are much less pronounced than with the commonly used tricyclic antidepressants. The risk of provoking epileptic seizures is small. Nevertheless, prescribing stimulants to children is a delicate matter. Therefore, and also because the possible long-term benefits of using stimulants have been poorly examined, stimulant treatment should be selected only for children with very severe DAMP problems and no major psychosocial problems. Stimulants should never be given as the only mode of treatment. Stimulants may also be a helpful adjunct in the treatment of attention deficit problems and autism spectrum problems. Contrary to old notions in the field, children on the autism spectrum who have mild mental retardation and severe ADHD often benefit from stimulant treatment. Side effects appear to be mild in most such cases.

The noradrenergic reuptake inhibitor atomoxetine has also been shown to have beneficial effects on ADHD in children and is used either as a second-line drug in cases needing medication treatment if stimulant treatment fails or, sometimes, as the preferred medication in children who have the combination of ADHD with tics and/or autism spectrum problems and/or major sleep problems. One study (Buitelaar et al. 2007) indicated that some children with ADHD who were treated for a year with atomoxetine were able to stay off medication thereafter (suggestive of remission of ADHD in those cases). Although clinical effects appear to be slightly less positive than with methylphenidate, there are advantages with this type of medication, firstly because it can usually be dosed once daily (with remaining positive 'core ADHD effects' the following morning), and, psychologically, because it is not a stimulant.

COGNITIVE BEHAVIOUR THERAPY (CBT)

Cognitive behaviour therapies comprise a whole range of interventions, and it is often difficult to tease out on the basis of individual studies exactly what type of treatment has been included for each individual. Some computer-based training programmes may be advertised as CBT. One recent study of such a training programme (Robo-MEMO) showed remarkably positive effects for core ADHD symptomatology (Klingberg et al. 2005), indicating that computer-training programmes should possibly be included in many intervention plans for children with ADHD and similar problems.

Various motor training programmes have not been documented to have a lasting effect on the overall clinical problems associated with ADHD/DAMP. For most children with DAMP, the motor coordination problems are those with seemingly the best prognosis, even without treatment. Therefore, it seems unwise to focus too much energy on this domain. However, the subgroup of about one in four with DAMP who have severe problems with clumsiness from an early age would need a more 'motor-focused' approach to intervention.

In the long term, problems associated with reading and writing can be the most handicapping, and every effort should therefore be made to help those children with ADHD who have early markers (including in the field of speech–language) of reading–writing disorders.

LONG-TERM OUTCOME

Some people who had ADHD in childhood and adolescence have overcome most or all of the severe problems by early adult life. However, about half have severe persisting problems, and many of the remainder have mild persistent problems. Criminal activity (e.g. arson, poisoning and bizarre violent behaviour – motivated by curiosity rather than malevolence) seems to be common, as do major psychiatric problems requiring in- or outpatient psychiatric treatment. Even among the many who outwardly appear to be doing relatively well, low self-esteem is common. Severe dyslexia, quite uncommon in adulthood in those who never had ADHD, is possibly present in 30–50% of cases. Even though the motor control problems appear to have the best prognosis of all, a substantial minority (probably about one in four) continue to have important problems with motor clumsiness well into adulthood.

REFERENCES

APA (1980) *Diagnostic and Statistical Manual of Mental Disorders, 3rd edn (DSM-III)*. Washington, DC: American Psychiatric Association.

APA (1994) *Diagnostic and Statistical Manual of Mental Disorders, 4th edn (DSM-IV)*. Washington, DC: American Psychiatric Association.

APA (2000) *Diagnostic and Statistical Manual of Mental Disorders, 4th edn, Text Revision (DSM-IV-TR)*. Washington, DC: American Psychiatric Association.

Arnold LE, Abikoff HB, Cantwell DP, et al. (1997) National Institute of Mental Health Collaborative Multimodal Treatment Study of Children with ADHD (the MTA). Design challenges and choices. *Arch Gen Psychiatry* 54: 865–70.

Aronson M, Hagberg B, Gillberg C (1997) Attention deficits and autistic spectrum problems in children exposed to alcohol during gestation: a follow-up study. *Dev Med Child Neurol* 39: 583–7.

Ayres AJ (1974) *Southern California Sensory Integration Test*. Los Angeles: Western Psychological Services.

Barkley RA (1990) *Attention Deficit Hyperactivity Disorder*. New York: Guilford Press.

Biederman J (2005) Attention-deficit/hyperactivity disorder: a selective overview. *Biol Psychiatry* 57: 1215–20.

Biederman J, Faraone SV (2005) Attention-deficit hyperactivity disorder. *Lancet* 366: 237–48.

Braun JM, Kahn RS, Froehlich T, et al. (2006) Exposures to environmental toxicants and attention deficit hyperacitivity disorder in U.S. children. *Environ Health Perspect* 114: 1904–9.

Buitelaar JK, Michelson D, Danckaerts M, et al. (2007) A randomized, double-blind study of continuation treatment for attention-deficit/hyperactivity disorder after 1 year. *Biol Psychiatry* 61: 694–9.

Carrey NJ, MacMaster FP, Gaudet L, Schmidt MH (2007) Striatal creatine and glutamate/glutamine in attention-deficit/hyperactivity disorder. *J Child Adolesc Psychopharmacol* 17: 11–7.

Cooke RW, Foulder-Hughes L (2003) Growth impairment in the very preterm and cognitive and motor performance at 7 years. *Arch Dis Child* 88: 482–7.

Denckla MB (1985) Neurological examination for subtle signs (PANESS). *Psychopharmacol Bull* 21: 773–800.

Ehlers S, Gillberg C (1993) The epidemiology of Asperger syndrome. A total population study. *J Child Psychol Psychiatry* 34: 1327–50.

Ek U, Fernell E, Westerlund J, et al. (2007) Cognitive strengths and deficits in schoolchildren with ADHD. *Acta Paediatr* 96: 756–61.

Faraone SV, Sergeant J, Gillberg C, Biederman J (2003) The worldwide prevalence of ADHD: is it an American condition? *World Psychiatry* 2: 104–113.

Gillberg C (1995) *Clinical Child Neuropsychiatry*. Cambridge: Cambridge University Press.

Gillberg C, Rasmussen P (1982) Perceptual, motor and attentional deficits in seven-year-old children: background factors. *Dev Med Child Neurol* 24: 752–70.

Gillberg C, Carlström G, Rasmussen P, Waldenström E (1983) Perceptual, motor and attentional deficits in seven-year-old children. Neurological screening aspects. *Acta Paediatr Scand* 72: 119–24.

Gillberg C, Melander H, von Knorring A-L, et al. (1997) Long-term stimulant treatment of children with attention-deficit hyperactivity disorder symptoms. A randomized, double-blind, placebo-controlled trial. *Arch Gen Psychiatry* 54: 857–64.

Gillberg C, Gillberg IC, Råstam M, Wentz E (2001) The Asperger Syndrome Diagnostic Interview (ASDI): a preliminary study of a new structured clinical interview. *Autism* 5: 57–66.

Gillberg IC (1987) Deficits in attention, motor control and perception: follow-up from pre-school to early teens. MD thesis, University of Uppsala.

Gillberg IC, Gillberg C (1988) Generalized hyperkinesis: follow-up study from age 7 to 13 years. *J Am Acad Child Adolesc Psychiatry* 27: 55–9.

Gillberg IC, Gillberg C, Groth J (1989) Children with preschool minor neurodevelopmental disorders. V: Neurodevelopmental profiles at age 13. *Dev Med Child Neurol* 31: 14–24.

Gillberg IC, Winnergård I, Gillberg C (1993) Screening methods, epidemiology and evaluation of intervention in DAMP in preschool children. *Eur Child Adolesc Psychiatry* 2: 121–35.

Hellgren L, Gillberg IC, Bågenholm A, Gillberg C (1994) Children with deficits in attention, motor control and perception (DAMP) almost grown up: psychiatric and personality disorders at age 16 years. *J Child Psychol Psychiatry* 35: 1255–71.

Hinshaw SP (2007) Moderators and mediators of treatment outcome for youth with ADHD: understanding for whom and how interventions work. *J Pediatr Psychol* 32: 664–75.

Jensen PS, Hinshaw SP, Swanson JM, et al. (2001) Findings from the NIMH Multimodal Treatment Study of ADHD (MTA): implications and applications for primary care providers. *J Dev Behav Pediatr* 22: 60–73.

Johansson S, Halleland H, Halmøy A, et al. (2007) Genetic analyses of dopamine related genes in adult ADHD patients suggest an association with the DRD5-microsatellite repeat, but not with DRD4 or SLC6A3 VNTRs. *Am J Med Genet B Neuropsychiatr Genet* (Epub ahead of print).

Kadesjö B, Gillberg C (1998) Attention deficits and clumsiness in Swedish 7-year-old children. *Dev Med Child Neurol* 40: 796–811.

Kadesjö B, Gillberg C (1999) Developmental coordination disorder in Swedish 7-year-old children. *J Am Acad Child Adolesc Psychiatry* 38: 820–8.

Kadesjö B, Gillberg C (2001) The comorbidity of ADHD in the general population of Swedish school-age children. *J Child Psychol Psychiatry* 42: 487–92.

Kadesjö C, Kadesjö B, Hägglöf B, Gillberg C (2001) ADHD in Swedish 3- to 7-year-old children. *J Am Acad Child Adolesc Psychiatry* 40: 1021–8.

Kadesjö B, Janols LO, Korkman M, et al. (2004) The FTF (Five to Fifteen): The development of a parent questionnaire for the assessment of ADHD and comorbid conditions. *Eur Child Adolesc Psychiatry* 13 Suppl 3: 3–13.

Klingberg I, Fernell E, Olesen PJ, et al. (2005) Computerized training of working memory in children with ADHD—a randomized, controlled trial. *J Am Acad Child Adolesc Psychiatry* 44: 177–86.

Landgren M, Pettersson R, Kjellman B, Gillberg C (1996) ADHD, DAMP and other neurodevelopmental/neuropsychiatric disorders in 6-year-old children: epidemiology and co-morbidity. *Dev Med Child Neurol* 38: 891–906.

Michelsson K, Ylinen A (1989) A neurodevelopmental screening examination for five-year-old children. *Early Child Dev Care* 29: 9–22.

Nydén A, Paananen M, Gillberg C (2000) [Neuropsychiatric problems among children are significantly underdiagnosed. Intervention programs result in better and less expensive care.] *Lakartidningen* 97: 5634–9, 5641 (Swedish).

Nydén A, Myrén KJ, Gillberg C (2008) Long-term psychosocial and health economy consequences of ADHD, autism, and reading–writing disorder: a prospective service evaluation project. *J Atten Disord* 12: 141–8.

Plessen KJ, Bansal R, Zhu H, et al. (2006) Hippocampus and amygdala morphology in attention-deficit/hyperactivity disorder. *Arch Gen Psychiatry* 63: 795–807.

Rapoport JL, Castellanos FX, Gogate N, et al. (2001) Imaging normal and abnormal brain development: new perspectives for child psychiatry. *Aust NZ J Psychiatry* 35: 272–81.

Rasmussen P, Gillberg C (2000) Natural outcome of ADHD with developmental coordination disorder at age 22 years: a controlled, longitudinal, community-based study. *J Am Acad Child Adolesc Psychiatry* 39: 1424–31.

Rasmussen P, Gillberg C, Waldenström E, Svenson B (1983) Perceptual, motor and attentional deficits in seven-year-old children: neurological and neurodevelopmental aspects. *Dev Med Child Neurol* 25: 315–33.

Rosenberg PB (1989) Perceptual–motor and attentional correlates of developmental dyscalculia. *Ann Neurol* 26: 216–20.

Rutter M (1982) Syndromes attributed to "minimal brain dysfunction" in childhood. *Am J Psychiatry* 139: 21–33.

Rutter M, Graham P, Yule W (1970) *A Neuropsychiatric Study in Childhood. Clinics in Developmental Medicine No. 35/36.* London: Spastics International Medical Publications.

Sandberg ST, Rutter M, Taylor E (1978) Hyperkinetic disorder in psychiatric clinic attenders. *Dev Med Child Neurol* 20: 279–99.

Sanson A, Prior M, Smart D (1996) Reading disabilities with and without behaviour problems at 7–8 years: prediction from longitudinal data from infancy to 6 years. *J Child Psychol Psychiatry* 37: 529–41.

Schachar R, Rutter M, Smith A (1981) The characteristics of situationally and pervasively hyperactive children: implications for syndrome definition. *J Child Psychol Psychiatry* 22: 375–92.

Schimmelmann BG, Friedel S, Christiansen H, et al. (2006) [Genetic findings in attention-deficit and hyperactivity disorder (ADHD).] *Z Kinder Jugendpsychiatr Psychother* 34: 425–33 (German).

Schonhaut S, Satz P (1983) Prognosis for children with learning disabilities: a review of follow-up studies. In: Rutter M, ed. *Developmental Neuropsychiatry.* New York: Guilford Press, pp. 542–63.

Spencer TJ, Biederman J, Mick E (2007) Attention-deficit/hyperactivity disorder: diagnosis, lifespan, comorbidities, and neurobiology. *J Paediatr Psychol* 32: 631–42.

Stevenson J, Graham P, Fredman G, McLoughlin V (1987) A twin study of genetic influences on reading and spelling ability and disability. *J Child Psychol Psychiatry* 28: 229–47.

Taylor EA, Sandberg S, Thorley G, Giles S (1991) *The Epidemiology of Childhood Hyperactivity. Maudsley Monographs No 33.* Oxford: Oxford University Press.

Touwen BCL (1979) *Examination of the Child with Minor Neurological Dysfunction, 2nd edn. Clinics in Developmental Medicine No. 71.* London: Spastics International Medical Publications.

Visscher PM, Medland SE, Ferreira MA, et al. (2006) Assumption-free estimation of heritability from genome-wide identity-by-descent sharing between full siblings. *PLoS Genet* 2: e41.

Weiss MD, Gadow K, Wasdell MB (2006) Effectiveness outcomes in attention-deficit/hyperactivity disorder. *J Clin Psychiatry* 67 Suppl 8: 38–45.

Whitmore K, Bax M (1986) The school entry medical examination. *Arch Dis Child* 61: 807–17.

WHO (1993) *The ICD-10 Classification of Mental and Behavioural Disorders. Clinical Descriptions and Guidelines.* Geneva: World Health Organization.

INDEX

Note: page numbers in *italics* refer to figures, those in **bold** refer to tables

CHILD disease (congenital hemidysplasia with ichthyosiform erythroderma and limb defects) 307
child protection 490
childhood, late *see* adolescence
childhood ataxia with CNS hypomyelination 334–335
childhood disintegration disorder 914
chin, familial trembling 357
chloride channel disorders 820
chloride deficiency 863
cholesterol
   biosynthesis *307*
   intracellular metabolism defects 306–307
   metabolic disorders 306–308
   Smith–Lemli–Opitz syndrome 157–158
cholesterol ester storage disease 308
chorea–acanthocytosis **345,** 346–347
choreas 344–347
   benign hereditary **345,** 346
   causes **345**
   Sydenham chorea 404–405, 460
chorein 346
choreoathetosis
   ataxia–telangiectasia 123
   paroxysmal 673, 674
      dystonic of Mount and Reback 673
      and infantile benign seizures 674
      kinesigenic 673
choreoathetotic dyskinesias 871
chorioamnionitis, periventricular leukomalacia 14
choroid, gyrate atrophy 716, *717*
choroid plexus carcinoma 194
choroid plexus papilloma 517, 522
   fourth ventricle 509
   infantile hydrocephalus 194
   viral DNA sequences 503
choroidoretinitis
   subacute sclerosing panencephalitis 419
   toxoplasmosis 429–430
chromosomal anomalies
   behavioural phenotypes 137–161
   epilepsy 587
chromosome 22q11 deletion syndrome 141
chronic infantile neurological, cutaneous and articular disease (CINCA) 460
chronic inflammatory demyelinating polyneuropathy 777–778
chronic positive airway pressure (CPAP), germinal matrix–intraventricular haemorrhage prevention 10
chronic renal failure 873
CINCA (chronic infantile neurological, cutaneous and articular disease) 460
cinchona alkaloids 429
circadian rhythm disruption 688
circle of Willis anomalies 555
circulation, head injuries 482
citrullinaemia 287
Claude Bernard–Horner syndrome 718
CLCN1 gene mutations 820
cleft lip/palate, Walker–Warburg syndrome 813
clonidine 681
Clostridium botulinum (botulism) 432
Clostridium tetani (tetanus) 431
cloverleaf skull **169,** 170, *171*

c-myc oncogene 502
coagulation defects 878
   subgaleal haemorrhage 28
coagulopathies **562,** 568
coarctation of the aorta, repair 871
Coats disease 715
cobalamin
   deficiency syndrome 291
   intracellular deficiencies 291
   metabolic pathway 289
cobblestone complex **69,** 72
   cerebellar cysts 88
   prognosis 74
cocaine use, maternal, fetal malformations 90
Coccidioides immitis 428
cochlear 725–726
cochlear implantation 734, 735–736
Cockayne syndrome 337
cocktail party syndrome 204
coeliac disease, occipital calcification 619
coenzyme Q10 293
   deficiency 297, 301, 831
Coffin–Lowry syndrome 688
Cogan disease, ocular motor apraxia 705
cognitive behaviour therapy 930–931
cognitive development 896
cognitive impairment 802, 803
   antiepileptic agents 642
   chronic lung disease 872
   diabetes mellitus 869
   head injuries 485
   hepatic failure 874–875
   lead poisoning 493
   leukaemia treatment 528
   muscle–eye–brain disease 813
   posterior fossa surgery 509
   see also learning difficulties; mental retardation
Cohen syndrome, Prader–Willi syndrome differential diagnosis 151
collicular plate, beaking 191
colloid cysts of third ventricle 517, 530
coloboma of optic nerve 711–712
colpocephaly 79, *80,* 83
coma
   barbiturate 534
   diabetic 868
   head injuries 478, 479–480
communication, support planning 735
communication problems
   cardiac surgery late sequelae 872
   cerebral palsy 235
compartmental syndromes 839
compassion development 899–900
complex neuropathies associated with CNS involvement 770–772
complex regional pain syndrome 783
compression injuries 473, 476
concentric sclerosis of Baló 452
concussion
   head injury 480
   spinal cord injury 491
conduct problems 929
cone dystrophy 716
cone–rod dystrophy 716
congenital adrenal hypoplasia 877
congenital central alveolar hypoventilation syndrome 686–687
congenital contractures 837–839

peripheral nerve disorders 839
congenital dislocation of the hip, prevention in cerebral palsy 232–233
congenital fibre-type disproportion 817
congenital fixation of the stapes footplate with perilymphatic gusher 729–730, 731
congenital heart disease 870–871
congenital hypomyelinating neuropathies 766
congenital hypothyroidism 875
congenital insensitivity to pain with anhidrosis 769
congenital laxity of ligaments 741
congenital muscular torticollis 839
congenital myasthenia syndromes **844,** 845
congenital myopathies 813–818
   Werdnig–Hoffmann disease differential diagnosis 746
congenital myotonic dystrophy 818–819, 838–839
   cerebral palsy differential diagnosis 229
congenital stiff-man syndrome 675
connexin-26 gene mutation 726, 728
Conradi–Hünermann syndrome 307
consciousness, paroxysmal disturbance 683–688
constraint-based therapy, cerebral palsy 233–234
continuous muscle fibre activity 824–826
continuous spike-wave of slow sleep 630–632
   drug choice **640**
contracture deformities, spina bifida cystica 53
contractures
   congenital 837–839
   Duchenne muscular dystrophy 802
   prevention in cerebral palsy 232–233
contusion injury 474
convergence palsy 705
convulsions
   benign familial infantile 623
   benign non-familial neonatal 623
   definition 583–584
   diphtheria–tetanus–pertussis vaccine 465
   febrile 593, 603–606
      clinical features 604
      differential diagnosis 604–605
      prognosis 605
      treatment 605–606
   focal infantile 603
   hemiplegia 560
   herpes simplex virus encephalitis 412
   MMR vaccine 465
   syndrome of focal neonatal and stroke 623
   tuberculous meningitis 396
copper
   deficiency and non-accidental injury differential diagnosis 490
   Menkes disease 311, 313
   metabolism disorders 247, 308–313
Cornelia de Lange syndrome 140–141
coronary artery disease 461–462
corpus callosum
   agenesis 79, *80,* 81–82
      with abnormal genitalia, familial syndrome 81
      Edward's syndrome 144

946